N. EDWARD ROBINSON, Ph.D., M.R.C.V.S.

Professor, Departments of Large Animal Clinical Sciences and Physiology,
Michigan State University College of Veterinary Medicine,
East Lansing, Michigan

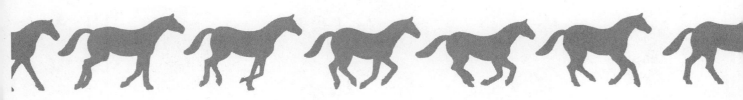

PHILADELPHIA, LONDON, TORONTO, MEXICO CITY, RIO DE JANEIRO, SYDNEY, TOKYO, HONG KONG

CURRENT THERAPY IN EQUINE MEDICINE

2

W. B. SAUNDERS COMPANY   1987

W. B. Saunders Company: West Washington Square
Philadelphia, PA 19105

Library of Congress Cataloging-in-Publication Data

Current therapy in equine medicine–2.
Includes bibliographies and index.

1. Horses—Diseases.   I. Robinson, N. E. (Norman Edward)
   [DNLM: 1. Horse Diseases—therapy. SF 951 C976]

SF951.C932 1987   636.1′089   86–4015

ISBN 0–7216–1491–4

Editor: Darlene Pedersen

Production Manager: Frank Polizzano

Manuscript Editor: Edna Dick

Indexer: Nancy Guenther

Current Therapy in Equine Medicine–2   ISBN 0–7216–1491–4

Last digit is the print number: 9   8   7   6   5   4   3   2

Dedicated to

My father
Norman Robinson
for high standards, a sense of humor, and my interest in horses

My mother
Sara Robinson
for energy, intellectual curiosity, and the desire to achieve

Current Therapy in Equine Medicine

CONSULTING EDITORS

JAMES L. BECHT
J. N. MOORE
Alimentary Tract Disease

KATHERINE A. HOUPT
Behavioral Problems

CHRISTOPHER M. BROWN
Cardiovascular Diseases

DAVID C. L. CHEN
Endocrine Diseases

CHRISTOPHER J. HILLIDGE
Foal Diseases

JOHN A. STICK
Foot Diseases

DEBRA DEEM MORRIS
Hematopoietic Diseases

R. P. HERD
Internal Parasites

JILL BEECH
Neurologic Diseases

H. F. HINTZ
Nutrition

MARY B. GLAZE
Ocular Diseases

REUBEN J. ROSE
*Problems of the Performance and
Endurance Horse*

SIDNEY W. RICKETTS
Reproduction

FREDERIK J. DERKSEN
Respiratory Diseases

T. MANNING
Skin Diseases

FREDERICK W. OEHME
Toxicology

W. M. BAYLY
Urinary Tract Diseases

CONTRIBUTORS

RAGAN ADAMS, M.A., D.V.M.

Resident, Department of Surgical Sciences, University of Florida College of Veterinary Medicine, Gainesville, Florida.

Neurologic Examination of the Newborn Foal; Acute Renal Failure

DOUGLAS ALLEN, Jr., D.V.M.

Assistant Professor of Large Animal Surgery, University of Georgia, College of Veterinary Medicine. Large Animal Surgeon, University of Georgia Veterinary Medical Teaching Hospital, Athens, Georgia.

Impaction of the Ileum

JENNIFER R. ALLEN, B.V.Sc.

Resident in Equine Medicine, Washington State University College of Veterinary Medicine, Pullman, Washington.

Physiological Responses to Exercise: Effects of Training

A. C. ASBURY, D.V.M.

Professor of Reproduction, University of Florida College of Veterinary Medicine. Clinician, University of Florida Veterinary Medical Teaching Hospital, Gainesville, Florida.

Failure of Uterine Defense Mechanisms

GORDON J. BAKER, B.V.Sc., Ph.D., M.R.C.V.S., Diplomate, A.C.V.S.

Professor and Head, Equine Medicine and Surgery, University of Illinois College of Veterinary Medicine, Urbana, Illinois.

Diseases of the Pharynx and the Larynx

BONNIE V. BEAVER, D.V.M.

Professor, Department of Small Animal Medicine and Surgery, Texas A & M University College of Veterinary Medicine, College Station, Texas.

The Use of Progestins for Aggressive and for Hypersexual Horses

JAMES L. BECHT, D.V.M., M.S.

Assistant Professor of Large Animal Medicine, University of Georgia College of Veterinary Medicine, Athens, Georgia.

Physical Examination of the Horse with Colic; Neonatal Isoerythrolysis; Blood and Plasma Therapy

JILL BEECH, V.M.D.

Associate Professor of Medicine, University of Pennsylvania School of Veterinary Medicine. Associate Professor of Medicine, The George D. Widener Hospital, University of Pennsylvania School of Veterinary Medicine, New Bolton Center, Kennett Square, Pennsylvania.

Tumors of the Pituitary Gland (Pars Intermedia); Equine Degenerative Myeloencephalopathy

G. MARVIN BEEMAN, B.S., D.V.M.

Associate Instructor, College of Veterinary Medicine and Biomedical Sciences, Colorado State University, Fort Collins, Colorado.

Distention Colic; Care of the Teeth

R. J. BELL, D.V.M.

Assistant Professor, University of Saskatchewan Western College of Veterinary Medicine, Saskatoon, Saskatchewan, Canada.

Feeding the Sick or Orphaned Foal

RONALD B. BLACKWELL, D.V.M.

Practitioner, Simpsonville, Kentucky.

Duodenitis—Proximal Jejunitis

JOHN C. BLOOM, V.M.D., Ph.D.

Adjunct Associate Professor of Clinical Laboratory Medicine, University of Pennsylvania School of Veterinary Medicine, New Bolton Center, Kennett Square. Assistant Director of Pathology, Smith Kline and French Laboratories, Philadelphia, Pennsylvania.

Evaluation of the Erythron

MURRAY G. BLUE, B.V.Sc., Ph.D., M.A.C.V.Sc., M.R.C.V.S., D.A.C.T.

Practitioner, Stratford, New Zealand.

Fungal Endometritis

CHARLES L. BOLES, D.V.M. Diplomate, A.C.V.S.

Alamo Pintado Equine Clinic, Los Olivos, California.

Enteroliths and Small Colon Obstruction

CONRAD H. BOULTON, D.V.M., Diplomate, A.C.V.S.

Assistant Professor of Surgery, Washington State University College of Veterinary Medicine. Equine Surgeon, Department of Veterinary Medicine and Surgery, Washington State University College of Veterinary Medicine, Pullman, Washington.

Alimentary Tract Neoplasia; Urinary Bladder Displacement

J. M. BOWEN, D.V.M.

Equine Extension Veterinarian, Virginia-Maryland Regional College of Veterinary Medicine, Virginia Polytechnic Institute, Blacksburg, Virginia.

Venereal Diseases of Stallions

KARL FREDERICK BOWMAN, D.V.M., M.S., A.C.V.S., and Diplomate, A.B.V.P.

Assistant Professor, Equine Surgery, Department of Food Animal and Equine Medicine, North Carolina State University School of Veterinary Medicine. Large Animal Surgeon, Veterinary Teaching Hospital, Raleigh, North Carolina.

Cleft Palate; Salivary Gland Disease

BARBARA D. BREWER, M.A., D.V.M.

Assistant Professor of Large Animal Medicine, University of Florida College of Veterinary Medicine, Gainesville, Florida.

Disorders of Calcium Metabolism; Equine Protozoal Myeloencephalitis; Neonatal Septicemia

F. BRISTOL, B.V.Sc., M.Sc.

Professor of Theriogenology, University of Saskatchewan Western College of Veterinary Medicine, Saskatoon, Saskatchewan, Canada.

Synchronization of Estrus

D. F. BROBST, D.V.M., Ph.D.

Professor of Clinical Pathology, Washington State University College of Veterinary Medicine, Pullman, Washington.

Normal Clinical Pathology Data

CHRISTOPHER M. BROWN, B.V.Sc., Ph.D., M.R.C.V.S., Diplomate, A.C.V.I.M.

Associate Professor, Large Animal Clinical Sciences, Michigan State University College of Veterinary Medicine, East Lansing, Michigan.

Acquired Disorders of Cardiac Blood Flow

CHRISTOPHER BUTTON, B.V.Sc., M.Med.Vet.(Med.), Ph.D.

Associate Professor of Veterinary Pharmacology, University of Pretoria, Faculty of Veterinary Science, Onderstepoort, South Africa.

Congenital Disorders of Cardiac Blood Flow

T. D. BYARS, D.V.M., Diplomate, A.C.V.I.M.

Hagyard-Davidson-McGee Hospital, Lexington, Kentucky.

Chronic Liver Disease; Warfarin Toxicosis; Disseminated Intravascular Coagulation; Hemophilia

G. KENT CARTER, D.V.M., M.S.

Assistant Professor, Department of Large Animal Medicine and Surgery, Texas A&M University College of Veterinary Medicine, College Station, Texas.

Gastric Diseases; Septic Arthritis and Osteomyelitis

GARY P. CARLSON, D.V.M., Ph.D.

Professor of Medicine, University of California School of Veterinary Medicine. Equine Clinician, Veterinary Medical Teaching Hospital, University of California School of Veterinary Medicine, Davis, California.

Thermoregulatory Problems; The Exhausted Horse Syndrome; Synchronous Diaphragmatic Flutter

DAVID C. L. CHEN, D.V.M., Ph.D.

Professor of Endocrinology, University of Florida, College of Veterinary Medicine. Chief, Clinical Endocrinology Laboratory, University of Florida Veterinary Medical Teaching Hospital, Gainesville, Florida.

Hypothyroidism

E. SUSAN CLARK, V.M.D.

Resident in Medicine, University of Pennsylvania School of Veterinary Medicine, New Bolton Center, Kennett Square, Pennsylvania.

Blood Loss Anemia

STEPHANE F. CLÉMENT, D.V.M.

Resident, Large Animal Medicine, University of Florida Veterinary Medical Teaching Hospital, Gainesville, Florida.

Peripheral Neuropathies

JAMES R. COFFMAN, D.V.M.

Dean, Kansas State University College of Veterinary Medicine, Manhattan, Kansas.

Deciding When to Refer the Horse with Colic

PATRICK COLAHAN, D.V.M.

Associate Professor, University of Florida College of Veterinary Medicine. Large Animal Surgeon, Chief, Large Animal Hospital, University of Florida Veterinary Medical Teaching Hospital, Gainesville, Florida.

Sand Colic

C. M. COLLES, B.Vet.Med., Ph.D., M.R.C.V.S.

Head, Equine Clinical Unit, Animal Health Trust (formerly Equine Research Station), Newmarket, U.K.

Fetal Electrocardiography

W. ROBERT COOK, F.R.C.V.S., Ph.D.

Professor of Surgery and Anatomy and Cellular Biology, Tufts University School of Veterinary Medicine, North Grafton, Massachusetts.

Diseases of the Auditive Tube Diverticulum (Guttural Pouch)

J. E. COX, B.Sc., B.Vet.Med., Ph.D., M.R.C.V.S.

Senior Lecturer, Division of Equine Studies and Farm Animal Surgery, University of Liverpool, Liverpool, England.

Cryptorchidism

SHARON E. CREGIER, Ph.D.

North American Editor, *Equine Behaviour*, Charlottetown, Prince Edward Island, Canada.

Trailer Problems and Solutions

MARK V. CRISMAN, D.V.M.

Resident; Equine Medicine, Washington State University College of Veterinary Medicine, Pullman, Washington.

Immune Deficiency Syndromes

KERSTIN DARENIUS, D.V.M.

Instructor in Obstetrics and Gynaecology, Swedish University of Agricultural Sciences, Uppsala, Sweden.

Early Fetal Death

RICHARD M. DEBOWES, D.V.M., M.S., Diplomate, A.C.V.S.

Assistant Professor of Equine Surgery, Department of Surgery and Medicine, Kansas State University College of Veterinary Medicine, Manhattan, Kansas.

Obstructive Urinary Tract Disease

FREDERIK J. DERKSEN, D.V.M., Ph.D.

Associate Professor of Internal Medicine, Michigan State University College of Veterinary Medicine. Internist, Veterinary Clinical Center, Michigan State University, East Lansing, Michigan.

Evaluation of the Respiratory System: Diagnostic Techniques; Chronic Obstructive Pulmonary Disease

CHARLES D. DIESEM, D.V.M., M.Sc., Ph.D.

Professor Emeritus of Veterinary Anatomy and Former Professor of Gross Anatomy, The Ohio State University College of Veterinary Medicine, Columbus, Ohio.

Anatomy of the Foot

STEPHEN DILL, D.V.M.

Assistant Professor, New York State College of Veterinary Medicine, Cornell University, Ithaca, New York.

Fibrinous Pericarditis

THOMAS J. DIVERS, D.V.M., Diplomate, A.C.V.I.M.

Associate Professor of Medicine, Department of Clinical Studies, University of Pennsylvania School of Veterinary Medicine, New Bolton Center, Kennett Square, Pennsylvania.

Acute Hepatic Failure (Theiler's Disease); Hepatic Disease in Foals; Chronic Renal Failure

K. F. DOWSETT, Q.D.A.H., B.V.Sc., Ph.D.

Senior Lecturer in Equine Reproduction, Department of Animal Production, University of Queensland School of Veterinary Science. Equine Unit, Veterinary School Farm, University of Queensland, St. Lucia, Queensland, Australia.

Seminal Abnormalities

ROLF M. EMBERTSON, D.V.M.

Surgeon, Rood and Riddle Equine Hospital, Lexington, Kentucky.

Parturient Perineal and Rectovestibular Injuries

ANNE G. EVANS, D.V.M.

Visiting Lecturer, University of California School of Veterinary Medicine, Davis, California.

Recurrent Urticaria Due to Inhaled Allergens

VALERIE A. FADOK, D.V.M.

Assistant Professor of Dermatology, University of Florida College of Veterinary Medicine, Gainesville, Florida.

Ectoparasites; Culicoides Hypersensitivity

CAROL S. FOIL, M.S., D.V.M., Diplomate, Am. Coll. of Veterinary Dermatologists

Associate Professor, Louisiana State University School of Veterinary Medicine. Veterinary Dermatologist, Veterinary Teaching Hospital and Clinics, Louisiana State University School of Veterinary Medicine, Baton Rouge, Louisiana.

Cutaneous Onchocerciasis

HARRY C. FRAUENFELDER, B.V.Sc., M.S., M.R.C.V.S., Diplomate, A.C.V.S.

Hahndorf Veterinary Hospital, Hahndorf, South Australia, Australia.

Cervical Abnormalities

DAVID E. FREEMAN, D.V.M.

Assistant Professor of Surgery, University of Pennsylvania School of Veterinary Medicine, New Bolton Center, Kennett Square, Pennsylvania.

Nutrition of the Sick Horse

SUSAN L. FUBINI, D.V.M.

Assistant Professor of Surgery, New York State College of Veterinary Medicine, Cornell University, Ithaca, New York.

Burns

MARY B. GLAZE, D.V.M., M.S., Diplomate, Am. Coll. of Veterinary Ophthalmologists

Associate Professor of Veterinary Ophthalmology, Veterinary Clinical Sciences, Louisiana State University School of Veterinary Medicine. Veterinary Ophthalmologist, Veterinary Teaching Hospital and Clinics, Louisiana State University School of Veterinary Medicine, Baton Rouge, Louisiana.

Examination of the Eye; Ocular Therapeutic Techniques

BRADLEY J. GORDON, D.V.M., M.S.

Graduate Student and Resident in Surgery, University of Georgia College of Veterinary Medicine, Athens, Georgia.

Blood and Plasma Therapy

RICHARD P. HACKETT, D.V.M., M.S.

Associate Professor of Surgery, New York State College of Veterinary Medicine, Cornell University, Ithaca, New York.

Colonic Volvulus and Intussusception

JOHN HALLEY, M.V.B., M.R.C.V.S.

Practitioner, Waterford, Eire.

Retained Meconium

THOMAS O. HANSEN, D.V.M.

Senior Resident in Medicine, University of Pennsylvania School of Veterinary Medicine, New Bolton Center, Kennett Square, Pennsylvania.

Narcolepsy and Epilepsy

J. PIERRE HELD, D.M.V., F.V.H., Diplomate, Am. Coll. of Theriogenologists

Associate Professor, University of Tennessee School of Veterinary Medicine. Attending Theriogenologist, University of Tennessee Veterinary Teaching Hospital, Knoxville, Tennessee.

Retained Placenta

R. P. HERD, M.V.Sc., Ph.D.

Professor of Parasitology, The Ohio State University College of Veterinary Medicine, Columbus, Ohio.

Diagnosis of Internal Parasites; Prophylactic Use of Anthelmintics; Chemotherapy of Migrating Strongyles; Anthelmintics and Drug Resistance; Pasture Hygiene; Monitoring Control Programs

DOUGLAS J. HERTHEL, D.V.M.

Alamo Pintado Equine Clinic, Los Olivos, California.

Enteroliths and Small Colon Obstruction

CHRISTOPHER J. HILLIDGE, B.Vet.Med., B.Sc., Ph.D., F.R.C.V.S.

Associate Professor of Medical Sciences, University of Florida College of Veterinary Medicine, Gainesville, Florida.

Corynebacterium Equi Lung Abscesses in Foals

ROBERT B. HILLMAN, A.B., D.V.M., M.S.

Senior Clinician, New York State College of Veterinary Medicine, Cornell University Veterinary Teaching Hospital, Ithaca, New York.

Induction of Parturition

RONALD W. HILWIG, D.V.M., M.Sc., Ph.D.

Associate Professor, Department of Veterinary Science, University of Arizona School of Veterinary Medicine, Tucson, Arizona.

Cardiac Arrhythmias

H. F. HINTZ, Ph.D.

Professor of Animal Nutrition, New York State College of Veterinary Medicine, Cornell University, Ithaca, New York.

Energy and Protein; Minerals; Vitamins; Feeding Programs; Sample Rations and Commercial Feeds

D. R. HODGSON, B.V.Sc., Ph.D.

Assistant Professor, Department of Veterinary Clinical Medicine and Surgery, Washington State University School of Veterinary Medicine, Pullman, Washington.

Exertional Rhabdomyolysis; Clinical Assessment of Performance Horses; Causes of Fatique; Rupture of the Urinary Bladder; Cystitis and Pyelonephritis

STEVEN M. HOPKINS, D.V.M., Diplomate, Am. Coll. of Theriogenologists

Associate Professor of Theriogenology, Veterinary Clinical Sciences Department, Iowa State University College of Veterinary Medicine, Ames, Iowa.

Ovulation Management

KATHERINE A. HOUPT, V.M.D., Ph.D.

Associate Professor, New York State College of Veterinary Medicine, Cornell University. Behavioral Consultant to the Large Animal Clinic and the Small Animal Clinic, New York State College of Veterinary Medicine, Cornell University, Ithaca, New York.

Foal Rejection

J. P. HURTGEN, D.V.M., M.S., Ph.D., Diplomate, Am. Coll. of Theriogenologists

Practitioner, New Freedom, Pennsylvania.

Evaluation of Stallion Fertility; Stallion Genital Abnormalities

B. HUSKAMP, D.V.M.

Tierklinik Hochmoor, Hochmoor, West Germany.

Displacement of the Large Colon

J. HYLAND, B.V.Sc., Ph.D., M.A.C.V.Sc.

Senior Lecturer, Melbourne Veterinary School, University of Melbourne, Werribee, Victoria, Australia.

Abortion

LEO B. JEFFCOTT, B.Vet.Med., Ph.D., F.R.C.V.S.

Professor of Veterinary Clinical Sciences, Chairman, Department of Veterinary Clinical Sciences, and Director, Veterinary Clinic and Hospital, Werribee, Victoria, Australia.

Passive Transfer of Immunity to Foals; Abortion

JANET JOHNSTON, D.V.M.

Resident, Large Animal Medicine, University of Pennsylvania School of Veterinary Medicine, New Bolton Center, Kennett Square, Pennsylvania.

Botulism; Tetanus

THOMAS J. KERN, D.V.M., Diplomate, Am. Coll. of Veterinary Ophthalmologists

Assistant Professor of Medicine, Section of Comparative Ophthalmology, New York State College of Veterinary Medicine, Cornell University, Ithaca, New York.

Intraocular Inflammation

M. KILEY-WORTHINGTON, B.Sc., D. Phil.

Associate Fellow in Applied Ethnology, School of Agriculture, University of Edinburgh, Edinburgh, Scotland, U.K.

Stereotypic Behavior

ERICH KLUG, Dr. Med. Vet. Habil.

Privatdozent für das Fach Fortpflanzung und Besamung der Haustiere, sowie Veterinärandrologie in der tierärztlichen Hochschule, Hannover, West Germany.

Ejaculatory Failure

NORBERT KOPF, Dr. Med. Vet., Univ.-Doz.

Universitätsdozent für Chirurgie und Augenheilkunde an der Universitätsklinik für Chirurgie und Augenheilkunde der Veterinärmedizinischen Universität Wien. Universitätslektor für "Abdominalchirurgie des Pferdes" an der Universitätsklinik für Chirurgie und Augenheilkunde der Veterinärmedizinischen Universität Wien; Praktischer Tierarzt, Privatpraxis in Wien, Breitensee, Austria.

Rectal Examination of the Colic Patient

ANNE M. KOTERBA, D.V.M., Ph.D.

Assistant Professor in Large Animal Medicine and Neonatology, University of Florida College of Veterinary Medicine. Veterinary Medical Teaching Hospital, Gainesville, Florida.

Identification, Diagnosis, and Treatment of the High-Risk Newborn Foal; Neonatal Septicemia; Respiratory Support for the Newborn Foal

PHILIP C. KOSCH, D.V.M., Ph.D.

Associate Professor of Physiology and Pediatrics, University of Florida College of Veterinary Medicine and College of Medicine, Gainesville, Florida.

Respiratory Support for the Newborn Foal

CLAIRE ANNE LATIMER, D.V.M., M.S.

Assistant Professor, Department of Veterinary Clinical Sciences, The Ohio State University College of Veterinary Medicine, Columbus, Ohio. Consulting Veterinary Ophthalmologist, Rood and Riddle Equine Hospital, Lexington, Kentucky.

Diseases of the Adnexa and Conjunctiva

J. D. LAVACH, D.V.M., M.S., Diplomate, Am. Coll. of Veterinary Ophthalmologists

Associate Professor, College of Veterinary Medicine and Biomedical Sciences, Colorado State University, Fort Collins, Colorado.

Ocular Emergencies

OLIVER W. I. LI, D.V.M., M.S.,

Department of Reproduction, University of Florida College of Veterinary Medicine, Gainesville, Florida.

Hypothyroidism

ALEXANDER LITTLEJOHN, B.V.Sc., D.V.Sc., M.R.C.V.S.

Research Fellow, Animal Health Trust, Newmarket, U.K.

Exercise-Related Cardiovascular Problems

IRWIN K. M. LIU, D.V.M., Ph.D.

Associate Professor, Department of Reproduction, University of California School of Veterinary Medicine, Davis, California.

Ovarian Abnormalities

DAVID H. LLOYD, B.Vet.Med., M.R.C.V.S.

Professor of Microbiology, The Royal Veterinary College, London, U.K.

Dermatophilosis

K. C. KENT LLOYD, D.V.M.

Resident, Equine Surgery, Veterinary Medical Teaching Hospital, University of California, Davis, California.

Western Equine Encephalomyelitis; Rabies

JOHN E. LOWE, D.V.M., M.S.

Associate Professor of Veterinary Surgery, New York State College of Veterinary Medicine. Director, Equine Research Park, New York State College of Veterinary Medicine, Cornell University, Ithaca, New York.

Large Colon Impaction

JILL J. McCLURE, D.V.M., M.S., Diplomate, A.C.V.I.M., A.B.V.P.

Associate Professor, Department of Veterinary Clinical Sciences, Louisiana State University School of Veterinary Medicine, Baton Rouge, Louisiana.

Acute Pancreatitis; Paralytic Bladder

RONALD J. MARTENS, D.V.M.

Professor, Department of Large Animal Medicine and Surgery, Texas A&M University College of Veterinary Medicine, College Station, Texas.

Septic Arthritis and Osteomyelitis

M. G. MAXIE, D.V.M., Ph.D., Diplomate, A.C.V.P.

Veterinary Pathologist, Veterinary Laboratory Services, Ontario Ministry of Agriculture and Food, Guelph, Ontario, Canada.

Peripheral Vascular Disease

A. M. MERRITT, A.B., D.V.M., M.S.

Professor of Medicine, University of Florida College of Veterinary Medicine. Large Animal Medicine Service, Veterinary Medical Teaching Hospital, Gainesville, Florida.

Diabetes Mellitus

NATHANIEL T. MESSER, IV, D.V.M.

Director of Medical Services, Littleton Large Animal Clinic P.C., Littleton, Colorado.

Distention Colic

POLLY MODRANSKY, D.V.M., M.S.

Assistant Professor, Large Animal Surgery, Virginia-Maryland Regional College of Veterinary Medicine, Virginia Tech, Blacksburg, Virginia.

Neoplastic and Anomalous Conditions of the Urinary Tract

CECIL P. MOORE, D.V.M.

Assistant Professor, Department of Surgical Sciences, University of Wisconsin School of Veterinary Medicine. Chief, Ophthalmology Section, Veterinary Medical Teaching Hospital, University of Wisconsin School of Veterinary Medicine, Madison, Wisconsin.

Diseases of the Cornea

J. N. MOORE, D.V.M., Ph.D.

Associate Professor, University of Georgia College of Veterinary Medicine, Athens, Georgia.

Endotoxemia

DEBRA DEEM MORRIS, D.V.M., M.S.

Assistant Professor of Medicine, University of Pennsylvania School of Veterinary Medicine. Internist in Large Animal Medicine, The George D. Widener Hospital for Large Animals, New Bolton Center, Kennett Square, Pennsylvania.

Immune-Mediated Thrombocytopenia; Hemolytic Anemias; Glomerulonephritis

WILLIAM W. MUIR, III, D.V.M., Ph.D.

Professor, Department of Veterinary Clinical Science, The Ohio State University, Columbus, Ohio.

Analgesics in the Treatment of Colic

MICHAEL J. MURRAY, D.V.M., M.S., Diplomate, A.C.V.I.M.

Assistant Professor, Virginia-Maryland Regional College of Veterinary Medicine, Virginia Tech, Blacksburg. Internal Medicine Clinician, Marion duPont Scott Equine Medical Center, Leesburg, Virginia.

Peracute Toxemic Colitis: Colitis X

JONATHAN M. NAYLOR, B.Sc., B.V.Sc., M.R.C.V.S., Ph.D.

Associate Professor, Veterinary Internal Medicine, University of Saskatchewan, Western College of Veterinary Medicine, Saskatoon, Saskatchewan, Canada.

Hyperlipemia; Feeding the Sick or Orphaned Foal; Nutrition of the Sick Horse

FRANK A. NICKELS, D.V.M., M.S.

Associate Professor of Equine Surgery, Michigan State University College of Veterinary Medicine, East Lansing, Michigan.

Hoof Cracks; Hoof Lacerations and Avulsions

MICHAEL W. O'CALLAGHAN, B.V.Sc., M.Sc.V., Ph.D., M.R.C.V.S.

Assistant Professor, Department of Surgery, Tufts University School of Veterinary Medicine, North Grafton, Massachusetts.

Echocardiography

FREDERICK W. OEHME, D.V.M., Ph.D.

Professor of Toxicology, Medicine, and Physiology, Kansas State University College of Veterinary Medicine. Director, Comparative Toxicology Laboratories, Veterinary Medical Hospital, Kansas State University College of Veterinary Medicine, Manhattan, Kansas.

Sample Collection for Diagnosis of Drug Abuse in Horses; Toxicoses Commonly Observed in Horses; General Principles in Treatment of Poisoning; Insecticides; Rodenticides; Snake Bite; Carbon Tetrachloride; Phenothiazine; Petroleum Products; Lead; Arsenic; Selenium; Plant Toxicities; Water Quality; The Etiologic Diagnosis of Sudden Death

JONATHAN E. PALMER, V.M.D.

Assistant Professor of Medicine, The George Widener Hospital for Large Animals, University of Pennsylvania School of Veterinary Medicine, New Bolton Center, Kennett Square, Pennsylvania.

Salmonellosis; Potomac Horse Fever

B. W. PARRY, D.V.M.

Lecturer, Department of Veterinary Clinical Sciences, University of Melbourne, Werribee, Victoria, Australia.

Normal Clinical Pathology Data

NOLTON PATTIO, V.M.D.

Resident, Large Animal Surgery, Department of Surgical Sciences, University of Florida College of Veterinary Medicine, Gainesville, Florida.

Wound Care and Excessive Granulation Tissue

H. PEARSON, B.V.Sc., Ph.D., F.R.C.V.S.

Professor of Veterinary Surgery, University of Bristol, Bristol, U.K.

Cesarean Section

LANCE E. PERRYMAN, D.V.M., Ph.D., Diplomate, A.C.V.P.

Professor, Department of Veterinary Microbiology and Pathology, Washington State University College of Veterinary Medicine, Pullman, Washington.

Immune Deficiency Syndromes

LLEWELLYN C. PEYTON, D.V.M., M.S.

Associate Professor, Large Animal Surgery, Department of Surgical Sciences, University of Florida College of Veterinary Medicine, Gainesville, Florida.

Wound Care and Excessive Granulation Tissue

P. W. PHYSICK-SHEARD, B.V.Sc., M.Sc., M.R.C.V.S.

Associate Professor of Large Animal Internal Medicine, Department of Clinical Studies, Ontario Veterinary College, University of Guelph, Guelph, Ontario, Canada.

Vectorcardiography; Peripheral Vascular Disease

DAVID G. POWELL, B.V.Sc., F.R.C.V.S.

Assistant Extension Professor, Department of Veterinary Science, University of Kentucky, Lexington, Kentucky.

Viral Respiratory Disease

SARAH L. RALSTON, V.M.D., Ph.D.

Mark Morris Chair of Clinical Nutrition, Assistant Professor, College of Veterinary Medicine and Biomedical Sciences, Colorado State University, Fort Collins, Colorado.

Feeding Problems

JOHN C. REAGOR, B.S., M.S., Ph.D.

Head, Department of Toxicology, Texas Veterinary Medical Diagnostic Laboratory, Texas A&M University College of Veterinary Medicine, College Station, Texas.

Cantharidin (Blister Beetle) Toxicity

WILLIAM C. REBHUN, D.V.M.

Associate Professor of Ophthalmology and Large Animal Medicine, Head, Large Animal Clinic, New York State College of Veterinary Medicine, Cornell University, Ithaca, New York.

Diseases of the Retina and Optic Nerve; Immunotherapy for Sarcoids

STEPHEN M. REED, D.V.M. Diplomate, A.C.V.I.M.

Associate Professor, Department of Veterinary Clinical Studies, The Ohio State University College of Veterinary Medicine, Columbus, Ohio.

Spinal Cord Trauma; Intracranial Trauma

VIRGINIA B. REEF, D.V.M.

Lecturer in Large Animal Medicine, University of Pennsylvania School of Veterinary Medicine. Head of Large Animal Cardiology and Diagnostic Ultrasonography, New Bolton Center, Kennett Square, Pennsylvania.

Vasculitis

SIDNEY W. RICKETTS, B.Sc., B.V.Sc., F.R.C.V.S.

"External" Lecturer, Universities of Cambridge, Bristol, and Liverpool Veterinary Schools. Practitioner, Rossdale and Partners, Newmarket, U.K.

Peritonitis; Perineal Conformation Abnormalities; Uterine Abnormalities

MALCOLM C. ROBERTS, B.V.Sc., Ph.D., F.R.C.V.S., F.A.C.V.Sc.

Professor of Equine Medicine, Department of Food Animal and Equine Medicine, North Carolina State University School of Veterinary Medicine. Equine Clinician, North Carolina State University, Raleigh, North Carolina.

Malabsorption Syndromes

STEPHEN J. ROBERTS, D.V.M., M.S.

Professor Emeritus of Large Animal Medicine, Obstetrics and Surgery, New York State College of Veterinary Medicine, Cornell University, Ithaca, New York. Practioner, Woodstock Veterinary Clinic, Woodstock, Vermont.

The Use of Progestins for Aggressive and for Hypersexual Horses

JAMES T. ROBERTSON, D.V.M., Diplomate, A.C.V.S.

Associate Professor of Equine Surgery, The Ohio State University College of Veterinary Medicine, Columbus, Ohio.

Small Intestinal Strangulation Obstruction; Parturient Perineal and Rectovestibular Injuries; Conditions of the Urethra

KATE A. W. ROBY, V.M.D.

Instructor, University of Pennsylvania School of Veterinary Medicine, New Bolton Center, Kennett Square. Fellow, Division of Biochemical Development and Molecular Diseases, The Children's Hospital of Philadelphia, Philadelphia, Pennsylvania.

Evaluation of the Erythron

REUBEN J. ROSE, B.V.Sc., Ph.D., F.R.C.V.S., Diplomate, M.A.C.V.Sc., F.A.C.B.S.

Associate Professor, Department of Veterinary

Clinical Studies, University of Sydney, Sydney, New South Wales, Australia.

Poor Performance Syndrome: Investigation and Diagnostic Techniques; Fluid, Electrolyte, and Acid-Base Disturbances Associated with Exercise

PETER D. ROSSDALE, M.A., Ph.D (Cantab), F.R.C.V.S., F.A.C.V.Sc., D.F.J.M.

Practitioner, Newmarket, U.K.

Neonatal Maladjustment Syndrome; Exogenous Control of the Breeding Season; Twin Pregnancy

VICKI J. SCHEIDT, D.V.M.

Assistant Professor of Dermatology, North Carolina State University School of Veterinary Medicine. NCSU Veterinary Teaching Hospital, Raleigh, North Carolina.

Dermatophilosis

GRETCHEN M. SCHMIDT, D.V.M.

Animal Eye Associates, Veterinary Specialty Clinic, Riverwoods, Illinois.

Algorithms for Ophthalmic Problems

D. G. SCHMITZ, D.V.M., M.S.

Associate Professor, Texas A & M University College of Veterinary Medicine, College Station, Texas.

Cantharidin (Blister Beetle) Toxicity; Toxic Nephropathies

ROBERT K. SCHNEIDER, D.V.M., M.S., Diplomate, A.C.V.S.

Practitioner, Allen-Schneider Equine Hospital, Gilbert, Arizona.

Orthopedic Problems of the Foot

H. F. SCHRYVER, D.V.M., Ph.D.

Equine Research Program, New York State College of Veterinary Medicine and New York State College of Agriculture and Life Sciences, Cornell University, Ithaca, New York.

Energy and Protein; Minerals; Vitamins

DANNY W. SCOTT, D.V.M.

Associate Professor of Medicine, Chief of Dermatology Service, Department of Clinical Sciences, New York State College of Veterinary Medicine, Cornell University, Ithaca, New York.

Demodicosis; Nodular Skin Disease

EDWARD A. SCOTT, B.S., D.V.M., M.S.

Equine Surgeon, Bergman Veterinary Medical Center, Cassosopolis, Mississippi.

Sinusitis

LEON SCRUTCHFIELD, D.V.M., M.S., Diplomate, A.C.V.I.M.

Associate Professor, Large Animal Medicine and Surgery, Texas A&M University College of Veterinary Medicine, College Station, Texas.

Chronic Diarrhea

ALVIN F. SELLERS, V.M.D., M.Sc., Ph.D.

Professor Emeritus, Department of Physiology, New York State College of Veterinary Medicine, Cornell University, Ithaca, New York.

Large Colon Impaction

SUSAN D. SEMRAD, V.M.D., M.S.

Resident, Large Animal Medicine, University of Georgia College of Veterinary Medicine, Athens, Georgia.

Endotoxemia

DAN C. SHARP, Ph.D.

Professor of Physiology, Animal Science Department, University of Florida College of Veterinary Medicine, Gainesville, Florida.

Photoperiod and Artificial Lighting

G. MICHAEL SHIRES, M.R.C.V.S., B.V.Sc., M.S., Diplomate, A.C.V.S.

Department Head and Professor of Surgery, Department of Rural Practice, University of Tennessee College of Veterinary Medicine, Knoxville, Tennessee.

Rectal Tears

DONALD J. SIMPSON, B. Vet. Med., M.R.C.V.S.

Practitioner, Newmarket, U.K.

Venereal Diseases of Mares

D. H. SNOW, B.Sc.(Vet.), B.V.Sc., Ph.D., M.R.C.V.S.

Head, Physiology Unit, Animal Health Trust, Newmarket, U.K.

Phenylbutazone Toxicity

IOANA M. SONEA, D.V.M.

Resident-Instructor, Large Animal Clinic, Michigan State University College of Veterinary Medicine, East Lansing, Michigan.

Strangles

EDWARD L. SQUIRES, B.S., M.S., Ph.D.

Professor and Director of Equine Reproduction Laboratory, College of Veterinary Medicine and Biomedical Sciences, Colorado State University, Fort Collins, Colorado.

Embryo Transfer

ANTHONY A. STANNARD, D.V.M.

Professor of Medicine and Professor of Pathology, University of California College of Veterinary Medicine, Davis, California.

Generalized Granulomatous Disease; Photoactivated Vasculitis; Hyperesthetic Leukotrichia

ROBERT R. STECKEL, D.V.M., M.S.

Assistant Professor of Surgery, Tufts University School of Veterinary Medicine. Staff Surgeon,

Tufts University Large Animal Hospital, North Grafton, Massachusetts.

Puncture Wounds, Abscesses, Thrush, and Canker

JOHN A. STICK, D.V.M.

Associate Professor, Michigan State University College of Veterinary Medicine. Head, Division of Equine Programs, Attending Surgeon, Veterinary Clinical Center, Michigan State University, East Lansing, Michigan.

Esophageal Disease; Laminitis

RUSS L. STICKLE, D.V.M.

Assistant Professor, Department of Large Animal Clinical Sciences, Michigan State University College of Veterinary Medicine, East Lansing, Michigan.

Radiology of the Foot; Orthopedic Problems of the Foot

SUSAN M. STOVER, D.V.M.

Department of Veterinary Pathology, University of California School of Veterinary Medicine, Davis, California.

Pre- and Postoperative Management of the Colic Patient

CORINNE RAPHEL SWEENEY, D.V.M.

Lecturer and Medicine Clinician, University of Pennsylvania School of Veterinary Medicine, New Bolton Center, Kennett Square, Pennsylvania.

Narcolepsy and Epilepsy; Pleuropneumonia; Exercise-Induced Pulmonary Hemorrhage

RAYMOND W. SWEENEY, V.M.D.

Lecturer, Large Animal Internal Medicine, University of Pennsylvania School of Veterinary Medicine, New Bolton Center, Kennett Square, Pennsylvania.

Lymphoproliferative and Myeloproliferative Disorders; Neurologic Examination; Cerebrospinal Fluid Collection

CYNTHIA M. TRIM, B.V.Sc.

Professor of Anesthesiology, University of Georgia College of Veterinary Medicine. Anesthesiologist, University of Georgia Teaching Hospital, Athens, Georgia.

Anesthesia of the Horse with Colic

TRACY A. TURNER, D.V.M., M.S.

Assistant Professor, Department of Surgical Sciences, University of Florida College of Veterinary Medicine. Large Animal Surgeon, University of Florida Veterinary Medical Teaching Hospital, Gainesville, Florida.

Rectal Prolapse

WENDY E. VAALA, V.M.D.

Lecturer in Medicine, University of Pennsylvania School of Veterinary Medicine, New Bolton Center, Kennett Square, Pennsylvania.

Anemia Due to Inadequate Erythropoiesis

M. VANDEPLASSCHE, D.V.M.

Ordinary Professor, Department of Reproduction and Obstetrics, Faculty of Veterinary Medicine, State University Clinic of Reproduction and Obstetrics, State University, Ghent, Belgium.

Prepartum Complications and Dystocia

PAMELA CARROLL WAGNER, D.V.M., M.S.

Associate Professor, Large Animal Surgery, Oregon State University College of Veterinary Medicine, Corvallis, Oregon.

Cervical Vertebral Malformation

ANGELINE WARNER, D.V.M., M.S.

Research Associate, Department of Environmental Science and Physiology, Harvard School of Public Health, Boston, Massachusetts.

Anhidrosis; Hemolytic Anemias; Equine Herpesvirus Type 1 Myeloencephalopathy

ALISTAIR I. WEBB, B.V.Sc., Ph.D., M.R.C.V.S., D.V.A., Diplomate, Am. Coll. of Veterinary Anesthesiologists

Associate Professor, Veterinary Anesthesiology, University of Florida College of Veterinary Medicine, Gainesville, Florida.

Restraint and Anesthesia of the Foal

NATHANIEL A. WHITE II, D.V.M., M.S.

Professor, Virginia-Maryland Regional College of Veterinary Medicine, Virginia Tech. Assistant Director, Clinical Services, Marion duPont Scott Equine Medical Center, Leesburg, Virginia.

Nonstrangulating Intestinal Infarction; Epizootiology, Risk Factors, and Prognostic Factors in Colic

STEPHEN D. WHITE, D.V.M., Diplomate, Am. Coll. of Veterinary Dermatology

Assistant Professor, Department of Medicine, Tufts University School of Veterinary Medicine, North Grafton, Massachusetts.

Photosensitivity

R. D. WHITLEY, D.V.M., M.S., Diplomate, Am. Coll. of Veterinary Ophthalmologists

Assistant Professor, Department of Comparative Ophthalmology, College of Veterinary Medicine, and Assistant Professor, Department of Ophthalmology, College of Medicine, University of Florida. Chief, Ophthalmology Services and Staff Veterinary Ophthalmologist, University of Florida Veterinary Medical Teaching Hospital, Gainesville, Florida.

Cataracts

ROBERT H. WHITLOCK, D.V.M., Ph.D.

Marilyn M. Simpson Professor of Equine Medicine, University of Pennsylvania School of Veterinary Medicine. Chief of Medicine Section, Department of Clinical Studies, The George D. Widener Hospital, New Bolton Center, Kennett Square, Pennsylvania.

Botulism

KATHERINE E. WHITWELL, B.V.Sc., M.R.C.V.S.

Deputy Pathologist, Pathology Unit, Animal Health Trust, Newmarket, U.K.

Fetal Membrane Abnormalities

MARTIN WIERUP, D.V.M., Ph.D.

Professor and State Epizootiologist, National Veterinary Institute, Uppsala, Sweden.

Intestinal Clostridiosis

JULIA H. WILSON, D.V.M., Dip., A.C.V.I.M.

Assistant Professor, University of Florida College of Veterinary Medicine. Faculty, Large Animal Medicine, Veterinary Medical Teaching Hospital, Gainesville, Florida.

Gastrointestinal Problems in Foals; Eastern Equine Encephalomyelitis

DON M. WITHERSPOON, B.S., D.V.M., Ph.D.

Director of Veterinary Services, Spendthrift Farm, Lexington, Kentucky.

Foal Heat Diarrhea

D. WOOD-GUSH, B.Sc., D. Phil.

Professor of Applied Ethology, School of Agriculture, University of Edinburgh, Edinburgh, U.K.

Stereotypic Behavior

WALTER W. ZENT, D.V.M.

Hagyard-Davidson-McGee Hospital, Lexington, Kentucky.

Postpartum Complications

JUAN-MANUEL L. ZERTUCHE, M.V.Z.

Resident, Large Animal Medicine, University of Florida College of Veterinary Medicine, Gainesville, Florida.

Corynebacterium Equi Lung Abscesses in Foals

ELLEN L. ZIEMER, D.V.M., M.S.

Lecturer in Diagnostic Medicine, University of Pennsylvania School of Veterinary Medicine. Cytologist and Instructor in Clinical Laboratory Medicine, University of Pennsylvania School of Veterinary Medicine, New Bolton Center, Kennett Square, Pennsylvania.

Renal Tubular Acidosis

PREFACE

It has been a pleasure to prepare this second edition of *Current Therapy in Equine Medicine*. The style of this edition is similar to the first and is designed to provide the practicing veterinarian and veterinary student with a concise description of recent information on the therapy of common medical problems of the horse. Each article contains a description of the disease and confirmatory diagnostic procedures. Therapy and prevention are emphasized and we have attempted to provide specific information on routes of administration and dosages of medications. Each article represents the author's opinion of the best current therapy.

Once again I have relied on section editors for their advice on the content of each section and for the selection of contributors. My editorial tasks were simplified by the exemplary performance of both section editors and authors. I owe them a very large vote of thanks.

This second edition is approximately 80 per cent rewritten to provide new opinions, and the whole book has been revised to update information. Because of the growth of knowledge on the treatment of diseases of foals and gastrointestinal and reproductive problems, these sections have been enlarged. New sections have been added on medical problems of the foot, behavioral disorders, and problems of endurance horses. Infectious diseases have been incorporated into the sections on organ systems.

Current Therapy in Equine Medicine is not meant to be a complete reference text on all the diseases of the horse and should not be judged as such. With each edition, the emphasis will shift depending on the development of new knowledge.

An editor of a book such as this has a large supporting cast. I have acknowledged the tremendous support of authors and section editors. Mary Herdt and Eileen Salmond typed the revised manuscripts; Heidi Immegart, Bob Ingersoll, and Liz Rosanski checked most of the references. I want to thank all of these people and the staff of W. B. Saunders for their invaluable assistance. Finally, I must acknowledge the help of my wife, Pat, and my children, Emily and Sarah, who cheerfully tolerated the accumulation of paper and the hours of reading and proofreading.

N. EDWARD ROBINSON

NOTICE

Extraordinary efforts have been made by the authors, the editors, and the publisher of this book to insure that dosage recommendations are precise and in agreement with standards officially accepted at the time of publication.

It does happen, however, that dosage schedules are changed from time to time in the light of accumulating clinical experience and continuing laboratory studies. This is most likely to occur in the case of recently introduced products.

It is urged, therefore, that you check the manufacturer's recommendations for dosage, especially if the drug to be administered or prescribed is one that you use only infrequently or have not used for some time.

In addition, some drugs mentioned have been used by the authors as experimental drugs. Others have been used in dosages greater than those recommended by the manufacturer. In these cases the authors have reported on their own considerable experience, but readers are urged to view the recommendations with discretion and precaution. Finally, within the United States, please check government regulations for U.S.D.A. approved drugs.

THE PUBLISHER

CONTENTS

Section 2 BEHAVIORAL PROBLEMS

Katherine A. Houpt, *Consulting Editor*

Section 3 CARDIOVASCULAR DISEASES

Christopher M. Brown, *Consulting Editor*

Section 4 ENDOCRINE DISEASES
David C. L. Chen, *Consulting Editor*

Section 5 FOAL DISEASES
Christopher J. Hillidge, *Consulting Editor*

Section 6 FOOT DISEASES
John A. Stick, *Consulting Editor*

Section 7 HEMATOPOIETIC DISEASES

Debra Deem Morris, *Consulting Editor*

Section 8 INTERNAL PARASITES

R. P. Herd, *Consulting Editor*

Section 9 NEUROLOGIC DISEASES

Jill Beech, *Consulting Editor*

Section 10 NUTRITION

H. F. Hintz, *Consulting Editor*

Section 11 OCULAR DISEASES

Mary B. Glaze, *Consulting Editor*

Section 12 PROBLEMS OF THE PERFORMANCE AND ENDURANCE HORSE

Reuben J. Rose, *Consulting Editor*

Section 13 REPRODUCTION

Sidney W. Ricketts, *Consulting Editor*

Section 14   RESPIRATORY DISEASES
Frederik J. Derksen, *Consulting Editor*

Section 15   SKIN DISEASES
T. Manning, *Consulting Editor*

Section 16 TOXICOLOGY

Frederick W. Oehme, *Consulting Editor*

Section 17 URINARY TRACT DISEASES

W. M. Bayly, *Consulting Editor*

Section 18   APPENDICES

Section 1

ALIMENTARY TRACT DISEASE

Edited by J. Becht and J. Moore

Cleft Palate

Karl Frederick Bowman, RALEIGH, NORTH CAROLINA

Cleft palate is an uncommon birth defect that results in postprandial bilateral nasal discharge, dysphagia, and aspiration pneumonia. The major types of orofacial clefts that occur in any species are clefts of the lip and anterior maxilla (regardless of palatal involvement), and clefts of the hard and soft palates. Clefts of the lip and maxilla are due to developmental defects of the primary palate in the embryo, and may be accompanied by clefts of the hard and soft palate as secondary anomalies. Failure of fusion of the secondary palate results in an isolated cleft of the hard or soft palate. All cases described in clinical reports have involved clefts of the hard and soft palate.

DIAGNOSIS

Classically, cleft palate in foals is manifested by bilateral nasal discharge containing milk or food, by dysphagia, and by aspiration pneumonia. In most cases, nasal regurgitation of milk becomes obvious soon after suckling, and its persistence prompts veterinary consultation. Confirmation of cleft palate is based upon clinical findings and observation of an orofacial cleft during oral or rhino-laryngoscopic examination. Cleft soft palate, especially involving the posterior portions only, can be difficult to detect by oral examination; therefore, the foal should be restrained appropriately and rhinolaryngoscopy performed. The lack of palatal tissue in contact with the inferior border of the epiglottis and the impression that the epiglottis has "dropped into the oral cavity" are confirmatory features. The dimensions and extent of clefting—and the possible presence of epiglottic entrapment, submucosal clefting, nasal septal deviation, and inflammation of the nasal passages—should be noted, because their presence will influence treatment. Submucosal clefting is dehiscence of the soft palatal muscles with most of the overlying mucosa intact; often this misplaced muscle is observed as two longitudinal ridges on either side of midline in the soft palate. Auscultation of the lungs, and in selected cases thoracic radiography, should be used to detect aspiration pneumonia. Microbiologic culture and antibiotic sensitivity testing of transtracheal aspirates are indicated to guide selection of appropriate antibiotic therapy for treatment of aspiration pneumonia. Additionally, dysphagia may contribute to several associated medical problems; namely, failure of passive transfer of

1

maternal immunoglobulin via colostrum (see p. 210) and chronic malnutrition, which may require specific therapy.

There have been isolated reports of cleft soft palate in otherwise normal adult horses that have exhibited postprandial nasal discharge since birth. Some of these horses were reported to be serviceable for intended use; however, one affected thoroughbred racehorse died soon after a period of exercise of fatal pulmonary hemorrhage, which was attributed to subclinical aspiration pneumonia. Signs of cleft palate can occur as a complication of excessive partial soft palate resection (staphylectomy), used to treat dorsal displacement of the soft palate.

TREATMENT

Cleft palate repair is done to alleviate postprandial nasal discharge, facilitate eating and drinking, and restore oronasopharyngeal function. Foals affected by cleft palate without aspiration pneumonia should be operated upon as soon as possible. Complicated cases may benefit from therapy to prevent and/or treat aspiration pneumonia, including muzzling, nasogastric or esophagostomy tube feeding, and antimicrobial therapy, prior to cleft palate repair. Most veterinary surgeons prefer to perform surgery prior to six weeks of age, because the depth of the surgical field is less than that encountered in older patients and the foal is still suckling, which allows coarse feed materials to be withheld from the diet.

There have been few reports of successful cleft palate repair in the horse. The surgical techniques that were used, especially the choice of suture material and patterns, have reflected the surgeon's preference. Since clinical cases must be treated individually, the surgical procedure should be selected on the basis of careful evaluation of the patient, clinical experience, and knowledge of documented techniques.

Surgical repair of cleft soft palate has a better prognosis than reconstructions involving the hard and soft palates; however, variability in tissue thickness and muscle in the remnant soft palate may complicate its repair. Large clefts of the hard palate, especially clefts that extend anteriorly to the level of the incisors, are often excessively wide, and incomplete development of the vomer bones precludes successful repair. Foals with these large defects usually have severe aspiration pneumonia.

The surgical approaches for cleft palate repair include the intraoral route, bilateral buccotomy, pharyngotomy, and mandibular symphysiotomy, or various combinations of these approaches. Oral approach for cleft palate repair is limited by inade-

quate exposure of the defect; however, in at least one case, ventral retraction of the tongue with a suture allowed successful repair. The standard approach, mandibular symphysiotomy, allows adequate exposure of the hard and soft palates, enabling repair with standard surgical instruments. Exposure of the posterior soft palate has been accomplished satisfactorily via pharyngotomy.

On the basis of current practice in the closure of cleft soft palate in humans, several recommendations can be made. Local injection of lidocaine hydrochloride with epinephrine (1:10,000 or more dilute) tenses the tissues and provides hemostasis during dissection. In addition to the use of lateral relief incisions, osteotomy and medial reflection of each hamulus of the pterygoid bone lessens the pull of the tensor veli palatini muscle and relaxes the soft palate. If the cleft of the soft palate involves greater than two-thirds of its length, the levator veli palatini muscle may need to be dissected free of its insertion at the posterior aspect of the hard palate. Recreation of the normal levator veli palatini muscle "sling" may help to restore pharyngeal function. Nasal mucosa should be apposed with absorbable suture material in an interrupted pattern. Suture knots should not be buried in the muscular layer; therefore, interrupted horizontal mattress sutures with knots in the oral cavity are recommended. Oral mucosa may be closed with an interrupted everting suture pattern. Use of this method of repair has improved results in several foals with cleft soft palate.

Small posterior defects of the hard palate can be repaired by a mucoperiosteal sliding-flap technique combined with cleft soft palate repair. Large clefts of the hard palate might be best repaired by the mucoperiosteal reflected-flap technique, which has been used successfully in dogs.

Postoperatively, patients should receive broad-spectrum antibiotic therapy and tetanus prophylaxis. Phenylbutazone may be indicated to alleviate swelling of the tongue, which is commonly encountered during the first three or four days after surgery. Foals should be encouraged to suckle the mare as soon as possible after surgery. In older animals, adequate nutritional intake may be provided by offering a water-soaked horse pellet gruel or by administering the gruel or other suitable semiliquid diet via nasogastric or esophagostomy tube. The oral incision should be inspected daily, and food material, which often becomes trapped between the teeth and tongue, should be washed out of the mouth. Palatoplasty sutures are not routinely removed. However, if indicated, they should be removed one to two weeks postoperatively to avoid the knots becoming buried in the healing palatal mucosa.

Healing of the cleft palate repair should be evaluated three to four weeks postoperatively, using the criteria of resolution of clinical signs and appearance of the repaired tissues. Further surgery to correct incomplete cleft palate repair may be unnecessary if normal oronasopharyngeal function has been restored. Some reported cases of incomplete resolution of clinical signs following closure may be related to physiologic dysfunction due to incomplete muscle reconstruction, to partial dehiscence of the posterior part of the soft palate, or to formation of a small oronasal fistula.

COMPLICATIONS

Serious complications of cleft palate repair in horses have not been overcome, and those complications may require euthanasia. Dehiscence of the palatoplasty, especially at the posterior aspect of the soft palate, and formation of oronasal fistula occur in 90% of cases followed by recurrence of clinical signs. Second attempts at repair are usually unsuccessful, because of lack of mucosa or palatal tissue for incorporation into the palatoplasty. Major complications directly associated with mandibular symphysiotomy are osteomyelitis and nonunion of the mandible. Although lower lip dehiscence may occur following mandibular symphysiotomy, it is not a major complication. There is a need to improve palatoplasty techniques in this species. At the onset of cleft palate repair, owners should be cognizant of the possible heritability of the condition, the low success rate and complications of reported procedures, and the period of intensive nursing care required in these patients.

ADDITIONAL COMMENTS

The prevalence and heritability of isolated cleft palate in horses are not known. There are reports of one case per 1,000 admissions to an equine referral center, two cases in 640 fetal and neonatal necropsies, and 53 cases in 144,348 university hospital admissions.

Clinicians should be aware of the 1984 opinion of the Judicial Council of the American Veterinary Medical Association: "Performance of surgical procedures in all species for the purpose of concealing genetic defects in animals to be shown, raced, bred, or sold as breeding animals is unethical. However, should the health or welfare of the individual patient require correction of such genetic defects, it is recommended that the patient be rendered incapable of reproduction." In my experience, all cases of cleft palate in horses required therapy for the animals' health and welfare, and cleft palate repair was selected as part of that therapy to optimize results. However, it is recommended that affected animals be excluded from breeding programs and that male horses be castrated. In the absence of data on maternal and/or paternal influences on incidence of cleft palate in horses, it is difficult to make recommendations for breeding of the dam and sire, especially since other nongenetic factors may cause cleft palate. Currently, I would advise against repeat breeding between the dam and sire.

The assistance, based upon their clinical experiences, of Drs. L. P. Tate, Jr. and J. T. Robertson is gratefully acknowledged.

Supplemental Readings

Bowman, K. F., Tate, L. P., Evans, L. H., and Donawick, W. J.: Complications of cleft palate repair in large animals. J. Am. Vet. Med. Assoc., *180*:652, 1982.
Jones, R. S., Maisels, D. O., DeGeus, J.J., and Lovius, B. B. J.: Surgical repair of cleft palate in the horse. Equine Vet. J., 7:86, 1975.
McIlwraith, C. W.: Equine digestive system. In Jennings, P. B. (ed.): The Practice of Large Animal Surgery, Philadelphia, W. B. Saunders Company, 1984, pp. 560–566.
Nelson, A. W., and Stashak, T. S.: Cleft palate. In Robinson, N. E. (ed.): Current Therapy in Equine Medicine, 1st ed. Philadelphia, W. B. Saunders Company, 1983, pp. 177–181.
Scott, E. A.: Surgery of the oral cavity. Vet. Clin. North Am. (Large Anim. Pract.), *4*:3, 1982.

Salivary Gland Disease
Karl Frederick Bowman, RALEIGH, NORTH CAROLINA

Salivary gland disease occurs uncommonly in the horse. Primary salivary gland conditions are sialadenitis, salivary calculi, salivary mucocele, trauma, and neoplasia. More frequently, the salivary glands and their ducts assume clinical significance when excess salivation occurs as a clinical sign or when the veterinarian performs surgery, including wound management, in the head and neck region.

DIAGNOSIS

Thorough examination of horses suspected of having salivary gland disease should include palpation of the glands and superficial portions of the parotid duct (Fig. 1), and detailed oral examination. Pain in the parotid region is associated with guttural pouch disease; therefore, endoscopic examination of the guttural pouches may be indicated. During oral examination, particular attention should be directed at the oral exits of the salivary ducts. The parotid salivary duct enters the oral cavity at its papilla opposite the third cheek tooth. The mandibular salivary duct opens into the oral cavity on the lateral aspect of the sublingual caruncle. The polystomatic sublingual salivary ducts, approximately 30 in number, are visible as small pores in the sublingual recess. Complete blood count (CBC) and microbiologic cultures are helpful in diagnosis of salivary gland infections. Determination of serum electrolytes and blood gas values are indicated when there is excess salivation or salivary loss such as may occur through a parotid duct fistula. Needle aspiration of swellings allows differentiation of abscessation, mucocele formation, and neoplasia; how-

ever, concern has been expressed regarding possible transplantation of neoplastic cells into adjacent tissues during needle withdrawal. Radiography has been used to diagnose and locate salivary calculi. Other diagnostic methods, primarily of academic interest but shown to be important factors in diagnosis and formulation of therapeutic regimens in humans and dogs, include sialography and radionuclide salivary scanning.

SALIVATION AS A CLINICAL SIGN

When salivation occurs as a clinical sign, it is necessary to differentiate between excess accumulation of saliva in the mouth, (sialism, ptyalism), and dysphagia. Heavy metal poisoning, parasympathomimetic poisoning, neurologic disease, and stomatitis can cause sialism. The first three conditions cause systemic signs of illness and additional laboratory testing such as serum lead determination or virus isolation may confirm the diagnosis. Stomatitis is often accompanied by malodorous breath and swollen tongue; successful treatment of its primary cause usually eliminates sialism.

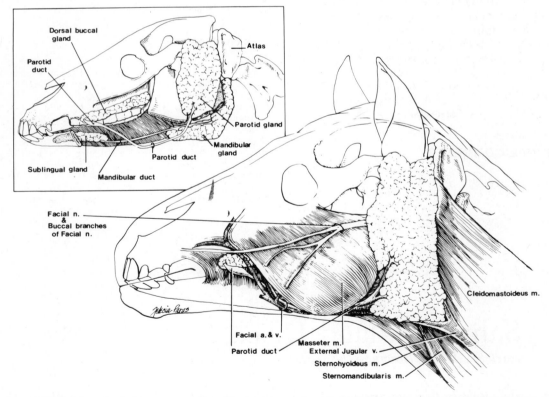

Figure 1. Facial anatomy of the horse. The mandible has been resected in the inset diagram. Three pairs of major salivary glands are present: the parotid, mandibular, and polystomatic sublingual salivary glands. Beneath the mucous membrane of the oral cavity and pharynx are numerous minor salivary glands, including the labial, buccal, and lingual glands. The minor salivary glands are of local importance and provide necessary moisture for their associated mucous membrane. Note the superficial locations of the parotid salivary duct and the facial artery and vein.

In horses, dysphagia results most commonly from esophageal obstruction, "choke;" therefore, a nasogastric tube should be advanced to ensure clear passage from the oropharynx to the stomach. Neurologic disease, either functional or infectious, can cause dysphagia. Although the signs of rabies in horses (see p. 364) are variable, they do not usually include salivation and dysphagia seen so commonly in other species. Protective gloves and handwashing are recommended for oral examination of horses with sialism.

A peculiar type of parasympathomimetic toxicosis is caused by ingestion of legume hay contaminated with *Rhizoctonia leguminicola*. This fungus produces a mycotoxin, slaframine ("slobber factor"), which causes sialism. Affected horses suffer no other ill effects from its ingestion, and sialism ceases when the tainted hay is no longer fed. Unfortunately, visual detection of the parasitized legume hay is not possible because the mycelial growth has the color and texture of the well-cured hay.

Hyponatremia, hypochloremia, and metabolic alkalosis occur soon after the onset of excess salivation or salivary loss in horses. Although the potential for potassium depletion during saliva loss is great, if the horse continues to eat, serum potassium may be only slightly lowered. Sodium chloride should be administered orally to correct electrolyte and acid-base imbalances. Equine diets usually provide adequate potassium.

TRAUMA

Lacerations usually involve the superficial portions of the parotid salivary gland and its duct. In fresh wounds of the salivary glandular tissue, cleansing, debridement, and primary closure of skin will usually be followed by satisfactory healing. When the duct is severed, the two ends should be located and repaired over a small plastic catheter that is allowed to emerge into the oral cavity. Infected wounds involving the salivary glands require local wound care and possibly parenteral antibiotic therapy to promote second intention healing. Liquid or moistened diets and isolation from other horses may benefit horses with salivary gland injury by reducing salivary flow.

Complications of salivary gland injury include salivary-cutaneous fistula or duct obstruction with acute enlargement (see under Salivary Mucocele). A salivary fistula that involves the glandular tissue has a good chance of spontaneous resolution, but salivary fistulas involving the duct usually do not heal. Reconstructive surgery may be employed to re-establish the continuity of the duct or to translocate the cutaneous fistula to an intraoral position. Perhaps the most simple solution to parotid duct

fistula is to perform ligation of its proximal, leaking end. In the absence of infection, atrophy of the parotid salivary gland occurs. In one report, a persistent salivary-cutaneous fistula purportedly involving the parotid salivary duct was treated successfully by resection of the parotid and mandibular salivary glands.

Many salivary-cutaneous fistulas in humans occur iatrogenically. Meticulous dissection of tissues is therefore essential during head and neck surgery in the horse. Abscess drainage, mandibular symphysiotomy, and the lateral approaches to the guttural pouches can all require displacement of salivary tissue.

SIALADENITIS

Sialadenitis occurs uncommonly. Although the salivary glands may become involved in any inflammatory process including infection, most commonly trauma causes sialadenitis of one gland. In the absence of infection or open wounds, symptomatic therapy aimed at relieving pain and inflammation is appropriate. Antimicrobial therapy may be indicated if culture and antibiotic sensitivity results indicate presence of infection. *Streptococcus equi* infection, "strangles," is rarely associated with sialadenitis.

Sialadenitis may result in salivary duct obstruction owing to accumulation of exudate and mucus; conversely, obstruction of the duct by an ingested foreign body may be the cause. In either case, salivary duct obstruction produces dilatation of the ductules, acinar swelling, and rupture. Clinically, the salivary gland becomes swollen, hot, and painful. Treatment consists of appropriate antimicrobial therapy and if necessary foreign body removal. Once inflammation subsides, the gland may atrophy and become replaced by scar tissue.

SALIVARY CALCULI

Chronic sialadenitis and partial duct obstruction may provide sufficient exudate and desquamated cells to form a nidus for calcium salt precipitation and calculus formation. Salivary calculi usually involve the parotid duct and become lodged at its orifice. If the salivary duct enlarges around the stone allowing salivary secretion, then clinical signs may be limited to discrete swelling along the course of the parotid salivary duct. However, since salivary calculi can become several centimeters in length and width, it is more likely that they will remain asymptomatic until duct obstruction and acute sialadenitis occur. Salivary calculi should be excised and sialadenitis treated appropriately.

SALIVARY MUCOCELE

A salivary mucocele is an accumulation of salivary secretions in single- or multiloculated cavities adjacent to a ruptured duct. Typically, a mucocele has brown, mucinous contents that may become inspissated. A ranula is a special type of mucocele that occurs secondary to obstruction of the sublingual salivary duct. Ranulae, at least in dogs, present as smooth, rounded, fluctuating prominences in the sublingual recess. These cystic distentions of the sublingual salivary duct are lined with epithelium and contain serous or thick mucus. Treatment requires creation of a salivary fistula into the oral cavity, or excision of the mucocele and associated salivary gland. Ranulae may respond to incision and marsupialization of the cyst.

SALIVARY GLAND NEOPLASIA

Salivary gland neoplasms are uncommon. However, benign mixed tumors, adenocarcinomas, and acinar cell tumors of the salivary glands have been reported in horses. Local invasion of a salivary gland by tumors originating in adjacent tissue or metastasis of melanomas to the parotid salivary gland occurs more frequently. Salivary gland neoplasms affect older horses, and the frequent site of occurrence is the parotid salivary gland. Clinical features, in addition to an enlarging mass in the parotid region, may include edema, pain, and fixation of the tumor to the overlying skin. Histopathologic diagnosis of the neoplastic cell type will facilitate design of the treatment regimen and help determine a prognosis.

Salivary gland neoplasms in humans and animals are similar in morphologic pattern and biologic behavior. Benign mixed tumors are locally invasive along peripheral vasculature; therefore, wide excision of the tumor is necessary. Recurrence of benign mixed tumors is common. Adenocarcinomas frequently metastasize to deep cervical and mediastinal lymph nodes and are not amenable to treatment. Acinic cell tumors are locally invasive but apparently do not exhibit metastasis; therefore, wide excision of tumor is indicated.

Melanomas are among the most common neoplasms of the horse and have a progressive and potentially malignant course over extended periods of time. As in humans, melanomas may metastasize to the parotid salivary gland. Affected horses should be evaluated for presence of a primary tumor and for any functional deficits, especially of the head and neck and gastrointestinal tract. On the basis of the natural biology of melanomas in the horse and reported lack of effectiveness of surgical resection of melanomas, no clear recommendation can be made for treatment of melanoma with parotid salivary gland metastasis, except serial observation of the mass and others for rate of enlargement. Rapid growth of a tumor is a poor prognostic sign.

Supplemental Readings

Koch, D. B.: The oral cavity, oropharynx, and salivary glands. *In* Mansmann, R. A., McAllister, E. S., and Pratt, P. W. (eds.): Equine Medicine and Surgery, 3rd ed. Santa Barbara, CA, American Veterinary Publications, 1982, pp. 473–475.

Stedham, M. A.: Neoplastic disease. *In* Jennings, P. B. (ed.): The Practice of Large Animal Surgery, Vol. 1. Philadelphia, W. B. Saunders Company, 1984, pp. 224–225.

Stick, J. A., Robinson, N. E., and Krehbiel, J. D.: Acid-base and electrolyte alterations associated with salivary loss in the pony. Am. J. Vet. Res., *42*:733, 1981.

Care of the Teeth

G. Marvin Beeman, LITTLETON, COLORADO

Dental problems that interfere with mastication or contribute to systemic infection should always be considered as a cause of chronic weight loss. Dental problems will often also affect performance when the horse is being directed by a bit in the mouth.

When a horse is presented with a history that suggests a dental problem, age, sex, use, diet, and eating habits should be considered in arriving at a diagnosis. Age is important because of the eruption of the various teeth and the shedding of the deciduous teeth, both of which are often accompanied by dental disease. Also, there are many dental problems that occur much more frequently in older horses. Sex is a consideration because the mare has fewer teeth than the stallion, which may dictate the type of problem encountered (such as presence of rudimentary lower canine teeth in the mare, which often do not erupt and may cause gingival irritation). Use is considered because a bit will often cause severe lacerations to the cheeks if forced against sharp enamel points of the premolars. Abnormal eating habits such as dropping of grain, excessive

TABLE 1. FORMULAS FOR DECIDUOUS AND PERMANENT TEETH

Deciduous Teeth
$2\left(\text{Di } \dfrac{3}{3} \text{ DC } \dfrac{0}{0} \text{ Dp } \dfrac{3}{3} \right) = 24$

Permanent Teeth
$2\left(\text{I } \dfrac{3}{3} \text{ C } \dfrac{1}{1} \text{ p } \dfrac{3 \text{ or } 4}{3} \text{ M } \dfrac{3}{3} \right) = 40 \text{ or } 42$

salivation, "quidding" of hay or grass, or tilting of the head are indications of painful dental problems. Because age and sex are significant factors when evaluating a dental condition, the formulas for deciduous and permanent teeth (Table 1), along with the eruption table (Table 2), should be known.

The canine teeth of the mare are very small or do not erupt, while those of the male are almost always present, are longer than the wolf teeth (P1), and are located in the rostral half of the interdental space. The lower canine teeth are more rostral than the upper ones. Canines should not be confused with the wolf teeth (P1), which are commonly found only in the upper arcade and vary from small, round (5 mm in diameter) needlelike structures just erupting from the gum to rather large (10 to 15 mm wide) concave teeth with the concavity on the lingual side. Even larger round wolf teeth have been encountered. Wolf teeth in the upper arcade may be located several millimeters rostral to or touching

TABLE 2. ERUPTION TIMES FOR THE TEETH

Deciduous	
Tooth	Eruption
1st incisor	Birth or first week
2nd incisor	4–6 weeks
3rd incisor	6–9 months
No deciduous canine	
No deciduous wolf teeth	
2nd premolar	
3rd premolar	Birth–first 2 weeks
4th premolar	

Permanent		
Tooth		Eruption
1st incisor	I1	2½ years
2nd incisor	I2	3½ years
3rd incisor	I3	4½ years
Canine	C	4–5 years
1st premolar (wolf tooth)	PM1	5–6 months
2nd premolar	PM2	2½ years
3rd premolar	PM3	3 years
4th premolar	PM4	4 years
1st molar	M1	9–12 months
2nd molar	M2	2 years
3rd molar	M3	3½–4 years

(Lowers may erupt about 6 months earlier — for PM3 and PM4)

the second premolar. When the lower P1 is present, it is quite small and needlelike and is adjacent to the lower P2.

Several anatomic factors influence dental wear and thereby the incidence of dental disease. The upper (maxillary) arcades of molars and premolars are more widely separated than the lower (mandibular) arcades, the distance between the mandibulae being least at the fourth premolar and first molar. The upper teeth, therefore, overlap the lower teeth on the buccal surface, and the lower teeth overlap the upper teeth on the lingual surface. The occlusal surfaces of the upper cheek teeth viewed from in front slope outward and downward, while those of the lower teeth angle inward and upward. This angulation of the occlusal surfaces, coupled with the overlapping of teeth described before and the side-to-side pattern of mastication, causes the development of sharp enamel points on the buccal surface (outside) of upper teeth and the lingual surface (inside) of lower teeth.

Prominent points occur on rostral and middle portions of the upper teeth. On lower teeth, points are evenly distributed. Upper points are more angled, while lower points are more vertical. These differences in points in upper and lower arcades determine the angle at which the float blade is applied to the points. Because of the anatomy and method of mastication, the upper fourth cheek tooth (first molar) is subject to most wear and is the most common site of serious dental disease.

Parrot mouth (brachygnathia of the lower jaw) or undershoot (prognathia of the lower jaw) cause long points on the rostral border of the upper second premolar and the caudal border of the lower third molar, respectively. This is especially true in horses older than seven years.

EXAMINATION OF TEETH

By correlating the history, particularly the age of the horse, with a thorough understanding of anatomy of the head and teeth, the examination routine is established. Before the oral cavity is examined, the exterior of the head should be examined for (1) any abnormal swellings and/or draining tracts over the maxilla or mandibles, (2) abnormal head tilt, and (3) unilateral, purulent, flaky nasal discharge with a fetid odor of necrotic bone. The exterior of the cheeks should be palpated over the upper cheek teeth for painful sites.

The majority of horses object to having the oral cavity examined and must be restrained. The degree of restraint should be determined by the horse's response. The examination should be done with the least amount of discomfort and restraint possible; however, if the dental lesions are quite painful, the examination may not be possible without the use of chemical restraining agents. Various agents such as xylazine* alone or in combination with acepromazine maleate† and/or pentazocine lactate injection‡ are very useful for this examination and certainly should be used before the horse is upset or abused.

The first step in the examination is to position the horse in optimal light so it cannot back away from the examiner. This is best done in a corner of a stall or in stocks with a darkened background. An assistant should be instructed in the way to hold the horse. Be certain the halter is large enough to allow the mouth to be opened to the maximal amount and without discomfort to the horse.

Rinse the mouth free of debris, preferably with cold water to elicit pain from a diseased tooth. In a fractious horse, warm water will be more readily tolerated. Evidence of halitosis should be noted also.

The incisor teeth are visually examined first for abnormalities and the determination of age. The interdental space, gums, and the cheek opposite the upper premolars are palpated and observed for injuries. Examination of the cheek teeth is most often accomplished without a dental speculum. However, if a speculum is necessary, care must be taken to prevent injury to the horse and/or the examiner. The left side of the dental arcade can be visually examined by inserting the fingers of the left hand through the right interdental space and grasping the tongue and withdrawing it out of the right side of the mouth. This will force the horse to open its mouth and to pull back. To avoid injury to the tongue if the horse should react violently, the little finger of the hand grasping the tongue should also grasp the halter. The mouth can be forced open further by applying pressure to the hard palate with a finger of the right hand. Visual examination is facilitated by a head lamp or pocket penlight. Palpation of the left arcade can be accomplished with the tongue held in the same manner and the right hand introduced into the left interdental space, forcing the tongue between the right cheek teeth with the back of the hand while palpating those of the left arcade. The examination of the right cheek teeth is done in the same manner by reversing all procedures.

If additional examinations are needed, further narcosis may be necessary and a dental speculum may be needed. Use of a short-acting general anesthetic is reasonable to facilitate a complete examination. A laryngoscope will facilitate close visual evaluation of an involved tooth. Extreme care must be taken to avoid damage to the laryngoscope. A dental pick is helpful in determining if an infundibulum is defective. Injection of a colored fluid into an external draining tract will determine if the lesion opens into the oral cavity (periodontal disease). Radiographs are quite helpful in determining the extent to which dental disease involves the periodontal tissue.

Since the age of the horse dictates to a large extent what might be the cause of dental disease, the diagnosis and therapy are categorized by age groups.

Age 10–18 Months

History. Not masticating well.

Examination. Reveals lacerations of cheeks from sharp points on upper premolars. This is not a common problem but may cause poor mastication in this age group.

Therapy. Float down the enamel points. The deciduous teeth are soft and will not require much rasping (see next section).

Age 18–24 Months

History. Poor mastication and bleeding from the mouth after riding with snaffle bit, objecting to bridle training, throwing head.

Examination. Ulcerated area of cheeks is present opposite the second upper premolar, tongue lacerations, small, very sharp points on all premolars, particularly the upper second premolar. Wolf teeth present.

Therapy

1. Remove wolf teeth. This should be done before the floating because they will likely be broken off or rasped down, thus making their removal difficult. In my opinion, this is the optimal time to remove these teeth because they are not as firmly embedded as they will be at an older age. Often the only restraint necessary to remove these teeth is a nose twitch; however, tranquilization and narcosis with or without local anesthesia may be indicated. The twitch and head must be held in a manner so that the wolf tooth can be seen. To do this, the twitch must be pushed toward the side being operated on while the head is held firmly. One method of removing the wolf teeth is to elevate the gingiva from the lateral, rostral, and caudal surface with an instrument specifically designed for this purpose or an orthopedic gouge (5 to 8 mm in width). The medial surface is left alone because of the danger of injuring the palatine artery. If the wolf tooth is quite close to the second premolar, forcing the instrument between the two teeth will loosen the wolf tooth sufficiently so that it can be pried out using the second premolar for support. If

*Rompun, Haver-Lockhart, Shawnee, KS

†Acepromazine Maleate-Injectible, Fort Dodge Laboratories, Inc., Fort Dodge, IA

‡Talwin-V, Veterinary Products Division, Winthrop-Breon Laboratories, New York, NY

this is not possible, the tooth can then be pulled with a pair of wolf tooth extraction forceps. It is advisable to remove the teeth intact, but if they are broken off well below the gum line, it is best to leave the fragment in place because it seldom will create a problem and unnecessary damage will be done to the alveolus by trying to remove it. Note should be made that the fragment may appear within a year's time and may be mistaken for another wolf tooth. Normally the fragment is easily removed when it appears. Removal of the wolf tooth without breaking it off is facilitated by grasping the tooth with forceps as deep into the gum and alveolus as possible. Apply traction straight down while rotating the tooth back and forth on its long axis rather than rocking the tooth medially and laterally. Also avoid the horse's mandibular movement, which will put lateral pressure on the forceps, causing the tooth to break off. When lower wolf teeth are present, they are removed in the same manner. They are usually small and easy to extract.

2. The sharp enamel points are rasped off. The floating procedure should be started with a minimal amount of restraint. Many horses can be floated completely with simple restraint; however, as objection increases, the level of restraint must be increased. A twitch is useful, but most horses will not tolerate it for the length of time necessary to complete the floating. In some horses, a lip chain applied to the upper incisor gingiva will provide better restraint than a twitch. It is much more desirable to use chemical restraint than it is to fight the horse (the same products or combinations thereof as mentioned previously are very helpful). Even the short-acting general anesthetics (such as xylazine and ketamine hydrochloride injection NF*) are preferred over excessive physical restraint to float or carry out a simple surgical procedure involving the teeth.

The noseband of the halter should be sufficiently large so that the horse's mouth can be opened to its maximum. The halter and assistant's arm should not put pressure on the horse's face, as this will cause the float to injure the cheeks. To enable the procedure to be carried out without excessive restraint, the teeth causing the most trouble should be floated first because most horses will tolerate some floating before objecting. Therefore, the upper cheek teeth are most often floated first (the premolars in young horses and molars in older horses). The lower cheek teeth are floated last because horses seem to object to this portion of the procedure more than any other and because horses are much more prone to chewing the float when doing the lower arcade. This can be prevented by

holding the tongue out of the side of the mouth opposite the side being worked on. However, as soon as the process is started, many horses will set their lower jaw and will actually stand quieter if the tongue is released.

In the actual floating process, the float (dental rasp) should be started on the teeth with relatively easy strokes until the rasps have established grooves. Then more pressure can be applied. Changing direction of the floats causes the most work; therefore, the longer the stroke, the better for the patient and the operator. Care needs to be taken to avoid injuring the mouth. One of the most vulnerable sites is beyond the last molar in both the upper and lower arcade. The rasp should be placed at approximately a 90° angle to the enamel points on the buccal surface of the upper cheek teeth and the lingual surface of the lower cheek teeth.

Buccal ulcerations are often caused by pressure from a snaffle bit against the sharp enamel points of the upper second premolar (either deciduous or permanent), particularly when a gag snaffle is used (as in polo ponies). In order to tolerate the bit, the upper and lower second premolars should have the rostral aspect rounded from the table surface to the gum line and from the lingual surface to the buccal surface. For the buccal surface of the uppers, a short-handled 30° float is inserted from the opposite side of the mouth through the interdental space. (Some operators prefer a file blade rather than a rasp.) A short straight float is used for the lingual side of the uppers and lowers from the same side of the mouth through the interdental space. Caution is necessary to avoid injuring the roof of the mouth. Occasionally the buccal side of the lowers is most easily reached with the same instrument from the opposite side.

There are many different types of floats and blades available today. The choice should be the one that best fits the operation. The blades should be sharp because the fewer strokes needed to remove the sharp points, the better it is for the horse and the operator. In my opinion, the blades that have carborundum pieces fixed to them* are the best because they are extremely sharp and stay that way with considerable use.

AGE 2½ YEARS THROUGH 4 YEARS

History. Same as in the preceding section. Often more obvious signs of painful mastication with a sudden onset and halitosis.

Examination. The problem is the same as in the preceding section, and the presence of retained

*Vetalar, Parke-Davis & Co., Morris Plains, NJ

*Jorgensen float blades, Jorgensen Laboratories, Inc., Loveland, CO

deciduous premolars (commonly called dental caps) should be anticipated. These horses present many different signs. Deciduous premolars (DcPm) should be considered retained when the permanent tooth has grown beyond the gum line and a definite demarcation between the cap and the permanent tooth can be seen. Often the infundibulae of DcPm are shallow or absent (this is a good identifying and differentiating feature of the DcPm). Occasionally the examination will reveal an upper cap that has split transversely or longitudinally with a portion missing or displaced laterally, causing buccal lacerations and facial swellings. One horse was observed in which buccal penetration from a cap fragment was complete, causing an oral fistula. Caps of the lower arcade occasionally split transversely but rarely displace medially or laterally. Retained caps commonly occur in pairs. The lower third and fourth premolars may erupt six months earlier than the corresponding uppers.

Chronic ossifying alveolar periostitis observed as swelling of the maxilla or more commonly the mandible over the roots of the cheek teeth is caused by impacted, overcrowded DcPms. The swelling may be accompanied by draining tracts. This condition is a common finding in three-year-olds of breeds with relatively small heads (such as Arabians).

Caps that are attached to gingiva entirely around their circumferences should be removed *only* if there is a definite indication that they are causing a problem. Not only will removal be difficult and result in excessive damage to the gum, but also it will be some time before the permanent tooth will erupt sufficiently to allow for proper mastication.

Therapy. Often buccal and/or lingual lacerations will be from the retained DcPms, which should be removed before any floating is done. Caps should also be removed if chronic ossifying alveolar periostitis is present to the extent that considerable irritation or a draining tract is evident. Mild alveolar periostitis will often recover with the normal loosening and loss of the caps. Therefore, a conservative approach to this condition is warranted. Caps should be removed before the permanent tooth is removed to treat the draining tract. The exterior swelling will be slow to disappear.

Removal of caps can be accomplished with a combination of a screwdriver (with a shaft 10 to 14 inches long and the tip rounded and bluntly wedged) and small dental equine forceps. The forceps are most useful for the lower caps and occasionally the upper second DcPm, while the screwdriver is the most efficient instrument for the upper three and four DcPms. The tongue is held out the contralateral side of the mouth. For the upper caps, the blade of the screwdriver is inserted between the permanent tooth and the cap at the rostrolingual

quarter by directing the shaft from the opposite interdental space. The instrument can often be forced between the cap and permanent tooth with little pressure, then rotated to cause the cap to be freed. Occasionally tapping the screwdriver with a solid object will be necessary to force the blade between the DcPm and the premolar to separate the two. Care must be taken to be certain the instrument is directed properly to avoid injury to the mouth. The lower DcPms three and four can often be removed with forceps, but the screwdriver will work quite well also. The site of insertion between the lower cap and the permanent premolar is more rostral than for the upper teeth. Sometimes it is necessary to direct the shaft of the instrument along the table surface of the teeth to loosen the lower DcPms three and four.

Retained deciduous incisors often cause displacement of the permanent incisors toward the lingual side. When retained, they are embedded in the buccal gingiva, and most often they can be removed with dental forceps. Occasionally they will have to be loosened as described for the wolf teeth. Fragments need to be removed unless excessive damage will result, and then they should be left for a time to allow the permanent teeth to further displace the fragments.

Following any interruption to the gingiva, the oral cavity should be rinsed two to three times daily with strong salt water for three to five days.

After removing those caps that are creating problems, floating of the remaining teeth may be necessary.

FIVE YEARS AND OLDER

History. Most commonly will be painful mastication and weight loss.

Examination. The examination may reveal a single entity or any combination of the following.

1. Sharp enamel points on upper cheek teeth (most commonly the molars) causing buccal lacerations; points on the lower cheek teeth (most commonly the third and fourth) causing lingual lacerations.

2. Canine teeth that are long and sharp (occasionally those that do not erupt cause a gingival cyst).

3. Brachygnathia of the lower jaw (parrot mouth) creates a long point on the rostral border of the upper second premolar and the caudal border of the lower third molar. If the lower jaw protrudes, points occur on the rostral border of the second lower premolar and the caudal border of the upper third molar.

4. Abnormally long cheek teeth (usually opposite the defect left by the loss of the corresponding tooth in the opposing arcade).

5. When dental pain is observed, periodontal disease is most likely to be the cause. Dental pain will be manifested by (a) slow and careful mastication that is exaggerated with pelleted feed and occasionally with grain (the affected horse will often leave grain but eat hay), (b) exaggerated tongue movements, (c) holding the head rotated with the affected side up (especially when eating pellets), (d) excessive drooling of saliva and grain, (e) dropping of feed boli (quidding), (f) avoiding cold water or showing pain when the mouth is washed with cold water, or (g) pain exhibited when the teeth are floated. Halitosis is further evidence of periodontal disease. The source can be identified by palpating the suspected tooth and getting the odor of necrotic bone from the palpating finger. The gum will recede from the affected tooth. A unilateral flaky purulent nasal discharge with a fetid odor is most commonly caused by advanced disease of the upper cheek teeth causing maxillary sinusitis. The roots of the third and fourth cheek teeth are usually located within the anterior maxillary sinus, and those of the fifth and sixth cheek teeth are within the posterior maxillary sinus. If the diseased alveolus ruptures to the exterior of the maxilla or mandible, a fistula results.

Therapy. A combination of the following may be necessary.

1. Rasping of enamel points may be necessary. In older horses, the upper molars will cause the most damage to the cheeks, so they should be floated first. There is a tendency to over-rasp the cheek teeth. The only rasping that is necessary is to remove the sharp enamel points. This is especially true in very old horses because their teeth can be inadvertently extracted by the rasp.

2. The canine teeth that are long, sharp, and perhaps are interfering with the bridle should be rasped down rather than removed. By grasping the horse's mandible at the level of the interdental space with the thumb on one side and the index and middle fingers on the other, the lower labia can be held down and away from the lower canines. The upper canines are done in the same manner by elevating the upper labia with the thumb of the free hand. They can be rasped or filed down by placing the instrument of choice directly over the tooth and at right angles to it. Most often this procedure is necessary to satisfy the owner rather than improve the horse's condition.

3. Elongation of the second upper premolar caused by parrot mouth can usually be corrected with a dental float, but often the elongation on the lower third molar will have to be cut off with molar cutters.

4. Excessively long cheek teeth that cause a masticating problem can be shortened by rasping at three- to six-month intervals. All the occlusal surfaces of the affected tooth must be rasped down. Sedation and a dental speculum will greatly enhance this procedure. Many times these cases are presented only after the affected tooth is quite long, and the only practical method of correction is cutting the tooth off with molar cutters or a similar instrument. Wire saws can also be used. There are various types of cutters. The compound molar cutter is the most effective, especially for large teeth. Extreme care must be taken in the proper placement of the instrument, and the pressure must be applied at 90° to the tooth with no rotational torque because the tooth can be fractured down into the alveolus. After the excess has been cut off, the buccal and lingual surfaces must be rasped smooth. This procedure can be done in the standing horse under sedation and local anesthesia. Even so, most horses will object to the pressure and excessive manipulation, which enhances the possibility of fracturing the tooth. Therefore, one of the short-acting general anesthetic regimens is indicated (an acepromazine, xylazine, and ketamine combination is very effective). A good dental speculum is also necessary. Care must be taken to prevent tooth fragments from being aspirated into the trachea in anesthetized horses.

5. The most common conditions causing dental pain are periodontal disease, defects of infundibulae, alveolar periostitis, and the resulting dental fistulas and/or sinus infections. These conditions are often seen in combination rather than as single entities. In my experience, they most commonly affect the fourth upper cheek tooth (first molar). Necrosis of the infundibulum is the commonest condition seen in our horse population. In many cases, the condition does not progress to the point that more serious sequelae develop. The affected tooth can be left in place and the entire arcade given regular examinations and conservative (floating) treatment at two- to four-month intervals to maintain normal mastication.

The lesion may progress to the point that the tooth splits, alveolar periostitis develops, and a sinus empyema occurs. When an upper cheek tooth splits, the fragment on the buccal side is displaced laterally, causing considerable cheek irritation. These fragments must be removed. Most often this can be accomplished with a small tooth extractor and dental speculum on the standing, sedated animal. That portion of the tooth left in place (usually on the lingual surface) is often quite stable, and the tooth will stay viable and will not require extraction. This has been successful in enough cases to warrant conservative treatment before removal of the entire tooth. If sinus empyema or a fistula does develop, removal of the tooth is necessary either by extraction or repulsion. Though less common, mandibular teeth can be affected with infundibular defects and can develop all of the previously mentioned sequelae. If a lower cheek tooth splits, the fragment on the lingual side most often will be displaced toward the tongue, causing considerable irritation and interference in mastication.

When periodontal disease causes empyema or fistulae, it is necessary to remove the tooth and establish drainage. However, it is possible to prevent the advancement of the disease if the initial lesions of gingivitis (hyperemia, edema, and open defects) are treated. Systemic antimicrobial and nonsteroidal anti-inflammatory medication in conjunction with frequent astringent mouthwashes and floating to maintain normal dental tables and mastication will correct the disease. Occasionally an early fistula will dry up if vigorously flushed with hydrogen peroxide and one of the tamed iodine products. Unfortunately, the early signs of the disease are often undetected.

The extraction or repulsion of the cheek teeth is adequately explained in the literature. In our hands, repulsion is the most efficient and satisfactory method of tooth removal. Extraction is very difficult, and sufficient drainage is difficult to establish for proper postoperative treatment and recovery. The very old horse is the most amenable patient for tooth extraction. A case can be approached by first attempting extraction, but if not successful, repulsion should be the final procedure. Inhalation general anesthesia is preferred because adequate ventilation is maintained while working in the mouth, and the head can be manipulated without interference with the airway.

Supplemental Readings

Baker, G. J.: Some aspects of equine dental disease. Eq. Vet. J., 2:105, 1970.

Baker, G. J.: Some aspects of equine dental radiology. Eq. Vet. J., 3:46, 1971.

Baker, G. J.: Surgery of the head and neck. In Catcott, E. J., and Smithcors, F. J. (eds.): Equine Medicine and Surgery, 2nd ed. Wheaton, IL, American Veterinary Publications, 1972, pp. 752–779.

Baker, G. J.: Some aspects of equine dental decay. Eq. Vet. J., 6:127, 1974.

Beeman, G. M.: Equine dentistry. Proc. 8th Annu. Conv. Am. Assoc. Eq. Pract., pp. 235–240, 1962.

Frank, E. R.: Affections of the teeth. In Frank, E. R. (ed.): Veterinary Surgery, revised ed. Minneapolis, Burgess Pub. Co., 1973, pp. 131–140.

Hofmeyr, C. F. B.: The digestive system. In Oehme, F. W., and Prier, J. E. (eds.): Textbook of Large Animal Surgery. Baltimore, Williams & Wilkins Co., 1974, pp. 364–382.

Clair, L. E.: Equine digestive system. In Getty, R. (ed.): Sisson & Grossman's Anatomy of the Domestic Animals, Vol. 1, 5th ed. Philadelphia, W. B. Saunders Company, 1975, pp. 460–470.

Vail, C. D.: Tips on equine dentistry. Lincoln, NB, Norden Laboratories, Norden News, 55(22):15, 1980.

Esophageal Disease

John A. Stick, EAST LANSING, MICHIGAN

Esophageal abnomalities in the horse include obstruction, or "choke," stricture, rupture, diverticulum, fistula, cyst, megaesophagus, and neoplasia. Of these, obstruction is the most common disorder with stricture formation as a possible sequela. This chapter discusses the diagnosis and medical management of these two common diseases of the equine esophagus. Readings pertaining to the surgical treatment of esophageal disorders may be found at the end of this chapter.

Clinical evaluation of the horse with esophageal disease may be completed with physical and radiographic examinations. Occasionally esophagoscopy may be necessary to recognize some disorders or to clarify the extent of some injuries of the esophagus, but clinical features and physical and radiographic techniques will permit identification of common disorders so that medical management may be instituted.

CLINICAL MANIFESTATIONS

Obstructive esophageal disease in the horse presents with regurgitation of food, water, and saliva through the mouth and nostrils, coughing, dysphagia, and excessive salivation. Attempts to eat are often followed by painful swallowing indicated by repeated extension of the head and neck, distress, and agitation. These signs may mimic those of abdominal pain. The time interval from swallowing until these signs are shown by the horse depends on the location of the obstruction within the esophagus. Retching and discomfort may occur 8 to 10 seconds after swallowing when the obstruction is in the lower esophagus, but when a cervical obstruction is present signs may occur immediately. Intermittent signs of choke followed by periods of relief may indicate a disease other than simple feed impaction, and further diagnostic procedures are warranted. Anorexia, electrolyte imbalances, and dehydration accompany cases of long duration. Aspiration pneumonia frequently follows esophageal obstruction and signs may be present as early as one day after the onset of choke.

PHYSICAL EXAMINATION

A thorough oral examination should be performed to rule out oral foreign body, dental disease, cleft palate, and oropharangeal neoplasms from the differential diagnosis. Observation and palpation of the neck in the area of the jugular furrows may reveal an enlargement in the cervical esophagus. Simple food impaction of the cervical esophagus may be localized in this manner. Crepitation or a diffuse firm enlargement may indicate a loss of integrity of the esophagus. Nasogastric tube passage often confirms luminal obstruction and localizes the site of involvement. Gentle lavage of warm water through the tube may permit material to be flushed free of the obstruction if feed or consumption of bedding is the cause of the problem. At this time, sedation of the animal with xylazine* (1.1 mg per kg intravenously) will lower the head and prevent further aspiration. Lavage may be continued until the obstruction is relieved and further diagnostic studies may be unnecessary. However, reobstruction is an indication that another esophageal disease may be present and a diagnosis should be pursued.

When esophageal disease has been present, auscultation and radiography of the thorax is indicated to monitor the development of aspiration pneumonia. This complication is common and should be treated when the primary problem is encountered.

RADIOGRAPHY OF THE ESOPHAGUS

Cervical esophagography in the adult horse is diagnostic in most instances and should be considered as part of the complete esophageal examination if reobstruction occurs. The thoracic and abdominal parts of the esophagus may also be successfully radiographed in foals. A survey film may establish the presence of feed impaction or foreign body. Frequently an area of dilatation will extend from the distal point of the obstruction to the upper esophageal sphincter after impaction of the esophagus has been relieved. Dilatation will present as air contrast in the esophagus, occasionally with a fluid line in the dilatation, and will serve to localize the lesion.

Barium paste† (120 ml) given by mouth will outline the longitudinal mucosal folds of the esophagus with the lumen undistended and will permit identification of the location of the obstruction or any disruption of the lumen. Feed will become coated with the barium, a complete obstruction will stop the barium at the site of the lesion, and rupture of the esophagus will permit barium to escape into the surrounding soft tissues. Sedation of the patient should be avoided if possible during this procedure because it suppresses the swallowing reflex and barium will be held in the mouth, reducing the amount available to coat the esophagus.

Liquid barium* (480 ml) administered under pressure by a dose syringe through a cuffed nasogastric tube to prevent reflux into the pharynx will demonstrate strictures and associated prestenotic dilatation of the esophagus. Liquid barium (480 ml) followed by air (480 ml) delivered by dose syringe under pressure provides a double-contrast study, permitting examination of mucosal folds with the esophagus distended. This latter technique gives the best definition of mucosal lesions such as circumferential mucosal ulcers following feed impaction. Although a diagnosis can often be made without using all three techniques, each technique will demonstrate lesions not seen with the other two.

Swallowing during contrast studies when the lumen is being distended will produce false signs of esophageal stricture. Xylazine (1.1 mg per kg intravenously) given five minutes prior to the barium-under-pressure or double-contrast esophagogram will help eliminate a swallow artifact by decreasing the reflex "secondary swallows" that follow luminal distention.

ENDOSCOPY OF THE ESOPHAGUS

Esophagoscopy may better define the severity and extent of esophageal lesions diagnosed on radiography and can be used as an ancillary diagnostic aid. However, endoscopic examinations always should be performed when radiographic findings are not diagnostic. If the endoscope is 150 cm or longer, the entire esophagus may be examined, and esophageal lesions in the thorax of the adult horse undetected on radiographic examination may be diagnosed. A flexible endoscope that allows irrigation and insufflation is necessary to provide good observation of mucosal disease and changes in luminal size.

Endoscopic examination may be safely performed on the restrained standing animal in most instances. Diagnostic observations are best made by starting with the endoscope fully inserted and the esopha-

---

*Rompun, Haver-Lockhart, Shawnee, KS
†Solo-O-Pake, (85% w/v with water), E-Z-EM Co. Inc., Westbury, NY

---

*Solo-O-Pake, (72% w/v with water), E-Z-EM Co. Inc., Westbury, NY

geal lumen insufflated and then by slowly withdrawing the endoscope tip craniad (toward the head). After each swallow, the endoscope should be cleared by irrigation and the esophagus dilated prior to further withdrawal. Several passes should be made over any area of suspected disease.

Normal longitudinal mucosal folds of the esophagus are seen when the endoscope tip is moved craniad and the esophagus is in the relaxed position. Insufflation flattens these folds and permits observation of luminal size. Transverse folds can be iatrogenically produced by moving the endoscope tip caudad (toward the stomach). When the cervical esophagus is insufflated, the outline of the trachea can often be seen through the esophageal wall. Swallowing produces changes in the lumen that give the appearance of diverticula and strictures to the untrained observer. The mucosa should appear white to light pink in color, with reddened colorations being signs of mucosal disease.

The cranial aspect of the cervical esophageal sphincter is difficult to examine because repeated stimulation of the swallowing reflex and the larynx directs the endoscope tip dorsally. Radiographic assessment of this area may be more diagnostic. Additionally, the longitudinal mucosal folds found along the rest of the esophagus are absent in this area.

Frequently, the endoscopic appearance of an esophageal obstruction is obscured by saliva mixed with ingesta that collects cranial to it. This fluid should be removed by suction through a nasogastric tube and the endoscope should be immediately reinserted to observe the obstruction.

An inability to insufflate the esophagus and flatten the longitudinal mucosal folds usually indicates a disease process. This will be noted cranial and caudal to a stricture. Additionally, transverse mucosal folds, when not iatrogenic from endoscope manipulation, are pathognomonic for mural lesions.

MANAGEMENT OF IMPACTION

The most common type of obstructive esophageal disease is impaction of ingesta. Nasogastric tube passage and gentle warm water lavage under xylazine sedation is usually successful in relieving the obstruction. Several alternative techniques may be necessary if gentle lavage meets with failure. A cuffed nasogastric tube* may be placed, the animal sedated, and water lavaged under pressure with a dose syringe or stomach pump. The tube helps prevent reflux of ingesta into the pharynx while permitting pressure of the water to push the obstruction distally. External massage and to-and-fro movement of the water will resolve most impactions. If this technique is not successful, the animal should be muzzled to prevent food and water intake, left alone for 8 to 12 hours, and the treatment should be repeated. Frequently, the initial treatment softens the impaction and it will become dislodged by swallowing or is easily relieved by a second treatment.

Refractory cases or intractable horses may benefit from general anesthesia and water lavage under pressure. This method has the advantages of providing some esophageal muscular relaxation, lessens chances of aspiration because the horse's head may be inclined downward, and decreases the risk of esophageal perforation with the tube in an intractable horse. Gentle manipulation is mandatory with this technique to avoid rupture of the esophagus.

Impactions that do not respond to conservative therapy should be definitively identified by radiographic and endoscopic examination, and if amenable should be relieved by longitudinal esophagotomy. Surgery is preferable to repeated trauma of the esophagus with a nasogastric tube. The use of the nasogastric tube as a probang is not recommended. Cervical esophagotomy can be performed standing or under general anesthesia (see supplemental readings). Distal obstructions can be lavaged through the incision if necessary. Primary closure will be successful if a soft diet* is fed for 10 days beginning 48 hours after surgery. Hydration and electrolyte balance is maintained parenterally for the first 48 hours.

One aftermath of simple impaction is fusiform dilatation of the esophagus that predisposes to reobstruction. This condition will resolve in 24 to 48 hours provided the dilatation is kept free of ingesta. Food should be withheld or only small quantities of a soft diet fed for two days after an episode of choke to permit the lumen to return to a normal diameter. An electrolye solution† for drinking should be provided in addition to fresh water so that electrolyte abnormalities secondary to salivary loss may be corrected.

Broad-spectrum antimicrobial therapy is indicated for five to seven days because the risk of aspiration pneumonia is high after choke. I prefer procaine penicillin G‡ (22,000 IU/kg twice a day) and gentamicin sulfate§ (2.2 mg per kg three times

---

*Bivona Inc, Gary, IN (special order)

---

*The Andersons, Maumee, OH (pellets + warm water = mash)

†Eltrad 4000, Haver-Lockhart, Shawnee, KS (8 oz. in 12 L water)

‡Pfizer, New York, NY

§Gentocin, Schering Corp., Kenilworth, NJ

a day). If pneumonia is not the major limiting factor in this disease, simple obstruction has a favorable prognosis.

When an obstruction has been present for several days or is refractory to the initial treatment, a postobstruction examination using radiography or endoscopy or both is warranted. Circumferential mucosal ulceration is not uncommon in these cases and usually results in esophageal stricture.

MANAGEMENT OF STRICTURE

Esophageal stricture is usually an annular lesion that may be classified into three types depending on location of the cicatrix. In order of decreasing prognosis for life, they are: type 1, esophageal rings or webs that involve only the mucosal and submucosal layers; type 2, mural lesions that involve only the muscularis; and type 3, annular stenosis that involves all layers of the esophageal wall.

The most common cause of mucosal strictures (type 1) are mucosal erosions secondary to long-standing impactions. Mucosal erosions usually cause the esophageal lumen to narrow and form a stricture by 15 to 30 days after injury. Episodes of choke will occur despite the type of feed used. However, if a soft diet is continually fed, the esophageal lumen will enlarge to normal diameter between 30 and 45 days after injury. Early recognition and management of this condition is mandatory for success. Prognosis for early cases is favorable; however, long-standing cases increase chances of refractory pneumonia and lack of client cooperation. Clients should be made aware that several episodes of choke may occur up to 40 days after injury, even when the soft diet is given. Because the diameter of the esophageal lumen may continue to enlarge up to 60 days after injury, surgical intervention should be delayed at least that long.

Mucosal strictures (type 1) that do not respond to the bougienage of eating a soft diet, and strictures of the entire esophageal wall (type 3), have been successfully managed by resection and anastomosis. Strictures that involve only the muscularis (type 2) may respond best to myotomy. Postoperatively, the former procedure is best followed by nasogastric tube-feeding while postmyotomy oral alimentation with a soft diet will suffice.

Esophageal obstruction should be treated as an emergency because early correction avoids the complication of mucosal erosion and subsequent stricture. Because the practitioner's success may depend in part on how much feed has been ingested and packed into the obstruction, clients should be advised to remove bedding, water, and food because many horses will continue to eat while choked. An attempt to ascertain the cause of obstruction may prevent recurrence and complications. Slowing of eating by placing rocks in the manger, regular dental care, and prophylactic therapy for bot fly larvae* may be indicated.

---

*Combot, Haver-Lockhart, Shawnee, KS

Supplemental Readings

Derksen, F. J., and Stick, J. A.: Resection and anastamosis of esophageal stricture in a foal. Equine Pract., 5:17, 1983.

Stick, J. A.: Surgery of the esophagus. Vet. Clin. North Am. (Large Anim. Pract.), 4:33, 1982.

Stick, J. A., Slocombe, R. F., Derksen, F. J., and Scott, E. A.: Esophagotomy in the pony; Comparison of surgical techniques and form of feed. Am. J. Vet. Res., 44:2123, 1983.

Todhunter, R. J., Stick, J. A., Trotter, G. W., and Boles, C.: Medical management of esophageal stricture in seven horses. J. Am. Vet. Med. Assoc., 185:784, 1984.

Epizootiology, Risk Factors, and Prognostic Factors in Colic

Nathaniel A. White, II, LEESBURG, VIRGINIA

Determining the incidence of a disease, the associated risk factors, or the specific etiology is difficult in the equine population because of the lack of a census or means to follow individual or herd problems for a prolonged period. Although most attempts at developing risk factors for equine colic have been completed at universities, individual investigators in certain practices have reported information on types of diseases, mortality, and geographic peculiarities.

Examining acute abdominal disease retrospectively for evidence of risk factors is also difficult because a majority of the patients are treated only one time. Often the record of the associated factors or the potential for a herd problem is insubstantial or nonexistent. Studies of colic have involved indi-

TABLE 1. FREQUENCY OF DISEASES CAUSING SIGNS OF COLIC

Type of Disease	% Total	Mortality (%)
Simple obstruction (includes tympany)	37.5	25.6
Strangulation obstruction	18.4	79.9
Nonstrangulating infarction	3.5	85.8
Peritonitis	4.4	81.4
Enteritis	4.7	57.1
Colic (no definitive diagnosis)	25.4	7.1

From 2385 cases of colic in the United States.

vidual cases presented to universities or practices over a period of time with the limits of small numbers of horses.

INCIDENCE OF COLIC

Twelve universities in the United States and two universities in England* are part of an ongoing retrospective study to generate three sets of data: (1) risk factors, (2) rates of diseases, and (3) prognostic clinical and laboratory findings from animals examined between 1979 and 1984. The goal of the study is to provide information that will help the practitioner decide on a therapy and predict the outcome in a case of equine colic. As of this writing, records have been examined from 2385 cases of colic in 12 university hospitals in the United States. The comparative information reported in this chapter comes from this study, two previous university studies, and one study from a practice in Germany.

Specific diseases have been assigned to one of six categories: simple obstruction, strangulation obstruction, nonstrangulating infarction, peritonitis, enteritis, and colic with no definitive diagnosis. The frequencies of each of the six types of disease are presented in Table 1. The small intestine and large colon were the segments of intestine involved most often in an acute abdominal problem (Table 2).

Colic caused by body systems other than the gastrointestinal tract and infections such as abdominal abscesses and primary peritonitis made up 7.8 per cent of the cases. The largest group listed as "unknown" in Table 2 included mild colic episodes or unconfirmed cases of colic in which the specific site of origin of pain could not be identified. It is perhaps surprising that no specific diagnosis was obtained in a large percentage of horses with colic examined at universities. Many diagnoses, which

were termed verminous arteritis or spasmodic colic, were based on signs rather than any confirmatory test or surgery that would indicate a definitive lesion. Although many patients respond to minimal symptomatic therapy, horses in this group had the least-understood type of abdominal disease.

The frequency of specific diseases causing colic is as follows. In the United States, large colon impactions make up 7.3 per cent, while large colon torsions and displacements combined represented 10.6 per cent of cases of colic. This is in agreement with other studies that indicate that most colic problems arise from the large colon. Of small intestinal diseases reported in the United States, small intestinal volvulus made up the greatest number with 4.3 per cent. This finding differs from a study in Germany in which ileal impaction was the commonest small intestinal disease.

The mortality in horses with acute abdominal disease treated in University hospitals was 39.6 per cent, greater than in a previous study by Tennant et al., which included cases of colic treated on the farm and in the hospital. Survival differs with the type of lesion (Table 3). Mortality was 25.6 per cent with obstruction, 79.9 per cent with strangulation obstruction, 85.8 per cent with nonstrangulating infarction, and 57.1 per cent with enteritis. The mortality rate was 7.1 per cent for cases diagnosed simply as "colic," which included unconfirmed cases of spasmodic colic, verminous arteritis, and indigestion. The mortality in some horses, particularly those requiring extensive treatment, may be influenced by the economic constraints that limit treatment.

Surgical mortality was a good predictor of survival in diseases requiring surgery. Mortality was predictably high (52.2 per cent) because horses with strangulating bowel lesions frequently die. The most common strangulating lesions were the large colon torsion and the small intestinal volvulus with surgical mortalities of 72.9 per cent and 80 per cent, respectively. Previous studies listed in Table 3 represent data from one locale. Survival differences may be due to differences in the speed of recognition of the disease and the time in different studies before hospital admission for surgery. The lower

United States: University of California, Colorado State University, Cornell University, University of Florida, University of Georgia, Kansas State University, Louisiana State University, Michigan State University, Ohio State University, Purdue University, Texas A & M University, Washington State University. *England*: Cambridge University, University of Liverpool.

TABLE 2. LOCATION OF LESION IN COLIC

Intestinal Segment	% Total	Mortality (%)
Stomach	2.3	73.7
Small intestines	19.0	70.2
Cecum	3.6	54.1
Large colon	25.4	40.2
Small colon	4.2	35.3
Rectum	0.8	81.0
Unknown	37.1	13.7

From 2385 cases of colic in the United States.

TABLE 3. MORTALITY IN DISEASES CAUSING SIGNS OF COLIC

Disease	Author	Year	Mortality of All Cases	Mortality of Surgical Cases
Small intestinal volvulus	Huskamp	1982	71.0%*	—
	BCRP	1985	85.9%	80.0%
Small intestine incarcerated in a mesenteric tear	Huskamp	1982	63.1%*	—
	BCRP	1985	83.4%	77.0%
Small intestine incarcerated in the epiploic foramen	Huskamp	1982	51.6%	40.8%
	Turner	1984	87.5%	83.8%
	BCRP	1985	96.0%	95.3%
Small intestine incarcerated in an inguinal hernia	Schneider	1982	25.9%	25.0%
	BCRP	1985	70.0%	62.6%
Ileal impaction	Huskamp	1982	16.8%	13.7%
	BCRP	1985	48.3%	42.9%
Cecal impaction	Huskamp	1982	66.6%	—
	Campbell	1984	66.6%	36.4%
	BCRP	1985	45.5%	74.0%
Large colon torsion	Huskamp	1982	57.8%	47.3%
	BCRP	1985	80.4%	72.9%
Large colon displacement	Huskamp	1982	3.5%	2.2%
	Hackett	1983	22.0%	—
	BCRP	1985	23.1%	19.5%
Enteroliths	Blue	1979	53.0%	—
	Huskamp	1982	0%	34.3%
	BCRP	1985	44.5%	—
Thromboembolic	White	1981	94.5%*	—
	BCRP	1985	85.8%	—

*All surgical cases
†Includes large colon cecum combined torsions
BCRP = Bolshoi colic research program (Univ. of Georgia)

mortality reported by Huskamp can be attributed to rapid referral of horses to surgery.

RISK FACTORS IN COLIC

Risk factors for the horse with acute abdominal disease include age, sex, and breed. Unfortunately, only two studies have compared the age, sex, or breed incidence to the base population of horses admitted to the respective university hospitals. Foals obviously have the greatest risk for meconium impaction with male foals being most commonly afflicted. Older horses have a greater susceptibility to incarcerations in the epiploic foramen, strangulating lipomas, and large colon torsions. The Standardbred, as compared to other breeds, has a higher incidence of inguinal hernia. Paint foals are predisposed to inherited colon hypoplasia, aplasia, or intestinal aganglionosis, and the paint breed appears to have a higher incidence of ileal impaction. Shetland ponies have a high incidence of small colon obstructions. Thoroughbreds appear to be at greater risk of having small intestinal incarcerations in the epiploic foramen. Mares are more susceptible to

gastrosplenic mesentery entrapment of bowel, abdominal abscess, and adhesions. The cause of these age and breed susceptibilities is unknown.

Geographic incidence of disease appears uniform except for a greater number of large colon problems in western United States and in Florida, and a greater percentage of small intestinal diseases in the eastern United States. There is a high incidence of ileal impactions and anterior enteritis (duodenitis and proximal jejunitis) in the South. Enteroliths are common in California, Florida, and Indiana. Ileal impactions and anterior enteritis are both reported from Germany, but neither have been observed at the universities in the United States or in England. There are obvious feed, seasonal, and habitat differences between these areas but none have been incriminated in the shift of emphasis from one intestinal segment to another.

Weather has also been incriminated anecdotally as a cause of colic in horses. In a recent three-year study of colic cases encountered in an ambulatory practice, daily barometric pressure, change in daily barometric pressure, daily temperature, and change in daily temperature were not associated with the frequency of colic. The etiology of colic was undiagnosed in most horses in this study.

TABLE 4. CLINICAL VALUES WITH
SIGNIFICANT DIFFERENCES
BETWEEN SURVIVORS AND NON-SURVIVORS

Diagnosis	Clinical Value		Mean of Value	Significance
Enteroliths	Temp‡	Surv*	100.6 °F	p<.05
		Nonsurv†	101.3°F	
	PeriTP‖	Surv	3.0 gm/dl	p<.025
		Nonsurv	4.2 gm/dl	
	Heart rate	Surv	67.6 BPM	p<.01
		Nonsurv	84.6 BPM	
Small Colon Obstruction	TP**	Surv	7.4 gm/dl	p<.05
		Nonsurv	6.9 gm/dl	
Large Colon Obstruction	PeriTP	Surv	2.7 gm/dl	p<.001
		Nonsurv	3.3 gm/dl	
	PCV§	Surv	38.1%	p<.001
		Nonsurv	44.5%	
	Heart rate	Surv	55.4 BPM	p<.001
		Nonsurv	73.7 BPM	
Cecal Impaction	Temp	Surv	99.7 °F	p<.001
		Nonsurv‡	101.6 °F	
	WBC‡‡	Surv	10199 /μl	p<.05
		Nonsurv	7715 /μl	
	Heart rate	Surv	50.00 BPM	p<.05
		Nonsurv	65.6 BPM	
Ileal Impaction	Temp	Surv	101.0 °F	p<.05
		Nonsurv	99.9 °F	
Large Colon Nephrosplenic Entrapment	PeriWBC	Surv	23638 /μl	p<.05
		Nonsurv	32351 /μl	
	Heart rate	Surv	60.5 BPM	p<.01
		Nonsurv	82.8 BPM	
Small Int. Volvulus	PeriTP	Surv	3.2 gm/dl	p<.05
		Nonsurv	4.5 gm/dl	
Large Colon Torsion	PeriTP	Surv	2.3 gm/dl	p<.05
		Nonsurv	3.2 gm/dl	
	PCV	Surv	39.5%	p<.05
		Nonsurv	49.6%	
Sand Colic	PCV	Surv	37.7%	p<.001
		Nonsurv	48.5%	
	TP	Surv	7.2 g/dl	p<.025
		Nonsurv	8.1 g/dl	
	Heart rate	Surv	51.2 BPM	p<.001
		Nonsurv	85.5 BPM	

*Survivor.
†Nonsurvivor.
‡Rectal temperature.
§Hematocrit.
‖Peritoneal fluid total proteins.
**Total plasma protein.
‡‡White blood-cell count.

PROGNOSIS

Determining the prognosis in a case of acute abdominal disease is difficult yet important to treatment and decision making by both veterinarian and horseowner. Blood lactate levels greater than 75 mg per dl are correlated with a high mortality. A blood anion gap greater than 25 mEq per L is also associated with high mortality.

$$\text{Anion gap} = (Na^+) + (K^+) - (Cl^-) - (HCO_3^-).$$

Clinical parameters are less valuable in providing a prognosis. If the definitive diagnosis is known, the outcome can be predicted (Table 3), but predictions must be adjusted according to the duration of colic and the speed of therapy. If a horse has signs indicating that abdominal surgery is required, the prognosis is worse than in a horse that does not require surgery. When considering horses with colic as a single group, systolic blood pressure lower than 60 mm Hg is associated with a mortality of 92 to 95 per cent. Heart rates of 40, 80, 100, and 120 beats per minute predict mortalities of 10 per cent, 50 per cent, 75 per cent, and 90 per cent, respectively. The hematocrit is also a predictor of survival; values of 30 per cent, 45 per cent, 60 per cent, and 65 per cent are associated with 7 per cent, 36 per cent, 80 per cent, and 90 per cent mortality.

When individual diseases are examined, different clinical parameters predict survival in different diseases. Heart rate, hematocrit, total serum protein, white blood cell count, peritoneal fluid total protein, and peritoneal white blood cell count were examined. These parameters did not predict survival in horses with ileal impaction or anterior enteritis. Several of the parameters were significantly different between survivors and nonsurvivors for specific diseases (Table 4). The heart rate and peritoneal total protein indicated survival more often than other values. These predictors are at a 95 per cent confidence level, meaning there is still at least a 5 per cent chance for error. Although reasons for the differences between diseases are unknown, these results emphasize the unreliability of measurements such as heart rate if used for all colic cases.

Recently, intraluminal pressure in obstructed small intestine has been correlated with mortality. Pressures above 10 cm of water (mean 15 cm of water) were associated with fatal lesions whereas pressures below this level (mean 6.0 cm of water) occurred in horses that survived.

These prognostic tools can be misleading, particularly when surgery is involved. A horse with a relatively low heart rate, low hematocrit, and normal peritoneal fluid may have a good chance of survival, but only if surgery is performed during this stage of the disease. If disease is allowed to progress until heart rate, hematocrit and peritoneal fluid protein, and white cell counts are elevated, the advantage is lost and the chance of survival is much less. The decision for surgery therefore is better made on the severity and recurrence of pain, and on the rectal examination. It has become apparent that horses with strangulating disease have a high mortality if surgery is not completed in four to six hours. Efforts at reducing the time for decision making will be the greatest means of increasing survival until more can be learned about the prevention of acute abdominal disease in the horse.

Supplemental Readings

Huskamp, B.: The diagnosis and treatment of acute abdominal conditions in the horse; the various types and frequency as seen at the animal hospital in Hochmoor. Proc. Equine Colic Res. Symp., University of Georgia, 1982; pp. 261.

Parry, B. W., Anderson, G. A., and Gay, C. C.: Prognosis in equine colic: A study of individual variables used in case assessments. Equine Vet. J., 15:337, 1983.

Sembrat, R. F.: The acute abdomen in the horse—epidemiologic considerations. J. Am. Coll. Vet. Surgeons, 4:34, 1975.

Tennant, B., Wheat, J. D., and Meagher, D. M.: Observations on the causes and incidence of the acute intestinal obstruction in a horse. Proc. 18th Ann. Conv. Am. Assoc. Eq. Pract., 1972, pp. 251.

Physical Examination of the Horse with Colic

James L. Becht, ATHENS, GEORGIA

Practitioners must often examine and assess the horse exhibiting signs of acute abdominal pain. Because this represents an emergency situation, the examination should be rapid, complete, and performed in a logical, organized manner. By examining every horse with acute abdominal pain in the same fashion, omission of important diagnostic and prognostic data is minimized. The veterinarian's responsibility is to provide the owner with answers to two questions: (1) Will this horse respond to conservative, on-the-farm (medical) therapy, or does the patient require referral for intensive therapy and/or surgical intervention? (2) What is the animal's prognosis? These questions can only be answered after examination of the patient's abdomen and an assessment of the level of systemic toxemia. Examination should determine the site and nature of the lesion causing pain. An attempt should be made to differentiate simple obstruction, strangulating obstruction, nonobstructive infarction, peritonitis, and enteritis.

MANAGEMENT AND MEDICAL HISTORY

Before the physical examination is started, or during its early stages, a history should be obtained. Because parasites are incriminated as the leading cause of colic, several questions should be raised about the anthelmintic schedule, products used, pasture rotation schedule, and animal density in paddocks or pastures. Repeated administration of ivermectin at eight-week intervals makes migratory damage by *Strongylus vulgaris* an unlikely cause of colic, whereas recent treatment of a poorly managed weanling with an organophosphate anthelmintic should alert the clinician to the possibility of *Parascaris equorum* impaction. The owner should be questioned about the occurrence and severity of previous colic episodes exhibited by the patient. Verminous arteritis, enterolithiasis, abdominal abscessation, muscular hypertrophy of the ileum, cholelithiasis and abdominal adhesions from previous surgery should be considered if episodes of abdominal pain have recurred.

The duration of the present painful episode should be established and considered when evaluating the degree of systemic toxemia. A horse that has exhibited pain for several hours but has obvious cardiovascular deterioration probably needs surgery; the prognosis for survival is rather poor.

Therapy administered by the owner is important, as analgesic agents may alter physical or laboratory parameters used to determine the nature of the lesion and prognosis for patient survival. Flunixin meglumine masks the early cardiovascular deterioration associated with endotoxemia and may delay intensive therapy or referral. Flunixin, like other nonsteroidal anti-inflammatory agents, exerts an antipyretic action that may mask the fever of a horse with enteritis or other systemic infection. Xylazine and acepromazine produce sedation that may be misinterpreted as depression; xylazine causes bradycardia that may alter the interpretation of the heart rate during the examination. Acepromazine also causes vasodilation and anemia and therefore may alter capillary refill time, mucous membrane color, pulse strength and heart rate.

INSPECTION OF THE PATIENT

Before the horse is handled, it is worthwhile to observe the patient in the stall or paddock or while being led by the owner. This brief inspection can provide valuable information pertaining to the type and severity of pain, mental status, and abdominal distention.

Visceral abdominal pain, evident in most horses with intestinal lesions, is manifested by restlessness, frequent movements, and attempts to roll. External pressure over the abdomen does not increase the animal's discomfort. Parietal peritoneal pain associated with peritonitis is reflected by a rather immobile animal that guards the abdomen. External pressure to the abdomen incites obvious discomfort in this patient. In the horse with advanced colic, both types of pain may be present as secondary peritonitis develops following intestinal devitalization. Generally, the more severe the visceral abdominal pain, the more likely the need for surgery, and the poorer the prognosis. A sudden disappearance of pain may result from spontaneous correction of the problem but unfortunately, in a horse with severe toxemia, it suggests gastric or intestinal rupture. Lesions that result in strangulating obstruction tend to cause constant, severe pain with rapid (several hours) development of systemic toxemia and cardiovascular deterioration. In contrast, pain that is mild to moderate and intermittent suggests simple obstruction, most often involving the large colon or cecum.

Because many horses require analgesic therapy to enable a thorough physical examination, the response to various analgesics must be considered. Pain that ceases following the administration of dipyrone is usually less serious than that which persists following administration of flunixin meglumine or xylazine. With the extensive use of potent analgesics, the decision to refer an animal must often be on physical and laboratory findings rather than the severity or persistence of pain. Successful control of pain does nothing to correct the underlying lesion. Repeated use of analgesics can mask pain in horses requiring the surgical intervention and therefore significantly worsen the prognosis for survival.

Depressed mental status is an important indicator of an infectious process such as enteritis, peritonitis, or pleuritis, or advanced systemic toxemia and cardiovascular deterioration associated with intestinal infarction. Horses exhibiting little or no depression tend to survive, whereas horses with severe depression have a poor survival rate, irrespective of the cause of colic. Infection is usually the cause of colic in depressed horses with good cardiovascular function.

Abdominal distention, or fullness in the paracostal and paralumbar regions, suggests the cecum and/or large colon as the site of the lesion. In the adult, small intestinal distention usually results in increased transdiaphragmatic pressure causing an increased respiratory rate, rather than abdominal distention. Acute diffuse peritonitis associated with gastric or intestinal rupture also causes obvious abdominal distention within several hours.

PHYSICAL EXAMINATION

System toxemia and cardiovascular deterioration are evaluated using body temperature, heart rate, respiratory rate, peripheral pulse strength, capillary refill time, mucous membrane color, and laboratory findings such as packed cell volume (PCV), total plasma protein (TPP), acid-base status, and possibly coagulation studies.

Rectal temperature can be increased by an elevated ambient temperature, excitement, muscular exertion, or an infectious process. Generally, a fever greater than 39.5° C suggests a primary infectious process such as enteritis, peritonitis, or pleuritis, rather than an intestinal accident. In retrospective studies, rectal temperature does not significantly differ between medical or surgical colic cases, nor does it differentiate survivors from nonsurvivors.

Heart or pulse rate varies widely in healthy horses due to variations in vagal tone and muscular fitness. In the colic patient, tachycardia results from anxiety, pain, and hypovolemia. Horses requiring surgical intervention have significantly higher heart rates than horses not requiring surgery. Likewise, nonsurvivors have significantly higher heart rates than survivors. On the basis of recent surveys, heart rates of horses that survive or respond to medical therapy are approximately 60 beats per min, those of horses requiring surgery approximate 80, and those of nonsurvivors exceed 100 beats/per min. Occasionally, however, horses with severe systemic toxemia or intestinal rupture have heart rates only slightly above normal (60 to 80 beats per min). In general, however, a drastic increase in heart rate indicates the need for surgery, but the prognosis is poor. However, the reverse is not always true, as a slightly increased heart rate does not necessarily indicate that the horse will respond to medical therapy or survive. As with other parameters, trends in the heart rate have more diagnostic and prognostic value than a single determination.

Conditions that result in an increased respiratory rate include metabolic acidosis, pain, respiratory infection, and increased pressure on the diaphragm from intestinal distention. Auscultation of the thorax while inducing deep breaths with a rebreathing bag, thoracic percussion, and assessment of acid-base status should identify the cause of the increased respiratory rate in the colic patient.

Peripheral pulse strength from palpation of the facial artery gives a reflection of cardiovascular function and tissue perfusion. Arterial pulse amplitude varies directly with systolic blood pressure, which is the most accurate prognostic indicator in colic patients. Generally, horses that survive have a normal pulse amplitude, whereas horses that do not survive have a weak or undetectable arterial pulse. Strength of arterial pulse does not differentiate horses requiring medical or surgical treatment.

Oral mucous membrane color reflects the quantity and quality of the circulating blood. Normal pale pink membranes can become bright red due to the vasodilation that occurs early in endotoxic shock. Later in endotoxic shock, vasoconstriction results in dark red, blue, "muddy," or perhaps more pale mucous membranes as blood is shunted to vital organs.

Capillary refill time is a means of assessing the status of peripheral tissue perfusion by providing information on the degree of hydration and vascular tone. By blanching the oral mucous membrane, the capillary refill time is determined by measuring the time for reperfusion to occur. A delayed capillary refill time (> 2 seconds) suggests decreased tissue perfusion most likely from hypovolemia. There is no significant difference in capillary refill time between medical and surgical colic cases, but nonsurvivors have significantly longer refill times than survivors.

LABORATORY EVALUATION

Packed cell volume and TPP values have diagnostic and prognostic significance and supply information on the magnitude of fluid needs. Packed cell volume alone is unreliable because of the wide range of normal values (30 to 45 per cent), which can be readily increased by splenic contraction. Horses requiring surgery generally have a higher PCV than horses responding to medical therapy. Similarly nonsurvivors have a higher PCV (approximately 55 per cent) than survivors (approximately 42 per cent). Although total plasma protein tends to be higher in horses requiring surgery, differentiation between nonsurvivors and survivors is difficult using this parameter. Horses with acute peritonitis, pleuritis, or enteritis tend to have subnormal TPP due to sequestration of protein in the affected body cavity or loss into the intestinal tract.

Blood gas analysis, serum electrolyte determinations, complete blood count, and coagulation studies can add valuable information, but their lack of availability to the practitioner limits their use.

EXAMINATION OF THE ABDOMEN

Diagnostic techniques used to assess the abdomen include auscultation, passage of a nasogastric tube, rectal examination and abdominocentesis.

Auscultation. Auscultation of the abdomen must be performed with patience. Correct interpretation of findings demands a basic understanding of intestinal motility patterns. Stomach or small intestinal contractions are not often detected during auscultation. Contractions of the cecum and large colon can be divided into mixing contractions between adjacent haustra and propulsive contractions. Mixing contractions are rather weak and last less than five seconds, whereas propulsive contractions last 10 to 20 seconds and are easily detected during auscultation. At any one site, mixing contractions occur in a series of approximately 10 contractions every three to five minutes. Propulsive contractions occur once every two to three minutes, but the recurrence is greatly affected by reflexes from other intestinal segments, intestinal irritation, or decreased blood perfusion. Generally, intestinal irritation and hypoperfusion result in decreased motility. Similarly, a factor causing decreased contractions in one area will adversely affect contractile activity in other areas. Luminal obstruction without decreased perfusion (simple obstruction) results in increased contractile activity in an attempt to move the obstruction more distally. Thus, normal contractile sounds suggest a mild, noninfarctive lesion as a cause of colic; increased contractile activity suggests a simple obstruction, most likely an impaction, and little or no contractile activity suggests intestinal irritation from an infectious process (enteritis, peritonitis) or hypoperfusion from a strangulating lesion. Auscultation of a horse with ileus associated with enterocolitis usually reveals high-pitched fluid sounds of short duration. In summary, horses that respond to medical therapy tend to have normal or increased intestinal sounds, whereas horses requiring surgery tend to have decreased sounds.

Nasogastric Intubation. Passage of a nasogastric tube should be performed on all horses with colic. A well-lubricated, large-diameter tube that fills the ventral meatus and has several holes in the gastric end is preferable. Following placement of the tube, negative pressure should be applied with a dose syringe, or a siphon should be established by filling the tube with water using a stomach pump. This practice should be repeated until gastric fluid is obtained or the veterinarian becomes confident that the stomach does not contain much fluid. Generally, the greater the volume of gastric reflux, the more proximal the lesion. Fluid containing feed material suggests gastric dilatation or stasis as the cause of colic. Yellow-green fluid reflects bile reflux originating distal to the common bile–pancreatic duct. Brown or reddish fluid indicates mucosal damage with hemorrhage and suggests small intestinal strangulation or hemorrhagic gastroenteritis. If fluid is obtained on several occasions, the stomach tube should, if possible, be left in place. Repeated reflux of fluid suggests small intestinal strangulation or duodenojejunitis (anterior enteritis). There is no correlation between the amount of fluid obtained and the need for medical or surgical management, but generally the greater the volume of gastric reflux, the greater the dehydration and the poorer the prognosis for survival.

Rectal Examination. Rectal examination is the single most important diagnostic technique in evaluating the abdomen of the equine colic patient. When performed correctly, the procedure demands adequate restraint of the patient, safety for the veterinarian, liberal lubrication of the examiner's arm and a sound knowledge of abdominal anatomy. The procedure should always be performed in the same fashion to minimize misinterpretation of findings. A complete description of rectal examination and findings is on page 23. Findings on rectal examination should be evaluated in light of other findings, but often the decision for referral or surgical intervention is based solely on this parameter. Early in the disease syndrome, systemic toxemia and cardiovascular deterioration may not yet be evident; therefore, accurate interpretation of rectal examination findings is important for the proper diagnosis and management of the colic case.

Abdominocentesis. Abdominocentesis is a valuable, simple technique that can be performed with minimal equipment. Although laboratory facilities to perform cytologic evaluation, measure protein content, and count nucleated cells are not usually available, assessment of color and transparency yields adequate information to make the technique worthwhile. A small area on the midline at the lowest point of the abdomen should be clipped and surgically prepared. Using a gloved hand, an 18-gauge, 1½ inch hypodermic needle is advanced approximately an inch through the skin into the peritoneal cavity. The needle is turned and gently maneuvered until peritoneal fluid is obtained. If this attempt is unsuccessful or results in hemorrhage or flow of intestinal fluid, the needle should be removed and another needle used in a different area. An alternative method involves local anesthesia of the skin and a small stab incision through the skin using a scalpel blade. A 2½- to 4-inch teat cannula is placed in the skin incision and advanced into the peritoneal cavity. The incidence of complications with either technique is extremely low.

Peritoneal fluid collected into a tube can be examined for color and transparency. Normal peritoneal fluid is clear or yellow and transparent or slightly turbid. As intestinal devitalization occurs, erythrocytes and protein are lost into the peritoneal fluid causing a reddish discoloration with increased turbidity. With advanced intestinal necrosis, the fluid becomes darkened and may be dark red to brown. Gastric or intestinal rupture results in fecal peritonitis, which is evidenced by flakes of ingesta in the peritoneal fluid. Unfortunately, when obvious changes occur in the peritoneal fluid, advanced intestinal disease is present in the abdomen. Therefore, if the veterinarian waits until the peritoneal fluid reflects intestinal necrosis before referring the horse for further evaluation and surgery, the prognosis for survival is poor.

During abdominocentesis, peritoneal fluid may be contaminated by peripheral blood from a vessel in the body wall. Very thick blood suggests puncture of the spleen. If a ruptured viscus is expected, abdominocentesis should be repeated several times if it yields ingesta.

Physical examination of the horse exhibiting acute abdominal pain is one of the most challenging tasks facing the equine practitioner. A thorough, organized approach and a logical assimilation of findings ensures that the patient will receive proper management. It is wiser to err and refer the horse for further evaluation unnecessarily rather than to refer the horse when the prognosis for survival is diminished!

Supplemental Readings

Adams, S. B., and McIlwraith, C. W.: Abdominal crisis in the horse: a comparison of presurgical evaluation with surgical findings and results. Vet. Surg., 7:63, 1978.

Parry, B. W., Gay, C. C., and Anderson, G. A.: Assessment of the necessity for surgical intervention in cases of equine colic: A retrospective study. Equine Vet. J., 15:216, 1983.

Parry, B. W., Anderson, G. A., and Gay, C. C.: Prognosis in equine colic: a study of individual variables used in case assessment. Equine Vet. J., 15:337, 1983.

Stashak, T. S.: Clinical evaluation of the equine colic patient. Vet. Clin. North Am. (Large Anim. Pract.), 1:275, 1979.

Rectal Examination of the Colic Patient

Norbert Kopf, VIENNA, AUSTRIA

Rectal examination is essential in each case of colic. Findings should always be considered in light of the results of physical examination, nasogastric intubation, abdominocentesis, and laboratory data. Rectal exploration always should be performed before paracentesis in order to recognize extremely enlarged portions of bowel and to prevent an accidental penetration of distended loops of intestine. To determine the type of intestinal obstruction, internal palpation is the most useful technique. Palpation findings usually give an indication of the need for surgical intervention or conservative treatment. The value of rectal examination depends on the experience of the examiner and cooperation of the patient. It is impossible to survey the peritoneal cavity completely by internal palpation, because only the pelvic cavity and the caudal portion, or approximately 40 per cent, of the abdominal cavity can be explored.

Frequently, rather subtle signs or hints found during examination yield information pointing to conditions in deeper abdominal regions. In other cases, the location and the type of the obstruction can be identified precisely—for example, incarcerated inguinal hernia and left dorsal displacement of the large colon.

TECHNIQUE

To minimize the risk of damage to the rectum, horses with unrelenting pain should be treated with analgesics or sedatives such as xylazine* (0.1 to 0.2 mg per kg). Use of a twitch is almost always necessary to prevent straining. An alternative method of restraint is the simple fixation of a hindleg with a rope attached to the pastern and led between the forelegs to the neck. If the veterinarian examines with the right arm the left hindleg is fixed, and vice versa. The anus of the horse and the gloved hand should be lubricated sufficiently to reduce resistance and mucosal irritation when the cone-formed hand is inserted. First, the mucosa of the ampulla should be examined for any lesions, and blood or clots on the withdrawn arm. Rectal mucus and the contents of the rectal ampulla are noted and fecal balls are eliminated. The next reinsertion of the arm should be as deep as possible when the rectum

*Rompun, Haver-Lockhart, Shawnee, KS

is flaccid to facilitate examination of deep regions. Initial manipulation of tissues with a half-inserted arm, and examination of the pelvic cavity first, usually causes tenesmus and propulsive contractions of the rectum. Consequently, thorough investigation of more cranial structures is prevented.

EXAMINATION FINDINGS

Normal Rectal Findings (Fig. 1). Rectal findings in the healthy animal include well-formed, soft fecal balls in the rectal ampulla that have an aromatic odor. Rectal mucosa is finely folded. The small colon is identified by fecal balls, which can be moved in all directions. At the right side, the cecum often can be recognized as a soft viscus containing some gas. The only portion of the cecum that always can be identified is the ventral taenia. In small horses ventral and medial taenia can be palpated. If the cecum contains some gas or ingesta its dorsal adhesion to the abdominal wall can be touched

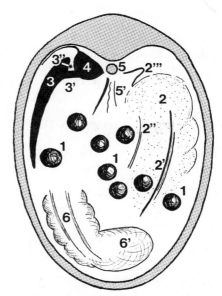

Figure 1. Normal rectal findings. 1, Fecal balls marking the small colon; 2, Cecal base containing some gas; 2′, Its ventral taenia; 2″, Its medial taenia; 2‴, Its adhesion to the dorsal abdominal wall; 3, Spleen; 3′, Its suspensory ligament; 3″, Nephrosplenic space; 4, Kidney; 5, Aorta; 5′, Cranial mesenteric root; 6, Large colon, bands of the ventral portion; 6′, Pelvic flexure.

going from the aorta to the right side. At the left flank the caudal edge of the spleen can be found. Usually the caudal pole of the left kidney and the suspensory ligament of the spleen or nephrosplenic ligament can be identified. Two or three fingers can be inserted into the nephrosplenic space between the dorsal part of the spleen and the left kidney. In small horses the cranial mesenteric root can be investigated by fingertips as a flaccid folded band running in a ventral direction. Parts of the large colon frequently cannot be identified. By passing the hand along the ventral abdominal wall, it is often possible to feel some bands or the pelvic flexure if it contains ingesta. The caudal part of the abdominal cavity can normally be reached in all directions without any resistance.

Pathological Findings. The common location of rectal tears is in the dorsal bowel wall at the cranial limitation of the rectal ampulla (see p.75). Lubricant on the glove with a sanguineous tinge after the first inspection of this area requires careful investigation. Bloody and malodorous brownish fluid is also found in all conditions that compromise the vascular supply of the small colon with or without compromise of its lumen. Injuries of the rectum are best explored by the more sensitive bare hand. The smooth mucosa disappears and the surface is rough.

In cases of intestinal obstruction the rectum frequently contains no fecal material and rectal mucus is inspissated. Small dry fecal balls coated with pasty mucus signify delayed transport of the feces. On the contrary, the chronic impaction of the cecum often causes a diarrhealike stool. In order to correctly interpret the findings of rectal examination, one must pay particular attention to the consistency, form, position, location, or tenseness of both the intestine and mesentery. The taenias are important structures for identification of specific segments of the large bowel. Intestinal impactions cause enlargement of the constipated parts of the bowel and have a pasty or doughy consistency. Digital impressions remain for some time.

In dilatations of the intestine caused by gas accumulation, impressions disappear at once. By pressing the bowels against the abdominal wall or pelvis, lesions such as edema and infarction that increase the thickness of the bowel wall can be identified. In this manner, localized intestinal pain can also be reproduced. In stallions and geldings the palpation of the vaginal ring should be a routine part of the examination.

Intravaginal inguinal herniation of the small intestine occurs if the peritoneal ring is large. Rectal findings in this condition are an enlarged loop of the small intestine with abnormal fixation at the abdominal wall in the inguinal region, acute pain, and a taut mesentery. External palpation of the scrotum completes this diagnosis.

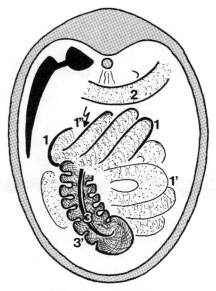

Figure 2. Rectal findings in small bowel obstruction. 1, Strangulated parts of small intestine, distended loops with thickened wall; 1′, Prestenotic loops of small bowel, tympanic without thickening of the wall; 1″(⟨), Painful area; 2, Caudal flexure of the distended duodenum; 3, Large colon containing solid ingesta; 3′, Its contracted sacculations.

Obstructions of the small bowel are characterized by distended loops of small intestine that are compressible to varying degrees. The diameter may vary from 5 to 12 cm depending on the duration of the condition. In cases of high obstruction or in late cases the dilated second flexure of the duodenum surrounding the dorsal adhesion of the cecum can be recognized. The strangulated part of the small bowel can be identified by the thickening of its wall. In all cases of small bowel obstruction the ingesta inside the large colon becomes more solid because of the dehydration. Dehydration also reduces the size of the large colon making the constrictions and sacculations of the ventral part of the large colon palpably more distinct (Fig. 2). Touching the strangulated intestinal or mesenteric parts may cause pain. In a high obstruction of the small intestine distended loops may not be within reach. In this situation, however, gentle traction on the ventral taenia of the cecum in a caudal direction is very painful. *Ileal impaction* can be diagnosed by rectal examination in early cases only. The obstipated ileum feels like a large sausage, the end of which is fixed in the right dorsal region at the base of the cecum, which is poststenotic and therefore empty and not palpable. Tension on the taut mesentery of the ileum produces pain. In late cases the constipated ileum cannot be palpated because the distended loops of the caudal portion of the prestenotic jejunum fill the caudal part of the abdominal cavity and the ileum may be dislocated in a cranial direction.

In cases of *ileocecal intussusception* a blunt mass can be felt in the right dorsal region. The mass is fixed at its dorsomedial pole and can be moved like a pendulum in transverse and sagittal directions. Touching the point of fixation is often painful. In all cases of small bowel obstruction *gastric dilatation* occurs. A dislocation of the spleen in the ventromedial and caudal direction is an indication of tremendous gastric dilatation.

Acute dilatation of the cecum produces obvious rectal findings as the form of the organ can be recognized very clearly. The ventral taenia, the large-caliber sacculations, and the deep constrictions can be felt. Impactions of the cecum can be diagnosed because of the typical form of this bowel, its dorsal junction to the abdominal wall, and the doughy consistency. Sometimes a relapsing spastic impaction of the overhanging part of the cecal base occurs. It can only be reached in medium-sized horses, can be recognized because of its oval form, and can be moved like a pendulum in a transverse direction. In severe cases of recurrent *impaction of the cecum* the hypertrophy of the circular layer of the smooth muscles of the base and the body of the cecum can be recognized even if the cecum is not well filled. In all cases of *strangulation of the large colon* characteristically there is a large amount of gas distention of the cecum proximal to the obstruction. When the cecum is distended with gas, its apex tends to "float up" and the ventral taenia becomes positioned in an oblique or transverse direction.

One of the most common findings in colic horses is *impaction of the left ventral portion of the large colon*. The colon is enlarged and the obstipation has a cone-formed end at the pelvic flexure (Fig. 3). The two free taenias of the ventral large colon can be felt as longitudinal grooves, separated by 90 degrees in relation to the circumference of the intestinal tube. The consistency of the obstipated ingesta depends on the tone of the intestinal wall and can change suddenly during the manual investigation. Because of the enlargement, the sacculations and constrictions are not recognizable. This is a very significant difference from cases of *pseudoimpaction* of the large bowels caused by the dehydration in cases of small bowel obstruction. This difference must be noted to prevent improper interpretation of cases in which the firmness of the contents of the large colon is increased.

Impaction of the ampulla of the right dorsal portion of the large colon has the shape and dimensions of a soccer ball, approximately 30 cm in diameter. Often it will not be within reach. Only in medium-sized horses in which the cranial mesenteric root can be investigated easily can the caudal

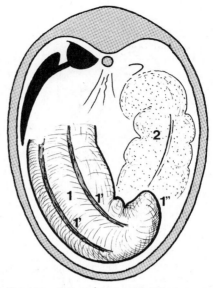

Figure 3. Rectal findings in impaction of the left ventral colon. 1, Enlarged large colon containing doughy ingesta; 1′, Its two free taenia (Distanced 90 degrees in relation to the circumference of the intestinal tube); 1″, Cone-formed end of the obstipation at the pelvic flexure; 2, Tympanic cecum.

part of the constipated ampulla coli be reached. The cranial mesenteric root can be pressed against the background of the domelike protrusion of the constipated dorsal colon and serves as a helpful guide to identify the location of the obstipated ingesta.

Occlusion of the large colon by enteroliths also occurs at the junction of the right dorsal and transverse colon. If the occluding stone can be touched, there is no question about the type of obstruction. The prestenotic parts of the large colon are greatly distended by gas as in all cases of strangulation and volvulus of the large colon in which the occlusion is total.

Extreme distention of the large colon with gas and tremendous tension on its taenias are the cornerstones in rectal identification of *torsion or flexion* of this intestinal part. After a few hours, the twisted bowels become edematous, and the thickened intestinal wall, haustra, and longitudinal bands are readily palpated. In some cases the ventral colon can be located dorsal to the dorsal colon. Because of the distention, the large bowel cannot be moved. In some cases, it is positioned in a transverse direction with the curvature of the pelvic flexure dislocated either toward the right flank or in a cranial direction. In dramatic cases of *torsion of the entire large colon* tympany may be so severe that it is impossible to explore the cranial regions of the abdominal cavity (Fig. 4).

A frequently observed condition is the *strangulation of the large colon by the suspensory ligament*

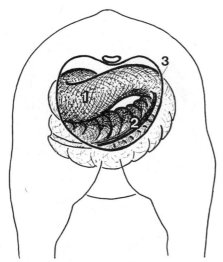

Figure 4. Rectal findings in torsion of the whole large colon. 1, Tympanic dorsal portion; 2, Edemous and gaseous distended ventral part of the large colon in transverse position with clearly contoured sacculations and constrictions; 3, Limitation of pelvic cavity (deeper regions cannot be explored).

of the spleen—the so-called left dorsal displacement of the large colon (Fig. 5). The location of the strangulation can be investigated by rectal palpation of these cases. If the dislocated portion of the colon is large, the bands (taenias) run diagonally to con-

verge at the nephrosplenic space on the left dorsal quadrant of the abdomen. By palpating from the caudal pole of the left kidney toward the left abdominal wall the taenias of the large colon can be palpated crossing dorsally to the nephrosplenic ligament. The spleen is almost always situated in its normal position but can be hidden by tympanic parts of the dislocated colon. In a few cases of left dorsal displacement of the large colon only the impacted pelvic flexure is strangulated over the suspensory ligament of the spleen. This condition can be recognized easily because of the wheellike form of this intestinal part with a diameter of the intestinal tube of 15 to 20 cm.

A similar condition is the *right dorsal displacement of the large colon* between the tympanic cecum and the right abdominal wall. The large colon is flexed in a right and caudal direction and covers the cecum. The edematous fat of the mesentery containing the large blood vessels between the ventral and the dorsal colon has a jellylike consistency.

Obstruction of the small colon by foreign bodies or fecal concretions can be diagnosed accurately by rectal examination (Fig. 6). The occluding body is usually situated at the ventral abdominal wall near the pelvic inlet and can be moved in all directions. The broad and prominent antimesenteric band of the small colon can be palpated and helps to identify this bowel section. The tympanic prestenotic loops

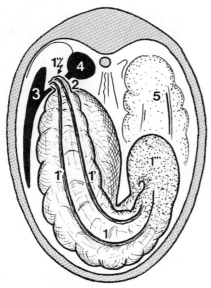

Figure 5. Rectal findings in left dorsal displacement of the large colon. 1, Enlarged large colon with accumulation of gas and ingesta; 1′, Tensed oblique sinistrodorsocranial converging taenia; 1″ (↯), Location of strangulation with pain on palpation; 1‴, Dislocated tympanic pelvic flexure; 2, Suspensory ligament of the spleen (covered by the large colon); 3, Spleen; 4, Kidney; 5, Prestenotic tympany of the cecum.

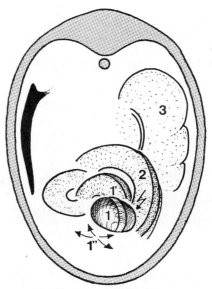

Figure 6. Rectal findings in occlusion of the small colon by an enterolith. 1, Obstructed bowel part with local pain on palpation (↯); 1′, prominent free taenia; 1″, Possible directions of manual displacement; 2, Tympany of the prestenotic part of the small colon; 3, Cecum.

of the small colon have a diameter of approximately 6 to 10 cm and are curved like wheels.

In cases of impaction or volvulus of the small colon, deep rectal examination is often not possible. Only the forearm can be inserted to touch the distended loops of the small colon. In such cases the caudal mesenteric root can be felt because it is tense. This is not found in any other condition because the free floating mesentery of the small colon normally is not noticeable.

Production of pain by palpation of the visceral surface of the abdominal wall is an indication of acute *diffuse peritonitis*. In cases in which rupture of an abdominal viscus has occurred the dorsal part of the abdominal cavity feels empty and there are floating flaccid intestinal loops in the ventral part. The peritoneum may feel rough because of adherent fecal particles, and in cases of gastric or cecal rupture there is evidence of emphysema in the supraperitoneal space.

To completely assess intestinal or intraperitoneal injury, rectal examination should always be complemented by abdominocentesis. In an analysis of 150 cases in our university, a definitive diagnosis was obtained in 75 patients by rectal palpation alone. In an additional 27 per cent an indication for surgical treatment was obtained by rectal exploration. Only in 6 per cent of these cases was there a false diagnosis caused by errors in interpretation of rectal findings. In 9 per cent of the horses rectal examination was not practicable because they were too small.

Supplemental Readings

Huskamp, B., Daniels, H., and Kopf, N.: Magen- und Darmkrankheiten. In Dietz, O. and Wiesner, E. (eds.): Handbuch der Pferdekrankheiten fur Wissenschaft und Praxis, Vol. 2, VEB. Gustav Fischer Verlag, Jena, 1982.

Huskamp, B., and Kopf, N.: Die Verlagerung des Colon ascendens in den Milzneirenraum beim Pferd (Hernia spatii lienorenalis coli ascendentis). Tierarztl. Prax. 8:327, 495, 1980.

Huskamp, B. and Kopf, N.: Right dorsal displacement of the large colon in the horse. Equine Pract., 5:20, 1983.

Kopf, N.: Rectal Findings in Horses with Intestinal Obstruction. Proc. 1st Colic Research Symposium, University of Georgia, 1982.

Kopf, N. and Huskamp, B.: Die rektale Untersuchung beim Kolikpferd. Prakt. Tierarzt, 59:259, 1978.

Analgesics in the Treatment of Colic

William W. Muir, III, COLUMBUS, OHIO

Colic produces a variety of behavioral and cardiopulmonary changes that are used to assess the severity of the disease process and to form a prognosis. The cause of abdominal pain in horses with colic is generally related to mechanical defects, such as distention, obstruction, and twisting of the abdominal viscera, or the production and release of chemicals that cause pain. Histamine, serotonin, kinins, potassium, prostaglandins (PGE_1, PGI_2), thromboxanes, leukotrienes, and various polypeptides are chemical substances capable of producing pain, causing hyperalgesia, and enhancing the susceptibility to pain. Ideally, the best treatment for pain is to remove its cause. In many instances, this can be accomplished by simple medical management. Severe colic can cause such extreme abdominal pain that a horse may become difficult to restrain resulting in harm to itself and its attendants. Patients with severe colic may require the administration of repeated doses of potent analgesics until surgery can be performed.

Nonsteroidal anti-inflammatory drugs, narcotic analgesics, non-narcotic analgesics, and sedatives are used to control colic in horses. These drugs produce analgesic effects by directly interfering with the production of the chemical mediators of pain, inhibiting the transmission of painful stimuli, and decreasing the central nervous system awareness of pain. Drugs that are commonly used to control colic in horses and their dosages are listed in Table 1.

An experimental model of visceral pain in horses utilizes a balloon inflated in the cecum. Cecal distention produces severe acute unrelenting pain that is variably responsive to analgesic drugs. Xylazine produces the most pronounced visceral analgesia for the longest period of time when this model is used. Butorphanol produces visceral analgesic activity that is less than, but second to, that of xylazine. Morphine, meperidine, methadone, and oxymorphone produce visceral analgesic effects that are highly variable and generally inferior to those of xylazine and butorphanol. Pentazocine, nalbuphine, and nonsteroidal anti-inflammatory drugs such as flunixin and dipyrone do not produce significant visceral analgesia in this visceral pain model. The extrapolation of this information to the clinical patient with colic must be done cautiously, although xylazine and perhaps butorphanol would be expected to produce the most pronounced visceral analgesic effects.

NARCOTIC AGONISTS AND AGONISTS—ANTAGONISTS

Narcotic analgesic drugs are frequently used and produce analgesia and other pharmacologic effects by combining with central and peripheral opioid receptors. The interaction of narcotic analgesic drugs with these putative opioid receptors is believed to be responsible for their sedative, analgesic, behavioral, locomotor, cardiorespiratory, and toxic effects.

The relative density and distribution of opioid receptors in horses are unknown, although the administration of narcotic receptor agonists to horses produces dose-related and reversible pharmacologic effects. Opioid receptor agonists used to treat colic in horses include morphine, meperidine, methadone, and oxymorphone. Several drugs both stimulate receptors and displace narcotic analgesics from opioid receptors. Pentazocine, butorphanol, and nalbuphine are examples of such drugs and are collectively referred to as narcotic agonist–antagonists. A potential clinical disadvantage of narcotic agonist–antagonists is their reversal or inhibition of previously administered narcotic agonists. Drugs that interact with opioid receptors producing only negligible stimulation and that displace narcotic agonist or agonist–antagonists are narcotic antagonists. Naloxone is a narcotic antagonist possessing high affinity for opioid receptors without producing analgesic, behavioral, or cardiorespiratory effects.

Wide variability exists in the ability of narcotic agonists or agonist–antagonists to produce visceral analgesia in horses. Although morphine, oxymorphone, and methadone produce visceral analgesia in horses, their ability to increase locomotor activity and induce behavioral side effects is great, particularly if repeated drug administrations are required. An increase in locomotor activity is typical in horses receiving large intravenous doses or repeated dosages of narcotics and is believed to be related to an

TABLE 1. DRUGS USED TO PRODUCE VISCERAL ANALGESIA IN HORSES

Drug	Recommended IV Dose (mg/kg)
Narcotic agonist	
Morphine	0.02 to 0.04
Meperidine	0.2 to 0.4
Methadone	0.05 to 0.1
Oxymorphone	0.01 to 0.02
Narcotic Agonist-Antagonist	
Butorphanol	0.02 to 0.05
Pentazocine	0.4 to 0.8
Non-narcotic analgesic	
Flunixin meglumine	0.6 to 1.1
Dipyrone (50%)	10 to 20 ml (slowly)
Sedative analgesic	
Xylazine	0.3 to 0.5

increase in central nervous system dopamine release. Acepromazine (0.02 to 0.04 mg per kg intravenously), xylazine (0.3 to 0.5 mg per kg intravenously), or naloxone (0.01 mg per kg intravenously) can be used to limit increases in locomotor activity and unwanted behavioral side effects. This finding supports the clinical observation that the combination of narcotic analgesics with phenothiazine tranquilizers or xylazine produces better chemical restraint and analgesia than the use of narcotics alone.

The clinical justification for the use of narcotic analgesics in horses is in their ability to produce visceral analgesia without significant cardiovascular depression. The clinical onset of action is within five minutes and the duration of visceral analgesic action is variable generally lasting for 30 minutes to four hours. Intravenous or repeated intramuscular dosages of narcotic analgesics increase heart rate, cardiac output, and blood pressure in pain-free horses. Apprehension, sweating, tachycardia, and ataxia, in addition to increased locomotor activity, are frequently observed following intravenous narcotic agonist or narcotic agonist–antagonist administration. Narcotic-induced respiratory depression is rare unless the patient is anesthetized. Mechanical support of breathing, however, is advisable during general anesthesia for the surgical treatment of colic in horses.

The cardiovascular effects of narcotics in horses with colic are dependent upon dosage and route of administraion, the relative degree of analgesia produced, and the severity of cardiovascular compromise. The narcotic analgesics and the dosages known to produce beneficial visceral analgesic effects in horses are listed in Table 1. Narcotic analgesics can mask the behavioral and cardiovascular effects of mild colic.

NON-NARCOTIC ANALGESICS

Flunixin meglumine* and dipyrone† are analgesic, antipyretic, nonsteroidal anti-inflammatory drugs (NSAIDs) used to treat abdominal pain in horses. These drugs are believed to produce their analgesic effects by inhibiting the production of prostaglandins. Their clinical effectiveness as analgesics in the treatment of colic in horses varies considerably. Flunixin is considered the most potent non-narcotic analgesic for the treatment of equine colic. The reason for flunixin's analgesic superiority over other NSAIDs remains unclear although it is known to be a relatively selective cyclo-oxygenase inhibitor. Flunixin, although not an effective analgesic in all types of equine colic, results in a good to excellent response when used in treating flatulent, spastic, and inflammatory causes of colic. Flunixin should be used cautiously in horses with suspected intestinal devitalization or endotoxemia because it may mask behavioral and cardiopulmonary signs associated with colic until it is too late to institute more specific therapy. The recommended dosage of flunixin for the treatment of colic is 1.1 mg per kg intravenously or intramuscularly (Table 1).

Horses that do not respond immediately to flunixin should receive a carefully conducted re-examination including abdominocentesis in order to rule out intestinal strangulation. When a specific condition has been identified that does not require surgical intervention, a dose may be repeated in two to four hours if pain returns or is incompletely controlled. The duration of flunixin's analgesic effects averages from four to 36 hours depending upon the cause and severity of abdominal pain. Toxic side effects have not been observed with doses up to 5 mg per kg for five days although the potential for gastrointestinal intolerance, protein-losing enteropathies, and blood dyscrasias exists.

Xylazine,‡ a non-narcotic analgesic, produces sedation and muscle relaxation in horses. Visceral analgesia is immediate in onset, more pronounced and of longer duration than that produced by NSAIDs, narcotic agonists, and narcotic agonist–antagonists. Sedation is characterized by lethargy, drooping and extension of the head and neck, and ataxia. The penis is usually extended in both stallions and geldings. Heart rate and respiratory rate are significantly decreased. Arterial blood pressure decreases although it may be increased initially. Xylazine is usually recommended to control visceral pain in horses that do not repond to other analgesic drugs or in horses that have become unmanageable. Xylazine will significantly mask the behavioral and hemodynamic effects of equine colic for short periods of time and is considered by some veterinarians to be used only as a final resort for this reason. Xylazine, however, may be the only drug that produces enough sedation and visceral analgesia to control severe abdominal pain or produce enough chemical restraint for shipment of the patient to a surgical facility. The recommended dosage of xylazine for the treatment of equine colic is 0.3 to 0.5 mg per kg intravenously (see Table 1). This dose can be repeated as necessary. Horses with colic that do not respond to repeated administration of xylazine should be seriously considered for exploratory laparotomy.

The clinical selection of an analgesic for the treatment of colic in horses should depend on the patient's clinical signs, the clinician's familiarity with the various analgesic drugs, and the patient's recent drug history. The recent administration of a narcotic agonist–antagonist, for example, precludes the use of a narcotic agonist. The frequent and repeated unsuccessful use of flunixin, dipyrone, or narcotic analgesics may indicate the need for a sedative analgesic drug such as xylazine. Because all drugs that produce visceral analgesia have the potential to mask the behavioral and cardiorespiratory signs of abdominal pain, the veterinarian must rely on rectal palpation, serum biochemical values, and analysis of peritoneal fluid for diagnosis and prognosis.

Supplemental Readings

Lumb, W. V., Pippi, N. L., and Kalpravidh, M.: Evaluation of analgesic drugs in horses. *In* Kitchell, R. L., and Erickson, H. H. (eds.): Animal Pain. Baltimore, Waverly Press, 1983, pp. 179–205.

Pippi, N. L., and Lumb, W. V.: Objective tests of analgesic drugs in ponies. Am. J. Vet. Res., 40:1082,1979.

---

*Banamine, Schering Corp., Kenilworth, NJ
†Novin, Haver-Lockhart, Shawnee, KS
‡Rompun, Haver-Lockhart, Shawnee, KS

Deciding When to Refer the Horse with Colic

James R. Coffman, MANHATTAN, KANSAS

It is important to separate the decision to refer a horse with an abdominal crisis to a surgical facility from the decision to perform surgery. All too often these two questions are addressed simultaneously and critical hours are lost. Centrally located modern clinical facilities have improved the surgical survival rate. Shorter transport time, provided by the proximity of such facilities, improved preoperative patient care, and improved communication between the referring veterinarian, surgeon, and owner have all served to improve the prognosis for a horse with colic. In contrast to academic institutions, which report survival rates of 40 to 60 per cent, it is common for these private practices to expect survival rates in excess of 75 per cent. This is a good example of how basic and clinical research and service at academic institutions can result in improvements that ultimately are more effectively applied in the private sector. The problem still exists, however, that a large number of horses with intestinal ischemia referred to either private clinics or university hospitals die in spite of surgical intervention. The delay in making the decision to refer may well represent the most critical problem in the chain of assessment, diagnosis, plan, and therapy.

ASKING THE RIGHT QUESTION

The same considerations are relevant, regardless of whether the horse is to be transported to a facility within the same practice, referred to another practice, or transported to an academic institution. The clinician must first determine the questions to ask, the answers to anticipate, and the pieces of information that are critical to indicate that the animal should be referred for possible surgery.

Certainly, at first examination, a definitive diagnosis is neither feasible nor necessary. An example of an inappropriate question is: "What is wrong with the horse?" The answer calls for a definitive diagnosis and often too much time is lost in reaching an answer. "Does the horse need surgery?" seems like an obvious question but is too broad and does not lead directly to definitive action. "Is irreversible tissue damage taking place?" is an effective question. When the answer is yes, the horse should be explored surgically at the earliest possible moment. This question relates well to modes of assessment commonly used by clinicians. These assessments are best organized into a problem-specific data base (PSDB) for initial characterization of abdominal pain. A decision to perform a celiotomy, or to outline therapy and monitor progress, will use a different and more extensive data base. The components of a PSDB for acute abdominal pain in horses are:

1. Signalment, history, and progress of the horse since the onset of signs of pain
2. Pulse or heart rate (HR), membrane color (MC), and capillary refill time (CRT)
3. Hematocrit (PCV) and total plasma protein (TP)
4. Body temperature
5. Results of nasogastric intubation
6. Thoracic and abdominal sounds
7. Results of rectal palpation
8. Composition of peritoneal fluid
9. Response to therapy

All too often the intense activity that accompanies the examination of a horse with abdominal pain can cause basic information to be ignored. Simple data such as age, reproductive status, and previous history of abdominal surgery may seem less important at this time than the immediate abnormal clinical findings. The attending veterinarian must, however, remember to ask these questions and keep that information in mind during the examination of the horse. It must be kept in mind that ileocecal intussusception and small intestinal volvulus tend to occur in younger horses; epiploic foramen incarceration, pedunculated lipomas, and cecal impaction occur in horses over seven years old; colonic torsions are common in recently foaled mares; inguinal hernias should be considered in every stallion showing signs of colic; and intra-abdominal adhesions may cause problems postoperatively. Consequently, if these basic aspects of the signalment are emphasized during the physical examination and data consistent with these conditions are obtained; the decision to refer the patient for possible surgery can be made more quickly. Similarly, it is vital that the veterinarian has an appreciation of the progress of the condition. When vital signs deteriorate in a matter of hours, immediate surgery is indicated in a high percentage of animals regardless of the definitive diagnosis. When the condition has a more protracted course, one must place additional importance on the findings of the rectal examination. Certain colonic displacements requiring surgical correction do not impair colonic function sufficiently to cause abrupt deterioration.

DIAGNOSTIC INDICATORS

Pulse, Heart Rate, Mucous Membrane Color, and Capillary Refill Time. Assessment of pulse, heart rate, membrane color, and capillary refill time provides a subjective insight into the animal's cardiac output and peripheral perfusion. Pulse deficit or variations in pulse amplitude suggest inconsistent stroke volume. Since stroke volume is determined by venous return, one must assume this is decreased if the myocardium is normal. The most likely reasons for decreased venous return are hypovolemia and increased total peripheral resistance, or both. Concomitantly, congested membranes are consistent with peripheral pooling of blood. Cyanotic, congested membranes suggest poor oxygen exchange, usually as a result of ventilation and perfusion mismatching in the lung. In either instance, hypovolemia and endotoxemia are usually contributing factors. Prolonged capillary refill time indicates hypovolemia, reduced cardiac output, and/or increased total peripheral resistance, which occurs concurrently in most instances. When these alterations in vital signs develop rapidly, they strongly indicate the presence of irreversible tissue damage and the need for possible surgery. Stabilization of the circulation and replacement of fluid losses should take place while arrangements are being made to transport the horse to a critical care and surgical facility.

Body Temperature. Body temperature is discussed separately because of its importance in detection of certain conditions that can elude the clinician and result in disastrous consequences. Unfortunately, many veterinarians overlook this basic step in the PSDB. Horses affected by pleuritis, peritonitis, and impending colitis commonly display clinical signs consistent with gastrointestinal obstruction or infarction. Body temperature greater than 39.5° C should always signal the clinician to consider these options, particularly if the degree of pain is mild or moderate. Fever is always cause for further immediate diagnostic tests such as a complete blood count. Neutropenia, particularly in the form of a degenerative left shift, is characteristic of acute colitis or pleuritis. Conversely, neutrophilia would more likely suggest the presence of an abdominal abscess.

Nasogastric Intubation. Without doubt, nasogastric intubation is the most important initial step in the assessment of horses affected with acute abdominal pain. Several circumstances may lead to gastric filling. Increased duodenal pressure mitigates against gastric emptying; therefore, distention of small intestine with fluid or gas or both results in life-threatening gastric distention. Nasogastric decompression can be life-saving if irreversible tissue changes are not present. Persistent distention of the colon due to impaction or enteroliths can also result in gastric distention. In most horses with gastric distension, decompression of the stomach results in obvious clinical improvement, especially if the small intestine is not distended with fluid. However, when gastric filling results from displacement of the colon, relief from pain is transient. Distention of the stomach as a result of small bowel disease may result from displacement of intestine, stasis, and hypersecretion of fluid with retrograde gastric filling, or from duodenitis-jejunitis. If the stomach is distended as a result of intestinal displacement, decompression via nasogastric intubation generally does not result in significant improvement. However, if response to nasogastric decompression is profound and tends to be lasting, irreversible morphologic changes are less likely to be present. Reflux via nasogastric tube is always a serious sign; if pain persists or recurs following decompression, surgery should be an immediate consideration. Logistics permitting, a horse with sequestration of fluid in the stomach should be considered for immediate transport to a surgical facility with the stomach tube taped in place.

AUSCULTATION OF THORAX AND ABDOMEN

Because horses affected with pleuritis may exhibit signs consistent with abdominal pain, the thorax should be examined thoroughly, particularly when pain is not severe. Auscultation should be coupled with thorough percussion as pleuritis is extremely painful in the early stages. The abdomen must be carefully auscultated on both sides. Generally speaking, borborygmi in the right flank reflect cecal and colonic activity, whereas those on the left are most consistent with sounds of the small intestine. If the abdomen is persistently silent, particularly in the presence of continued pain, the horse should be transported to a surgical facility.

Rectal Palpation. Rectal palpation is the most definitive diagnostic procedure in the PSDB (see p. 23). Certain lesions can be diagnosed definitively, such as dorsal displacement of the colon, 180-degree rotation of the left colon, impaction, fecalith, enterolith, inguinal hernia, small bowel entrapment, volvulus, and intussusception. This fact justifies careful exploration of the abdomen by rectal palpation, provided the examiner is vigilant to the risks of trauma to the rectal wall (see p. 75). The identification of the large colon dorsal to the nephrosplenic ligament, distended loops of small bowel, confluence of bowel with an internal inguinal ring, presence of a concretion in contrast to an impaction, and palpation of severely distended large bowel warrant immediate referral.

Abdominal Paracentesis. Viewed within the context of the question of whether irreversible tissue damage is taking place, abdominal paracentesis is extremely helpful to detect an increased protein concentration or red blood cells in the peritoneal fluid. Extravasation of blood should always be considered cause for immediate referral if the owner understands that the prognosis is already poor. Conversely, elevated protein concentration without the presence of red blood cells is suggestive of morphologic change with a somewhat better prognosis. The decision to perform surgery should not be based solely upon increased protein concentration, even in the presence of persistent pain. Duodenitis-jejunitis and cantharadin intoxication (p. 120) both result in the elevation of protein concentration in peritoneal fluid. Cantharadin poisoning is usually accompanied by urine dribbling or frequent urination and by hypocalcemia; duodenitis-jejunitis is more difficult to diagnose. Acute peritonitis also results in an increase in peritoneal fluid protein levels; however, the accompanying increase in neutrophils, of which many are toxic, usually leads to an accurate diagnosis. Although laboratory evaluation of peritoneal fluid certainly provides important information for the assessment of the patient's condition, the prognosis for survival will be improved if the animal can be transported to a referral clinic before significant alterations in peritoneal fluid composition occur.

RESPONSE TO THERAPY

Persistent pain is a reliable indicator for surgical intervention. Certain factors must be considered when interpreting response to various forms of therapy. Clinical response to potent nonsteroidal anti-inflammatory drugs such as flunixin meglumine may be misleading. These agents inhibit the production of prostaglandins and mask the early clinical responses to endotoxemia. Consequently, these drugs should be used with caution and not be given repeatedly to a patient unless all other physical examination findings indicate that irreversible tissue damage is not occurring. Some horses experience a profound sympathoadrenal response to pain, which apparently alters gastrointestinal function causing persistent violent pain. Interruption of pain breaks this cycle; this is the only means of avoiding unnecessary surgery on these horses. In some instances, basal narcosis is necessary to achieve complete analgesia. One means of approaching this problem is to administer a profound short-acting analgesic or combination of analgesics having minimal effect on cardiopulmonary function. In such instances recurrence of pain is just as meaningful as persistent pain in the presence of less profound analgesia. Most clinicians agree that horses responding to dipyrone rarely have a lesion requiring surgery, except for those horses having either fecaliths or enteroliths.

Response to fluid therapy is also meaningful. Moderate pain and hemoconcentration are common in horses with impending colitis, peritonitis, and impaction, none of which necessitate surgery. Generally speaking, correction of hemoconcentration results in progressive improvement in these horses, whereas pain may become more evident in horses with a surgical problem.

ANCILLARY CONSIDERATIONS

In most instances veterinarians examine and treat horses affected with abdominal pain while the horse is held by an attendant. Horses restrained by halter will exhibit signs if pain is severe. However, if the degree of pain is slight or moderate, many of these same horses will stand quietly as long as they are held. However, when turned loose, in a box stall for example, they may exhibit signs of pain. Because of this, the veterinarian should always observe the horse loose in the stall for 10 to 15 minutes after it appears to have responded to therapy.

Early transport of horses in abdominal crisis to a surgical facility does not constitute a decision for surgery—it serves only to get the horse to a location where surgery can be performed with minimal delay. The decision to operate should be made by the surgeon. A large majority of veterinarians become extremely effective at detecting those horses that have life-threatening problems. That ability can serve the public well if it leads to early referral of the horse that may require surgery.

Pre- and Postoperative Management of the Colic Patient

Susan M. Stover, DAVIS, CALIFORNIA

Gastrointestinal lesions may produce major alterations in fluid, electrolyte, and acid-base balance. Metabolic abnormalities vary with the duration, location, nature, and severity of the gastrointestinal lesion. In general, intestinal obstruction results in intestinal distention, and increased secretion and reduced absorption of water and electrolytes. Fluid accumulates within the intestinal lumen at the expense of the intravascular compartment resulting in hypovolemia. Hypovolemia and lowered blood pressure result in reduced tissue perfusion, which may lead to tissue hypoxia, anaerobic metabolism, and lactic acidosis. If intestinal integrity is compromised, for example by strangulating obstruction, bacteria and toxins are absorbed systemically. Septicemia and endotoxemia exacerbate hemodynamic alterations and tissue injury. Hypovolemia, hemoconcentration, and electrolyte and acid-base imbalances develop and if uncorrected, may progress toward irreversible shock. Clinically, these conditions are recognized by tachycardia, altered mucous membrane color and prolonged capillary refill time (CRT), weak pulse, delayed jugular distensibility, cold extremities, hypotension, and oliguria.

The following discussion assumes that the colic patient is a surgical candidate and that a physical examination and other procedures essential to the diagnosis have been performed. Management of the surgical colic patient includes resolution of the intravascular fluid deficit and metabolic abnormalities as well as correction of the gastrointestinal lesion. Complete resolution of metabolic abnormalities is generally not possible until the gastrointestinal lesion has been corrected. Therefore, the principal goals of preoperative colic management are the rapid restoration of intravascular fluid volume and peripheral tissue perfusion in order to improve the ability of the patient to tolerate anesthesia and surgery.

PREOPERATIVE MANAGEMENT

Examination and treatment of the surgical patient must be performed quickly and efficiently to minimize the time interval to surgical correction of the gastrointestinal lesion. A temporal record (Fig. 1) should be utilized to record clinical parameters systematically, organize therapy and evaluate the patient's condition and response to therapy.

It is often necessary to restrain the colic patient for safe examination and treatment. If chemical restraint is required, xylazine* (0.2 to 0.5 mg per kg intravenously) is preferred because of its rapid onset of action (within 1 minute), profound sedation and short duration of action (15 to 40 minutes). Administration of xylazine may be repeated for recurrent pain. Xylazine is capable of producing bradycardia, second-degree heart block, hypotension, and decreased gastrointestinal motility. These effects should be considered during clinical evaluation.

Three procedures that should be performed on the colic patient soon after arrival are gastric decompression, blood sampling, and initiation of intravascular fluid volume replacement. After these steps have been taken, careful physical examination and laboratory evaluation of the patient are completed. Occasionally, exceptions must be made for horses with intractable pain such as a horse with a 360-degree torsion of the large colon, which may require immediate general anesthesia and surgical correction for safe management.

Gastric Decompression. Gastric decompression is accomplished by nasogastric intubation. If passive reflux of gastric contents does not occur, the nasogastric tube should be primed with water and repositioned within the stomach to promote removal of gastric fluid. Removal of excess fluid will relieve pain due to gastric distention and decrease the possibility of gastric rupture. The nasogastric tube should remain in place, secured to the halter.

Blood Samples. An anticoagulated blood sample is obtained for immediate determination of packed cell volume (PCV) and plasma protein concentration (PP). Blood is also obtained for sodium (Na^+), potassium (K^+), and chloride (Cl^-) concentration determinations, complete blood count (CBC), and blood gas analyses. Although these results may not be available prior to surgery, they are useful for establishing patient baseline values and for evaluating the patient's response to therapy when this is measured serially.

Fluid Therapy. Fluid should be administered

---

*Rompun, Haver-Lockhart, Shawnee, KS

Veterinary Medical Teaching Hospital
University of California, Davis

EQUINE INTENSIVE CARE FLOW SHEET

Owner's Name: _____

Horse's Name: _____   Sheet # _____

Stall No.: _____

Date: _____   Duty Intern Phone: _____

Time					
Temperature					
Respiration Rate					
Heart Rate & Character					
Mucous Membranes					
Perfusion Time					
P.C.V.					
Plasma Proteins					
Total W.B.C.					
Attitude/Degree of Pain					
Gut Motility					
Feces (character)					
Urine (volume)					
Digital Pulse					
Medication					
Fluid Therapy					
Flush Catheter					
Appetite					
Water Consumption					
Exercise					
(Clinician Only) Rectal/Paracentesis					
Comments					

D3091 (10/79) Form #76

Figure 1. *Equine Intensive Care Flow Sheet*

intravenously at a rapid rate to replenish the intravascular volume and improve tissue perfusion. Since the initial intravascular fluid loss in most colic patients is the result of a compartmental shift of isotonic sodium containing fluid into the gastrointestinal tract, lactated Ringer's solution or one of the other balanced polyionic solutions is the replacement fluid of choice. These fluids provide electrolytes in approximately physiologic concentrations, are effective in increasing intravascular volume, and provide a substrate for bicarbonate production. Warm lactated Ringer's solution is initially administered at a rate of 10 to 20 L per hr (20 to 45 ml per kg per hr). After fluid replacement has been initiated, the clinical examination is completed, the patient's condition is assessed, and treatment is modified accordingly. If surgery must be delayed, the patient is reassessed hourly.

Precise estimation of the intravascular fluid deficit is difficult because the presurgical patient has continuing gastrointestinal losses. Although not entirely accurate, it is useful to relate clinical signs of dehydration and hypovolemia to a percentage loss of body weight. Thus, if dehydration is clinically apparent evidenced by altered skin turgor, dry mucous membranes, weak pulse, and prolonged CRT, the patient is assumed to be at least 4 to 6 per cent dehydrated. In this example a 450 kg horse will require at least 18 L of fluid.

Fluid deficit [L] = clinical dehydration [%] × body weight [kg]

More severe clinical signs are associated with fluid deficits of 10 per cent (45 L) or more.

Sequential determinations of PCV and PP, heart rate (HR), CRT, pulse pressure, urinary output, and clinical appearance of the horse provide the most useful guides to the adequacy of fluid therapy. Reductions in HR and CRT, and increased pulse pressure and urinary output, are indicative of improved intravascular volume and tissue perfusion. Generally the PCV and PP increase proportionally in response to reduced plasma volume. However, PCV may be affected by catecholamine release and splenic mobilization of red blood cells or blood loss. The PP may be normal or low if protein is lost into the intestine, peritoneal cavity, or interstitial spaces. In general, fluids are given to effect, with the objective of reducing the PCV to approximately 40 per cent and PP to 7.0 gm per dl. Surgical correction of the gastrointestinal lesion may be necessary before complete resolution of the hemodynamic abnormalities can be achieved.

Although metabolic acidosis may be seen with progression of disease, it is not an invariable finding in colic patients. Correction of hypovolemia will improve peripheral tissue perfusion and promote renal acid-base compensatory mechanisms and may thus result in improvement of metabolic acidosis. Since the inappropriate administration of sodium bicarbonate may produce persistent metabolic alkalosis and depress cardiac output, sodium bicarbonate is not administered unless acidosis is substantiated by a pH less than 7.30 and base deficit greater than 10 mEq per L. If laboratory support is unavailable clinical suspicion of metabolic acidosis is indicated by severe shock or marked elevation of the heart and respiratory rates.

Antibiotics. Prophylactic broad-spectrum antibiotic therapy in the colic patient is indicated. Enteric bacteria are able to pass through compromised intestinal wall within hours, and peritoneal contamination should be anticipated in surgical patients because it inevitably attends trocharization, enterotomy, and anastomoses. Antibiotic regimens effective against gram-positive, gram-negative, and anaerobic bacteria are indicated. In our hospital, penicillin and gentamicin are instituted prior to abdominal surgery or are given intraoperatively at a dosage rate of 40,000 IU per kg aqueous penicillin* four times a day and 2.2 mg/kg gentamicin† three times a day intravenously. The anesthetist should be advised of gentamicin therapy because aminoglycosides have been reported to potentiate neuromuscular blockade and depress cardiovascular function. This has not been a significant problem for horses in my experience. If either neuromuscular complications or penicillin- and gentamicin-resistant organisms are recognized, selection of other broad-spectrum antibiotics should be considered.

Anti-inflammatory Drugs. Flunixin meglumine‡ (1 mg per kg intramuscularly or intravenously), a nonsteroidal anti-inflammatory drug, is administered preoperatively. Analgesic and anti-inflammatory effects are mediated through inhibition of prostaglandin formation. Flunixin is effective for relieving visceral pain and has been shown to prevent some of the detrimental effects of endotoxin when administered early in experimental disease. It has minimal effect on gastrointestinal motility but has the potential to mask some of the signs of systemic disease.

POSTOPERATIVE MANAGEMENT

During the anesthetic recovery period, the nasogastric tube is removed to prevent reflux of fluid on the recovery room floor. Tracheal intubation is maintained until the horse stands. Oxygen is ad-

---

*Pfizerpen, Pfizer, Inc., New York, NY
†Gentocin, Schering Corp., Kenilworth, NJ
‡Banamine, Schering Corp., Kenilworth, NJ

ministered at 10 to 15 L per min through an insufflation tube inserted in the endotracheal tube to increase the inspired oxygen concentration. Horses that remain recumbent for 60 to 90 minutes or longer are evaluated for hydration and electrolyte and acid-base status and examined for neuromuscular complications. After standing, tetanus toxoid prophylaxis is given. Within 12 hours, blood is drawn for CBC (including PCV, PP, and fibrinogen), electrolyte (Na^+, K^+, Cl^-, and calcium [Ca^{++}]), acid-base, blood urea nitrogen (BUN), creatinine, and serum enzyme determinations to aid in evaluation of the patient's postsurgical metabolic status.

NURSING CARE

The intensity of nursing care will vary with the patient's systemic condition and gastrointestinal function. Initially all colic patients are evaluated at two- hour intervals with careful monitoring of the PCV and PP. Either a nasogastric tube is left in place or gastric decompression is performed periodically or following any significant increase in HR or pain. Patients should be walked for five to 10 minutes every two hours; this may aid in the prevention of laminitis, it may improve their mental attitude, and it may possibly aid in the initiation of gastrointestinal motility. Monitoring intervals are lengthened as the patient's condition becomes stable. Patients that have minor gastrointestinal lesions and are in good physical condition may require less intensive monitoring and can be quickly returned to routine feeding and management. Patients that have compromised intestine remaining in the abdomen or are in poor physical condition are monitored frequently and require intensive care.

Horses are not allowed to eat or drink for at least four hours after surgery. Salt (NaCl) is freely available. When water is tolerated orally, hay is offered in small amounts and the horse is allowed to graze when walked. If hay and water are consumed without complications the horse is gradually returned to full feed. The time course of events varies greatly with the individual patient, according to resumption of normal gastrointestinal function.

If gastric reflux is present, oral intake is restricted and it is usually necessary to maintain hydration with intravenous fluids. Fluids are given to effect, with the objective of maintaining the PCV at 40–45 per cent, PP at 7.0 gm per dl, HR at 40 beats per min, CRT less than 2 sec, and normal pulse pressure and urinary output. Patients with compromised gastrointestinal function or ileus accompanied by continued gastric reflux may require more than 40 L of fluid per day. Plasma protein will decline

disproportionately if protein is lost into the gastrointestinal tract or peritoneal cavity. If PP is less than 5.0 gm per dl, fluid administration is slowed to prevent further decrease of plasma osmotic pressure and loss of intravascular fluid into the interstitium. If PP decreases below 4.0 gm per dl, four to six liters (10 ml plasma per kg body weight) of compatible plasma (see p. 317) can be given and may benefit the patient but often may have a negligible effect on the observed plasma protein concentration.

Selection of an appropriate replacement fluid is based on the patient's hydration and electrolyte and acid-base status. Provided that renal function is adequate, many patients can correct mild abnormalities such as Na^+ of 120–150 mEq per L, Cl^- of 90–110 mEq per L, K^+ of 2.5–5 mEq per L, pH of 7.3 to 7.45 when given balanced polyionic fluids. Fluids should be supplemented with potassium chloride (10 to 20 mEq per L), provided that hyperkalemia is not present. Since these patients are generally off feed, their K^+ intake is markedly reduced while renal K^+ excretion continues. The rate of K^+ administration should not exceed 0.2 to 0.3 mEq per kg per hr since normal cardiac and neuromuscular function is dependent on normal serum K^+ (3 to 5 mEq per L). Electrolyte concentration should be serially monitored during electrolyte supplementation.

Acid-Base Balance. Acid-base imbalances are most commonly metabolic in origin in the colic patient. Metabolic acidosis has been associated with increasing severity and progression of disease; however, metabolic alkalosis has been associated with some disorders including obstructive lesions of the proximal small intestine. Therefore, laboratory determination of the patient's acid-base status is desirable. Arterial samples are preferred for acid-base analysis; however, useful information can be obtained from venous blood, since blood pH and bicarbonate are of primary interest. The base deficit is a useful guide for assessing acid-base requirements.

Base deficit can be used to estimate the bicarbonate requirement in the following way:

$$\text{bicarbonate deficit (mEq HCO}_3^-) = \text{base deficit} \text{ (mEq per L)} \times 0.4 \text{ body wt* (kg)}$$

Alternatively, the approximate bicarbonate content can be estimated from the total venous carbon dioxide content measured with a Harleco CO_2 analyzer.† Bicarbonate accounts for over 95 per cent of

---

*Some authors recommend the use of 0.3 as an estimate of this fluid space.

†Harleco CO_2 Analysis Set, American Scientific Products, McGaw, IL

the total carbon dioxide measured in this fashion. The bicarbonate requirement can be estimated by substituting total carbon dioxide for the measured bicarbonate concentration in the formula:

bicarbonate deficit (mEq HCO_3^-) = (normal-measured HCO_3^- conc.) (mEq per L) × 0.4 body wt* (kg)

The normal bicarbonate concentration in venous blood of horses is 24 to 28 mEq per L. These formulas provide a conservative estimate of the bicarbonate deficit.

Sodium bicarbonate supplementation is indicated for treatment of the patient with marked metabolic acidosis indicated by pH less than 7.30 and base deficit greater than 10 mEq per L. Sodium bicarbonate may be administered as a 5 per cent solution in water (50 gm sodium bicarbonate per L water). Five per cent sodium bicarbonate is hypertonic, supplying approximately 600 mEq sodium and 600 mEq bicarbonate per liter of solution. If the bicarbonate deficit was calculated to be 1200 mEq, 2 liters of 5 per cent sodium bicarbonate solution would be required to replace the deficit. This solution should not be administered faster than 1 to 2 L per hr. It is important to remember that horses with colic that are severely acidotic also tend to be very dehydrated. It may be preferable to administer bicarbonate as an isotonic (150 mEq per L) solution in water. Isotonic saline (0.9 per cent NaCl) is indicated as a volume replacement fluid in horses with a hypochloremic alkalosis (pH greater than 7.45). Isotonic saline supplies 154 mEq sodium and 154 mEq chloride per liter of fluid. In instances of hypokalemic hypochloremic metabolic alkalosis as would be caused by proximal small intestine obstruction, potassium supplementation of saline may be indicated.

If urinary output increases in the face of persistent evidence of hypovolemia, inappropriate fluid composition, administration rate, persistent intestinal disease, and renal dysfunction should be considered. Evaluation of PCV, PP, serum and urine electrolytes, BUN, creatinine and serum enzymes, and a urinalysis and abdominocentesis may be indicated to identify the causal factors.

When gastric reflux is no longer obtained, the patient should be offered small amounts of water (1 to 2 L) at hourly intervals. If gastric reflux does not recur, the horse may then be allowed access to both water and electrolyte† supplemented water.

If surgery was uncomplicated, antibiotics are discontinued after 24 hours. If significant contamination has occurred, if intestine of questionable via-

bility remains in the patient, or if peritonitis, septicemia, or endotoxemia is present, antibiotic therapy should be continued as needed. Flunixin meglumine is normally discontinued after 48 hours, unless complications warrant continuation of therapy.

Anticoagulants. Anticoagulant therapy has been advocated for the prevention of venous and pulmonary thrombosis and treatment of consumptive coagulopathies. Heparin* (40 to 100 U per kg subcutaneously twice a day) is thought to indirectly decrease fibrin deposition, enhance phagocytosis by the reticuloendothelial system, and decrease platelet aggregation. Although these postulated actions may be beneficial, clinical efficacy has not yet been proved in the horse. Nonsteroidal anti-inflammatory drugs may also be beneficial in this regard as they may inhibit platelet aggregation. In our hospital, heparin therapy has been used in patients with peritonitis, septicemia, and endotoxemia. A marked drop in PCV may accompany heparin therapy, but the PCV usually increases toward normal following heparin withdrawal.

Paralytic Ileus. Ileus is managed with nasogastric decompression, fluid, electrolyte, and acid-base support, and exercise. If hypokalemia (K^+ less than 2.5 mEq per L) is present, intravenous fluids are supplemented with KCl (20 to 30 mEq per L). If hypocalcemia (Ca^{++} less than 10 mEq per L) is present, calcium is administered as calcium gluconate† (23 per cent solution; 50 to 100 ml slowly intravenously). During K^+ or Ca^{++} supplementation, the heart should be monitored for arrhythmias and serial measurements of electrolyte concentrations should be performed. Therapy should be discontinued if arrhythmias become apparent or electrolyte concentrations become elevated. Neostigmine‡ is a parasympathomimetic drug that has been shown to stimulate contractions of the large intestine. Neostigmine (2 to 4 mg subcutaneously every two hr) may be administered after correction of large bowel displacement to promote intestinal contractions and may aid in reduction of intestinal edema. Neostigmine is discontinued when gastrointestinal motility returns. Neostigmine may be harmful when given in small intestinal disease because it may increase secretion into the gastrointestinal tract and has been shown not to be effective in producing progressive contractions of the small intestine.

Aftercare. Alternating skin sutures should be removed from abdominal incisions at two weeks in uncomplicated cases. The remaining sutures should

---

*Some authors recommend the use of 0.3 as an estimate of this fluid space.
†Eltradd, Haver-Lockhart, Shawnee, KS

*Heparin, Elkins-Sinn, Inc., Cherry Hill, NJ
†Calcium Gluconate, Quality Plus Products Co., Fort Dodge, IA
‡Stiglyn, Pitman-Moore, Inc., Washington Crossing, NJ

be removed two days later. In order to minimize herniation and evisceration, exercise should be restricted by confining the horse in a large stall or small paddock and hand walking the horse for one month. The horse may then be confined in a larger paddock for an additional two months. The owner should be advised not to ride the horse for a period of four to six months after surgery.

Acknowledgement

The author would like to thank Gary P. Carlson, DVM, PhD for assistance in preparation of this manuscript.

Supplemental Readings

Donawick, W. J.: Fluid, electrolyte, and acid-base therapy in large animal surgery. *In* Jennings, P. B., Jr. (ed.): The Practice of Large Animal Surgery. Philadelphia, W. B. Saunders Company, 1984, pp. 99–128.

Kohn, C. W.: Preparative management of the equine patient with an abdominal crisis. Vet. Clin. North Am. (Large Anim. Pract.), *1*:289, 1979.

Rose, R. J.: A physiological approach to fluid and electrolyte therapy in the horse. Equine Vet. J., *13*:7, 1981.

Anesthesia of the Horse with Colic

Cynthia M. Trim, ATHENS, GEORGIA

Intestinal obstruction results in changes that alter the animal's response to anesthetic drugs. Preoperative treatment to correct these abnormalities reduces the risk of complications associated with general anesthesia.

PREPARATION FOR ANESTHESIA

Fluid loss into the gastrointestinal tract results in decreases in blood volume and in cardiac output. The hypovolemia should be corrected before induction of anesthesia because anesthesia causes a severe decrease in cardiac output, even in the healthy horse. In a study of 341 operations for colic, the survival rate was decreased when the hematocrit (PCV) exceeded 45 per cent and plasma protein concentration (PP) was less than 5.4 gm per dl at the time of induction. The concentration of plasma protein should be serially monitored during fluid replacement.

Metabolic acidosis, hypokalemia, and hypocalcemia may also occur in the colic patient and adversely affect cardiovascular function under anesthesia. The metabolic status of horses with colic ranges from alkalosis to acidosis. An arterial pH of less than 7.20 decreases myocardial contractility and reduces myocardial responsiveness to catecholamines. Therefore, if metabolic acidosis is suspected, sodium bicarbonate can be given at 1.5 mEq per kg intravenously over 30 minutes. Large doses of sodium bicarbonate should be administered only after metabolic status has been determined using total CO_2 (TCO_2) or pH and blood gas analysis.

When available, laboratory determinations of blood potassium and calcium concentrations should be included in the preoperative assessment. Hypokalemia that may occur from loss of potassium into the lumen of distended bowel results in decreased myocardial contractility and predisposes to hypotension and ventricular dysrhythmias. Potassium chloride should be added to the intravenous fluids of hypokalemic patients and infused at a rate not exceeding 0.5 mEq per kg per hr. Hypocalcemia is associated with hypotension and dysrhythmias and therefore should be corrected before induction of anesthesia.

Increased intra-abdominal pressure severely decreases the cardiac output in dogs, and this appears to be true also for horses. Ventilation is also restricted. Therefore, the abdominal pressure should be reduced as much as possible before anesthesia by removing gastric fluid and gas by stomach tube, and by cecal trocharization if necessary.

EQUIPMENT

Two important aspects of anesthesia of the colic patient are inserting an endotracheal tube to produce an airtight seal in the trachea and enriching the inspired air with oxygen. The first is necessary because passive regurgitation of gastric fluid may occur during anesthesia, and aspiration into the lungs results in fatal pneumonia. Oxygen supplementation is essential because the anesthetized horse on its back is unable to maintain adequate arterial oxygenation while breathing air. This hypoxemia is the combined result of anesthetic depression of ventilation and circulation, interference with chest expansion, and endotoxin-induced changes in pulmonary function. Ventilation can be assisted using a demand valve attached to an oxygen cylinder, and anesthesia maintained with injectable drugs. It is more usual and advisable, however, to connect the horse to an anesthesia machine and maintain anesthesia with an inhalation agent such as halothane in oxygen. Artificial ventilation can then be provided by manual compression of the rebreathing bag, or by the use of a mechanical ventilator.

Because severe cardiovascular depression is common in anesthetized colic patients, the measurement of arterial blood pressure can be a valuable guide to the administration of anesthetics and adjunct drugs. Equipment to monitor blood pressure indirectly can be purchased relatively inexpensively,* or more sophisticated units† are available. Since it is easy to insert a needle or catheter into a facial artery, direct measurement of blood pressure offers the additional advantage of visual observation of second-by-second changes. Although mean arterial pressure can be measured inexpensively using an aneroid manometer, veterinarians in practices with a high case load would find investment in an electrical transducer with oscilloscopic display worthwhile.‡

An electrocardiogram is of additional help by giving early warning of dysrhythmias. Increased size or reversed polarity in the T wave, or ST segment depression, may indicate a deterioration in ventricular function and the need for a change in the anesthetic management.

ANESTHESIA TECHNIQUES

A variety of drug combinations have been used successfully for anesthesia of the colic patient. Anesthesia for horses with little physiologic change from normal is similar to that used for elective surgery. In other patients, it is extremely important to assess the degree of central nervous system and cardiovascular depression, and reduce drug dosages from those normally used in a healthy horse. Acepromazine is usually avoided because its alpha-blocking properties increase the difficulty of treating hypotension under anesthesia. Atropine is not used, except to treat bradycardia, because it decreases intestinal motility. In our clinical setting, tractable

---

*Parks Electronics, Aloha, OR

†Dinamap, Critikon, Tampa, Florida; Accutorr, Datascope, Paramus, NJ

‡Datascope, Paramus, NJ; Space Labs (Tektronix), Chatsworth, CA

colic patients having minor physiologic abnormalities are most frequently anesthetized with guaifenesin and thiopental or thiamylal. The horse receives no premedication, or is lightly sedated with xylazine, 0.35 to 0.5 mg per kg intravenously. Anesthesia is induced by intravenous infusion of a mixture of 1 gm thiobarbiturate and 50 gm guaifenesin in 500 ml of water. Up to 110 mg per kg of guaifenesin is usually necessary for induction. This barbiturate dosage is half of that used in a healthy horse.

Very sick animals do not receive barbiturates; neuroleptanalgesia is used for premedication. Xylazine, 0.35 to 0.6 mg per kg, is given intravenously with either pentazocine, 0.3 mg per kg, butorphanol, 0.03 to 0.05 mg per kg, or oxymorphone, 0.01 to 0.02 mg per kg. Recumbency is induced by an infusion of guaifenesin, sufficient to allow endotracheal intubation. The addition of a narcotic deepens the sedation, thus reducing the amount of halothane required for anesthesia, without further depressing the cardiovascular system.

When ketamine is used for induction of anesthesia, the dose of xylazine usually used to prevent the excitement induced by ketamine may cause an excessive decrease in cardiac output. A more satisfactory alternative is to incorporate guaifenesin, thus allowing a reduction in the xylazine dose. An example would be premedication with xylazine, 0.45 to 0.6 mg per kg intravenously followed by guaifenesin, 50 mg per kg, and ketamine, 1.7 mg per kg.

In each case, anesthesia is usually maintained by halothane in oxygen; however, either enflurane or isoflurane is occasionally substituted for halothane in the sicker animals. Isoflurane does not decrease the cardiac output as much as halothane, although the arterial blood pressure will be equally depressed. Recovery from isoflurane anesthesia is usually quicker than from halothane.

Balanced anesthesia, incorporating a nondepolarizing neuromuscular blocking drug such as pancuronium, may be used. Some anesthesiologists have experienced difficulty in reversing neuromuscular blockade following pancuronium in horses with colic. Two new drugs, atracurium and vecuronium, are currently being investigated in the horse and may prove more useful than pancuronium.

Abortion occurring after anesthesia in a pregnant mare may be attributed to factors arising from colic, such as catecholamine release from pain, reduced uterine blood flow from hypovolemia, endotoxemia, and metabolic acidosis. Anesthesia may result in abortion if oxygen delivery to the fetus is inadequate due to decreased uterine blood flow or low arterial PO_2 in the mare. Xylazine has been demonstrated to cause uterine contractions in the cow. Use of nitrous oxide in late pregnancy has been associated with premature parturition. In late pregnancy, when the mare is on her back, the weight of the uterus may compress the caudal vena cava and result in decreased venous return and cardiac output. The blood pressure should be monitored as the mare is thus positioned, and if necessary, the mare tilted to shift the weight of the uterus off the vena cava.

Anesthesia in foals may be induced and maintained with halothane or isoflurane. The foal may be premedicated with low doses of xylazine (0.5 mg per kg) and pentazocine (0.3 mg per kg), or diazepam (0.05 mg per kg) and pentazocine (0.3 mg per kg) to facilitate induction.

ANESTHETIC MANAGEMENT

Gastric fluid should be removed by stomach tube immediately before the start of anesthesia to minimize the risk of regurgitation before tracheal intubation. The stomach tube should be left in place to act as a conduit for gastric fluid should regurgitation occur. Horses producing large volumes of gastric reflux may be supported on the sternum after induction of anesthesia, until the trachea is intubated and the cuff inflated, to reduce the risk of regurgitation and aspiration.

Extremely depressed patients will benefit from preoxygenation. Using rubber tubing inserted six inches up the nose, oxygen is delivered for a few minutes before and during induction of anesthesia at a rate of 15 L per min for a 450-kg horse. This maneuver produces higher than normal arterial oxygen concentration during induction of anesthesia and partially compensates for the decreases in ventilation and cardiac output produced by the anesthetic drugs. When the horse is anesthetized, oxygen is then supplied through the endotracheal tube.

In colic patients anesthesia should begin with a lower vaporizer setting than is usually used on a healthy horse. The patient's tolerance of anesthesia should be closely observed, particularly during the first ten minutes. Frequently colic patients have a lower requirement for anesthetic drugs than would be expected from the clinical assessment.

The arterial blood pressure or strength of the peripheral pulse should be monitored closely after the horse is rolled onto its back. The weight of full, distended bowel can compress the abdominal aorta or vena cava and cause sudden hypotension.

During anesthesia, the mucous membrane color and capillary refill time, pulse rate and rhythm, and arterial blood pressure must be monitored. Animals with brick-red mucous membranes preoperatively may have a normal or high cardiac output. They may initially need a much higher dosage of anesthetic drugs than expected, but the cardiovascular function of these animals may deteriorate suddenly.

Horses with pale pink or pale blue membranes probably have a low cardiac output and will need cardiovascular support during anesthesia.

Adequate cardiac output and blood pressure are produced by keeping the administration of anesthetic drugs to a minimum, maintaining blood volume, and avoiding acidemia, and through the use of cardiac stimulating drugs. Balanced electrolyte solutions such as Ringer's lactated solution should be infused intravenously at 10 ml per kg per hr, or at a rate to maintain the PCV below 45 per cent. The PCV and PP should be checked every hour. When available, plasma should be given to prevent PP decreasing below 4 gm per dl. If arterial pressure and peripheral perfusion remain poor, intravenous infusion of dopamine or dobutamine (3 to 5 μg per kg per min) may be indicated. These drugs increase cardiac output by increasing myocardial contractility and also cause peripheral vasodilation. If the heart rate increases more than a few beats per minute, the infusion should be stopped until the heart rate slows, then resumes at a slower rate. In some instances the arterial pressure may be slow to rise, but evidence of increased cardiac output should be present in the improved mucous membrane color and more rapid capillary refill time. These drugs are extremely potent and the infusion rate should be carefully monitored. These drugs are not very effective in the presence of metabolic or respiratory acidosis or hypovolemia and will not take the place of adequate preoperative preparation of the patient.

The rate and depth of breathing should be assessed repeatedly during anesthesia. Mild hypoventilation may not be deleterious because increased arterial carbon dioxide concentration stimulates the sympathetic nervous system resulting in increased cardiac output and blood pressure. Light anesthesia with spontaneous breathing is therefore likely to result in a higher cardiac output and blood pressure than occurs with controlled ventilation. Severe hypoventilation on the other hand causes acidosis and decreases the cardiac output. Many colic patients have distended bowel and increased abdominal pressure, which limit spontaneous breathing; artificial ventilation is required in these instances. Although recommendations for respiratory rate and tidal volume vary, a rate of 10 breaths per minute with 11 ml per kg per tidal volume is usually effective in achieving an arterial carbon dioxide concentration of 40 mm Hg. In healthy horses this tidal volume is provided using a peak inspiratory pressure of about 22 cm of water. Horses with abdominal distention will require a higher pressure to deliver an adequate volume. Pressures exceeding 40 cm H_2O are avoided because they usually cause severe cardiovascular depression.

Adverse cardiopulmonary effects from the release of vasoactive substances should be anticipated if ischemic bowel is observed when the abdomen is opened. Unless recently administered, flunixin meglumine (1 to 2 mg per kg intravenously) should be given before the bowel is manipulated and the anesthetic administration should be decreased. Hypotension often follows the handling of severely ischemic intestine and metabolic acidosis may develop. If facilities for pH and blood gas analysis are available, it is advisable to submit arterial blood for analysis every 20 to 30 minutes. Sodium bicarbonate should then be administered according to the results, using the following formula: base deficit × 0.3 × kg body weight = mEq to be infused.

CARE DURING RECOVERY

At the end of surgery, the horse may become hypoxemic when disconnected from the anesthesia machine and allowed to breathe room air. The transition from controlled ventilation to spontaneous breathing should occur when the depth of anesthesia has been lightened and while the animal is still attached to 100 per cent oxygen. After the horse is disconnected from the anesthesia machine, oxygen can be insufflated (15 L per min for a 450-kg horse) through tubing placed first inside the endotracheal tube, and after extubation in the ventral nasal meatus. An oxygen demand valve can be used while the endotracheal tube is in place. The nasal turbinates should be checked for edema before extubation of the trachea. If swelling is present, a clear airway can be provided by inserting a small endotracheal tube through the ventral nasal meatus into the trachea. The edema is primarily the result of congestion from the effects of gravity, and can be relieved by propping up the nose at 45 degrees to the horizontal for 15 to 30 minutes.

Recovery may be smoother in excitable animals if xylazine, 0.1 to 0.2 mg per kg, is injected intravenously at the time of extubation. Depending on the facilities available, the horse may be left alone to stand by itself or assisted with the use of a tail rope. The rectal temperature should be checked after the horse is standing, and a blanket applied if it is less than 36.4° C (97.5° F). Medical management of fluid and electrolyte balance should be resumed.

Supplemental Readings

McDonell, W. N.: General anesthesia for equine gastrointestinal and obstetric procedures. Vet. Clin. North Am. (Large Anim. Pract.), 3:163, 1981.
Pascoe, P. J., McDonell, W. N., Trim, C. M., and Van Gorder, J.: Mortality rates and associated factors in equine colic operations—A retrospective study of 341 operations. Can. Vet. J., 24:76, 1983.
Trim, C. M., Moore, J. N., and White, N. A.: Cardiopulmonary effects of dopamine hydrochloride in anaesthetized horses. Equine Vet. J., 17:41, 1985.

Gastric Diseases

G. Kent Carter, COLLEGE STATION, TEXAS

GASTRIC DILATATION

Dilatation of the equine stomach, which is often encountered in horses suffering from abdominal crises, may be either primary or secondary. Primary gastric dilatation is most commonly observed following overeating of highly fermentable feeds, particularly concentrated grain rations, although pelleted and cubed rations have also been incriminated. Dilatation associated with grain overload is further complicated by an increased osmotic pressure within the stomach and resulting fluid accumulation. Gastric dilatation may result from excessive consumption of water following strenuous exercise or a period of water deprivation. Less severe gastric dilatation may be observed following aerophagia while cribbing or eating immediately after strenuous exercise.

Secondary gastric dilatation occurs more frequently than primary dilatation and results from intestinal reflux into the stomach. Although all cases of intestinal obstruction can evolve into gastric dilatation, it occurs most commonly with small intestinal obstructions or ileus. In general the higher the obstruction, the greater the amount of reflux. Secondary gastric dilatation also occurs in horses with acute necrotizing pancreatitis, most likely due to concurrent proximal small intestinal damage.

Clinical Signs. The most consistent clinical observation is abdominal pain. The severity of pain and clinical deterioration are proportional to the severity and duration of dilatation. In cases of secondary gastric dilatation, clinical signs are often dependent upon the primary intestinal lesion. Clinical signs include increased heart and respiratory rates, sweating, rolling, depression, and other signs referable to gastrointestinal pain. Abnormal postures such as "dog sitting" are frequently described but not commonly observed.

Although retching and vomiting are uncommon in horses, they may be observed in cases of gastric dilatation. Eructation, retching, vomiting, or the presence of ingesta at the nostrils warrant consideration of severe gastric dilatation. Other causes of ingesta at the nostrils such as pharyngeal paralysis or esophageal choke, should be ruled out.

Signs of hemoconcentration, dehydration, and decreased tissue perfusion will vary depending upon the severity and duration of intestinal disease. Laminitis may occur in conjunction with gastric dilatation, particularly in those cases associated with overeating of concentrates.

Diagnosis. Gastric dilatation is best confirmed by passage of a nasogastric tube and the subsequent reflux of a variable volume of gastric fluid and gas. The largest diameter stomach tube that can be comfortably passed should be used. If the animal shows resentment or exhibits pain during passage, or resistance is encountered at the cardia, use a smaller diameter tube. The tube should not be forcibly inserted, since esophageal or gastric perforation may occur. The anatomic arrangement of the distal esophagus and cardia may be altered because of the gastric distention so that patience and persistence are often necessary to pass the nasogastric tube. If pain or resistance is encountered at the distal esophagus, infusion of 35 to 50 ml of 2 per cent lidocaine may be helpful.

When the distended stomach is entered, gastric fluid and gases usually flow spontaneously. However, the nasogastric tube may require repositioning to locate pockets of fluid. Movement of the tube, aspiration, and initiation of a siphon by administering small volumes of water and lowering the end of the tube may be necessary to initiate flow.

Differentiating primary from secondary gastric dilatation is important in evaluation and management of the patient. If the dilatation is secondary to small intestinal obstruction, decompression of the stomach will only partially and temporarily alleviate the problem. Gastric decompression in primary dilatation should achieve a cure, if secondary metabolic abnormalities and serious complications such as laminitis and gastric rupture have not occurred.

A history of management problems such as acute concentrate or water overload or habits such as cribbing will be helpful in identifying causes of primary gastric dilatation. Complete gastric decompression and evaluation of the contents may be helpful in identifying overeating as a cause. Determining pH of the reflux fluid may be misleading; therefore, a complete evaluation of the patient should be done to determine the source of gastric reflux.

On rectal palpation, distended loops of small intestine suggest that gastric dilatation is secondary to intestinal obstruction. Some conditions produce minimal rectal palpation changes yet result in significant gastric reflux. The spleen may be displaced caudally by the distended stomach and palpated in the caudal abdomen. Since the spleen can be palpated in most horses and its location may be affected by other conditions, this finding is not diagnostic for gastric dilatation.

Duration of gastric reflux may be helpful in differentiating primary from secondary gastric dilatation. Reflux from a primary gastric dilatation is generally of shorter duration than that of secondary causes. In cases of secondary dilatation, an exploratory laparotomy might be necessary to determine the cause.

Therapy. Initial therapy for either primary or secondary gastric dilatation should be decompression via nasogastric tube. If it is not possible to decompress the stomach with a nasogastric tube, surgical intervention may be considered. Removal of gas from the distended stomach during the laparotomy may allow passage of a nasogastric tube and enhance decompression of the stomach. Although surgical approaches to the equine stomach have been described, it is relatively inaccessible and gastrotomy may produce significant peritoneal contamination.

If copious amounts of reflux are obtained, the stomach tube should be left in place and the exteriorized portion taped to the halter. The animal should be checked for reflux every one to four hours, depending on the volume of fluid being obtained. The tube should be manipulated and a small amount of water administered to initiate a siphon each time the tube is checked because even when the tube is left indwelling, assistance is often required to achieve adequate evacuation. Most horses will tolerate an indwelling tube; however, in some individuals it is necessary to insert the tube each time that monitoring for reflux is done.

Administration of mineral oil or other medications via the nasogastric tube is contraindicated when gastric reflux is present. The administration of medications into the stomach may aggravate the gastric dilatation and make the removal of gastric fluids more difficult.

Primary gastric dilatation usually subsides fairly rapidly following removal of the cause. Secondary gastric dilatation usually subsides when the intestinal obstruction or cause of ileus is corrected. However, adynamic ileus may persist for several days and require decompression of the stomach at two- to four-hour intervals. There is individual variation and careful patient monitoring is important. An increasing heart rate or signs of pain usually indicate the need for decompression.

Intravenous fluids and electrolyte maintenance are important for supportive care of the patient. Most horses with gastric dilatation and reflux have variable degrees of hemoconcentration, dehydration, hypokalemia, hyponatremia, and hypochloremia. In contrast to most other gastrointestinal diseases, gastric dilatation and reflux are often associated with alkalosis due to intraluminal sequestration and loss of electrolytes and hydrogen ions. Metabolic acidosis can occur in gastric dilatation following intestinal obstruction. Therefore, acid-base and electrolyte evaluations are helpful in selecting and monitoring fluid and electrolyte therapy for cases of persistent gastric reflux. Intravenous nutritional support should be an adjunct to therapy, but it is difficult and expensive to meet the nutritional requirements of an adult horse by intravenous hyperalimentation. For further information, specific chapters on these subjects should be consulted (see p. 33 and 424).

Therapy with various pharmacologic agents that stimulate gastric emptying and small intestinal motility is often attempted to decrease the amount and duration of gastric reflux. Neostigmine is an anticholinesterase drug that has been used extensively to treat nonobstructive ileus in the horse. However, in a recent study neostigmine did not increase propulsive motility in the jejunum, and it was concluded that clinical use of the drug for promoting motility in horses with adynamic ileus of the jejunum is not warranted. Panthenol is an alcohol analogue of pantothenic acid that is a precursor of coenzyme A. Theoretically this drug should increase the formation of acetylcholine and thereby stimulate intestinal smooth muscle. Panthenol is often used to stimulate intestinal motility in horses with adynamic ileus. However, in an experimental model panthenol had no effect on intestinal motility and cannot be recommended for use as an intestinal stimulant in the horse. Metoclopramide, a derivative of procainamide that stimulates gastric emptying in humans, has been used to stimulate gastric emptying in the horse. However, no data have been generated to determine the proper dosage and benefit of metaclopramide in the horse.

Secondary gastric dilatation due to intestinal obstruction warrants surgical correction. Persistent gastric reflux is only one of several parameters consistent with intestinal obstruction, and findings from other diagnostic procedures must be considered in making a decision for surgical intervention.

Prognosis. The prognosis for primary gastric dilatation depends on the etiology, severity, and duration of the disease. Most horses with primary gastric dilatation do well if treated before development of complications such as laminitis or gastric rupture. The prognosis for secondary gastric dila-

tations is determined by the cause of intestinal reflux.

GASTRIC RUPTURE

Gastric rupture is a not uncommon serious complication of severe or untreated gastric distention. Rupture may occur from overdistention and inability of the horse to vomit efficiently, or secondary to falling to the ground in abdominal pain or in terminal movements. A distended stomach may also be perforated during nasogastric tube manipulation. Sudden relief of pain followed by anxiety, profuse sweating, and hemoconcentration suggest gastric rupture. Deterioration is rapid with profound tachycardia, severe nonresponsive hypovolemic shock, cyanotic mucous membranes, and a prolonged capillary refill time. Death follows rapidly.

Antemortem diagnosis of gastric rupture is made from the history, clinical signs, and finding of intestinal contents in the peritoneal cavity. Ingesta obtained during abdominocentesis is not diagnostic for gastric rupture, as intestines are commonly punctured during the procedure. Fluid obtained by abdominocentesis following bowel rupture will usually have more inflammatory cells than a sample obtained by inadvertent intestinal puncture. However, this observation may not be true in cases of acute rupture. Rectal palpation may reveal a gritty feel to the serosa of the bowel and peritoneal lining if a viscus has ruptured and peritonitis has occurred. Some horses will develop rectal and intestinal emphysema following gastric rupture. If abdominocentesis findings are equivocal and other parameters suggest that surgical intervention is necessary, gastric rupture may be confirmed by laparotomy. Therapy for gastric rupture in the horse has been universally unsuccessful.

An antemortem rupture examined at necropsy almost always is seen to occur along the greater curvature of the stomach, to have hemorrhagic margins, and to be accompanied by diffuse peritonitis. Postmortem ruptures lack the diffuse peritonitis and hemorrhagic tear line and may occur anywhere on the stomach. Perforations made by a nasogastric tube are usually small holes, whereas tears are extensive.

GASTRIC IMPACTIONS

Gastric impaction due to accumulation of dry ingesta in the stomach has been described in horses. Although abnormal diets are often incriminated, cases of gastric impaction have also been reported in horses eating normal diets. Abnormally coarse roughages are most often incriminated in gastric impactions but impactions of persimmon seeds and mesquite beans have also been identified. Gastric impaction due to pyloric stenosis and foreign bodies have also been described.

Clinical signs vary depending on the cause and severity of gastric impaction; acute abdominal pain temporarily responsive to systemic analgesics is common. Chronic recurrent colic, weight loss, and inappetence are observed with pyloric stenosis or gastric foreign bodies. Bruxism and excessive salivation have also been observed in horses with pyloric stenosis.

Diagnosis is based upon clinical signs and ruling out of other causes of colic. Gastroscopy may be beneficial if adequate visualization of the stomach is possible. The reported cases of primary gastric impaction have been diagnosed at surgery during an exploratory laparotomy. Lesions such as pyloric stenosis or gastric foreign bodies are often identified at necropsy.

Therapy. Therapy is best achieved during surgery after the diagnosis of gastric impaction is made.

Infusion of from one to four liters of distilled water into the impacted mass through a 12-gauge 3″ needle and manual massage may break up the impaction. Gastric lavage via a nasogastric tube may also soften the impaction. Surgical relief of a gastric impaction by gastrotomy has been described in a pony. The prognosis for such a procedure in an adult horse would be less favorable due to the relative inaccessibility of the stomach and the potential for peritoneal contamination.

Supplemental Readings

Adams, S. B., Lamar, C. H., and Masty, J.: Motility of the distal portion of the jejunum and pelvic flexure in ponies: Effects of six drugs. Am. J. Vet Res., 45:795, 1984.

Barclay, W. P., Foerner, J. J., Phillips, T. N., and MacHarg, M. A.: Primary Gastric Impaction in the Horse. J. Am. Vet. Med. Assoc., 181:682, 1982.

Becht, J. L.: Gastric diseases. In Robinson, N. E. (ed.): Current Therapy in Equine Medicine. Philadelphia, W. B. Saunders Company, 1983, pp. 196–200.

Whitlock, R. H.: The stomach and forestomach, part I, Equine stomach diseases. In Anderson, N. (ed.): Veterinary Gastroenterology. Philadelphia, Lea & Febiger, 1980, pp. 392–395.

Duodenitis–Proximal Jejunitis

Ronald B. Blackwell, WINTERVILLE, GEORGIA

Duodenitis–proximal jejunitis describes a clinical syndrome previously referred to as anterior enteritis. Colic is a prominent early clinical sign. Other clinical signs include gastric reflux, distention of the small intestine, lack of borborygmi, and dehydration. An etiologic agent has not been identified, however, clostridial toxins are thought to be involved in the pathogenesis of the syndrome.

Gross pathologic lesions observed during surgery or at necropsy are limited to the proximal small intestine. Distention of the small intestine with a reddish-brown fluid, and multifocal petechial and ecchymotic hemorrhages of the serosal surface are the cardinal lesions. The hemorrhagic areas are interspersed with paler serosa varying in color from pale pink to light yellow with white or darker yellow streaks. Although similar changes occur in the stomach, no lesions are observed distal to the jejunum.

HISTORY AND CLINICAL SIGNS

The syndrome occurs most commonly in adult horses. Signs of mild to severe abdominal pain are most often reported. The signs of colic are generally acute in onset and are followed by depression.

Signs of severe depression or mild to severe abdominal pain are usually present. Most horses have an increased body temperature (over 38.5° C) and an elevated pulse rate (over 60 per min). Relief of signs of pain is often provided by nasogastric intubation and removal of a large volume (>12 L) of orange-brown tinged gastric reflux.

Signs of insufficient peripheral perfusion are prominent. Pulse rate is elevated, capillary refill time is prolonged, and mucous membranes are injected. Loss of skin turgor indicates 8 to 10 per cent dehydration.

Rectal palpation identifies distended small intestine in most affected horses. Small bowel distention has also been identified by radiography. Lack of borborygmi is a consistent finding.

CLINICAL LABORATORY FINDINGS

Elevation of the packed cell volume (>42 per cent) and total plasma protein (>8.0 gm per dl) reflect the animal's fluid losses. The white blood cell count is variable.

Blood pH most commonly is normal but metabolic acidosis may occur with severe dehydration. Early in the syndrome, gastric reflux may produce metabolic alkalosis.

When there is necrosis of the intestinal wall, the peritoneal fluid becomes serosanguinous to hemorrhagic. In most peritoneal fluid samples, however, the fluid is yellow and clear or cloudy. Generally, peritoneal white blood cell counts are normal. In one report, 18 of 19 horses had peritoneal white blood cell counts less than 10,000 cells per μ. Elevation of protein levels in the peritoneal fluid is consistent. In the study of 19 cases, 17 horses had peritoneal protein levels greater than 3.0 grams per dl.

THERAPY

Acute Disease. Because the etiologic agent is unknown, management of horses with a diagnosis of duodenitis-proximal jejunitis remains symptomatic. Supportive therapy centers on gastric decompression, fluid and electrolyte replacement, analgesia, antimicrobials, and ancillary therapy.

Constant and efficient removal of fluids sequestered in the stomach is essential. This prevents gastric or intestinal rupture and provides relief from pain caused by visceral distention. Large volumes of fluid are generally gathered with repeated attempts at gastric decompression. The nasogastric tube should be sutured in place and regular attempts at decompression made. Manipulation of the tube and siphoning is recommended to initiate the flow of gastric reflux.

The movement of large volumes of fluid into the gastric and intestinal lumina results in severe extracellular fluid losses, which must be replaced by intravenous fluid therapy. A balanced electrolyte solution should be used. Administration of sodium bicarbonate solution will be dictated by evaluation of the acid-base status of the patient.

Immediate relief of pain is provided by gastric decompression. In the early phase of the syndrome when colic is severe, xylazine may be needed. In most horses, adequate analgesia is provided by the administration of flunixin meglumine.

Penicillin in large doses is thought to be beneficial. Addition of an aminoglycoside antibiotic broadens the antimicrobial spectrum and may prove useful in avoiding complications such as septicemia. Heparin is administered in an attempt to stimulate the monocyte-macrophage system during the possible period of bacterial and/or endotoxin absorption. Clostridial antitoxins provide no benefit.

Chronic Disease. Even in the absence of abdominal pain, gastric reflux can continue for several days. During this time, the attitude of the patient generally improves but the continued reflux necessitates gastric decompression and rehydration by intravenous fluid therapy.

Surgical procedures to provide for gastric decompression and rehydration include intestinal bypass by either duodenocecostomy or duodenojejunostomy. Complications of these surgical procedures include the development of intraperitoneal adhesions producing signs of colic. The symptomatic supportive therapy of the patient with chronic disease often offers a more favorable prognosis than does surgical management.

MORTALITY

The mortality rate is 50 to 70 per cent, even with supportive therapy. Duodenitis-proximal jejunitis presents several signs that have traditionally been interpreted as indicative of intestinal strangulation and obstruction. These signs include acute onset of severe pain, gastric reflux, absence of borborygmi, intestinal distention, and changes in the peritoneal fluid. Attention must be paid to signs seen in duodenitis–proximal jejunitis and not generally associated with the diseases of the abdomen requiring surgery. These signs include fever, depression in the absence of or following pain, leukocytosis, and elevation in the total protein of the peritoneal fluid without a concomitant rise in white blood cell count. The mortality increases substantially when horses with duodenitis–proximal jejunitis undergo general anesthesia for exploratory laparotomy.

COMPLICATIONS

Laminitis occurs commonly in horses surviving the initial phase of the syndrome. Other complications include pneumonia and pleuritis, hepatitis, multifocal abscessation of lymph nodes, and intraperitoneal adhesion formation. With the high mortality rate and incidence of complications, duodenitis–proximal jejunitis is a fatal syndrome. In the absence of a specific test for the syndrome, duodentis–proximal jejunitis must be included in the differential diagnosis in any horse presenting with signs of small intestinal obstruction. Early recognition of affected horses leads to initiation of supportive symptomatic therapy, which provides the best prognosis for survival of the patient without development of complications.

Supplemental Readings

Blackwell, R. B., and White, N. A.: Duodenitis-proximal jejunitis in the horse. Proc. Equine Colic Res. Symp., University of Georgia, 1982, p 106.

McClure, J. J.: Anterior enteritis. *In* Robinson, N. E. (ed.): Currrent Therapy in Equine Medicine. Philadelphia, W. B. Saunders Company, 1983, p 214.

Acute Pancreatitis

Jill J. McClure, BATON ROUGE, LOUISIANA

Both acute and chronic pancreatitis have been described in horses. Chronic pancreatitis is generally associated with failure of the endocrine functions of the pancreas and the development of diabetes mellitus, whereas acute pancreatitis is characterized by a fulminating syndrome of abdominal pain, gastric distention, and shock.

Acute pancreatitis is rarely diagnosed in horses, and the prevalence may be underestimated for several reasons. Antemortem diagnosis is difficult on the basis of clinical and laboratory findings, the pancreas is not easily visualized by routine surgical approaches to the abdomen, and the pancreas is easily overlooked at necropsy, particularly if gastric rupture has occurred. Whereas a spectrum of pathologic changes with variable mortality rates is recognized in pancreatitis in humans, only the most severe cases that result in death are likely to be confirmed as pancreatitis in horses.

ETIOLOGY

The cause of naturally occurring acute pancreatitis in horses is unknown. In other species, pancreatitis has been associated with the administration of drugs such as furosemide and corticosteroids, pancreatic duct obstructions, vitamin E–selenium deficiencies, vitamin A deficiency, methionine deficiency, vitamin D intoxication, bacterial and viral infections, toxins, migrating parasites, immune-mediated damage, and reflux of enteric juice into the gland secondary to small intestine obstructions.

CLINICAL SIGNS

Hallmark clinical features of acute pancreatitis are moderate to severe abdominal pain and hypovolemic shock. Gastric distention, which contributes to pain, and cardiovascular compromise are typically present and voluminous amounts of gastroenteric fluid are often recovered via nasogastric tube. Release of vasoactive substances from the pancreas and loss of blood and body fluids either into the gastrointestinal tract or into the abdominal cavity also contribute to shock and dehydration. Signs of cardiovascular compromise including tachycardia, tachypnea, prolonged capillary refill time, congested mucous membranes, decreased temperature of the distal extremities, and sweating may all be present. Abdominal sounds on auscultation are variably present. Rectal examination is generally unremarkable.

Peritoneal fluid varies from brownish-colored flocculent fluid to frank hemorrhage. Increased numbers of neutrophils may be present as a result of inflammation. The gross or microscopic appearance of fat globules in peritoneal fluid is common in human acute pancreatitis and may be a useful diagnostic feature in evaluating equine peritoneal fluid.

LABORATORY TESTS

Antemortem confirmation of pancreatitis is difficult in all species, and a diagnosis is often reached by excluding other causes of abdominal pain. Laboratory tests that may be of value in the horse include serum amylase and lipase activity, peritoneal fluid amylase activity, and fractional excretion of amylase (FEam), also called per cent creatinine clearance ratio of amylase. Reference values should be established for each laboratory because testing methods vary widely. The following values are given to serve as a basis for discussing expected changes in pancreatitis and may not be directly applicable to all laboratories. Serum amylase activity for normal horses generally ranges from 15 to 20 IU per L and values less than 50 IU are considered within normal limits. Peritoneal fluid amylase activity is usually slightly lower than serum activity. Normal horses have serum lipase activity of less than 0.2 Sigma-Teitz (S-T) units per L.

The fractional excretion of amylase (FEam) is calculated by the following formula:

$$\frac{urine\ amylase}{serum\ amylase} \times \frac{serum\ creatinine}{urine\ creatinine} \times 100 = FEam$$

FEam in normal horses is less than 1 per cent.

Hyperamylasemia, hyperlipasemia, increased peritoneal fluid amylase activity, and increased

FEam are expected laboratory findings in pancreatitis. However, pancreatic enzyme activity can be difficult to interpret for several reasons. The enzymes are not exclusively of pancreatic origin and increased activities may reflect damage of other organs. Various insults to the gastrointestinal tract, especially the small intestine, may result in leakage of enzymes into the general circulation from the lumen of the bowel. Renal dysfunction may result in decreased urinary excretion of amylase and therefore may contribute to elevated serum activity. The pancreas may suffer secondary ischemic damage as a result of bowel distention or hypovolemia or chemical damage from reflux of duodenal contents via the pancreatic duct into the gland in cases of small intestine distention.

The magnitude of increase in serum amylase and lipase activity may be helpful in differentiating increases due to pancreatitis from increases associated with other causes. In documented cases of pancreatitis confirmed at necropsy, amylase activity is often greater than 700 to 1000 IU per L and lipase activity may be greater than 3.5 S-T units per L, whereas serum enzyme activities in other gastrointestinal disease, although elevated, are generally less than this. Amylase activity may be elevated only transiently in humans with pancreatitis even though the inflammatory process is ongoing. Although the kinetics of the hyperamylasemia in horses has not been examined, samples for enzyme activity will probably be most informative when collected early in the course of the disease. Increased renal clearance of amylase may result in rapid return of serum amylase activity to normal. The use of FEam circumvents this problem; however, an increase in this ratio, like serum enzyme activity, is not specific for pancreatitis. Serum lipase activity remains elevated somewhat longer than serum amylase activity.

Other laboratory tests that are of value for monitoring the general condition of the patient include serum calcium, packed cell volume and/or hemoglobin, serum electrolytes, blood gases, serum urea nitrogen and creatinine, total and differential white blood cell counts.

MANAGEMENT

Management of acute pancreatitis is symptomatic. Continuous gastric decompression with a large-bore nasogastric tube is one of the most important therapeutic measures to prevent gastric rupture and minimize respiratory distress. Large volumes of intravenous fluids and electrolytes are required to maintain hydration and combat shock. Hypocalcemia may result from the deposition of calcium salts in tissues following fat necrosis. Calcium-containing solutions are indicated if serum calcium concentrations are low. Secondary bacterial infections are potentially a problem and prophylactic antimicrobial therapy is probably beneficial. Aminoglycosides should perhaps be avoided in light of hypovolemia and potential hypocalcemia. Analgesics are indicated for control of abdominal pain.

PROGNOSIS

The prognosis for patients with acute pancreatitis is apparently poor, although this may reflect bias in that most cases are diagnosed at necropsy. Wider use of appropriate laboratory tests may subsequently confirm that some medically responsive colics are indeed the result of pancreatitis.

Small Intestinal Strangulation Obstruction

James T. Robertson, COLUMBUS, OHIO

Interruption of the blood supply to the bowel with simultaneous luminal blockage produces intestinal strangulation obstruction (ISO) characterized by congestion and edema of the wall, accumulation of hemorrhagic fluid in the lumen, and loss of mucosal integrity of the affected segment of bowel. Damage to the mucosal barrier, which may be severe after only three hours of strangulation obstruction, allows penetration of bacteria and endotoxin through the bowel wall and their release into the peritoneal cavity. Left untreated, the horse becomes hypovolemic, develops endotoxemia and metabolic acidosis, and suffers circulatory collapse. Death will follow within 24 to 48 hours. Obviously, early recognition of a strangulating lesion is paramount for successful treatment.

TABLE 1. CLINICAL FINDINGS IN SMALL INTESTINAL STRANGULATION OBSTRUCTION

Pain: moderate to severe, intermittent to unrelenting, can be accompanied by depression

Cardiovascular status:
  a. Heart rate–> 60/minute and elevating
  b. Pulse–weak, thready, or not palpable
  c. Mucous membranes–injected, muddy, or cyanotic
  d. Capillary refill–> 2.5 to 3 seconds
  e. Packed cell volume–> 50 and increasing
  f. Plasma protein–> 8.0 gm/dl or decreased if protein is lost into the bowel or peritoneal cavity

Intestinal motility: hypomotile or amotile

Nasogastric tube: continuous small intestinal reflux; tube should be fixed in place to allow gastric decompression and prevent rupture

Rectal: distended loops of small intestine

Paracentesis: serosanguinous, cloudy fluid
  > 5–10,000 WBC, > 2.5 gm/dl protein
  Intracellular or free bacteria
  Ingesta in repeated taps indicates rupture

Blood gases: metabolic acidosis, increased blood lactate

Response to Medication: short-lived analgesia, lack of auscultable peristalsis, increased PCV and total protein despite intravenous fluids and bicarbonate

CLINICAL FINDINGS AND DIAGNOSIS

The clinical signs and findings associated with ISO are variable and their severity is dependent on the location of the lesion, the length of bowel involved, and the stage of the disease. The potential masking effects of potent analgesics and anti-inflammatory medications must be considered. Evaluation of a horse with a suspected ISO should include physical and rectal examinations, passage of a nasogastric tube, a complete blood count (CBC) with particular attention to packed cell volume (PCV) and total plasma protein (TP), peritoneal fluid analysis, and assessment of the degree of pain and the response to medication (Table 1).

The temperature is usually normal or slightly elevated as a result of increased exertion in response to abdominal pain. A subnormal temperature may be seen with shock. A fever greater than 39.4° C, combined with a marked neutrophilia or neutropenia, may signal a medical cause for ileus such as duodenitis and proximal jejunitis or *Salmonella* enteritis. Surgical intervention in these instances should be avoided. In some cases of anterior enteritis, in addition to the voluminous gastric reflux, there are distended loops of small intestine on rectal examination and peritoneal fluid changes that make differentiation from strangulating obstructions difficult.

Nasogastric intubation should be considered both a diagnostic and a therapeutic measure. Large volumes of fluid, two to three gallons with a pH greater than 6.0, can accumulate rapidly following severe small intestinal obstruction. Decompression of the stomach provides immediate relief of pain and prevents stomach rupture. A nasogastric tube, as large a diameter as possible, should be fixed in place to allow continuous drainage of reflux.

Normal abdominal fluid is clear, straw-colored, and has a white blood cell (WBC) count of 500 to 5000 per cu mm with a total protein content of less than 2.5 gm per dl. In the early stages of ISO, the peritoneal fluid becomes serosanguinous and slightly cloudy because of red cell leakage and increases in the WBC count (5,000 to 20,000 per cu mm) and TP content (more than 2.5 gm per dl). Initially, it appears that an elevated TP level may be the most sensitive indicator of peritoneal inflammation. As the disease progresses the WBC count becomes elevated in response to loss of the mucosal barrier and passage of bacteria and endotoxin into the peritoneal cavity. The TP level increases above 4.0 gm per dl as peritoneal inflammation becomes severe. At this point, the fluid is serosanguinous and quite cloudy.

An abdominocentesis yielding ingesta should be repeated because it is possible to inadvertently puncture a segment of bowel. Ingesta present in repeated taps indicates rupture of the stomach or intestine and a grave prognosis.

The decision to perform an exploratory celiotomy is based on an assessment of the composite of the variables examined. Although too much importance should not be placed on any single parameter, occasionally the decision to operate may be made on the weight of one finding such as intractable pain, abnormal findings on rectal examination or abdominocentesis.

SURGICAL MANAGEMENT

Volvulus and strangulation. Table 2 lists conditions that can cause small intestinal strangulation obstruction. The rotation of a segment of small intestine around the long axis of its mesentery produces a volvulus and strangulation obstruction. Predisposing lesions include small intestinal incarceration, infarction, fibrous adhesions, and the congenital remnant of a Meckel's diverticulum or a mesodiverticular band. In the absence of an obvious causative lesion other factors to be considered include dramatic dietary changes and verminous arteritis. The length of bowel involved is variable but the ileum is frequently incorporated because of its fixed position at the ileocecal junction. The direction of the twist can be determined by palpation of the affected mesentery. In severe cases, the twist is located at the root of the mesentery. The affected bowel is exteriorized, untwisted, and resected if necessary.

TABLE 2. EXAMPLES OF SMALL INTESTINAL STRANGULATION OBSTRUCTIONS

I. Volvulus
II. Intussusception
III. Internal hernias
    A. Epiploic foramen
    B. Mesenteric defect
    C. Gastrosplenic ligament
    D. Nephrosplenic ligament
    E. Cecocolic ligament
    F. Broad ligament
    G. Omental defect
    H. Fibrous bands and adhesions
IV. Diaphragmatic hernia
V. External hernias
    A. Inguinal hernia
    B. Umbilical hernia
VI. Pedunculated lipoma

Evaluation of intestinal integrity is based on the return of color to the affected bowel, peristalsis in response to pinching, and mesenteric artery pulsation. The margins of most strangulating lesions are distinct because of the obvious discoloration of the bowel. If the viability is in question, an enterotomy may be useful to evaluate the color and condition of the mucosa. Intravenous fluorescein may be of some clinical value for predicting intestinal viability. However, if the viability of a segment that can be safely resected is in question—particularly the ileum—resection is indicated.

The entire segment to be resected should include at least six to 12 inches of normal bowel at each end of the lesion to ensure normal vascularity at the anastomotic site. End-to-end anastomosis is used for anastomosis of the jejunum. Because of its blood supply, resecting of a segment of ileum and anastomosing it to the remaining portion of ileum is impossible. When ileum is resected, the terminal portion, which cannot be exteriorized, is blind stumped and an end-to-side or side-to-side jejunocecal anastomosis is performed. When the distal stump of the ileum is devitalized peritonitis or abscess formation is likely.

If more than 35 to 40 feet of small intestine is devitalized, euthanasia should be considered. Experiments in ponies have shown that there is a point, somewhere between resection of 40 and 60 per cent of the small intestine, at which malabsorption, weight loss, and liver damage will develop.

Intussusception. Jejunal, ileal, and ileocecal intussusceptions are seen most frequently but not exclusively in young horses and are the result of abnormal peristalsis. The invagination of the intussusceptum and its mesentery into the distal intussuscipiens usually produces an acute, complete luminal obstruction, although subacute and chronic forms of intestinal intussusception have been reported. Congestion and edema in the invaginated bowel leads to infarction and necrosis. Proposed causes include dramatic dietary changes, enteritis, ascarid infection, verminous arteritis, and tapeworm attachment at the ileocecal orifice. Intussusception can also follow small bowel enterotomy or anastomosis. Signs of complete small intestinal obstruction usually develop. If the horse is large enough to examine rectally, palpation of the ileocecal region may elicit pain in cases of ileocecal intussusception. Devitalization of the intussusception is reflected in peritoneal fluid changes associated with strangulation. With an ileocecal intussusception, however, the ileum is contained within the cecum and peritoneal fluid changes may not reflect the degree of necrosis.

Although there are reports of successful correction of intestinal intussusception by simple reduction, there is reason to recommend resection and anastomosis, particularly if the ileum is involved. Although the serosal surface of the bowel may appear viable and the blood supply adequate after reduction, there may be mucosal necrosis. Resection and anastomosis may also prevent stricture or recurrence of intussusception. After reduction of an ileocecal intussusception the ileum is blind stumped, resected, and a jejunocecal anastomosis is performed. If the intussusception is not reducible the ileum is amputated near the cecum and a jejunocecal anastomosis is performed or a side-to-side jejunocecal bypass is created and the intussusception is left in the cecum to slough. The prognosis for successful correction of the nonreducible ileocecal intussusception is poor when compared with prognoses of those that can be reduced and resected.

Mesenteric Incarceration and Herniation. Epiploic foramen and mesenteric defect incarcerations of bowel are examples of internal herniation; that is, the displacement of small intestine through a normal or pathologic opening within the abdominal cavity, without the formation of a hernial sac. Horses older than six or seven years of age are predisposed to epiploic foramen herniation because atrophy of the right caudate lobe of the liver, occurring as the horse ages, enlarges the potential opening. Small intestine can pass from the peritoneal cavity through the epiploic foramen into the omental bursa in a right-to-left fashion or, less frequently, from left to right, either rupturing the omentum or pushing it through the foramen. A recent report showed that epiploic foramen incarceration does not always produce the signs typical of ISO. Many horses showed only slight pain and had no gastric reflux or no bowel distention on rectal palpation. Peritoneal fluid analysis was the most useful aid for determining the necessity of surgery.

At surgery, the foramen can be carefully dilated manually and the hernia reduced following intestinal decompression. Because the caudal vena cava and portal vein form part of the boundaries of the foramen, excessive trauma in this area can produce fatal rupture of either of these veins. The prognosis for successful surgical correction is poor.

Congenital or acquired tears in the mesentery, the nephrosplenic, gastrosplenic, cecocolic, and broad ligaments, and the greater omentum as well as fibrous bands and adhesions provide openings for internal herniation. A mesodiverticular band, formed from an anomalous persistent vitelline artery, can predispose to rupture of the jejunal mesentery with subsequent herniation and strangulation of small intestine. Volvulus of the herniated loop of bowel may follow. Mesenteric tears produced while handling bowel at surgery should always be repaired. Foals with peritonitis and distended loops of small intestine have very friable mesentery that tears easily and splits up to the root of the mesentery, making repair almost impossible.

Diaphragmatic Hernia. Diaphragmatic herniation may occur through congenital or acquired defects and produce abdominal pain, tachypnea, or dyspnea as a result of intestinal incarceration and obstruction and respiratory compromise. The clinical signs depend on the size of the hernial orifice and the extent and duration of visceral herniation into the thorax. Although a presumptive diagnosis can be made on physical findings and thoracocentesis, a definitive preoperative diagnosis is made with thoracic radiography. Positive-pressure ventilation is necessary to ensure adequate ventilation during surgery. In most adult horses the prognosis for surgical repair of a diaphragmatic hernia is poor because of inadequate exposure, inability to adequately retract the viscera, and friability of the diaphragmatic tissue. If there is an intestinal strangulation, septic pleuritis will develop. If repair is attempted, the approach is through a ventral midline incision and is often facilitated by the use of a mesh implant to bridge the defect in the diaphragm.

Inguinal Hernia. Acquired inguinal hernia in the stallion almost always produces acute small intestinal obstruction that requires rapid surgical intervention. Within hours, the bowel displaced through the vaginal ring and contained within the common vaginal tunic can become strangulated. Almost all are unilateral and the diagnosis is confirmed on rectal examination. An interesting finding, however, in a review of horses with acquired inguinal hernia was that only half of the cases were diagnosed before referral. This emphasizes the obligation of the veterinarian to rectally examine the internal inguinal region in all stallions with colic. In the very early stages of the disease, before the herniated loop becomes strangulated, attempts may be made to reduce the hernia per rectum. Palpation of the scrotum usually reveals a swollen, firm, cool testicle

on the affected side. There appears to be a higher incidence of inguinal herniation in Standardbred stallions, and it often follows recent breeding activity or strenuous exercise. Large internal inguinal ring openings may also predispose to herniation.

Inguinal laparotomy is indicated and resection and anastomosis of jejunum can be accomplished through this approach. However, a second abdominal incision, either ventral midline or right paramedian, is necessary for ileal resection and jejunocecal anastomosis. The affected testicle is usually removed and the external inguinal ring is sutured closed. If the herniated bowel is not strangulated, if the testicle is viable, and if salvage is desired, the testicle can be saved. The prognosis for life is good if surgical repair is achieved within a few hours of the herniation.

Most inguinal hernias in foals become corrected spontaneously as the foal grows. Owners should be cautioned, however, to observe these foals and reduce the hernia on a daily basis. Occasionally, the herniated bowel will break through the common tunic and migrate subcutaneously producing severe scrotal and preputial swelling and abdominal discomfort. The hernia is no longer reducible and surgical repair is indicated. A skin incision over the inguinal ring exposes the intestine, which is then decompressed and replaced into the peritoneal cavity. The testicle is removed and the external inguinal ring is closed with simple interrupted absorbable suture material. A ventral incision should be made in the scrotum to allow for drainage.

Lipomas. Pedunculated lipomas should always be considered as a cause of ISO in older horses (mean age of 15 years). Although often found incidentally, lipomas that are suspended on mesenteric pedicles have the potential to knot around a loop of intestine or break through the mesentery and wrap around the bowel causing obstruction and strangulation. Surgical correction is achieved by severing the pedicle of the lipoma and releasing the affected bowel, which is then resected.

PROGNOSIS

It would appear that ISO is encountered in approximately 30 to 40 per cent of cases of surgical colic, and the reported survival rates after correction range from 27 to 70 per cent. The horse that is diagnosed and treated early in the course of the disease has fewer operative and postoperative complications and the best prognosis for survival.

Problems after surgery include gastrointestinal distention and ileus, peritonitis, and adhesion formation at the operative sites. Technical errors can lead to hemorrhage from the mesenteric stump following resection and obstruction or leakage at the anastomotic site.

Supplemental Readings

Huskamp, B.: The diagnosis and treatment of acute abdominal conditions in the horse: The various types and frequency as seen at the animal hospital in Hochmoor. *In* Proceedings Equine Colic Res. Symp., University of Georgia, 1982, pp. 261–272.

Moore, J. N., and White, N. A.: Acute abdominal disease: Pathophysiology and preoperative management. Vet. Clin. North Am. (Large Anim. Pract.), *4*:61, 1982.

Schneider, R. K., Milne, D. W., and Kohn, C. W.: Acquired inguinal hernia in the horse: A review of 27 cases. J. Am. Vet. Med. Assoc., *180*:317, 1982.

Sullins, K. E., Stashak, T. S., and Mero, K. N.: Evaluation of flourescein dye as an indicator of small intestine viability in the horse. J. Am. Vet. Med. Assoc., *186*:257, 1985.

Tate, L. P., Ralston, S. L., Koch, C. M., and Everett, J. I.: Effects of extensive resection of the small intestine in the pony. Am. J. Vet. Res., *44*:1187, 1983.

Tulleners, E. P.: Small bowel obstruction. *In* Robinson, N. E. (ed.): Current Therapy in Equine Medicine, 1st ed. Philadelphia, W. B. Saunders Company, 1983, pp. 224–231.

Turner, T. A., Adams, S. B., and White, N. A.: Small intestine incarceration through the epiploic foramen of the horse. J. Am. Vet. Med. Assoc., *184*:731, 1984.

White, N. A., Moore, J. N., and Trim, C. A.: Mucosal alterations in experimentally induced small intestinal strangulation obstruction in ponies. Am. J. Vet. Res., *41*:193, 1980.

Impaction of the Ileum

Douglas Allen, Jr., ATHENS, GEORGIA

The ileum is the segment of small intestine most commonly involved with impactions leading to colic. It is located in the left caudal abdomen, courses to the right at the level of the third or fourth lumbar vertebra, and passes upward to the lesser curvature of the cecal base, ending at the ileal orifice. Although a true ileal sphincter muscle at the ileocecal orifice is not present, the horse does have a functional valve composed of two components. First, the ileal mucosa protrudes slightly into the cecal lumen, forming an annular fold or papilla, the submucosa of which is richly supplied with vasculature. Second, the ileal muscularis is thicker and more contractile than the remainder of the small intestine. During contraction, the ileum shortens and thickens, the mucous membrane becomes folded, and the annular fold distends due to engorgement of the vasculature. The ileum can then deliver small intestinal contents into the cecum against a pressure gradient. Closure of the ileal opening, as a result of vascular engorgement, prevents a backflow of ingesta.

The pathophysiology of ileal impactions is not well understood. Several clinical entities are associated with impactions. Ileal muscular hypertrophy, which is recognized in man, pigs, and horses, narrows the ileal lumen. The condition is ascribed to an abnormality of the autonomic nervous system that permits uncontrolled propulsive contractions of the ileum, resulting in work hypertrophy. Hypertrophy also results from increased workload caused by stenosis due to mucosal lesions or partial obstructions. Regardless of the mechanism involved, work hypertrophy results in thickening of the ileal wall, especially in the circular layer, and narrowing of the intestinal lumen.

Other causes of ileal impactions include thrombotic mesenteric vascular disease and spasmodic contractions of the ileum around finely ground feedstuffs. Bermuda grass hay, fed in the southeastern part of the United States, has been incriminated in the pathogenesis of the latter condition.

CLINICAL SIGNS

The clinical signs of ileal impaction include sudden, severe abdominal pain due to distention and tonic spasm of the gut at the impaction site. This initial colic may subside after the first few hours with the horse becoming depressed. The systemic effects of impaction are mild initially with little if any change in temperature, pulse, respiratory rate, packed cell volume (PCV), or plasma proteins. After 6 to 10 hours, fluid, gas, and ingesta begin to accumulate proximal to the ileum, and the small intestine and stomach distend. As the condition progresses, the horse again shows signs of abdominal pain. The first signs of cardiovascular collapse are recognized by a PCV greater than 45 per cent and increased plasma proteins. This is due, in part, to failure of fluid passage into the colon preventing water absorption and in part to depletion of the circulating plasma volume caused by increased secretion into the proximal small bowel and stomach. At this time, pulse and respiratory rates increase as a reflection of shock and pain. Peripheral white blood cell counts (WBC) usually reflect a neutrophilia and lymphopenia consistent with stress.

Peritoneal fluid analysis is probably the most helpful in differentiating a simple impaction from a strangulation obstruction, because abnormal peritoneal fluid total protein levels, and leukocyte counts tend to develop earlier in the case of strangulation. With ileal impaction, the peritoneal total protein level and leukocyte count early in the course of the disease are less then 2.5 gm per dl and 4000 per μl, respectively. As the duration of obstruction lengthens, both parameters increase.

In the early stages of disease, the impacted ileum can often be felt by rectal palpation as a smooth sausage-shaped tube 3 to 5 cm in diameter extending from left of midline obliquely upward to the cecal base, ending blindly in a cone. The cecum is usually empty and distention of the small intestine is not detected. The pelvic flexure is usually palpable in the lower left caudal abdomen. With prolonged ileal impaction, the proximal small intestine secretes and gastric reflux develops. As the disease progresses, more distended loops of small intestine displace the impaction cranially until it is no longer palpable per rectum. Definitive diagnosis of an impacted ileum is based on identification by rectal examination of the impacted sausage-shaped ileum. If rectal findings are inconclusive, a presumptive diagnosis of small intestinal impaction can be made by noting the duration and course of the disease, the presence of gastric reflux, and the peritoneal fluid characteristics.

Differential diagnosis of ileal impactions must include strangulation obstructions, anterior enteritis (proximal duodenitis-jejunitis), and obstruction by extraluminal or intramural masses.

TREATMENT

Most horses with small intestinal distention require surgery. There are two notable exceptions. One is the horse with proximal jejunitis (see p. 44). The second exception is the horse with normal to slightly elevated pulse, respiratory rate, and total protein. Rectal examination may reveal distended loops of small intestine. However, the animal shows no sign of pain. These animals should be monitored closely by serial measurements of hematocrit and plasma proteins and by rectal examinations. Some horses with the latter signs respond well to supportive medical therapy. Presumably, a small bowel obstruction either from malposition of a segment of the intestine or intraluminal obstruction resolves spontaneously.

The medical therapy of ileal impaction is supportive and consists of intravenous fluids, analgesics, and gastric and proximal intestinal decompression via nasogastric tube. Mineral oil may be given at the onset of pain only after rectal examination reveals no distended loops of small intestine and attempts at removal of gastric reflux are unrewarding. If conservative therapy fails and the impaction does not soften, the small intestine and stomach will distend and surgery is indicated. If pain continues during diagnostic procedures and gastric or small intestinal distention persist, early surgery improves the prognosis. The average time from onset of signs to surgery in horses that survive is 17 hours compared with 25 hours in nonsurvivors. The reported survival rates for surgically managed ileal impactions varies from 50 to 67 per cent.

SURGERY AND POSTOPERATIVE THERAPY

Surgery should be performed with the horse under general anesthesia and in dorsal recumbency. A ventral midline laparotomy provides the best exposure for abdominal exploration and correction of the lesion. Upon entrance into the abdominal cavity, distended loops of jejunum are generally present in the surgical field. Deeper exploration of the abdomen will usually reveal the impacted ileum adjacent to the dorsal abdominal body wall. The ileum and cecum should be exteriorized as much as possible to permit reduction of the impacted mass. The ileocecal valve must be palpated to ensure that the impaction is not secondary to ileocecal intussusception. The impaction should then be milked into the cecum. When the impaction is very dry and firm, sterile saline can be infused into the impacted mass through a needle to facilitate reduction of the impaction. Once the impaction has been reduced and the small intestinal contents moved into the cecum, the ileum should be evaluated for morphologic changes. If changes such as thickening of the bowel wall or vascular thrombotic disease are present, the ileum should be bypassed or resected. Resection of the terminal ileum is impractical because of its inaccessibility, as it attaches firmly to the cecum and dorsal abdominal body wall. Therefore, approximately 10 to 15 cm of ileum must be blind-ended and left attached to the cecum. The remainder of the ileum can be easily resected and a side-to-side anastomosis of jejunum to cecum performed between the dorsal and medial cecal bands as close to the cecal base as possible. An alternative to resection is bypassing the ileum by a side-to-side jejunocecostomy, leaving the ileum in situ. This should cause a shunting of ingesta into the cecum.

Postoperatively, a nasogastric tube should be passed and gastric reflux removed every 90 minutes to two hours. Postoperative ileus and gastric reflux can last from a few hours to four to five days, depending on the interval between onset of colic and surgical intervention. The fluid removed from the stomach is a plasma dialysate, and the horse must be maintained on intravenous fluid to prevent dehydration and cardiovascular collapse. Heparin therapy has been advocated in severe cases to prevent the development of postoperative adhesions although its efficacy is unproven.

Once the gastric reflux has stopped, small amounts of hay can be fed over the following two days and the animal returned to normal feeding regimen after five to seven days. The animal should be monitored closely for signs of dehydration and abdominal pain during the initial feeding period. Postoperative complications include reimpaction of ileum or impaction of the anastomotic site, adhe-

sions, and unrelenting gastric reflux and dehydration. These problems are generally encountered in horses that have a prolonged interval between onset of the condition and surgical repair.

Supplemental Readings

Embertson, R. M., Colohan, P. T., Brown, M. P., et al.: Ileal impaction in the horse. J. Am. Vet. Med. Assoc., *186*:570, 1985.

Gabella, G.: Hypertrophy of smooth muscle. J. Physiol., *249*:183, 1975.

Nickel, R., Shumner, A., and Sirferle, E.: The viscera of the domestic animals. Berlin, Paul Parey, 1973, pp. 186–187.

Stelling, C. B., and Straus, F. H.: Roentgenographic findings in work hypertrophy of the muscularis propria of the terminal ileum. Digest. Dis., *22*:1117, 1977.

Large Colon Impaction

Alvin F. Sellers, ITHACA, NEW YORK
John E. Lowe, ITHACA, NEW YORK

Impactions of the large intestine are encountered frequently by the practitioner. In one series of 453 cases of intestinal obstruction, impaction was the cause in 112 cases. The large colon is most frequently involved, usually at the sites where it narrows, such as the pelvic flexure and the termination. Fortunately, the majority of large colon impactions are diagnosed and treated successfully. Cecal impactions are difficult to treat successfully.

PATHOPHYSIOLOGY

Normally, digesta are milked in long columns, in oral and caudal directions, near the pelvic flexure pacemaker. This separates the less well-digested particulates that are propelled backward into the left ventral colon from the finer particulates that are propelled aborally. The strong muscular efforts give rise to loud, long-duration sounds (15 to 30 seconds) on the left side of the abdomen and cause shortening of the bowel accompanied by narrowing of the lumen. These two processes cause extensive movement of the pelvic flexure.

The myenteric plexus coordinates the motor events in the colon contiguous to the pelvic flexure. These motor events are driven by the pelvic flexure pacemaker. An ectopic pacemaker or anything that lessens myenteric plexus control of the physical separation of digesta in this area tends to cause accumulation of digesta in the terminus of the left ventral colon. The subsequent distention extends

cranial and caudal to the original accumulation, and at first excites large, strong, repeated propulsive contractions, occurring in groups. Contractions are heard as louder than normal, prolonged (30 seconds or more) sounds over the left flank. Coincident with these sounds the animal goes down and gets up, rolls, paws, makes violent head and neck movements, and shows other evidence of episodic pain, i.e., "spasmodic colic." Alpha$_2$-adrenergic receptor stimulation may be one cause of loss of myenteric plexus control of the highly specialized equine colon. Contractile efforts of the left ventral colon become dissociated from those of the left dorsal large colon; ileus and impaction follow. The etiology of cecal impactions is more obscure but likely involves a malfunction in the extrinsic and/or intrinsic nerve supply to that organ.

ETIOLOGY

Impactions can occur when coarse, poor-quality hay is the primary feed, when nutrition is marginal, when water is supplied infrequently, when care of teeth is poor, when teeth are diseased or missing or worn out from old age leading to incomplete mastication, or when horses gorge themselves on bedding or roughage to which they are unaccustomed. Parasitic disease can interfere with blood supply and nerve transmission, leading to poor muscular force or poorly coordinated gut motility, which then predisposes to impaction. More uncommonly, partial obstruction can occur from abscesses or neoplasms in the intestinal wall that predispose to impactions. With abdominal surgery practiced more frequently today, the chance of adhesions interfering with lumen size or gut motility is greater. Good management means good preventive medicine and that means very few colics including impactions. Thus, in spite of the acute need for diagnosis, therapy, and/or surgery, preventive measures are the real key to stopping impactions before they start.

CLINICAL SIGNS

Impactions typically are low-grade colics. They start with a horse showing partial or complete anorexia, slight depression, and decreased fecal production. The horse typically has a normal rectal temperature, a normal to slightly above normal pulse rate (36 to 48), and a normal respiratory rate. The horse kept in a box stall or slip stall is much more likely to be observed to be "off" at this time than is the horse in a group feeding situation. Unwellness in the group-fed horse is usually first noticed because it hangs back and does not come up at grain feeding time, or if no grain is being fed, it is observed to be lying down while the others are eating.

The horse may look at its flanks occasionally, stretch its neck and curl its upper lip up (flehmen), or may stretch more often than usual to urinate. These signs may be obvious or subtle.

Capillary refill is less than two seconds, the conjunctivae may show slight reddening and appear "injected." A penlight should be used routinely to examine the conjunctivae rather than relying on lights in the stall. It should be remembered that the conjunctivae of some ponies normally look "injected" compared to horses.

Feces are scant, often mucus covered, totally formed, light in color, and have a dry texture. Rectal examination may reveal a firm doughy pelvic flexure, helping to make a diagnosis, or it may reveal nothing. Early in an impaction, if a stomach tube is passed, no gastric reflux will be found.

Auscultation may reveal decreased sounds or if one listens long enough or at the right time in the course of the problem some long, loud contractions may be heard over the colon. As the impaction persists, intestinal sounds decrease in rate and intensity. As the impaction breaks up, intestinal sounds become more frequent and more intense.

Diagnosis is often based on elimination of other causes of colic or other diseases producing similar low-grade signs. Mild pain and mild generalized illness allow time for a conservative approach, which is usually successful.

THERAPY

Therapy involves pain control, laxatives and wetting agents to resolve the impacted mass, fluid therapy when needed, intestinal stimulants when appropriate, and surgery or euthanasia when conservative measures fail or when pain becomes too intense or impaction is diagnosed as secondary to a life-threatening primary problem.

Impactions usually produce low-grade pain. We prefer flunixin meglumine* 1.1 mg per kg repeated at 12-hour intervals if necessary to relieve pain. Since shock is not a problem, alpha-adrenergic blockers such as acepromazine can be used for their relatively prolonged sedative effect. Xylazine† is preferred in doses of 100 to 300 mg per 500 kg for more intense pain. However, if repeated doses of xylazine need to be used, the primary diagnosis of impaction needs to be reassessed. Xylazine is an $alpha_2$-adrenergic agonist that almost eliminates large intestine contractions. This may in the short run be beneficial for pain relief; however, with repeated doses it could be detrimental. For a discussion of the broad range of analgesics used in the colic patient, see p. 27.

Laxatives are essential for impactions. Heavy mineral oil (USP) administered via stomach tube in doses of two to four quarts and repeated every 12 to 24 hours is the drug of choice. It may take as much as five gallons of mineral oil before a stubborn impaction is resolved. Mixing one to two quarts of warm water with the mineral oil makes it easier to administer and provides some more fluid for the horse. Pumping the mineral oil in at a moderate speed does not endanger the horse with impaction and is much preferred to gravity flow.

The wetting agent, dioctyl sodium sulfosuccinate, is useful to help resolve impactions. In theory, it should not be administered with mineral oil for fear of promoting absorption of emulsified mineral oil from the intestine. The dose is 7.5 to 30 gm orally. One of us has used 3 to 5 gm simultaneously with mineral oil routinely over the past 20 years with no observed ill effects. If a choice has to be made, mineral oil is by far the more important of the two drugs.

Saline and irritant cathartics should be used with caution or avoided. If the impaction is mild or breaking up, the hypertonic and irritant properties of these products may be effective and tolerated. However, if a solid impaction still exists, serious consequences such as dehydration, shock, and bowel rupture may occur.

Most impactions do not usually require fluid therapy. However, when impaction persists for

---

*Banamine, Schering Corp., Kenilworth, NJ
†Rompun, Haver-Lockhart, Shawnee, KS

more than 24 hours, assessment of oral consumption of fluids and consideration of whether fluids by stomach tube are being utilized are necessary. When warranted by the value of the horse, intravenous fluids are very helpful to resolve an impaction. Monitoring of dehydration and acid-base state by laboratory tests is nice but not essential.

Intestinal stimulants such as neostigmine, carbachol, and panthenol are sometimes utilized once an impaction begins to break up. In protracted cases of impaction, the bowel wall may be weakened or even necrotic and stimulants may cause rupture. The problem with stimulants is the inability to control their site of action or predict the degree to which they will work in any given case. They can also cause intense pain in the horse with obstruction. Therefore, caution is needed when considering their use.

Surgery or euthanasia is a last resort in horses with impaction. Fluid therapy, administration of broad-spectrum antibiotics, and adequate pain control are essential to maintain the horse until surgery can be performed. The quicker the decision for surgery, the better the surgical risk will be. At surgery, the impacted mass can be injected with wetting agents or fluids or both, or it can be manually disintegrated, especially if it is already softened by previous therapy. If the bowel is accessible, it can be exteriorized and evacuated.

Signs consistent with a favorable response to therapy include passage of feces and/or gas, increasing intestinal sounds including peristaltic rushes without pain accompanying them, a brighter attitude in the horse, and improved appetite.

A horse should not be overfed for 24 hours after recovery from an impaction—only half the usual hay ration should be fed. The horse should not be allowed to eat bedding. Bran mashes are given for one or two days, and pasture or hand grazing should be available for restricted periods.

If euthanasia is necessary, a postmortem examination should be done to confirm the diagnosis and to learn.

Supplemental Readings

Lowe, J. E., Sellers, A. F., and Brondum, J.: Equine pelvic flexure impaction. A model used to evaluate motor events and compare drug response. Cornell Vet., 70:401, 1980.

Sellers, A. F., Lowe, J. E., Rendano, V. T., and Drost, C. J.: Guest Editorial: The reservoir function of the equine cecum and ventral large colon—Its relation to chronic nonsurgical obstructive disease with colic. Cornell Vet., 72:233, 1982.

Sellers, A. F., and Lowe, J. E.: Visualization of auscultation sounds of the large intestine. Proc. 29th Annu. Meet. Am. Assoc. Eq. Pract., 1983, pp. 359–364.

Sellers, A. F., Lowe, J. E., Drost, C. J., Rendano, V. T., Georgi, J. R., and Roberts, M. C.: Retropulsion-propulsion in equine large colon. Am. J. Vet. Res., 43:390, 1982.

Sellers, A. F., Lowe, J. E., and Cummings, J. F.: Trials of serotonin, substance P, and alpha$_2$-adrenergic receptor effects on the equine large colon. Cornell Vet., 75:2, 1985.

Sand Colic

Pat Colahan, GAINESVILLE, FLORIDA

Irritation or obstruction of the gastrointestinal tract is a problem when sand is ingested by horses. Sand is consumed when it becomes mixed with hay fed on the ground, when horses graze grass covered by silt after flooding, when they graze the roots and attached soil of plants uprooted in short or overly grazed pastures, and when they drink from shallow muddy pools at times of fresh water unavailability. Some horses will deliberately eat sand. In adult horses this habit has been attributed to boredom or salt deficiency. This behavior has been observed frequently in foals as young as two to three days of age. However, no definite cause for eating sand has been demonstrated.

Although the prevalence of the sites of irritation or obstruction has not been documented, the stomach, ileocecal junction, cecum, large colon, and transverse colon have been mentioned. The large colon, and in particular the right colons, pelvic flexure, and transverse colon, are by far the most common sites of obstruction. In the absence of scientific data, one can conjecture that the sand collects in the large colon because it is a fermentative area of reduced flow and the sand consequently settles out of the ingesta. The pelvic flexure and transverse colon become obstructed when masses of accumulated sand become lodged in these narrowed segments.

CLINICAL SIGNS

Sand in the intestine causes both mucosal irritation and mechanical obstruction. The mucosal irritation results in diarrhea, which may precede mechanical obstruction of the bowel by several days.

When obstruction occurs, the bowel orad becomes distended with gas, fluid, and ingesta. Pain results from stretching of the bowel wall.

The weight of the impacted mass or distention of the bowel or both can result in two acutely severe sequelae: twisting or other displacement of the impacted segment of bowel, and necrosis of the bowel wall at the site of the impaction. Although there may be little change in signs accompanying the necrosis of the wall of the bowel until perforation occurs, both perforation and mechanical displacement of the bowel will be accompanied by increased signs of pain and the development of shock.

DIAGNOSIS

The diagnosis of sand colic depends upon the history, careful observance of clinical signs, and a thorough physical examination. Simple observations of feeding practices and the environment will reveal the opportunity for ingestion of sand. A history of diarrhea followed in several days by colic, the appearance of mild to moderate colic acutely or intermittently, and mild colic followed by an acute increase in severity are typical of sand obstruction of the gastrointestinal tract. Pulse and respiratory rate, capillary refill time, and mucous membrane color vary with the duration and severity of the condition and the accompanying shock. Abdominal distention and gastric reflux are the results of complete obstruction or displacement or both and are signs of a severe condition requiring surgery.

Rectal palpation for sand impaction is not conclusive as impactions occur most frequently in areas that are not within reach. When they do occur in segments of bowel that are normally palpable, the weight of the sand causes the bowel to rest, out of reach, in the ventral abdomen. Upon palpation, sand impactions feel extremely hard and do not indent easily.

During rectal palpation, samples of feces should be examined for the presence of sand. Six fecal balls can be broken up into a quart pitcher of water and the sand allowed to settle. More than a teaspoon of sand in the container is abnormal. A more convenient, but less quantitative, method is to collect two to four fecal balls in the gloved hand during rectal palpation. As the disposable glove is removed it is inverted over the fecal material. Enough water is added to make a slurry of the feces. The glove is then suspended for several minutes thus allowing the sand to separate from the slurry. More than one fourth of an inch of sand remaining in the fingers of the glove is indicative of excessive sand in the feces. All horses in regions with sandy soil may have some sand in their feces and differing soil types may be more pathogenic than others. The practitioner must therefore use judgment in interpreting the results of any measurement of the quantity of sand in feces.

The presence of large quantities of sand in the gastrointestinal tract is frequently detected accidentally. Occasionally during paracentesis the bowel is penetrated and sand is obtained. The penetration of sand-impacted bowel can occur easily because the weight of the sand presses the impacted bowel against the ventral abdominal wall. Although such accidental paracentesis diagnoses the presence of sand in the intestinal tract, it also causes at least a localized peritonitis. In some cases severe sequelae such as generalized septic peritonitis or abscessation occur, therefore, deliberately attempting to tap a sand impaction is not advisable.

TREATMENT

Treatment of sand impaction depends on the severity of the condition. If pain is mild to moderate and can be controlled with analgesics, and the horse is still passing stool, even if it is diarrhea, then medical therapy is indicated. Medical therapy should include laxatives, fluids to maintain hydration, and a diet of high-quality roughage. All the common laxatives available for impaction colics, including mineral oil, dioctyl sodium sulfosuccinate (DSS), and saline cathartics, have been used to treat sand impaction in horses. Mineral oil is not as effective as water-based laxatives because it does not penetrate the water-soaked sandy mass and does little to remove the accumulated sand. The saline cathartics ($MgSO_4$, $NaSO_4$) and DSS will bring more fluid into the bowel and help prevent dessication of the mass but will do little to promote passage of the sand. The laxative of choice is *Psyllium hydrophilia mucilloid*.* This is a lubricating bulk laxative that becomes gelatinous in the intestinal tract. The jelly collects the sand and lubricates its passage through the digestive tract. The initial regimen is to administer 0.5 kg of mucilloid in 6 to 8 L (1 pound in 1½ to 2 gallons) of water via nasogastric tube. This can be repeated as necessary during the acute phase of the colic as long as fluid does not build up in the horse's stomach and the horse continues to pass stool.

Administration of mucilloid via stomach tube can be difficult if the water and mucilloid granules or flakes are mixed too long before they are pumped into the tube. When mucilloid comes into contact with water, it becomes gelatinous and cannot be pumped. To administer it with a nasogastric tube and pump, mucilloid must be mixed into the water as the mixture is pumped into the tube. Pouring

---

*Metamucil, Searle and Co., San Juan, PR

the measured amounts of water and mucilloid simultaneously into a bucket as the mixture is pumped from the bucket into the tube is a more manageable method of administration. After the initial treatment, mucilloid can be added to each feeding. It is usually palatable up to 125 gm per feeding if mixed dry with a small amount of grain or sweet feed. Horses refusing to eat any amount of mucilloid in their feed will require repeated tubing for continuous therapy.

It is important not to discontinue therapy for sand colic too soon. These obstructions usually develop over a prolonged period of time and the amount of accumulated sand is considerable before clinical signs develop. The cessation of the overt signs does not mean that the sand has been eliminated. Usually a considerable amount of sand remains and will lead to recurrence of signs unless treatment is continued.

Maintenance of hydration is critical for sand colic. Sufficient fluid must be taken to replace the fluid lost by normal body processes such as urination, defecation, sweating, breathing, and skin evaporation as well as pathologic processes such as diarrhea. Provision of insufficient fluid leads to fluid absorption from intestinal contents, making impactions drier and more difficult to break up and pass. Fluid supplement is therefore a critical part of the treatment.

Both the oral and intravenous route of fluid administration are available. If no gastric fluid buildup occurs, 8 to 10 liters of warm water or electrolyte solution can be administered via nasogastric tube hourly until fluid requirements are met. Intravenous supplementation with sterile, balanced polyionic solution is essential for the horse in shock or when the stomach is not emptying. Occasionally catheterization and intravenous administration are more convenient than repeated nasogastric intubation.

SURGICAL MANAGEMENT

Surgical treatment of sand colic is indicated when the pain is uncontrollable, abdominal distention or distention of bowel on rectal examination becomes marked, the condition does not respond to intensive medical therapy within 48 to 72 hours, or the condition suddenly becomes markedly worse. Delaying surgery can result in necrosis and rupture of the bowel. In the surgical treatment of sand colic it is important to remember that the impaction is heavy, the bowel is usually markedly distended, the bowel wall is compromised and mechanically weakened, and most or preferably all of the sand must be removed. A ventral midline or paramedian incision is preferred for easy delivery of the bowel from the abdomen. The bowel must be lifted from the abdomen preferably over one or both arms rather than by grasping with the hands. The wall of the bowel may rupture if not maximally supported during delivery.

The sand must be removed via enterotomy. Massage of sand impaction whether injected with fluid and DSS or not is usually unsuccessful, as the sand simply settles in the bowel again after manipulation. Also, there is considerable risk of rupturing the weakened bowel wall during massage. The sand is most safely and effectively removed by flushing large volumes of water through the bowel via an enterotomy. Since the most common sites of impaction are in the large colon, the easiest way to flush the bowel is to place the colon between the rear limbs, perform the enterotomy in the pelvic flexure and flush the dorsal and ventral colons with a hose and large volumes of tap water. If the impaction is in the right colon and cannot be readily flushed because the bowel cannot be delivered from the abdomen, a siphon can be created using a large stomach tube placed through the enterotomy in addition to the hose. To remove the sand and flush water, the siphon and flush hoses can be manipulated through the bowel wall by the member of the surgical team not contaminated by doing the enterotomy.

Following closure of the enterotomy the bowel and the abdominal cavity should be lavaged with large volumes (more than 30 L) of sterile isotonic fluids containing 2000 units sodium heparin per liter to reduce bacterial contamination and remove blood and food particles. Thorough lavage and the pre- or intraoperative initiation of broad-spectrum antibiotic therapy is important in preventing peritonitis. The addition of heparin to the lavage solutions helps to prevent the precipitation of fibrin clots on the bowel and in the abdomen.

The prognosis for horses that respond to medical therapy is fair. If surgery is required, the prognosis must be considered guarded because of the dangers of intraoperative rupture, postoperative peritonitis, and adhesion formation.

PREVENTION

The ultimate solution to sand colic is prevention. In sandy environments, management must prevent the ingestion of sand. Hay should be placed in feed racks, nets, or bunks and not on the ground. Pastures must be seeded, fertilized, and irrigated to produce lush grass growth. When pasture growth is seasonally slow, supplemental feeding or stall confinement must be instituted. When sand eating is a vice in individual horses, stall confinement or muzzling must be used.

In sandy areas some sand ingestion is unavoidable. To assist in reducing sand buildup, many horsemen feed a moist bran mash once or twice a week. Although there is no scientific data to support the efficacy of bran in preventing sand accumulation, bran feeding is widely practiced and reputed to be effective and is harmless.

Supplemental Readings

Kohn, C. W.: Acute diarrhea. *In*: Mansmann, R. A., McAllister, E. S., and Pratt, P. W. (eds.): Equine Medicine and Surgery, 3rd ed. Santa Barbara, CA, American Veterinary Publications, 1982, pp. 528–542.

McIlwraith, C. W.: Equine digestive system. *In* Jennings, P. D. (ed.): The Practice of Large Animal Surgery, Philadelphia, W. B. Saunders Company, 1984, pp. 554–664.

Meagher, D. M.: Obstructive disease in the large intestine of the horse: Diagnosis and treatment. Proc. 18th Annu. Meet. Am. Assoc. Equine Pract., 1972, pp. 269–279.

Merritt, A. M.: Chronic diarrhea. *In*: Mansmann, R. A., McAllister, E. S., and Pratt, P. W. (eds.): Equine Medicine and Surgery, 3rd ed. Santa Barbara, CA, American Veterinary Publications, 1982, pp. 542–547.

Robertson, J. T.: Obstructive diseases. *In*: Mansmann, R. A., McAllister, E. S., and Pratt, P. W. (eds.): Equine Medicine and Surgery, 3rd ed. Santa Barbara, CA, American Veterinary Publications, 1982, pp. 559–579.

Distention Colic

Nathaniel T. Messer, IV, LITTLETON, COLORADO

G. Marvin Beeman, LITTLETON, COLORADO

Distention colic describes a nonsurgical colic usually lacking a definitive etiologic diagnosis and responding to conservative medical therapy. Included in this category are spasmodic colic, gas or flatulent colic, impaction colic with partial luminal obstruction, and certain verminous colics. Although little statistical or epidemiologic data are available, this type of colic is one of the more common colics seen in equine practice.

By virtue of the self-limiting nature of most distention colics and their response to a variety of therapeutic regimens, the pathophysiologic mechanisms involved must be transient and reversible. Just as in other types of colic, alterations in gastrointestinal motility play a significant role in distention colic. Ineffective peristaltic activity secondary to spasm or adynamic ileus rapidly leads to distention of the intestines with gas or fluid or both. This distention increases intramural tension in the gut wall, resulting in pain. The inciting causes of this disturbance in gastrointestinal motility are poorly defined; however, in some way they are influenced by disturbances in blood flow or changes in the neuroendocrine control to the bowel. Historically, they have been attributed to many factors, including: internal parasites, inappropriate feeding and management, stress or excitement, sudden changes in weather, and administration of certain medications including anthelmintics.

CLINICAL SIGNS

The clinical signs associated with distention colic vary with the degree of distention and the portion of the intestine involved. Typically, the horse has intermittent episodes of pain characterized by the signs associated with any type of abdominal discomfort, such as reluctance to eat, pawing, kicking at the abdomen, stretching, lying down, looking back at the flank, and mild sweating. Because of this, it is extremely important to include in the initial examination as many parameters as necessary to satisfactorily rule out the presence of a surgical type of colic.

The temperature, heart rate, and respiratory rate will usually be normal as will the color of the visible mucous membranes and capillary refill time. During episodes of pain there may be transient elevations in heart rate and respiratory rate proportional to the degree of pain. These elevations return to normal as the pain subsides.

Auscultation of the abdomen is valuable to determine the presence, absence, and character of intestinal sounds. Although in most cases of distention colic borborygmi are decreased or even absent during episodes of pain, gas and fluid sounds are prominent. In between bouts of pain, active peristaltic sounds are often heard. Percussion of the abdomen identifies areas where gas is accumulating in large amounts.

Passage of a nasogastric tube will provide information regarding the upper portion of the gastrointestinal tract. In distention colic usually there is minimal reflux of fluid from the tube. There may be enough gaseous reflux to produce a pungent fermentative odor. In unusual cases a large volume of gas or fluid reflux will escape from the tube, and following decompression of the stomach the horse may return to normal with no further treatment required.

At this point in the examination, depending on the severity of pain being exhibited by the horse, it may be necessary to administer some form of analgesic medication to control the pain and to safely proceed with the examination. With distention colic, response to treatment provides further diagnostic information. In most cases the animal will respond to minimal analgesia.

Rectal examination is an important part of evaluating a horse with colic. It is imperative to ensure that the size and temperament of the animal allow rectal palpation, that proper restraint is utilized, and that a careful and systematic examination is performed. In distention colic, rectal examination can be misleading if not correlated with previous physical findings because often gas or fluid distention of segments of bowel is present similar to that which occurs in strangulating obstructions or displacements. However, the other parameters in distention colic point toward a less severe problem. Abdominal paracentesis reveals normal peritoneal fluid.

TREATMENT

Treatment of distention colic should be directed toward re-establishment of normal gastrointestinal motility. Much evidence has accumulated to suggest that the basic mechanism for ileus is an overactivity of the sympathetic nervous system. Acepromazine (.04 to .06 mg per kg), as an alpha-adrenergic blocker may increase perfusion of the intestine in a well-hydrated horse and may help increase ingesta transport in addition to reducing anxiety. Dipyrone (22 mg per kg), an antiprostaglandin and mild pain reliever, decreases nonpropulsive intestinal spasms with minimal effects on peristalsis. In most cases of distention colic adequate pain relief is obtained following treatment with acepromazine and dipyrone. Xylazine (1.1 mg per kg), a more potent analgesic, has adverse effects on gastrointestinal motility and should, therefore, be used to control pain in distention colic only when acepromazine and dipyrone are ineffective.

The administration of oral medication by stomach tube is indicated in distention colic except in those rare cases in which there is a large amount of fluid reflux from the tube. Either mineral oil (2 to 4 L) or simply warm water will stimulate the gastrocolic reflex and help initiate some peristaltic activity, as well as lubricating and softening ingesta to aid in its movement through the digestive tract.

In cases of colic with excessive gas distention, mechanical decompression by stomach tube or percutaneous trocarization of the distended viscus often restores motility. The site of trocarization should be clipped, shaved, and surgically prepared. A local anesthetic is used to block the site and a No. 15 scalpel blade to pierce the skin. A 14-cm trocar or 12- to 14-gauge biopsy needle is used to pierce the abdominal wall, enter the abdominal cavity, and proceed into the lumen of the bowel. A rush of gas from the needle will occur immediately, and the trocar should be left in place until gas is no longer free-flowing. From 10 to 20 ml of a broad-spectrum antibiotic is injected through the trocar as it is withdrawn as an aid to the prevention of local peritonitis. Systemic antibiotics may further suppress diffuse peritonitis or generalized infection.

PROGNOSIS

The prognosis for the majority of patients with distention colic is good to excellent, because there is seldom any serious underlying cause predisposing to future problems. Although the clinical signs seem mild compared to those seen in cases requiring surgery, it is just as important to treat these cases, as the alterations in gastrointestinal motility that do occur could easily progress to more serious problems.

Supplemental Readings

Adams, S. B., Lamar, C. H., and Masty, J.: Motility of the distal portion of the jejunum and pelvic flexure in ponies: Effects of six drugs. Am. J. Vet. Res., *45*:795, 1984.

Becht, J. L., and Richardson, D. W.: Ileus in the horse: Clinical significance and management. Proc. 27th Annu. Meet. Am. Assoc. Eq. Pract., pp. 291–297, 1981.

Bennett, D. G.: Predisposition to abdominal crisis in the horse. J. Am. Vet. Med. Assoc., *161*:1189, 1972.

Byars, T.D.: Flatulent colic. *In* Robinson, N. E. (ed.): Current Therapy in Equine Medicine, 1st ed. Philadelphia, W. B. Saunders Company, 1983, pp. 236–238.

Rollins, J. B., and Clement, T. H.: Observations on incidence of equine colic in a private practice. Equine Pract., *1*:39, 1979.

Shideler, R. K., and Bennett D. G.: Medical management of colic. *In* Robinson, N. E. (ed.): Current Therapy in Equine Medicine, 1st ed. Philadelphia, W. B. Saunders Company, 1983, pp. 220–224.

Tulleners, E. P.: Small bowel obstruction. *In* Robinson, N. E. (ed.): Current Therapy in Equine Medicine, 1st ed. Philadelphia, W. B. Saunders Company, 1983, pp. 224–231.

Displacement of the Large Colon

B. Huskamp, HOCHMOOR, WEST GERMANY

The equine large colon is 3 to 4 meters long, double horseshoe shaped, and has a capacity of 60 to 130 liters. Apart from its attachment at the root of the great mesentery it is freely movable in the abdominal cavity. Colonic contents vary in consistency and can be fluid, firm, or gaseous. Consequently, changes in the amount of colonic contents can cause an increase or decrease in the size of the colon. A constant state of balance between the large colon and other portions of the large and small intestines is achieved by the reciprocal (frictional) influence of individual parts of the intestines on each other. This balance within the abdominal cavity can be disrupted by changes in the intestinal contents. Obstructed portions of gut tend to sink ventrally whereas gas-filled portions of gut tend to rise dorsally. Hyperperistalsis or paralysis of the gut can also predispose to intestinal displacements. A reduction in the force of friction between different portions of the gut due to the presence of exudates or transudates in the abdominal cavity can also facilitate intestinal displacement. Lastly, intraluminal pressure caused by increased gas production may be so elevated that other abdominal organs are displaced from their original position.

Left- and right-sided dorsal displacements of the large colon are the two most common forms of colonic displacement. In both instances large-framed horses seem to be predisposed, and the larger the horse, the greater the risk of these displacements.

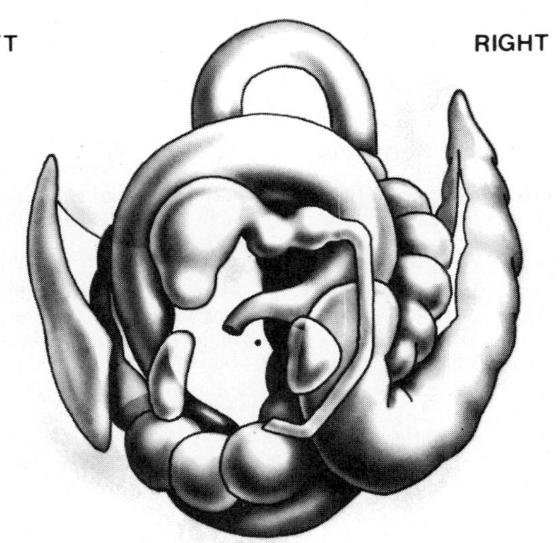

LEFT DORSAL DISPLACEMENT OF THE LARGE COLON

In the case of left-sided dorsal displacement of the large colon, the colon is usually trapped cranially (in rare cases caudally) in the nephrosplenic (reno-splenic) space. Consequently, the colon lies between the left kidney and the nephrosplenic ligament, the dorsal pole of the spleen, and the dorsal abdominal wall. As a consequence, the colon is twisted approximately 180 degrees at the site of constriction, so that the ventral side of the entrapped portion of the colon lies dorsally and the dorsal side lies ventrally (Figs. 1 and 2). In mild cases, only the pelvic flexure and a small part of the ventral and dorsal colon are trapped by the nephrosplenic ligament (Fig. 3).

In more severe cases, when there is considerable gas accumulation, the enlarged entrapped loop can take up more than two thirds of the colon. This enlargement also results in an equivalent decrease in the size of the prestenotic portion (Fig. 1). As a result of the combination of incarceration and torsion, two sites of obstruction form. The first occurs in the prestenotic portion of the ventral colon anterior to the site of the incarceration, so that gas accumulation occurs that can extend as far proximal as the cecum. In the entrapped portion of the colon

CRANIAL

LEFT   RIGHT

CAUDAL

Figure 1. Displacement of the large colon over the renosplenic ligament (dorsal view): Two thirds of the large colon is incarcerated; the pelvic flexure is in front of the diaphragm.

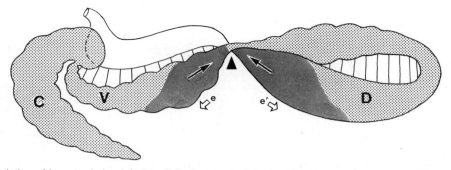

Figure 2. Accumulation of ingesta during left dorsal displacement of the large colon. The first impaction is a prestenotic one in the ventral part of the large colon and the second impaction is also prestenotic, but in the dorsal large colon. Proximal to these two impactions is an accumulation of gas. C: Cecum; V: Ventral part of the large colon; D: Dorsal part of the large colon. The white-bordered arrows show the direction of the peristalsis. The white arrows (e and è) show the effects of peristalsis on the intestinal tube.

obstruction occurs in the dorsal colon posterior to the site of strangulation, so that gas buildup occurs in the remaining entrapped region. The poststenotic portion of the dorsal colon is usually empty. As a

CRANIAL

LEFT   RIGHT

CAUDAL

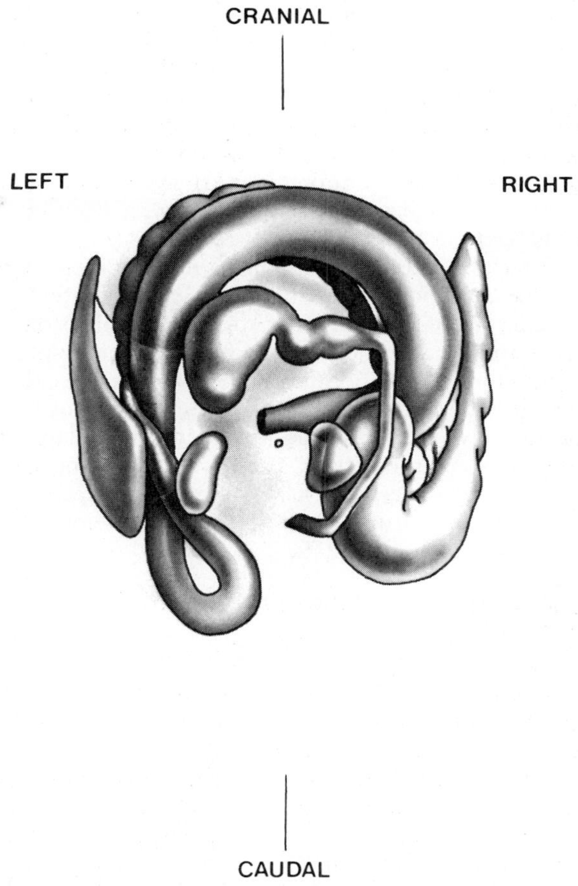

Figure 3. Displacement of the pelvic flexure over the nephrosplenic ligament.

result of these changes in the region of the large colon, the spleen is displaced medially, venous drainage is slightly impaired, and congestion of the spleen occurs.

In cases in which more than two thirds of the colon is trapped by the nephrosplenic ligament, the pre- and poststenotic loops of the colon can be further displaced between the filled stomach and liver, so that they are also trapped by the gastrophrenic ligament. In such extreme cases, the largest portion of the large colon lies caudal to the site of constriction. The longitudinal parts of the colon in front of the pelvis are bent cranially so that the pelvic flexure may lie as far forward as the diaphragm.

Etiology and Pathogenesis. Since the condition occurs primarily in large-framed geldings, and recurrences are sometimes seen, an individual predisposition is probable. It is still not clear which route the colon takes when displaced into the nephrosplenic space. One theory is that the colon moves dorsally on its side between the left abdominal wall and spleen (Fig. 4). To support this theory, on rectal examination I have often found intermediate stages in which the colon lies halfway up between the left abdominal wall and the spleen.

Especially in cases of gastric distention, when the congested spleen is displaced medioventrally, a narrow split is formed between the spleen and the left lateral abdominal wall, into which the colon can ride up sideways, in particular when the colon is filled with gas.

It is conceivable that such a buildup of gas could occur anterior to an obstructive plug present at the pelvic flexure. Initially the left ventral portion of the colon would move up between the lateral abdominal wall and spleen. The empty left dorsal portion of the colon anterior to the site of the obstruction would be pulled with it. If both portions

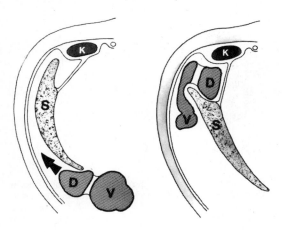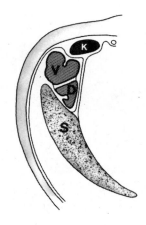

Figure 4. Proposed pathogenesis of left dorsal displacement of the large colon into the nephrosplenic space. S: Spleen; K: Kidney; D: Dorsal part of the large colon; V: Ventral part of the large colon.

of the colon are eventually forced into the nephrosplenic space, then the dorsal pole of the spleen traps them like a carabiner hook used by mountain climbers. The subsequent course of the condition depends on the degree of intestinal filling in the trapped portion of colon. Due to peristalsis at the site of the obstruction and the buildup of gas, more of the prestenotic portion of the colon is drawn into the site of constriction.

Clinical Signs. The course of the condition is usually protracted. Over a considerable period of time only slight changes or none are seen in the animal's general condition. Moderate to mild colic develops periodically. There is anorexia, moderate abdominal distention, and abdominal sounds seem shortened. Signs of shock occur only in severe cases; usually, the pulse rate is slightly increased and the pulse strength is normal. Quite often secondary distention of the stomach occurs. Findings on rectal examination are so characteristic that further tests and investigations are usually unnecessary. Diagnosis can be made on rectal examination alone (see p. 23).

The course of the conditions depends directly on the length of the entrapped portion of the colon and volume of its contents. Thus in exceptional cases in which more than two thirds of the colon is incarcerated, a severe form of colic may result. The greater the length of the trapped colon and the volume of its contents, the greater the tension on the root of the mesentery, with ensuing development of severe colic pain. If considerable gas accumulates in the entrapped and prestenotic portions of the colon, this causes congestion and edema of the intestinal wall and occurrence of considerable transudation. The congestion is usually not severe enough to cause necrosis.

Treatment

CONSERVATIVE. When a relatively undistended portion of the pelvic flexure is trapped, fasting of the patient usually leads to spontaneous resolution of the condition. The use of intravenous fluids can help to soften the ingesta. Trocharization of the cecum via the right flank and the large colon via the rectum removes the gas, and removal of gas and fluid from the stomach with a nasogastric tube facilitates the spontaneous repositioning of the colon. A wait-and-see approach is also advisable when the colon lies laterally between the spleen and lateral abdominal wall and the dorsal pole of the spleen has not performed its carabiner hooklike action. In my experience, cases of trapped colon may resolve spontaneously when the patient is placed in dorsal recumbency during positioning for surgery; therefore, rolling of the horse in a clockwise direction can be a successful treatment (Fig. 5).

SURGICAL. If conservative treatment is ineffective or the condition is too severe to contemplate this, surgery is recommended. After decompression of the entrapped portion of the large colon, the spleen is lifted ventrally and medially over the large colon, which is pushed dorsolaterally. Surgical repositioning can also be performed using a left flank laparotomy in which the 18th rib is resected. This approach has the advantage that the nephrosplenic space can be closed by suturing and recurrence prevented.

RIGHT DORSAL DISPLACEMENT OF THE LARGE COLON

Right dorsal displacement of the large colon in the horse has received little attention in the literature but is a distinct syndrome.

Etiology and Pathogenesis. The etiology of right dorsal colonic displacement is unknown. The roles of various feeding and overall husbandry practices are unclear, although they may be important. In this condition, the large colon passes between the right body wall and the cecum (Fig. 6). The displacement arises cranially and can move laterally or

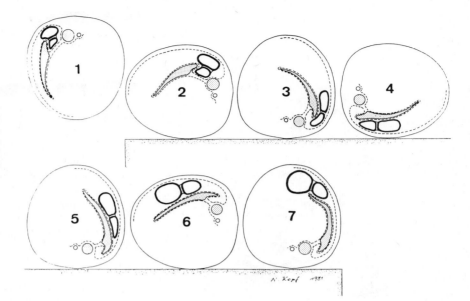

Figure 5. The mechanism of reposition in cases of left dorsal displacement of the large colon during rolling the horse. 1, Standing position; 2, 6, Right lateral recumbency; 3, 5, 7, Dorsal recumbency; 4, Left lateral recumbency.

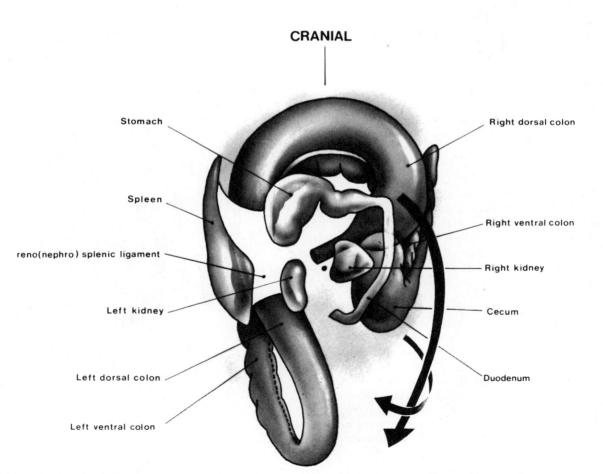

Figure 6. Normal position of the large colon in the horse (dorsal view) showing the typical direction taken by the large colon as right dorsal displacement develops (large arrow). Torsion of the bowel during each displacement may also occur (small arrow).

CRANIAL

LEFT

RIGHT

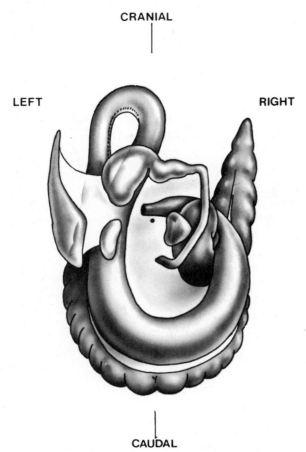

CAUDAL

Figure 7. Right dorsal displacement of the colon with flexion (dorsal view).

of the right flank due to gaseous accumulation in the colon is evident. Passage of the nasogastric tube is normally negative for reflux of fluids and ingesta and abdominal paracentesis produces small amounts of grossly normal-appearing fluid. In the more typical acute cases, signs of shock are evident. The flanks are considerably more distended with gas. The hematocrit is typically between 45 and 50 per cent and blood pH determination reveals a mild acidosis. In such cases there is often a gastric reflux. Abdominal paracentesis will reveal fluid containing erythrocytes and leukocytes. The rectal examination allows the diagnosis of the different states of dislocation, flexion, and torsion (see p. 23). The main differential diagnoses for right dorsal displacement are torsion, volvulus, and retroflexion of the large colon.

Treatment

Conservative. This is indicated only when the bowel is relatively empty and there is no torsion of the entrapped portion. Starvation and continuous

medially around the cecum. The proportion of medial to lateral displacements is approximately 1:15. Invariably a flexure of the colon occurs at the beginning and end of the large colon. The pelvic flexure is nearly always diplaced as far forward as the diaphragm, so that it cannot be felt on rectal examination. At the site of flexure, torsion (180 to 360 degrees) can occur, although a 180 degree torsion is more common. The degree of torsion and the volume of the colonic contents dictates the course of the disease, intensity of pain, rate of development of signs of shock, as well as the degree of circulatory disturbance in the involved bowel. If only a flexion without torsion is present (Figs. 7 and 8), then movement of ingesta through the lumen of the bowel is only partially halted and circulatory disturbances are slight. If, however, a torsion completely closes the bowel (Fig. 9), an impaction forms in the dorsal colon and severe circulatory disturbances follow.

Clinical Signs and Diagnosis. In the relatively mild case, when signs of colic are slight, distention

CRANIAL

LEFT

RIGHT

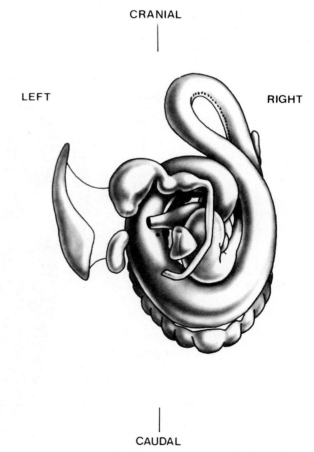

CAUDAL

Figure 8. The relatively rare right dorsal displacement of the large colon with medial flexion (dorsal view).

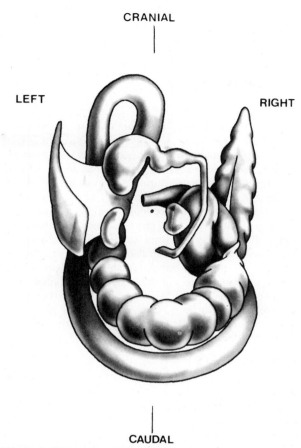

CRANIAL

LEFT   RIGHT

CAUDAL

Figure 9. Right dorsal displacement of the large colon with flexion and torsion (dorsal view).

infusion of intravenous fluids together with rectal trocharization of the gas-filled colon usually leads to resolution of the condition.

Surgical. Surgery is the treatment of choice in cases of right dorsal displacement of the large colon when signs of shock are present. Without operation, these animals eventually succumb to bowel infarction and necrosis.

Following a midline incision, an enterotomy is performed and the large colon is emptied of gas and ingesta. Care must be taken during manual repositioning of the bowel to prevent rupture. Compared with strangulating volvulus or torsion of the large colon, right dorsal displacement has a relatively good prognosis for survival.

MEDIAL DISPLACEMENT OF THE LARGE COLON

A medial displacement of the large colon can occur in heavily pregnant mares. Due to the capacious uterus, the large colon is pushed medially and caudally. This results in a flexion proximal to the cecum and a prestenotic impaction in the dorsal colon. The condition is similar to right dorsal displacement but differs in that the colon does not move around the cecum, but remains in the center of the abdomen. A stomachlike enlargement can be felt in an unusually caudal location on rectal palpation. The cecum is freely accessible.

FLEXION OR RETROFLEXION OF THE LARGE COLON

This condition arises as a result of a cranial displacement of the pelvic flexure in which the pelvic flexure lies in a lateral, medial, dorsal or ventral position, and is normally secondary to impaction or tympany of the large colon. The signs resemble those already described for the other displacements. In cases in which conservative treatment is unsuccessful or not indicated, surgery must be performed.

Supplemental Readings

Foerner, J. J.: Diseases of the large intestine. Vet. Clin. North Am. (Large Anim. Pract.), *4:*141, May, 1982.

Huskamp, B., and Kopf, N.: Die Verlagerung der Colon ascendens in den Milznierenraum beim Pferd (1 und 2). Tierarztl. Prax., *8:*327, and 495, 1980.

Huskamp, B., and Kopf, N.: Right dorsal displacement of the large colon in the horse. Equine Pract., *5:*20, 1983.

Huskamp, B., et al.: Diseases of the Horse. A Handbook for Science and Practice. New York, S. Karger, 1984, pp. 203–207 and 221.

Milne, D. W., Tarr, M. J., Lochner, F. K., et al.: Left dorsal displacement of the colon in the horse. J. Equine Med. Surg., *1:*47, 1977.

Colonic Volvulus and Intussusception

Richard P. Hackett, ITHACA, NEW YORK

COLONIC VOLVULUS

The large colon of the horse is anatomically predisposed to displacement. The horse's colon is extremely large compared with that of other species and is fixed in position only by attachments at the right ventral and right dorsal colon. The mesocolic axis functions as an axis about which the dorsal and ventral colons can rotate. It has been suggested that other predisposing factors are rolling of the horse that has colic of other causes, thromboembolic bowel ischemia, and feeding practices that induce abnormal intestinal motility or intestinal tympany.

Two forms of volvulus are encountered. The most common type is volvulus of the large colon and cecum. The site of rotation is the base of the cecum and the right dorsal colon as it narrows to form the transverse colon. The direction of this volvulus is typically counterclockwise as viewed from the ventrum. Volvulus of the large colon without involvement of the cecum may occur anywhere between the pelvic flexure and the level of the origin of the right ventral colon. This volvulus may be either clockwise or counterclockwise. There appears to be a predisposition for colonic volvulus in brood mares and in horses eight years of age or older. In one study, colonic volvulus constituted 135 of 785 cases of surgical colics (17 per cent) presented over a three-year period. Colonic volvulus was diagnosed in 11 per cent of all surgical colic cases in another practice.

CLINICAL SIGNS

The effects of volvulus on colonic function depend upon the degree of rotation, the location and duration of volvulus, and the length of the intestinal segment over which rotation occurs. Mild to moderate volvulus results in simple intestinal obstruction or partial obstruction with signs of impaction that progress slowly. Mild to moderate abdominal pain accompanies good cardiovascular status, reduced intestinal sounds, and normal peritoneal fluid. The balance of this discussion is limited to the signs of severe volvulus, a condition that results in obstruction and vascular impairment of the large colon or large colon and cecum. Clinical signs are acute in onset and are rapidly progressive. Affected horses exhibit signs of extreme abdominal pain caused by ischemia of large segments of bowel and subsequent intestinal distention. Profound shock is indicated by tachycardia, cool extremities, weak pulse, dehydration, and poor mucous membrane color and refill time. Marked abdominal distention is a conspicuous feature of this disorder. Large areas of tympanitic resonance ("pings") may be identified by simultaneous auscultation and percussion of the abdomen.

Rectal examination reveals colonic edema and tympany within a few hours of onset of clinical signs. It is rarely possible to determine the exact location of volvulus but findings such as inability to identify the pelvic flexure or palpation of distended colon oriented transversely strongly suggest the diagnosis (see p. 23). Colonic and cecal tympany are consistent findings. Exploration of the abdomen may be very difficult if markedly distended colonic segments occupy the pelvic cavity.

LABORATORY FINDINGS

The composition of peritoneal fluid is compatible with strangulation obstruction of intestine. Early in the course of the disease fluid is increased in volume and more turbid than normal due to elevation of total protein and a mild elevation of white blood cells. In more prolonged cases, fluid is serosanguineous. Hemoconcentration, a stress leukocytosis, and metabolic acidosis are typical.

TREATMENT

Colonic volvulus should be treated surgically as rapidly as possible. In no other form of colic is the prognosis as directly related to the time between onset of the disease and surgical intervention. Presurgical percutaneous trocharization of tympanitic cecal and colonic segments reduces attendant respiratory and cardiovascular embarrassment. Intravenous fluid and electrolyte therapy should be instituted at presentation. Severe dehydration in many cases mandates use of a mechanical roller pump to deliver a large fluid volume intravenously in a short period of time. Additional preoperative medication includes broad-spectrum antibiotics and flunixin meglumine. Presurgical preparations should not unduly delay surgical intervention. Mechanical ventilatory assistance is indicated during anesthesia.

A liberal ventral midline celiotomy is performed to ensure adequate exposure for colonic manipulation. Needle decompression of exposed segments of colon or cecum is performed immediately upon opening the peritoneum before exploration of the abdomen is attempted. This process is expedited by using a length of sterile latex tubing to allow suction aspiration of intraluminal gas. The abdomen is manually explored to determine the site of volvulus, to evaluate the degree of colonic vascular compromise, and to define the amount and type of colonic content. The pelvic flexure and left colon are identified and are exteriorized as completely as possible. It is essential that the colon be thoroughly emptied before correction of volvulus is attempted. Failure to do so entails a substantial but avoidable hazard of colonic rupture. In some cases needle aspiration of tympanitic colonic segments provides satisfactory colon emptying but in most cases accumulated fluid and ingesta mandates enterotomy. The pelvic flexure is removed from the celiotomy incision as far as possible and thoroughly isolated with water-impervious draping materials. An enterotomy is performed near the pelvic flexure and fluid and ingesta in the colon are milked out. If there is substantial solid ingesta in the colon, lavage with warm water delivered by a garden hose passed through the enterotomy is recommended. The amount of bleeding from the enterotomy incision and the appearance of the colonic mucosa is noted. Mechanical stapling instruments are useful for closing the enterotomy.

The most common type of volvulus, that of the large colon and cecum, occurs at the base of the cecum and termination of the right dorsal colon. The volvulus is readily apparent when these areas are palpated. Correction is preceded by exteriorizing as much of the free portion of the colon as possible so that the remaining intra-abdominal portion of the colon is nearly vertical. The base of the cecum and the right dorsal colon are then rotated to effect correction. In most cases, because volvulus is counterclockwise as viewed from the ventrum, rotation should be clockwise. Volvulus of the colon alone is corrected by exteriorizing as much colon as possible and rotating the free portion of the colon as necessary to effect correction. Colonic volvulus may be either clockwise or counterclockwise. Correction of either type of volvulus is confirmed by exteriorizing the cecal apex and tracing the cecocolic fold onto the right ventral colon and by ensuring that the transition from right dorsal colon to transverse colon is free of abnormality.

PROGNOSIS

The prognosis is directly related to the severity of vascular impairment induced by volvulus. The degree of impairment ranges from moderate interference with venous return to obvious devitalization of the affected segment. The prognosis is favorable in the former situation; in the latter, the horse should be euthanized on the table. For the group between these extremes the decision to allow or not allow recovery from anesthesia is based upon

the surgeon's best estimate of the degree of ischemic damage to the colon and the likelihood that colonic function will return after surgery. Objective indicators of intestinal perfusion and viability as measured by fluorescein dye, Doppler ultrasound, thermography, and surface oximetry have not been described from the equine large colon. Standard visual criteria therefore must be used to evaluate the effects of vascular impairment on the colon. The determinations should be made after volvulus has been corrected. An unfavorable prognosis is indicated by severe colonic edema, serosal cyanosis and congestion, venous thrombosis, mucosal necrosis, and lack of reflex motility. However, it must be recognized that such determinations are subjective and hence are not consistently reliable. In equivocal cases the patient must be given the benefit of such doubts and allowed to recover.

The extent of damage precludes resection in cases of volvulus of the large colon and cecum, but this may be an option in cases of volvulus of the colon. Resection is possible in cases of left colon volvulus and in cases of right colon volvulus in which adequate exposure of the affected site can be achieved for successful resection and anastomosis. Each limb of the colon is oversewn, preferably with mechanical stapling equipment, and a side-to-side colocolostomy is performed to re-establish colonic continuity. As much as 75 per cent of the colon may be removed with no apparent effects on digestive function.

The prognosis for colonic volvulus is unfavorable. In one study 42 of 106 horses died or were euthanized during surgery. Of 64 horses recovered from anesthesia, 57 (89 per cent) survived. The overall survival rate was 42.2 per cent. In another study, 16 of 25 horses died or were euthanized during or shortly after surgery. Of the nine horses that survived surgery, only four were long-term survivors. One horse died of unrelated causes. Recurrence of volvulus was documented in two horses.

INTUSSUSCEPTION OF THE COLON

Intussusception of the large colon is an unusual cause of intestinal obstruction in horses. It has been reported most frequently in young horses less than three years old but has been seen in older animals.

Clinical signs of this disease resemble those of impaction or nonstrangulating colon displacement early in the course of the disease. Signs include mild to moderate signs of colic, slow progression, reduced or absent fecal output, reduced intestinal sounds, slight tachycardia, mild dehydration, and reasonably normal mucous membrane appearance and capillary refill time. Rectal examination usually reveals a gas- and ingesta-filled left colon. In rare cases, the intussusception itself may be palpated rectally. However, in most cases such mild clinical signs lead to initial medical management until lack of response to therapy, progressive intestinal tympany, or increasing severity of abdominal pain dictate surgical exploration.

All recently reported colonic intussusception cases have involved the left colon—one in the left ventral colon, two involving the pelvic flexure, and one in the left dorsal colon. In two of these cases, the intussusception was treated by manual reduction, but in the other two, the intussusception could not be reduced. An intussusception of the left dorsal colon was treated by resection and end-to-end colocolotomy. A pelvic flexure intussusception was resected using mechanical stapling equipment. A side-to-side colocolotomy was then performed. All four animals reportedly survived the disorder.

Supplemental Readings

Barclay, W. P., Foerner, J. J., and Phillips, T. N.: Volvulus of the large colon in the horse. J. Am. Vet. Med. Assoc., *177*:629, 1980.

Hackett, R. P.: Nonstrangulated colonic displacement in horses. J. Am. Vet. Med. Assoc., *182*:235, 1983.

Huskamp, B.: The diagnosis and treatment of acute abdominal conditions in the horse: the various types and frequency as seen at the animal hospital at Hochmoor. Proc. Eq. Colic Res. Symp., 1982, pp. 261–272.

Wilson, D. G., Wilson, W. D., and Reinertson, E. L.: Intussusception of the left dorsal colon in a horse. J. Am. Vet. Med. Assoc., *183*:464, 1983.

Enteroliths and Small Colon Obstructions

Charles L. Boles, LOS OLIVOS, CALIFORNIA
Douglas J. Herthel, LOS OLIVOS, CALIFORNIA

ENTEROLITHS

Enteroliths are mineralized aggregates of ingesta salts that form slowly in the large colon, usually the right dorsal colon. They consist primarily of ammonium magnesium phosphate (59 per cent to 93 per cent) with traces of calcium, chromium, nickel, copper, and lead. Small particulate materials such as metallic objects or pebbles usually serve as the nidus for the progressively layered mineral deposition. All enteroliths of one study contained a nidus of chert, a common flintlike stone of silicon dioxide. Cross-sectioning or in vitro radiography will usually reveal the nature of the object at the center of the enterolith. Enteroliths probably form over many months or years. They are clinically significant as intraluminal intestinal obstructions of the large, transverse, or small colon. They can also be found as incidental necropsy findings that have not caused apparent clinical intestinal disturbances.

Epidemiology. The incidence of enteroliths is greatest in the western and southwestern United States. Within this large geographic region, small locales and specific farms experience an even higher incidence rate. Water and soil are usually the only common factors; this incriminates them as significant contributors to enterolith formation. The increasing occurrence of enteroliths suggests that changes or modifications in horse management or other unknown factors may contribute to their formation. A possible predisposition toward enterolith formation may exist in Arabian and part-Arabian horses. Within the Arabian breed a familial predisposition has been recently recognized. Clinical reports have documented the occurrence of enteroliths in all age groups over four years of age.

Pathogenesis. The presence of a developing enterolith does not cause intestinal dysfunction. They are of clinical significance when their size or change in location in the bowel creates an obstruction to the flow of ingesta or gas or both. Two clinical syndromes are generally recognized. A moderate-sized enterolith having formed asymptomatically in the large colon can result in a sudden obstruction as it passes into and obstructs the transverse or small colon. The obstruction is usually complete and allows no passage of ingesta and little or no gas passage. Signs associated with obstruction are more acute and more pronounced than signs usually associated with large enteroliths. Large enteroliths usually create obstructions at the origin of the transverse colon from the dorsal right colon. They are too large to pass into the transverse colon and thus serve as "ball" valves restricting the normal flow. Gas and small amounts of ingesta can escape around the enterolith, allowing for milder clinical signs of incomplete and intermittent obstruction.

History and Clinical Signs. Many affected horses have a history of recurrent bouts of colic. This suggests a large enterolith or enteroliths in the right dorsal colon that is producing an intermittent and spontaneously regressing obstruction at the origin of the transverse colon. The affected individual or other horses on the farm may even have a history of intermittently passing enteroliths in the stool with or without evidence of intestinal obstruction.

Clinical findings are consistent with any functional obstruction of the large or small colon and not specific for an enterolith obstruction. On the basis of history, signalment, and presence in a high incidence area, a tentative diagnosis can be made. Abdominal pain is mild to moderate. The degree of cardiovascular impairment is a reflection of the degree and duration of the enterolith obstruction.

Rectal examination findings will usually depend on site of obstruction. If the obstruction is incomplete gaseous distention may not be evident. Complete enterolith obstruction usually results in a moderate gaseous distention of the large colon and is detectable by rectal examination and as abdominal distention. Incomplete obstruction may allow the passage of mineral oil producing a rectal finding of scant, oily, mucus-containing feces. If the individual has not been treated with mineral oil, then the rectum may be devoid of fecal material or have a small amount of feces with mucus accumulation. Seldom can the enterolith be specifically identified on rectal examination.

Peritoneal fluid findings are also a reflection of the degree and duration of the intestinal obstruction. Fluid protein levels and white cell numbers are usually only slightly increased early in the course of the obstruction and in incomplete obstructions. Higher peritoneal fluid protein levels and white cell numbers will usually be found when the enterolith obstructs the transverse colon or small colon, producing local intestinal ischemia. Pronounced changes in peritoneal fluid indicative of significant bowel wall compromise are usually found only in protracted cases.

Abdominal radiography has proved very satisfactory for the definitive diagnosis of enterolithiasis in horses up to 559 kg and with an abdominal width of 75 cm. The necessary radiographic technique requires rare earth screens, compatible film, and a machine capable of at least 600 mA and 120 kV. If available, abdominal radiography should be considered in horses with recurrent bouts of colic if enterolithiasis is a possibility.

Surgery. An animal with intestinal obstruction failing to respond to medical therapy must be considered for surgical exploration of the abdomen with or without a tentative diagnosis of an enterolith obstruction. As previously described (see p. 33), hydration deficits, electrolyte imbalances, acid-base disturbances, and significant gastric distention should be corrected before anesthetic induction.

Abdominal distention seldom necessitates percutaneous decompression. However, if necessary for temporary relief during transport or induction of anesthesia, it is most effectively performed on the right side. The presence of distended bowel necessitates a gentle and controlled induction of anesthesia to minimize any possibility of viscus rupture.

A ventral midline celiotomy allows the greatest exposure of and access to the abdominal viscera where enteroliths may be encountered. Aspiration of gas distention proximal to the site of the obstruction greatly facilitates exploration of the abdominal cavity and exposure of any involved viscus. The distal limits of the right dorsal colon cannot be exteriorized. The large colon is exteriorized to the maximum extent and evacuated via a longitudinal pelvic flexure enterotomy off to the side of the animal. If possible, the obstruction is milked to and removed through the pelvic flexure enterotomy. If the enterolith is too large to be milked to the pelvic flexure, it must be removed via a second enterotomy at a location to which it can be manipulated, as far from the ventral midline incision as possible.

Enteroliths obstructing the transverse colon cannot be exteriorized beyond the abdominal incision because of the short mesenteric attachment of the transverse colon. Often thorough gas decompression or exteriorization and evacuation of the large colon will allow exposure of the transverse colon obstruction, which is then meticulously "packed off" with sterile, moistened surgical towels and maintained in position by an assistant. A longitudinal enterotomy through the antimesenteric band over the enterolith allows its removal. When evacuated, the empty transverse colon is much more difficult to keep exposed, and the risk of fecal contamination of the abdomen is greatest during closure of the enterotomy site. This technique should only be utilized by a surgical team having considerable expertise with intra-abdominal operations.

Enterolith obstruction of the small colon usually allows greater exteriorization of the obstructed segment. Removal of these enteroliths also requires careful isolation of the enterotomy site to avoid spillage of any bowel contents. Large, transverse, and small colon enterotomies are closed with two layers of absorbable suture in a Cushing pattern.

Consideration must be given to the multiple nature of enteroliths. Surgical exploration of the abdomen must include thorough examination of the colon, transverse colon, and small colon for the presence of additional enteroliths after the primary obstructing enterolith has been identified. If a flat-sided enterolith or an enterolith with a highly polished area on a rough surface is identified, there probably was or is at least one other enterolith present. All enteroliths present should be removed.

If the incidence of enteroliths is high in a particular environment, consideration should be given to selective deionization of the animal's drinking water.

FIBROUS FOREIGN BODY OBSTRUCTIONS

Indigestible fibrous material can produce obstructions of the pelvic flexure, right dorsal colon, transverse colon, or the small colon, especially in horses less than three years old. The materials are most commonly rubber fencing or rubber tires used as feeders, but can be miscellaneous objects such as blankets, feed sacks, feed tubs, and tarpaulins.

The synthetic polyester or nylon fibers of the rubber fencing are usually ingested one at a time. The fibers probably then accumulate and amalgamate into an entangled mass in the right colon. Small mineralized concretions form over much of the surface of the mass. Materials from the rubber tires may be either individual fibers or pieces of rubber with fiber; collectively they form obstructive masses or serve as the loose nidus for mineral accumulations.

Horses with foreign body obstructions present very similarly to horses with enterolith obstructions. However, most present acutely without previous colic episodes. A history of exposure to rubber fencing or rubber tires can be significant if there is reason to expect foreign body obstruction. One should be aware that the horse may be removed from the source of foreign material for some time before signs of obstruction are evident. In one report a horse was removed from rubber fencing for two years before developing an obstruction. Similar histories have been reported with rubber tires.

The surgical principles for removing the fibrous foreign material are the same as for enterolith removal. Because of the potentially large fibrous entangled nature of the rubber fence obstructions, up to 90 cm in length and 6.9 kg, numerous enterotomies may be required to remove the mass if it involves the right dorsal colon, transverse colon, small colon or any combination of these. Also the rough irregular surface of these concretions frequently precludes manipulation anterograde or retrograde within the bowel.

Supplemental Readings

Blue, M. G.: Enteroliths in horses—a retrospective study of 30 cases. Equine Vet. J. *11*:76, 1979.

Blue, M. G., and Wittkopp, R. W.: Clinical and structural features of equine enteroliths. J. Am. Vet. Med. Assoc., *179*:79, 1981.

Boles, C. L., and Kohn, C. W.: Fibrous foreign body impaction in young horses. J. Am. Vet. Med. Assoc., *171*:193, 1977.

DeGroot, A.: The significance of low packed cell volume in relation to the early diagnosis of intestinal obstruction in the horse, based on field observations. Proc. 17th Ann. Conv. Am. Assoc. Eq. Pract., 309, 1972.

Evans, D. R., and Trunk, D. A.: Diagnosis and treatment of enterolithiasis in equidae. Comp. Cont. Ed. 3:383, 1981.

Rose, J. A., Rose, E. M., and Sande, R. D.: Radiography in the diagnosis of equine enterolithiasis. Proc. 26th Ann. Conv. Am. Assoc. Eq. Pract., 211, 1981.

Nonstrangulating Intestinal Infarction

Nathaniel A. White, II, LEESBURG, VIRGINIA

Nonstrangulating intestinal infarction (NSI) has been identified in two forms in the horse. The first is known as thromboembolic colic, or thrombotic or thromboembolic infarction, and is associated with the thrombotic lesion produced by the migrating fourth and fifth stage larvae of *Strongylus vulgaris*. The severity of the lesion of arteritis is determined by the number of migrating larvae and the horse's acquired resistance. Thrombus formation reduces mesenteric blood flow and produces ischemia with subsequent intestinal damage. The reduction of blood flow is thought to result from the physical obstruction by the thrombus or by vasoconstriction due to the active coagulation process that is present at the site of the arterial lesion.

The other cause of NSI is reduced blood flow that may result from local causes other than arteritis or may be caused by decreased cardiac output. This is usually observed in horses in shock following intestinal strangulation obstruction and is due to reduced circulating blood volume. Reduction of intestinal blood flow caused by hypovolemia, systemic hypotension, or intestinal distention produces lesions throughout the bowel. The result of the reduced blood flow is ischemia with focal or generalized infarction, which produces bowel dysfunction such as ileus, tympany, impaction, and diarrhea.

CLINICAL SIGNS

The signs of NSI produced by verminous arteritis are most common in yearling and young adult horses, although NSI has been observed in foals less than two months of age. Verminous arteritis is expected in horses in environments in which measures for control of *Strongylus vulgaris* are poor and the parasite is prevalent. However, the disease can also occur in horses being treated routinely with anthelmintics (see p. 328). One or two migrating larvae can incite arteritis sufficient to cause NSI. Because NSI can affect single or multiple parts of the intestinal tract, clinical signs are determined by the bowel segments involved and the extent of the lesion.

Infarction associated with verminous arteritis is most common in the large colon and cecum. When these organs are involved, ileus and tympanic distention are often chronic. The greater the distention the greater the pain. Small intestinal infarction is usually associated with gastric reflux and rapid dehydration. Unfortunately, the signs are variable and mimic signs occurring with simple obstruction, strangulation obstruction, arteritis, and peritonitis.

Pain can be mild to severe and normally disappears as the disease progresses and produces peritonitis. Depression then becomes predominant. Pain can be intermittent or can recur at intervals of days and weeks. The temperature and heart rate are not helpful in determining the severity of NSI, nor do they help discriminate between other types of disease and NSI. Gastric reflux when present is a sign of small intestinal involvement, but because the bowel is usually unobstructed, there can be severe small intestinal ischemia or infarction and minimal gastric reflux. Borborygmi are almost always reduced with NSI; gas and fluid sounds may be present but there is little or no progressive bowel motility. Chronic arteritis may produce diarrhea, weight loss, and chronic depression.

If the bowel is distended, rectal examination can help to determine the segment of intestine involved. Unfortunately, rectal examination cannot determine if verminous arteritis is the cause of distention. Neither fremitus, thickness, nor pain in the mesenteric stalk are valid indicators of the presence or the severity of arteritis.

The skin elasticity, hematocrit (PCV), and total plasma protein can help evaluate the animal's hydration and the severity of shock. There is no consistent pattern of fluid or protein loss in NSI. In severe disease, peritonitis may induce a leakage of protein into the peritoneal cavity or intestine, but

this process is similar to other diseases that produce shock or peritonitis. Dehydration is usually mild. Over a long period of time, dehydration can result from lack of fluid intake rather than from acute fluid shifts to a third compartment. If bowel infarction is severe and results in endotoxemia, the signs of shock are rapidly progressive.

Peritoneal fluid can be of help in identifying NSI. The fluid can be normal or can be opaque and yellowish or serosanguineous. Often the peritoneal fluid contains increased numbers of white blood cells resulting from degeneration of bowel and transmural escape of endotoxin and bacteria. Peritoneal fluid protein levels are commonly elevated over 3.0 gm per dl. Peritoneal white blood cell counts as high as 200,000 per cu mm have been observed. If red blood cells are present in the peritoneal fluid they do not differentiate strangulation obstruction from NSI. Peritoneal fluid analysis is evidence of the severity of the disease and surgery is elected to determine the diagnosis. When the peritoneal fluid white blood cell count and total protein level are elevated, but there is minimal pain or shock, medical therapy for peritonitis may be indicated rather than surgical exploration of the abdomen.

A peripheral white blood cell count does not distinguish NSI from other diseases. Neutropenia may be present if peritonitis is severe.

There is no test that specifically identifies verminous arteritis or NSI caused by verminous arteritis. Even the fecal examination for strongyles can be negative if all worms are prepatent. Electrophoretograms of blood can reveal an elevation of the beta$_2$-globulin fraction in horses with verminous arteritis. However, this elevation can occur from other parasitic infections and chronic disease processes.

The NSI caused by hypoperfusion as a result of hypovolemia or secondary to severe bowel disease usually becomes a problem following surgery for acute strangulating bowel disease. The condition has also been observed when hypovolemia results from severe enteritis and heat exhaustion. The primary signs are ileus and shock.

THERAPY

Treatment for NSI is symptomatic. If the ischemia is severe enough to produce infarction, surgery is necessary to remove the affected bowel segment. Because of the large areas of the cecum, large colon, or small intestine involved, total removal of the affected bowel may not always be possible. Once the disease has progressed to the stage at which surgery is required, the mortality rate can be as high as 90 per cent.

Ischemia of the small intestine is indicated by

gastric reflux, distended loops of small intestine palpable on rectal examination, abnormal peritoneal fluid resulting from bowel degeneration, uncontrollable pain, and lack of response to medical therapy. Surgery is required to remove infarcted segments. Progressive NSI is a common sequel, so the prognosis is grave.

Treatment of the verminous arteritis may be helpful in chronic mild colic. Three anthelmintics kill the third and fourth stages of *Strongylus vulgaris* larvae during their migration; thiabenzadole* (440 mg per kg orally on two successive days), fenbendazole† (10 mg per kg orally daily for five days or 50 mg per kg orally daily for three days), and Ivermectin‡ (200 μg per kg orally as a single dose). These drugs kill larvae slowly so that larvae remain in the artery for days to weeks before they are removed and the endothelium heals. The use of these anthelmintics during acute NSI is not advisable because intestinal disease may prevent drug absorption.

Medical therapy for NSI with bowel necrosis is aimed at maintaining normal tissue perfusion, preventing further thrombus formation in cases of arteritis, preventing and treating peritonitis, and controlling pain. Blood volume replacement with a polyionic isotonic fluid is important for combating shock. If possible, acid-base status should be determined (see p. 36) because the horse may be either alkalotic as a result of gastric reflux or acidotic as a result of shock. Bicarbonate replacement can be calculated once acid-base status is determined (see p. 36). Because of chronic lack of food intake and the changes in electrolyte absorption from the bowel, serum levels of potassium and calcium need to be monitored and values corrected by administration of intravenous fluids with potassium chloride or calcium chloride added in the appropriate levels to replace the deficit (see p. 37). Administration of calcium requires monitoring of the heart, best done with electrocardiography.

Ileus is often present and may be helped by maintaining normal blood levels of calcium and potassium. Neostigmine§ (2 to 4 mg subcutaneously every 30 minutes) may help stimulate the large bowel; however, if the intestine has ischemic lesions the bowel often will not respond. Relief of bowel distension is indicated using either cecal trocharization for large bowel tympany or nasogastric intubation for small bowel distention.

In severe or chronic NSI, antimicrobial therapy is necessary because degenerating bowel results in peritonitis. Gram-negative organisms and some gram-positive organisms such as Streptococcus and anaerobes can be involved. Penicillin* (20,000 units per kg four times a day intravenously) or ampicillin† (11 mg per kg three times a day intravenously) combined with an aminoglycoside such as gentamicin‡ (2 mg per kg three times a day intravenously) provides an optimal combination of drugs. Because of the risk of renal tubular damage by hypovolemia and aminoglycoside therapy, renal function should be monitored before and during therapy. A trimethoprim-sulfamethoxazole combination§ has also been useful in peritonitis and can be given orally at a dosage of 2 mg per kg (trimethoprim) twice a day. It should not be used if ileus is present. Peritoneal lavage can also be useful (see p. 77).

Plasma protein replacement should be considered as part of therapy for peritonitis. The goal is to maintain serum albumin levels and to replace needed opsonins and gamma globulins. Estimates of plasma replacement are based on the plasma volume (5 per cent of body weight) and the protein deficit.

Analgesic therapy is necessary in some cases of NSI to relieve pain, comfort the animal, and prevent reflex ileus. Flunixin meglumine‖ (.25 mg per kg twice a day or four times a day) is the most useful drug; its cyclooxygenase inhibitor activity helps to control the effects of endotoxemia and in so doing provides relief from pain. Xylazine¶ (.06 to 0.22 mg per kg intravenously) as repeated small doses also provides effective analgesia. Xylazine should be used as sparingly as possible as it can reduce large bowel activity. Butorphanol# is a narcotic with good analgesic properties and is effective at dosages of 0.05 to 0.1 mg per kg.

Laxatives can be used to help lubricate or soften large intestinal masses or food impactions that may complicate NSI. Five per cent dioctyl sodium succinate** (250 ml per 450 kg once daily) helps water to soften the mass. Mineral oil may help prevent endotoxin absorption and acts as a lubricant.

Anticoagulation has been attempted to help reduce the effects of thrombus formation. Minidose heparin†† therapy (40 units per kg intravenously or subcutaneously three times a day) does not alter coagulation but has been reported to prevent laminitis subsequent to endotoxemia. Anticoagulant heparin therapy (100 units per kg intravenously four times a day) has not been proved to increase survival. Nonsteroidal anti-inflammatory agents are useful in inhibiting platelet activity. This type of

---

*Omnizole, MSD-AGVET, Rahway, NJ
†Panacur, American Hoechst Corp., Somerville, NJ
‡Equivalen, MSD-AGVET, Rahway, NJ
§Stiglyn, Pitman Moore, Inc., Washington Crossing, NJ

---

*Pfizerpen, Pfizer Inc., New York, NY
†Omnipen, Wyeth Laboratories, Inc., Philadelphia, PA
‡Gentocin, Schering Corp., Kenilworth, NJ
§Cotrim, Lemmon Co., Sellersburg, PA
‖Banamine, Schering Corp., Kenilworth, NJ
¶Rompun, Haver-Lockhart, Shawnee, KS
#Stadol, Bristol Laboratories, Syracuse, NY
**Cerusol, Burns-Biotec, Oakland, CA
††Heparin, Elkins-Sinn, Inc., Cherry Hill, NJ

therapy with flunixin meglumine, phenylbutazone (4 mg per kg daily), or aspirin (25 mg per kg orally once daily) should help reduce thrombus formation at the site of arteritis, but the clinical benefits are not proved. Dextran 70%* administered intravenously at 5 to 15 mg per kg of a 6 per cent solution per day has been reported to benefit horses with verminous arteritis.

Medical therapy for NSI is relied upon whenever possible because anesthesia and abdominal surgery can exacerbate the ischemia and increase mortality. If surgery is necessary, dopamine† (2.5 to 5 μg per kg per minute intravenously) in conjunction with blood volume replacement during and after surgery will help maintain cardiac output and provide increased mesenteric blood flow.

PROGNOSIS

The prognosis for NSI associated with verminous arteritis is determined by the severity of shock. The most commonly used prognostic indicators are increases in heart rate, PCV, and the degree of anaerobic metabolism as indicated by plasma lactate or the anion gap. Peritoneal fluid analysis may reveal marked elevations in the white blood cell count and protein level; however, horses may survive this severe peritonitis.

*Dextran 70, Travenol, Deerfield, IL
†Intropin, Arnar-Stone, Inc., Aquadilla, PR

Supplemental Readings

Drudge, J. H.: Clinical aspects of *Strongylus vulgaris* infection in the horse. In Symposium on Gastroenterology. Vet. Clin. North Am. (Large Anim. Pract.), *1*:251, 1979.

Sellers, A. F., Lowe, J. E., Prost, O. J., et al.: Retropulsion-propulsion in equine large colon. Am. J. Vet. Res., *43*:390, 1982.

White, N. A.: Intestinal infarction associated with mesenteric vascular thrombotic disease in the horse. J. Am. Vet. Assoc., *178*:259, 1981.

White, N. A., Moore, N. N., and Douglas, M.: SEM study of *Strongylus vulgaris* larva-induced arteritis in the pony. Equine Vet. J., *15*:349, 1983.

White, N. A.: Thromboembolic Colic in Horses. Compend. Cont. Ed., 7:S156, 1985.

Rectal Prolapse

Tracy A. Turner, GAINESVILLE, FLORIDA

Rectal prolapse is a relatively uncommon problem in horses, with a higher incidence in mares than in male horses. Predisposing factors leading to rectal prolapse may include loss of anal sphincter tone, loose attachments of the mucous membrane to the muscular coat of the rectum, and loose attachments of the rectum to perirectal tissues. Prolapse can accompany any condition that causes tenesmus, such as constipation, diarrhea, proctitis, intestinal parasitism, infectious enteritis or colitis, rectal foreign body, neoplasia, dystocia, urethral obstruction, and colic.

CLINICAL SIGNS

Rectal prolapse is an evagination of mucous membrane and associated structures through the anus. Four types of rectal prolapse are recognized. Mucosal prolapse (type 1) produces a circular swelling, resembling a large doughnut, at the anus. The protrusion results from the mucosa and submucosa sliding backward on the muscularis of the rectum (Fig. 1A). A complete prolapse (type II), which everts all or part of the ampulla recti (Fig. 1B), is generally larger and more cylindric than a type I prolapse. The ventral portion of this type of prolapse is usually larger and thicker than the dorsal portion. The third type of prolapse (type III) may appear like a complete prolapse but it is usually firmer and thicker because of the invagination of small colon into the rectum (Fig. 1C). A type IV prolapse is an intussusception of peritoneal rectum or small colon through the anus (Fig. 1D). This type of protrusion results in a palpable trench that may extend for several meters into the rectum depending on the length of the intussusception.

TREATMENT

The first aim of therapy is identification and alleviation of the cause. If the prolapse is small and recent, conservative therapy is often successful. Manual reduction of the prolapse is facilitated by epidural anesthesia. Edema in the prolapsed tissues

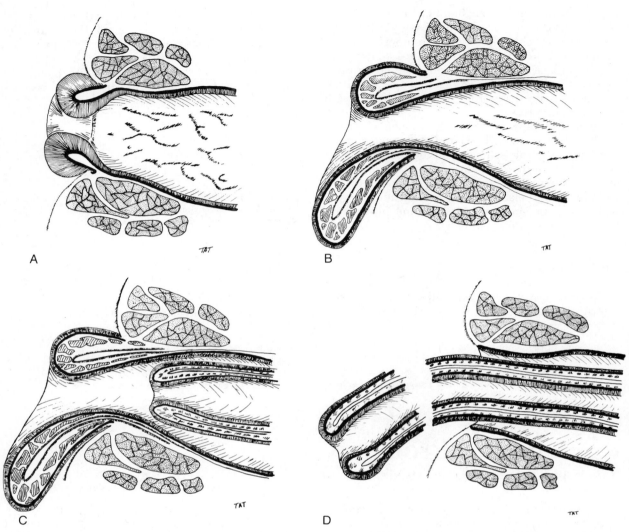

Figure 1. *A,* Type I rectal prolapse. Mucosal prolapse involving only mucosa and submucosa of the rectum. *B,* Type II rectal prolapse. Complete prolapse involving full wall thickness of the rectum. *C,* Type III rectal prolapse. Complete prolapse plus intussusception of peritoneal rectum or small colon. *D,* Type IV rectal prolapse. Intussusception of the peritoneal rectum or small colon or both.

can be reduced with topical glycerin, sugar, or magnesium sulfate. Once the prolapse is reduced a pursestring suture can be placed in the anus to prevent recurrence of the prolapse. Lidocaine enemas (12 ml of 2 per cent lidocaine in 50 ml water) will desensitize the rectal tissue and may prevent straining for a short time. Nonirritant laxatives such as mineral oil may also be beneficial to prevent obstipation and to soothe irritated tissues.

Unique problems are encountered when conservative therapy is used to treat rectal prolapse. Pursestring sutures may not be suitable because the horse's feces are too large and dry to readily pass through the sutured anus. The sutures also cause

anal irritation and the horse may tend to strain against the suture. Repeated epidural anesthesia to prevent prolapse may result in temporary paralysis of the hind limbs and decreasing effectiveness of analgesia.

Type I and type II prolapses are usually amenable to conservative treatment. If not, or if the mucosa becomes severely inflamed, traumatized, cyanotic, or necrotic, the prolapse should be corrected by submucosal resection. Type III rectal prolapse can be partially treated using either conservative methods or submucosal resection. Celiotomy is usually necessary to reduce the intussusception in both type III and type IV prolapses. Since vascular integrity of the small colon may be lost if excessive tension is placed on the mesentery, colostomy may be indicated.

PROGNOSIS

Generally, the prognosis for type I or type II prolapse is favorable, but complications may arise. Rectal strictures are possible if extensive areas of denuded rectal mucosal are allowed to heal by epithelialization and contraction. Obstipation is a common problem, but it can be alleviated by laxatives and manual evacuation. While pararectal abscesses are a potential problem, they have not been encountered in the horse as a result of rectal prolapse. This absence of abscesses is attributed to good vascularity and natural resistance to infection.

Types III and IV prolapses have a more guarded prognosis. Prognosis depends on vascular integrity of the intussusception. This must be determined by visual examination of the mesentery and bowel.

Supplemental Readings

Brown, M. P.: Conditions of the rectum. Vet. Clin. North Am. (Large Anim. Pract.), 4:185, 1982.
Johnson, H. W.: Submucous resection, surgical correction for prolapse of the rectum. J. Am. Vet. Med. Assoc., 102:113, 1963.
Turner, T. A., and Fessler, J. F.: Rectal prolapse in the horse. J. Am. Vet. Med. Assoc., 177:1028, 1980.

Rectal Tears

G. Michael H. Shires, KNOXVILLE, TENNESSEE

Rupture of the equine rectum is a potentially life-threatening disaster that should be evaluated as soon as it is suspected. A high percentage of patients with intraperitoneal rectal tears die from peritonitis despite treatment.

The causes of rectal tears are varied and the commonest of these are listed in Table 1. The greatest number of tears occur as a sequel to rectal palpation and are most commonly caused by veterinarians. Inexperience and vigorous exploration during palpation, a disparity between the size of the palpator's arm and the horse's rectal tube, and insufficient lubrication predispose to problems. Nervous and restless horses improperly restrained are more likely to incur rectal tears, and it is also reported that rectal tears occur more frequently in the Arabian breed. Rough objects such as seams in rectal sleeves can also initiate tears in the rectal mucosa. The consequences of such accidents are serious and may be costly to the practitioner. The severity and prognosis of these lesions depends on their size and location, the number of tissue layers torn, and the length of time between occurrence, diagnosis, and treatment.

In the event of this occurrence, it is essential to communicate with the owner or agent from the start, explaining the problem and potential outcome completely. Full disclosure and vigorous treatment with the client's thorough understanding will help to reduce the possibility of legal issues should the patient succumb.

DIAGNOSIS

The first sign of a break in the rectal mucosa is red-tinged feces or lubricant on the rectal glove. While a slight amount of blood-tinged feces on the hand might not indicate a serious problem, it indicates the necessity for precautions. Fresh, clotted blood on the glove and in the feces indicates a considerable tear in the mucosa and should be treated as a potentially serious problem to be fully evaluated without delay. Other evidence of rectal tears ranges from the presence of a palpable lesion or break in the mucosa, usually on the dorsal area of the rectum, to sudden relaxation of the rectum and easy palpation of extrarectal structures. Restlessness of the animal with concurrent straining may signal discomfort secondary to rectal damage.

Signs of discomfort, straining, or difficulty in advancing the hand into the rectal tube should

TABLE 1. COMMON CAUSES OF RECTAL TEARS

Rectal palpation	Dystocia
Breeding accidents	Pelvic and other fractures
Enema	Spontaneous rupture
External trauma	Sphincter abnormalities

caution the palpator to inspect for the presence of any blood. If signs of a tear should not be recognized during palpation and if the horse starts to evidence colic or tenesmus—even discomfort and sweating—soon after the palpation, the possibility of a rectal tear must be investigated.

Proper treatment of rectal tears requires an accurate and early diagnosis. If circumstances preclude this possibility, then the animal should be referred to more suitable facilities. To minimize complications and offer the animal the best chance of survival, the following procedures are necessary.

INITIAL AND GENERAL MANAGEMENT

A realistic prognosis and rational treatment regimen require early recognition of the problem and procurement of a data base. When a tear is suspected, the patient should be sedated, the lesion should be evaluated by palpation, and the rectum must be emptied, cleaned, and inspected carefully. Epidural anesthesia or a smooth muscle relaxant, such as propantheline bromide (0.05 mg per kg intravenously), and a speculum facilitate examination. Baseline values of temperature, pulse and respiration rate should be taken as well as a blood sample for measurement of a complete blood count, total protein, and packed cell volume, and abdominocentesis for cytologic examination, smear, and cell counts.

If necessary, booster tetanus immunization is administered. In all but hopeless cases antibiotic therapy is initiated using a systemic bactericidal with a gram-positive, gram-negative, and anaerobic spectrum. Most practical choices would be therapeutic doses of procaine penicillin coupled with gentamicin, neomycin, or similar drugs. The newer sulfa combination drugs would also make an excellent choice, especially as they can be administered orally once a suitable blood level has been obtained by an initial systemic administration. Fluid therapy is instituted if there is evidence of dehydration. If possible, fluids should be administered orally to rehydrate the animal and keep the feces soft.

Should tenesmus be a problem, parasympatholytic drugs such as atropine or propantheline bromide could be used as long as the effect of drugs on gastrointestinal function is taken into account. The concomitant use of fecal softeners such as dioctyl sodium sulfosuccinate or emollients such as mineral oil will reduce the likelihood of constipation and obstructive colic.

Although straining can also be overcome by use of an epidural anesthetic, the procedure cannot be repeated over a period of time for a variety of reasons, not the least being the risk of injury due to improper function of the hind legs.

To be able to monitor the animal's progress intelligently, the person caring for the horse should be made aware of potential clinical signs including sweating, straining, colic, increased pulse, respiration and temperature, shock, and collapse. In most cases, it is wise to change the patient's feed for a day or two in an effort to keep the feces soft. Handlers must also note the quantity and color of voided feces for a few days. If it is impossible to monitor the animal's progress, the horse should be moved to a more suitable place for adequate care.

A presumptive diagnosis made from blood on the hand or ease of palpation should be followed by a definitive diagnosis as quickly as possible. This may require referring the patient to a veterinary hospital. If this is the case, the initial clinical and laboratory data should be sent with the horse. If shock is imminent, treatment for this as well as initial antibiotic therapy should be initiated before the animal is transported. A complete and accurate history, especially relating to the time of injury and any treatment initiated, should accompany the horse. Heroic attempts at suturing rectal tears in the standing patient are not usually successful. Most tears cannot be visualized sufficiently to enable even the most skilled surgeon to suture them suitably via the anus. Partial closure of the mucosa over a contaminated lesion potentiates infection, abscessation, and peritonitis.

SPECIFIC MANAGEMENT

The repair of rectal tears includes several therapeutic and surgical options varying with the severity of the lesion. Choices can only be properly made once an accurate diagnosis has been established and the client fully appraised (Fig. 1).

Assessment of the type and severity of lesions should categorize the rectal tear into one of four grades (Table 2). Prognosis and treatment both depend to a great extent on the type and location of lesion (Tables 3 and 4). Even when the immediate danger is passed, there is the possibility of complications following peritonitis. These vary from abscesses and septicemia to obstruction and recurrent colic resulting in cachexia and death.

Attempts to suture grade 1 tears in the standing animal should only be made in the rare case in which these lesions are easily visualized via the anus. Most grade 1 tears can be treated successfully with aggressive antimicrobial therapy coupled with a diet that keeps feces soft for a few days. Drugs such as flunixin meglumine or butazolidin may be used to reduce inflammation and subsequent straining. Since by definition grade 2 tears do not include the mucosa or submucosa, it is most unlikely that this type of tear will be recognized following pal-

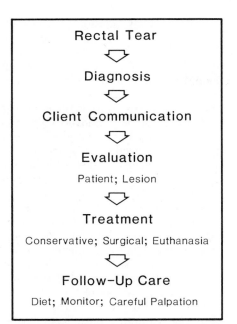

Rectal Tear

⇩

Diagnosis

⇩

Client Communication

⇩

Evaluation

Patient; Lesion

⇩

Treatment

Conservative; Surgical; Euthanasia

⇩

Follow-Up Care

Diet; Monitor; Careful Palpation

Figure 1. Disposition of a case of rectal tear.

TABLE 3. TREATMENT CHOICES FOR RECTAL TEARS

Grade I	Close to anus	Conservative therapy, monitor, suture standing?
	Not visualized from anus	Conservative therapy, monitor
Grade II		Usually not recognized; treat subsequent abscessation or fistula
Grade III		Medical therapy, peritoneal lavage and/or surgery.
Grade IV	With local peritonitis	Surgery, vigorous medical therapy, and peritoneal lavage
	With diffuse peritonitis	Heroic treatment and surgery? Euthanasia usually most suitable

for cytologic examination and cell count. The procedure may be repeated two or three times and the cell count monitored. It is unnecessary to include antibacterials in this fluid if the patient is being given systemic antimicrobials. The catheter can be sealed and bandaged to the abdomen using a belly band in a sterile manner so that the procedure can be repeated subsequently without having to introduce catheters repeatedly.

Surgical Treatment of Grades 3 and 4 Tears. If abdominal contamination is minimal, most grade 3 tears are best treated by vigorous medical treatment combined with peritoneal lavage. Surgical repair of grades 3 and 4 tears can be attempted via a number of approaches that visualize the lesion. If tears are far from the anus in the small colon, they may be exteriorized through an abdominal incision. Most tears, however, must be sutured intra-abdominally with very limited visualization and exposure using a ventral midline laparotomy or a paramedian approach. Alternatively, an abdominal incision may be used to prolapse the rectum sufficiently for another surgeon to suture the prolapsed lesion. If prolapse is the choice, speed is essential to avoid thrombosis of the mesenteric vessels. This is a real concern, even in animals with a moderate amount of mesenteric fat.

pation. Evidence of grade 2 tears is found either when pararectal or paravaginal abscesses or fistulas occur, or at necropsy, usually as a secondary finding.

Peritoneal Lavage. Peritoneal lavage is a successful adjunct to surgery when contamination of the peritoneal cavity is suspected. Using sterile technique, a Foley catheter of medium diameter (10 to 12 Fr) is placed through a stab incision on the ventral midline into the peritoneal cavity. The catheter is fixed in place after inflating the balloon, and 6 to 10 L of warm normal sterile saline or balanced electrolyte solution is run through the catheter into the peritoneal cavity using gravity flow. A pump may be used but care must be taken to avoid too-rapid fluid administration. The horse often shows some mild discomfort when sufficient fluid is placed in the abdomen. The catheter is then clamped and the horse walked vigorously for 10 to 15 minutes. The clamp is removed and fluid is drained from the abdomen. An early sample is taken

TABLE 2. CLASSIFICATION OF RECTAL TEARS

Grade I
  Tear of mucosa or submucosa
Grade II
  Tear of muscular layers but not mucosa or submucosa
Grade III
  Mucosa, submucosa, and muscular layers torn—usually retroperitoneal
Grade IV
  All layers torn and extending into peritoneal cavity

TABLE 4. SURGICAL CHOICES FOR RECTAL TEARS

Grade I
  Clean and debride
  Suture standing
Grade II
  Flush and drain abscess
Grades III and IV
  Laparotomy and suture
  Laparotomy and prolapse
  Temporary colostomy
  "end-on" or loop

Colostomy. When neither prolapse of the lesion nor an abdominal approach allow adequate visualization for surgical closure, it may be preferable to divert fecal material using a colostomy and allow the lesion to heal under less adverse conditions.

A temporary diverting colostomy is created with the animal either standing under sedation and local anesthesia or in lateral recumbency under general anesthesia. The incision is made in the left flank in a position low enough to allow feed material to flow with gravity but high enough to minimize soiling and trauma when the animal lies down. A suitable section of the small colon is then exteriorized. The surgeon may choose one of two procedures.

In the first procedure, the small colon is transected and the distal stump closed and sealed. The section of the small colon containing the lesion is replaced into the abdominal cavity. The proximal stump of the small colon is sutured to the skin at the ventral margin of the incision and the dorsal part of the incision closed so that the proximal small colon is sutured to the skin around its entire circumference. Feces are thus voided via this colostomy on the flank and diverted from the more distal rectal tear. After a suitable period to allow healing of the primary lesion, the colostomy is carefully dissected from the incision, which is then closed, and the small colon is anastomosed. Since the distal stump usually shrinks considerably, reanastomosis is best done via a ventral midline incision. Automatic stapling instruments may facilitate this difficult anastomosis.

The second method for creation of a temporary diverting colostomy requires a left flank incision. A suitable section of the small colon proximal to the rectal tear is exteriorized and secured to the flank incision so that the antimesenteric band projects from the flank. The colon is arranged so that the proximal end descends to the incision and the distal end ascends toward the segment containing the lesion. An incision is made through the middle of the antimesenteric band into the lumen of the small colon for about four inches. The skin incision is closed incorporating the mucosa, submucosa, and muscularis tissues circumferentially. The small colon now has an exit for the passage of fecal material proximal to the lesion. Very careful gravity flow of sterile electrolyte solutions via the anus will clean the distal segment through this colostomy, and if fluids are allowed to flow through the distal segment periodically, this segment will be kept functional. After a period of about 14 days to allow healing of the original lesions, the circumferential sutures are removed. The incision into the antimesenteric band of the small colon is exteriorized slightly, debrided, cleaned, and closed using at least a two-layer closure. The repaired small colon is replaced into the abdomen and the flank incision closed routinely. This loop colostomy is functionally similar to the first procedure described but does not involve reanastomosis of the small colon nor does it require a second abdominal incision to return the small colon to its normal function.

Whatever surgical procedure is selected, vigorous medical therapy must be employed to control peritonitis. While it has been stated that "end on" colostomy (the first procedure described) is the only way to ensure diversion of the fecal stream, the complicated and costly surgical procedures required for reanastomosis makes the loop colostomy a more practical and workable choice in the horse.

Creation of a colostomy, temporary as it may be, is a surgical choice resorted to only for lesions that are life-threatening. Complications of either procedure include self-mutilation of the colostomy site, prolapse of bowel through the colostomy, peritonitis, obstipation, and scalding of the skin below the colostomy site. Careful postoperative care and dietary control can minimize these complications so that the surgical creation of a temporary colostomy is a realistic treatment of the life-threatening rectal tear.

Euthanasia. In cases of severe grade 4 tears and significant fecal contamination of the peritoneal cavity, euthanasia must be included in the discussion with the client. Heroic attempts to save the animal's life without success but with considerable cost may only serve to alienate the client. Communication from the start regarding all aspects of the problem, including the cause and a realistic prognosis, should minimize problems with most clients. Honest acknowledgment of the etiology combined with complete and realistic evaluation of the situation and excellent care will go a long way in protecting the veterinarian's reputation, and at the same time should be looked upon favorably should any litigation result.

PREVENTION

It should be emphasized to the owner that any animal that has had a rectal tear may be predisposed to another tear. This fact should be made clear to anyone attempting rectal palpation of this animal in the future. Preventive measures should always be taken to preclude the occurrence of this serious problem. Proper restraint of the animal, tail wraps to prevent tail hairs from entering the rectum, seamless or soft gloves, adequate nonirritating lubricant, careful and gentle clearing of the feces, intelligent manipulation of the rectal tube, and relaxing for peristaltic waves and straining should be employed at all times.

In animals with a small rectal tube and those that resist palpation, a choice has to be made as to the importance of the examination related to the potential for disaster. If rectal palpation is essential, sedatives and/or drugs to relax the anus and distal rectum can be employed. It may also be possible to allow someone with a smaller arm to palpate animals with a narrow rectal tube.

Supplemental Readings

Arnold, J. S., and Meagher, D. M.: Management of rectal tears in the horse. J. Equine Med. Surg., 2:64, 1978.

Arnold, J. S., Meagher, D. M., and Lohse, C. L.: Rectal tears in the horse. J. Equine Med. Surg., 2:55, 1978.

Azzie, M. A. J.: Temporary colostomy in the management of rectal tears in the horse. J. South Africa Vet. Assoc., 46:121, 1975.

Stashak, T. S., and Knight, A. P.: Temporary diverting colostomy for the management of small colon tears in the horse: A case report. J. Equine Med. Surg., 2:196, 1978.

Scott, E. A.: Rectal tears. 7th Ann. Surg. Forum, Am. Coll. Vet. Surg., Proc. Eq. Gastrointestinal Seminar No. 4, 1979.

Shires, G. M. H.: The temporary loop colostomy: Another choice. Proc. Eq. Colic Res. Symp., September 1982, p. 293.

Peritonitis

Sidney W. Ricketts, NEWMARKET, ENGLAND

Inflammation of the peritoneum of the horse is a potentially fatal or permanently incapacitating condition. It may occur as a primary condition or, more commonly, as a secondary complication and may be associated with either infectious or noninfectious disease. Treatment depends upon an early precise diagnosis, which frequently presents a challenge to the clinician.

CLINICAL SIGNS AND PATHOGENESIS

Clinical signs vary widely, depending on the cause. Animals with peracute peritonitis following intestinal rupture may be found dead, those with acute disease may have pyrexia, acute colic, depression, and constipation or diarrhea, and those with chronic disease may show gradual weight loss with little or no sign of abdominal discomfort.

Peritonitis can be a complication of a variety of conditions (Table 1) when the peritoneum is exposed to infection by invading microorganisms. Peritoneal fluid provides an ideal culture medium, and the continual movement of the intestinal tract and diaphragm ensures rapid dissemination of the infection throughout the cavity. Fibrin is rapidly precipitated, either diffusely as in septicemia or following intestinal perforations with diffuse contamination or focally around an intestinal perforation. In focal peritonitis, spread throughout the cavity is sometimes limited by the formation of fibrous adhesions.

The inflammatory response mobilizes leukocytes and immunoglobulins and causes a profound relocation of proteins, fluids, and electrolytes from plasma. These fluid shifts may be sufficient to cause cardiovascular collapse. If the response is less acute, the toxic products of microbial multiplication and tissue catabolism may cause systemic toxemia.

DIAGNOSIS

The clinical signs are too varied to be confirmatory. A definitive diagnosis can usually be made simply and efficiently by the examination of a peritoneal fluid sample obtained by abdominal paracentesis. With the horse bridled and restrained in the standing position, a 4 cm 18- to 19-gauge hypodermic needle may be passed through the prepared skin and linea alba at the lowest point of the abdomen, which is approximately six inches behind the xiphisternum. With careful manipulation, fluid is collected by free drip.

Peritoneal fluid is normally clear to slightly opalescent and is slightly yellow to straw colored. In peritonitis, the fluid may be turbid and off-white in color suggesting a high cell count, homogenously blood-stained suggesting hemoperitoneum or intestinal vascular embarrassment, or turbid and brown-green in color suggesting intestinal content contamination or an intestinal tap.

Peritoneal fluid normally has a nucleated cell count of 1000 to 10,000 per μl in adult horses and less than 5000 per μl in foals less than four months of age. In peritonitis, nucleated cell counts are greater than 10,000 per μl and in septic peritonitis greater than 50,000 per μl. Nucleated cell counts less than 1,000 per μl in adult horses suggest a peritoneal transudate rather than an exudate. Transudates sometimes occur in diarrhea and hepatic disease.

Peritoneal fluid of adult horses usually contains

TABLE 1. CONDITIONS ASSOCIATED WITH PERITONITIS

Septicemia (e.g. neonatal foals)
Peritoneal abscess (e.g. *St. equi, Rh. equi*)
Penetrating abdominal wounds
Laparotomy repair, complications (e.g. wound dehiscence)
Castration complications (e.g. scirrhous cord)
Peritoneal neoplasia (e.g. mesothelioma)
Vaginal injury (e.g. at coitus)
Uterine injury (e.g. at parturition, dystocia)
Ovarian adenocarcinoma
Bladder rupture (e.g. neonatal foals)
Urachal infection (e.g. neonatal foals)
Urinary blockage (e.g. calculi, neoplasia)
Nephritis
Hepatitis
Biliary leakage
Pancreatitis
Splenitis
Esophageal injury (e.g. choke)
Ruptured diaphragm
Gastric rupture (e.g. acute tympany, grass sickness)
Gastric or duodenal ulceration (e.g. foals)
Gastric neoplasia (e.g. carcinoma)
Gastric perforation (e.g. bots)
Intestinal infarction, torsion, intussusception, volvulus,
  incarceration, strangulation, ulceration
Intestinal perforation (e.g. Ascariasis)
Intestinal parasitism (e.g. *Strongylus vulgaris*)
Enteritis
Enterolith
Ileus
Intestinal neoplasia (e.g. lymphosarcoma)
Cecal rupture (e.g. at parturition)
Cecal impaction (e.g. with sand)
Colonic infarction, torsion, displacement, ulceration
Colitis
Rectal injury (e.g. tears, perforations, or retroperitoneal
  abscess)

more than 90 per cent polymorphonuclear leukocytes, the remaining 10 per cent being mesothelial cells and mononuclear leukocytes including lymphocytes and some macrophages. In peritonitis, toxic, pyknotic and actively phagocytic polymorphonuclear cells, degenerate mesothelial cells, and active macrophages are seen in large numbers. In cases of peritoneal or intestinal neoplasia, exfoliation of abnormal cells often permits diagnosis from analysis of peritoneal fluid (see page 107).

Gram stain will sometimes identify bacteria within macrophages or free in the fluid, and this may help to guide treatment. Even with the best bacteriologic techniques, cultures are not always obtained although infection is present. The use of enrichment media available commercially* is recommended. Three to five ml of peritoneal fluid is inoculated into the medium, which is then incubated for 24 hours before being plated out using standard techniques.

Peritoneal fluid cannot be obtained from all horses, and this occurrence is not necessarily significant. However, dehydration and diffuse peritoneal fibrosis with adhesion formation usually precludes fluid collection. Meaningful samples cannot usually be obtained if the splenic capsule is penetrated during abdominocentesis.

Further characterization of the degree, severity, and significance of the peritonitis may be obtained by laboratory estimations of fluid and electrolyte balance, blood gas analysis, and hematological examinations. Profound leukopenia with neutropenia and hypoproteinemia is often a feature of acute peritonitis, whereas leukocytosis with neutrophila and sometimes monocytosis and hyperproteinemia with hypergammaglobulinemia is usually seen in chronic peritonitis. Dehydration with acidemia, hypoalbuminemia, and electrolyte imbalance may be seen in cases complicated by diarrhea. Azotemia and elevations in liver enzymes may suggest renal and hepatic failure in toxemic horses with tissue catabolism.

A careful review of the clinical history and a full physical examination is required to determine the cause of the peritonitis (see Table 1). An early exploratory laparotomy may be indicated for diagnostic, therapeutic, and prognostic reasons, and is best performed while the horse is a reasonable anesthetic risk. As they become more widely used, ultrasound echography and laparoscopy may be of diagnostic value.

TREATMENT

Treatment must correct the cause if possible, and the infection and effects of inflammation. Pain relief and the correction of fluid, electrolyte, and acid-base disturbances, and cardiovascular and endotoxic shock may be all necessary. Medical treatment for peritonitis is unlikely to be successful without surgical correction of the cause, when possible.

Infectious peritonitis may be caused by any of the aerobic and anaerobic bacteria normally found in the intestinal tract of the horse. Alternatively, in cases of abscess, specific organisms such as *Streptococcus equi* and *Rhodococcus equi* may be found in pure culture. Antibiotic treatment must be started early, before culture results are available. Penicillin is first choice as it is well tolerated, is known to produce peritoneal fluid levels in excess of the minimum inhibitory concentration, and is bactericidal against most of the gram-positive aerobic organisms (except *Rh. equi*), and most of the anaerobic organisms (except *Bacteroides fragilis*). For gram-negative aerobic organisms and *Rh. equi*,

---

*Blood grow, Medical Wire and Equipment Co., Ltd. Corsham, Wilts, England

gentamicin is recommended. Gentamicin achieves peritoneal fluid levels in excess of the minimum inhibitory concentrations. When gentamicin is not available, trimethoprim-potentiated sulphonamides or oxytetracyclines are recommended, bearing in mind the risk of colitis.

The rapid precipitation of fibrin, either diffusely or in the form of localized abscesses, has a limiting effect on antibiotic penetration and thus therapeutic success. When antibacterial activity is required in the face of fibrosis, sodium iodide (0.4 ml per kg, 16 per cent solution, intravenously twice weekly for four weeks) may be used.

Peritoneal lavage with 5 to 10 L of a warmed Ringer's lactate solution containing 1 to 3 per cent povidone iodine via a Foley or improvised catheter placed through the linea alba at the lowest point of the abdomen has been recommended for the treatment of peritonitis in horses (see p. 77 for a detailed description of the technique). It provides a form of fluid debridement, helping to remove bacteria, toxins, cellular debris, and intestinal contents when present. Prior correction of the causal factors is essential if treatment is to be worth attempting. When large-scale fibrin deposition has occurred or when there is abscess formation, adequate circulation of the lavage fluid within the cavity does not occur. Nevertheless, in spite of the absence of controlled studies, experience suggests that this technique may have value.

Flunixin meglumine is recommended for pain relief and for the control of endotoxic shock. Short-acting corticosteroids, isotonic fluids, electrolytes, and bicarbonate should be used to control cardiovascular shock and acid-base imbalance, as indicated by frequent laboratory examinations. Larvicidal anthelmintics such as ivermectin are indicated when intestinal parasitism is thought to be the cause of the problem.

PROGNOSIS

When the causal lesion can be rapidly corrected, the prognosis is fair to good. If, however, there is intestinal penetration, the prognosis is very poor. Exploratory laparotomy, even when performed early and under optimal anesthetic and surgical conditions, frequently reveals a lesion that cannot be corrected or else the degree of peritoneal contamination is too great. Few cases of localized adhesion formation or abscessation have a successful outcome, especially when *Rh. equi* is involved. Even if the immediate crisis is overcome, chronic ill-thrift and recurrent colic, frequently with a secondary crisis, often follows. When there is diarrhea, the prognosis is poor.

Peritonitis is a diagnostic and therapeutic emergency; even the best-managed cases may not respond to treatment. We as veterinarians must make our best attempts with each case, but we must also recognize our responsibilities to avoid unnecessary suffering by making an early decision that further medical or surgical treatment is inappropriate.

Supplemental Readings

Bach, L. G., and Ricketts, S. W.: Paracentesis as an aid to the diagnosis of abdominal disease in the horse. Equine Vet. J., 6:116, 1974.

Dyson, S.: Review of 30 cases of peritonitis in the horse. Equine Vet. J., 15:25, 1983.

Schneider, R. K.: The peritoneum. In Mansmann, R. A., McAllister, E. S., and Pratt, P. W. (eds.): Equine Medicine and Surgery, 3rd Ed., Vol. 1. Santa Barbara, CA, American Veterinary Publications, 1982, pp. 620–633.

Scrutchfield, W. L.: Peritonitis. In Robinson, N. E. (ed.): Current Therapy in Equine Medicine. Philadelphia, W. B. Saunders Company, 1983, pp. 241–244.

Vaughan, J. T.: Peritonitis and acute abdominal diseases. In Anderson, N. V. (ed.): Veterinary Gastroenterology. Philadelphia, Lea & Febiger, 1980, pp. 651–673.

Endotoxemia

Susan D. Semrad, ATHENS, GEORGIA

James N. Moore, ATHENS, GEORGIA

Endotoxin, also called lipopolysaccharide, phospholipolysaccharide, and endotoxin phospholipopolysaccharide, is a heat-stable complex (mw > 100,000) extracted from gram-negative bacteria. It is an integral, structural component of the outer bacterial wall that accounts for many of the antigenic and toxic properties of the bacterium. The endotoxin complex is composed of two polysaccharide conglomerates, phospholipid, and a variable amount of protein. The outer O-specific polysaccharide is unique to each strain of bacteria and imparts antigenic properties and serologic specificity to the molecule. Lipid A, which is located in the inner region and binds the molecule to the outer wall of the bacterium, is biologically active and confers the toxic properties to the molecule. The structure of lipid A is similar in all gram-negative bacteria. Endotoxin can be extracted and purified by chemical means, thus making it possible to study the pathophysiology of clinical endotoxemia.

The intestinal flora of healthy horses includes a relatively stable population of gram-negative bacteria. During normal bacteriolysis and rapid growth phases, endotoxin is released into the surrounding environment. Detection of endotoxin in the lumen of the intestine, cecum, and colon is therefore considered normal. Endotoxin levels of up to 80 μg per ml have been measured in the cecal fluid of clinically healthy horses.

Two biologic adaptations, the intestinal mucosal barrier and the hepatic reticuloendothelial cells, function in concert to prevent bacteria and bacterial endotoxin from entering the systemic circulation. The physical and chemical components of the intestinal mucosal cell barrier limit transmural movement of these substances. The mucosal epithelial cells and the adjacent layer of oxygen-sensitive resident bacteria serve to discourage penetration by potential bacterial invaders. Evidence of a chemical barrier, composed of primarily acid hydrolases secreted by the epithelial cells, has been demonstrated in cell cultures in vitro. The local importance of these hydrolases as well as secretory IgA, complement, lysozymes, and leukocyte secretions in vivo has yet to be substantiated. The efficacy of the barrier is variable and depends on both intraluminal (pH) and extraluminal factors such as blood flow. Although very efficient under normal conditions, the mucosal barrier does not completely inhibit movement of endotoxin into the portal circulation. The Kupffer cells of the hepatic reticuloendothelial system rapidly clear endotoxin from portal blood, thus preventing its entrance into the systemic circulation.

PATHOPHYSIOLOGY AND CLINICAL SIGNS

Endotoxemia potentially is a component of several equine diseases such as enteric disease, laminitis, and retained placenta. Even though there has been a vast amount of clinical investigation and research devoted to endotoxemia in the last 10 years, our understanding of the pathophysiologic mechanisms involved is still in its infancy. It is known, however, that in order to exert its adverse effects, endotoxin must gain access to the general circulation by either of two methods: (1) entering a mucosal barrier damaged by ischemia, mechanical derangement or obstruction, parasitic vasculitis, thrombotic disease, or disruption of gastrointestinal

TABLE 1. EFFECTS OF ENDOTOXIN

Early	Late
Hypoxemia	Pyrexia
Hyperpnea	Leukocytosis
Pulmonary hypertension	Hypoglycemia
Respiratory alkalosis	Systemic hypotension
Tachycardia	Dehydration
Leukopenia	Metabolic acidosis
Thrombocytopenia	Hepatic dysfunction
Hyperglycemia	Coagulation abnormalities
Hemoconcentration	Abortion

internal environment, or (2) overwhelming the ability of the reticuloendothelial system to clear endotoxin from the portal circulation. After gaining access to the general circulation, endotoxin may cause cardiovascular compromise, pulmonary hypertension, damage to respiratory vascular endothelium, leukopenia, thrombocytopenia, interference with carbohydrate, lipid or protein metabolism, lactic acidosis, hepatic renal and nervous system dysfunction, gastrointestinal disturbances and coagulopathies (see Table 1).

In the horse, clinical signs following endotoxin challenge include tachypnea, tachycardia, alterations in mucous membrane color and moistness, pyrexia, abdominal discomfort, and softened feces. These signs are reproducible and closely reflect or mimic the changes seen in clinical cases of endotoxemia or endotoxic shock. Although not completely defined, several mechanisms for endotoxin-induced damage have been proposed: (1) a direct toxic effect of endotoxin on vascular endothelial cells, platelets, and leukocytes, (2) plasma complement activation resulting in activation of the blood coagulation system and plasma bradykinin generation, (3) initiation of cellular prostaglandin–producing systems, and (4) a wide range of effects on endothelium mediated through generation and release of other vasoactive substances such as leukotrienes, catecholamines, and histamine.

Currently, in the equine species, much emphasis has been placed on the role of prostaglandin mediators, as many of the early effects of endotoxemia are mediated by arachidonic acid metabolites. The roles of two of these vasoactive metabolites, thromboxane A_2 and prostacyclin, have recently been documented in equine endotoxemia. Agents that inhibit the production of these mediators, e.g., cyclooxygenase inhibitors (NSAID) including flunixin meglumine, dipyrone, and phenylbutazone, have been shown to be of some benefit in treating clinical endotoxemia. These agents, however, have no effect on the leukopenia or granulocytopenia accompanying endotoxemia.

PYROGENIC EFFECT. The temperature response to endotoxin appears to be mediated by at least two mechanisms. Endotoxin may have a direct effect on the thermoregulatory center in the brain and an indirect action on a variety of body cells such as granulocytes, monocytes, and reticuloendothelial macrophages, causing them to release "endogenous pyrogens." Endogenous pyrogens are thought to act on the anterior hypothalamus resulting in the formation of prostaglandins and cyclic AMP (cAMP), which either reset the thermoregulatory centers or alter heat redistribution or production. Experimentally, the pyrogenic response has been triggered by minute amounts of endotoxin and may be only partially attenuated by the use of NSAIDs. The pyrogenic response may be monophasic or biphasic depending upon the amount of endotoxin exposure. Clinically, it is important to realize that fever frequently occurs as a result of endotoxemia, that the intestinal mucosal barrier usually has been damaged, and that administration of NSAIDs may not affect the febrile response.

HEMODYNAMIC EFFECTS. The hemodynamic effects of endotoxemia can be devastating and may lead to serious and possibly fatal shock. The extent of damage and course of the disease are related to the underlying causes of endotoxemia, the amount of endotoxin absorbed, and the rapidity and accuracy of therapy. The underlying feature of either experimental or clinical circulatory shock is inadequate perfusion of vital organs. Several vasoactive compounds such as histamine, bradykinin, catecholamines, prostaglandins, and myocardial depressant factor have been implicated in the cardiovascular alterations that accompany endotoxemia. Following endotoxin administration, there is an abrupt reduction in cardiac output and systemic arterial pressure while pulmonary arterial pressure increases transiently. Blood pressure and cardiac output continue to decline as a result of decreased vascular resistance, venous pooling, and decreased venous return to the heart. Blood flow is maintained or increased in noncritical organs such as those of the gastrointestinal tract. Tissue perfusion is compromised by vascular sludging following splenic contraction and hemoconcentration.

LEUKOPENIA AND LEUKOCYTOSIS. Leukopenia is a very sensitive diagnostic signal of endotoxemia and may be present even when other clinical signs are not evident. Neutropenia is an important early sign of gram-negative bacterial sepsis. The leukopenic response is due to a shift of cells from the circulating leukocyte pool to the marginal pool and sequestration of cells in the pulmonary capillaries. Increased margination of neutrophils and inhibition of migration of neutrophils to extravascular sites of injury is thought to be secondary to endotoxin-induced complement activation.

The secondary leukocytosis following exposure to endotoxin is characterized by an increased release of immature leukocytes from the bone marrow. This rebound leukocytosis is thought to be associated with an increase in production of a granulocyte-releasing factor.

THROMBOCYTOPENIA. The lowering of platelet numbers during endotoxemia may be caused by various mechanisms: (1) binding of endotoxin directly to platelets causing aggregation, (2) platelet aggregation and adhesion to damaged vascular endothelium with resultant thrombus formation, (3) sequestration of platelet aggregates in the pulmonary vasculature, and (4) stimulation of the extrinsic coagulation system. Thrombin and fibrin produced with coagulation system activation are known to induce platelet aggregation. Clinically it is important to remember that although platelet numbers may return to normal, platelet function may be impaired.

HEPATIC EFFECTS. Endotoxin has multiple effects on liver function and may interfere with carbohydrate, protein, and lipid metabolism. Endotoxin can act as a "false messenger" to activate hepatic membrane–bound enzymes, which stimulate glycogenolysis and produce the initial hyperglycemia seen following exposure to endotoxin. Secondary hypoglycemia is caused by depletion of carbohydrate stores, decreased glucose production, and increased glucose metabolism. Conversion by the liver of lactic acid to glucose is inhibited by endotoxin, resulting in further cellular compromise and systemic lactic acidosis.

COAGULATION. Endotoxin may initiate intravascular coagulation and thrombogenic disorders through several mechanisms: (1) direct activation of Hageman factor (XII); (2) direct platelet damage with release of procoagulant constituents; (3) endothelial damage with subsequent activation of factor XII and platelet aggregation; (4) direct or indirect activation of complement; (5) complement-mediated platelet damage; (6) release of tissue thromboplastin and activation of extrinsic pathways; (7) decreased levels of factor VII; and (8) platelet damage and release of platelet factor 3. This activation of the blood clotting system and intravascular clot formation adversely affects both the macro- and microcirculations and may result in the development of disseminated intravascular coagulation.

Clinically, coagulopathies may be characterized by petechial or ecchymotic hemorrhages on the mucous membranes, conjunctivae, and nictitans or hematoma formation or prolonged bleeding following venipuncture or abdominoparacentesis. Confirmation of consumptive coagulopathy may be made through demonstration of decreased circulating platelets, increased prothrombin time, increased activated partial thromboplastin time, and increased circulating levels of fibrin degradation products.

THERAPY

The choice of therapy will be determined by assessment of the horse's status, recognition of the underlying disease processes, concurrent illnesses, and response to previous therapy. The central aims of therapy include prevention or correction of circulatory shock, control or elimination of the initiating cause of shock, restoration of adequate blood volume, and amelioration of the detrimental effects of tissue hypoxia.

Restoration of adequate blood volume should be undertaken with consideration for the need to correct concurrent acid-base and/or electrolyte imbalances. The immediate fluid needs are determined by evaluating the packed cell volume (PCV) and total plasma proteins. In the field situation, the degree of dehydration (loss of total body water) may be estimated by determination of skin turgor, mucous membrane color, capillary refill time, temperature of extremities, mental attitude, and moistness of mucous membranes and cornea. Further evaluation of the cardiovascular status may include assessment of strength and regularity of peripheral pulses, ease with which the jugular vein is raised, and blood pressure measurement from the coccygeal artery.

In early stages of endotoxemia or when exposure to endotoxin has been at a low level, alterations in plasma volume and metabolic balance may be minimal. In mild cases of endotoxemia or when the gastrointestinal tract is not disturbed, oral replacement of fluids may be possible. In the majority of cases, however, intravenous therapy may be required. Fluid replacement with a polyionic solution such as acetated Ringer's solution or lactated Ringer's solution is usually sufficient. The aim of fluid replacement is to decrease the viscosity of blood and break up aggregates of red blood cells that form during low blood flow states, thus improving capillary perfusion and enhancing oxygen transportation in tissues. Response to fluid therapy can be used as a guide to the need for further laboratory workup. In cases of severe or prolonged endotoxemia, closer evaluation of the electrolyte, acid-base, and plasma protein status are essential.

Derangements in tissue metabolism, tissue perfusion, and capillary permeability lead to special therapeutic concerns. As a result of damage to the vascular endothelium, plasma proteins may be lost into the tissues or intestinal lumen and result in relative hypoproteinemia in clinically dehydrated animals. This is evidenced by elevated PCV with disproportionately normal or low total plasma protein values. Rapid rehydration with large fluid volumes in such instances will result in hypoproteinemia with possible edema development in the gastrointestinal mucosa or pulmonary system. Con-

sequently, poor response to fluid therapy occurs and is shown by a continued elevation in PCV in the face of a declining total protein. Administration of plasma intravenously may increase the protein content of the blood, allowing for intravenous administration of polyionic fluid to correct the fluid deficit. Whenever plasma is used, the animal must be carefully monitored. Heart rate, respiratory rate, muscle fasciculations, and general attitude are observed for signs of adverse reaction or compromise.

Experimentally, administration of endotoxin results in an early hyperglycemia and later hypoglycemia. Glucose labsticks* can rapidly provide an estimate of the blood glucose levels. Since glucose administration increases survival rates in some species, the administration of 2½ or 5 per cent dextrose in water by intravenous drip may be advisable if hypoglycemia is present. Administration of glucose to the point of diuresis, however, may further compromise the hydration status of the animal and should be avoided unless signs of renal insufficiency exist.

In animals with moderate to severe acidosis determined by blood gas or total carbon dioxide measurement, bicarbonate therapy is indicated. Half of the amount required for correction may be given over 60 to 90 minutes and the remainder over the next 12 to 24 hours, depending on the severity of the condition. If the animal fails to show improvement following therapy for electrolyte and acid-base deficits, these parameters should be re-evaluated. In animals with moderate to severe acidemia, the acidemia may be enhanced by administration of large volumes of polyionic solutions without consideration for bicarbonate replacement. As the circulation is restored and capillary beds in the ischemic tissues are perfused, lactate produced during anaerobic glycolysis may enter the systemic circulation, resulting in a lowering of blood pH. Shock at this stage is usually accompanied by lactate accumulation and some compromise in the conversion of lactate to bicarbonate equivalents. In such situations, the use of bicarbonate replacement or acetated Ringer's solution is preferred. Bicarbonate should not be added to fluids containing calcium (such as lactated Ringer's) because some of the bicarbonate will be lost as precipitated calcium carbonate. To more accurately control bicarbonate replacement therapy, a sterile 5 per cent solution in distilled water may be given.

Nonsteroidal anti-inflammatory agents (NSAIDS) are currently believed to be of benefit in treatment of endotoxemia due to their ability to block production of vasoactive arachidonic acid metabolites and thus many of the early metabolic and hemodynamic

---

*Chemstrip bG, Boehringer Mannheim, Indianapolis, IN

alterations seen in endotoxemia (Fig. 1). Flunixin meglumine (1.0 mg per kg) appears to be more effective than phenylbutazone or dipyrone at suppressing prostaglandin-mediated effects of endotox-. emia in the horse. Consequently, this agent is used extensively in clinical instances of intestinal ischemia and endotoxemia.

Concern has been expressed regarding both the potential toxicity of NSAIDs (see p. 118), and the ability of flunixin meglumine to mask clinical signs. NSAIDs have been associated with gastrointestinal ulceration and renal papillary necrosis in compromised and hypovolemic horses. Recent research has shown that reduced dosage of flunixin meglumine (0.1 mg per kg to 0.25 mg per kg intravenously) allows clinical assessment of the horse's status while effectively inhibiting prostaglandin production and attenuating some clinical signs of endotoxemia.

Broad-spectrum antibiotics with gram-negative effectiveness are indicated whenever there is evidence of bacteremia or when an underlying focus of infection is associated with endotoxemia. Penicillin, due to its effect against anaerobes, should be included in the antibiotic regimen. Blood for aerobic and anaerobic culture and sensitivity determination should be obtained aseptically before antibiotic administration if possible. Occasionally, clinical signs of endotoxemia appear more severe after antibiotic therapy is initiated due to the lysis of gram-negative bacteria resulting in endotoxin release. To avoid potential nephrotoxicity, assessment of renal function and adequate hydration should be achieved before aminoglycosides are used. Research indicates that nephrotoxicity occurs more rapidly when aminoglycosides and NSAID agents are used concurrently than when either agent is used alone. Therefore, careful monitoring of renal function is advised when using a combination of these agents in volume-deficient horses.

The use of heparin in endotoxic shock in horses is controversial. The beneficial effects attributed to heparin include (1) activation of a plasma enzyme system capable of degrading circulating toxins, (2) inhibition of the coagulation process, (3) facilitation of clearance of endotoxin by the reticuloendothelial system, and (4) prevention of laminitis. Factors XII,

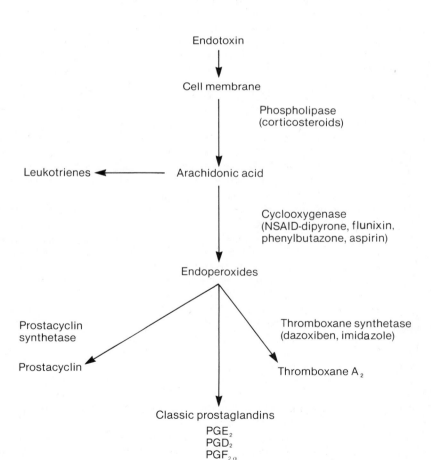

Figure 1. Arachidonic acid cascade: Pharmaceutic agents modifying specific enzyme activity included in parentheses.

Endotoxin

Cell membrane

Phospholipase (corticosteroids)

Leukotrienes ◄───── Arachidonic acid

Cyclooxygenase (NSAID-dipyrone, flunixin, phenylbutazone, aspirin)

Endoperoxides

Prostacyclin synthetase

Thromboxane synthetase (dazoxiben, imidazole)

Prostacyclin

Thromboxane A_2

Classic prostaglandins
PGE_2
PGD_2
$PGF_{2\alpha}$

XI, IX and activated factor X are inhibited by low molecular weight heparin and cofactor antithrombin III, consequently decreasing the risk of activation of the intrinsic coagulation pathway and subsequent development of disseminated intravascular coagulation in endotoxic shock. Increased clearance of endotoxin is due to the potent opsonizing effect of heparin in combination with fibronectin, which aids phagocytosis by the reticuloendothelial system. Heparin in minidoses (40 IU per kg intravenously or subcutaneously two or three times a day) is often recommended to achieve these effects and may forestall the development of microthrombi in the vessels of the gastrointestinal tract and hoof (laminitis). Additional studies are needed to test these claims. Higher dosages of heparin have been recommended but should be used with caution in the event that bleeding should develop. Potential side effects of heparin therapy include edema at the site of subcutaneous injection, thrombocytopenia, and anemia as reflected in a decreased packed cell volume and red blood cell count. These effects are usually reversible by discontinuation of heparin therapy.

The use of corticosteroids in endotoxic shock is controversial. In cases in which bacteremia or an underlying septic process is present, steroid use is questionable. Proposed benefits derived from corticosteroids include improved integrity of capillary endothelium, peripheral vasodilation, improved tissue perfusion, inhibition of complement activation, decreased activation of clotting cascade, decreased neutrophil aggregation, stabilization of lysosomal membranes and decreased release of proteolytic enzymes, protection of hepatic gluconeogenesis and tissue glycolysis, increased efficiency of glycolytic enzymes, and improved survival in experimental shock in dogs. Detrimental effects have centered on suppression of neutrophil function and decreased ability to withstand bacterial or viral invasion. While these benefits are proposed, the use of steroids in equine experimental shock models has met with only limited success. If given before or early after inducing endotoxemia, steroids attenuate lactic acidosis, prevent alterations in the coagulation system, and maintain or increase blood pressure. No advantage, however, over the use of NSAIDs has been documented. In one study the adverse effects of endotoxemia and survival rate were more favorably altered by flunixin meglumine than either dexamethasone or prednisolone.

Animals in severe or advanced endotoxic shock with circulatory collapse or hypoxia may require oxygen supplementation. Oxygen from a portable tank may be administered via face mask, via nasal insufflation using a stomach tube or soft urinary catheter placed into the pharynx, or via an intratracheal catheter. An oxygen flow rate of 15 L per minute is recommended for an adult horse.

Vasoactive amines have been used in septic or endotoxic shock to improve cardiovascular status and perfusion to the viscera. Dopamine, the immediate precursor of norepinephrine, has mild alpha- and beta-adenergic activity and a specific dopaminergic vasodilatory action in mesenteric, cerebral, renal, and coronary vessels. In the dog and in humans, low doses of dopamine increase blood flow to these vascular beds and have a positive ionotropic effect on the heart with little change in heart rate. Dopamine has been evaluated both in conscious ponies and anesthetized horses. In the ponies, 3.75 μg per kg per minute intravenously increased cardiac output by 27 per cent. In the anesthetized horses 2.5 μg per kg per minute intravenously and 5 μg per kg per minute intravenously increased cardiac output 44 per cent and 68 per cent, respectively. Adverse effects at the higher dose rate included tachycardia and supraventricular premature contractions that subsided upon withdrawal of the drug. In endotoxic horses, dopamine may be an aid in maintaining blood flow to the kidney and visceral organs as well as improving cardiac output and systemic blood pressure. Administration of dopamine 2.5 μg per kg per minute intravenously to the standing awake horse has appeared beneficial clinically. Dopamine HCl (200 mg) dissolved in 500 ml normal saline or 5% dextrose in water and administered at a rate of 30 drops per minute (assuming 10 drops per ml) provides a dose rate of 2.5 μg per kg per minute in a 450-kg horse. In order to derive beneficial effects from dopamine administration, however, hypovolemic horses should be rehydrated before its administration. Proper fluid therapy and careful monitoring of the animal's status must accompany use of this drug.

Recent investigations into the treatment of endotoxemia have been aimed at modulation of prostaglandin production and development of a specific antiendotoxin antiserum. Specific thromboxane synthetase inhibitors to block generation of thromboxane A_2 have improved survival rates in some species. In preliminary work in horses and ponies, however, a specific inhibitor of thromboxane generation failed to modify the clinical signs of endotoxemia. Prostacyclin, the arachidonic acid metabolite with vasodilator properties, is beneficial during endotoxemia in other species. In anesthetized normal and endotoxic horses, however, prostacyclin (30 to 100 ng per kg per minute) infused intravenously caused progressive tachycardia, hypotension, hypoxemia, enhanced lactic acidosis, and hemoconcentration.

Research directed toward the development of a vaccine or antiserum against gram-negative core antigens has shown promising results in several species. Clinical trials have shown that antibodies directed against the *E. coli* J$_5$ mutant improved survival in human patients with gram-negative bacteremia. Results of those trials suggest that the J$_5$ antibody does not prevent gram-negative infection but rather acts as an antitoxin against endotoxin. The use of J$_5$ antiserum is presently under investigation in the equine species. Field reports have cited the beneficial effects of antiendotoxin antisera against colitis X and equine endotoxemia. Research studies to confirm the efficacy of antiendotoxin antisera against experimentally induced endotoxemia have to date been disappointing.

Rapid and complete resolution of the endotoxemia is paramount to ensure survival of the animal and reduce the occurrence of harmful sequelae. Animals surviving the toxic crisis may eventually succumb to possible sequelae, including laminitis, renal or gastrointestinal infarction, and coagulation abnormalities.

Supplemental Readings

Bottoms, G. D., Templeton, C. B., Fessler, J. F., Johnson, M. A., Roesel, O. F., Ewert, K. M., and Adams, S. B.: Thromboxane, prostacyclin I$_2$ (epoprosterol), and the hemodynamic changes in equine endotoxin shock. Am. J. Vet. Res., *43*:999, 1982.

Culbertson, R., and Osburn, B. I.: The biological effects of bacterial endotoxin: A short review. Vet. Sci. Comm., *4*:3, 1980.

Gans, H.: Mechanism of heparin protection in endotoxin shock. Surgery, 77:602, 1975.

Lees, P., and Higgins, A. J.: Clinical pharmacology and therapeutic uses of nonsteroidal anti-inflammatory drugs in the horse. Equine Vet. J., *17*:83, 1985.

Moore, J. N.: Endotoxemia: Part II Biological reactions to endotoxin. Comp. Cont. Ed., *3*:S392,1981.

Trim, C. M., Moore, J. N., and White, N. A.: Cardiopulmonary effects of dopamine hydrochloride in anaesthetized horses. Equine Vet. J., *17*:41, 1985.

Foal Heat Diarrhea

Don M. Witherspoon, LEXINGTON, KENTUCKY

A self-limiting diarrhea commonly occurs in foals between four and 14 days of age and thus usually coincides with the mare's first postparturient estrus. The etiology of foal heat diarrhea has been debated for years. Proposed etiologies include hormonal changes within the mare, changes in milk composition, overengorgement of milk by the foal, bacterial or viral enteritis, coprophagy, ingestion of genital discharges, ingestion of roughage and irritants, strongyloidosis, and physiologic changes within the foal's gastrointestinal tract.

Recently, research has disproven or cast doubt on several of these factors as contributing significantly to foal heat diarrhea. There is no appreciable change in milk volume or composition during the period when foal heat diarrhea occurs in foals. Milk production fluctuates during the early postpartum period and often decreases during the mare's first estrus. It therefore seems unlikely that milk overengorgement is involved. It is interesting to note that most foals separated from the dam at birth and fed a controlled volume of an artificial milk replacer having a consistent composition still develop a self-limiting diarrhea between nine to 13 days of age. Although diarrhea has been reported in older foals following sand ingestion and accumulation in the large colon, there is no evidence that coprophagy or ingestion of sand or other possible irritants produce diarrhea in young foals. There is little proof that *Strongyloides westeri* produces diarrhea in foals less than 14 days old. In fact, a recent study that involved larvae removal from mares revealed no significant difference in the incidence of foal heat diarrhea in infected and noninfected foals. Several studies to identify rotavirus, coronavirus, and cryptosporidia in feces of foals with foal heat diarrhea have been inconsistent and largely disappointing. Presently, remaining viable explanations for the etiology of foal heat diarrhea are that it is physiologic in nature and is related to alterations in intestinal microbial flora or perhaps is associated with increased quantities of roughage in the large intestine, which is not yet sufficiently developed to digest it properly. Even though the etiology remains to be determined, conscientious farm management and proper veterinary attention are usually sufficient to sustain the affected foal.

CLINICAL SIGNS AND DIAGNOSIS

The foal usually exhibits soft to watery feces but is bright, alert, and nurses. Rectal temperature is almost always within normal limits, and rarely exceeds 39° C. When diarrhea is present, however, it is important to monitor both the nursing habits of the foal and its rectal temperature. Failure of the foal to nurse results in enlargement of the mare's udder and periodic streaming of milk from the teats. If this occurs, or if the foal's temperature exceeds 39° C or watery diarrhea persists for longer than 36 hours, further laboratory monitoring and diagnostic work-up are indicated. Clinical assessment of hydration determined by skin turgidity, sunken eyes, and moistness of oral mucous membranes will alert the veterinarian to developing dehydration. Periodic packed cell volume and total plasma protein determinations will also be of benefit in assessing how the foal is handling the diarrhea-associated fluid loss. If it becomes apparent that the foal is suffering systemically from the diarrhea, more sophisticated measurements should be taken. A complete blood count, serum electrolytes (Na^+, Cl^-, K^+, and HCO_3^-), and fecal culture using gram quantities of feces and antibiotic sensitivity should be performed. An effort should be made to inquire about the history of similar problems on the farm, or more specifically in the particular barn housing the affected foal.

THERAPY

If the foal remains bright, alert, afebrile, and continues to nurse, no therapy is indicated. Mineral oil or petrolatum applied topically to the perineal region help prevent scalding. Administration of an intestinal inoculant* may have some benefit in shortening the duration of the diarrhea. If the diarrhea persists but the foal remains normal in other respects, an anthelmintic such as cambendazole† may be administered. Other approaches to treatment consist of 180 gm mineral oil and 30 gm castor oil by stomach tube to evacuate the gastrointestinal tract, or administration of intestinal protectants, orally. If the diarrhea persists for longer than several days, or the foal deteriorates systemically, parenteral antibiotics, intravenous fluids, and electrolytes and a more energetic schedule of monitoring should be instituted. Along with this, fecal and blood samples should be submitted for culture and further diagnostic workup. Regardless of the approach to therapy, the importance of frequent monitoring of the foal for fever, hydration, and nursing activity cannot be overemphasized.

---

*Probiocin, Pioneer Hi-Bred International, Portland, OR
†Camvet, MSD-AGVET, Rahway, NJ

Salmonellosis

Jonathan E. Palmer, KENNETT SQUARE, PENNSYLVANIA

Salmonellosis is a common cause of acute enterocolitis in the horse accounting for more than half the acute diarrhea cases in patients admitted to our referral hospital. Horses of all ages and in all management situations may be affected. Although acute diarrhea is the most common clinical manifestation, Salmonella infections cause several clinical syndromes.

A susceptible horse exposed to a virulent type of Salmonella may not develop clinical disease. The determinants of a successful infection are the exposure dose, the virulence of the bacterium, and the susceptibility of the host. Under experimental conditions, 10^8 or more organisms are required for successful infection. However, under natural conditions as few as 100 to 1000 bacteria may result in disease. The virulence of Salmonella varies between substrains within serotypes. Intestinal motility and normal intestinal flora are the primary lines of host defense. Progressive intestinal motility expells luminal contents, including pathogens. The normal flora appears to produce a hostile environment for Salmonella, protecting the host through competitive exclusion of the pathogen. Changes in intestinal motility or flora may decrease the host's resistance and result in infection. Equine salmonellosis is commonly associated with stressful conditions, such as advanced pregnancy, adverse weather conditions, transportation, recent surgery, and therapy with antibiotics. Many of these stressful situations result in changes in food intake, which alter intestinal motility and the normal intestinal flora.

CLINICAL SYNDROMES

Salmonella infection produces eight clinical syndromes. The most common, acute diarrhea, can occur at any age but is most prevalent in weanlings and young performance horses. The first signs are often fever, severe depression, abdominal pain, and injected mucous membranes. Diarrhea, which may not develop for two to four days, is usually projectile, profuse, and foul-smelling. Despite all therapeutic efforts the diarrhea may persist for three to four weeks; however, most frequently it resolves within a week. The onset of diarrhea often marks an improvement of the other clinical signs, such as abdominal pain and depression. The horse may continue to eat despite the severe endotoxemia and profuse diarrhea.

Occasionally adult horses will develop a peracute syndrome resembling colitis X with a course of 6 to 12 hours. Often the horse will die before the development of diarrhea. A bacteremic-septicemic syndrome of foals closely mimics other neonatal septicemias. Older foals may have severe enteritis followed by physitis, pneumonia, nephritis, or meningitis. Chronic diarrhea is rarely caused by Salmonella infections. The chronic diarrhea reflects the long recovery time required in some cases in which damage is extensive.

Mild to severe abdominal pain is an important finding in four clinical syndromes. In the first, colic is mild and the prominent signs are depression and fever. Without a high index of suspicion, the enteritis may not be diagnosed unless the feces are loose and leukopenia is present.

Some horses infected with Salmonella initially appear to have impaction colic. The only indications that the horse has more than a pelvic flexure impaction are fever and leukopenia. The first feces obtained contain Salmonella. As the impaction resolves, the horse may develop a very mild diarrhea as would be expected after an impaction colic or may develop a diarrhea more typical of an enteritis.

Occasionally horses with salmonellosis have severe abdominal pain that can be controlled only with heavy sedation. No feces are passed. Fever and leukopenia, along with negative rectal findings, may be helpful diagnostically. The pain is difficult to manage until diarrhea develops.

Proximal or anterior enteritis is uncommonly caused by Salmonella. These cases appear to follow the same course as other proximal enteritis cases (see p. 44). Diarrhea may or may not develop.

Complications occasionally seen in cases of equine salmonellosis include laminitis, thrombophlebitis, hepatitis, nephritis, and disseminated intravascular coagulopathy. Thrombophlebitis often affects veins containing indwelling catheters. When the jugular vein is affected, head edema may develop and may become life-threatening if the phlebitis is bilateral. Nephritis may be a serious complication in some cases. A prerenal azotemia is common and must be distinguished from a renal azotemia. If renal function deteriorates despite adequate rehydration, the prognosis is poor. Hepatitis frequently occurs but usually is subclinical and reversible. Dependent edema may rarely develop and become quite extensive.

DIAGNOSIS

Diagnosis of Salmonella infection depends on the isolation of the microbe. Ten grams of feces, approximately two thirds of a fecal ball, should be cultured using an enrichment technique. At least five cultures should be obtained because Salmonella species are inconsistently shed in horse feces even during the acute disease. Some horses seem to begin to shed when the feces first become normal. When the microbe cannot be found in fecal cultures, a small rectal biopsy can be obtained using a uterine biopsy punch and cultured in an enrichment medium.

Approximately 40 per cent of horses with positive antemortem cultures will have negative postmortem cultures. Conversely, some horses with negative antemortem fecal cultures will have positive necropsy cultures. I recommend culturing the cecal wall, colonic wall, ileal wall and contents, mesenteric or colonic lymph nodes, and bile postmortem. Culturing all these will maximize the probability of isolating the pathogen. The tissues may be "pooled" and one culture performed. It is important to culture tissue and not just bowel contents.

TREATMENT

Fluid Therapy. The most important therapeutic consideration is fluid and electrolyte replacement. Horses with colitis frequently are hyponatremic, hypokalemic, hypochloremic, and acidotic. Although the fluid loss through the colon is isotonic, the hyponatremia and hypochloremia are primarily due to replacement of fluid loss with fresh water. The hypokalemia is caused by a combination of decreased intake and gastrointestinal loss. The acidosis is a result of the combination of gastrointestinal loss, hypovolemic shock, and endotoxemia. If diarrhea began recently, the deficits can be corrected rapidly. However, if the hyponatremia (115–125 mEq per L) is long-standing, rapid replacement of the deficits may result in neurologic signs and death due to cerebral hemorrhage.

The fluid and electrolyte needs should be met with isotonic balanced replacement fluids. Horses with profuse dehydrating diarrhea frequently require intensive intravenous fluid therapy. The fluids should be given rapidly but not to the point that there is excess urination, which may occur even in the face of dehydration. Some of the fluid and electrolyte needs may be met by oral therapy in horses that continue to eat and drink. The horse should always be offered the choice of fresh water and isotonic electrolyte solutions rather than only one. Many commercial electrolyte mixes of varying quality are available for use in large animals. A simple inexpensive electrolyte mix can be made with baking soda (one half teaspoon approximately equals 20.9 mEq $NaHCO_3$), salt (one half teaspoon approximately equals 60 mEq NaCl), and salt substitutes (one half teaspoon NoSalt* approximately equals 35 mEq KCl, one half teaspoon Lite Salt† approximately equals 24 mEq NaCl and 19 mEq KCl). Two teaspoons of salt, two teaspoons NoSalt, and two tablespoons baking soda dissolved in one gallon of water results in a solution with 90 mEq Na^+, 95 mEq Cl^-, 35 mEq K^+, 30 mEq HCO_3^- and an osmolarity of 250 mOsm. The solution can be tailored to the patient's needs by adding more baking soda or NoSalt, but the solution should not become hypertonic. Occasionally a horse will have an excessive thirst and will drink 20 gallons of water or more per hour. Such excessive intake will exacerbate the diarrhea.

Although body weight is the best monitor of fluid therapy, weighing the horse is often impractical. Initial assessment of dehydration is by observation of decreased skin turgor, capillary refill time, and the moistness of mucous membranes. However, except in the extremely dehydrated animal, these signs can be quite variable between individuals. Packed cell volume and total plasma protein are quite useful; however, pain associated with enteritis may cause splenic contraction, elevating the packed cell volume. There may also be a protein-losing enteropathy resulting in a fall in total plasma protein in the face of dehydration. The urine specific gravity cannot be used as a good monitor of hydration, because with intensive fluid therapy the urine may be dilute before complete rehydration. Prerenal azotemia is common and its resolution is a good measure of hydration. However, renal disease, which is common in horses with severe enteritis, may complicate the interpretation of BUN and creatinine values.

Protein-losing enteropathy is a common problem associated with acute salmonellosis. The decrease in total plasma protein may be profound and rapid, total plasma protein dropping below 5 gm per dl and occasionally below 3 gm per dl. Despite the low protein, dependent or pulmonary edema is not common. Because of the large protein deficit, a large volume of plasma is required for effective replacement. Horses receiving plasma transfusion (see p. 317) often subjectively appear better. Anecdotal experience indicates some benefit despite the fact that the total plasma protein is only transiently increased. Cross-matching to ensure compatibility of plasma is important, especially in a horse that has received biologics of equine origin.

Antidiarrheals. Certain antidiarrheal medications may help in acute salmonellosis but others can cause harm. Diarrhea, which is a protective mechanism, occurs when the transit rate of ingesta through the gastrointestinal tract is rapid and there is either a lack of absorption or active secretion of fluid. The short transit time allows rapid expulsion of bacteria and toxins; diarrhea is harmful only when the fluid loss is excessive. Fluid loss rather than the rate of transit of the ingesta should be the focus of therapy. Slowing transit with antimotility drugs is contraindicated because it may allow for multiplication of the microbe in the lumen. Pharmacologic modulation of diarrhea should decrease active secretion and enhance fluid absorption. Effective "gut protectants" probably modulate the absorptive and secretory mechanisms rather than acting as a physical barrier between the intestinal tract and irritants. Bismuth subsalicylate* is effective in some cases of Salmonella diarrhea. Thirty-two to 64 oz is given to a mature horse via nasogastric tube twice a day. If the drug is effective, fecal consistency changes within 72 hours. The drug should be continued until the horse produces normal fecal balls or for at least 24 hours. Bismuth oxidizes within the gastrointestinal tract and produces black feces, which may be confused with melena. Other gut protectants such as kaolin and pectin or activated charcoal are not consistently beneficial. Activated charcoal is an effective absorber of luminal toxins and thus may be useful; however, it has little direct antidiarrheal activity.

Antimicrobials. The use of antimicrobials in acute salmonellosis is controversial. They do not speed the resolution of the diarrhea or change the course of the enteric infection but may prevent the seeding of other tissues with bacteria, which occurs most frequently in foals less than six months old. Bacteremia may occasionally occur in adults, but uncommonly is there seeding of other tissues. Thus, I believe that antibiotics are only indicated in foals less than six months of age and adults that are severely compromised. Antibiotics may have a role in preventing catheter sepsis when intravenous catheters are maintained for prolonged periods.

Salmonella can receive resistance factors as plasmids from other Enterobacteriaceae. Thus, an endemic strain of Salmonella is unlikely to be susceptible to antibiotics that are commonly used on the farm. In the past, chloramphenicol, gentamicin, amikacin, trimethoprim-sulfa combination drugs, and ampicillin have been the antibiotics of choice in treating acute salmonellosis. However, with the prevalence of resistant strains, the sensitivity of

---

*NoSalt, Norcliff Thayer Inc., Tuckahoe, NY
†Morton Thiokol, Inc., Chicago, IL

---

*Pepto Bismol, Norwich Eaton Pharmaceuticals, Inc., Norwich, NY or Bismusal Suspension, Veterinary Laboratories, Inc., Lenexa, KS

each isolate should be determined. Oral nonabsorbable antibiotics offer no benefit for the host and may exacerbate the disease by disrupting the gastrointestinal flora.

Antiinflammatory and Analgesic Drugs. Nonsteroidal anti-inflammatory drugs may offer some benefit because prostaglandins are mediators of the signs of endotoxic shock and mediate secretion in Salmonella enteritis. However, because antiprostaglandin drugs such as phenylbutazone and flunixin meglumine can themselves cause enteritis and diarrhea they should be used with moderation at reduced dose (e.g., 0.22 mg per kg flunixin meglumine every eight hours).

If an analgesic is necessary to control pain, nonsteroidal anti-inflammatory drugs should be used with moderation at the aforementioned low dose. If the horse is not manageable with these drugs, other analgesics such as butorphanol and xylazine or sedatives such as chloral hydrate may be used. These drugs should also be used sparingly as they may interfere with intestinal motility. They should be used only when essential to manage pain.

PROGNOSIS

Because of the variable syndromes caused by Salmonella, prognosis for survival varies greatly between individuals. Severe diarrhea may last two to three weeks, and attempting to maintain intravenous fluid therapy is costly and difficult. Horses with prolonged diarrhea may not fully recover for four to six months, but if there are no devastating complications such as laminitis, most horses will return to the same level of work as before the illness.

Although some recovered horses shed Salmonella in their feces for more than a year, most have a short shedding period. After recovery from the diarrhea, the horse should not be returned to the herd before five serial negative cultures have been obtained at weekly intervals. One third of the horses with acute enteritis will continue to shed for a month following recovery and only 10 per cent will shed for more than 120 days. An unknown percentage of horses that continue to carry the organism but do not shed it in the feces may be a reservoir of infection.

CONTROL AND PREVENTION

Salmonella outbreaks should be controlled by isolating sick animals early in the disease; minimizing stress from such causes as shipping, overcrowding, changes of feed, and weaning; disinfecting and cleaning contaminated areas; and monitoring all exposed animals and isolating at the first sign of disease. Horses infected with Salmonella may begin to shed the organism before development of diarrhea, and the shedding rate seems to be quite high early in the disease. Thus, when Salmonella is a problem on a farm, isolation should begin with the first signs of depression and fever. Movement of people, other domestic animals, wild animals, and equipment between isolated animals and the rest of the herd should be eliminated. Care should also be taken in carefully disinfecting contaminated areas. Poor cleaning is the most common cause of ineffective disinfection because disinfectants are inactivated by organic material. Although Salmonella does not grow well in the environment, the best growing conditions occur when excretions such as feces and urine are diluted with water. The most effective disinfectants are the phenolics* and 2 per cent formaldehyde; however, they are the most toxic. Quaternary ammonium compounds† and sodium hypochlorite are also effective. Most disinfectants will kill Salmonella; however, care must be taken to use them properly. Some quaternary ammonia compounds do not work in hard water, whereas others are designed for such water. After disinfection, environmental cultures should be taken to measure the effectiveness of the procedure. When routine disinfection seems to be inadequate, formaldehyde gas should be considered. However, it is extremely toxic and should only be used as a last resort.

Prevention is best achieved through preventive health management and avoidance of high-risk situations. The level of stress on individual animals should be kept to a minimum. High-risk situations may be minimized by developing suitable traffic patterns within the farm. Breeding animals and performance animals should be separated. Transient performance horses and brood mares should not be mixed with resident mares and foals. Minimizing frequent movement of farm personnel, tractors, and feed from one area of the farm to another may also be helpful. Vaccination, using a killed bacterin, has not been successful and is certainly not a substitute for good management and sanitation practices.

Supplemental Readings

Morse, E. V., Duncan, M. A., Page, E. A., and Fessler, J. F.: Salmonellosis in equidae: A study of 23 cases. Cornell Vet., 66:198, 1976.

Palmer, J. E.: Update in equine diarrheal diseases: salmonellosis

---

*O-Syl, Lehn & Fink Industrial Products, Montvale, NJ or One-Stroke-Environ, Vestal Laboratories, St. Louis, MO

†A33 or A99, Airwick Industries, 40 Seaview Dr., Secaucus, NJ or Roccal-D, Winthrop-Breon Laboratories, New York, NY.

and Potomac Fever. Proc. 12th Annu. Sci. Program, Am. Coll. Vet. Int. Med., 1984, pp. 126–132.

Palmer, J. E., and Benson, C. E.: Salmonella shedding in the equine. Proc. 1st International Symp. Salmonella, 1984.

Smith, B. P.: Salmonella infections in horses. Compend. Cont. Educ., 3:S4, 1981.

Potomac Horse Fever

Jonathan E. Palmer, KENNETT SQUARE, PENNSYLVANIA

Potomac horse fever is an acute enteric disease of adult horses that was first recognized in Montgomery County, Maryland, in 1979. It has also been referred to as Potomac Valley fever, Potomac fever, acute equine diarrheal syndrome (AEDS), midatlantic diarrhea syndrome, equine monocytic ehrlichiosis, and acute equine ehrlichial enterocolitis.

EPIDEMIOLOGY

The epidemiology of Potomac horse fever is quite unique and differs from the epidemiology of other acute toxic enteric diseases of horses. Outbreaks seem to occur within close proximity of large rivers such as the Potomac, the Susquehanna in Pennsylvania, and the Snake River in Idaho. In the past several years, however, the disease has occurred as far as 20 miles from the Potomac. The outbreaks show a seasonal pattern. Cases are seen as early as May and become more frequent after the middle of June, with the majority occurring in July and August. Occasional cases may be seen as late as October or November. Although there may be "epizootics" in endemic areas, the disease is actually sporadic. Many animals develop the disease within the endemic area, but large outbreaks do not necessarily occur on any one farm. This pattern differs significantly from the epizootics caused by other enteropathogens, such as Salmonella and rotavirus.

There is no breed or sex predilection for the disease; however, there may be a predilection for pleasure horses. Disease may occur in horses of any age. There appears to be no significant age-related immunity, with a number of horses over the age of 20 developing the disease.

Direct contact with a sick or recovered horse is not necessary for the development of disease. There is no indication that this disease is directly transmitted from horse to horse and experimentally it is difficult if not impossible to transmit using the fecal-oral route. There is no evidence for a point source infection, both stable and pastured horses being affected.

Because the etiologic agent is a Rickettsia and other rickettsial agents are transmitted by arthropods, an arthropod vector has been suggested. The epidemiologic pattern suggests that a reservoir exists outside the horse. Mice, which can develop the disease after experimental inoculation, or other small mammals may be the reservoir. Multihost blood-sucking arthropods such as the American dog tick may be responsible for transmitting the disease to horses. Although the American dog tick has been found on horses in endemic areas, as of this writing there is no supporting evidence for this theory.

CLINICAL SIGNS

The disease typically begins with mild depression and anorexia. The horse usually has a temperature of 39.5 to 41.5° C with mildly injected mucous membranes. Borborygmi are noticeably decreased or absent. In 24 to 48 hours the horse develops profuse watery diarrhea, which may last up to 10 days. Signs of laminitis may begin a few days after the diarrhea.

Although the disease in the majority of horses follows the typical course, in a few it does not. Some develop transient depression and fever as their only signs. Others are febrile, have decreased borborygmal sounds, very injected mucous membranes, abdominal distention, and severe abdominal pain and frequently die before diarrhea develops. The most consistent sign in all horses is the decrease in borborygmi. In 1983, laminitis occurred in 25 per cent of the cases reported in the Potomac region of Maryland, and occasionally resulted in euthanasia.

There is no clinical distinction between Potomac horse fever and acute toxic enterocolitis due to other causes. Salmonellosis, clostridiosis, antibiotic associated enteritis, nonsteriodal anti-inflammatory drug toxicity, and idiopathic enterocolitis may all produce clinical syndromes that are indistinguishable from Potomac horse fever.

ETIOLOGY

An Ehrlichia antigenically related to *Ehrlichia sennetsu* and to a lesser degree to *Ehrlichia canis* has been isolated from the blood of horses with Potomac horse fever. The agent that has been observed in blood monocytes and the intestinal tract of infected horses can be grown in tissue culture and will produce the typical disease syndrome. Potomac horse fever is the only rickettsial disease producing enterocolitis, and it is also the only enteritic disease not transmitted by the fecal-oral route.

DIAGNOSIS

Clinical diagnosis is based on appropriate clinical signs in an endemic area. Definitive diagnosis is achieved by isolation of Ehrlichia in tissue culture, by animal inoculation, and by measurement of seroconversion using an indirect fluorescent antibody test. The organism can be grown in tissue culture from peripheral blood monocytes obtained during the acute phase of the disease and in some cases for an extended time after recovery. This technique is difficult and not practical. Animal inoculations will also confirm the presence of the disease. Fresh blood (50 to 500 ml) transfused into normal ponies will result in the reproduction of clinical signs in 10 to 14 days. Intraperitoneal injection of a buffy coat preparation into weanling mice will also result in reproduction of the disease. The organism can be identified in the spleen and peripheral blood of the mice using an indirect fluorescent antibody test.

The most practical method of diagnosis is by use of paired antibody titers. Single samples are meaningless because horses may carry a titer as high as 1:640 for a year or longer. A fourfold change in titer over a period of three to four weeks is diagnostic. Sera taken within the first few days of clinical signs will have a positive titer, which will rise dramatically over two to three weeks. Low titers (1:20, 1:40) may be meaningless and should not be overinterpreted. Therapy with drugs, such as oxytetracycline, does not interfere with the development of an antibody titer.

Clinical laboratory findings in cases of Potomac horse fever are similar to those of other cases of acute toxic enterocolitis. Although severe leukopenia with neutropenia and lymphopenia may occur, it is not consistently found in experimental animals. Hyponatremia, hypokalemia, hypochloremia, and acidosis are common findings as is azotemia, which is most frequently prerenal but may be renal. Secondary enteric bacterial infection is common and may result in additional clinical laboratory abnormalities.

THERAPY

As with other diseases resulting in acute enteritis, the most important aspect of therapy is correction of fluid, electrolyte, and acid-base imbalances. Fluid losses should be replaced with polyionic balanced electrolyte solutions, special attention being paid to the potassium and acid-base status. Aggressive intravenous fluid therapy is often required initially because of the rapid dehydration. Severely affected horses may require well in excess of 100 liters of intravenous fluids per day.

Survival rate is optimal when fluid therapy is combined with trimethoprim-sulfa* (5 mg per kg twice a day orally or intravenously) heparin† (20 to 40 units per kg twice or three times a day subcutaneously) and nonsteroidal anti-inflammatory drugs. Although most Rickettsia are sensitive to tetracyclines, the therapeutic value of this drug in treatment of Potomac horse fever has not been tested. Tetracyclines cannot therefore be recommended as of this writing.

PROGNOSIS, PREVENTION, AND CONTROL

The fatality rate of Potomac horse fever ranges from 17 to 36 per cent, some horses dying from secondary complications such as acute or chronic laminitis. Some horses remain unthrifty for prolonged periods of time, and there is apparently a high incidence of large colon displacements in recovered cases.

Effective prevention and control will only be possible when the full epidemiology of the disease is understood, including the method of transmission and the natural reservoirs of the pathogen. Although the fecal-oral route is an unlikely method of transmission, horses with Potomac horse fever may have secondary bacterial infections, including salmonellosis. Acutely affected animals should therefore be isolated, fecal contamination kept to a minimum, and cultures for Salmonella obtained. Attempts to control possible blood-sucking arthropod vectors have not prevented Potomac horse fever.

---

*Tribrissen, Burroughs Wellcome Co., Kansas City, MO or Bactrim, Roche Laboratories, Nutley, NJ
†Heparin Na Injection, USP, Elkins-Sinn, Inc., Cherry Hill, NJ

Supplemental Readings

Palmer, J. E.: Update on equine diarrheal diseases: Salmonellosis and Potomac fever. Proc. 12th Annu. Sci. Program, Am. Coll. Vet. Int. Med., 1984, pp. 126–132.
Perry, B. D., Palmer, J. E., Birch, J. B., Magnusson, R. A., Morris, D., and Troutt, H. F.: Epidemiologic characterization of an acute equine diarrheal syndrome: the case-control approach. Proc. Soc. Vet. Epid. Prev. Med., 1984, pp. 148–153.
Whitlock, R. H., Palmer, J. E., Benson, C. E., Acland, H. M., Jenney, A., and Ristic, M.: Potomac horse fever: Clinical characteristics and diagnostic features. Proc. 27th Annu. Mtg. Am. Assoc. Vet. Lab. Diagnosticians, 1984, pp. 103–124.

Peracute Toxemic Colitis: Colitis X

Michael J. Murray, ATHENS, GEORGIA

Peracute toxemic colitis is a highly fatal inflammatory condition of the cecum and large colon characterized by the sudden onset of profuse watery diarrhea, alterations in cardiovascular parameters, and derangements in metabolic homeostasis. The condition has previously been termed exhaustion shock and colitis X. The term colitis X has been used to describe cases of colitis in which a specific etiologic agent was not identified or as an umbrella term for all cases of peracute colitis with diarrhea and shock. Peracute toxemic colitis is sporadic and has been associated with stress, antibiotic administration, and experimental anaphylaxis. The condition also occurs in horses that have not been stressed, have not received antibiotics, and have been healthy until the onset of clinical signs. The condition cannot be clinically differentiated from acute salmonellosis and many undiagnosed cases of peracute colitis probably are salmonellosis. The condition also resembles some cases of the acute equine diarrhea syndrome (Potomac fever) recently associated with an organism of the Ehrlichia genus.

The association of peracute colitis with stresses such as strenuous exercise, transportation, surgery, and deworming and with antibiotic administration suggests that alterations in the cecal and colonic microflora may be a common factor contributing to the condition. Such an alteration could lead to decreased numbers of volatile fatty acid–producing bacteria, (primarily anaerobes), increased numbers of gram-negative enteric organisms (including Salmonella species), and decreased anaerobic fermentation of soluble carbohydrates into volatile fatty acids, leading to an increased fermentation of carbohydrates into lactic acid and a lowering of cecal and colonic pH. This latter change could damage cecal and colonic mucosal epithelium and allow endotoxin absorption from the lumen. Experimental administration of endotoxin in ponies produces changes similar to those seen in horses with peracute colitis.

CLINICAL SIGNS AND DIAGNOSTIC PROCEDURES

The clinical course of peracute colitis is characterized initially by inappetance, depression, and fever. Signs of abdominal pain are frequently present and often severe. The onset of diarrhea is sudden, with large volumes of watery stool produced. Diarrhea may be hemorrhagic and contain protein casts. Auscultation of the abdomen may indicate increased fluid and gas in the cecum and large colon with borborygmi of varying character and intensity. Dehydration is evidenced by decreased skin turgor and dry mucous membranes, which are frequently injected and congested. The pulse is usually rapid and often weak, and the respiratory rate is increased.

Characteristic hematologic changes include an elevated packed cell volume (PCV) and total protein (TP), indicative of dehydration and hemoconcentration. The PCV is usually greater than 50 per cent and may be as high as 70 to 80 per cent. Concurrently, TP will range from 8 to 12 gm per dl. As the condition progresses, TP can rapidly fall because of protein loss through the cecum and colon. Total protein and albumin can decrease to 3.5 gm per dl and less than 1.0 gm per dl, respectively, within 48 to 72 hours. Plasma fibrinogen may be increased to 600 to 800 mg per dl and can be used to estimate the degree of inflammation.

Leukopenia is characteristic of peracute toxemic colitis and can be attributed to neutrophil migration to the cecum and colon, diapedesis across the inflamed mucosa into the lumen of the bowel, and endotoxin-mediated margination of neutrophils on the vascular endothelium. As the condition progresses, the neutrophil count steadily decreases—to zero in some cases—and the band neutrophil count increases. Juvenile forms of the neutrophil series may be seen and toxic changes in neutrophils are common.

Blood urea nitrogen and creatinine are increased by dehydration and possibly also by renal mechanisms. Blood glucose is frequently increased to more than 150 mg per dl, presumably due to an increase in circulating catecholamines. Aspartate aminotransferase (SGOT) can be increased due to hepatocyte damage from endotoxin delivered in the portal circulation. Hyponatremia, serum sodium levels of 120 to 135 mEq per L, and hypochloremia, serum chloride levels of 80 to 90 mEq per L, are present because of decreased cecal and colonic absorption and possibly increased secretion of these electrolytes. Initially, serum potassium levels may be increased secondary to metabolic acidosis but typically decrease to 1.5 to 2.5 mEq per L because of decreased colonic absorption of potassium and lack of intake. Metabolic acidosis is reflected by a decreased total carbon dioxide in the blood or decreased serum bicarbonate (7 to 15 mEq per L). Total carbon dioxide in the blood can be measured with a Harleco CO_2 apparatus* and is a reliable estimate of serum bicarbonate. If available, arterial blood gas analysis should be performed, because many horses will have arterial hypoxemia (PaO_2 less than 80 mm Hg) secondary to endotoxemia. Additionally, venous blood gas analysis may reveal an increased venous Po_2 (greater than 60 mm Hg), indicating poor capillary perfusion and poor oxygen extraction by tissues.

Fecal cultures should be routinely submitted for isolation of Salmonella spp. (see p. 89). Gram quantities of feces should be submitted, and selenite enrichment broth can be used to enhance the chances of isolation of *Salmonella* from watery feces. Culturing fecal samples obtained on five consecutive days enhances the possibility of isolating *Salmonella*. Even if *Salmonella* is not isolated in the feces, salmonellosis cannot be completely ruled out. With the recent identification of an Ehrlichia sp. as the causative agent of Potomac fever (see p. 92), efforts should be made to identify this agent in cases of peracute colitis.

PATHOLOGIC FINDINGS

Gastrointestinal lesions are generally confined to the cecum and large colon, which appear reddish blue on the serosal surface. The mucosa is hyperemic and edematous, and may be sloughed over a large area of the cecum and colon. Luminal contents are fluid in consistency and rarely may contain blood. The cecocolic and mesenteric lymph nodes are frequently hyperemic and edematous and the adrenal glands have varying degrees of cortical hemorrhage. Petechial and ecchymotic hemorrhages are often found on the peritoneum and pleura as well as on the epicardium and in the myocardium. These changes are not specific and are also characteristic of salmonellosis and other systemic gram-negative infections.

PATHOPHYSIOLOGY

The pathophysiology of peracute colitis remains speculative. Endotoxin, through its local and systemic effects, appears to have a central role in peracute colitis both directly and by induction of other mediators. Signficant quantities of endotoxin are normally present in the lumen of the cecum and large colon but are prevented from entering

---

*Harleco CO_2 Apparatus, American Scientific Products, Obetz, OH

the circulation by impermeability of the mucosal cells. The events by which endotoxin gains access to the circulation are not known; however, many effects of endotoxin, once it passes the mucosal barrier, are known. Locally, endotoxin can damage cell membranes and thus provide substrate for prostaglandin synthesis. Prostaglandin E_2, prostacyclin, and thromboxane are produced normally in the colonic tissue of humans, and in inflammatory colitis PGE_2 and prostacyclin production are increased. PGE_2 can stimulate fluid and electrolyte secretion in the colon, and has been experimentally shown to promote protein exudation into the bowel lumen. Precursors of prostaglandin synthesis alternatively may be metabolized via the lipoxygenase pathway to leukotrienes. Leukotrienes are a family of compounds with a variety of biologic activities. The leukotriene 5-HETE promotes fluid and electrolyte secretion by the small and large intestine and leukotriene B_4, a potent chemotactic agent, is thought to play a role in human colitis. Endotoxins can increase vascular permeability to macromolecules, and may promote fluid and protein leakage from the microvasculature of the cecum and colon.

Systemically, endotoxin induces depression, abdominal pain, fever, leukopenia, congested mucous membranes, elevated heart and respiratory rates, arterial hypoxemia and mild transient diarrhea. Endotoxin-like substances have been identified in blood from patients with clinical cases of colitis, both Salmonella positive and negative. Coupled with similarities between experimental endotoxemia and peracute colitis, the findings of endotoxin in blood suggest a significant role for endotoxin in peracute colitis. Other mediators such as bradykinin, oxygen radicals from leukocyte infiltration in the large intestine, and catecholamines may contribute to the complex pathophysiology of this condition.

THERAPY

Therapy should be directed toward correction of clinical abnormalities. Dehydration and shock are the most immediate life-threatening problems, requiring vigorous intravenous fluid therapy. Initially, the amount of fluid given depends on the degree of dehydration. Horses with decreased skin elasticity and PCV greater than 60 per cent can be estimated to be at least 8 to 10 per cent dehydrated. A 450-kg horse requires at least 40 liters of fluid initially and more as fluid losses continue. In practice, complete rehydration is not possible as long as profuse diarrhea persists, and once the dehydration is moderated, continued rapid administration of intravenous fluids may exacerbate the diarrhea.

The choice of fluids used depends on the specific

electrolyte and acid-base disturbances present. Selection of the type of fluids and electrolyte supplementation to be used is based on the needs of the horse, route of administration, compatibility of constituents in the solution, and osmolality of the solution. In critically ill horses, adjustments in composition of fluids and rate of infusion must be made on the basis of frequent evaluation of hydration, electrolyte, and acid-base status.

Lactated or acetated Ringer's solution can be administered to most horses with colitis. Potassium can be added to these solutions, up to 3 gm KCl per liter, to provide a final potassium concentration of 44 mEq per L. Solutions with this potassium concentration can be infused at a rate of 1 L per 100 kg per hour. If more potassium supplementation is required, isotonic potassium chloride solution may be administered by stomach tube, up to 700 mEq (50 gm) per dose. Because serum potassium concentration decreases as serum pH increases, potassium should be re-evaluated as metabolic acidosis is treated. Initially, metabolic acidosis should be treated with isotonic sodium bicarbonate solution intravenously, the amount given depending on the base deficit (see p. 36). Oral bicarbonate supplementation, up to 100 gm in two gallons of water, can be used in addition to intravenous administration.

Administration of antibiotics is usually indicated in horses showing signs of endotoxemia and sepsis. The choice of antibiotics is determined by the efficacy of an antibiotic against the suspected pathogen (suspect Salmonella until proved otherwise), route of administration and serum levels achieved, potential toxicity of the antibiotic, and cost. Intravenous administration of antibiotics is preferred in peracute colitis in order to ensure complete delivery of the drug to the circulation. I prefer a combination of potassium penicillin, 22,000 to 44,000 units per kg intravenously four times a day, and gentamicin, 2.2 mg per kg intravenously three times a day. This combination gives broad-spectrum coverage, and the two antimicrobials act synergistically against gram-negative organisms. Adequate renal perfusion should be established and maintained during gentamicin therapy. In lieu of gentamicin, trimethoprim-sulfadiazine, 4.4 mg per kg intravenously twice a day, can be used. It has good activity against most Salmonella spp. prevalent in horses and can be used in combination with potassium penicillin. Chloramphenicol has frequently been advocated in treatment of equine salmonellosis but has several disadvantages. The injectable form for intravenous administration is very expensive and the serum half-life is quite short. The drug can be given orally, but should be administered by stomach tube to achieve adequate blood levels.

Pretreatment of experimental ponies with flunixin meglumine before endotoxin administration minimizes many of the adverse effects. Flunixin meglumine* is thus recommended for use in horses with peracute colitis and endotoxemia. Flunixin meglumine, and other nonsteroidal antiinflammatory drugs, inhibit prostaglandin synthesis and may have antisecretory activity in the colon. The dosage should not exceed 1.1 mg per kg twice a day, and a dosage of 0.55 mg per kg twice a day may be effective. If a dosage greater than 1.1 mg per kg is administered to a severely dehydrated horse, toxic effects identical to those produced by phenylbutazone administration can occur (see p. 118). Sodium heparin, 20 to 40 units per kg intravenously or subcutaneously three times a day, appears to be a useful treatment in horses with gastrointestinal disturbances and endotoxemia. This dosage is not an anticoagulatory dose. Heparin may prevent or minimize the occurrence of laminitis, a frequent complication in peracute colitis. The PCV may fall 25 to 35 per cent with this treatment, and thus lose its effectiveness as a reflection of hydration status.

Hypoproteinemia can contribute to intestinal and peripheral edema, and in itself promote diarrhea. Hypoproteinemia also complicates vigorous fluid administration and the dosage of drugs that are extensively protein bound, such as nonsteroidal anti-inflammatory drugs and gentamicin. Intravenous plasma therapy is valuable in enhancing plasma oncotic pressure and may also provide serum factors that are depleted in the toxemic horse. In horses with severe and progressive hypoproteinemia, 1 to 2 L per 100 kg may be required. Plasma may be obtained by collecting blood from a donor horse and separating plasma from red cells by gravity sedimentation. With this method, red cell contamination of plasma is unavoidable, and donor red cells should be cross-matched with recipient plasma before administration. Commercially produced equine plasma has recently become available and, although expensive, is free of red cell contamination; cross-matching is not required.†

Pharmacologic support of the cardiovascular system may be necessary in some horses. Most drugs that affect the sympathetic system should be avoided because undesirable cardiovascular effects usually outweigh the desired effects. Dopamine hydrochloride, however, can be effective in increasing cardiac output and perfusion to vital splanchnic organs without significantly altering systemic arterial pressure. Dopamine should be infused in normal saline, 3 to 5 μg per kg per minute, intravenously. The heart should be monitored for any increase in rate or any rhythm disturbance. If either

---

*Banamine, Schering Corp., Kenilworth, NJ
†Plasmate, Applied Technologies and Pharmaceuticals, Inc., Atlanta, GA

of these occurs, or the horse becomes anxious or excited, dopamine infusion should be discontinued. Infusion may be resumed at a lower dose after signs of adverse reaction abate. The use of corticosteroids in support of the cardiovascular system in horses with endotoxic shock is controversial. Many of the beneficial effects of corticosteroids in endotoxin shock can be achieved or surpassed with flunixin meglumine. Adverse effects of corticosteroids are widely documented and so their use in this context is questionable.

If analgesia is required, flunixin meglumine, 1.1 mg per kg twice a day, can be used. Short-term analgesia may be obtained with xylazine, 0.4 to 0.6 mg per kg, but xylazine may adversely affect cardiovascular performance in horses with endotoxic shock. Butorphanol tartrate may provide adequate analgesia at a dose of 0.1 to 0.2 mg per kg.

Intestinal protectants such as activated charcoal and preparations containing bismuth subsalicylate may be administered but are usually ineffective in peracute colitis.

Horses that survive the first 72 hours of illness will usually require medical attention for 7 to 10 days. It is not uncommon for complicating problems such as vascular thrombosis and laminitis to require longer treatment. Horses should be encouraged to eat grass hay. Grain should be avoided for several days because the normal flora of the cecum and colon are still likely to be decreased in number. Parenteral B-vitamin supplementation is recommended. When the horse's hydration and metabolic status are stabilized, oral fluid, electrolyte, and bicarbonate supplementation may be adequate.

Supplemental Readings

Ewert, K. M., Fessler, J. F., Templeton, C. B., et al.: Endotoxin-induced hematologic and blood chemical changes in ponies: Effects of flunixin meglumine, dexamethasone, and prednisolone. Am. J. Vet. Res., 46:24, 1985.

Musch, M. W., Miller, R. J., Field, M., et al.: Arachidonic acid metabolism and colonic secretion. Gastroenterology, 84:1062, 1983.

Rooney, J. R., Bryans, J. T., Prickett, M. E., et al.: Exhaustion shock in the horse. Cornell Vet., 56:220, 1966.

Smith, B. P.: Salmonella infection in horses. Comp. Cont. Ed., 3:S4, 1981.

Sprouse, R. F., and Garner, H. E.: Normal and perturbed microflora of the equine colon. Proc. Eq. Colic Res. Symp., University of Georgia, 1982, pp. 53–61.

Intestinal Clostridiosis

Martin Wierup, UPPSALA, SWEDEN

Equine intestinal clostridiosis (EIC) was first described in the 1970s in Sweden and later in other countries, including the United States. The typical case is characterized by diarrhea and toxemia in stressed horses. An intestinal dysbacteriosis with abnormally high counts of *Clostridium perfringens* type A is pathognomonic for EIC. Strong evidence exists that EIC is an enterotoxemia caused by that microbe.

EPIDEMIOLOGY

The disease affects all ages but rarely occurs in horses less than one year of age. No sex or breed predisposition has been observed. Horses have often been subjected to stress, usually in the form of hard training but also in the form of infections, surgery, deworming, or recent antibiotic therapy. The disease is usually sporadic, but occasionally several cases may occur in one stable within a limited period of time. The prognosis is dependent on the degree of intoxication. In one study of 31 consecutive cases, 12 (39 per cent) died.

CLINICAL SIGNS

Typically the disease has a peracute onset, the most prominent signs being profound depression, diarrhea, and discolored mucous membranes. The diarrhea is often projectile, watery, dark-colored, and foul-smelling. Occasionally the first sign is depression followed by diarrhea a few hours later. Rarely diarrhea may not be present, but there may be colic. Conjunctival and scleral vessels are usually congested as a result of toxemia. Capillary refill is delayed accordingly. Severely affected horses stand or move only with great difficulty and usually lie down.

The heart rate varies with the severity of the illness. In severe cases, the heart rate is elevated to 75 to 140 beats per minute. Especially in severe cases, a decreased skin temperature indicates failing circulation (shock). The respiratory rate seems to be related to the severity of metabolic acidosis. The temperature may be normal but in most cases increases to 39 to 40° C. Dehydration is an important clinical feature. Laminitis may occur in prolonged cases. On rectal examination no abnormal observation is made apart from the watery rectal and intestinal contents.

The disease usually runs a rapid course. Occasionally death is apoplectic. Some horses have fallen dead during races. Among terminal cases, however, it is most common that the horse dies within 24 hours after an acute onset with severe signs. Intensive therapy at an early stage of the disease may prolong the course. In milder cases, the course is often more prolonged. Horses surviving the disease appear to recover full health and racing capacity. Only in very few cases has recurrence been observed.

NECROPSY FINDINGS

Necropsy findings are characterized by widespread capillary damage with hyperemia, edema, and hemorrhages. The blood clots poorly. Acute inflammatory lesions are present in the intestinal tract. Acute hemorrhagic or necrotizing typhlitis and colitis of varying severity are consistent findings in subacute to chronic cases. The peracute cases may show only minor lesions. In the small colon and rectum, similar lesions are seen only in prolonged cases. In about two thirds of the patients, the small intestine is affected as well. Only in rare cases is the stomach the site of lesions. The intestinal contents of the cecum and large colon are watery, dark-colored, often mixed with blood, and usually foul-smelling.

Myocardial degeneration is occasionally observed histologically. The lungs consistently exhibit extensive hyperemia, edema, hemorrhage, and hyperinflation. Hemorrhage is also common in the adrenal glands, which may show necrosis. The liver is severely hyperemic in most cases and in horses with prolonged disease also has degenerative changes. The majority of the cases have hyperemic splenomegaly and congested intestinal lymph nodes. Bacteriologic examination of lymph nodes and organs reveals no specific aerobic or anaerobic organism.

CLINICAL PATHOLOGY

Increased serum levels of ornithine carbamyl transferase (up to 18.2 IU per L) and aspartate aminotransferase indicate liver damage. Liver injury and reduced liver function have also been verified by demonstration of extensive parenchymatous de-

generation in liver biopsies and by increased retention of sulphobromophthalein. In the majority of the cases, there are high (up to 2004 IU per L) alkaline phosphatase levels, which mainly reflect lesions of the biliary tree. Elevated values of urea nitrogen can also be observed, most probably as a result of prerenal azotemia. Dehydration is indicated by elevated total protein values and a rise in the hematocrit. Leukopenia (WBC down to 2.5×10^3) appears early, and leukocytosis (WBC up to 25.9×10^3) occurs later in the disease. ECG usually demonstrates abnormalities suggesting myocardial myopathy.

ETIOLOGY

Evidence clearly indicates that EIC is an enterotoxemia caused by *C. perfringens* type A. The disease is associated with an intestinal dysbacteriosis as shown by abnormally high counts of *C. perfringens*. Moreover, if the disease regresses, the *C. perfringens* counts decrease to normal levels. Numbers of *C. perfringens* in the feces are correlated with the severity of illness. In healthy horses in both Sweden and the United States, *C. perfringens* is not isolated or in rare cases is detected only in counts less than or equal to 10 colony-forming units (CFUs) per gm of feces.

The clinical and pathoanatomic findings resemble those characteristically seen during clostridial enterotoxemias in other animal species. Indeed, many of the prominent signs and the clinicopathologic changes can be construed as being indicative of physiologic disturbances or tissue damage caused specifically by toxins of *C. perfringens*. Immunologic investigations have revealed that EIC horses and those fed *C. perfringens* experimentally possess precipitating antibodies against an extracellular antigen elaborated by an equine isolate of *C. perfringens* type A. Although it has proved difficult to mimic enterotoxemias caused by *C. perfringens* under experimental conditions, horses given broth cultures of *C. perfringens* type A orally revealed signs similar to spontaneous cases of EIC, although usually less pronounced. It can be concluded that other predisposing factors must coincide with the rise in the *C. perfringens* counts in order to trigger the disease.

DIAGNOSIS

EIC should be suspected primarily in stressed horses developing acute signs of intoxication and diarrhea but also in cases of apoplectic deaths. However, for the confirmative diagnosis, clinical signs or pathologic changes must be found in connection with an abnormal rise in fecal or intestinal *C. perfringens* counts. The specimen, simply feces in a plastic bag, should be subjected to serial dilutions and *C. perfringens* identified primarily by Nagler reactions on egg yolk agar. Regularly, cultures should also be made for detection of Salmonella. Cultures should preferably be made within four hours of sampling, but within 24 hours is also acceptable when specimens are kept under cool conditions. *C. perfringens* counts greater than 10^2 CFUs per gm of feces in most types of horses can be judged as abnormal, but during the acute phase of EIC, the corresponding value usually is 10^4 to 10^5 CFUs. Bacteriologic examination thus is essential. If this is not performed, cases of EIC might be diagnosed as colitis X, a term likely inclusive of various causes of acute colitis.

THERAPY

The primary treatment is directed at stopping the toxin production of *C. perfringens*. The basic therapy for this purpose is the immediate use of "sour milk." This milk product is derived from lactic acid–producing strains of Streptococcus and is available in every grocery store in Sweden.* A horse weighing 400 to 500 kg should be given 4 to 6 L by stomach tube. Treatment should be repeated at least once after six hours. Many cases of EIC are often dramatically improved within two hours. Although the clinical effect of sour milk is quite clear, its pharmacologic action is not fully understood. However, in vitro studies have demonstrated that sour milk has a strong antibacterial effect against *C. perfringens* but not against several other bacteria belonging to 12 genera, including Salmonella. As yet, research has not demonstrated a corresponding result for buttermilk or yogurt. It has also been reported that cases diagnosed as EIC have been successfully treated with *C. perfringens* types C and D antitoxin, 250 ml given intravenously diluted in 2 L of lactated Ringer's solution.

Treatment must also be directed to replacement of the loss of water and electrolytes and correction of the metabolic acidosis. This is done by intravenous infusions of lactated Ringer's and $NaHCO_3$ solutions (p. 36).

---

*Note: Sour milk is not generally available in the United States.

In severe cases, 40 to 60 L of fluid are needed. Conventional shock therapy with corticosteroids (1 to 4 mg per kg dexamethasone) may also be considered.

As no bacteremia occurs, any antibiotic used should be active in the intestine, but experience has shown antibiotics to be of little or no value. Neomycin and tetracycline must not be used because of the adverse effect on gut flora. If sour milk is not available or where such a therapy does not improve the condition, chloramphenicol may be used.

After recovery from severe EIC, a convalescence of at least one month is needed, and preferably no training should be started until an ECG examination has excluded myocardial lesions.

CONTROL

Clinical and experimental studies have clearly demonstrated that tetracycline therapy can result in an intestinal overgrowth of *C. perfringens* resulting in diarrhea and death. However, a history of tetracycline therapy exists only for a minority of the spontaneous cases of EIC, and in the rest the underlying cause of the rise of the intestinal *C. perfringens* count is not known. Tetracycline should, therefore, be used with care, and long-term treatment with the drug should be avoided. It has been demonstrated experimentally that high doses of lysine and methionine can alter the intestinal flora of horses, as indicated by abnormally high, up to 10^5, *C. perfringens* CFUs per gm of feces. This observation should be kept in mind when these amino acids are included in feed additives given to intensively fed and trained racehorses.

Supplemental Readings

Andersson, G., Ekman, L., Mansson, I., Persson, S., Rubarth, S., and Tufvesson, G.: Lethal complications following administration of oxytetracycline in the horse. Nord. Vet. Med., 23:9, 1971.

Anderson, N. V.: Veterinary gastroenterology. Philadelphia, Lea & Febiger, 1980.

Vaughan, J. T.: The acute colitis syndrome, colitis "X." Vet. Clin. North Am., 2:301, 1973.

Wierup, M.: Equine intestinal clostridiosis. An acute disease in horses associated with high intestinal counts of *Clostridium perfringens* type A. Acta Vet. Scand., Suppl 62, AVSPAC, 62:1, 1977.

Wierup. M., and DiPietro, J. H.: Bacteriological examination of equine fecal flora as a diagnosis tool for equine intestinal clostridiosis. Am. J. Vet. Res., 42:2167, 1981.

Chronic Diarrhea

Leon Scrutchfield, COLLEGE STATION, TEXAS

Chronic diarrhea is one of the more frustrating conditions encountered by the equine practitioner. Causes include *Strongylus vulgaris* larval migrations, trichonema infections, chronic salmonellosis, enteric *Corynebacterium equi* infections in young animals, granulomatous enteritis, aseptic peritonitis, viruses, gastrointestinal neoplasia, chronic liver disease, and sand enteropathy. A specific cause is determined in only a small percentage of cases; consequently, therapy is usually nonspecific and results are rarely rewarding.

CLINICAL EXAMINATION

A complete physical examination should be performed because multiple systems may be involved. Except in the situation described, insufficient information is gained by routine rectal examination of patients with chronic diarrhea to warrant the risk of rectal tears. These horses tend to have friable rectal mucosa and there is considerable risk of rectal injury. Rectal examination should be performed if granulomatous enteritis is suspected on the basis of moderate to severe hypoalbuminemia, mild to moderate hypoglobulinemia, and a history of abdominal pain. Rectal examinations may be indicated in Standardbreds with diarrhea because they apparently have a greater incidence of granulomatous enteritis than other breeds. If a rectal examination is performed the general condition of the rectum should be observed, and abnormal masses noted in the areas of the cranial and caudal mesenteric roots, gut wall, mesentery and abdominal cavity. If suspicious areas are close enough to the anus, granulomatous enteritis can be confirmed by rectal biopsy obtained by carefully removing a pinch of rectal mucosa with a uterine biopsy instrument.

LABORATORY EVALUATION

Laboratory test may include complete blood counts (CBC), total plasma protein and fibrinogen, serum biochemical profile, serum protein electrophoresis, serum electrolytes, blood gases, peritoneal fluid examination, and fecal examination including direct smear, flotation, and culture. A xylose or glucose absorption study may also be performed.

The CBC is usually within normal limits. An elevated total white blood cell (WBC) count with an absolute neutrophilia may be due to stress or bacterial infection. Eosinophilia may indicate parasitism. Total plasma protein may be low because of malabsorption or excessive gastrointestinal protein loss or both. The fibrinogen level gives an indication of the degree of inflammation. The serum biochemical profile helps evaluate kidney and liver status. The serum protein electrophoresis may indicate protein-losing enteropathy if the albumin, beta, and gamma fractions are decreased, liver disease if there is hypoalbuminemia with elevated beta and gamma fractions or infection if there is an elevated gamma globulin fraction.

Most chronic diarrhea patients are metabolically compensated and have blood pH and serum electrolytes within normal ranges. However, some patients will require sodium bicarbonate or electrolyte supplementation or both.

Peritoneal fluid examination will indicate the presence or absence of peritonitis. Parasite migration is suggested if eosinophils comprise greater than 5 per cent of WBC present.

The number of trichomonads found on direct fecal smears varies greatly, and this does not indicate a cause of the diarrhea. Salmonella rarely causes chronic diarrhea except as a sequel to acute salmonellosis; however, it has been suggested that 15 per cent of chronic diarrhea patients shed Salmonella organisms. Since Salmonella shedders are potentially dangerous to other animals and humans, fecal cultures should be done (see p. 89).

TREATMENT

A treatment plan should be developed for any specific problems revealed by the history, physical, and/or laboratory examination.

Intestinal Parasites. If there is evidence of strongyle larva migrans such as cranial and/or caudal mesenteric arteriopathy on rectal palpation, eosinophils in the peritoneal fluid, elevated serum beta globulins, or large numbers of strongyle eggs in the feces, a larvicidal dose of an anthelmintic should be given (see p. 331).

Chronic diarrhea due to infection with Trichonema has been reported in England in the spring. The diarrhea may be caused by simultaneous maturation of previously inhibited larvae in the gut wall. Signs include intermittent diarrhea, mild colic, anorexia, and weight loss. Only a few small strongyle eggs are found in the feces. Larvicidal doses of thiabendazole, fendendazole, or ivermectin are indicated.

Bacteria. There is no good treatment program for the chronic diarrhea patient that is shedding salmonella organisms in the feces. Systemic antibiotics have questionable value even when sensitivity test results are followed. There seems to be a greatly increased resistance to the commonly used antibiotics chloramphenicol, trimethoprim-sulfa, and gentamicin. Some salmonella shedders seem to respond to treatment with 5 to 10 gm iodochlorhydroxyquin* orally per day. However, there are reports that some shedders become worse and may even die when placed on iodochlorhydroxyquin treatment. Salmonella shedding can continue for several months and these animals are a potential health hazard to other animals and humans. Affected animals should be isolated and treated symptomatically.

Rhodococcus equi can cause chronic diarrhea in foals with or without respiratory disease. Thoracic radiography may reveal circular areas of pulmonary consolidation suggestive of *Rh. equi* "abscesses," even when there are no clinical signs of respiratory disease. Treatment may be futile, but the same antibiotics suggested for the respiratory form of the disease could be tried (see *Rhodococcus equi*, p. 231).

Granulomatous Enteritis. Some patients with granulomatous enteritis have chronic diarrhea but most have weight loss, depression, and anorexia without diarrhea. The cause is unknown. Rectal examination findings include enlarged lymph nodes and/or nodules in the mesentery or around the cranial mesenteric root. The rectal wall may be thickened and friable. Moderate to severe hypoalbuminemia and mild to moderate hypoglobulinemia are often present. Definitive treatment regimens for granulomatous enteritis are not available since the cause has not been determined. It has been suggested that prednisolone in decreasing doses may be effective.

Sand Ingestion. Sand enteropathy (see p. 55) may cause chronic or acute diarrhea. Signs of abdominal pain may or may not be present. Attempts at abdominocentesis often result in accidental puncture of the ventral colon and collection of a sample that contains sand. Sand may be felt during rectal palpation of the ventral colon, or the horse may be passing considerable amounts of sand in the feces. Management and feeding practices need to be changed to prevent the ingestion of sand. Treatment suggestions vary, but usually involve the use of a

hemicellulose product* at a dose of 250 to 500 gm in 8 L of water via nasogastric tube. Hemicellulose may also be added to the horse's feed (125 to 175 gm daily) until sand is no longer passed in the feces. Some horse owners feed bran on a regular schedule such as 2 pounds twice a day Mon., Wed., and Fri. as a prophylactic measure.

Nonspecific Causes. Many regimens have been attempted in the treatment of nonspecific chronic diarrhea, which indicates that none are particularly effective as of this writing. The advisability of performing an expensive in-depth work-up on a chronic diarrhea patient that is thin but maintaining a stable body condition is questionable. Seldom can a specific and effective therapeutic regimen be prescribed.

Thiabendazole (TBZ) at a dosage of 66 to 100 mg per kg body weight may decrease the severity of the diarrhea, probably due to TBZ's anti-inflammatory action. The improvement following TBZ administration is usually temporary.

Iodochlorhydroxyquin, 10 gm orally per day in a 450-kg horse, helps many chronic diarrhea patients. It may take a week of therapy before improvement is seen. If the diarrhea improves or stops while the horse is being treated the dose should be reduced very gradually. It is not known why iodochlorhydroxyquin helps many horses. Unfortunately, a high percentage of the patients that respond will have resumption of the diarrhea when iodochlorhydroxyquin treatment is stopped.

Transfaunation with fresh-strained cecal and large bowel contents may be indicated when no ciliates are in the feces and the stools are soft and pasty. The cecal and large bowel contents are collected from recently killed horses and filtered to remove the colonic liquor. If possible, 5 to 6 L of liquor are collected and given to the patient immediately by stomach tube. It is impossible to determine which patients will respond favorably, and some horses become worse after transfaunation. There is a slight risk that the transfaunate could be from an apparently normal horse that is a Salmonella shedder.

Grass pasture seems to be beneficial to some horses with chronic diarrhea. Fresh water as well as water spiked with electrolytes should be available. Commerical electrolyte preparations may be used. One suggested formulation includes:

NaCl	117 gm (4 oz)
KCl	150 gm (5 oz)
NaHCO$_3$	168 gm (5.5 oz)
KHPO$_4$	135 gm (4.5 oz)

60 to 90 gm (2 to 3 oz) is mixed into a 12-L bucket of water.

While some chronic diarrhea patients do lose condition to the point of dying, hope should not be

---

*Rheaform, Squibb, Princeton, NJ

*Metamucil, Searle Pharmaceuticals Inc., Chicago, IL or Mucilose, Winthrop-Breon Laboratories, New York, NY.

abandoned too early. Unless destroyed for humane or economic reasons, many a "walking skeleton" has returned to normal use after a few months to two years on pasture and/or grass hay.

Supplemental Readings

Chiejina, S. N., and Mason, J. A.: Immature stages of trichonema spp. as a cause of diarrhoea in adult horses in spring. Vet. Rec., *100*:360, 1977.

Merritt, A. M.: Chronic Diarrhea. *In*: Mansmann, R. A., and McAllister, E. S. (eds.): Equine Medicine and Surgery, 3rd ed. Santa Barbara, CA, American Veterinary Publications, 1982, pp. 542–547.

Merrit, A. M.: Chronic Equine Diarrhea—Differential Diagnosis and Therapy. Proc. 21st Annu. Conv. Am. Assoc. Eq. Pract., 1975, p. 401.

Malabsorption Syndromes

Malcolm C. Roberts, RALEIGH, NORTH CAROLINA

The term malabsorption refers to impaired digestion and absorption of dietary constituents arising from structural or functional disorders of the small intestinal tract and associated organs—the pancreas, liver, and biliary tract. Malassimilation would be a more appropriate description. The resulting pathophysiologic changes may adversely affect large intestinal functions. Although the incidence is unknown, malabsorption syndromes appear to be far less common in horses than in humans and small animals. Malabsorption is not synonymous with diarrhea in any species, although diarrhea may be a feature. Chronic equine diarrhea, predominantly a large bowel problem, may be considered to represent a malabsorption of water and electrolytes.

Primary small intestinal disease can compromise normal large bowel function and precipitate transient or protracted diarrhea through the presence of abnormal quantities of bile acids, fatty acids, and carbohydrates entering the large bowel in ileal effluent. These substances directly or indirectly enhance secretion and/or decrease absorption rates, thereby overwhelming colonic salvage capacity. This is exacerbated in pre-existing large bowel disease, in which concomitant changes in the microbial flora, gut peptides, and neurotransmitters could further affect regulation of motor activity, secretion, and absorption.

The clinical investigation of malabsorption must be directed at attempting to define and localize a functional or structural derangement, or both, to a specific region of the gastrointestinal tract or associated organ, and to determine which dietary constituents are principally involved. Human syndromes can be described in terms of fat, carbohydrate, and more uncommonly, protein malabsorption. This scheme is not applicable to herbivores. Consequently, a proposed classification of malabsorption syndromes in the horse is based on functional and pathologic factors (Tables 1 and 2). Chronic weight loss is invariably the predominating clinical feature. Other more commonly encountered causes of wasting must be excluded before a diagnosis of malabsorption is made. Frequently, enteric protein loss may coexist with and prove more debilitating than malabsorption.

CLINICAL FINDINGS AND INVESTIGATION

The history should elucidate the duration of the condition, precipitating factors, nature of the ration, deworming and routine health care programs, previous or intercurrent disorders, and the number, age, and proximity of other affected animals.

A thorough physical examination should be performed. Clinical signs are not pathognomonic for malabsorption and include poor condition, muscle wasting, reduced performance, normal or reduced demeanor, variable appetite and thirst, and changes in the size, volume, color, and odor of feces. Vital signs are usually normal until later stages of the disease. Pyrexia may be attributed to mediators released from inflamed tissues. Abdominal pain may reflect inflammation, mesenteric or mural abscesses, adhesions, or partial obstruction. Flatulence and abdominal distention may be present. Dependent edema, cachexia, and weakness tend to appear later.

Systemic or extraintestinal manifestations, including skin and ocular lesions, vasculitis, arthritis, hepatitis, and renal disease, may indicate immunologic reactions, particularly with inflammatory bowel disease. Other malabsorption-related dermatoses, characterized by thin hair coat, patchy alopecia, and focal areas of scaling and crusting, are often symmetrically distributed. These have been

TABLE 1. PROPOSED CLASSIFICATION OF MALABSORPTION SYNDROMES
IN THE HORSE—MALDIGESTION

Condition	Example (Recognized or Putative)
A. Gastric disorders	
B. Deficiency or inactivation of pancreatic lipase	
1. Exocrine pancreatic insufficiency	Chronic pancreatitis: pancreatic carcinoma
C. Reduced intestinal bile salt concentration (with impaired formation of micellar lipid)	
1. Hepatic dysfunction	Parenchymal liver disease; cholestasis
2. Interrupted enterohepatic circulation of bile salts	Ileal inflammatory disease or resection
3. Abnormal bacterial proliferation in the small bowel	Stagnant (blind) loops, adhesions, fistulas, strictures. Incompetent ileocecal valve, surgical bypass, resection; hypomotility
4. Drug-induced (sequestration of bile salts)	Neomycin, cholestyramine, calcium carbonate
D. Small intestinal brush border enzyme deficiency	

observed with strongylosis and in suspected zinc deficiency. Foals with malabsorption may show diarrhea and abdominal discomfort; more severe systemic signs supervene with bacterial infection, especially if passive transfer is inadequate.

CLINICAL PATHOLOGY

The clinical pathology profile should be selective to aid differential diagnosis, provide valid information, and avoid unnecessary expense. The range of specific tests is limited in comparison to those available for humans and small animals. There is no biochemical or other test specific for the presence or severity of malabsorption. An initial data base could include a complete blood count; fibrinogen, total protein, albumin, amino aspartate transferase, gamma glutamyl transpeptidase, alkaline phosphatase, creatinine, and glucose levels; urinalysis; and fecal examination for parasite ova, larvae, protozoa, and occult blood. A carbohydrate absorption test should be performed if an intestinal problem is indicated. Additional procedures may include abdominocentesis, plasma protein electrophoresis, fecal culture and leukocyte count, immunologic studies, and biopsy of rectal or intestinal mucosa, lymph node, or liver.

Many animals with gastrointestinal problems have subnormal or low albumin and total protein levels attributed to enteric protein loss. Hypoalbuminemia can occur in the presence of normo- and hyperproteinemia due to increased beta and gamma globulin levels. A marginal to moderate, normocytic, nor-

TABLE 2. PROPOSED CLASSIFICATION OF MALABSORPTION SYNDROMES
IN THE HORSE—MALABSORPTION

Condition	Example (Recognized or Putative)
A. Inadequate absorptive surface area	Intestinal resection; villous atrophy
B. Cardiovascular disorders	Congestive heart failure; intestinal ischemia
C. Primary mucosal absorptive defects	
1. Inflammatory or infiltrative disorders	Granulomatous enteritis. Chronic eosinophilic gastroenteritis. Alimentary lymphosarcoma; amyloidosis. Tuberculosis; histoplasmosis; *Rhodococcus equi*. Invasive enterocolitis—*Salmonella* sp. Large and small strongyle larval migration
2. Biochemical or genetic abnormalities (± histological changes)	Acquired lactase deficiency. Dietary-induced enteropathy. Monosaccharide transport defect
D. Lymphatic obstruction	Lymphosarcoma; mesenteric lymphadenopathy. Intestinal lymphangiectasia; abscessation. Thoracic duct obstruction
E. Miscellaneous	Parasites—large and small strongyles, *Strongyloides westeri* (foals). Endocrinopathies. Partial chronic bowel obstruction—adhesions, abscesses. Drug-induced; heavy metal toxicity. Zinc deficiency

mochromic anemia is not uncommon. Lymphopenia may appear if lymphocyte-rich lymph is lost into the intestinal lumen in abnormal amounts. Other serum components, such as iron, copper, calcium, and lipids, may accompany leaking protein.

The investigational objective should be to select a logical sequence of tests to localize defects to a particular phase of digestion and absorption.

CARBOHYDRATE ABSORPTION TESTS

Four screening tests (glucose, D-xylose, starch, and lactose) have been devised to assess small intestinal function. These are simple to perform and assays are within the scope of most practice laboratories. An abnormal flattened absorption curve is suggestive of small intestinal dysfunction and may reflect extensive pathophysiologic changes, considering the vast absorptive surface area. However, the shape of the absorption curve does not always correlate with the presence of gross and microscopic lesions of the small bowel.

The oral glucose tolerance test (1 gm glucose per kg body weight as a 20 per cent solution) produces a maximum plasma glucose rise in normal animals at 120 minutes, approximately double the resting level, which is regained by six hours. The absorptive phase of the curve depends upon the rate of gastric emptying, mucosal cell function, intestinal transit time, and previous dietary history. Glucose tolerance curves are steeper in pasture-fed horses than in those fed a higher energy ration.

The D(+)xylose absorption test is becoming widely adopted, since endogenous factors do not influence plasma xylose levels. In humans, the pentose is absorbed preferentially in the jejunum by active transport utilizing the glucose carrier and by facilitated diffusion. This may apply to horses, although abnormal curves have been recorded with significant lesions of the distal small bowel. Peak blood levels are attained 60 to 90 minutes after oral administration of either 0.5 or 1.0 gm xylose per kg body weight as a 10 per cent solution. The test has proved discriminatory at the lower dose. The shape of the absorption curve is influenced by the rate of gastric emptying, intestinal motility, intraluminal bacterial overgrowth, renal clearance, and the immediate dietary history. Horses on low-energy rations have higher peak plasma xylose levels than those receiving high-energy diets. Xylose absorption was decreased in 73 per cent of horses with actual or recent signs of gastrointestinal disease. Abnormal absorption has been found in inflammatory bowel disease, and with villous atrophy, edema, or necrosis of the lamina propria in the small bowel, associated with evidence of *Strongylus vulgaris* larval migration. Abnormal xylose curves

were demonstrated in ponies with 40 per cent, 60 per cent, and 80 per cent distal small bowel resection, presumably due to reduced surface area and intestinal bacterial overgrowth. Malabsorption is a potential complication of extensive surgical resection to relieve small intestinal obstruction.

Theoretically, the starch tolerance test (2 gm cornstarch per kg body weight as a 20 per cent solution) could assess small bowel and exocrine pancreatic function. Pancreatic secretion is profuse (9 to 12 L in 24 hours) and apparently continuous, although the content and output of digestive enzymes, including α-amylase, is low. Advantages of the starch tolerance test have not been documented; however, the presence of intestinal glucoamylase activity may detract from its specificity, unless both pancreatic and small bowel dysfunction coexist.

The oral lactose tolerance test (1 gm lactose per kg body weight as a 20 per cent solution) has been used to evaluate nonsystemic diarrhea with malabsorption in the suckling or artificially reared foal. Normally, the peak plasma glucose level is reached 90 minutes after oral dosing. A reduced tolerance curve may predicate the need to restrict or prevent milk access for a short period to prevent colonic overload, with consequent osmotic diarrhea and abdominal discomfort, and facilitate epithelial regeneration. Epithelial regeneration can be monitored by repeating the test.

OTHER PROCEDURES

Under research conditions, enteric protein loss concomitant with malabsorption can be confirmed and quantitated using radiolabeled albumin. Reduced tritiated oleic acid uptake indicative of fat malabsorption has been shown in one granulomatous enteritis case. Regulations governing the use of such radiolabeled substances limit their availability.

Serum vitamin B_{12} and serum and red cell folate determinations may prove beneficial in assessing small intestinal integrity. Rectal biopsy may reveal focal or diffuse inflammatory infiltration. Culture of the biopsy and fecal examination for leukocytes and epithelial cells may aid in confirming the presence of Salmonella or other invasive organisms. On occasions, exploratory laparotomy may be justified to establish or confirm the diagnosis. Several intestinal and lymph node biopsies should be obtained for histopathology, enzymology, and immunology. Immunologic techniques, such as direct and indirect immunofluorescence for immune-mediated disorders and immune complex deposition, should be performed on serum and tissue samples. Contrast radiography of the bowel may be feasible in foals and small ponies, while ultrasonography using external or rectal probes could delineate intra-abdominal masses in larger animals.

SPECIFIC CONDITIONS

Maldigestion. Maldigestion per se is difficult to evaluate and is probably rare (see Table 1), in contrast to its prevalence in other species, exemplified by pancreatic enzyme deficiency. However, digestive disturbances cannot be discounted and may contribute to the pathophysiology of some chronic weight loss conditions. Pancreatic enzyme deficiency has not been demonstrated in the few cases of exocrine pancreatic insufficiency. Intestinal bile salt concentrations may be reduced in hepatic and ileal dysfunction, and while this may not impair digestion in the adult herbivore, diarrheal states in the milk-fed foal may be exacerbated. Surgical resection or bypass of the distal small bowel may facilitate bacterial overgrowth, with associated bile salt deconjugation and fatty acid hydroxylation, potentially affecting large bowel function.

Malabsorption. Malabsorption syndromes can result from a variety of functional and structural changes (see Table 2). Most are probably multifactorial. Distinctive features include changes in mucosal and submucosal morphology with associated absorptive defects in the small intestine and lymphatic obstruction. The large intestine may be involved. However, overt signs of malabsorption do not correlate always with gross and histopathologic changes, emphasizing the existence of functional disorders and the need to devise more sophisticated diagnostic techniques than are currently employed.

Despite recognition of idiopathic villous atrophy, the most significant mucosal absorptive defects are attributed to severe inflammatory bowel infiltration in horses, usually over one year of age. Inflammatory bowel disease (IBD) is exemplified by granulomatous enteritis, chronic eosinophilic gastroenteritis, alimentary lymphosarcoma, tuberculosis, and histoplasmosis. The first two may represent different stages rather than exclusive conditions. Pathologic lesions are rarely distributed uniformly and may be more florid at particular sites in the small or large bowel with apparently normal tissue between. Regional lymph nodes can be involved, and to a lesser extent the stomach, associated organs, and occasionally distant organs and tissues.

Some inflammatory bowel disorders of horses may be immunologically mediated if analogies can be drawn with human conditions showing remarkably similar pathology. Unfortunately, detailed immunologic studies have rarely been undertaken and the existence of hypersensitivity reactions or immune complex deposition remains speculative but highly probable. Putative antigens include intestinal wall components, dietary constituents, infectious agents (bacterial cell wall), and internal parasites, particularly migrating *Strongylus vulgaris* larvae.

Granulomatous Enteritis. Granulomatous enteritis has been reported in horses from the United States, Canada, South Africa, Australia, and Sweden. The condition principally affects Standardbreds one to five years of age. The upper recorded age is 11 years. Clinical signs include weight loss (progressive or rapid in onset), poor condition, lethargy, variable appetite, dependent edema, and occasionally diarrhea, intermittent abdominal pain, periods of pyrexia, and alopecia. Rectal exploration may reveal enlarged mesenteric lymph nodes, other intra-abdominal masses, and thickened bowel wall. Pathologic lesions are most evident in the small intestine. The granulomatous reaction in the gut wall is marked by diffuse and patchy infiltrates and distinct granulomas, composed of epithelioid, lymphoid, and occasional giant cells, and macrophages. Accompanying features include lymphoid hyperplasia, perilymphatic and transmural inflammation, lymphangiectasia, villous atrophy, mucosal ulceration, fibrosis, crypt abscesses, and serosal fibrosis. Granulomatous changes are often demonstrated in alimentary tract tissues beyond the small bowel and its lymph nodes and even multisystemically.

The condition is unresponsive to therapy. Abnormal carbohydrate absorption is common; lipid malabsorption has been demonstrated in one animal, and enteric protein loss confirmed. Although specific pathogens have not been implicated, the role of cell wall defective organisms or atypical mycobacteria cannot be excluded. *Mycobacterium avium* has been identified on occasion in tissue or feces, and screening for acid-fast organisms should be undertaken.

Chronic Eosinophilic Gastroenteritis. Chronic eosinophilic gastroenteritis has been described in Australia in horses 2 to 12 years of age, most being under 6 years old. The condition is manifested by chronic weight loss, variable appetite and fecal consistency, dependent edema, dullness and occasional pyrexia and oral ulceration. Skin lesions were frequently the major presenting complaint, particularly ulcerative coronitis, and alopecia, hyperkeratosis, and exudative dermatitis distributed symmetrically over the muzzle, face, and limbs, accompanied by intense pruritus, self-mutilation, and secondary infection. Rectal examination may reveal enlarged mesenteric lymph nodes and thickened mesentery, and bowel wall. Reduced carbohydrate absorption, hypoalbuminemia, and hypoproteinemia were consistent findings. There is diffuse and focal eosinophilic infiltration of the alimentary tract, regional lymph nodes, adjacent organs, and extra-intestinal tissues, especially the skin. The location and severity of gastrointestinal lesions are not uniform; they predominate in the proximal duodenum, distal ileum, and cecum, with discontinuous lesions elsewhere. Microscopic changes are more widespread. The cellular infiltrate usually comprises lymphoid, epithelioid, plasma, and mast cells, macrophages, an occasional giant cell and abundant eosinophils associated with villous atrophy, mucosal to transmural (and serosal) thickening and fibrosis, mucosal ulceration, and surface-raised nodules with caseous centers. Parasite involvement is unremarkable and no significant bacteria are recovered. There is no therapy.

Alimentary Lymphosarcoma. Horses with alimentary lymphosarcoma are mature, aged five years and older, and can present with weight loss, edema, variable appetite and demeanor, occasional pyrexia, diarrhea, and colic. Weight loss can be relatively rapid in onset or progressive. Intra-abdominal masses, including enlarged mesenteric lymph nodes, may be palpated. Malabsorption has been demonstrated on the basis of abnormal carbohydrate absorption, villous morphologic changes, disaccharidase deficiency, and lymphatic obstruction. Major pathologic changes occur in the small intestine and associated lymph nodes, although neoplastic infiltration is found elsewhere in the gastrointestinal tract, and in adjacent and distant organs. Hypoalbuminemia is frequently associated with hyperproteinemia due to increased beta and gamma globulin levels. Lymphocytosis is extremely rare. No therapy exists at present.

Lactase Deficiency. Acquired lactase deficiency of suckling foals exemplifies a biochemical functional abnormality in which brush border disaccharidase enzymes are decreased following loss or damage of mature enterocytes at villous tips. Congenital lactase deficiency has not been identified. Morphologic changes may involve partial villous atrophy, crypt hyperplasia, and lamina proprial infiltration. The condition may result from infection with rotavirus, coronavirus, possibly adenovirus, or the protozoa cryptosporidium. Salmonella and other invasive bacteria may exacerbate the problem. This range of pathogens could provoke malabsorption states in older animals.

Foals with lactose intolerance may develop osmotic diarrhea and exhibit abdominal discomfort. Ideally, the lactose load should be reduced by restricting or withholding milk for at least three to five days to allow replenishment of normal enterocytes. All disaccharidase enzymes are depressed but lactase activity remains lowered for a much longer period. Other brush border–related functions may be affected, for instance assimilation of fat micelles. Enterokinase and dipeptidase enzyme deficiencies have not been detected. Lactase deficiency is not a problem of mature horses.

Migrating Parasites. Migrating *Strongylus vulgaris* larvae may contribute to malabsorption by altering rates of blood flow, even without overt vascular damage, impairing perfusion at the mucosal level, and consequently secretory and absorptive processes. Although pathologic lesions manifested by extensive ulceration and erosion in the cecum and colon have been related to chronic diarrhea and enteric protein loss, functional changes induced by perturbations in the mucosal vasculature may underlie many cases of malabsorption and diarrhea. Extensive mucosal lesions caused by Cyathostominae sp. larvae emerging en masse from nodules can precipitate enteric protein loss and malabsorption.

TREATMENT AND MANAGEMENT

Horses suffering from true malabsorption present difficulties in management, support, and therapy. As the condition is usually well advanced when identified, the prognosis is grave and treatment usually proves unrewarding. There is a better outcome in parasitic conditions and functional disorders of the large bowel. Many animals are hypophagic and in protein-calorie malnutrition. Therapeutic objectives are to address protein, calorie, water, and electrolyte imbalances, thus enhancing the compromised immune system, and attend to any existing anemia and vitamin and mineral deficiencies. This necessitates providing palatable, easily assimilated high-energy and protein sources, restoring and maintaining mineral balance (calcium and magnesium, and to a lesser extent, zinc, copper, and iron) and supplementing fat- and/or water-soluble vitamins. Good-quality alfalfa hay, chaff or meal, with sweet feed for energy is beneficial. Nevertheless, some animals, even those that are hyperphagic, appear unable to sustain their current maintenance condition by oral intake. Sporadic grazing will not suffice.

Alimentation, via an indwelling nasogastric tube, may be justified for animals with poor appetites to immediately restore protein and energy balance and stimulate normal feeding habits (see p. 424).

Animals with chronic diarrhea may improve steadily as the microbial flora and bidirectional fluid and electrolyte fluxes revert toward normal. Intensive parasite control initiated by larvicidal anthelmintic therapy with avermectins or benzimidazoles can promote a marked clinical improvement, weight gain, cessation of diarrhea, and increased albumin and protein levels.

A diagnosis of chronic inflammatory bowel disease (IBD) invariably carries a grave prognosis. The owner should understand that intensive nutritional and symptomatic support may be unable to maintain the present status, and continued professional efforts and expenditure are unjustified. Therapy has been attempted with various combinations of corticosteroids, adrenocorticotrophic hormone (ACTH), azothioprine, metronidazole, sulfasalazine, prostaglandin inhibitors, anabolic steroids, antithrombotics, vitamins, minerals, and anti-diarrheal preparations, together with fluids, electrolytes, anthelmintics, and antimicrobials. The outcome has been consistently unsuccessful. Antimicrobial administration may alleviate clinical signs in cases in which anaerobic or aerobic bacterial overgrowth is a problem. Adequate penetration of antimicrobials into inflammatory bowel lesions including those caused by *Rhodococcus equi* in foals is doubtful.

Milk access should be restricted for lactose-intolerant foals by muzzling, stripping the udder, or providing alternative energy sources—glucose electrolyte solution or nonlactose (soybean) milk replacer. The latter may be a valid option for an orphan foal. It may be possible to pretreat collected mare's milk or more practically, a commercial milk replacer with a yeast-derived lactase enzyme,* widely used in human pediatrics. Most nonsystemic foal diarrheas with lactose intolerance resolve spontaneously or with symptomatic therapy. Antimicrobial therapy should be instituted together with fluid therapy and/or serum to augment passive immune transfer in systemic infections.

*Lactaid, SugarLo Company, Pleasantville, NJ

Severely afflicted animals, particularly those with IBD, should be destroyed at the earliest stage and subjected to complete autopsy examination. Malabsorption cases provide a diagnostic challenge, the pursuit of which will be limited by economic realities. Many available tests do not sufficiently discriminate structural or functional defects, and maldigestion cannot be differentiated. More sophisticated screening and diagnostic criteria are required. At present, therapy is largely supportive and symptomatic. More specific therapy must await medical advances to identify, and then to develop pharmacologic agents to enhance or suppress the biochemical factors acting directly or indirectly in the intestinal lumen or wall.

Supplemental Readings

Roberts, M. C.: Protein-losing enteropathy in the horse. *In* Grunsell, C. S. G. and Hill, F. W. G. (eds.): The Veterinary Annual 24. Bristol, Scientechnica, 1984, p. 52.

Roberts, M. C.: Malabsorption syndromes in the horse. Comp. Contin. Educ. Pract., 7:S637, 1985.

Roberts, M. C., and Hill, F. W. G.: The oral glucose tolerance test in the horse. Equine Vet. J., 6:28, 1974.

Roberts, M. C., and Norman, P.: A re-evaluation of the D(+)xylose absorption test in the horse. Equine Vet. J., 11:239, 1979.

Roberts, M. C., and Pinsent, P. J. N.: Malabsorption in the horse associated with alimentary lymphosarcoma. Equine Vet. J., 7:166, 1975.

Alimentary Tract Neoplasia

Conrad H. Boulton, PULLMAN, WASHINGTON

Primary gastrointestinal neoplasia in the horse is rare. There are limited retrospective necropsy studies available from which the incidence is estimated at less than 0.1 per cent of examined horses. When the population becomes narrowed to cases characterized by acute or chronic signs referable to the abdomen, the incidence increases to approximately 5 per cent.

The most common forms of primary neoplasia are squamous cell carcinoma of the stomach, and the alimentary form of lymphosarcoma. There are no reports of successful treatment in either case. Other isolated types of neoplasia can be found in the veterinary literature including lipoma of the mesentery, leiomyoma, adenocarcinoma, and ameloblastic odontoma. Metastatic involvement of the alimentary tract is noted in cases of malignant melanoma, transitional cell carcinoma, multicentric lymphosarcoma, teratoma, and many others but, again, is infrequently observed. The most frequent locations and types of reported primary neoplasia are presented in Figure 1.

CLINICAL SIGNS AND THERAPY

The presenting complaint and clinical signs of alimentary tract neoplasia to some degree depend upon the location and type of neoplasm. The majority of cases present as progressive weight loss or exercise intolerance or both. The weight loss can occur for a variety of reasons but is most often the result of "cancer cachexia" associated with possible impairment of ingestion, digestion, absorption, and

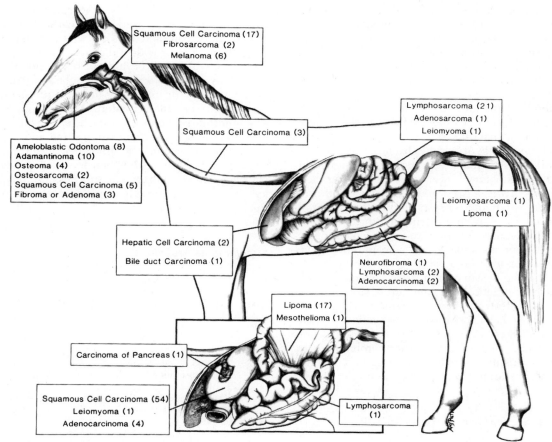

Figure 1. The most common types and locations of primary alimentary tract neoplasia reported in the literature (217 cases).

utilization of nutrients or excessive energy requirements of the host and tumor. Depending upon the location, size, and number of tumors, varying degrees of bowel occlusion or impairment may be produced. While the most common presenting sign is weight loss, this may be overshadowed by a variety of signs, including dysphagia in pharyngeal, esophageal, or gastric neoplasms, acute abdominal crises in cases of strangulating lipoma or intussusception incited by a small intestinal tumor, chronic abdominal pain where intestinal adhesions have formed, and chronic diarrhea secondary to neoplastic infiltration of the intestinal walls. This variability causes the tentative diagnosis of neoplasia to begin relatively low on a list of differential diagnoses in cases involving alimentary tract signs, and to slowly rise in the index of suspicion as the many more commonly encountered pathologies are eliminated.

Generally, definitive diagnosis of alimentary tract neoplasms is made at postmortem examination. Reports of successful treatment have been cases in which complete surgical resection of neoplastic tis-

sue could be achieved. Availability of antineoplastic drugs, knowledge of toxic effects, ability to provide supportive therapy during treatment, and financial support to treat these lesions as practiced in human medicine have not existed in the horse. The notable exception has been radiation therapy of accessible peripheral lesions.

OROPHARYNGEAL NEOPLASIA

Odontogenic and osteogenic tumors are infrequently seen in the horse. All present as firm immobile swellings of the mandible or maxilla and require radiography or biopsy for diagnosis. Among those possible are ameloblastic odontomas, which occur as congenital lesions in foals, and adamantinomas, which occur in older animals. Osteomas and osteosarcomas may occur at any age, although most osteomas are noted in younger horses.

The prognosis of these tumors and other forms of neoplasia is guarded to poor. If left untreated they have the potential to cause dental malocclusion and starvation. Successful resection of both an osteoma and two cases of adamantinoma do offer hope. A recent report of successful radical mandibular resection in a Thoroughbred stallion illustrates an aggressive endeavor in reconstructive surgery that warrants further exploration in other cases of oral neoplasia.

Pharyngeal neoplasia shares the guarded prognosis of oral neoplasia. The most common types are squamous cell carcinoma and fibrosarcoma. Although surgical extirpation might be theoretically possible, it is seldom realistic when the limited surgical exposure and difficulty in defining neoplastic borders are considered. Radiation therapy may be a possibility but is unreported. Short-term salvage may be possible through the use of tracheostomy and/or esophagostomy when complete pharyngeal obstruction becomes imminent.

Gastric Squamous Cell Carcinoma

Squamous cell carcinoma is the most common form of alimentary tract neoplasia in the horse. The history is usually one of progressive weight loss of one to two months' duration in a middle-aged or older animal. Horses are generally thin or emaciated at presentation. There is approximately a 4:1 male to female ratio in reported cases. A common presentation would include anorexia when the horse is alert and responsive to presentation of feed but eats only sparingly and then walks away. The same may be true with water. Occasionally horses will be dysphagic or present for chronic thoracic choke if the cardia is grossly involved.

Physical and laboratory examination may reveal a low-grade fever, a normochromic and normocytic anemia, and slight elevation of peritoneal fluid protein. Rarely are neoplastic cells found in peritoneal fluid. The most rewarding examination is rectal, in which two thirds of cases involve palpable abdominal masses or adhesions around the cranial mesentery or in the left half of the abdomen.

The most rewarding definitive diagnostic procedure is an exploratory laparotomy with either local or general anesthesia and associated biopsy of suspected lesions. In this way the stomach and lymph nodes may be directly palpated and metastatic nodules appreciated. This, however, may be preempted by the less frequently rewarding technique of gastric lavage to obtain exfoliative neoplastic cells, or possibly by endoscopic examination of the stomach via esophagostomy. Ultrasonography is a diagnostic mode that may acquire more reliability with increasing experience by operators.

Ultimately gastric squamous cell carcinoma results in death or euthanasia due to the inaccessibility of the lesion for surgical resection or other possible treatment, and due to the likely presence of metastasis.

Intestinal Lymphosarcoma

Intestinal lymphosarcoma, the second most commonly diagnosed form of alimentary tract neoplasia, generally shares the same clinical presentation and dismal prognosis as gastric squamous cell carcinoma. Differences in presentation may include chronic diarrhea, ascites, and the rare leukemia. If the more common subcutaneous and lymph node syndromes of the disease result in metastatic spread to the abdomen then additional clues may be obtained by peripheral biopsy of suspect lesions. Difficulty is encountered in differentiating this disease from granulomatous enteritis because both can cause mesenteric lymphadenopathy, anemia, diarrhea, hypoalbuminemia, and malabsorption. The definitive way to differentiate the conditions is biopsy of suspected lesions. This most often is possible only with exploratory laparotomy. There is no recognized successful treatment of lymphosarcoma in the horse as of this writing.

Other forms of primary alimentary tract neoplasia are listed by type and location in Figure 1. Practically speaking there is no successful treatment except the occasionally possible surgical extirpation. Alimentary tract neoplasia may mimic a variety of treatable syndromes. The reader is urged to review those chapters on dental care, gastric disease, impactions, enteroliths and small colon obstruction, bowel displacement, peritonitis, malabsorption syndromes, chronic diarrhea, and chronic liver disease, to name a few. Because of the poor prognosis associated with alimentary tract neoplasia, the thrust of equine veterinary care in these cases should be toward a definitive diagnosis by biopsy.

Supplemental Readings

Cotchin, E.: A general survey of tumours in the horse. Equine Vet. J., 9:16, 1977. (117 references)
French, D. A., Fretz, P. B., Davis, G. D., Holmberg, D. L., and Doige, C.: Mandibular adamantinoma in a horse, radical surgical treatment. Vet. Surg., 13:165, 1984.
Newfeld, J. L.: Lymphosarcoma in the horse: A review. Can. Vet. J., 14:129, 1973.
Tennant, B., Keirn, D. R., White, K. K., Bentinck-Smith, J., and King, J. M.: Six cases of squamous cell carcinoma of the stomach of the horse. Equine Vet. J., 14:238, 1982.
Theilen, G. H., and Madewell, B. R. (eds.): Veterinary Cancer Medicine. Philadelphia, Lea & Febiger, 1979.
Traub, J. L, Bayly, W. M., Reed, S. M., Modransky, P. D., and Rantanen, R. W.: Intra-abdominal neoplasia as a cause of chronic weight loss in the horse. Comp. Cont. Ed., 10:S526, 1983.

Acute Hepatic Failure (Theiler's Disease)

Thomas J. Divers, KENNETT SQUARE, PENNSYLVANIA

The occurrence of hepatic disease may be frequent, but the great majority of affected horses never develop hepatic failure. Hepatic failure occurs only when greater than 60 per cent of the liver function is lost from an acute or chronic process. Regardless of the disease duration, however, the onset of clinical signs is usually acute. Because the majority of horses with acute hepatic failure are diagnosed as having Theiler's disease, this is the major focus of the chapter.

ETIOLOGY

Theiler's disease is an acute or subacute hepatitis of unknown etiology and occurs only in adult horses. The outbreak of the disease may be sporadic or affect several horses on a farm during a two- to three-month period, mostly between the months of August and November. Theiler's disease is also termed "serum hepatitis" because it frequently occurs in outbreaks 4 to 10 weeks after the administration of a biologic of equine origin. The use of such biologics has declined, but a similar syndrome of hepatic failure still frequently occurs when there is no history of their administration. The association with equine serum administration, multiple horse involvement on some farms, and the apparent seasonal incidence suggest infectious blood-borne etiologic agents. Experimental transmission using blood or tissue inoculation from affected animals has not been rewarding. No incriminating agent has been identified and serologic testing of the affected horses for human hepatitis virus has not proved positive.

Mycotoxins and pyrrolizidine alkaloid–contaminated feeds have on rare occasions produced acute hepatic failure, poor diet, and prior exposure increasing susceptibility. The toxin of *Penicillin rubrum* (rubratoxin) has also been reported to cause liver failure in horses ingesting corn contaminated with the toxin.

Obese ponies and on a rare occasion a horse with anorexia may develop severe hyperlipemia with fatty infiltration of the liver and hepatic dysfunction (see p. 114). The lipemia is usually grossly visible in the patient's serum. Suppurative cholangitis, portal vein thrombosis, and obstruction of the biliary system by adhesions or intestinal displacement are other causes of acute hepatic failure. A large number of toxins may cause hepatic disease but hepatic failure does not generally occur.

CLINICAL SIGNS AND PATHOPHYSIOLOGY

The clinical signs of hepatic failure occurring with Theiler's disease usually do not differ from those occurring with hepatic disease of other etiology. Signs occur because the liver is unable to perform its vital functions, which include gluconeogenesis, production of clotting factors II, VII, IX, and X, production of essential proteins, conversion of ammonia to urea, metabolism of amino acids, fats and carbohydrates, conjugation of bilirubin, production of bile, and metabolism of a variety of toxins and drugs.

Horses are usually examined when changes in behavior are observed. Depression, head pressing, uncontrolled circling, propulsive walking, seizure, and coma are the most common neurologic signs. Ataxia and excessive yawning may also be observed. Spontaneous bleeding is not a common sign, but excessive hemorrhage from self-inflicted wounds may occur. Horses with suppurative cholangitis may be febrile and demonstrate mild abdominal pain. Signs of abdominal pain may occur whenever biliary obstruction causes hepatomegaly.

The onset of clinical signs may be insidious over a few days or may be peracute. Horses are often examined because of self-inflicted trauma, which may lead to the erroneous diagnosis of abdominal pain. In some horses, photosensitization or pruritius or both may be the first clinical sign. Although icterus becomes intense with Theiler's disease, it may not be noted at the onset of the behavioral signs.

DIAGNOSIS

The diagnosis of Theiler's disease is based upon history, clinical and laboratory findings, and microscopic examination of the liver. Administration of equine-origin antiserum within the previous 4 to 10 weeks supports the diagnosis as does the occurrence of the disease in several adult horses. However, aflatoxicosis and pyrrolizidine alkaloid toxicity might also cause liver failure in more than one horse on the same farm. A history of chronic illness and chronic liver disease does not support a diagnosis of Theiler's disease or other acute hepatic failure.

Clinical laboratory findings are summarized in Table 1. Serum concentration of enzymes originating in the liver are elevated as is the serum bilirubin concentration. Prothrombin time and partial thromboplastin time may serve as prognostic indicators. A liver biopsy may help to confirm the diagnosis of the liver disease. The biopsy should be attempted from the right 12th intercostal space between lines drawn from the olecranon to the tuber coxae and from the point of the shoulder to the tuber coxae. Bleeding associated with the biopsy is rare. Because of a sometimes marked decrease in liver size with Theiler's disease, a successful biopsy might be difficult without prior ultrasonic examination to outline the liver. Even with an ultrasound examination, it might be difficult to visualize the liver from the right, but it can almost always be imaged from the lower left and most rostral portion of the abdomen. Ultrasonic examination might be helpful in determining hepatomegaly often found with any primary obstruction of the biliary tract.

The liver from a horse with Theiler's disease typically has moderate-to-severe hepatocellular degeneration throughout the lobule with the most severe changes noted in the centrilobular and midzonal areas. Hepatocellular ballooning with lipid-filled vacuoles or moderate necrosis and blood-filled sinusoids are consistent changes. The cellular reaction is mild to moderate and consists largely of lymphocytes and macrophages. Biliary hyperplasia

may be observed. Many toxic hepatopathies may cause lesions similar to Theiler's disease. Microscopic examination of liver tissue is also helpful in defining fatty infiltration, suppurative hepatitis, and biliary obstruction.

THERAPY

The initial aim of therapy is to control the abnormal behavior and support liver function. Dextrose (5 per cent) is administered intravenously at 1 L per hour. If laboratory findings confirm severe hypoglycemia, a higher concentration of dextrose may be given. The horse should be fed a low-protein, high-energy diet. Sorghum or beet pulp, which are rich in branch-chain amino acids, are ideal foodstuffs and can be mixed with molasses to improve palatability and caloric content. Stomach tubing with high caloric feeds is recommended for anorexic horses (see p. 424). If a high-protein feed was consumed prior to onset of clinical signs, 10 grams of neomycin or 200 ml of lactulose may be administered by stomach tube every six hours for two days to reduce ammonia production. Correction of the acidosis should be gradual. Seizures or maniacal behavior can often be controlled with xylazine. Plasma exchange transfusions may be attempted if the other medical therapies have failed to alleviate the hepatoencephalopathy. If excessive bleeding is noted from self-inflicted lacerations or from needle punctures, fresh plasma can be administered. Balanced electrolyte solutions should be provided along with the dextrose to maintain normal

TABLE 1. SUMMARY OF MAJOR CLINICAL LABORATORY FINDINGS IN HORSES WITH ACUTE LIVER FAILURE (THEILER'S DISEASE)

Laboratory Test	Observation
Aspartate amino transferase (AST, SGOT)	Usually elevated but not specific for liver disease. Released early in hepatic failure. Long half-life in serum; stable when serum is frozen.
Carbamyl transferase (OCT)	Usually elevated and specific for liver disease. Short half-life in serum; unstable.
Gamma glutamyl transferase (GGT)	Persistently elevated in most liver disease especially with biliary tract disease. Relatively specific for liver disease; stable in frozen serum.
Sorbitol dehydrogenase (SDH)	Usually elevated and specific for liver disease. Short half-life in serum; unstable.
Serum bilirubin	Elevated in liver failure, indirect comprising 70–90% of total. Elevated with biliary disease, indirect comprising about 50% of total.
Prothrombin time	Prolonged in liver failure; good prognostic indicator.
Partial thromboplastin time	Prolonged in liver failure; good prognostic indicator.
Bilirubinuria	Occasionally observed.
Hemoglobinuria	Occasionally observed.
Blood glucose	Hypoglycemia not infrequent.
pH	Profound acidosis not infrequent.
Blood urea nitrogen (BUN)	May initially be elevated, but soon decreases to very low concentrations.
Blood ammonia	May be elevated. Not a useful measurement in devising therapeutic plan.
Packed cell volume (PCV)	Elevated and often unresponsive to IV fluids.
White cell count	Leukocytosis with suppurative cholangitis.
Bile acids	Elevated

intravascular volume. Supplementation with B complex vitamins is recommended.

If suppurative cholangitis is suspected, a combination of trimethoprim-sulfa or penicillin and an aminoglycoside is administered, unless a specific etiologic agent has been identified and its sensitivity determined. Photosensitization can be prevented by eliminating exposure to sunlight.

Many horses that stabilize with therapy and continue to eat will recover rapidly. Declines in prothrombin time, serum concentration of hepatic enzymes, and bilirubin, are all favorable laboratory findings.

Supplemental Readings

Carlson, G. P.: The liver. *In* Mansmann, R. A., McAllister, E. S., and Pratt, P. W. (eds.): Equine Medicine and Surgery, 3rd Ed. Santa Barbara, CA, American Veterinary Publications, 1982, p. 633.

Divers, T. J.: Liver disease and liver failure in horses. Proc. 29th Annu. Conv. Am. Assoc. Eq. Pract., 1983, pp. 213–223.

Gulick, B. A., Liu, I. K.M., Qualls, C. W., et al.: Effect of pyrrolizidine alkaloid-induced hepatic disease on plasma amino acid patterns in the horse. Am. J. Vet. Res., *41*;1894, 1980.

Rico, A. G., Braun, J. P., Bernard, P., et al.: Tissue distribution and blood levels of gamma glutamyl transferase in the horse. Eq. Vet. J., *9*:100, 1977.

Tennant, B. C., and Hornbuckle, W. E.: Diseases of the liver. *In* Anderson, N. V. (ed.): Veterinary Gastroenterology. Philadelphia, Lea & Febiger, 1980, p. 593.

Chronic Liver Disease

T. D. Byars, LEXINGTON, KENTUCKY

Horses with chronic liver disease are usually presented with signs of either chronic weight loss or acute liver failure. These clinical signs represent the cumulative loss of hepatic tissue beyond the organ's functional reserve capacity. Chronic insults to the liver can be direct to hepatic cells or can be the result of posthepatic cholestasis.

Chronic liver disease is most commonly observed in areas where hepatotoxic plants are relatively abundant. Crotolaria, Heliotropium, Amsinckia, and Senecio are examples of plants containing pyrrolizidine alkaloids capable of causing megalocytic hepatopathy. These plants can contaminate hay and pelleted feeds. Clinical signs occur during prolonged ingestion of contaminated feed or at some time following exposure.

Mycotoxins such as aflatoxins infrequently cause liver disease in the horse. Liver neoplasia, most commonly hepatic carcinomas, can affect adult horses of any age. Fatty infiltration of the liver, which occurs in horses and particularly ponies, is usually associated with obesity and anorexia. A more rare hepatorenal syndrome characterized by fatty liver failure and anuria occurs in mares after foaling.

Chronic active hepatitis is usually caused by drugs or bacteria. Black disease caused by *Clostridium novyi* is considered an acute hepatopathy although a chronic infection may occur. Chronic liver infection may result in chronic cholangitis, multiple abscesses, or obstructive lesions of the biliary tract. Obstructive cholelithiasis may be localized to the bile duct or generalized throughout the liver canaliculi in association with chronic generalized abscessation. Serum hepatitis (Theiler's disease) may represent a chronic hepatic insult but is generally observed as an acute hepatopathy (see p. 110).

The final stage of all forms of chronic liver disease is fibrosis. Once fibrosis occurs, determining the etiology of liver disease is virtually impossible.

CLINICAL SIGNS

The clinical signs of chronic liver disease can vary from weight loss through subtle changes in behavior to fulminant hepatic coma. Most horses are presented merely as having chronic weight loss. Behavioral changes can include belligerence, somnolence, and excessive yawning. Head pressing, circling, aimless walking, blindness, and infrequent seizures are additional central nervous signs of hepatic origin. Muscular weakness can result in incoordination, toe dragging, dysphonia, dysphagia, and upper airway obstruction.

Gastrointestinal signs include partial to complete anorexia, decreased borborygmi, intermittent soft stools, and infrequently ascites. Colic may be associated with these abdominal disorders. Icterus is an inconsistent clinical sign.

Additional clinical signs can include pruritus, photophobia, keratitis, and photosensitization of nonpigmented skin. Polydipsia and polyuria may also be observed.

DIAGNOSIS

Results of laboratory tests in horses with chronic liver disease are variable. Hematology may demonstrate a variable white cell count and occasionally an increased hematocrit. Blood levels of liver enzymes such as sorbitol dehydrogenase (SDH), ornithine carbamyl transferase (OCT), gamma glutamyl transpeptidase (GGT), and aspartate aminotransferase (AST, formerly SGOT) are increased by active hepatocellular degeneration or cholestasis or both. The simultaneous elevation of the GGT and alkaline phosphotase (AP) should alert the clinician to cholestatic disease such as cholangitis or cholelithiasis. The blood urea nitrogen and blood glucose are often subnormal. Bilirubin levels can be normal but blood ammonia levels are usually elevated especially in the horse exhibiting signs of hepatic coma. Hypoproteinemia is not a consistent finding in chronic liver disease. Electrophoresis may reveal slight hypoalbuminemia and elevation of beta or gamma globulins or both. Elevated alphafetoprotein occurs in horses with hepatic carcinoma. A relative increase in aromatic amino acids and decrease in branch chain amino acids can occur in conjunction with liver disease.

Tests such as the Bromsulphalein (BSP) and indocyanine green clearance provide accurate assessments of liver function. However, the former has limited availability to the practitioners in the United States and the latter is expensive. Urinalysis may reveal isosthenuria, bilirubinuria, and the presence or absence of urobilinogen.

The liver biopsy remains the major diagnostic and prognostic aid. The biopsy aids in determining the cause and extent of liver disease. Coagulation tests are recommended prior to biopsy; however, they are seldom abnormal. The biopsy is performed with a biopsy needle by using ultrasound for guidance or between the 11th and 12th right intercostal space three inches below a line drawn from the tuber coxae to the point of the shoulder. The biopsy specimen should be cultured for microorganisms before being placed in formalin.

Ultrasound diagnosis is useful in determining liver size, focal changes in tissue consistency, the presence or absence of choleliths, and the presence of ascites.

TREATMENT

Chronic liver disease offers a guarded-to-poor prognosis. The clinician should provide as accurate an assessment as possible primarily on the basis of the results of liver biopsy. It is pointless to treat a horse with end-stage liver disease. Euthanasia may be a wise decision to prevent suffering and needless expenditure. The treatment of chronic liver disease is similar to that of acute liver disease: removal of the offending cause and supportive care.

Treatment should begin with a high-carbohydrate, low-protein diet. B-complex vitamins should be supplemented by parenteral injection. Glucose (dextrose) should be given orally as a 20 per cent solution or intravenously as a 5 to 10 per cent solution. Approximately 15 to 20 calories per pound of body weight (4 to 5 gm per pound) is needed to meet the daily maintenance requirements in an anorexic horse.

In cases of chronic active hepatitis of bacterial origin, parenteral antibiotics should be used after culture results are obtained from the liver biopsy. Oral neomycin (50 to 100 mg per kg) is used to decrease intestinal generation of ammonia by bacterial fermentation. Cathartics are recommended to purge the gastrointestinal tract of existing ammonia, and lactulose (150 to 200 ml, four times a day) is used to acidify the colonic contents for conversion of ammonia to nonabsorbable ammonium. Anticonvulsants and sedatives are indicated whenever the horse is likely to injure itself. The half-life of these drugs is prolonged in patients with liver disease.

The use of steroids remains controversial. They do not inhibit fibrosis and may facilitate formation of ascites. Low doses should be used as steroids are metabolized by the liver. Colchicine may provide a future therapy to inhibit fibrosis.

Supplemental Readings

Gay, C. C., Sullivan, N. D., Wilkinson, J. S., McLean, J. D., and Blood D. C.: Hyperlipidemia in ponies. Aust. Vet. J., 54:459, 1978.

Gulick, B. A., Rogers, Q. R., and Knight, H. D.: Use of plasma amino acid patterns of liver disease of the horse. Calif. Vet., 33:21, 1979.

Tennant, B. C., and Hornbuckle, W. E.: Diseases of the liver. *In* Anderson, N. V., (ed.): Philadelphia, Lea & Febiger, 1980, pp. 593–620.

Hyperlipemia

Jonathan M. Naylor, SASKATOON, SASKATCHEWAN, CANADA

Hyperlipemia and hyperlipidemia are conditions in which blood lipids are elevated. Hyperlipemia traditionally describes a severe clinical syndrome characterized by fatty infiltration of the liver and elevations of blood lipids sufficient to cause grossly visible changes in the blood. Hyperlipidemia is used to describe subclinical elevations of blood lipids that can only be detected using laboratory tests and that are not associated with fatty liver.

LIPID METABOLISM

Most cases of hyperlipemia and hyperlipidemia are seen in equids with a reduced food intake. During fasting, adipose tissue triglycerides are broken down into free fatty acids and glycerol, which are released into the blood (Fig. 1). Some free fatty acids are used directly by peripheral tissues such as muscle, but a significant portion is taken up by the liver. In the liver, fatty acids may be oxidized completely to provide energy or partially to provide ketone bodies. Some fatty acids are reesterified to triglycerides and phospholipids, which either accumulate within the liver or are released back into plasma as part of the very low density lipoproteins (VLDL). In equids, triglyceride production is emphasized over ketone formation; therefore, lipemia rather than ketosis dominates the response to pro-

longed fasting. Triglyceride accumulation in plasma is thus a normal response to a few days of complete food deprivation. These changes can initially only be detected in the clinical chemistry laboratory and are indicative of hyperlipidemia. In ponies, prolonged food deprivation results in the progressive accumulation of lipid in the blood. Lipid also accumulates in the liver and fatty liver develops, accompanied by signs of illness. The syndrome is called hyperlipemia. Horses can tolerate fasting better than ponies and lipid does not accumulate in the high concentrations characteristic of hyperlipemia. An exception to this is in horses that are both azotemic and eating poorly. Azotemia inhibits the peripheral removal of triglycerides, possibly by inhibiting lipoprotein lipase, an enzyme that plays a critical role in the uptake of lipid by peripheral tissue. In aphagic azotemic horses, hyperlipemia occurs because of concomitant lipid mobilization and blockage of lipid removal from blood.

HYPERLIPIDEMIA

Many sick aphagic horses and ponies have mild elevations of serum lipids. There is no visible opacity to the plasma, and laboratory tests record serum triglyceride values of less than 5 gm per L. In the absence of clinicopathological evidence of liver dam-

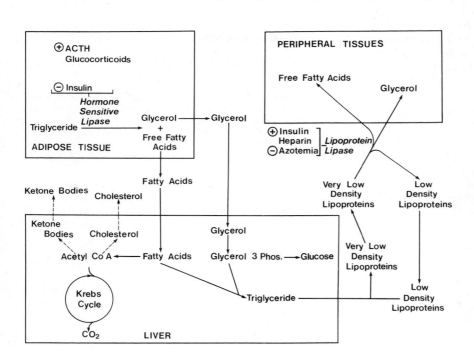

Figure 1. A simplified diagram of lipid metabolism in the horse. Inhibitors are indicated by −, activators by +.

age, this mild lipemia signals the need for nutritional supportive therapy.

THE HYPERLIPEMIA SYNDROME

Clinical Findings. There are no clinical findings specific for the hyperlipemia syndrome. Affected horses are moderately to severely depressed. Weakness, muscle fasciculations, ataxia, and terminal recumbency can occur. The tongue may have a gray-white coating and the breath a fetid odor. There are reports of ventral edema, possibly related to fat embolism and vascular thrombosis. Diarrhea has been reported in some affected ponies, but it is unclear to what extent this reflects concurrent parasitism. Some healthy horses and ponies denied food develop diarrhea after more than three to five days of food deprivation. This suggests that imbalances in gut function brought on by lack of food may produce diarrhea and may account for some instances of diarrhea in hyperlipemic horses. Jaundice occurs in some cases of hyperlipemia, presumably as a result of the combined effects of food deprivation and liver dysfunction.

The hyperlipemia syndrome is most common in ponies but has also been reported in donkeys and horses. Affected ponies are often fat, but this is not an invariable finding. Affected horses are in good-to-thin body condition. Pregnant and lactating ponies are particularly susceptible, and because of this, most cases are seen in the spring in the Northern Hemisphere. Transport can also predispose to the development of the condition.

Affected ponies often suffer from a primary disease process that depresses food intake. Heavy parasite burdens are a common inciting cause, with parasites both depressing food intake and competing for available nutrients. The condition is also seen as a sequela to underfeeding, usually in ponies wintered at pasture. In horses, negative energy balance does not result in the hyperlipemic disease unless the affected horse is also azotemic.

An unusual presentation of hyperlipemia in ponies is in association with pituitary tumor. These animals often eat readily, and the hyperlipemia is thought to be secondary to prolonged fat mobilization in response to hormonal imbalances.

DIAGNOSIS

Diagnosis is based on examination of the blood. Lipemic blood tends to have a blue tinge, and serum or plasma is opaque and varies in color from white to yellow, depending on the relative degrees of hyperlipemia and hyperbilirubinemia. Early cases of hyperlipemia are characterized by a faint cloudiness to serum or plasma; this is easier to see in a test tube than in a microhematocrit tube. Sometimes normal plasma can appear slightly hazy and may be confused with hyperlipemia. Repeated centrifugation at high speed will clear the opacity, probably caused by residual platelets, from normal plasma. Hyperbilirubinemia is common in anorectic horses and imparts a yellow color to plasma or serum which are nevertheless clear. Opacity indicates hyperlipemia.

When the hyperlipemia syndrome is diagnosed on the basis of clinical signs and the appearance of the blood, serum can be submitted for triglyceride assay to quantify the degree of lipemia. Early cases will have serum triglyceride concentrations of 5 to 10 gm per L; in severe cases triglyceride concentrations rise to 50 gm per L or more. It is also important to conduct liver function tests, particularly the Bromsulphalein (BSP) clearance test, to determine the degree of liver dysfunction. Tests of serum enzyme activities, such as sorbitol dehydrogenase, and gamma glutamyl transferase, help quantify the degree of active liver destruction. The blood glucose concentration may be low and should be measured. Serum creatinine should be determined because azotemia can contribute to the pathogenesis of the condition. Some commercially available laboratory screening tests offer an inexpensive method of measuring triglyceride, glucose, creatinine, and enzyme activities in serum.

Metabolic acidosis may develop in severe cases of the syndrome, and attempts should be made to quantify this; base deficits as large as 24 mEq per L have been reported.

At necropsy, lipemic changes may be grossly visible in unclotted blood. The liver is often swollen, greasy in texture, and light tan to yellow in color. In severe cases, liver samples will float in formalin, and the liver may have ruptured. The kidneys may be pale. These changes are often more marked in hyperlipemic ponies than in horses. Histologically, fatty change is seen in liver, kidney, and sometimes muscle. Thrombosis of blood vessels, possibly secondary to lipid embolism has also been reported.

TREATMENT

The first priority is to treat the inciting cause of hyperlipemia and to attempt to improve feed intake. Ponies that are febrile or in pain may benefit from the administration of antipyretics or analgesics. Feed intake may also be improved by offering a variety of feeds and allowing the patient to choose. Patients that eat bedding may prefer poor-quality hay to better hays. Fresh grass is often the last food to be refused by a sick horse; allowing ponies to graze has been used as part of some successful therapeutic regimens. Patients that refuse all food should be fed gruels of dried grass or a complete feed by stomach tube. Supportive therapy should include maintenance of the patient's hydration in order to avoid prerenal azotemia.

There are a number of therapeutic regimens aimed at speeding the removal of lipids from the blood. On a long-term basis, these treatments may also decrease lipid accumulation in the liver. The treatments fall into two categories: those that inhibit mobilization of lipids into blood from adipose tissue stores and those that speed the removal of triglycerides from blood. Insulin and glucose decrease mobilization of adipose tissue lipids, whereas heparin speeds the removal of triglycerides from the circulation.

Limited information is available on the dosage of heparin. One recommendation is that ponies be given from 100 to 250 USP units per kg body weight twice daily. We have used somewhat lower dosages (40 USP units per kg) and have observed a temporary beneficial effect on the severity of the hyperlipemia. Heparin inhibits blood clotting in vivo, and this danger should not be overlooked.

Insulin therapy is usually combined with carbohydrate administration. Combinations of glucose and insulin can be used successfully, but there are reports of this therapeutic regimen resulting in a severe lactic acidosis and a poor recovery rate. A treatment in which insulin administration is combined with glucose and galactose administration on alternate days is reported to give better results than either glucose and insulin or heparin treatments. Using this regimen, a 200-kg pony would be given 30 IU protamine zinc insulin intramuscularly with 100 gm of glucose orally twice daily on the first and succeeding odd days. On even days, 15 IU protamine zinc insulin is given intramuscularly twice daily with 100 gm of galactose orally once daily. Treatment is administered until the serum is no longer grossly lipemic, although insulin can be administered in decreasing doses for an additional three days if required.

Acidosis may be corrected with a replacement solution fortified with sodium bicarbonate as necessary. Acid-base status, blood glucose concentration, and the degree of lipemia should be monitored during therapy. If heparin therapy is used, blood clotting studies should be performed during therapy, and the patient should be monitored for bleeding problems.

The success rate in treatment of hyperlipemia is usually low. Cases in which the inciting disease process is responsive to therapy and in which the hyperlipemia is less than 20 gm total lipids per L have the best prognosis. Foaling or abortion during treatment may also improve the prognosis. The prognosis for horses with hyperlipemia is very poor unless the associated azotemia can be corrected.

PREVENTION

Most cases of hyperlipemia in ponies can be avoided by maintaining feed intake. Adequate food should be available, and supplemental feeding is necessary for animals wintered at pasture. Ponies that are being transported long distances should be rested periodically and allowed to eat. The development of hyperlipemia secondary to disease-induced aphagia can be prevented by tube feeding. These precautions are particularly important if the pony is pregnant or lactating. Prolonged restriction of feed intake for therapeutic purposes, such as in overweight laminitic ponies, should be done with care. The risk of hyperlipemia may be reduced by feeding a half-maintenance ration rather than using complete feed withdrawal.

Supplemental Readings

Baetz, A. L., and Pearson, J. E.: Blood constituent changes in fasted ponies. Am. J. Vet. Res., 33:1941, 1972.
Bauer, J. E.: Plasma lipids and lipoproteins of fasted ponies. Am. J. Vet. Res., 44:379, 1983.
Gay, C. C., Sullivan, N. D., Wilkinson, J. S., McLean, J. D., and Blood, D. C.: Hyperlipemia in ponies. Aust. Vet. J., 54:459, 1978.
Naylor, J. M., Kronfeld, D. S., and Acland, H.: Hyperlipemia in horses: Effects of undernutrition and disease. Am. J. Vet. Res., 41:899, 1980.
Schotman, A. J. H., and Wagenaar, G.: Hyperlipemia in ponies. Zbl. Vet. Med., 16:1, 1968.
Wensing, T. H., Schotman, A. J. H., and Kroneman, J.: A new method in the treatment of hyperlipemia (hyperlipoproteinaemia) in ponies. Neth. J. Vet. Sci., 5:145, 1973.

Retained Meconium

John Halley, COOLMORE STUD, IRELAND

From midgestation onward, fecal material consisting of digested cellular debris accumulates in the foal's rectum and small colon, to make up the meconium. Thus, meconium is the first fecal material that the newborn foal normally evacuates soon after parturition. Meconium is usually in pellet form, brown to black in color and very firm. Under stressful conditions, such as anoxia, the foal can pass the meconium during or before foaling.

Retained meconium is a common condition in foals that results from either the impaction of these fecal pellets in the rectum or colon or both, or hypomotility of the colon. Colts are more often affected than fillies, possibly due to the narrower pelvic cavity. It has been suggested that foals over 340 days of gestation are more prone to meconium retention.

CLINICAL SIGNS

Clinical signs that usually appear during the first 24 hours of life can vary from mild abdominal discomfort to a colic violent enough to alarm personnel. Initially, the foal exhibits signs of abdominal discomfort, with the tail raised and swishing from side to side. It repeatedly attempts to defecate and backs into the dam. In more severe cases the foal repeatedly gets up and down, rolls and may assume unusual positions while down, such as lying on its back with the head towards its abdomen or on its back with a front leg over the head. Foals usually continue to nurse between bouts of colic and are afebrile. The pulse, although rapid during spasms, remains full and strong.

DIAGNOSIS

Diagnosis is usually not difficult and is based on clinical signs or palpation of meconium at the anal sphincter. This condition must be differentiated from ruptured bladder, intestinal atresia, acute intestinal crisis, septicemia, and prematurity. Although bladder rupture also occurs predominantly in male foals, clinical signs usually become evident after 24 hours of age. Stance of the foal for defecation differs from that for urination. During defecation, the foal stands with the four feet close together and the back arched dorsally, whereas during urination the hind legs are usually widespread with the back dipped or ventroflexed. Serum and plasma electrolytes, usually normal in foals with retained meconium, show profound changes in the foal with a ruptured bladder.

TREATMENT

Treatment is symptomatic with most foals responding readily. However, correction of the condition can sometimes be difficult or protracted. Enemas with surface tension–reducing agents such as, sodium biphosphate and sodium phosphate, which are now readily available in individual soft flexible dispensers, can help to resolve some cases. Five hundred milliliters of mineral oil (liquid paraffin) or a combination of equal amounts of mineral oil and glycerin may be administered by stomach tube in 3 oz doses. Foals continuing to show signs of discomfort require analgesics to suppress pain. Flunixin meglumine* (2.2 mg per kg), meperidine† (5 ml of a 10 per cent solution), and dipyrone‡ (44 mg per kg) are very effective, safe analgesics.

Warm soapy water enemas administered through flexible rubber tubing such as a foal stomach tube can be very effective in aiding evacuation of the offending impaction. These should be given with great care to avoid ballooning or rupture of the rectum. Up to two quarts of warm soapy water can be allowed to flow by gravity. This procedure can be repeated several times until the condition is resolved. Mineral oil or glycerin or both can be added to this type of enema. Care should be taken not to pass the tube forcefully and to only administer fluid by gravity flow.

Other treatments that have been recommended include castor oil in 6 oz doses by stomach tube, repeated as necessary, and combinations such as 8 oz of mineral oil and 4 oz of milk of magnesia and 2 oz of castor oil.

Mechanical extractors such as spoons or forceps are not recommended, and in most cases are not necessary. In extremely refractory cases surgical intervention should be considered.

The average duration of meconium retention is about 24 hours, but the condition can last for up to three days. Once the meconium has been evacuated there is a complete remission of signs and an immediate return to normal.

---

*Banamine, Schering Corp., Kenilworth, NJ
†Demerol, Winthrop-Breon Laboratories, New York, NY
‡Novin, Haver-Lockhart, Shawnee, KS

PREVENTION

In our practice my colleagues and I recommend that an enema with surface tension–reducing properties be given to every foal soon after birth. Since the introduction of this procedure in our foaling units some years ago, the incidence of retained meconium needing veterinary attention has fallen dramatically. It may also be prudent to turn out the mare and foal the day after foaling as exercise may aid the foal in evacuation of any remaining meconium.

Supplemental Readings

Cosgrove, J. S. M.: The Veterinary Surgeon and the newborn Foal. Vet. Rec., 86:961, 1967.
Petersdorf, R. G., et al. (eds.): Harrison's Principles of Internal Medicine, 10th Ed. New York, McGraw-Hill, 1983.
Pouret, E.: A clinical approach to diseases and abnormalities of the foal in the first month of life. Proc. British Equine Vet. Assoc. Congress, 1965.
Rossdale, P. D.: Differential diagnosis and treatment of equine neonatal diseases. Vet. Rec., 91:581, 1972.
Rossdale, P. D.: Modern concepts of neonatal disease. Equine Vet. J., 4:117, 1974.

Phenylbutazone Toxicity

David H. Snow, NEWMARKET, ENGLAND

Following nearly 30 years of use, phenylbutazone (PBZ), a nonsteroidal anti-inflammatory drug, is believed to be an extremely safe and effective therapeutic agent. It is widely used in horses of all ages and occasionally is administered in excessive dosages. Since the first report of toxicity of PBZ in 1979, further experimental and clinical findings have confirmed that the drug has a low therapeutic index and in certain circumstances caution is necessary in its usage. Two types of toxicity have been described. The first primarily affects the gastrointestinal tract, and the second is associated with dehydration, resulting in renal damage. However, both syndromes can occur in some animals. Pony breeds and foals rather than larger breeds are more susceptible to the gastrointestinal syndrome, which is most likely to occur following oral rather than intravenous administration.

Toxicity described for PBZ may also occur with excessive dosage of other nonsteroidal anti-inflammatory agents such as meclofenamic acid, naproxen, and flunixin. Combination therapy with members of this group of drugs should be avoided.

PATHOGENESIS

PBZ, like other nonsteroidal anti-inflammatory drugs, inhibits the enzyme cyclooxygenase (prostaglandin synthetase), which is responsible for the synthesis of a variety of prostaglandins. By blocking cyclooxygenase, PBZ alleviates many of the signs of inflammation. This antiprostaglandin activity may also be responsible for the toxic manifestations. Various suggestions have been presented to explain the loss of gastrointestinal integrity, which is characteristic of toxicity.

The initial lesion is damage to junctions between mucosal cells leading to a loss of protein into the gastrointestinal tract. Such loss occurs in the absence of gross or microscopic lesions. With time, erosions develop, progressing to ulceration. The antiprostaglandin activity of PBZ is thought to prevent either normal turnover of mucosal cells or enteric secretions. It may also constrict small vessels causing ischemia. Whatever the cause, toxicity results from a local (rather than a systemic) effect, because only very high intravenous doses produce gastrointestinal lesions, and oral ulceration is greater when PBZ is given as a powder rather than in capsule form. Intestinal lesions seen following large intravenous doses may result from local concentration of the drug by the biliary system.

Renal crest necrosis is considered to arise from the synergistic effects of PBZ and reduced water intake. The inhibition of renal prostaglandins is thought to cause a reduced blood supply in the vasa recta leading to ischemia, while reduced water intake may result in reduced urine flow in the loops of Henle causing extreme hypertonicity in the papillary interstitium.

CLINICAL SIGNS

In susceptible animals clinical signs of PBZ toxicity can develop immediately, gradually, or suddenly at a later stage. The first signs are usually thirst and a decrease in appetite, which may progress to complete anorexia. Animals become depressed, lethargic, and listless. Anorexia and loss of plasma protein lead to progressive weight loss and emaciation. Diarrhea is only an occasional finding, with reduced fecal output being more common. The decrease in plasma proteins and fall in oncotic pressure may cause ventral edema, especially in the abdominal and preputial areas. Examination of the oral cavity may reveal areas of ulceration. In the terminal stages the animal becomes recumbent. Death is preceded by the development of signs consistent with toxic shock.

DIAGNOSIS

Phenylbutazone-induced protein loss has to be differentiated from other causes of protein-losing gastroenteropathy. A history of PBZ therapy should suggest the diagnosis when typical clinical and laboratory findings occur.

Laboratory Findings. The most consistent findings are a progressive decrease in total plasma protein concentration and an increase in blood urea nitrogen. The extent of these changes is closely related to the degree of toxicity, with very pronounced alterations occurring in animals that die. In parallel with the decrease in total plasma protein there is a fall in plasma calcium concentration. In the later stages of toxicity, plasma creatinine rises reflecting either muscle wasting or compromised renal function. Terminal shock elevates the hematocrit.

The white blood cell profile alters during toxicity. A decrease in leukocyte numbers occurs as neutrophils emigrate into tissue. In severely affected animals there is toxic vacuolation of the neutrophils and a left shift with the appearance of precursor cells.

Necropsy Findings. Following oral PBZ administration, necropsy findings are generally restricted to the gastrointestinal tract. Oral ulceration involves the buccal, palatine, and lingual mucosa. Erosions and ulcers may be found in the stomach and small and large intestine. Within the cecum and colon, the predilection sites for ulceration are along the mesenteric border. Microscopically the erosions show necrosis and desquamation of the mucosa and exposure of the lamina propria. The necrotic areas are invaded by bacteria. In areas of ulceration there is vasculitis, thrombosis of submucosal venules, submucosal edema, and gross thickening of the intestinal wall. In foals, gastric ulceration is more prominent than intestinal ulceration.

In most studies in which gastrointestinal pathology has been demonstrated, no gross or microscopic lesions were reported in other organs, including the kidney. Recently renal medullary crest (papillary) necrosis has been described. This is considered to occur more readily if the animal is dehydrated.

TREATMENT

Therapy with PBZ and other nonsteroidal anti-inflammatory drugs must cease immediately. No other specific treatments have been described, but appropriate symptomatic therapy should be instituted. Cimetidine may be useful in the treatment of gastric ulceration. An easily digestible high-protein diet should be given to compensate for the protein losses (see p. 424).

Following PBZ removal, recovery should occur in all but the most severe cases. A gradual regeneration of the gastrointestinal mucosa occurs, and there is a slow return of normal plasma protein concentrations. Recurrence of signs has been observed; peritonitis, adhesions, and abscessation within the abdominal cavity apparently result from intestinal perforation.

RECOMMENDATIONS ON PHENYLBUTAZONE DOSAGE

These recent findings of PBZ toxicity have led to a revision of the recommended dosage by the main marketer of PBZ in the United Kingdom. Efficacy can be attained using a therapeutic dose of 4.4 mg per kg body weight twice on day 1, then 2.2 mg per kg twice daily for 4 days and 2.2 mg per kg once daily thereafter. In ponies the dose rates are 4.4 mg per kg once daily for four days, then 4.4 mg per kg on alternate days.

Although prolonged therapy with low doses is safe, regular determinations of total plasma protein concentrations are recommended in those animals most at risk for toxicity, i.e., ponies and foals. Dehydrated animals should not receive PBZ.

Supplemental Readings

Gunson, D. E., and Soma, L. R.: Renal papillary necrosis in horses after phenylbutazone and water deprivation. Vet. Pathol., *20*:603, 1983.

Snow, D. H., Bogan, J. A., Douglas, T. A., and Thompson, H.: Phenylbutazone toxicity in ponies. Vet. Rec., *105*:26, 1979.

Snow, D. H., Douglas, T. A., Thompson, H., Parkins, J. J., and Holmes, P. H.: Phenylbutazone toxicoses in Equidae: A biochemical and pathophysiologic study. Am. J. Vet. Res., *42*:1754, 1981.

Snow, D. H., and Douglas, T. A.: Studies on a new paste preparation of phenylbutazone. Vet. Rec., *112*:602, 1983.

Traub, J. L., Gallina, A. M., Grant, B. D., Reed, S. M., Gavin, P. R., and Paulsen, L. M.: Phenylbutazone toxicosis in the foal. Am. J. Vet. Res., *44*:1410, 1983.

Cantharidin (Blister Beetle) Toxicity

David G. Schmitz, COLLEGE STATION, TEXAS

John C. Reagor, COLLEGE STATION, TEXAS

Cantharidin toxicosis results from ingestion of dead blister beetles that during harvesting become entrapped in alfalfa hay or its products. Over 200 species of blister beetles (family Meloidae) occur throughout the continental United States, the genus Epicauta commonly causing disease in the southwest, and the three-striped blister beetle, *Epicauta lemniscata*, being most often encountered in Texas. The adult beetle is slender, 1 to 1.5 cm long, and the head and prothorax or "neck" are narrower than the body. It is brownish yellow in color with three black stripes on each wing cover.

Cantharidin, the sole toxic principle, is contained in the hemolymph, genitalia, and possibly other tissues of the beetles. It is a highly irritating substance that causes acantholysis and vesicle formation when in contact with skin or mucous membranes. Cantharidin is absorbed from the gastrointestinal tract and is rapidly excreted by the kidney.

The increased frequency of poisoning in recent years may be related to modern forage harvesting techniques. Simultaneously cutting and crimping forage incorporates swarms of beetles into the hay. Since the beetles live in clusters, baling results in many insects in one small area of harvested forage. Storage of hay does not decrease the toxicity of cantharidin.

CLINICAL SIGNS

The severity of clinical signs produced by ingestion of blister beetles depends on toxin dosage. The concentration of cantharidin varies from less than 1 per cent to greater than 5 per cent of the insect's dry weight and as little as 4 to 6 gm of dried Epicauta beetles may be fatal to a horse.

The clinical signs are those of shock, gastrointestinal and urinary tract irritation, renal insufficiency, myocardial failure, and hypocalcemia. Onset and duration of signs varies from hours to days. The most commonly observed clinical signs include varying degrees of abdominal pain, anorexia, depression, and submerging the muzzle in water or frequently drinking small amounts of water. Rectal temperature is initially elevated, as are respiratory and cardiac rates. Cardiac contractions tend to be forceful and the heartbeat can be observed through the thoracic wall. Mucous membranes are congested and capillary refill time is prolonged. The feces tend to be watery in consistency but rarely contain blood. Profuse sweating may reflect severe abdominal pain. Horses that live longer than six to eight hours make frequent attempts to void small amounts of urine that is usually grossly normal, although a few horses will pass blood-tinged urine or urine that contains blood clots. Gross hematuria may occur during the later stages of disease.

Other less commonly observed signs include contraction of the diaphragm with each heartbeat and erosions of gingival and oral mucosal surfaces. Occasionally, affected horses will exhibit a stiff, short-strided gait that resembles the gait seen with acute myositis. Sudden death has also been reported.

DIAGNOSIS

Laboratory Findings. Routine clinical laboratory analyses yield no findings specific for cantharidin toxicosis. Packed cell volume is generally elevated and accompanied by a normal to elevated serum protein concentration. Neutrophilic leukocytosis is frequently present. The acid-base and serum sodium chloride and potassium values are usually within normal limits.

In the early stages of illness, blood urea nitrogen is frequently moderately elevated but seldom exceeds 50 mg per dl. Serum creatine phosphokinase may be elevated in more severely affected patients and suggests a deteriorating prognosis. Hyperglycemia is almost always present in the initial stages of the disease.

Significant decreases in serum calcium and magnesium occur in most horses. Total serum calcium may be as low as 4.5 mg per dl and the low calcium concentration may be responsible for the synchronous diaphragmatic flutter observed in some affected horses. Serum magnesium is generally less than 1.5 mg per dl. Profound hypocalcemia and hypomagnesemia will persist for longer than 48 hours if untreated.

Tests for blood in urine are positive. Epithelial cells are occasionally seen but casts are seldom present. The urine specific gravity may range from 1.003 to 1.006 even though the horse is dehydrated. The cause of the low specific gravity is undetermined, although it is thought due to decreased permeability of the collecting ducts to water. Feces are generally positive for occult blood.

Other Phases of Diagnosis. When signs of abdominal pain are exhibited by horses ingesting alfalfa hay or other feed prepared from alfalfa, blister beetle toxicosis should be considered. A definitive test has been developed for cantharidin in urine and stomach contents. Fresh urine, 500 ml minimum, should be mailed in a refrigerated container. At least 200 gm of solid stomach contents can also be refrigerated and submitted for analysis.* The concentration of cantharidin in urine becomes negligible four to five days following consumption of blister beetles, so urine collected early in the disease will be most diagnostic.

A tentative diagnosis can be made when horses exhibit clinical signs, when laboratory findings are compatible with cantharidin toxicosis, and when blister beetles are found in the hay. A thorough inspection should be made of all hay recently available to the affected animals. However, the beetles can be difficult to identify and are often not found because they may be present in only a small portion of a bale.

Although not diagnostic, laboratory findings of prolonged hypocalcemia, hypomagnesemia, and elevated serum creatine phosphokinase may be helpful in differentiating cantharidin toxicosis from other causes of acute abdominal crisis.

PATHOPHYSIOLOGY

Cantharidin is a potent irritant to many tissues and causes acantholysis and epidermal vesication when in contact with mucous membranes and skin. Within the intestinal tract, exposure results in mucosal degeneration and necrosis, and submucosal edema and hemorrhage. Cantharidin causes varying degrees of renal tubular damage, excessive mucus secretion by the glands of the renal pelvis, and ulceration and hemorrhage of the bladder mucosa. Its mechanism of action at the cellular level is unknown.

Because of extensive necrosis and sloughing of the mucosal lining of the proximal gastrointestinal tract, hypovolemic shock and pain develop rapidly. The normal transfer of fluid, nutrients, and electrolytes across the mucosal lining is disrupted and at necrospy affected horses often have an abnormally large amount of fluid filling the small and large intestines.

Renal lesions are generally not severe enough to be the cause of death. Renal tubular damage may however be important in the development of fluid, acid-base, and electrolyte abnormalities.

The cause of hypocalcemia and hypomagnesemia has not been elucidated. Hypocalcemia may play a role in the myocardial failure observed in some horses, but myocardial necrosis is probably caused by the direct effect of cantharidin. Damaged mitochondria within the myocardium are evident upon examination with electron microscopy even when no lesions are observed with light microscopy. These findings may help explain the occurrence of sudden death, although cardiac arrhythmias have not been reported.

TREATMENT

Although there is no specific antidote for cantharidin, prompt and conscientious symptomatic therapy is necessary to remove the toxic source, evacuate the gastrointestinal tract, maintain fluid balance, and control pain. If toxicity is suspected, all hay—particularly alfalfa—should be destroyed, as cantharidin is toxic to other animals. Hay subsequently fed should be examined carefully for the presence of blister beetles.

Horses should be given repeated doses of mineral oil (2 to 4 L) via nasogastric tube. Mineral oil is not only a mild laxative that will help in evacuation of the bowel but also binds some of the lipid-soluble cantharidin. All exposed horses in a group should be prophylactically treated with mineral oil.

Intravenous fluid to combat dehydration and promote diuresis should be maintained throughout the course of disease. A balanced polyionic solution is most suitable unless other specific therapy is indicated. Fluid therapy is of prime importance in treating existing hemoconcentration or dehydration and in minimizing renal tubular damage.

Diuretics are of value early in the disease because cantharidin is excreted via the kidney. Furosemide* (1 mg per kg intravenously or intramuscularly) should be used sparingly because overzealous use may result in electrolyte alterations. Dimethyl sulfoxide† (DMSO) is a potent diuretic that may be given intravenously. One ml of 90 per cent DMSO (0.90 gm) per kg body weight diluted to 10 per cent in a balanced polyionic solution is a suggested dosage, but we have given 100 to 120 ml of 90 per cent DMSO diluted in 1 L of a balanced polyionic solution to 450-kg horses with good success. This regimen can be repeated two to three times at 12- to 24-hour intervals. Concentrations greater than 20 per cent should not be used because they may cause hemolysis.

---

*Laboratory specimens may be mailed to the Texas Veterinary Medical Diagnostic Laboratory, College Station, TX 77843.

*Lasix, American Hoechst Corp., Somerville, NJ
†Domoso, Diamond Laboratories, Des Moines, IA

Acepromazine maleate and other alpha-adrenergic blockers are contraindicated because they may precipitate or potentiate hypovolemic shock.

Analgesics are required because most horses exhibit some degree of abdominal pain. Flunixin meglumine* may be given at a dosage of 1.1 mg per kg intravenously or intramuscularly. In our experience, xylazine† (0.5 to 1.0 mg per kg intravenously or intramuscularly) provides better analgesia, although it has the disadvantage of being relatively short-acting. Pentazocine‡ may be used at a dosage of 0.4 mg per kg intravenously. Other suitable analgesics are described on page 27.

Calcium gluconate§ is indicated for treatment of hypocalcemia, particularly when synchronous diaphragmatic flutter is present. While it is best to measure serum calcium and calculate the deficit, good results have been obtained with 500 ml of a calcium gluconate–magnesium solution given intravenously to average-sized adult horses. This preparation is given slowly or diluted in a balanced polyionic solution or saline. This dosage regimen may be repeated if necessary. Foals or smaller-sized horses should receive proportionately less.

Broad-spectrum antibiotic therapy may be useful to minimize complications from the disease process. If antibiotics are employed, those that have potential for nephrotoxicity, such as the aminoglycoside group and sulfonamiades, should be avoided.

PROGNOSIS AND PREVENTION

The prognosis is poor in all cases of cantharidin toxicosis. Early and vigorous treatment is impera-

---

*Banamine, Schering Corp., Kenilworth, NJ
†Rompun, Haver-Lockart, Shawnee, KS
‡Talwin, Winthrop-Breon Laboratories, New York, NY
§Cal-Dextro No. 2, Fort Dodge Laboratories, Inc., Fort Dodge, IA or Calcium gluconate injection, American Quinine Co., Shirley, NY

tive if a successful outcome is to be obtained. In horses that remain alive for several days, persistence of an elevated heart rate and respiratory rate and increasing serum creatine phosphokinase are associated with a worsening prognosis. While no long-term cardiac or renal dysfunction has been demonstrated in horses that recover, the heart and kidneys should be monitored.

Every effort should be made to inspect alfalfa for the presence of blister beetles before feeding. Because it is impossible to examine all hay given to horses, prevention is more appropriately aimed at conscientious harvesting of alfalfa hay.

In Texas, beetles should not occur in significant numbers until June. Hay harvested before that time should be relatively free of beetles. Hay fields, especially the field margins, should be inspected before harvesting. If any "pockets" of blister beetles are identified, hay should not be harvested from that particular area. The problem may occur more frequently in areas or during given years when grasshoppers are in abundance, because the larvae of the blister beetle live in the soil and feed extensively on grasshopper eggs.

Supplemental Readings

Rabkin, S. W., Friesen, J. M., Ferris, J. A. J., and Fung, H. Y. M.: A model of cardiac arrhythmias and sudden death: Cantharidin-induced toxic cardiomyopathy. J. Pharmacol. Exp. Ther., *210*:43, 1979.

Ray, A. C., Post, L. O., Hurst, J. M., Edwards, W. C., and Reagor, J. C.: Evaluation of an analytical method for the diagnosis of cantharidin toxicosis due to ingestion of blister beetles (*Epicauta lemniscata*) by horses and sheep. Am. J. Vet. Res., *41*:932, 1980.

Schoeb, T. R., and Panciera, R. J.: Blister beetle poisoning in horses. J. Am. Vet. Med. Assoc., *173*:75, 1978.

Schoeb, T. R., and Panciera, R. J.: Pathology of blister-beetle (*Epicauta*) poisoning in horses. Vet. Pathol., *16*:18, 1979.

Shawley, R. V., and Rolf, L. L., Jr.: Experimental cantharidiasis in the horse. Am. J. Vet. Res., *45*:2261, 1984.

BEHAVIORAL PROBLEMS

Edited by K. A. Houpt

Feeding Problems

Sarah L. Ralston, FORT COLLINS, COLORADO

Horses are physiologically and psychologically adapted to a herbivorous diet that, although usually available, may be seasonal in nutritional content. If accustomed to free access to a diet, horses devote 10 to 12 hours each day to eating, rarely fasting for more than three to four hours. They rapidly alter total feed intake in response to changes in palatability, ease of consumption, and external stimuli such as the presentation of fresh feed or extreme environmental temperatures. It takes days to weeks, however, for horses and ponies to respond to changes in nutritional content of their rations. The size and/or duration of a single meal is governed primarily on the basis of palatability, time since the last meal, and external stimuli, such as the presence of other horses and environmental conditions. Many situations created by modern management of horses predispose to aberrant or pathologic feeding activities. The more common of these are discussed.

OVEREATING

Horses will overeat on a long-term basis leading to obesity, or within a single meal causing founder, colic, or other forms of gastrointestinal distress. This apparent lack of control is closely related to the natural regulation of feed intake.

The horse that overeats and becomes obese is not demonstrating a pathologic behavior. These animals are adapted to a diet seasonally variable in nutritional content and relatively low in soluble carbohydrate content. It is adaptive to store body fat during the summer months to endure throughout the leaner winter months. Unfortunately, the horse has not adjusted to present management techniques wherein food is continually available. Most horses given free access to a nutritious and palatable feed will become obese. The provision of highly palatable, nutritious feeds in large quantities, frequent feeding, decreased roughage (hay), and restriction of exercise are feeding practices predisposing to obesity. "Cold-blooded" horses and ponies are more prone to obesity than "hot-blooded" animals.

Treatment of obesity should be limited to the restriction of feed and increased exercise. It is not advisable to starve an obese horse to reduce its body weight because of the danger of hyperlipemia (see p. 114). The prevention of obesity in horses should include a regular exercise program, feeding primarily loose hay of moderate- to low-energy content, and restricting high-energy density feeds.

The horse that overeats within a single meal is also demonstrating normal feeding behavior. Over evolutionary time, horses were not exposed suddenly to large amounts of highly nutritious and palatable feeds and consequently are not adapted to regulating their intake of high-energy feeds on a short-term basis. Horses will not engorge in a single meal if offered only grass hay. Gastrointestinal stimuli such as gastric fill and nutrient feedback cues from the ingestion of feed do not normally regulate the size of a given meal. These stimuli come into play only when the cues received by the animal are those of pain. At this point it is usually too late since the horse does not usually regurgitate. A horse governs its ingestion of a single meal on the basis of: (1) the taste, smell, and texture of the feed; (2) ease of consumption (grain, grain mixtures, and small pellets are eaten more rapidly than long-stem hay); (3) duration of time the horse has fasted (the longer the fast, the more it will eat); and (4) environmental stimuli such as the presence or absence of other horses and climatic conditions (hot weather will decrease feed intake, cold temperatures will increase eating activity).

The following measures should be taken to prevent grain overload in horses: (1) store all grain concentrates and pelleted feeds where horses cannot gain access to them; (2) make hay available throughout the day or night to prevent prolonged fasting periods; (3) if the horse has experienced a fast of more than six hours, limit access to high-energy density feed; (4) avoid sudden changes to high-energy feedstuffs.

ANOREXIA

Anorexia is the lack of eating by a horse that should, on the basis of previous dietary history, be hungry and seeking feed. It has a variety of causes, some of which are pain, fever, anxiety, fear, metabolic disturbances, and extremes of environmental temperature. Anorexia may be treated by many methods, all of which are predicated upon understanding why the animal is not eating. If the horse is in pain, the obvious solution is to remove the source of pain. Phenylbutazone and flunixin meglumine at therapeutic levels have been effective in increasing feed intake in animals suffering painful conditions such as pleuritis or limb fractures. The febrile horse will dramatically reduce feed intake. Antipyretics such as dipyrone are effective in increasing feed intake in febrile sheep after endotoxin administration. It has been my clinical experience that febrile, anorectic horses will often resume eating when given antipyretic and analgesic preparations. Anxiety is a major cause of reduced feed intake in many hospitalized horses. A horse may be distressed by separation from its herd companions, restriction of exercise, and/or suffering of painful procedures by strangers. Reduction of anxiety may increase feed intake by the hospitalized horse. If the animal normally is stabled with a companion

(horse, pony, goat), it is best that the animal accompany the horse during hospitalization. The site and sound of other horses eating may also stimulate appetite.

Antianxiety drugs such as diazepam have been recommended as appetite stimulants although they are not in common use at this time. Extremely low doses (0.2 mg per 100 kg body weight) may be used in a horse that is distressed or anxious due to chronic low-grade pain. Extreme caution should be exercised when using diazepam. The animal must be observed carefully throughout the period of treatment for signs of excessive tranquilization or excitement. The drug is given intravenously and will take effect immediately, if it is effective at all. Feed must be available to the horse at the time of injection. Distractions such as loud noises and disturbances must be kept to a minimum. Diazepam has a short period of action, the stimulatory effect lasting only 10 to 15 minutes. If it effectively stimulates feeding activity, only two to three treatments in a 24- to 48-hour period are usually necessary to reinstate normal eating activity.

Other methods of stimulating anorectic horses to eat include: (1) presentation of small amounts of very palatable food at frequent intervals; (2) offering small amounts of foods considered to be treats, such as carrots, sugar, and apples, with the normal rations; and (3) allowing the animal access to fresh grass. A horse refusing to graze is usually a strong candidate for extraoral supplementation of nutrients (see p. 424).

It is of utmost importance to note that horses do not have "nutritional wisdom." They will not "balance" their diets for nutrients other than energy, water, and sodium. A horse should not be relied upon to select a diet that is balanced in protein, phosphorus, calcium, or other trace minerals. These must be provided in a balanced diet that is palatable to ensure adequate intake.

VICES RELATED TO FEEDING

Woodchewing. Woodchewing is one of the most common and destructive vices of the horse. Although a normal activity, woodchewing may be enhanced by a lack of fiber or protein or both in the diet, wet, cold weather, the feeding of a complete pelleted diet and no hay, and perhaps boredom. Horses will chew more wood when the weather is wet and cold than when fed the same rations under dry, warm conditions. The association of woodchewing with pelleted feeds has been well documented. The actual cause of woodchewing associated with these feeds is unknown, although reduced cecal pH and relative lack of fiber or "chewing time" or both have been incriminated.

Problems associated with woodchewing include destruction of property and ingestion of nails or other foreign materials with the wood and subsequent development of enteroliths.

In prevention of woodchewing, underlying dietary causes should first be ruled out. Low protein or energy levels or both in the ration may also be predisposing factors. If the animal is receiving a complete pelleted feed, provision of five to six pounds of hay per day may reduce the desire to chew wood. The animal should be receiving adequate amounts of feed for the environmental condition, its age, and its reproductive status (see p. 419). If the animal's exercise has been restricted and woodchewing occurs from boredom, increased exercise or the provision of toys or a companion may alleviate the problem.

Unfortunately, woodchewing becomes a habit for some horses and requires more dramatic measures to prevent its occurrence. The most common method employed is the covering of all wooden surfaces with a noxious substance such as carbolineum, lemon-flavored oils, or hot pepper. Wood treated with fire retardants is chewed less frequently than untreated woods. Although often impractical, electrified wiring strung along wood surfaces also prevents woodchewing. If all else fails, the provision of a pine or aspen log containing no nails and untreated with chemical substances may reduce the damage to treated wooden structures.

Coprophagy. The eating of feces (coprophagy) is a normal activity in foals less than three months of age and should not be discouraged. In the older horse, however, it is usually an indication of a dietary imbalance, either in the past or present. Diets inadequate in energy or protein cause animals to seek out and consume fecal material. Unfortunately, this habit may develop into a vice that is difficult, if not impossible, to correct. If the animal has just started to consume feces, the diet should be examined carefully and any necessary alterations made. If the diet appears to be balanced and complete in all respects, the horse may have developed this behavior because of boredom or a previous dietary imbalance. Muzzling the animal between feedings or confining it to a tie stall will prevent coprophagy, but the necessity of such drastic measures is debatable. Coprophagy results in the ingestion of parasites, but if an adequate parasite control program is established (see p. 328), parasitism should not be a problem. The esthetics of this behavior appears to be the major complaint.

Pica. Pica, the ingestion of abnormal substances such as dirt or rocks, includes some forms of woodchewing, coprophagy, and chewing or sucking on metal surfaces. Because pica may be due to a dietary imbalance, the diet should be examined carefully for energy, protein, or mineral deficiencies. Psy-

chologic stress also should be considered a potential cause of pica because this vice is most common in intensively managed racehorses and show horses.

Windsucking (*Cribbing*). During windsucking or cribbing, horses grab a fixed surface with the upper teeth, arch their necks, and suck in air. The terminology is somewhat confusing since windsucking and cribbing also refer to other problems. Cribbing is also a synonym for woodchewing, and windsucking also has been used to describe a vaginal disorder in mares. Here I will discuss only the behavior wherein the horse grabs a fixed surface with its incisors and sucks in air. This is an abnormal behavior probably brought on by boredom or frustration, by observing other horses windsucking, or accidentally discovering the action when playing with rubber tires or other such objects. Windsucking apparently creates a pleasurable sensation. Horses not bored or frustrated, such as foals in a large pasture with their dams, will learn to perform the movement and continue to do so unless aversive stimuli, such as cribbing straps, are used to prevent the activity. The major problems associated with windsucking are owners objecting to the noise and hypertrophy of the sternocephalicus muscle (esthetics), excessive wear on the incisor teeth and ill thrift secondary to decreased feed intake. Most horses referred to veterinary clinics for the surgical treatment of windsucking are in good health and presented primarily for esthetic reasons. There is no scientific evidence that windsucking causes an increase in flatulent colic or decreases the ability of the animal to digest its diet. Windsuckers suffering chronic colic and weight loss do not improve physically after surgical intervention to prevent the behavior.

The prevention of cribbing is traditionally by physical methods such as the use of cribbing straps. These straps, made of leather or a combination of leather and metal, are placed around the neck just behind the jaw. They allow the ingestion of feed and water but prohibit the animal from arching its neck and sucking air. Cribbing straps put on too tightly restrict breathing or eating or both. If the straps are not tight enough, however, they will not serve the purposes for which they are intended. Coating fixed surfaces with noxious substances prevents the vice in horses that have just begun to windsuck, but is of no benefit in established cribbers. Increasing exercise and reducing boredom and/or stress may be beneficial for those horses beginning to crib. Companions, such as a goat or pony, and the provision of metal mirrors in the back of the stall may reduce the frequency of windsucking by nervous, confined horses.

Surgery that physically prevents the animal from cribbing is available and is described on page 181 of the first edition of this book. The procedure involves the sectioning of the ventral branch of the accessory nerve and/or sternohyoideus, sternothyroideus, and omohyoideus muscles involved in arching the neck. It may be cosmetically acceptable, and a 70 to 80 per cent success rate in preventing the activity has been reported. In a follow-up survey of 10 horses in which this surgical procedure was used, it appears that "cured" horses tended to be young animals that had engaged in the activity for less than one year. Those that did stop windsucking did not engage in other aberrant activities, supporting the idea that cribbing or windsucking is not due solely to boredom or frustration. In eight of the ten horses, the management of the horses had not been altered after surgery.

Supplemental Readings

Hintz, H. F.: Horse Nutrition: A Practical Guide. New York, Arco Press, 1983.
Houpt, K. A.: Oral vices of horses. Equine Pract., 4:16, 1982.
Kiley-Worthington, M.: Cause, function and prevention of stereotypies in horses. Equine Pract., 34:34, 1983.
Laut, J., Houpt, K. A., Hintz, H. F., and Houpt, T. R.: The effects of caloric dilution on meal patterns and food intake in ponies. Physiol. Behav., 35:549, 1985.
Ralston, S. L.: Common behavioral problems in horses. Comp. Cont. Educ., 4:S142, 1982.
Ralston, S. L.: Controls of feeding in horses. J. Anim. Sci., 59:1354, 1984.
Turner, A. S., White, N. A., and Ismay, J. A.: Modified Forsell's operation for crib biting in the horse. J. Am. Vet. Med. Assoc., 184:309, 1984.

Foal Rejection

Katherine A. Houpt, ITHACA, NEW YORK

Although foal rejection can be responsible for serious financial losses to the horse breeder, its incidence is unknown. The rejected foal may be killed by its dam, but it is usually saved to be fostered onto a nurse mare, or hand raised. Hand-rearing foals is not only costly and time-consuming, but hand-reared foals are often difficult to train, probably because they are not as submissive to humans as are normal horses.

The physiologic control of maternal behavior has not been investigated in mares. The abrupt decline in both estrogen and progesterone, accompanied by a transient increase in oxytocin, may sensitize the central nervous system to sight, sound, and particularly the smell and taste of a newborn foal. In sheep, a high percentage of virgin animals will exhibit maternal behavior toward newborns if they are treated with the proper ratio of estrogen, progesterone, and corticosteroids. Recreating the hormonal conditions that exist during the immediate postpartum period would probably also stimulate normal maternal behavior in mares. It is likely that the proper hormonal relationships are present in the foal-rejecting mare, but that the central nervous system does not respond normally. The lack of response may be innate, caused by some genetically determined aberrant behavior. This seems particularly likely in Arabians, which have a greater incidence of foal rejection than other breeds.

Maternal behavior can also be modified by experience. Of the 42 cases of foal rejection reported to the New York State College of Veterinary Medicine in a recent two-year period, few occurred in mares reported to have themselves been rejected, but almost all mares (37 of 42) were primiparous (Table 1). The experience of being a mother, even a poor mother, is apparently important. The sex of the foal is not important. Older mares reject foals more commonly than younger ones. The importance of licking the placenta is unknown, but one mare accepted her foal after it was rubbed with the placenta. Exposure to foals both during development and as an adult may also determine the reaction of a mare to her own newborn foal. Dams that reject their foals are often those that had been isolated during their youth. As foals they were rarely turned out with other mares and foals but rather were stalled and pastured with their dam or after weaning were kept alone.

In summary, hormonal and neural factors, plus experience, influence maternal behavior in horses (Fig. 1). An abnormality or deficiency of any of

TABLE 1. SURVEY OF 42 CASES OF FOAL REJECTION (ANIMAL BEHAVIOR CLINIC, NEW YORK STATE COLLEGE OF VETERINARY MEDICINE)

	Yes	No	Unknown
Arabian or 50% Arabian	24	18	
Foal rejection by mare's dam	2	12	27
Primiparous	37	5	
Mare older than 4 years	33	8	1
Placenta removed from stall within first hour of birth	25	12	9
Foal subsequently accepted	13	26	3

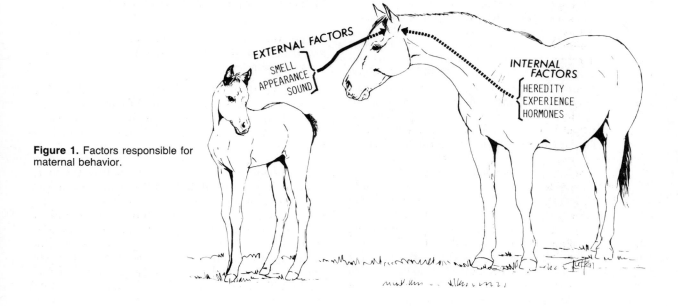

Figure 1. Factors responsible for maternal behavior.

these factors may lead to foal rejection, although the lack of prior maternal experience seems to be the most important cause. Mares predisposed to foal rejection are primiparous, Arabian, and/or those that previously rejected foals.

Foal rejection can be classified into three types: mares that accept their foals but will not allow them to nurse, mares that do not accept their foals and are actively aggressive toward them at all times, and mares that are frightened of their foals.

THERAPY

Refusal to Allow Nursing. The mare should be restrained to allow the foal to nurse. If restraint is not possible by placing a pole across the stall, she should be handheld. In some cases that is all that is necessary. Foals nurse every 15 to 20 minutes during the first week of life. This probably optimizes absorption of colostrum during the first 24 hours of life as well as strengthening the mare-foal bond by frequently rewarding the foal with milk and the mare with the relief of udder tension. The more often the foal suckles a mare that initially refuses to allow nursing, the more quickly she will accept the foal. One or two days of restraining the mare while the foal suckles is usually sufficient. The owner or barn manager will be rewarded for a few sleepless nights with a foal that is raised by its mother rather than bottle fed or fostered.

The mare should not be twitched when the foal attempts to suckle. If she is punished she may associate the pain with nursing. Twitching releases endogenous opiates, but that is probably secondary to pain produced by stimulation of the numerous sensory receptors on the equine upper lip. Tranquilization with acepromazine* or xylazine† is often helpful, but the tranquilizing drugs may be excreted into the milk. If the foal appears sedated or uncoordinated, the mother should not be given more of the drug.

Mares That Attack Their Foals. The attacking mare will usually bite the foal on its withers. This behavior is similar to that of the foal-savaging stallion and may indicate a masculinization of the brain either during development or during pregnancy. The aggressive mare may spontaneously attack her foal. She may allow it to suckle, but attack it whenever it walks in front of her, especially if she is eating. She may attack it only when it stands, or more rarely, only when it lies down.

Some mares respond to punishment, usually whipping, and subsequently accept their foals. Punishment must occur as the mare begins to attack, because she must be stopped before injuring the foal. It is important that the punishment be closely associated with the undesirable behavior. A remotely operated shock collar could also be used as a punishing tool.

Close confinement in box stalls could precipitate foal savaging by some mares. Mares are more apt to accept their foals if they are in a more natural

---

*Promace, Fort Dodge Laboratories, Inc., Fort Dodge, IA
†Rompun, Haver-Lockhart, Shawnee, KS

environment such as paddocks. Great care must be taken to ensure that the foal is protected when therapy is unsuccessful.

Sometimes the presence of horses in adjacent stalls will redirect aggressive behavior toward the foal. However, in other cases, mares will show normal maternal behavior only when turned out with other horses against which they protect the foal. Dogs have been used to threaten foals, to arouse normal maternal defense behavior in mares. Occasionally separating the foal from the dam briefly will initiate normal maternal behavior.

The most safe and effective method of treating foal rejection is to restrain the mare so she is unable to injure the foal. A pole can be placed across the box stall converting it into a straight stall for the mare and a larger area for the foal. The pole must be at the proper height so as to allow the foal access to the udder. The mare can still bite the foal if it approaches her head, although most foals learn to avoid the mare's head. Care must be taken that the foal cannot get between the mare's hindquarters and the wall of the stall. Bales of hay can be used to prevent this. Ten days of restraint may be necessary before a mare will accept the foal. If a mare has a history of foal rejection, the pole should be constructed before parturition and the mare accustomed to it. This will obviate the need for emergency carpentry at the time of foaling. A device for this purpose is commercially available.* A more elaborate straight stall can also be constructed with a solid wall and a cutout area in the flank region so the foal can nurse. Cross-tying the mare and/or hobbling can serve the same function, but the mare will not be restrained so well.

The Frightened Mare. The most important differential diagnosis of foal rejection is between mares attacking their foals and those that are frightened of them. The frightened mare will stay as far from the foal as possible, may kick when it attempts to suckle, and will most likely cause injury by running over the foal in attempting to avoid it. Posture, tucked tail, and ears turned to the side indicate fear. The frightened mare should not be punished, but instead be rewarded for allowing the foal to approach and suckle. Tranquilization, particularly with anti-anxiety agents such as diazepam,† is more likely to be therapeutically successful in these frightened mares than in those that attack their foals. Removal of the foal for a brief period is more likely to initiate normal maternal behavior in a frightened mare than in those that are aggressive.

---

*Safoal Nurser, Newington, CT
†Valium, Roche Laboratories, Nutley, NJ

PREVENTION OF FOAL REJECTION

The following recommendations should be followed in managing the prepartum mare to reduce risks of foal rejection.

1. Move the mare into the foaling stall several weeks before the expected date of parturition.
2. Eliminate visual contact with other horses.
3. Desensitize primiparous mares to udder contact.

Two people are necessary to desensitive the mare to udder contact—one to hold the mare and reward her, the other to handle the udder. Touch the mare's flank. If she does not flinch she should be given a food reward of grain or sugar immediately. If she does not object to flank contact, touch the udder gently as she is given a food reward. If the mare does not flinch at udder contact, touch a teat. Again, give the mare a food reward for not flinching or kicking. Repeat many times, gradually increasing udder and teat contact until it approximates that of a foal's butting. Squeeze and pull the teats as a suckling foal would, each time rewarding the mare for passive acceptance. If the mare's sensitivity to udder contact does not decrease rapidly, do not attempt to continue desensitization. Improper timing can aggravate the mare's intolerance to udder contact.

If the mare has a history of foal rejection, she should be placed in a restraining stall daily several weeks before parturition so that she becomes accustomed to the restraint. She should also be fed there. She should not, of course, be restrained during parturition.

In summary, foal rejection can be prevented in some cases and treated when it occurs in others. Mares to be used for breeding should be bred to foal at four or five years of age, because primiparous mares older than five years are more likely to reject their foals. Primiparous mares should not be used as embryo transplant recipients. Foal rejection may be even more of a problem with cross-species embryo transplantation. For example, one mule mare rejected her donkey foal whereas two others accepted their horse foals.

Supplemental Readings

Houpt, K. A.: Foal rejection and other behavioral problems in the postpartum period. Compend. Cont. Ed., 6:S144, 1984.
Waring, G. H.: Horse Behavior. Park Ridge, NJ, Noyes Publications, 1983.

The Use of Progestins for Aggressive and for Hypersexual Horses

Stephen J. Roberts, WOODSTOCK, VERMONT

Bonnie V. Beaver, COLLEGE STATION, TEXAS

Aggression in horses can be subdivided into aggression against other horses and aggression toward people. Aggression among horses can be further subdivided into normal and abnormal aggression. The types of normal aggression seen are dominance-related aggression, maternal aggression, and sex-related aggression either between a mare and a stallion or among stallions. Dominance-related aggression is most likely to lead to injury under normal management practices. Aggression toward people is more difficult to classify but is mostly dominance-related. Proper handling and training should be used to establish dominance and control over the horse, but when the owner is having difficulty in establishing dominance or control, progestin therapy may be helpful. In cases of extreme aggression euthanasia is the safest solution.

NORMAL MATERNAL AGGRESSION

Maternal aggression is the sexually dimorphic pattern of a mare protecting her foal from intruders. In a herd environment, the dam prevents other mares from approaching the foal or from standing between her and the foal. In a stall or pasture environment the unfriendly greeting can be extended to humans as well. Maternal aggression is a normal, innate response that can be modified by learning. It should be considered as possessiveness or protection of the foal.

A mare rapidly bonds to her own foal and will usually reject approaches by strange foals, although she is more tolerant of the presence of other foals than of other mares. As her own foal gets older, a mare's protectiveness of it tends to decrease. Even though she may allow the foal to nurse well past its first birthday, the aggressive protection is usually gone.

Variations in maternal aggression occur in individuals. At one extreme is the mare attacking its newborn foal, which probably reflects stress during parturition or poor learning experiences (see p. 127). Other mares may pay little attention to their foals and do not react when their foals are taken away. The extremely protective mare represents the other extreme. For her, any separation, regardless of the age of the foal, produces an exaggerated amount of whinnying and pacing.

NORMAL SEX-RELATED AGGRESSION

Sex-related aggression is usually exhibited by the anestrous mare toward an investigating stallion. In the teasing, this individual will often squeal and strike with a front foot or turn and lash out with both hind feet. The behavior is intensified because the restrained mare cannot escape as she could on pasture. Stallions have been severely injured by nonreceptive mares, and this has prompted use of mare breeding hobbles and mounting phantoms and limiting or eliminating pasture breeding. During late proestrus the mare will accept an increasing amount of solicitation by the stallion. Only in full behavioral estrus will the normal mare not show aggression.

Occasional variations do occur. A mare has been known to reject the advances of a specific stallion but allow mounting by other stallions. The basis of this selection is unknown. It does occur in other species as well. Other mares, especially maiden mares, may be frightened and react by kicking, but this cannot be considered aggressive. A few mares have been known to continue resistance toward a stallion throughout estrus. It is interesting to speculate that the hormone levels are such to permit ovulation but may not reach the necessary threshold to affect the behavior centers of the hypothalamus. Another speculation is that the latter centers are relatively unresponsive to the hormones.

HORMONAL ABNORMALITIES

There is little definitive knowledge about gonadal and adrenal hormones and their interactions with the central nervous system in horses. Hypertestosteronism has been implicated as a cause of aggression in mares. Granulosa cell tumors are frequently associated with aggression and stallionlike behavior. A pathologic cause of aggression in mares should be considered before a purely behavioral explanation is sought.

Testosterone in mares is normally produced in both the adrenal cortex and ovaries. In the adrenal cortex, cholesterol is converted to pregnenolone, which can produce progesterone. This is converted to 17-hydroxyprogesterone, and it to testosterone. Testosterone is the precursor of estradiol. Impairment of enzymatic transformations along this pathway can result in an accumulation of intermediates or in an increased production of products such as testosterone.

Ovarian thecal cells produce testosterone, which is converted to estradiol by the granulosa cell. Proliferation of the thecal cells or a deficiency in the granulosa cells could also result in the build-up of serum testosterone. The hypothalamopituitary axis can also elevate serum testosterone by the secretion of adrenocorticotropic hormone (ACTH) and gonadotropin. ACTH stimulates the conversion of cholesterol to pregnenolone in the adrenal cortex, while gonadotropin accomplishes the same in gonadal tissue.

Lesion location can be determined through three different endocrine tests. An ACTH stimulation test should raise all adrenal cortical steroid levels except that of aldosterone, unless an adrenal tumor is already causing maximum secretion. Dexamethasone administration reduces ACTH at the pituitary. If serum testosterone values decrease with dexamethasone, a hypothalamic and pituitary origin would be expected. If serum testosterone values do not change, the high levels could be of ovarian origin or from an adrenal tumor not under pituitary control. A gonadotropin stimulation test would help define an ovarian origin when a tumor was not palpable.

PHYSIOLOGY OF PROGESTINS

Natural progestins, progesterone, and other progestational compounds are produced principally by the corpus luteum and the placenta of mares. They act to control and regulate the estrous cycle, suppressing sexual activity and receptivity during diestrus, even when follicular development and ovulation may occur. The progestins prepare the uterus for the nutrition and maintenance of the zygote and fetus through gestation as well as playing a role in preparing the udder for lactation. Before 90 days of gestation progesterone from the corpora lutea maintains equine pregnancy, and after 90 days, progestins from the placenta maintain it.

ROLE OF PROGESTINS IN TREATING BEHAVIOR PROBLEMS

Progestins administered to male animals produce an antagonistic effect and possibly neutralizing and antiandrogenic effects similar to the antiestrogenic effects of progestins in females. These effects in males are characterized by an inhibition of luteinizing hormone (LH) from the anterior pituitary gland resulting in a reduction in Leydig cell activity, plasma testosterone levels, ejaculate volume, libido, and spermatogenesis. In females this suppression of LH results in failure of follicular growth, estrus, and ovulation. There is evidence that progestins may also block central and peripheral androgen- and estrogen-sensitive receptor sites. These progestational effects are reversible when the exogenous or endogenous progestins are withdrawn.

.Furthermore, in domestic male animals and in humans there is definite clinical, physiologic, and psychologic evidence that progestins produce a tranquilizing, or possibly a narcotic, effect on the central nervous system. It is axiomatic that pregnant mares have a more quiet, relaxed, and placid attitude than nonpregnant mares. These actions or effects of progestins have been utilized in the relatively short-term treatment of a variety of aggressive, psychotic, antisocial, and deviant sexual behavioral problems in dogs, cats, cows, horses and humans. Castration or gonadectomy was and is the more radical, irreversible approach to such problems.

Besides the natural progestin progesterone, a large number of synthetic progestins have been produced, some of which are commercially available for veterinary use in horses. The more commonly used progestational products are:

1. Progesterone–available in an oil base at concentrations of 50 mg per ml; injected intramuscularly in doses of 0.4 mg per kg of body weight daily.

2. Altrenogest (allyl-trenbolone)*–available in a 0.22 per cent solution; given orally or in the grain ration at a dose rate of 0.02 ml per kg body weight daily.

3. Megestrol acetate†–available in 5 and 20 mg tablets; given orally or in the grain ration at a dose of 65 to 85 mg daily for a 500-kg horse.

4. Repositol progesterone‡–available in an alcohol and propylene glycol solution in a concentration of 50 mg per ml; given intramuscularly at a dose rate of 1000 or 2000 mg at four- or seven-day intervals, respectively, for a 500-kg horse.

Some less commonly used progestins for horses

---

*Regumate, American Hoechst Corp., Somerville, NJ
†Ovaban, Schering Corp., Kenilworth, NJ
‡Progesterone Injection Repository, Med-Tech Laboratories, Elwood, KS

include melengestrol acetate (MGA), chlormadinone acetate (CAP), cyproterone acetate, and medroxyprogesterone acetate (MPA or MAP). The latter two progestins are currently being used commonly in humans.

Exogenous progestins are often used in reproductive management, and there is no evidence that prolonged judicious use of approved exogenous progestins is permanently harmful to mares, fetuses, or stallions. In mares and stallions it may require up to six months or more to re-establish normal reproductive capabilities and fertility after the prolonged administration of progestins or other exogenous gonadal or anabolic steroids. Long-term use of progestins in the latter part of the third trimester of gestation in mares may cause a prolonged gestation period with parturient complications including fetal death, as has occurred in cows.

Several days to several weeks of short-term, progestational therapy at the doses mentioned has, in our experience, had "tranquilizing" antiandrogenic and antiestrogenic effects in nervous, hypersexual, aggressive stallions and mares, permitting them to be more easily transported, handled, and shown without the depression or incoordination associated with use of tranquilizers or sedatives. In mares these undesirable behavioral traits are seen most commonly during the estrous or estrogenic period and in stallions during the breeding season. Because of its calming and tranquilizing effect, progestin therapy might possibly be indicated in those mares that reject their foals.

In the past, castration or spaying has been recommended for the highly nervous, excitable, flighty, neurotic, self-mutilating, aggressive mare or stallion. If this operation is performed before severe vicious, violently aggressive behavior toward other horses and the human handlers has been well established, a satisfactory behavioral response is often achieved. Progestin therapy in the early stages of such behavior in the nymphomaniac, aggressive mare or the hypersexual, aggressive stallion is often indicated together with judicious, firm, but not abusive handling or retraining of the animal. Once these highly undesirable, deviant, vicious, aggressively dominant psychotic attitudes are ingrained in an animal, correction by progestins or even castration is unlikely. As in dogs and men, inter-male aggression or hypersexuality is often reduced by progestin therapy but other types of aggressive behavioral dominance are not affected by progestins or even castration.

Supplemental Readings

Beaver, B. V., and Amoss, M. S., Jr.: Aggressive behavior associated with naturally elevated serum testosterone in mares. Appl. Anim. Ethol., 8:425, 1982.

Hart, B. L.: Progestin therapy for aggressive behavior in male dogs. J. Am. Vet. Med. Assoc., *178*:1070, 1981.

Houpt, K. A., and Wolski, T. R.: Domestic Animal Behavior for Veterinarians and Animal Scientists. Ames, Iowa State University Press, 1982.

Neely, D. P., Liu, I. K., Hillman, R. B., and Hughes, J. P.: Equine Reproduction. Nutley, NJ, Hoffman-La Roche Inc., 1983.

Stabenfeldt, G. H.: Physiologic, pathologic and therapeutic roles of progestins in domestic animals. J. Am. Vet. Med. Assoc., *164*:311, 1974.

Waring, G. H.: Horse Behavior: The Behavioral Traits and Adaptations of Domestic and Wild Horses, Including Ponies. Park Ridge, NJ, Noyes Publications, 1983.

Stereotypic Behavior

M. *Kiley-Worthington*, ISLE OF MULL, SCOTLAND
D. *Wood-Gush*, EDINBURGH, SCOTLAND

There is considerable confusion in the veterinary profession between "stable vices" and stereotypic behavior (stereotypies). Stereotypies are repetitive behaviors that are constant in form and serve no apparent purpose, such as weaving. Stable vices are behavior patterns that interfere with management and are a nuisance to the owner and trainer. While stable vices include some stereotypic behaviors, they also include excessive aggression, biting, kicking, and ingestion of bedding materials.

Table 1 lists some stereotypies, many of which are more common than generally recognized. We have visited racehorse stables in which all of the horses were performing stereotyped behavior. In another stable, 26 per cent of the horses performed a stereotypy within a half hour of observation. Most horse owners and trainers consider stereotypies esthetically displeasing and sense that the behavior indicates the horse's lack of interest in the environment.

TABLE 1. LIST OF STEREOTYPIC BEHAVIORS

Origin of Behaviors			
Eating	*Locomotion*	*Cutaneous Irritation*	*Aggression*
Chewing	Pacing	Box-kicking (hind feet)	Head-extending, ears back and nodding
Lip-licking	Weaving	Self-rubbing	Kicking stall (hind feet)
Licking environment	Pawing	Self-biting	
Cribbing	Tail-swishing	Head-tossing	
Windsucking	Door-kicking (front feet)	Head-circling	
Woodchewing		Head-shaking	
		Tail-swishing	

ETIOLOGY

Although there is no evidence that stereotypic behaviors are inherited, they may be learned by foals from their dams. This behavior is more common in "hot-blooded" horses such as Thoroughbreds and Arabians than in heavier breeds such as the draft horse. This may be due to the housing of "hot bloods" in restricted environments rather than to an inherited predisposition.

Brain damage has been suggested as a cause of stereotypic behavior, although this is unlikely in most cases. Stereotypic behavior in the young may affect brain development, however. Although dietary causes of stereotypic behavior are unlikely, the presentation of prepacked food of low fiber content could lead to abnormal behavior.

The psychologic causes of stereotypies are more easily identified. These include frustration when something is required but unattainable, conflict between approach to an object and withdrawal from it in fear, and fear of objects or personnel. Stereotypies are often reinforced by handlers giving attention to the horse during abnormal behavior. "Establishing stereotypic behaviors" are performed only at key times such as before feeding or upon the appearance of the handler. Although these behaviors can develop at any age, they usually develop in young horses subjected to sudden environmental changes. Weaning, stabling after living at pasture, change in location or stablemates, and change in personnel may all precipitate abnormal behavior. Proper attention given to the environment, housing, nutrition, and social interaction can prevent the establishment of abnormal behavior. Stereotypic behaviors are probably learned and self-rewarding. For example, a horse that head tosses due to nasal irritation may be returned home. Thereafter, the horse considers head tossing a way to terminate the ride. When stereotypic behaviors are self-rewarding they become established and are performed frequently and often in seemingly inappropriate situations. Established behaviors are difficult to cure. Horses, as a species, develop fixated habits quite readily. While this aids training, it also favors established stereotypic behavior.

The more important causes of stereotypic behavior, along with some preventive and corrective measures, are described in the next section. Usually abnormal behavior patterns are a summation of several major etiologies and some minor ones. The total environment of the animal, its past experiences, and its genetic make-up must be considered in both establishing the cause and searching for the cure.

WEANING

The mare and foal have a particularly close bond, foals staying near to their dams until six months of age or older. The closest bonds between individuals in horse groups tend to be between generations. As a result, weaning is a particularly traumatic occurrence for the young horse and its dam, particularly if the foal is kept in isolation. Weaning foals in pairs is one management technique that may reduce stress. These foals show less distress than those kept in isolation. Alternatively, foals need not be weaned but could remain with the group. Horses raised in this manner are easily integrated into groups and require less training for saddling and mounting. Other management techniques for weaning foals include the following:

1. A handler or other person can be substituted for the dam. This might be the best approach for raising easy-to-train horses but requires six to 10 hours a day and is therefore often impractical.

2. Foals can be gradually weaned and familiarized with groups of horses with which they will be living.

3. Another adult horse, previously familiar with and tolerant of young foals, can be substituted for the dam. A barren mare can accompany several foals.

CONFINEMENT FOR PROLONGED PERIODS

The development of stereotypic behavior is to some extent associated with the degree of confinement. Those horses tied in stalls for long periods, confined in box stalls, fed restricted fiber diets, and limited to less than two hours' exercise a day are more likely to develop stereotypic behavior. The design of stable facilities is important in the prevention of stereotypic behavior. Attention must be given to the amount of activity in the horse's visual field and its contact with other horses.

Modern box stalls, separated from others by bars and with sliding barred doors that do not allow the horse to look into the passage, tend to increase the likelihood of developing stereotypies. Due to insufficient environmental stimuli, the animal turns to rewarding self-stimulation.

Placement of the stables is important to provide visual "interest" and stimuli for the horse. Traditional stables with half doors facing blank walls are no improvement over loose boxes with barred doors. Stables should be positioned to allow visibility of activity such as that around the arena or close to paddocks or yards. There should be plenty of activity throughout the day, with long quiet periods of time avoided. Unfortunately, although there is much advice available about stable design and construction to ensure physical health, rarely, if ever, do advisers consider the psychologic needs of the horse.

FEEDING

It is now widely recognized that feeding fiber to horses is nutritionally important since they have evolved a gastrointestinal system for cellulose digestion. The feeding of fiber is also psychologically important. Feral, or pastured, horses eat approximately 16 hours per day. This time period varies only by two or three hours, whether food is scarce or abundant. If pasture grass is scarce, horses stop eating before consuming maintenance requirements and become malnourished. At the other extreme, when large amounts of nutritionally rich pasture are accessible, they will overeat, become overweight, and may develop laminitis. The stabled horse may eat for only two hours a day. For the extra 12 hours stabled horses tend to stand immobile (Tables 2 and 3) and this may lead to performance of a stereotypic behavior.

Solutions to this problem include:
1. Turning the horse out for at least part of the day, even if there is little to graze.
2. Providing the horse with access to roughage at all times by providing hay or straw.
3. Feeding a high-quality fiber diet such as hay ad libitum and less grain.
4. Keeping horses in groups in corrals or yards where social interactions can be freely performed.

Owners of racing horses and competitive horses may not wish to feed horses fiber ad libitum. Horses

TABLE 2. PERCENTAGE OF TIME SPENT BY FERAL AND DOMESTIC ANIMALS IN VARIOUS ACTIVITIES

Activity	Feral Horses*		Stabled Horses
	Summer (%)	Winter (%)	
Eating	56.17	61.55	25
Standing	22.50	24.20	65
Lying	11.60	7.90	10
Walking	9.50	6.20	0

Domestic horses were unable to easily see or touch another horse and were fed a restricted fiber diet (5 lb hay/day, 15 lb complete feed pellets and oats).

*Data adapted from Duncan (1980) for Camargue horses. Stabled horse data from anecdotal evidence.

eating too much fiber may be unable to consume the concentrated foods needed for their work. Nevertheless, it is possible to offer animals access to fiber without the occurrence of overeating. A hay net having small holes makes the horse work for long periods to obtain even a small amount of food. Such nets can be purchased or made according to need. Provision of these types of nets can reduce woodchewing and various other stereotypic behaviors by approximately half.

ISOLATION

Social isolation in a gregarious species such as the horse may have profound effects on many aspects of behavior. Stallions—in particular, Thoroughbreds—may be weaned at four months and then have no more free social contact with other horses. When treated in this way, they frequently if not always become "difficult," sometimes severely pathological, always socially inept, and frequently perform stereotypic behaviors.

Keeping horses in groups reduces stereotypic behavior, but the custom of housing animals in isolation is traditional in horse husbandry and therefore difficult to change. The cost of inappropriate behavior resulting from isolation may outweigh any

TABLE 3. PERCENTAGE OF TIME SPENT IN VARIOUS ACTIVITIES BY EIGHT HORSES IN A GROUP AND THREE INDIVIDUALLY STABLED HORSES*

	Group Stabled	Individually Stabled
Eating	53.2	50.3
Standing	28.1	48.3
Dozing	10.0	19.2
Lying	4.2	6.1
Walking	1.2	0
Drinking	0.7	0.5
Performing and receiving social interactions	4.6/hr	4.7/hr

*Totals are more than 50 per cent because horses can perform two or more activites simultaneously.

potential risk of injury resulting from living in groups. In fact, horses living together for the majority of their lives in familiar groups rarely injure each other. Visual contact through bars, although better than no contact, is apparently not sufficient to prevent stereotypic behavior. Horses in groups able to hear, touch, and smell each other interact frequently, on average 4.5 times per hour (Table 3).

Isolation can be avoided in all types of horses by maintaining them outside in freely associating groups or with family groups in free-housing systems. Several family groups can be kept together, which has the added advantage of reducing labor costs. Pilot work indicates that horses raised in this way require less training time before mounting than those weaned and isolation-reared. Allowing free contact with other individuals for some part of each day in exercise rings or yards, or allowing the maximum amount of contact between animals in their boxes, also prevents stereotypic behavior. Designing the boxes with partitions allowing horses to touch, smell, and see each other helps in this respect. In the 325 horses studied to date, no cases of stereotypic behavior in animals kept in family groups with freedom of movement and access to fiber have been observed.

LACK OF EXERCISE

Horses have evolved to move fast and freely over a considerable area. Even when food is plentiful, feral horses move over their entire "home range" and spend half an hour of each day moving freely. The finely tuned physiology enabling the horse to move quickly and efficiently is obtained by free movement and exercise sporadically throughout a 24-hour day and not by enforced sudden hard work for short periods followed by enforced immobility in confinement for long periods. Group-housed animals move around for longer periods and further distances than the single stabled animals allowed the same space per individual. Individual stabling therefore seems a poor way to create a conditioned animal. Many long-distance competitive horses are now kept at pasture during the competitive season in order to achieve the highest standards of fitness and endurance. One possible solution to lack of movement is to allow the horse access to exercise corrals. The horse can also be allowed prolonged periods of less strenuous exercise by training to harness and performing routine chores around the stable. If increased activity is not possible and the horse merely requires maintenance, feed should be reduced and only free access to roughage allowed.

PREVENTION AND CURE

Because stereotypic behaviors are safety valves that allow animals to survive stress without life-threatening psychosis, attempts to curb the behavior may be more harmful than the behavior itself. If harmless behaviors such as stall walking and weaving are prevented, the unacceptability of the environment is further enhanced and more pathological behavior may result. If genetic selection is avoided, stereotypic behaviors will be selected because they tend to allow survival in the psychologically difficult modern stable environment.

It is essential that clinicians understand the multifactorial causes and adaptive function of stereotypic behavior before recommending therapies and preventions. The first step in prevention is designing an environment to accommodate the animal's needs. Without major changes in stable design, stereotypic behaviors will become more common as horses become more confined. Environmental change may not remedy established behavior, and habit-breaking procedures may be necessary. Devices such as cribbing collars to prevent certain behaviors work only while they are in place. Aversive therapies such as electric shocks are being studied but have not, to our knowledge, been successfully used to prevent established stereotypic behavior.

It is quite possible to design environments in which competing and racing horses can be housed without development of stereotypies. Those who use the modern practice of surgery to prevent behaviors such as cribbing and windsucking make no attempt to understand their cause. Without proper environmental redesign such procedures are to be condemned. It would take only one generation to eliminate stereotypies with proper environmental design.

Supplemental Readings

Carson, K., and Wood-Gush, D. G. M.: Equine behaviour. II. A review of the literature on feeding, eliminative and resting behaviour. Appl. Anim. Ethol., *10*:179, 1983.

Houpt, K. A., Hintz, H. F., and Butler, W. R.: A preliminary study of two methods of weaning foals. Appl. Anim. Behav. Sci., *12*:177, 1984.

Kiley-Worthington, M.: The behaviour of horses in relation to management and training. London, J. A. Allen, 1986.

Singer, P.: Animal Liberation. A New York Review Book distributed by Random House, 1975.

University Federation of Animal Welfare. Behavioural needs. The results of a workshop on behavioral needs, Potters Bar, 1983, 1985.

Waring, G. H.: Horse behavior: The behavioral traits and adaptations of domestic and wild horses, including ponies. Park Ridge, NJ, Noyes Publications, 1983.

Trailer Problems and Solutions

Sharon E. Cregier, CHARLOTTETOWN, PRINCE EDWARD ISLAND

Motor transport is a stress that can adversely affect the horse's behavior and performance—loading, travel, and unloading all being foreign to the horse's structure and behavior. A panicking or unstable horse threatens its own life and the lives of other passengers, and can contribute to the loss of control of a vehicle. Equally important, horses that superficially adapt satisfactorily to transport may nevertheless suffer stresses that endanger performance and health.

Successful transport of horses requires knowledge of the ailments common to transport, the treatment of injuries that might be incurred during transport, and horse behavior patterns that are exacerbated by transport, as well as those that can be utilized for the horse's benefit. Awareness of equine physical and behavioral needs helps the veterinarian and handler to maintain the horse's physical, psychological, and functional integrity, ensuring improved performance.

A variety of factors can make transport a traumatic experience for the horse. Transport separates the animal from familiar surroundings, disrupting eating, sleeping, and social behavior. The horse confronts changes in temperature, ventilation, group size, and handlers and is subjected to engine, tire, and traffic noise in a confined, jolting, and vibrating environment. Rapid movement, braking, and long waits alternate unexpectedly. The animal is also exposed to fumes from dung, urine, and vehicle exhaust.

LOADING AND TRAVEL PROBLEMS

Conventional trailer transport requires the horse to be loaded into a darkened interior, often up an unstable or hollow-sounding ramp. If the trailer entry is low, the horse meets the edge of the roof as it steps up the ramp. To avoid entering, the horse may step off the ramp, rear, or rush backward.

Once loaded, the animal must be secured by chains or a barrier at head and buttocks. Securing the buttocks restraint necessitates activity in the horse's rearward blind spot, contributing to its feelings of apprehension. In spite of restraining devices, horses may strain against the bars or reverse beneath the bars, injuring the legs or spinal column.

As the vehicle accelerates, the horse senses the ground moving from its rear to its forequarters. It may try to leap away from the sensation, sometimes wedging its forequarters into the manger area.

Typically, acceleration moves the horse's center of gravity toward its hindquarters, which normally maintain only 35 to 40 per cent of body weight. Abducting the hindlimbs to support the increased weight places strain on pelvic structures. Directional changes, magnified in the area ahead of the trailer's axles, increase forequarter instability while braking pitches the head and forequarters forward, risking collision with the bulkhead. To avoid collision the horse lifts its head, causing fatigue of neck muscles.

"POOR" AND "GOOD" TRAVELERS

Poor travelers exhibit extreme behavioral response to transport. These responses include vocalizing, kicking, head-tossing, tail-wringing, lying down, leaning against the trailer side or partition, scrambling to the opposite side of the trailer, and becoming nonresponsive to stimuli. Padded skull caps, shipping boots, halter nose bands, and tail wraps provide limited protection against the hazards of loading, traveling, and unloading. Although good travelers show few behavioral problems, much effort is required to adapt to the physical and mental rigors of transport. Maintaining this effort for prolonged periods is a stress that can decrease the animal's resistance to disease and its ability to compete.

Trembling, increased defecation, and rapid heart rate are all indications of apprehension. Although the apprehensive horse sweats, sweat may evaporate rapidly into the air that flows over the horse, leaving no indication of the degree of water loss. Dehydration can also be exacerbated by failure to drink during a journey. Under severe transport tension, some horses will refuse to eat or will grab at hay or grain. Dehydration coupled with improper mastication can cause choke. Another common behavioral manifestation of transport stress is energetic, aggressive biting.

Decreased serum calcium, neutrophilia, and elevated blood cortisol and glucose levels are associated with transport of a few hours' duration. Elevated creatine phosphokinase (CPK) can be attributed to the muscular effort required to remain upright during conventional transport. This postural effort may contribute to myositis or cramping of the back muscles, and to sacroiliac and sacrolumbar strain.

Travel stress may also aggravate viral or bacterial infections and activate latent disease states. Medical problems associated with transport include lamini-

135

tis, salmonellosis, respiratory disease, spasmodic colic, impaction colic, and transit tetany. Mares in estrus transported as few as 32 km to a breeding farm may arrive out of estrus. Brood mares transported close to foaling may exhibit abnormal maternal behavior.

Many of the problems associated with transport are considered routine or unavoidable. Rope burns, abrasions, lacerations, kicks, and lameness are frequent findings. Shoulder stiffness and a sore chest result from being thrown against the breast bar during braking. Horses backed out of transport risk leg and head injuries. An animal attempting a forceful rearward exit before its head is released may panic, struggle, and injure the poll or neck.

REMEDIAL METHODS

Chemical Restraints. Chemical restraint is not generally recommended for horses in transport. The sedated animal cannot cope well with mechanical restraints, its thermoregulatory behavior may be disrupted, and it may become incoordinated. Chemical restraint may heighten the horse's response to lights, moving objects, and noises, causing it to overreact.

New Transport Designs. A major factor contributing to the sense of insecurity is the conventional trailer's failure to accommodate the horse's psychological needs and its anatomy and balancing system. Recently, trailers have been designed that address these needs. These design modifications allow transport of the horse facing away from the direction of travel with its head toward a back exit and its rear toward the engine. Following loading, a chest-high door or bar is secured in front of the animal. These design changes, which are coming into increasing use by transporters, may be adapted to other means of transport, including aircraft. Table 1 compares the reactions of the horse in conventional and rear-facing transport.

Rear-face trailer transport design necessitates a change in axle placement. Axles must be moved about 1.22 m forward from their position in a conventional trailer. This change accommodates the weight placement of the cargo: the horse's forequarters and its center of gravity are placed directly over, or within centimeters of, the trailer's steadiest spot, its center of gravity.

Removable interior partitions allow a foal access to its dam. As the subadult horse is accustomed to propping itself for balance, it can readily travel for short distances facing the direction of travel as it nurses. It then usually resumes lying beneath the dam's nose for much of the trip.

Horses in various physical conditions have been transported nonstop in well-ventilated rear-face

conveyances for 1930 km. At their destination, they have passed veterinary inspection within 30 minutes of arrival and have been able to immediately enter and win competitive events such as endurance riding, dressage, and showjumping.

Stock Trailers. Horses transported without restraint in stock trailers may travel side-on to the direction of travel. More usually they face a rear corner of the stock trailer with buttocks oriented to the diagonally opposite corner. To prevent piling up in the event of emergency braking or collision, horses traveling unrestrained in groups should be divided into pens within the trailer according to condition, age, sex, size, and compatibility.

Bloodstock shippers, racehorse trainers, and show horse competitors may cater to the travel orientation preference of their animals by designing stalls either diagonally rear-facing or facing directly to the rear.

THE CONVENTIONAL TRAILER

Conventional Front-Face Trailers. Conventional front-face, double-axle, two-horse trailers can be converted to rear-face design if the interior width is at least 165 cm and the interior length at least 284.5 cm. The manger, escape door, and forward windows must be removed and the double axles shifted forward until the loaded trailer registers a hitch weight between 40.8 kg and 49.4 kg. A 132 cm-long platform with an adjustable support replaces the conventional trailer's entry system.

A single horse may be hauled diagonally front-facing in an unmodified 1.83 m to 2.44 m wide conventional front-facing trailer if the center partition is removed. The horse's forequarters must, however, remain in the front half of the trailer. Small horses and ponies may be transported rear-face in a conventional two-horse trailer provided the driver brakes conservatively. Under no circumstances should large animals be hauled rear-face in an unmodified conventional trailer. The additional weight over the rear axles increases the danger of sway during traffic maneuvers and of jackknifing during braking.

Loading and Traveling in the Conventional Trailer. There are ways to minimize the difficulties of loading horses into conventional trailers. Ramps can be raised to rest level on a ground slope so that the horse walks from solid ground directly onto the platform and into the trailer. This method encourages low head carriage, minimizing the chances of the horse hitting the edge of the trailer's roof. While a step-in trailer may give the horse a more solid feeling during entrance than the usual sloped ramp entry, it is more likely to injure the horse's fetlocks during entry and exit.

Horses may enter a conventional trailer more

TABLE 1. EFFECTS OF TRANSPORT PRACTICES ON THE HORSE

Equine Behavioral Requirements	Rear-face Transport	Conventional Transport
Clear visual field	Headfirst entry eliminated or lighted passageway provided	Horse faces shadows, dark interior
Security from activity in blind area and kicking zone	One man loads/unloads at horse's head; horse faces all activity from security of its stall	Need for coercive tactics or activity in horse's blind area and kicking zone; horse unable to monitor activity from its stall
Secure footing	Horse unloads forward; pasterns, hocks at no risk	Horse must be backed into unseen activity onto uncertain footing; pasterns, hocks frequently injured
Effortless balance	Horse in transit has sensation of substrate moving normally from front to rear; no need to brace. No scramble marks on trailer sides. Low head carriage, hipshot resting stance assumed. Gimbal action of thoracic sling maintained	Horse feels like a man on a rug being snatched out from the front. Horse must brace or scramble; damage sustained by equipment, muscle strain or injuries sustained by horse. Tiring, unstable, head-up, weight-back stance must be maintained. Gimbal action of thoracic sling negated
Freedom to clear respiratory passages	Withers-level tether allows clearing of respiratory passages at will	Short tether, transport movement discourage clearing of respiratory passages
Stable substrate	Horse's center of gravity automatically retained over trailer's center of gravity	Need for continuous shifting for balance contributes to sway, jackknifing, engine and hitch wear
Need to void wastes at will	Male horses can stretch and urinate at will in transit	Male horses discouraged from stretching to urinate in transit
Maintenance of upright, stable posture during potentially threatening maneuvers	Horse automatically leans away from point of forward impact to maintain natural balance; fleshy buttocks presented to impact area.	Horse thrown forward at original speed of conveyance; vulnerable head, throat, chest presented to impact area
	Driver meets braking regulations, stops within 9 m at 32 km/hr without throwing horse, jackknifing trailer, initiating sway, or losing steering control	Driver cannot meet braking requirements for emergency stops without endangering cargo, losing steering control
	Hitch weight remains stable	Hitch weight fluctuates

readily if preceded by a stable companion such as a dog or goat. Apprehensive horses have been calmed by the use of soft, rhythmic sound. Classical music with a low, understated, regular beat and flowing melody is played in association with pleasant activities such as grooming, feeding, or idling and then used to establish calmness during training and tense or novel situations. Transporters might consider wiring their conveyance for such music. Recommended are Mozart concertos, the works of Haydn and Bach, the Canon de Pachelbel, and violin, flute, or clarinet pieces.

Where highway regulations allow, an attendant should travel in a protected area with the horse. The attendant should be skilled in assessing the horse's mental and physical state and be prepared to reposition the horse, change shipping equipment, and act in an emergency.

SELF-MONITORED DRIVING SKILLS

A driver should eliminate abrupt driving tactics likely to upset the horse. A capped, clear plastic glass filled with water to 1.3 cm below a marked line can be placed on a level area of the cab dash within the driver's sight. Careless braking and steering will frequently send the water above the 1.3 cm mark. Skilled drivers who can maintain a steady speed and maneuver their rig without allowing the water to rise repeatedly over a .64 cm mark offer the smoothest ride to their horses. The best hauling practices minimize dependence on the brakes.

EMERGENCY PROCEDURES

Poor ventilation, high humidity, isolation, noise, irritation by insects, blowing fodder or bedding, poor footing, prolonged sleeplessness, and poor driving habits contribute to "van fits." The animal becomes frenzied and unresponsive to normal handling tactics.

A control method used to immobilize frenzied horses in crushes might be utilized in these instances. A length of rope is secured on the bottom off-side wall or partition, passed over the horse's neck in front of its withers, and then drawn downward sharply to bite into the ligamentum nuchae. Pressure in this area may transfix the horse long enough for additional remedial action to be taken. It is a contingency procedure worth providing for.

EFFICIENT TRANSPORT

The following list identifies some practices worth integrating into shipping routine.

1. Obtain the owner's written authorization to administer emergency veterinary treatment.

2. Give horses prone to fecal impaction mineral oil by stomach tube before a journey of eight hours or longer.

3. Do not transport exhausted horses until they are cool and rehydrated (see p. 477).

4. Put electrolytes in the feed or water before as well as during transport; they may alleviate the effects of travel fatigue and dehydration (p. 479).

5. Condition the horse to drink water mixed with molasses or other flavoring before transport. The same flavoring can disguise foreign water offered during the trip.

6. Ensure access to clean, fresh water at least once every 12 hours and preferably more often. Horses will drink more readily from a tank than a bucket. Turn the vehicle engine off to prevent vibration when offering water in the trailer.

7. Allow a weanling at least one month to adjust to a solid diet before transport.

8. Sprinkle a liter mix of vinegar in water on the bedding to neutralize ammonia in conveyances that are unclean or poorly ventilated.

9. If possible, transport the horse with a preferred companion, such as another horse, goat, donkey, hen, or dog.

10. Paint the interior of the conveyance a non-glare, light color.

11. Avoid coercive loading tactics such as shouting, prodding, whipping, or using dogs.

12. Avoid transporting horses in a conventional trailer more than 643 km without an overnight rest, even if horses are in good athletic shape.

13. Stop at quiet, uncrowded places. A feeling of insecurity in a strange place may prevent a horse from lying down and a foal from sleeping. Make provision for increased lying-down time for subadult horses that lack the adult ability to doze standing.

14. Classical music during transport masks tire and traffic noise and induces relaxation.

15. Ensure plentiful ventilation at all times. Closed-cell urethane spray foam insulation on the trailer ceiling minimizes condensation and maintains cool temperatures in summer and warmer ones in winter.

16. Transport mares to stud farms at least 30 days before their foaling date.

17. Use artificial insemination when possible to avoid transport hazards.

18. *Do not* transport a large horse rear-face in a conventional trailer. Unless the axles have been moved forward to accommodate changed weight placement, too much weight will be at the rear of the trailer, increasing its tendency to sway and jackknife.

Supplemental Readings

Cregier, S. E.: Reducing equine hauling stress: A review. J. Equine Vet. Sci., 2:6, 186, 1982.

Cregier, S. E.: Road transport of the horse: An annotated bibliography, 7th Ed. Charlottetown, P.E.I., Equine Behaviour Journal, 1984.*

Hails, M. R.: Transport stress in animals: A review. Animal Regulation Studies, 1:4, 289, 1978.

Hoffmann, K.: Pferde sicher transportieren [Safe Transport for Horses]. Stuttgart, Albert Müller, 1975.

Houpt, K. A.: Misbehavior of horses: Trailer problems. Equine Pract., 4:2, 12, 1982.

*Available from Word Wizards, PO Box 170022, Atlanta, GA 30317.

CARDIOVASCULAR DISEASES

Edited by C. M. Brown

Echocardiography

Michael W. O'Callaghan, PALMERSTON NORTH, NEW ZEALAND

(on leave at DAVIS, CALIFORNIA)

Echocardiography is now a well-established diagnostic procedure in both human and veterinary medicine. Several features of this technique have contributed to its growing popularity in both general and specialist cardiology practice. Ultrasound is noninvasive, produces no known harmful effects in the diagnostic form, and provides images of soft tissue structures that are not readily attainable using other techniques such as radiology. Recent technologic advances, particularly in solid-state components, have not only significantly reduced the price but greatly improved the flexibility of available equipment. Incorporation of highly sophisticated microcomputer components into even the cheapest modern echocardiographs and the addition of amplifiers for recording electrocardiograms (ECGs), phonocardiograms, and cardiac impulse tracings provides clinicians with diagnostic information previously attainable only with more invasive techniques.

Despite the outwardly complicated appearance of many echocardiograph machines the basic principles behind the operation of ultrasound apparatus are relatively simple. The greatest complexity is in the methods of displaying the resulting echoes as images rather than in the generation and reception of the ultrasound beam.

EQUIPMENT

The sound waves used in echocardiography and other medical diagnostic apparatus possess frequencies in the range of 1 to 10 MHz; that is, 1 to 10 million cps. In this frequency range a proportion of the sound waves projected into tissue are reflected at tissue interfaces of differing acoustic impedance or density. Since the projected beam and the reflected waves travel through solid tissue at a finite speed (1540 m per sec), the reflected signals provide information on tissue depth and characteristics. Ultrasound, however, is not transmitted through air or gas, and is ineffective in bone because of multiple reflection and attenuation of the beam.

Figure 1 illustrates in graphic form the basic design of an echocardiographic machine with some of the more commonly employed image recording apparatus. The hand-held transducer contains the piezoelectric crystal, which determines the frequency of the ultrasound beam produced and also acts as receiver for the ultrasound waves returning from the tissues. When a small, rapidly fluctuating voltage is applied to the piezoelectric crystal it undergoes periodic deformations causing sound waves of a specific wave length to be emitted. Conversely, sound waves returning from the tis-

139

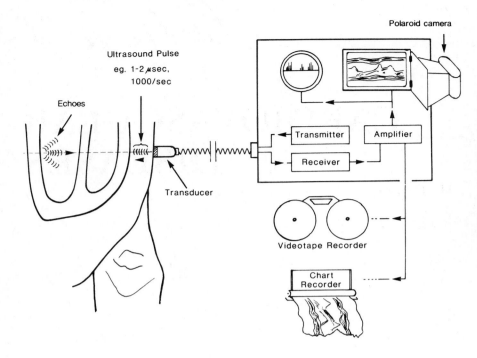

Figure 1. Graphic representation of echocardiograph design. The transducer, containing the piezoelectric crystal of a specific frequency (generally 1.8, 2.25, 3.0, 3.5, or 5 mHz), emits brief pulses of ultrasound repetitively and then acts as a receiver for the returning echoes. Signals produced by the returning echoes are amplified and displayed either in A mode (*upper left oscilloscope*) or as two-dimensional images (in this case M mode) (*upper right*).

sues, by deforming the crystal, cause it to generate small surface voltage changes proportional to the degree of deformation, which when suitably amplified and displayed produce the diagnostic image. In order to accommodate the transmission and reception functions, the piezoelectric crystal emits sound only in short bursts, usually only 1 microsecond in duration (one millionth of a second), then remains silent for 999 microseconds in order to receive the reflected sound waves. This basic cycle is then repeated 1000 times per second. Owing to the very small proportion of time spent in transmission, very little energy is transferred to the tissues. This in part accounts for the innocuous nature of the procedure.

Image Production. According to the manner in which the signals received from the crystal are processed and displayed, a variety of visual images may be obtained. With a single, fixed crystal transducer, three basic forms of image are possible, A mode (amplitude), B mode (brightness), and M mode (motion) (Fig. 2).

In A mode, individual echoes are represented on an oscilloscope by a series of spikes along a graduated horizontal axis, representing depth or distance from the transducer. Echo strength is shown by the height of the spikes.

B mode employs the same horizontal axis, but individual echoes are represented on the screen as dots rather than spikes, their intensity proportional to echo strength.

M mode images are created either by moving the time base of the B mode display across the oscilloscope or by moving light-sensitive paper over a B-mode illuminated platen. Images may be recorded as hard copy by one of the following three methods:

1. Polaroid photographs taken from the face of the oscilloscope. (Poorest quality but cheapest option.)

2. On light-sensitive paper. (The chart recorders are relatively expensive.)

3. In more modern machines photographed in a variety of ways from the digitized, freeze-frame mode of the monitor screen, either directly or after replay from a video taperecorder incorporated in the apparatus (Fig. 1). Polaroid photographs in this case give good-quality images and are relatively cheap whereas multiformat cameras, another option, produce multiple images on ultrasound film at much higher cost.

M mode has significant application only in cardiology, in which it still remains the most widely used ultrasound technique for reasons of cost and for the accuracy of dimension measurements.

Two-Dimensional Images. By using a transducer constructed either with multiple parallel aligned crystals (linear array) or by rapidly rotating a single or multiple crystal mechanically or electronically through an arc of multiple positions (sector scanning), visual displays of tissue slices in motion can be obtained (Figs. 3A–D). This type of image is termed *real time*.

Alternatively, a single-beam transducer can be moved through an arc or over the skin, and with the aid of either a storage oscilloscope or digital

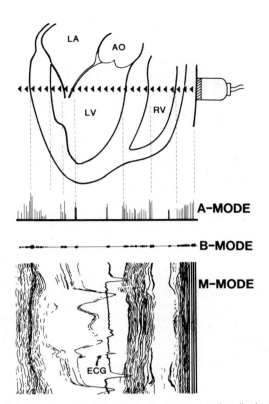

Figure 2. Echoes returning from the heart may be displayed along a horizontal axis representing tissue depth, either as spikes proportional in height to echo strength (A mode) or as points of light of varying intensity (B mode). M-mode images are created by adding a time dimension to the B-mode signals either on the oscilloscope or with light-sensitive paper on a chart recorder. (AO = aorta, LA = left atrium, LV = left ventricle, RV = right ventricle, ECG = electrocardiogram.)

circuitry a composite image of the plane examined can be displayed (Fig. 3*E*). This technique, widely used in human obstetric and abdominal examinations, does not permit real time images and is therefore of little value in cardiology. This system is sometimes called a *B-scan system*, and although it uses the B-mode dots to create the image, the two should not be confused.

Choice of Equipment. While simple M-mode echocardiographs are readily available, most ultrasound machines now on sale to veterinarians are the so-called real time variety. These machines acquire images using either linear array or sector-scanning transducers and circuitry. For two-dimensional echocardiography in the horse, sector scanners are essential because of the need to project the ultrasound beam between rib spaces and avoid attenuation by bone. Linear array scanners are more suitable for abdominal or rectal scanning. Sector scanning equipment is however generally more expensive owing to the complexity of the transducers. Some machines have both facilities and are

now becoming more readily available at reasonable prices. Most sector scanners are also sold with M mode and freeze-frame options, both highly desirable features for satisfactory echocardiographic examinations. Incorporation of a video taperecorder is also useful for obtaining hard copy of recording sessions (Fig. 1).

Transducers. A wide range of transducers is available for M-mode echocardiography at relatively low cost. For the horse's thorax a 2.25-MHz transducer is generally satisfactory although 1.8 MHz may be necessary for very large animals. High-frequency transducers provide better detail, but attenuation of the beam may prevent penetration to the left ventricular wall. In M mode, it is initially preferable to begin with a nonfocused transducer since structures are more easily detected with this type. However, focused transducers are preferable for accurate measurements since more limited divergence of the beam reduces the incidence of margin artifacts arising from objects lateral to the central beam axis.

For sector scanning the choice will probably be

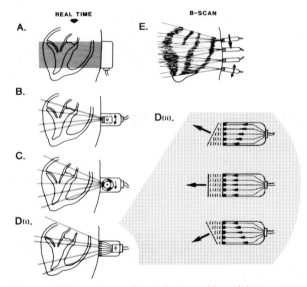

Figure 3. Various types of transducers, with real time systems illustrated in the left column. *A*, Linear array transducer made up of multiple parallel elements. *B*, Mechanically oscillating single transducer for sector scanning, with limited arc of movement (older type). *C*, Rotary sector scan transducer. Contains three- or four-element rotating head, providing variable sector angles from 45 to 120 degrees (most common system currently available). *D*(i), Phased array sector scan transducer containing 32 to 64 multiple elements cut from one piezoelectric crystal. *D*(ii), Phased array transducers operate on Van Huygen's principle, in which the angle of a wave front composed of multiple wavelets determines the direction of the single resulting sound wave. The ultrasound wave is made to oscillate rapidly in an arc by sequentially varying the arrival of the electrical impulses at each crystal element as illustrated. *E*, B-scan image obtained with a single transducer moved or rotated through an arc covering the organ of interest.

limited by the cost of the transducer, often a substantial proportion of the price of the apparatus. Once again 2.25 MHz is the ideal; unfortunately many sector scanners are only sold with standard transducers of 3.0, 3.5, or 5 MHz. It is important when considering sector scanning equipment for echocardiography to ensure that the transducer and amplifier permit imaging of the left ventricular free wall, which is sometimes 35 to 40 cm from the transducer. Most available apparatuses only permit imaging to depths of 20 to 25 cm. The maximum displayable depth is not only determined by the oscillation frequency of the crystal but also by the pulse rate of the transducer; for example, at 1000 pulses per sec (1 msec cycle) the maximum depth that can be displayed by the system is 75 cm, while at 2000 pulses per sec (0.5 msec cycle) it is 37.5 cm.

Doppler Echography. Doppler facilities are offered with some echocardiographs for blood flow measurements. Operating on the Doppler shift phenomenon produced when ultrasound waves are reflected from moving objects such as red blood cells, the technique is theoretically capable of providing noninvasive measurements of blood flow in major vessels or in the heart. Unfortunately technical difficulties in standardizing the procedure and obtaining meaningful measurements currently seriously restrict the clinical application of this technique.

ECHOCARDIOGRAPHIC TECHNIQUE

To obtain artifact-free echocardiograms requires a precise appreciation of the cross-sectional anatomy of the thorax and heart and a significant degree of learned skill in manipulating the transducer and controlling the settings of the recording apparatus, especially the gain and reject controls.

PREPARATION. It is an advantage to clip the skin over the site of examination. Acoustic coupling must also be provided between the face of the transducer and skin with proprietary gels liberally applied to the site. Gels made up from methyl cellulose are equally effective.

M Mode. For both M mode and sector-scan examination of the horse's heart, the recommended site for placing the transducer is on the right side at the fourth or fifth intercostal space at approximately the level of the olecranon. In this position there is no lung tissue interposed between the chest wall and the heart. It is helpful to have the right leg held forward. This position corresponds to the standard left parasternal "window" in humans in which the central beam traverses the chest wall, part of the right ventricle cavity, the interventricular septum, and then either the left ventricle or

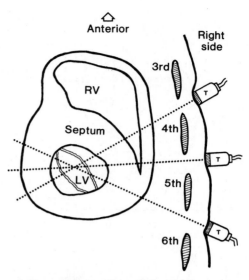

Figure 4. Transducer position relative to the heart and rib spaces in an adult horse, viewed from above. The diagram was drawn from a section of a horse's thorax frozen in situ, then sectioned in the horizontal plane. (*Note:* In the living animal the left ventricle will be very much larger, extending caudally over the fifth and sixth rib space.) (LV = left ventricle, RV = right ventricle.)

left atrium and aortic root depending on angulation of the beam (Figs. 4 and 5). From the fourth or fifth rib space the transducer should be angled inward and slightly backward. Initially the operator should attempt to find the mitral valve leaflets, very easily identified by their characteristic motion. In the normal animal they are identified as thin line densities rapidly flicking in and out of the plane of the beam, creating an M-shaped pattern on the tracing (Fig. 5C). By adjustment of the beam angle the anterior leaflet should be visible throughout the entire heart cycle, while behind it the posterior leaflet, less apparent, should produce the reversed pattern. At this level the septum should show as a broad density changing in thickness with each heartbeat. Behind the posterior mitral leaflet the left ventricular wall close to the atrioventricular ring is visible, and behind it the very echogenic pericardial reflection. If only the anterior mitral leaflet is identified, the anechoic space and wall echoes behind are part of the left atrium.

When the beam is directed further ventrally until the mitral valve leaflets disappear, the septal wall will appear to thicken slightly and the left ventricular wall will also appear to thicken appreciably. Within the left ventricular cavity dense line echoes close to the ventricular free wall are the *chordae tendinae*. In this position (that is, above the papillary muscles and below the thinner muscle bordering the atrioventricular ring), measurements of wall thickness and main left ventricular cavity dimen-

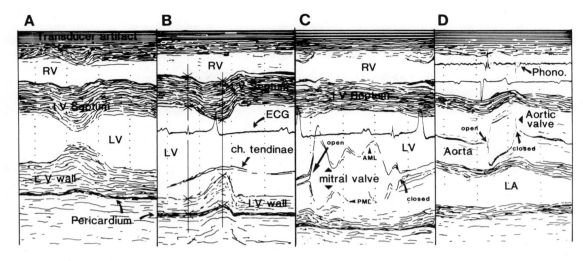

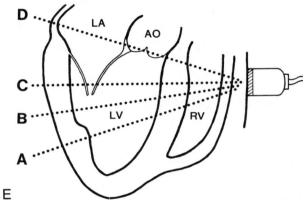

Figure 5. M-mode echocardiograms (*A–D*) obtained with the transducer orientated as in the accompanying diagram (*E*). *A*, Lower level of left ventricle through the papillary muscle. *B*, Standard position for measuring left ventricular dimensions between mitral valve leaflets and papillary muscles. Diastolic values are taken at the R-wave peak and systolic values at peak wall thickening as indicated by the vertical lines. *C*, Mitral position–The mitral valve is easily recognized by its characteristic motion. *D*, Aortic root study–The aortic semilunar valves are indicated. (Phono = phonocardiogram, ECG = electrocardiogram, LV = left ventricle, RV = right ventricle, LA = left atrium, AO = aorta, AML = anterior mitral valve leaflet, PML = posterior mitral valve leaflet.)

sions should be made (Fig. 5*B*). Farther downward angulation of the beam produces apparent thickening of the ventricle walls as the beam encounters the papillary muscles (Fig. 5*A*). Farther apically the left ventricular cavity disappears, the apex showing as a thick band on the M mode image.

If the beam is angled upward from the mitral position the outflow tract of the left ventricle becomes evident with the left atrium behind. Further dorsal angulation will show the densely echogenic walls of the aorta, easily recognized as two thick, dense lines moving in a sawtooth, parallel manner midway between the left atrium and the chest wall. Careful positioning of the transducer at the aortic root will show the aortic semilunar valves as a very thin line in midaorta during diastole, opening and closing very rapidly into a skewed parallelogram during systole (Fig. 5*D*).

Other positions for the transducer are possible in the horse, for example, from the left side. The reader is also referred to the standard human texts for detailed explanations of other techniques and the anatomic considerations for their use.

Sector or Two-Dimensional Scanning. Sector scanning images are initially easier to interpret than M mode patterns since the image displayed is a recognizable anatomic cross-section of the heart. Essentially the same position and technique of conducting the scans is employed except that instead of a single pencil-like beam, the sector, radiating in an arc from the transducer, demonstrates a slice of tissue that may vary not only according to the orientation of the axis but also the plane of the slice (Fig. 6).

Initially, the transverse plane through the heart at the level of the chordae tendinae is the easiest to recognize because the left ventricle is seen as a thick-walled circular structure, beating rhythmically. Slices in this plane may be examined by angling the transducer either toward the apex to demonstrate the chordae tendinae and papillary muscles or toward the base of the heart where the mitral valves, aorta, and pulmonic root become visible (Figs. 6*A* and 7*A*). If the transducer is then rotated 90 degrees on its axis, a series of slices of the heart along its long axis may be obtained. This

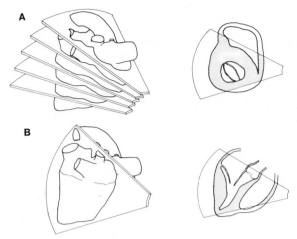

Figure 6. Two-dimensional scanning of the heart from the right side of the thorax with horizontal (A) and vertical orientation (B) of the sectors. On the right of the diagram representative slices obtained with each orientation are illustrated.

is also superior to images obtained with sector scanning, making it more accurate for size measurements, provided that structures are accurately identified and images are correctly interpreted. Simple M mode machines are also much cheaper than other types of echocardiograph. Their major disadvantage is the greater difficulty experienced in interpreting the images and being sure that artifacts are avoided, especially when dimensions are being measured.

Sector scan echocardiography has several advantages over M mode for clinical purposes. Visualization and recognition of the continuity of confluent structures is better, mass lesions are more easily demonstrated, and flow and distribution of contrast materials is more readily appreciated. However, it has the disadvantage of poor temporal resolution, making it of limited value for measuring the timing of events, and poor spatial resolution especially laterally, making measurement of dimensions less accurate. Improvements in design of transducers, especially the phased array types, will no doubt remedy some of these deficiencies. Sector scanners however are still relatively expensive.

view is extremely useful for demonstrating the mitral valve in profile, the left ventricular outflow tract, the aortic root, and the left atrium (Figs. 6B and 7B). In human cardiology the third orthogonal plane is displayed with the transducer placed over the apex of the heart to produce the "four-chamber view." This view is particularly valuable in contrast studies of congenital defects but is difficult to obtain in the horse.

Technique Comparison. M mode has the advantage of excellent temporal resolution for the timing of events, especially when ECGs are recorded simultaneously. Spatial resolution of M mode images

CLINICAL APPLICATION

Echocardiography provides the means of confirming the diagnosis of a number of cardiac conditions that by other clinical means would remain tentative. Several of these conditions in the horse have been described in some detail; however, the list is by no means exhaustive. The reader is therefore directed to the relevant human texts in the supplemental readings list since the same basic principles of

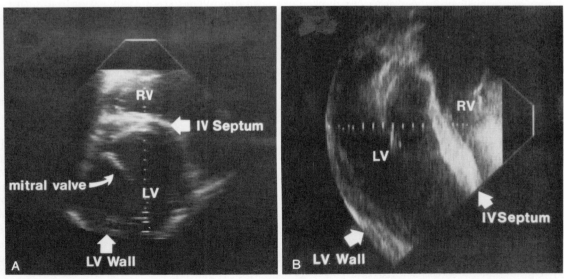

Figure 7. Sector scans of a normal horse's heart demonstrating the horizontal (A) and vertical planes (B). Major structures are labeled. (LV = left ventricle, RV = right ventricle, IV = interventricular septum.)

interpretation apply to all species. The key to accurate interpretation of echocardiographic images in any individual case rests heavily on understanding the exact anatomy of the section of the heart through which the beam has passed and understanding the physical changes produced in blood flow, valvular action, and cardiac dimensions in the pathologic processes under consideration.

In the assessment of murmurs, M mode echocardiography will often demonstrate the vibrating structure either generating the murmur or being acted upon by turbulence or abnormal flow patterns (Fig. 8). Similar turbulence is sometimes more difficult to appreciate with sector scanners. Examples of these conditions are:

1. Downward deviation and vibration of the anterior mitral leaflet by the backflow of blood into the left ventricular outflow tract in aortic regurgitation.

2. Vibration of the chordae tendinae during systole in mitral or tricuspid regurgitant murmurs (Fig. 8A).

3. Vibration of the chordae tendinae of the tricuspid valve septal cusp caused by flow of shunted blood in interventricular septal defects (IVSD) (Fig. 8B).

4. Vibration of the aortic semilunar valves in aortic outflow murmurs caused by small nodules on the cusp margins or as a result of anemia causing hemic murmurs (Fig. 8C).

Abnormal motion of the heart valves, especially the mitral valve leaflets, may be apparent in conditions such as prolapse of the mitral valves, atrial fibrillation, and vegetative bacterial endocarditis. In the latter, vegetations on the valves cause multiple dense echoes and apparent gross thickening of the mitral or tricuspid leaflets, with markedly reduced excursion of the leaflets. Care must be exercised, however, since inappropriate gain settings may lead to image artifacts mimicking this condition. Mass lesions such as vegetations are often easier to identify and measure on sector scans than with M mode.

Cardiac dimensions are often significantly altered in disease. Both M mode and sector scans allow direct measurements of wall thickness, cavity diameters, and aortic root dimensions for comparison with normal values. Although little published data are available at present for normal animals, more widespread use of echocardiography should provide appropriate figures in the near future. A correlative study in the horse has demonstrated the value of some M mode measurements for predicting wall thickness and heart mass; however, more studies of this kind are required to provide useful clinical data. Some conditions affecting the cardiac silhouette in the horse have been described such as enlargement of the aortic root and left atrium in aortic regurgitation. Pericardial effusion is also readily demonstrated on M mode or sector scans as a nonechogenic space between the ventricular walls and the densely echogenic pericardium.

CONTRAST ECHOGRAPHY

Echocardiography has revolutionized the diagnosis and study of congenital cardiac defects in both human and veterinary medicine. These improvements have been due not only to the characteristics of the ultrasound image but to the development of contrast techniques on the basis of injections of air microbubbles to opacify the normally anechoic heart cavities (Fig. 9).

Microbubbles are formed when certain fluids are injected into the bloodstream from a syringe and needle. Initially, cavitation at the needle tip was considered the most likely source of the bubbles, but more recent views favor the microbubbles being present in the injectate. Agents used vary according to personal preference of the clinician. Dextrose 5 per cent, 0.9 per cent saline, and the patient's own blood are readily available, cheap, and quite effective, especially if saturated with air by rapidly aspirating and injecting the solution in and out of the syringe just before injection. Indocyanine green dye is the most widely employed and one of the most effective agents by virtue of its surfactant qualities, which stabilize the microbubbles. However, it is expensive. For the horse, equal volumes of indocyanine green dye (5 mg per ml) with 0.9 per cent saline, to make 10 to 15 ml of injectate, have been recommended. Other agents such as carbon dioxide gas (1 to 3 ml in 5 to 8 ml of saline) and hydrogen peroxide (5 ml diluted 1:10) have been tested in other species, the latter with some adverse reaction.

Microbubbles injected into the blood are identified as dense clouds of echoes following the flow of blood through the heart (Fig. 9). Recirculation does not occur since bubbles larger than 8 to 10 microns in diameter lodge either in the pulmonary capillaries with venous injection or in the systemic capillaries if injected on the left side. Right-to-left shunting is easily diagnosed by injecting the contrast into a peripheral vein, or by catheter into the anterior vena cava, and watching the echoes appear in either the left atrium or the ventricle. However, most congenital defects in the horse involve left-to-right shunting. To demonstrate interventricular septal defect, the most common, requires either left ventricular catheterization or direct needle puncture of the heart.

Alternate ways of introducing the contrast material into the left circulation have been described. Pulmonary wedge injections in animals and humans

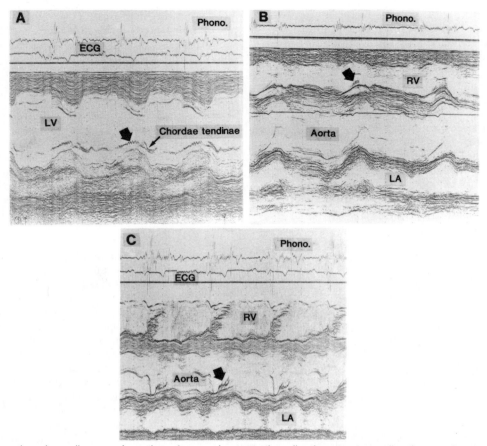

Figure 8. M-mode echocardiograms from three horses demonstrating vibrating structures directly associated with murmurs. Phonocardiograms are shown at the top of each record. *A,* Chordae tendinae vibration in mitral disease. *B,* Vibration of tricuspid chordae in interventricular septal defect with left-to-right shunt. *C,* Fluttering movement of an aortic cusp as a result of a small nodule on the valve margin causing a systolic outflow murmur. (ECG = electrocardiogram, LA = left atrium, LV = left ventricle, RV = right ventricle, Phono = phonocardiogram.)

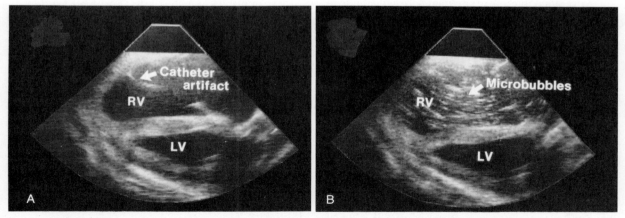

Figure 9. Microbubble contrast introduced into the grossly dilated right ventricle of a horse by catheter injection. *A,* Preinjection–the enlarged right ventricle is evident in the upper part of the echocardiogram. *B,* During injection microbubbles appear in the right ventricle but not in the left ventricle, indicating the absence of right-to-left shunt. Further echocardiograms in this horse revealed tricuspid insufficiency, with bubbles returning to the right atrium from the right ventricle. (RV = right ventricle, LV = left ventricle.)

with 7-gauge Swan-Ganz balloon-tipped catheters have resulted in sufficient contrast in the left heart to demonstrate left-to-right shunts. More recently newer agents, utilizing minimicrobubbles less than 10 microns in diameter capable of passing through the pulmonary capillary bed, have been developed. The most promising material on in vitro tests appears to be ultrasonically generated bubbles of a 70 per cent sorbitol solution with bubbles of a mean size of 6 microns. While the latter technique has yet to be tested on clinical cases, the potential for virtually noninvasive contrast scans of both left and right sides of the heart in the near future appears to be very promising.

NEGATIVE CONTRAST. Using sector scanning equipment, left-to-right shunts can sometimes be demonstrated with simple right-sided injection of the contrast agent. Contrast-free blood flowing across a shunt into a right-sided chamber filled with contrast medium will sometimes indent the echo-filled chamber with bursts of echo-free blood. Similarly, regurgitant or incompetent valves may be demonstrated by backflow of echo-free blood into a contrast-filled chamber.

LIMITATIONS

Operator skill in performing an ultrasound examination has an extremely important and direct influence on the quality of the image obtained. In addition because of the very subjective nature of interpreting images, especially in M mode, echocardiography is open to quite serious potential abuse. This is particularly so in the measurement of dimensions and attempts to predict performance potential from these measurements without adequate control data. Nonetheless, echocardiography has been shown to be a very valuable diagnostic aid in equine cardiology with the potential to become even more so with development of clinically applicable contrast techniques and accumulation of data on cardiac parameters.

Supplemental Readings

Bonagura, J.D., and Pipers, F.S.: Diagnosis of cardiac lesions by contrast echocardiography. J. Am. Vet. Med. Assoc., 182:396, 1983.
Chang, S.: Echocardiographic techniques and pattern recognition. Philadelphia, Lea & Febiger, 1976.
Feigenbaum, H.: Echocardiography, 3rd ed. Philadelphia, Lea & Febiger, 1981.
Morganroth, J., Parisi, A., and Pohost, G.M.: Noninvasive Cardiac Imaging. Chicago, Year Book Medical Publishers Inc., 1983.
O'Callaghan, M.W.: Comparison of echocardiographic and autopsy measurements of cardiac dimensions in the horse. Equine Vet. J., 17:361, 1985.
Pipers, F.S., and Hamlin, R.L.: Echocardiography in the horse. J. Am. Vet. Med. Assoc., 170:815, 1977.
Pipers, F.S., Hamlin, R.L., and Reef, V.: Echocardiographic detection of cardiovascular lesions in the horse. J. Equine Med. Surg., 3:68, 1979.
Reale, A.: Contrast echocardiography: Transmission of echoes to the left heart across the pulmonary vascular bed. Am. J. Cardiol., 45:401, 1980.
Roelandt, J.: Contrast echocardiography. Ultrasound Med. Surg., 8:471, 1982.
Wingfield, W.E., Miller, C.W., Voss, J.L., and Bennett, D.G., and Breukels, J.: Echocardiography in assessing mitral valve motion in 3 horses with atrial fibrillation. Equine Vet. J., 12:181, 1980.

Vectorcardiography

Peter W. Physick-Sheard, GUELPH, ONTARIO, CANADA

Applications of the ECG in clinical medicine include: (1) documentation and analysis of arrhythmias, (2) monitoring of heart rate during anaesthesia, intensive care, and exercise and training, and (3) detection and monitoring of changes in heart size, workload, or distribution of muscle mass. The first two can satisfactorily be achieved by the use of a simple bipolar lead (two electrodes, one positive, one negative). The only requirement in the selection of electrode positions is that the method used should provide a large, easily read deflection as free as possible from artifact and simple to apply in a consistent manner.

Uniformity in the choice of leads (electrode positions) allows rapid and accurate comparison between collection events and between horses. Limb lead II has traditionally been used for rhythm monitoring in the conscious animal. However, I have found the Y lead (positive electrode on the xiphoid, negative on the manubrium), to be very satisfactory, providing a large, easily read signal that is relatively free from muscle tremor and baseline drift. The diagnosis of arrhythmias may be assisted in some cases by the use of additional leads, particularly when low amplitude waveforms are difficult to discern from baseline noise, and in the further interpretation of ventricular arrhythmias. Any ECG machine can be used for these applications of electrocardiography in the horse simply by selecting one lead pair and setting the lead selection dial to the appropriate position.

MULTIPLE-LEAD SYSTEMS AND VECTORCARDIOGRAPHY

During electrical systole (myocardial depolarization) there is a constantly changing, three-dimensional or spatial pattern of electrical activity both within and surrounding the heart. Multiple-lead systems employ a variable number of electrode positions to view this pattern from several different directions. Information as to the probable magnitude and direction of wavefronts of myocardial depolarization can then be derived from the polarity and magnitude of the ECG signal and a knowledge of the location and polarity of electrodes. In clinical medicine the results are usually evaluated in scalar terms by measurement of the height (voltage) and duration of different waveforms in each of the leads. Abnormality is then expressed in terms of deviation from determined normal ranges. When the potential difference measured in each lead is resolved into vectors (either a single, two-dimensional resultant vector as in the use of the Bailey hexaxial system, or a series of instantaneous spatial vectors the tips of which describe a vector loop), the technique is described as vectorcardiography. Since scalar interpretations depend upon vectorcardiographic concepts, the term *vectorcardiography* is used here to refer to all applications of multiple lead systems other than their use in the evaluation of arrhythmias.

The majority of published information concerning equine vectorcardiography employs Einthovens' system of limb leads or systems derived therefrom. Adaptations involve the addition of electrodes on the dorsal midline or sides of the thorax to add a third dimension to the two-dimensional (horizontal) plane of the limb leads. Einthovens' system was not designed for the horse however and studies suggest major shortcomings in its ability to accurately detect the true pattern of electrical activity. A lead system specifically designed for use in the horse was developed by Holmes and Darke and Holmes and Else, and its clinical application reported upon. The system is referred to as semiorthogonal. More recent studies have identified some deficiencies in this system. Systems derived from limb leads such as that described by Grauerholz appear to lead to similar diagnostic conclusions as the semiorthogonal system but offer no advantage and are likely to be less sensitive.

In the clinical application of vectorcardiography many assumptions are made, notably that the pattern can be accurately measured by a minimal (manageable) number of body surface electrodes, and that changes in chamber size will be associated with detectable changes in the temporospatial distribution of electrical activity. In fact, the lead systems used never fully meet the electrical criteria upon which the technique of vectorcardiography is based, while the vectorcardiogram (VCG) is often a very insensitive indicator of chamber enlargement. The procedure of extracting scalar values and summaries from the ECG rather than instantaneous vectors introduces further error. Analysis therefore always involves significant approximation.

For accurate measurement of the VCG the distribution of electrodes should be based upon the true pattern of electrical activity. This approach is particularly important in the horse, because the majority of the ventricular myocardium depolarizes spontaneously and is electrically silent so far as the body surface ECG is concerned. Only the apical and basal third of the interventricular septum appears to make any significant contribution to the ECG. A change in chamber size may not necessarily influence the VCG pattern; therefore, in attempting VCG analysis it is extremely important that these shortcomings be kept in mind.

APPROACH TO VCG ANALYSIS

In humans the sensitivity and specificity of ECG changes for the diagnosis of changes in chamber size and load rarely exceed 60 to 70 per cent. This level of diagnostic accuracy has been achieved by the concurrent use of numerous diagnostic aids and the accumulation over many years of correlative data from large numbers of patients. In the horse variation in lead systems, small numbers of horses, limited exchange of information between referral centers, and lack of opportunity to apply many of the diagnostic procedures available in humans have precluded the establishment of dependable diagnostic criteria. While the literature contains a number of clinical papers in which VCG patterns derived from limb leads are related to clinical abnormality, the majority of publications that present normal ranges for scalar values for limb leads do not attempt to provide guidance in interpretation. Such guidance as is provided is mainly extrapolated from humans and can be reviewed by reference to any standard human text on electrocardiography. No comprehensive study of the diagnostic sensitivity and specificity of limb leads in the horse has been performed, and the diagnostic value of the technique is essentially unknown.

In terms of clinical correlation the most definitive studies have been performed by Holmes, using the semiorthogonal system, and Grauerholz, using a three-dimensional modification of the limb lead system. The findings I have made using the semi-orthogonal system are in general agreement with these earlier studies. These findings are briefly summarized below to stimulate interest in the application of the system in the hope that experience will help determine its clinical value. It must be emphasized that the specificity and sensitivity of the observations has not been determined and normal ranges are not yet established. There is considerable overlap in populations, and the influence of such confounding variables as age, breed, and sex has not been determined. Fundamental and presently unresolved questions regarding the validity of clinical vectorcardiography in evaluation of the QRS in the horse have been raised.

Practical Application. The semiorthogonal system is depicted in Figure 1, together with a listing of electrode positions. It consists of three bipolar leads, designated X, Y, and Z. For all except lead X the actual electrode can be a copper alligator clip permanently attached to the patient cable. For the X lead large electrodes are used to defeat proximity effects. I use 15 cm square anodized silver electrodes contoured to fit the triceps area and chest wall. Other workers have used small plate electrodes attached to both forelimbs (essentially lead I of the limb lead system).

To collect the three leads on a machine designed for limb leads (which includes almost all ECGs made for clinical use), the lead selection switch is set to lead I, when the black (left arm) cable will be the positive electrode, the white (right arm) cable the negative electrode. These two electrodes are attached with the polarity as shown in Figure 1 for each lead (X, Y, Z) in succession. The green (brown) ground cable may be attached somewhere over the shoulder and left there for each lead. The remaining electrodes are not used. The horse must stand square during recording. The floor should be dry and the horse should stand on a rubber mat to isolate it from the ground. Heart rate should ideally be in the resting range.

CLINICAL INTERPRETATION

Previous studies of the equine VCG have suggested that the extent to which electrical activity is directed backward may relate to the relative size of the left and right ventricles. In my study groups of

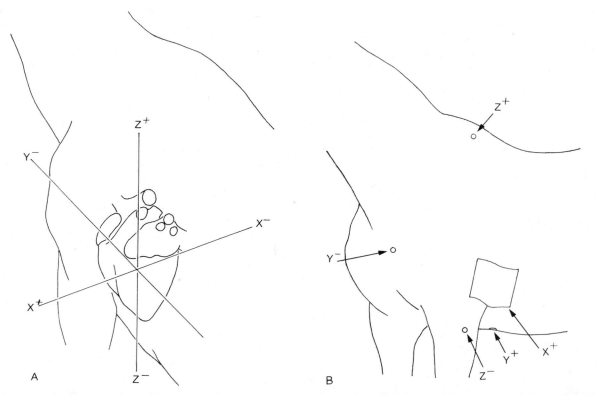

Figure 1. *A,* Theoretical relationship of lead axes to the heart and *B,* Electrode locations for the semi-orthogonal lead system. X⁺, left triceps area above elbow and adjacent thorax. X⁻, same area on the right side. Y⁺, ventral midline directly over the xiphoid cartilage. Y⁻, midline directly over the bony prominence of the manubrium. Z⁺, left side of the withers directly above the left forelimb. Z⁻, lateral aspect of the left forelimb directly over the bony prominence of the lateral tuberosity of the humerus at the elbow.

animals with clinical findings consistent with probable left ventricular hypertrophy (ventricular septal defect [VSD], mitral insufficiency, pandiastolic murmurs isolated to the aortic valve), showed a significantly higher incidence of extensive backward and leftward vectors than horses not so affected. In scalar terms this is equivalent to large Z_Q and Y_R, large Y_R/Y_S ratio, and prolonged duration of Y_R. Z_R tends to be small and the peak of X_R tends to occur with or just after the peak of Y_R. Z_Q is prolonged or occurs late so that the Z lead is still negative while Y_R is rising. Although the changes do not appear to result in any change in total QRS duration, there is a prolongation of the time to the maximum value of the Y lead (peak of Y_R), and minimum value of the Z lead (peak of Z_Q).

The VCG pattern for right ventricular change is undefined and cannot presently be separated from the effects of overall cardiac mass (see later discussion). Horses with large VSD with major left-to-right shunt and horses with severe chronic respiratory disease generally showed very limited Y_R or an absence of that waveform and variable Y_S. Cases of cor pulmonale tend to show large X_Q and Z_R and small or absent Y_R. Horses with severe respiratory distress show marked swings in conformation of waveforms.

The results from a small series of postmortem cases (n = 21) support the broad conclusions just outlined, but reveal the confounding effect of heart mass upon all associations. It would appear that absolute heart mass (regardless of body weight) may need to be used to control parameters before attempting to interpret the significance of changes in VCG pattern. The specificity and sensitivity of vector patterns for particular clinical conditions cannot be determined until a much greater amount of clinical and postmortem material has been examined. Definition of the relationship between VCG parameters and heart mass may allow regression techniques to be used in the detection of deviation from normal.

T-WAVE CHANGES

The T wave in the horse is notoriously labile, spontaneous changes occurring in the resting animal, often in response to environmental stimuli. Persistent changes in waveform and polarity are also found in apparently healthy animals and as of this writing cannot be consistently associated with any particular clinical entity. Despite its lability the waveform does tend to vary within limits, while the frequency of particular waveform conformations under a given circumstance allows inferences to be made as to the probable abnormality of observed changes. While such observations rarely have any

diagnostic specificity, their presence, in conjunction with the overall clinical picture, may help the clinician decide about further investigation or therapeutic intervention.

Resting, relaxed horses generally exhibit a biphasic (negative then positive) T wave in the Y lead (Y_T), with a similarly biphasic (though smaller amplitude) or negative waveform in the X lead. In the Z lead the T wave is usually low amplitude and may be negative, positive, or biphasic. In fully relaxed, normal horses, the negative component of Y_T may be greater in amplitude than Y_S. In such cases the ST segment is almost invariably positive (i.e., elevated above the isoelectric line). Y_T is rarely totally negative.

When the horse is not relaxed, in the case of electrolyte disturbance, in animals experiencing increased myocardial workload, and during many arrhythmias, the negative component of Y_T becomes smaller and the positive component larger, Y_T often becoming entirely positive. The presence of the relatively normal, biphasic, and predominantly negative T wave under such circumstances would thus be unusual. The T wave in the X lead usually remains biphasic or negative during nonspecific T wave changes, even when Y_T is positive. If the resting positivity of the Y lead is clearly associated with clinical disease, then increasing positivity of X_T is often found. These changes are usually associated with minimal or inconsistent changes in Z_T. Under conditions of severe myocardial stress (myocardial failure, hypoxia), X_T and Y_T both become large and positive. A large, positive X_T is rarely seen under normal resting conditions.

Under anesthesia Y_T is usually positive. Under conditions of hypotension or hypoxemia the wave may become distinctly spiked, not necessarily in association with tachycardia. A negative Y_T is sometimes seen under anesthesia, occasionally in animals that subsequently get into difficulties. The precise significance of the change is unclear.

The changes described are not necessarily associated with changes in heart rate. However, significant change in the T wave does occur as heart rate increases. In scalar terms the change consists of increasing positivity of Y_T to a tall, spiked T wave. At the same time the ST segment becomes less elevated, then blends into the S and T waves. X_T similarly becomes progressively more positive.

During postexercise deceleration T wave changes vary. An overshoot has been described in which Y_T becomes more negative than at rest, slowly returning to normal as heart rate falls. The magnitude of this overshoot is less if the horse is recovering from steady-state as opposed to short-term exercise. In some animals the overshoot may be absent, the positive Y_T of exercise returning smoothly to the resting conformation. It has been suggested that exercise-related changes in T-wave polarity will subside within four minutes in most horses, although return to normal amplitude is unlikely to occur until heart rate approaches normal. The relationship between exercise and T-wave changes requires further investigation.

P-WAVE CHANGES

In scalar terms the P wave in the horse is most often bifid (showing two peaks) and positive in the Y lead and the X lead, and bifid and negative in the Z lead. In many cases an early negative component to Y_P will be observed. The two peaks of Y_P, usually referred to as P_1 and P_2, can be loosely related to the pattern of atrial depolarization, P_1 arising during depolarization of the right atrium and the cranial edge of the left atrium, P_2 mainly arising during depolarization of the left atrium.

Interpretation of P-wave changes is complicated by simultaneous depolarization of areas of both atria. Caution is also required since some horses exhibit variations in P-wave conformation in the absence of clinical signs. In some cases these changes are intermittent, and are described as *wandering pacemaker*. In other cases they are persistent, e.g., a biphasic negative then positive waveform, or a monophasic, positive Y_P.

It has been observed that increased magnitude of P_2 can occur in association with left atrial enlargement in cases of mitral insufficiency, and that P_2 may become more positive in the X lead and smaller in the Z lead in chronic respiratory disease, although once again the sensitivity and specificity of these changes has not been investigated. Cardiac pathology has not been convincingly associated with P-wave changes in the horse and at this time the diagnostic value of the waveform is undetermined. However, the associations between P-wave changes and left and right atrial enlargement generally accepted in humans and the dog appear to hold in the horse, although atrial pathology needs to be quite advanced before P-wave changes become diagnostic.

HEART SCORE

The heart score theory proposes a relationship between heart mass and QRS duration whereby aerobic work capacity can be predicted. This theory has found application in man, the greyhound, and the horse. The probable validity of the mass-to-duration relationship has been demonstrated, as has the confounding influence of numerous variables, in particular age, breed, sex, and pattern of depolarization. The effect of the latter and its relationship to cardiac mass suggest a means of increasing the predictive power of the relationship.

However, although cardiac work capacity is a major determinant of aerobic capacity, numerous other variables must be taken into consideration in the evaluation of race potential. Adherence to a single measurement is naive and an oversimplification` of the situation. It has been demonstrated repeatedly that the predictive power of the theory as currently applied is very limited. It should be used only with great caution, and with allowance being made for confounding variables.

Supplemental Readings

Grauerholz, G.: Untersuchungen uber den QRS-Komplex im EKG des Pferdes. Berl. Munch. Tierarztl. Wschr., 93:301, 1980.

Holmes, J.R.: Spatial vector changes during ventricular depolarization using a semi-orthogonal lead system—A study of 190 cases. Equine Vet. J., 8:1, 1976.

Holmes, J.R., and Rezakhani, A.: Observations on the T wave of the equine electrocardiogram. Equine Vet. J., 7:55, 1975.

Lalezari, K., and Kroneman, J.: Comparison of different lead systems in the horse. Proceedings of the Fifth Meeting of the Academic Society for Large Animal Veterinary Medicine, Glasgow, 1980, p 65.

Muylle, E., and Oyaert, W.: Atrial activation pathways and the P wave in the horse. Zentralbl. Veterinaermed., 22:474, 1975.

Muylle, E., and Oyaert, W.: Equine electrocardiography: The genesis of the different configurations of the "QRS" complex. Zentralbl. Veterinaermed., 24:762, 1977.

Physick-Sheard, P.W., and Hendren, C.: Heart score: Physiological basis and confounding variables. *In* Snow, D.H., Persson, S.G.B., and Rose, R.J. (eds.): Equine Exercise Physiology. Cambridge, Granta Editions, 1983, pp. 121–134.

Steel, J.D.: Studies on the Electrocardiogram of the Horse. Sydney, N.S.W., Australasian Medical Publishing Co., 1963.

Fetal Electrocardiography

Christopher M. Colles, NEWMARKET, ENGLAND

Fetal electrocardiography in the mare is a simple technique to confirm the presence of twin fetuses, to confirm that a fetus is alive, and to monitor the fetus for signs of distress such as may occur during protracted foaling. In addition it may be of value for confirmation of pregnancy in small horses. Although the first recordings of fetal electrocardiograms were made in 1921, detailed descriptions were not reported until 1977 and 1978.

RECORDING TECHNIQUE

Only a bipolar lead system is required. This may be a specialized monitoring system, or alternatively a conventional four-lead electrocardiogram (ECG) apparatus may be used, making use of only two of the four leads. The electrodes are positioned in the midline on the midlumbar region of the back and in the midline 15 to 20 cm in front of the udder. This latter electrode may be placed to the left hand side of the midline if this is preferred. It is normally easiest to use hand-held electrodes with a fairly large surface area (3-cm diameter is ideal). Smaller electrodes are more difficult to hold and maintain good contact with the skin. Self-adhesive electrodes can be used quite satisfactorily. The skin under the electrodes should be clipped and degreased using 70 per cent alcohol. A normal electrode gel is used to give good contact. Self-adhesive electrodes are satisfactory for short periods, but when monitoring protracted parturition, sweating of the mare may cause these electrodes to detach. This can be overcome by using a standard human antiperspirant spray over the area where the adhesive contacts the skin, masking off the area of electrode contact.

When a standard ECG machine is used, the "left arm" electrode should be used in the dorsal position and the "left leg" electrode in the ventral position. A sensitivity of 20 mm per mV minimum and a chart speed of 25 mm per second are recommended. With most equipment, it is not necessary to use a ground lead to the mare; however, practical circumstances and the type of equipment used may make this lead necessary.

RESULTS

Using the system described, both the maternal and fetal ECG will be recorded. The amplitude of the maternal electrocardiogram can be modified by repositioning the electrodes, rotating them around the trunk of the mare. The minimal maternal influence is seen when the electrodes are placed almost horizontally across the abdomen. Because of difficulty in interpreting the significance of some deflections on the trace, however, it is generally recommended that the maternal P, QRS, and T waves should be located on the trace and marked off at their regular intervals before location of the fetal QRS complex is attempted (Fig. 1).

Usually the P and T waves of the fetal ECG are not visible, except shortly before term (when the T wave is occasionally seen). The QRS complex is seen as a distinct regular deflection. It may be positive, negative, or bipolar, depending largely on the position of the fetus. Early in pregnancy (150 to 200 days) the fetal deflection is normally bipolar, and occasionally spontaneous reversal of the fetal cardiac vector may be detected without alteration in the fetal position. Late in gestation the deflection is usually of opposite polarity to the maternal QRS complex but tends to be at least slightly bipolar. The maternal heart rate rises slowly through pregnancy and the fetal heart rate decreases (Fig. 2).

The amplitude of the fetal ECG is extremely variable and is affected by many factors. Amplitude becomes greater in later stages of pregnancy. The spatial arrangements of the fetus relative to the electrodes is important; at the present time it is not possible to relate amplitude to any clinical findings. A marked increase in the size of the fetal deflections has been seen as the fetal chest engages the birth canal in second-stage labor. This is thought to be normal if it is not persistent. The birth of the fetus should follow rapidly at this point.

Although pregnancy has been confirmed with electrocardiography as early as the 42nd day of gestation, pregnancy diagnosis before the 150th day is not recommended because a number of false negatives will result. The detection of fetal heartbeats even at 150 days may be difficult, and if no fetal deflection is evident it is recommended that the mare be given gentle exercise (walking and trotting when led in hand) for 5 to 10 minutes before a further trace is made. This will often result in repositioning of the fetus and a detectable fetal heartbeat. Twin fetuses may be detected by the presence of two fetal QRS complexes. The heart rate of the two fetuses is invariably different. Slight differences in position result in fetal deflections of different size or character, giving pairs of peaks that converge and separate along the trace (Fig. 1).

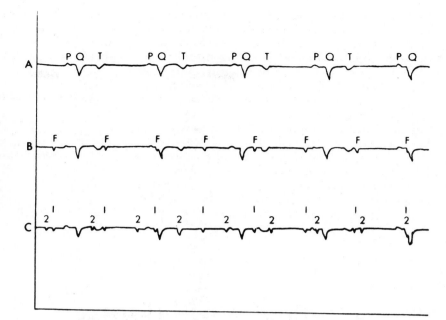

Figure 1. Diagrammatic appearance of fetal electrocardiographic traces. *A,* Nonpregnant; *B,* Singleton pregnancy; *C,* Twin pregnancy; *P,* Maternal P wave; *Q,* Maternal QRS complex; *T,* Maternal T wave; *F,* Singleton fetal QRS complex; *1,* Twin 1 fetal QRS complex; *2,* Twin 2 fetal QRS complex.

SIGNIFICANCE OF FETAL ECG FINDINGS

Tachycardia. Fetal tachycardia is a heart rate of more than twice the standard deviation from the mean for the defined stage of gestation (Fig. 2).

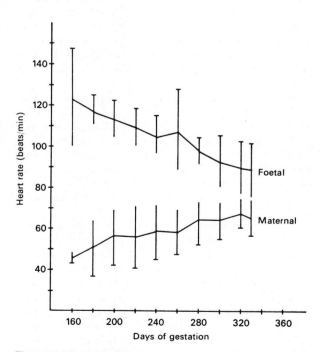

Figure 2. Mean maternal and fetal heart rates through normal pregnancy in pony mares.

Intermittent fetal tachycardia is a frequent finding after 150 days' gestation. It is a normal finding associated with periods of fetal activity, often occurring at similar times of day on successive days. Gentle exercise of the mare returns the fetal heart rate to normal.

During parturition persistent fetal tachycardia is abnormal. Although it is not generally seen in natural parturition, during induced first stages of labor with strong maternal contractions, fetal tachycardia may be recorded. Transient tachycardia is probably not significant. Heart rates of up to 200 beats per minute are probably not clinically important, provided that they are present only for short periods (up to one minute). A heart rate of 300 beats per minute has been associated with fetal maladjustment syndrome after birth.

A transient tachycardia is probably present in all fetuses in the latter part of second-stage labor, as the fetal chest is engaged in the pelvic canal of the mare. A marked increase in the size of the deflections of the fetal ECG has also been seen at this point. A persistent tachycardia, with a heart rate rising slowly for two hours or more, is probably a sign of fetal distress. It has been associated with abortion in Thoroughbred and pony mares. In twin pregnancies, persistent tachycardia of one fetus should be regarded as evidence of distress to that fetus, and may be followed by fetal death.

Fetal Bradycardia. Fetal bradycardia is five consecutive heartbeats of more than two standard deviations below the mean heart rate for a stated stage of gestation (Fig. 2). Bradycardia is abnormal and has been seen following tachycardia in an aborting mare. During normal foaling some slowing of the fetal heart rate is seen, but bradycardia does not develop. Bradycardia during foaling should be regarded as a sign of fetal distress and appropriate action taken according to the clinical circumstances. This may mean assisting parturition or carrying out cesarean section.

Fetal Cardiac Arrhythmia. Fetal arrhythmia has been associated with fetuses that have subsequently aborted, but has also been seen in normal pregnancies. The arrhythmia consists of two fetal QRS complexes in quick succession (usually about 0.12 seconds between the deflections). The possibility that an apparent arrhythmia is due to failure to detect a fetal deflection or interference from some external source must be ruled out very carefully. If an arrhythmia is confirmed, then the pregnancy should be regarded as being at risk.

Supplemental Readings

Colles, C.M., Parkes, R.D., and May, C.J.: Fetal electrocardiography in the mare. Equine Vet. J. *10*:32, 1978.

Hon, E. H.: The electronic evaluation of the fetal heart rate. Am. J. Obstet. Gynecol. 75:1215, 1958.

Norr, J.: Foetale elektiokardiogramme vom Pferd. Z. Biol., 73:123, 1921.

Parkes, R.D., and Colles, C.M.: Fetal electrocardiography in the mare as a practical aid to diagnosing singleton and twin pregnancy. Vet. Rec., *100*:25, 1977.

Cardiac Arrhythmias

Ronald W. Hilwig, TUCSON, ARIZONA

The most important consideration in the treatment of cardiac arrhythmias in horses is an accurate diagnosis of the arrhythmia coupled with an assessment of its significance. Corrective therapy should not be attempted without first determining the probable cause of the arrhythmia. The horse has a relatively higher incidence of cardiac arrhythmias at rest than other domestic livestock species owing primarily to autonomic nervous system influences. Arrhythmias in a healthy resting horse should not immediately be looked upon as abnormal, since autonomic-induced arrhythmias almost invariably disappear when the heart rate is elevated by exercise, excitement, or administration of anticholinergic drugs. Numerous organic diseases and underlying physiologic imbalances as well as myocardial disease may precipitate resting cardiac arrhythmias. Frequently, treatment of the primary disease or correction of imbalances corrects the arrhythmia.

Postexercise or excitement alterations in cardiac rhythm, excluding simple increased heart rate, should be viewed with suspicion, especially if accompanied by reduced performance, weakness, or dyspnea. Many changes occur in normal electrocardiogram (ECG) waveforms at increased heart rates, and these must not be confused with abnormalities. A thorough ECG examination must include tracings obtained at rest, immediately after exercise, and during the cool-down period, since some arrhythmias may be evident only transiently or during one of these periods.

The majority of arrhythmias are initially detected by careful auscultation of the patient, and some can be adequately diagnosed by this means alone. Signs and symptoms that may accompany an abnormal cardiac arrhythmia include lack of exercise tolerance and poor performance, labored breathing, pulmonary edema, ascites and dependent edema, abnormal arterial pulses, and jugular vein pulsations. A thorough physical examination should be performed on the animal suspected of having an abnormal heart rhythm.

The most reliable means of diagnosing normal and abnormal cardiac arrhythmias is with the ECG. Treatment, if any, should be deferred until the ECG and physical examinations are completed. A simple single-channel recorder is adequate for routine arrhythmia diagnosis. Chart speeds of 25 mm per sec and 50 mm per sec are preferable, but a single speed of 25 mm per sec will suffice for most cases.

If the limb leads are used, muscle tremor and subtle shifting movements to maintain body position may result in ECG recordings that are of little value. Various "monitor" leads have come into use for evaluation of cardiac electrical activity. These have the advantages of minimizing movement artifacts and allowing the generation of relatively larger waveforms. One such lead system that I have found satisfactory places the right forelimb electrode on the right side of the neck along the jugular groove about one third of the way up the neck from the

TABLE 1. DURATION IN MILLISECONDS OF ECG WAVEFORMS AND INTERVALS FROM NORMAL ADULT HORSES AND PONIES

	P Wave	P–R Interval	QRS Complex	Q–T Interval
Horses				
Range	80–200	220–560	80–170	320–640
Mean	140	330	130	510
Ponies				
Range	85–106	209–226	66–86	420–483
Mean	100	217	78	462

torso. The left forelimb electrode is placed on the ventral midline under the apex of the heart. Alligator clips, preferably copper, are used with suitable electrode paste to attach the electrodes to the skin. The ground electrode (right hindlimb) may be placed at any site remote from the heart. Lead I is selected on the recorder. This monitor lead has the advantages of being relatively indifferent to limb position and positional changes and provides large amplitude waveforms that allow the sensitivity of the recorder to be reduced, thereby reducing muscle tremor artifacts. All tracings below, except Figure 5C, were recorded using this monitor lead. Figure 5C utilized the conventional Lead I.

The duration of ECG waveforms and time intervals for normal adult horses and ponies are shown in Table 1. All time durations are shortened at higher heart rates. Resting ECG durations should be determined at heart rates greater than 22 but less than 50 beats per min. Resting rates outside these limits should be considered as bradycardia and tachycardia, respectively, except in ponies, which may have resting rates exceeding 50.

Postexercise or excitement alterations in the ECG include increased amplitude and peaking of the P and T waves, shifting of T wave polarity, and deviation of the S–T segment. Figure 1 shows the normal resting ECG and the changes following exercise. The S–T segment usually slopes toward the initial limb of the T wave. S–T segment deviations greater than 0.2 mv above or below baseline in the resting ECG are considered abnormal and may indicate myocardial hypoxia or electrolyte imbalances. Deviations greater than this may be seen in postexercise or excitement tracings.

DETECTION AND SIGNIFICANCE

SUPRAVENTRICULAR ARRHYTHMIAS

Sinus Arrhythmia (Fig. 2). This normal resting arrhythmia appears on the ECG tracing as a varying P–P or R–R interval and missed beats. This arrhythmia is attributed to waxing and waning of vagal tone and is abolished by increased heart rates or admin-istration of anticholinergic drugs such as belladonna alkaloids (e.g., atropine).

Wandering or Shifting Atrial Pacemaker (Fig. 2). This arrhythmia appears as a progressive or abrupt alteration in P wave contour that may be accompanied by changes in the P–R interval. Sinus arrhythmia or missed beats or both may accompany this condition. The wandering pacemaker cannot be detected by auscultation, but the missed beats are diagnosed as a silent period during the time a beat is expected. Occasionally the fourth (atrial) heart sound alone can be heard during a missed beat. While some authors consider this condition abnormal, most believe that it is a normal shifting of the pacemaker within the sinoatrial node. Approximately 30 per cent of normal resting horses exhibit this wandering pacemaker, but during excitement or exercise when vagal tone is overridden, it is abolished. No treatment is indicated with either sinus arrhythmia or wandering atrial pacemaker.

Supraventricular Premature Beats (Figs. 3 and 9). Spontaneous discharge of a pacemaker located within the SA node, the atria, or the atrioventricular junction before the normal pacemaker discharges may elicit a supraventricular premature beat. The P wave may or may not appear and be different from normal, but the QRS complexes are similar to those of the basic rhythm. The P wave may be superimposed on the trailing edge of the preceding T wave, thereby distorting its configuration. SA node and atrial premature beats are not usually followed by a compensatory pause, although atrioventricular junction premature beats may occasionally be followed by a compensatory pause. Most authors view this condition as being indicative of cardiac disease.

Careful auscultation can detect the presence of premature beats, but the focus of origin cannot be determined without use of the ECG machine. Most premature beats of supraventricular origin result in first and second heart sounds of less than normal intensity. The arterial pulse for the premature beat is weaker than normal, and the beat following the premature beat may produce a pulse of increased amplitude.

Tachycardias (Fig. 3). Short bursts of supraventricular premature beats are termed paroxysmal nodal, atrial, or junctional tachycardia. If the tachycardia persists, the term paroxysmal is dropped. These conditions can be detected by auscultation as an abrupt change in heart rate accompanied by rapid and relatively weak arterial pulsations. The differentiation between supraventricular and ventricular origin cannot be made by auscultation alone. The supraventricular tachycardias are indicative of myocardial disease or electrolyte imbalances predisposing to atrial fibrillation and should be treated to prevent its onset.

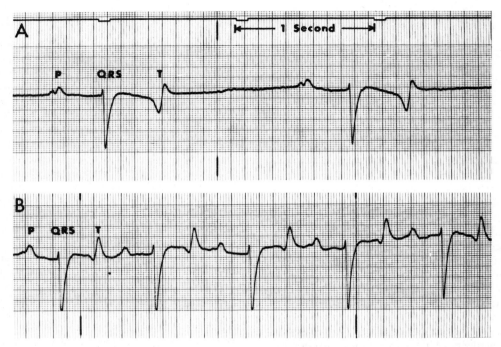

Figure 1. Recording from a normal horse at a resting heart rate of 33 BPM (*A*) and the same horse after light exercise at a rate of 80 BPM (*B*). At increased heart rates, all time intervals and waveforms are abbreviated, and the two positive components of the P wave are less evident. The T wave has lost much of its negative component and is of higher positive amplitude. Paper speed 50 mm per sec.

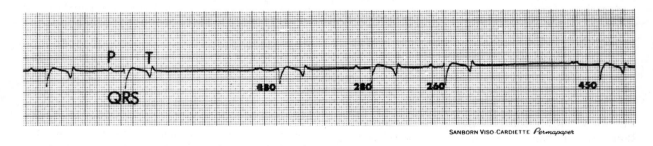

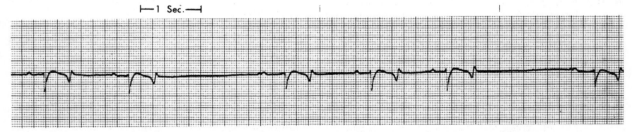

Figure 2. Continuous recording from a normal horse showing sinus arrhythmia and wandering atrial pacemaker. This rhythm was correlated with respiratory activity. The long pauses between sets of three beats occurred during expiration. The P–R (P–Q) interval, shown in milliseconds, is longest on the beat following the pause, and the P wave configuration is much different for that beat. One might argue that SA block had occurred during the long pause, since another beat would almost fit perfectly into the rhythm during this period. The simple surface ECG recording could not detect this condition if it occurred. Paper speed 25 mm per sec.

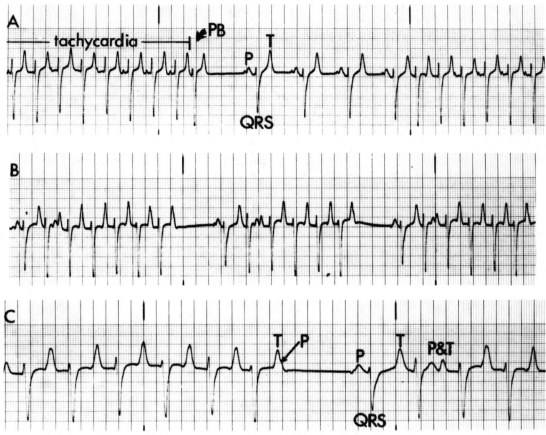

Figure 3. Supraventricular tachycardia. Tracing *A* (paper speed 25 mm per sec) shows paroxysmal atrial tachycardia with a heart rate of 180 BPM, with a short period of relatively rapid sinus rhythm having a heart rate of 80 BPM, followed again by the tachycardia. A supraventricular premature beat (PB) interrupts the tachycardia and is followed by a compensatory pause, which allows the sinus node pacemaker to capture the rhythm for four beats before another supraventricular premature beat precipitates a bout of tachycardia. Tracing *B* shows atrial tachycardia with a heart rate of 160 BPM interrupted by an occasional sinus beat. Tracing *C* was recorded at twice the speed (50 mm per sec) as *B* to show the P wave superimposed upon the T wave preceding the sinus beat. The P wave blocked the tachycardia pacemaker and allowed the sinus node to capture the ventricle for a beat before the atrial pacemaker assumed control again. Note the P wave between the QRS complex and T wave of the first post-sinus beat.

Atrial Fibrillation (Fig. 4). Atrial fibrillation is characterized by an absence of discrete P waves preceding each QRS complex. The P waves are replaced by fine, coarse, or variable atrial waves known as F waves, flutter waves, or fibrillation waves. The frequency of occurrence of these waves may be as high as 500 per minute. The ventricles are not able to respond this frequently, and the QRS complex occurs irregularly at 50 to 120 beats per minute at rest. Occasionally a relatively slow but irregular QRS frequency of 25 to 35 beats per minute may appear with this arrhythmia. At higher ventricular rates, S–T segment deviation from baseline and T wave peaking may be observed on the ECG. A variable intensity of heart sounds, absence of the fourth (atrial) heart sound, an irregular heart rate, and arterial pulsus alternans and pulse deficit are usually observed with this condition. Occasion-

ally this arrhythmia produces a relatively regular heart rate, but no fourth heart sound is heard on auscultation. Some horses at rest have no outward signs of the arrhythmia, whereas others exhibit dyspnea, dependent edema, ascites, and jugular pulsations. Animals with atrial fibrillation have reduced exercise or work performance, and this is sometimes the only complaint that initiates the cardiac examination.

An unfavorable prognosis should be given if a murmur of atrioventricular valve insufficiency is auscultated in the presence of this arrhythmia. Occasionally, atrial fibrillation develops for no apparent reason or is secondary to organic disease or electrolyte imbalance. Most horses with this type of fibrillation can be converted to sinus rhythm, and many will return to equal or better than pre-arrhythmia performance. Those with valvular dis-

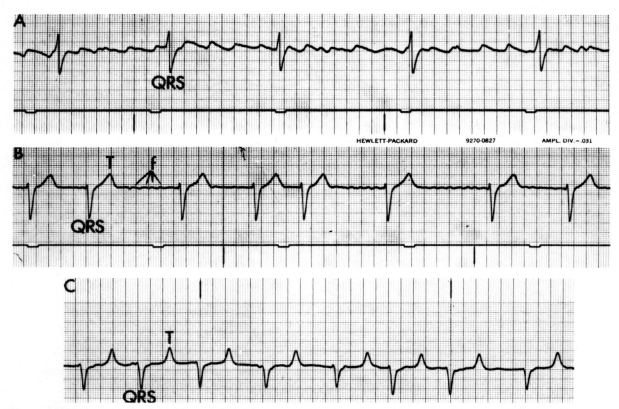

Figure 4. Tracings of atrial fibrillation from three different horses showing the variability of this arrhythmia. Tracing *A* shows coarse undulations of the baseline, which represent the electrical activity of the atria. QRS complexes occur at quite regular intervals at 60 BPM. T waves cannot be distinguished from the atrial waves. Tracing *B* shows fine undulations of atrial activity and a relatively fast, irregular heart rate of approximately 98 BPM. Both QRS complexes and T waves are readily observed. Tracing *C* shows atrial fibrillation with almost no baseline undulations of atrial origin and a rapid, quite regular heart rate of 120 BPM. QRS complexes and T waves are well defined. Paper speed in all tracings was 50 mm per sec.

ease–caused fibrillation may be more difficult to convert to sinus rhythm and have a relatively higher incidence of reverting to atrial fibrillation.

Cases of paroxysmal atrial fibrillation have been reported in young racehorses. They performed poorly in a race and were found to be fibrillating immediately afterward. They converted to sinus rhythm within 24 hours. Some then returned to normal performance. The incidence of this condition in racehorses is unknown.

Atrioventricular (AV) Block (Figs. 5 and 6). This arrhythmia takes three major forms: (1) first degree, which is seen as a prolonged P–R interval; (2) second degree, in which some P waves are not followed by a QRS complex; and (3) third degree, in which P waves and QRS complexes occur independently from each other. First-degree AV block is due to waxing and waning of vagal tone. Second-degree block is of two types, type 1 or Wenckebach phenomenon and type 2. The type 2 block is uncommon and appears as a missed QRS complex without impending ECG signs. The type 1 block is characterized by progressive lengthening of the P–R in-terval until a P wave is not followed by a QRS complex. Minor variations of this progressive-type block have also been reported. The first postblock beat is characterized by a decreased Q–T interval and diminished T wave amplitude and high-ampli-tude arterial pulse. The missed beats are detected on auscultation as described previously. If missed beats appear infrequently, no treatment is indi-cated, since this is thought to be vagally induced. First- and second-degree blocks normally disappear at elevated heart rates.

Third-degree AV block is a pathologic condition characterized by a relatively slow heart rate that may not be altered by excitement or exercise. Pauses between beats of three to 50 seconds have been observed, and fainting or staggering bouts may occur especially upon exertion. The QRS com-plexes may appear quite normal or may be bizarre, depending upon the location of the pacemaker. First and second heart sounds are altered only minimally, if at all. In some cases, discrete fourth (atrial) sounds are audible but are not correlated with the first and second sounds. Cardiac diseases cannot always be demonstrated in animals with this arrhythmia, and treatment is frequently unsuccessful.

Ventricular Arrhythmias

Ventricular Premature Beats (Fig. 7). Spontaneous discharge of a latent pacemaker located in the specialized conduction tissue of the interventricular septum or ventricular myocardium results in a bizarre-appearing ventricular ECG waveform. Premature ventricular beats appear earlier than expected and are characterized by prolonged and relatively large QRS and T waves. The beat may be either interpolated, wherein it falls between two normal beats (a true extrasystole), or noninterpolated, wherein the abnormal beat is followed by a compensatory pause with little or no change in heart rate. The origin of the premature beat may be determined by the polarity of the QRS complex. Using the monitor lead system described previously, a beat originating from the right ventricle will have a positive QRS complex, and one originating from the left ventricle will have a negative QRS complex. Presence of ventricular premature beats at rest is indicative of myocardial disease or cellular electrolyte imbalances. This arrhythmia is frequently noted during inhalation anesthesia, especially if surgery is being performed on the gut for obstruction or torsion.

Auscultation alone is not sufficient to differentiate this arrhythmia from supraventricular premature beats, although several circumstances may suggest a ventricular origin. In many cases, the extraventricular beat results in louder than normal first, second, or first and second heart sounds, and the arterial pulse is weak or absent. Compensatory pauses more frequently accompany ventricular premature beats than atrial premature beats. The first beat following the premature ventricular beat produces louder than normal heart sounds and a stronger than normal arterial pulse. Premature supraventricular beats frequently produce less than normal intensity first and second heart sounds and only a slight change in arterial pulse amplitude on the first beat following the premature beat. These circumstances are only

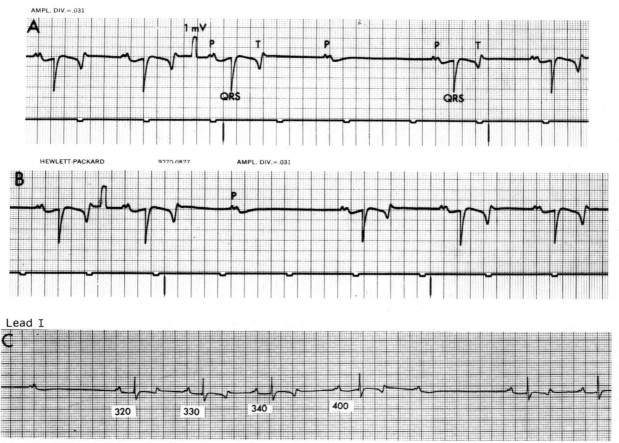

Figure 5. Tracings *A* and *B* are continuous and show type 2 second-degree atrioventricular block wherein the electrical signal from the atria is not conducted to the ventricle. This type of block has no pattern and appears as a random P wave that is not followed by a QRS complex. Tracing *C* shows type 1 second-degree atrioventricular block, which is characterized by an increasing P–R (P–Q) interval (shown in milliseconds) until a P wave is not followed by the QRS complex. Paper speed 25 mm per sec.

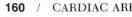

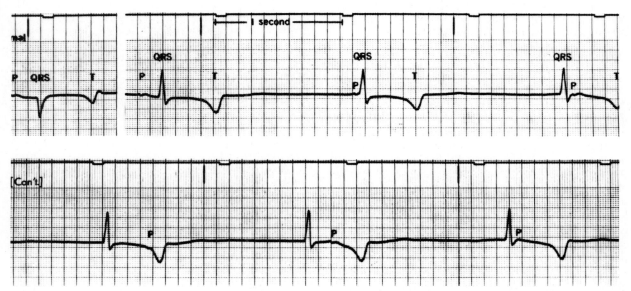

Figure 6. Continuous recording showing complete or third-degree atrioventricular block. A normal waveform is shown as a reference on the upper left. P waves occur at regular intervals but are not conducted to the ventricle. A right ventricular focus has assumed pacemaker function at a relatively fixed rate of 40 BPM. Paper speed 50 mm per sec.

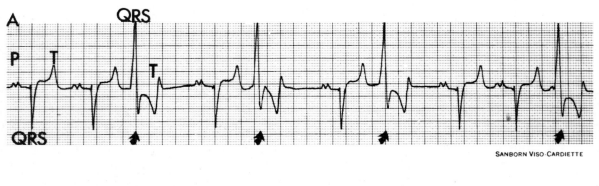

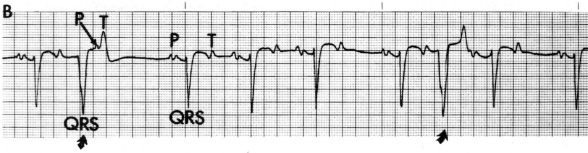

Figure 7. Tracing *A* shows ventricular premature beats or extrasystoles (*arrows*) originating from the right ventricle. The QRS complexes of these ectopic beats are large and wide and are followed by a large, opposite-polarity T wave. Tracing *B* shows ventricular premature beats (*arrows*) originating from the left ventricle. The QRS complexes of the ectopic beats are large and wide and are followed by a large, opposite-polarity T wave. The ectopic beat on the left of this tracing is noninterpolated, since it is followed by a compensatory pause, whereas the ectopic beat on the right of this tracing is interpolated and does not disrupt the basic rhythm. Paper speed 25 mm per sec.

presumptive, and ECG diagnosis must be established prior to treatment if any is to be undertaken.

Ventricular Tachycardia (Fig. 8). Short or long bursts of ectopic ventricular depolarizations may periodically appear on the ECG tracing. This condition, known as paroxysmal ventricular tachycardia, may be accompanied by premature ventricular beats. If long-standing over several seconds or minutes, the term paroxysmal is dropped. Paroxysmal ventricular tachycardia and ventricular tachycardia are ominous signs of cardiac disease and predispose to ventricular fibrillation, a terminal event. During a bout of tachycardia, the ECG may show occasional P waves, normal QRS complexes, and fusion beats (a normal beat superimposed upon an ectopic beat) that are inscribed during a relatively quiet period of electrical activity. The ectopic focus of activity may be unifocal or multifocal, giving one or more types of ventricular waveforms. Multifocal ventricular tachycardia is highly suggestive of myocardial

disease but also appears as a result of a combination of inhalation anesthetic administration and electrolyte imbalance. This arrhythmia must be treated vigorously to prevent its progression to ventricular fibrillation. Auscultation alone cannot differentiate this condition from paroxysmal supraventricular tachycardias since both are heard as abrupt changes in heart rate. More frequently in a ventricular-induced tachycardia, the first and second heart sounds become much louder and the heart rate much higher than in supraventricular-induced tachycardias. Exceptions to this generality, of course, exist.

Ventricular Fibrillation (Fig. 8). This arrhythmia is terminal, and all organized electrical and contractile activity of the heart ceases. The ECG shows irregular oscillations of varying amplitudes and frequencies. No heart sounds are heard, and arterial pulsations are absent. Treatment other than electrical defibrillation is universally unsuccessful.

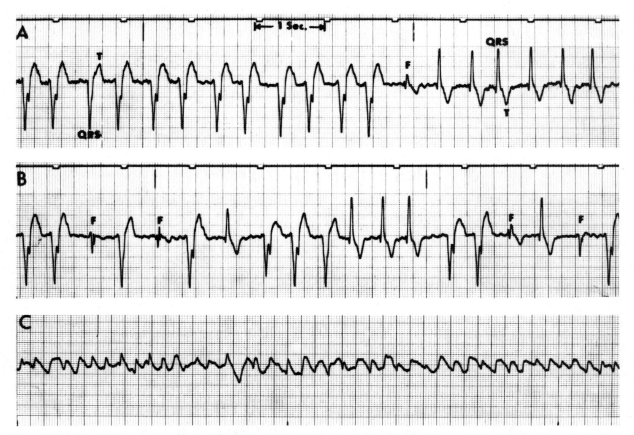

Figure 8. Tracing *A* illustrates ventricular tachycardia from a left ventricular focus in the left two thirds of the tracing. A fusion beat (F) is seen at the end of this section of the recording wherein two pacemakers discharged at the same time, giving rise to two different ventricular waveforms that summated in the fusion beat. Immediately following this beat, a right ventricular pacemaker assumed control, resulting in tachycardia. Tracing *B* shows multifocal ventricular tachycardia with fusion beats interspersed. A suggestion of P waves or other atrial electrical activity can also be observed on the baseline and T waves in both tracings. Tracing *C* shows ventricular fibrillation in which no organized activity occurs. Paper speed 25 mm per sec.

COMPLEX ARRHYTHMIAS

Complex arrhythmias with several ECG abnormalities are also seen occasionally (Fig. 9). Multiple pacemaker sites can be demonstrated by the variations in waveforms. These types of arrhythmias may pose a therapeutic problem, since it is sometimes difficult to determine which particular arrhythmia is most significant and what agent should be employed without making the condition worse.

TREATMENT

Treatment of abnormal cardiac arrhythmias is not always successful and may be only temporary. Arrhythmias may arise secondarily to another disease state that, when corrected, will result in spontaneous disappearance of the arrhythmia. The potential hazards of treatment must be weighed against those of not treating, and the subsequent decision should be made jointly with the owner and attending veterinarian. After initiation of therapy, the arrhythmia sometimes appears worse for a period before it gets better and therefore requires good judgment and confidence in diagnosis and choice of therapeutic agents. Frequent ECG evaluation and clinical monitoring must accompany the antiarrhythmic therapy, especially in complex arrhythmias, to guard against undesired outcomes.

It is assumed in this section on therapy that most conditions that could have precipitated cardiac arrhythmias have been corrected or ruled out by careful clinical examinations or assessment of what was being done to the animal at the time. Unless otherwise stated, dosages have been calculated for the adult 450 kg horse and should be adjusted as necessary on the basis of the weight of the animal being treated.

QUINIDINE

Quinidine sulfate has been used to treat ventricular arrhythmias, including frequent supraventricular premature beats, paroxysmal atrial tachycardia, atrial tachycardia, and atrial fibrillation, frequent ventricular premature beats or extrasystoles, paroxysmal ventricular tachycardia, and ventricular tachycardia. Possible undesirable side effects from the administration of quinidine include swelling of the nasal mucosa, which may become extensive enough to close off the nasal passages, development of urticarial wheals, laminitis, gastrointestinal upset, cardiovascular collapse, atrioventricular block or other arrhythmias, and sudden death. For these reasons, a small test dose of 5 gm is administered orally to observe adverse reactions, if any, before treatment is undertaken. Quinidine should not be given to animals that are showing signs of advanced congestive heart failure or those having atrioventricular block on the ECG. The negative inotropic effects on the myocardium and the slowed atrioventricular conduction time resulting from quinidine therapy may accentuate both of these conditions. Digitalis glycosides have been used prior to, or simultaneously with, quinidine in congestive states. The glycosides have a positive inotropic action upon the myocardium, but they should not be used in the presence of advanced second degree or complete atrioventricular block. Limited experience indicates that intravenous dihydroquinidine gluconate or quinidine gluconate can be used successfully to abolish arrhythmias, but because of their greater toxicity hazard, they should not be used for long-term therapy.

Several therapeutic regimens using quinidine have been employed to abolish arrhythmias, and the choice depends upon the circumstances. Two methods are presented here as starting points only.

ORAL ADMINISTRATION OF QUINIDINE SULFATE (BY STOMACH TUBE OR IN LARGE GELATIN CAPSULES)

Method 1

Day 1: 5 gm test dose
Days 2 and 3: 10 gm twice a day
Days 4 and 5: 10 gm three times a day
Days 6 and 7: 10 gm four times a day
Days 8 and 9: 10 gm every five hours
Day 10 and thereafter: 15 gm four times a day

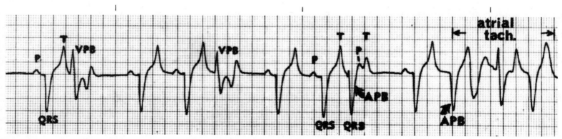

Figure 9. This tracing shows a variety of abnormalities, including ventricular premature beats (VPB), atrial premature beats (APB), and atrial tachycardia as well as some normal sinus beats. Paper speed 25 mm per sec. (From Hilwig, R.W.: Cardiac arrhythmias in the horse. J. Am. Vet. Med. Assoc., *170*:153, 1977.)

Method 2

Day 1: 5 gm test dose

Day 2: 10 gm every two hours until a total dose of 80 gm or less has been given.

Once the arrhythmia is abolished the total dose can be reduced by one half every two days until a maintenance dose that prevents re-establishment of the arrhythmia is reached. In cases of atrial fibrillation, quinidine administration can usually be discontinued one or two days after conversion to sinus rhythm. Oral doses of quinidine exceeding 40 gm per day predispose to undesirable side effects.

INTRAVENOUS ADMINISTRATION OF QUINIDINE GLUCONATE OR DIHYDROQUINIDINE GLUCONATE

These preparations are about 10 times more soluble in water than the sulfate form and should be diluted to a 1 per cent solution in glucose or physiologic saline solution for intravenous administration via slow drip at a rate not exceeding 40 to 50 ml per minute. Very frequent ECG monitoring is required, and administration should be stopped if the P–R interval or QRS complex elongates beyond 125 per cent of the pretreatment values. Atrial fibrillation has been reported to convert to sinus rhythm after a total of 5 to 20 gm of intravenous quinidine. If a maintenance dose is required, the animal should receive oral quinidine sulfate.

Some arrhythmias, particularly paroxysmal atrial tachycardia, may transiently appear to get worse before getting better, but for the confident and courageous, continued administration of quinidine often results in beneficial effects on cardiac rhythm.

PROPRANOLOL

Some investigators have employed propranolol for controlling tachyarrhythmias. Its quinidine-like action and beta-adrenergic blockade properties may result in slowed atrioventricular conduction time and reduced myocardial contractility. For these reasons, it should not be used in the presence of advanced atrioventricular block or congestive heart failure. Digitalis glycosides have been used in conjunction with propranolol in congestive states to overcome negative inotropic effects. The efficacy of propranolol therapy is dependent upon the intrinsic adrenergic activity at the time of administration, and the beneficial results are thus not predictable. Propranolol has not received the high acclaim of quinidine in converting atrial fibrillation to sinus rhythm. Beneficial results are obtained using propranolol for controlling ventricular extrasystoles and tachycardias, and it is quite effective in slowing ventricular rate even in the presence of atrial fibrillation.

ORAL ADMINISTRATION OF PROPRANOLOL

Days 1 and 2: 175 mg three times a day

Days 3 and 4: 275 mg three times a day

Days 5 and 6: 350 mg three times a day

INTRAVENOUS ADMINISTRATION OF PROPRANOLOL

Days 1 and 2: 25 mg twice a day

Days 3 and 4: 50 mg twice a day

Days 5 and 6: 75 mg twice a day

Atropine (0.045 mg per kg) should be available for intravenous administration in the event of excessive ventricular slowing or atrioventricular block.

LIDOCAINE

The local anesthetic lidocaine may be employed as an antiarrhythmic agent for short-term control of some arrhythmias and as a relatively simple presumptive diagnostic aid in differentiating a supraventricular tachyarrhythmia from a ventricular tachyarrhythmia. Do not use preparations of lidocaine that contain epinephrine. An intravenous bolus of 1 to 1.5 mg per kg is usually temporarily effective in slowing ventricular rate during a bout of ventricular tachyarrhythmia but has no such effect on a supraventricular tachyarrhythmia. This fact allows its use for presumptive diagnosis when an ECG is unavailable. The antiarrhythmic effects are lost within a few minutes. Convulsions have been reported to occur after administration of a bolus of lidocaine. A slow intravenous drip of lidocaine is useful in controlling ventricular arrhythmias that may develop during some surgical procedures involving the gastrointestinal tract or extensive muscle trauma.

DIGITALIS GLYCOSIDES

Digitalis glycosides have been used successfully for the treatment of congestive heart failure and for certain cardiac arrhythmias. The best antiarrhythmic responses occur with supraventricular tachyarrhythmias, since the glycosides slow atrioventricular conduction and thus effect ventricular slowing. Atrial fibrillation does not convert to sinus rhythm with these drugs; in fact, atrial electrical activity may increase, but the reduced ventricular rate and increased contractility of the myocardium often result in remission of signs of congestive heart failure. Signs of digitalis intoxication include increased P–R interval and atrioventricular block, prolongation of the QRS complex, and additional cardiac arrhythmias, particularly ventricular extrasystoles. Mental depression, lack of appetite, and diarrhea may also indicate intoxication.

ORAL ADMINISTRATION OF DIGITALIS GLYCOSIDES

Digitalization is accomplished by five to six doses at eight-hour intervals. The dose is dependent upon the product used. Powdered digitalis or digitoxin is given at 0.03 to 0.06 mg per kg, digoxin at 0.06 to 0.08 mg per kg, or digitalis tincture at 0.3 to 0.6 ml per kg. These dosages may be increased by one fourth to one half every two days until the arrhythmia is abolished or signs of intoxication develop. The daily maintenance dose after digitalization usually consists of one eighth to one fourth of the digitalizing dose.

INTRAVENOUS ADMINISTRATION OF DIGITALIS GLYCOSIDES

Rapid digitalization may be effected by intravenous administration of 2.5 to 3.0 mg of ouabain every one and one half to two hours until heart rate slows, a total dose of 10 mg has been given, or signs of intoxication develop. Frequent ECG monitoring is required during this interval. When digitalization has been achieved, a maintenance dose not to exceed one fifth of the digitalizing dose may be used. Usually oral administration of another digitalis glycoside is used for maintenance. Daily doses of digitalis should be adjusted as dictated by clinical and ECG signs.

ATROPINE

This drug is usually employed as a diagnostic or short-term palliative agent to remove parasympathetic influences on the heart to effect increased heart rate. It will usually abolish first- and second-degree atrioventricular blocks and bradycardias that are vagally induced but is not effective in increasing the rate of idioventricular rhythm in the event of third-degree atrioventricular block. Long-term administration is not done because of the undesirable side effects, which include drying of mucous membranes and alterations in gastrointestinal motility and secretory activity. The parenteral dose is 0.045 mg per kg.

Supplemental Readings

Amada, A., and Kurita, H.: Five cases of paroxysmal atrial fibrillation in the racehorse. Exp. Rep. Equine Health Lab., No. 12, 89–100, 1975.

Buss, D. D., Rawlings, C. A., and Bisgard, G. E.: The normal electrocardiogram of the domestic pony. J. Electrocardiog., 2:229, 1969.

Hilwig, R. W.: Cardiac arrhythmias in the horse. J. Am. Vet. Med. Assoc., 170:153, 1977.

Proceedings Academy of Veterinary Cardiology: Standards for Equine Electrocardiography. Boston, 1977.

Senta, T., Smetzer, D. L., and Smith, C. R.: Effects of exercise on certain electrocardiographic parameters and cardiac arrhythmias in the horse. A radiotelemetric study. Cornell Vet., 60:552, 1970.

Acquired Disorders of Cardiac Blood Flow

Christopher M. Brown, EAST LANSING, MICHIGAN

When evaluating an equine heart the veterinarian faces a major challenge: What is the significance of abnormal auscultatory findings? There is usually no problem if a murmur is extremely loud or widely radiating or if an arrhythmia is extremely bizarre and frequent. The problem exists when the changes are subtle. In these situations horses rarely have sufficiently severe problems to warrant euthanasia, and hence are rarely available for detailed necropsy examination. Currently it is unknown how clinical findings, athletic performance, and necropsy findings are related for horses. Holmes and Else established the incidence of cardiac lesions in 1557 horses consigned for slaughter. They auscultated them prior to death and correlated their pre- and post-mortem findings. However, they had no clinical histories and therefore had little or no data available to establish the clinical significance of their findings. This study, however, is the most extensive undertaken in order to solve the clinician's dilemma. Ideally, a study encompassing all aspects of the cardiovascular evaluation would include history, physical findings, detailed cardiologic findings including ECG, and echocardiograms, and finally a detailed necropsy examination. The lack of such a comprehensive study leaves many questions unanswered. As a result, much of what follows is based on opinion and speculation, and at times is necessarily vague.

The methods used to evaluate the equine heart are covered in other parts of this section, and in the previous edition of this book (pp. 121–126). The majority of acquired flow disorders in horses are detected, or suspected, on the basis of auscultatory findings. This section deals with the etiology, evaluation, and significance of murmurs arising from these flow disorders. They will be considered primarily under two separate groups, systolic murmurs and diastolic murmurs. This division is somewhat artificial but reflects the presentation of the problem, rather than a more formal consideration of the diseases of each valve individually.

SYSTOLIC MURMURS

Intracardiac phonocardiographic studies in horses have shown that flow in the aortic root and pulmonary artery is sufficiently turbulent to produce ejection murmurs. Some of these probably radiate to the chest surface and may be audible over their respective sites. It is my impression that similar murmurs, over the pulmonic valve, are more common in horses with chronic lung disease, and may be a product of the altered right-sided hemodynamics in these horses. Turbulence in the aortic root is probably the origin of the ejection murmur detected in some severely anemic horses.

In 1557 horses, Holmes and Else found 356 with valvular lesions. Of these 74 had a single valvular lesion, and systolic murmurs were detected from mitral incompetence in 15, from tricuspid incompetence in 6, and from aortic stenosis in 21. No case of valvular pulmonic stenosis was recorded as a source of a systolic murmur. In addition, 22 horses with systolic murmurs had lesions of both the mitral and aortic valves, and the origin of the murmur could not be determined. This series of systolic murmurs varied in intensity, but all were audible at some location on the left thorax, and many were also audible on the right. The location of the site of maximum intensity gave some indication of the possible origin of the murmur.

The majority of systolic murmurs detected in horses are associated with mild chronic valvular changes. The murmurs are usually low in intensity and fairly localized. Clinical signs associated with these valvular lesions, and their resultant murmurs, are generally very vague and difficult to confirm. Many animals are presented with a history of poor or reduced athletic performance, but others have no history suggestive of abnormal cardiac function. It is often very difficult to determine the significance of these abnormal cardiac sounds, and ancillary aids (ECG, echocardiogram) may not shed any further light on the situation. In general, a soft localized murmur probably arises from a less severe lesion than a loud, widely radiating murmur. However, since many variables can affect the audibility and radiation of a murmur, this is only a rough guide.

It is wise to make an exhaustive search for other reasons for reduced performance before ascribing the blame to a low-amplitude localized systolic murmur.

On the other hand a loud, widely radiating systolic murmur will develop with severe mitral insufficiency resulting from rupture of the chordae tendineae of the mitral valve. This is apparently a fairly rare event but has been well documented, and produces an apparently consistent clinical syndrome. At the time of rupture there is often sudden onset of respiratory distress, presumably due to the development of severe pulmonary edema. There is a loud, widely radiating systolic murmur, often with a palpable thrill. The persistent pulmonary hypertension eventually leads to right heart failure and resulting peripheral venous congestion with edema. Some horses have a persistent cough and markedly reduced exercise tolerance. Not all cases involve severe signs. One horse was reported to have atrial fibrillation, presumably secondary to the left atrial distention that resulted from the mitral regurgitation. Echocardiographic assessment of the mitral valve may identify the lesion. Once their condition is diagnosed, little can be done for these horses. Diuretics may help reduce the pulmonary edema, but the long-term prognosis is poor.

The pathophysiologic findings in seven horses with mitral insufficiency have been described in detail. Three had signs of left and right heart failure, and of these, two had atrial fibrillation. The signs in these three cases were similar to those described in cases involving ruptured mitral chordae tendineae. The other four horses had less severe signs, although one had atrial fibrillation. Hemodynamic abnormalities were marked in the first three horses, with elevated left ventricular end-diastolic pressures, pulmonary hypertension, and elevated right ventricular pressures. The other four cases had essentially normal intracardiac pressures. At necropsy all had intact mitral chordae tendineae but all had moderate to severe mitral valvular lesions typically thickening and rounding of the free borders of the valve. Four animals had jet lesions in the left atrium. In addition, the three severely affected horses had evidence of tricuspid dysfunction.

Systolic murmurs may be detected in cases involving clinical signs suggestive of valvular endocarditis. However, these murmurs may not appear until late in the course of the disease, and other clinical signs may predominate. These will vary depending upon the valve or valves involved; they include recurrent fever, venous distention, and laboratory data consistent with a chronic infection. A blood culture may be positive if taken during a febrile episode. Echocardiographic assessment may also be helpful in suspected cases. Although aggressive appropriate antibiotic therapy may bring about temporary remission of some of the signs, confirmed cures are rare.

Occasional and unusual lesions may develop that give rise to systolic murmurs. These include rupture of the roots of the great vessels, particularly the aorta. This may be associated with sudden death or if the animal survives the development of aneurysms that cause turbulence and audible murmurs. In addition, there may be signs of severe cardiovascular dysfunction.

In the horses examined by Holmes, 23 had isolated mid to late systolic clicks on auscultation with no other abnormal noises. These horses had no visible cardiac lesions at necropsy. The origin of these clicks has not been determined, but they appear to be benign, and should not be considered as evidence of significant cardiac disease.

DIASTOLIC MURMURS

These could potentially arise from pulmonic or aortic incompetence, or from stenosis of the atrioventricular valves. In horses, the commonest cause by far appears to be acquired aortic incompetence, and this was detected in 32 animals by Holmes' group. An additional 17 horses had diastolic murmurs and had lesions of both the aortic and mitral valves. Thus the murmur could have arisen from either aortic incompetence or mitral stenosis. Pulmonic incompetence and tricuspid stenosis appear to be rare causes of diastolic murmurs in horses.

The murmurs of aortic incompetence vary. They are often pandiastolic but may end in middiastole. There may be presystolic accentuation of the murmur following atrial contraction. In some cases the murmur is not present during every cardiac cycle. The nature of the murmur also varies from one horse to another. In some the murmur is musical, almost a pure tone, but in others the murmur is very noisy and contains a wide range of frequencies. The very noisy, widely radiating murmurs are usually associated with more severe lesions than the musical tonal ones.

The murmurs are usually audible over the area of the left ventricle on the left, and often on the right side of the thorax as well. Clinical signs vary, but many athletic horses have reduced performance. The impact of the aortic valvular dysfunction depends upon several factors, including the severity of the lesion, the rate in which it develops, and the expected use of the horse. In some animals there may be no significant effect from the lesion, while in others it may render the animal unsuitable for its intended purpose. Auscultation is still the most valuable means for assessing the significance of a diastolic murmur, although the use of the semiorthogonal lead ECG may be of some value in assessing the change in heart size that could ensue from aortic incompetence (see page 147).

In some young horses, particularly racehorses, a diastolic noise is often detected. It occurs in early diastole and is possibly an accentuated third heart sound. The colloquial name "three-year-old squeak" adequately describes the nature of this noise. It is not associated with any clinical problems and appears to become inaudible when the animals mature.

The aortic valve and others may be involved in vegetative endocarditis, and diastolic murmurs may ensue. As in the case when systolic murmurs arise from endocarditis, signs may vary and will be similar to those described in the section on systolic murmurs.

Supplemental Readings

Brown, C.M., and Holmes, J.R.: Phonocardiography in the horse: I. The intracardiac phonocardiogram. Equine Vet. J., *11*:11, 1979.
Brown, C.M., Bell, T.G., Paradis, M-R., and Breeze, R.G.: Rupture of the mitral chordae tendineae in two horses. J. Am. Vet. Med. Assoc., *182*:281, 1983.
Else, R.W., and Holmes, J.R.: Cardiac pathology in the horse. 1. Gross pathology. Equine Vet. J., *4*:9, 1972.
Else, R.W., and Holmes, J.R.: Cardiac pathology in the horse. 2. Microscopic pathology. Equine Vet. J., *4*:57, 1972.
Holmes, J.R., and Else, R.W.: Cardiac pathology in the horse. 3. Clinical correlations. Equine Vet. J., *4*:195, 1972.
Holmes, J.R., and Miller, P.J.: Three cases of ruptured mitral valve chordae in the horse. Equine Vet. J., *16*:125, 1984.
Miller, P.J., and Holmes, J.R.: Observations on seven cases of mitral insufficiency in the horse. Equine Vet. J., *17*:181, 1985.
Wagenaar, G., Kroneman, J., and Breukink, H.: Endocarditis in the horse. Blue Book Vet. Prof., *12*:38, 1967.

Congenital Disorders of Cardiac Blood Flow

Christopher Button, ONDERSTEPOORT, REPUBLIC OF SOUTH AFRICA

INCIDENCE AND ETIOLOGY

The incidence of congenital disorders of cardiac blood flow in horses is low in comparison with that found in other domestic animals. In one survey four cases were diagnosed in approximately 2500 equine necropsies, giving an incidence of one in 625. Since a percentage of foals born with these defects probably die in the perinatal period without diagnosis, the true incidence may be higher than this figure indicates. Likewise, when inbreeding has occurred, one might expect the incidence to increase.

The etiology of equine congenital cardiac blood flow disorders has not been established scientifically. Increasing incidence with inbreeding and apparent over-representation of the Arabian breed in published case reports make it likely that genetic factors are involved. The possible role of embryonic viral infection and teratogenic xenobiotics has not thus far been established. Morphogenesis of the equine heart is complete by the 49th day of gestation so that, to induce such disorders as ventricular septal defect, tetralogy of Fallot, and tricuspid atresia, potential agents would have to be active before this time. Congenital disorders such as patent ductus arteriosus occur when prenatal flow channels fail to close postnatally. The latter defect could be influenced by maternal and fetal factors occurring in late gestation or by factors affecting foals soon after birth.

DIAGNOSIS

In humans, and to a lesser extent in dogs and cats, it is important to diagnose and categorize these cardiac defects so that appropriate therapeutic and surgical procedures can be instituted. For the following reasons, however, it is doubtful whether surgical correction can be justified in horses:

1. Assuming a possible genetic basis for some lesions, it is possible that defects could be propagated if surgically "cured" animals are used for breeding.

2. In most instances the cost of surgery far exceeds the value of the patient.

3. Given that surgical teams seldom perform open heart surgery on horses, the probability of successful correction of lesions is low. In the available literature no instances of successful cardiac surgery in horses could be found.

The importance of recognizing congenital cardiac flow disorders in horses can be summarized as follows:

1. Horses with such congenital disorders must be distinguished from normal horses with innocent signs that may mimic some congenital disorders, as in foals and horses with innocent flow murmurs.

2. Individuals with established congenital cardiac disorders can be prevented from breeding, and repeat mating between two individuals that have produced a foal affected by these conditions can be avoided.

3. Diagnosis of the exact nature of the disorder will permit an accurate prognosis and rational choices concerning the future of affected animals.

It is beyond the scope of this chapter to detail all the methods used in the diagnosis of congenital cardiac flow disorders. Table 1 lists the modalities that may be employed. Many of the procedures listed can be used in private veterinary practices. Techniques such as selective angiography and echocardiography are best left to veterinary institutions with the necessary equipment and expertise.

VENTRICULAR SEPTAL DEFECT

Ventricular septal defect (VSD) is the most common equine congenital cardiac disorder. The defect is usually high in the septum just below the aortic valve on the left and opens under the septal leaflet of the tricuspid valve on the right. A number of complex defects include a VSD. These are described elsewhere. The following discussion refers to isolated VSD.

When there is a VSD, the usual flow pattern is from the left ventricle to the right ventricle, resulting in pulmonary overperfusion and volume overload of both ventricles. In rare instances pulmonary hypertension severe enough to reverse the shunt may occur, so that blood flows from the right to the left ventricle. Pulmonary hypoperfusion and cyanosis then result.

Horses with a small-diameter VSD may be well grown and, apart from a murmur, asymptomatic. The majority of affected animals are stunted and in poor condition. Exercise tolerance is usually reduced and respiratory distress or even syncope may follow exertion. A grade III or IV or louder holosystolic murmur is audible on both sides of the

TABLE 1. MODALITIES USED IN DIAGNOSING CONGENITAL DISORDERS
OF CARDIAC BLOOD FLOW

Item	Evaluate and Record
1. Signalment	Owner details, patient individual markings, breed, age, sex, color.
2. Anamnesis	*Patient ancestry:* breeding, affected siblings or ancestors.
	Patient signs: age when noted, coughing, dyspnea, exercise intolerance, growth rate, staggering, syncope.
	Dam influences: diseases, vaccinations, deworming, other treatments during early pregnancy.
3. Clinical examination	*Observation:* respiration, bodily condition, discharges, mucous membranes, veins, dependent edema.
	Palpation: arterial pulse, cardiac impulse left and right, thrills.
	Auscultation: both lung fields; mitral, aortic and pulmonic areas on left side; tricuspid area on right side; cardiac rate, rhythm, intensity of sounds; murmurs grade I–V, systolic, diastolic, continuous; point of maximal intensity.
4. Radiography	*Lateral view:* cardiomegaly, chamber enlargement (left atrial or ventricular), increased prominence of ascending aorta, increased or decreased pulmonary vascular markings.
5. Laboratory aids	*Hemogram:* anemia or polycythemia, leukocytosis.
	Carotid blood: oxygen saturation, oxygen tension, acid-base status.
	Serum biochemistry: Liver, kidney function.
6. Electrocardiography	Leads I, II, III, aVR, aVL, aVF, V10, CV6LU, CV6LL, CV6RU, CV6RL, semiorthogonal lead Y.
	Cardiac rate, rhythm, duration/amplitude of P wave, PQ interval, QRS complex, S–T segment, T wave on lead II (young foals in right lateral recumbency, others standing).
7. Phonocardiography	Mitral, aortic, pulmonic and tricuspid areas, various frequencies, atrial sound, first, second and third heart sounds, "shape" and timing of murmurs.
8. Cardiac catheterization	*Right side:* jugular, anterior vena cava, right atrium, right ventricle, pulmonary artery, pulmonary artery wedge.
	Left side: carotid, aorta, left ventricle.
	At each site: blood gases including oxygen saturation, pressure measurement, selective injections of radiopaque contrast medium.
9. Echocardiography	M mode, with or without contrast (microbubble) techniques, numerous measurements possible, e.g., wall thicknesses, indices of contractility, valvular movements.

thorax but is classically loudest over the right anterior thorax (second to fourth intercostal spaces). A palpable thrill may be present over the point of maximal intensity of the murmur. Mucous membranes are pink unless there is shunt reversal or severe pneumonia.

The cardiac silhouette on a lateral radiograph is normal if the defect is small. When the defect is large, there may be generalized cardiomegaly and prominence of the pulmonary artery and pulmonary vascular markings. The electrocardiogram is usually within normal limits.

Diagnosis can be confirmed by catheterization. Oxygen saturation is greater in the pulmonary artery and right ventricle than in the right atrium or great veins. Pulmonary arterial and right ventricular systolic pressures may be elevated. Angiographic confirmation of VSD requires injection of radiopaque contrast medium into the pulmonary artery or left ventricle. Provided that the shunt is left to right, simultaneous opacification of the left and right ventricles will occur.

The prognosis for isolated VSD is fair for smaller diameter defects. Of the cases described, most have been diagnosed in horses 18 months or older. Nevertheless it is probably wise to recommend that such animals not be ridden or used for breeding. Large-diameter defects result in exercise intolerance and may progress to frank cardiac failure.

TETRALOGY OF FALLOT AND RELATED CONDITIONS

Tetralogy of Fallot (TOF) and its variants comprise probably the second most common group of congenital cardiac disorders in horses. In TOF the aorta and its orifice are displaced to the right, overriding a VSD. In addition there is pulmonary stenosis, usually valvular or infundibular, and secondary right ventricular hypertrophy. A variant, pentalogy of Fallot, consists of the aforementioned four lesions with the addition of patency of the ductus arteriosus (PDA). In a second variation, pseudotruncus arteriosus plus PDA, the pulmonary artery is atretic and reduced to a fibrous cord.

In TOF, pulmonary stenosis and the VSD result in right ventricular hypertension with the greater proportion of combined ventricular output ejecting into the aorta, which is dilated in consequence. There is relative pulmonary hypoperfusion, resulting in arterial hypoxemia sometimes severe enough to produce cyanotic mucous membranes.

In pentalogy of Fallot, aortic blood shunts into the pulmonary artery by way of the PDA, reducing the degree of pulmonary hypoperfusion and tendency to develop cyanosis. In fact, a palliative surgical procedure used in humans with TOF is to create an artificial shunt between the aorta and pulmonary artery. In pseudotruncus arteriosus plus

PDA, all pulmonary perfusion is by way of the PDA.

These diagnostic features refer to TOF, but some features may be shared by the two variants. Affected foals may have difficulty in suckling. They are usually stunted and have reduced exercise tolerance. Respiratory distress, polypnea, cyanosis, unsteadiness, or even syncope may occur at rest or, more commonly, following mild exercise or excitement. A loud systolic murmur, which may be accompanied by a palpable thrill, is usually loudest over the left heart base but radiates widely. The electrocardiogram is unfortunately not a reliable diagnostic aid in TOF. The mean electrical axis of the QRS complex in the frontal plane is normally directed forward in neonatal foals and swings leftward as they mature. The most that can be said is that ventricular hypertrophy should be suspected if QRS complexes are large (more than 2.5 millivolts).

Plain radiographs may show right ventricular enlargement and prominence of the ascending aorta. TOF can be confirmed by catheterizing the right heart. There is right ventricular hypertension and a distinct pressure gradient across the area of pulmonary arterial stenosis, right ventricular systolic pressures being greater than pulmonary arterial systolic pressures. Contrast medium injected into the right ventricle clears simultaneously by way of the pulmonary artery and left ventricle and aorta.

The prognoses for TOF and pseudotruncus arteriosus plus PDA are poor, and euthanasia is probably the rational course to follow once a diagnosis has been confirmed. In pentalogy of Fallot the short-term prognosis may be slightly more favorable, but it is still unlikely that an affected animal will reach maturity.

PATENT DUCTUS ARTERIOSUS

The ductus arteriosus shunts blood from the pulmonary artery to the aorta in the fetus. In the early postnatal period, pulmonary vascular resistance decreases and systemic vascular resistance increases, with the result that the shunt is reversed. The murmur of the ductus arteriosus can be auscultated in most foals up to approximately four days postpartum. Patency of the ductus after this time is referred to as patent ductus arteriosus (PDA), a well-recognized equine congenital cardiac flow disorder.

The usual left to right shunting PDA results in pulmonary hyperperfusion and volume overload of the left atrium and ventricle. Flow across the PDA is greatest during late systole but continues throughout diastole. Older horses with PDA may develop pulmonary hypertension. Flow across the PDA may then decrease and in rare instances may even revert to the fetal pattern of pulmonary artery to aortic shunting.

Horses with PDA may grow normally and occasionally live to old age. More often, affected individuals are poorly grown and have reduced exercise tolerance. The mucous membranes are pink and the arterial pulse bounding. Typically the murmur of PDA is continuous and machinelike. The murmur is heard most clearly over the left thorax in the third or fourth intercostal spaces but radiates widely to include the right side of the thorax. The murmur may be accompanied by a palpable thrill. In adult horses with PDA the diastolic component of the murmur may be less distinct or even absent. The decline of the diastolic component is likely to be the result of elevated pulmonary artery pressures and reduced shunting.

The electrocardiogram and plain radiograph findings of equine PDA have not been adequately described. On catheterization, oxygen saturation in the pulmonary artery exceeds that in the right ventricle, atrium, and great veins. Right ventricular and pulmonary arterial pressures may be normal or elevated. Injection of radiopaque contrast medium at the aortic root results in opacification of both the aorta and the pulmonary artery, provided that there is no shunt reversal.

The prognosis of PDA varies with the degree of shunting and other factors. In general, the younger the age at which an affected horse becomes symptomatic the poorer will be the prognosis. Although PDA is potentially operable without open heart surgery, no case reports of successful repair could be found in the equine literature. A potential lethal complication of PDA is rupture of one of the branches of the pulmonary arteries secondary to pulmonary arterial hypertension.

TRICUSPID ATRESIA

Tricuspid atresia (TA) is a well-recognized, relatively uncommon complex equine cardiac disorder. The defect is characterized by atresia of the tricuspid (right atrioventricular) valve, patency of the foramen ovale, eccentric hypertrophy of the left ventricle, VSD, and hypoplasia of the right ventricle. The pulmonary artery may be normal or stenosed, or have valvular abnormalities such as a bicuspid pulmonic valve.

In TA, blood drains from an enlarged right atrium through the patent foramen ovale into the left atrium and then into the left ventricle. Left ventricular blood is ejected, partly through the aorta and partly via the VSD, to the right ventricle and pulmonary artery. Pulmonary perfusion is often inadequate, so that cyanosis is a likely clinical finding. Clinical signs have been described for a

TABLE 2. SOME OTHER CONGENITAL DISORDERS OF FLOW

Disorders	Features
Patent foramen ovale	Patency beyond postnatal period. Isolated defect results in left to right shunt with volume overload of right ventricle. Part of complex defects, e.g. tricuspid atresia.
Tricuspid valve dysplasia	Various examples, e.g. tricuspid stenosis; aplasia of parietal papillary muscle resulting in tricuspid insufficiency; tricuspid atresia.
Pulmonic valve dysplasia	Bicuspid pulmonic valve, valvular pulmonic stenosis; isolated or as part of complex defects.
Aortic valve dysplasia	Aortic valve with 2 cusps or 5 cusps; incomplete aortic valve commissure with aortic insufficiency.
Dysplasia of coronary arteries	Many variants described, e.g. single coronary artery, common origin of left and right coronary arteries. Isolated lesion or may accompany more complex defects.
Interruption of aortic arch	Congenital aplasia of aortic arch, accompanied by atrial and ventricular septal defects and PDA. Descending aorta receives pulmonary arterial blood via PDA.
Transposition of great arteries	Aorta originating from right ventricle, pulmonary artery from left ventricle, ventricular septal defect.
Persistent truncus arteriosus	Single primitive vessel, the truncus arteriosus, overrides a ventricular septal defect. Pulmonary arteries branch off the truncus arteriosus, which continues as the aorta.
Persistent right aortic arch	Esophageal entrapment by ligamentum arteriosum usually but not always resulting in dysphagia.
Three-chambered heart	Large common atrium, atresia of tricuspid valve, ventricular septal defect, right ventricular hypoplasia. Possibly an extreme variant of tricuspid atresia.

few foals and may include stunting, respiratory distress, cyanosis, and exercise intolerance. Polycythemia may develop secondary to hypoxemia. A systolic murmur with or without precordial thrill may be auscultated. Antemortem diagnosis can be confirmed only by employing the full range of diagnostic aids listed in Table 1. This is a serious defect and affected foals described in case reports have died before one year of age. Euthanasia is advocated once the diagnosis has been confirmed.

Some other types of congenital cardiac disorders are listed in Table 2. The clinical features of these disorders either are not documented or are inadequately described. Their anatomic features are described in the table. Diagnosis of these disorders requires a full cardiologic investigation, and in most instances these defects have been diagnosed at necropsy.

MANAGEMENT

Medical management may be used to support affected horses before and during diagnostic investigations. Long-term medical management of these conditions is normally neither necessary or desirable.

If signs of congestive heart failure such as subcutaneous or pulmonary edema are noted, digoxin may be administered once daily at a maintenance dose of 0.007 mg per kg intravenously or 0.035 mg per kg orally. One should monitor the patient daily for signs of digitalis overdosage such as anorexia, depression, and arrhythmias. Diuretics such as furosemide may be needed to help control edema formation and should be administered at a paren-

teral dose rate of up to 2 mg per kg three times daily. Serum potassium should be checked intermittently and corrected if necessary. Antimicrobials may be used to control concurrent respiratory infection. Excitement and exercise should be minimized. Tranquilizers should be used with caution as most have adrenolytic properties that may severely affect individuals with compromised cardiovascular dynamics. Fluids should be given sparingly since the kidney avidly conserves sodium, chloride, and water in congestive heart failure.

It is unwise to breed from horses affected by congenital cardiac disorders even if the lesion is minor or has been corrected surgically. There are reasonable grounds to suspect that genetic factors are involved in some cases. Similarly, it is considered unwise to recommend that horses with these defects, even if they are otherwise clinically sound, be used for riding. Injury to a rider resulting from death or collapse of a horse with a confirmed congenital cardiac disorder would have potentially serious legal implications.

Supplemental Readings

Button, C., Gross, D. R., Allert, J. A., and Kitzman, J.V.: Tricuspid atresia in a foal. J. Am. Vet. Med. Assoc., *172*:825, 1978.

Fregin, G. F.: The cardiovascular system. *In* Mansmann, R. A., McAllister, E. S., and Pratt, P. W. (eds.): Equine Medicine and Surgery, 3rd ed. Santa Barbara, CA, American Veterinary Publications, 1982.

Huston, R., Saperstein, G., and Leipold, H. W.: Congenital defects in foals. J. Equine Med. Surg., *1*:146, 1977.

Rooney, J. R., and Franks, W. C.: Congenital cardiac anomalies in horses. Path. Vet. *1*:454, 1964.

Vitums, A.: The embryonic development of the equine heart. Zbl. Vet. Med. C. Anat. Histol. Embryol., *10*:193, 1981.

Fibrinous Pericarditis

Stephen Dill, ITHACA, NEW YORK

Inflammation of the pericardium occurs secondary to pneumonia, pleuritis, septicemia, and viral infections. Pericardial effusion may occur with neoplastic metastasis to the pericardium or epicardium. Fibrinous pericarditis is infrequent in the horse. It may be caused by bacterial infection, occasionally secondary to a foreign body penetrating the thorax and pericardial sac. Rarely, a foreign body may penetrate the diaphragmatic flexure of the colon, diaphragm, and pericardium, resulting in septic pericarditis. Frequently, the precise etiology of fibrinous pericarditis cannot be determined.

HISTORY AND CLINICAL SIGNS

Horses are initially presented for a gradual onset of exercise intolerance, depression, ventral edema, and often weight loss. The clinical signs vary, depending upon the amount of pericardial effusion and the severity of the heart failure. The rectal temperature may be normal but is often mildly elevated. Heart rate is increased to between 50 and 100 beats per minute. Respiratory rate is elevated and some horses display respiratory distress. Peripheral pulse quality is weak.

Cardiac auscultation early in the course of illness may reveal pericardial friction rubs. Rubs may occur at any phase of the cardiac cycle; they are usually heard consistently with each heartbeat. As pericardial fluid and fibrin accumulate, cardiac sounds become muffled bilaterally and may become completely inaudible. Unilateral muffling of heart sounds is more suggestive of a tumor, an abscess, or fibrin accumulation unilaterally between the heart and thoracic wall. Gas is not present in the pericardial sac of horses with fibrinous pericarditis unless there has been a penetrating wound to the pericardium or pericardiocentesis has been performed, hence splashing sounds are uncommon.

Dorsal displacement of the ventral lung border can be determined on both thoracic auscultation and percussion. The lung is displaced dorsally by pleural fluid accumulation and by enlargement of the pericardial sac. Therefore, lung sounds are absent ventrally. The absence of lung sounds ventrally is also a common finding in primary pleuritis with pleural effusion. Pleuritis can be differentiated from pericarditis by the presence of widely radiating heart sounds in pleuritis cases, and by the absence of other signs of cardiac disease.

Bilateral jugular vein distention is present. Central venous pressure (CVP) values are elevated up to 45 cm of water (normal = <10 cm). A bilateral jugular pulse is evident. Arterial blood pressure is decreased. Edema develops in the pectoral and ventral abdominal areas. As heart failure progresses, limb edema and ascites also occur. Mucous membranes vary from pale to congested or cyanotic. Capillary refill time may be normal or significantly prolonged.

Echocardiography reveals a thickened, fibrin-covered pericardium and epicardium. Pericardial effusion is apparent. For further information on echocardiography, see p. 139.

The most consistent finding with electrocardiography is a decrease in amplitude of QRS complexes in all leads. This finding is not diagnostic for pericardial effusion, as QRS amplitudes also decrease with pleural effusion and obesity.

If pericardial effusion is minimal, thoracic radiographs may be normal. In more severely affected cases, on lateral thoracic radiographs there is an enlarged cardiac silhouette and dorsal displacement of the trachea. In cases with pleural effusion, drainage of the pleural fluid may allow visualization of the cardiac silhouette.

Clinical laboratory abnormalities are nonspecific and may include a stress leukogram, hypoalbuminemia, prerenal azotemia, and hyponatremia.

Pericardiocentesis should be performed at the sixth to ninth intercostal space at the level of the costochondral junction following a surgical prep and local infiltration of anesthetic. A stab incision will decrease tissue resistance on the needle and allow more sensitivity as the needle is passed through tissues. A syringe should be attached to the needle to prevent the occurrence of a pneumothorax. After the needle is passed through the intercostal muscle, resistance will be met as the needle contacts the pericardium. Rhythmic movements of the pericardium synchronous with cardiac contractions can be perceived as they are transmitted along the needle. The needle is then advanced through the pericardium, and fluid is obtained for cytology, aerobic and anaerobic culture and sensitivity, and viral isolation. Inaccurate direction of the needle could result in myocardial laceration and hemorrhage or ventricular fibrillation. An echocardiogram is useful to verify the presence and amount of pericardial fluid and to determine the correct placement of the needle. Electrocardiography will show a premature ventricular contraction if the needle inadvertently contacts the myocardium. If echocardiography or electrocardiography is unavailable, pericardiocentesis can be performed after a diagnosis of pericarditis has been made on clinical signs, but should not be attempted if it is suspected that pericardial effusion is small in volume.

TREATMENT

The survival rate of horses with fibrinous pericarditis is low. Therapy should be based on the determination of a specific etiology when possible. Antibiotics are indicated in cases of septic pericarditis. The choice of antibiotic is determined by culture and sensitivity. If culture results are unavailable, then broad-spectrum antibiotics are indicated. Nonsteroidal anti-inflammatory drugs may decrease the rate of pericardial fluid formation. Furosemide* (2 mg per kg intravenously three times a day) should be utilized to decrease the total intravascular fluid volume in the management of congestive heart failure. Sodium intake should be restricted.

Excessive pleural effusion should be removed by thoracocentesis. Pericardial fluid should be removed by pericardiocentesis. A No. 5 to 12 French size Argyle trocar† is useful for this purpose. Drainage of pericardial fluid should be performed slowly over several hours. The procedure should be stopped if the pericardial fluid suddenly contains an excessive amount of blood. Care should be taken to ensure that the drain is placed in the pericardial space and not inadvertently placed in the pleural space. Echocardiography and radiology are helpful in confirming the removal of pericardial fluid. If these ancillary procedures are not available, proper positioning of the drain can be verified by physical examination. If sufficient pericardial fluid is removed, then there should be a variable degree of improvement in cardiac function. The heart rate should decrease, the CVP should decrease, and heart sounds may increase in intensity. Improvement in these parameters is variable because they are determined by both the amount of pericardial

*Lasix 5%. American Hoeschst Corp., Somerville, NJ
†Argyle Trocar Catheter, Argyle Division of Sherwood Medical, St. Louis, MO

effusion and the dense granulation tissue covering the epicardium.

Corticosteroid therapy along with pericardiocentesis and drainage of pericardial fluid has been reported to be successful in some early cases of eosinophilic pericarditis.* Corticosteroids should be avoided in cases with a possible bacterial etiology.

An eosinophilic pericarditis has been recognized in areas of California and Nevada. Horses with eosinophilic pericarditis have clinical signs indistinguishable from fibrinous pericarditis. Diagnostic features of this disease include peripheral eosinophilia and the presence of many eosinophils in the pericardial fluid. The prognosis with eosinophilic pericarditis is good. The most important treatment is pericardiocentesis and drainage of excessive pericardial fluid. Corticosteroids have been used successfully in conjunction with pericardial fluid removal.‡

Pericardectomy and pericardial stripping are performed in people affected with constrictive pericarditis. Pericardectomy would prevent further pericardial effusion and allow fibrin to be stripped off the epicardium. Surgical treatment of horses with fibrinous pericarditis would probably be unsuccessful unless attempted early in the course of disease. The thick, dense granulation tissue layer is tightly adhered to the epicardium, making its removal very difficult.

*Personal Communication with John Freestone, B.V.Sc., VMTH, Davis, CA

Supplemental Readings

Dill, S. G., Simoncini, D. C., Bolton, G. R., Rendano, V. T., Crissman, J. W., King, J. M., and Tennant, B. C.: Fibrinous pericarditis in the Horse. J. Am. Vet. Med. Assoc., *180*:266, 1982.

Fregin, G. F.: The cardiovascular system. *In* Mansmann, R. A., McAllister, E. S., and Pratt, P. W. (eds.): Equine Medicine and Surgery, 3rd ed. Santa Barbara, CA, American Veterinary Publications, 1982.

Wagner, P. C., Miller, R. A., Merritt, F., Pickering, L. A., and Grant, B. D.: Constrictive pericarditis in the horse. J. Equine Med. Surg., *1*:242, 1977.

Peripheral Vascular Disease

Peter W. Physick-Sheard, GUELPH, ONTARIO, CANADA

M. Grant Maxie, GUELPH, ONTARIO, CANADA

DISEASES OF VEINS

THROMBOSIS AND THROMBOPHLEBITIS

Spontaneous venous thrombosis may occur in association with disseminated intravascular coagulation (DIC), aortoiliac thrombosis, and systemic viral diseases such as equine viral arteritis. However, the specific and local effects of such obstruction are often not evident, and specific therapy is not applied. Spontaneous deep vein thrombosis such as is seen in humans and the cow in association with deep trauma or enforced recumbency is not a commonly recognized clinical entity in the horse.

Thrombosis of a superficial vessel, particularly the jugular vein, is often seen in the horse and is almost invariably associated with venipuncture. A hypercoagulable state, prolonged use of indwelling catheters, and intravenous infusion of irritant or concentrated solutions with resultant endothelial damage all predispose to thrombosis.

Inflammation (thrombophlebitis) may be a direct sequel to spontaneous thrombosis, but more often precedes or accompanies venous obstruction. Thrombophlebitis is the usual outcome when an irritant has been injected perivascularly. Involvement of the jugular vein and thrombosis accompanies an extensive inflammatory response, which may involve the entire ventral neck and lead to necrosis and sloughing of tissue. The carotid artery may become involved, although damage to the vagosympathetic trunk and recurrent laryngeal nerve with resultant Horner's syndrome or laryngeal paralysis is a more common sequel. These complications are more likely when the irritant is deposited beneath the jugular vein. In some cases there is minimal perivascular swelling; the vein is hard and corded and initially painful. Such cases reflect thrombophlebitis without primary perivascular involvement. Thrombophlebitis is frequently complicated by sepsis, which should be suspected when systemic signs are observed, such as pyrexia, depression, and neutrophilia with left shift. Extensive sloughing and suppuration may occur.

Additional complications of thrombophlebitis include extensive edema in distal parts, endocarditis, and pulmonary thromboembolism. When jugular thrombosis is unilateral or develops slowly, collateral venous drainage compensates and no swelling is evident, although all superficial veins on the affected side are distended. Severe edema follows rapid, total venous occlusion, and is exacerbated by the animal's tendency to hold its head down and by extension of inflammation by gravity. In both acute and chronic thrombosis there is the possibility that the tail of the thrombus may break off and pass into the pulmonary artery. Such pulmonary thromboemboli can cause pulmonary hypertension, and also give rise to bacterial endocarditis and pulmonary abscessation if the emboli are septic. Emboli can predispose to aneurysm formation and arterial rupture. The risk of embolization is increased in cases of septic thrombophlebitis when the septic process tends to break down the thrombus.

TREATMENT

In the case of recent perivascular injection, local infiltration with saline should be attempted to dilute the irritant. Concurrent infiltration with a diluted solution of local anesthetic (*without* epinephrine) to reduce vascular spasm and provide local analgesia has also been recommended. In the case of severe perivascular reaction every attempt should be made to control the inflammation. Thrombosis of the vein should be assumed. Application of hot packs may be of help, as may the use of gentle massage and application of antiphlogistic salves, although care should be taken that the combination of treatments does not promote further damage to compromised skin.

Nonsteroidal anti-inflammatory agents are indicated. An oral route should be used for maintenance therapy, especially when thrombosis results from a hypercoagulable state. If sepsis is suspected, systemic antibiotic therapy should be administered. In the case of tissue necrosis and abscess, surgical drainage of the area may be required. When thrombophlebitis occurs in the absence of severe perivascular and subcutaneous reaction a similar approach to therapy may be appropriate. The approach to thrombosis without obvious inflammation will depend upon the inciting cause, since such thrombosis usually occurs as an accompanying feature of systemic disease.

Healing usually results in the vessel changing to a firm, fibrous cord. A recurrence of the inflammation indicates residual infection that may be best treated by surgical removal of the vessel. Use of anticoagulation therapy is rational in the early stages of disease to control the extent of thrombosis and to reduce the repeated formation and detachment of tail thrombi. Because the treatment is not without danger, warfarin and heparin should not be used unless clotting function can be monitored daily.

PREVENTION

Irritant and concentrated solutions should be diluted with isotonic fluids before intravenous administration. Injection of irritant material in a bolus should be avoided. Intravenous technique should be atraumatic, and when an animal's temperament or the lack of adequate facilities for restraint make injection difficult, the installation of an indwelling catheter should be considered. Injections into veins should never be made with a needle less than 4 cm long, and as much of the shaft as possible should be positioned in the lumen of the vessel. When frequent intravenous injection is required, the site should be changed often.

When indwelling catheters are installed, a totally aseptic technique, including the use of surgical gloves and full surgical skin preparation, should be employed. Using long catheters that can be tunneled for several centimeters beneath the skin before entering the vein helps reduce the incidence of secondary sepsis, while the use of catheters that extend to the thoracic inlet will help reduce the incidence of thrombosis. No catheter should be allowed to extend into the heart because of the risk of trauma to the valves and resulting endocarditis. When infusion is not continuous the catheter should be flushed frequently with heparinized saline. If infusion rates are low a small-bore catheter should be used to maintain sufficient flow velocity through the catheter to maintain patency. Blocked catheters should be changed, not forcibly flushed. No matter how effective the catheterization technique, no catheter should be left in place longer than three days. Once thrombosis of a vessel has occurred, bacteriologic swabbing of the tip of the catheter on removal may reveal the presence of infection and facilitate rational therapy.

Intravenous therapy of animals in actual or potential hypercoagulable states should be approached with circumspection. Such cases would include DIC, shock, toxemia, dehydration and hypovolemia, any low cardiac output condition, animals with partial obstruction to venous flow (heart failure, anterior thoracic mass), and mares in mid to late gestation, especially if they are experiencing toxic and septic processes. Jugular thrombosis may occur in a matter of hours. Oral therapy is preferable to intravenous therapy in such cases, while atraumatic intravenous technique is essential. It may be profitable to administer parenteral treatments through fine-gauge needles in such cases to minimize vessel trauma. Some success has been achieved by infusing fluids via a catheter placed in the lateral thoracic vein behind the elbow. Although it is not quite so easy to keep this site clean, thrombosis occurs less readily, possibly because of the higher flow rate that can be maintained in this smaller vessel.

DISORDERS OF ARTERIES

Arterial Rupture. Rupture of the ascending aorta between the right coronary sinus and the brachiocephalic trunk is observed particularly in stallions during periods of activity such as racing or breeding. Rupture occurs when systemic arterial pressure is high, but no structural abnormalities of the aorta have been consistently observed.

Aortic rupture causes sudden death either as a result of hemopericardium or interruption of and hemorrhage into the atrioventricular node and bundle. In some cases a dissecting fistula is formed between the coronary sinus and the right ventricle (cardioaortic fistula). Clinical signs include obvious distress, ventricular tachyarrhythmias, and a very characteristic, continuous murmur that is particularly intense during diastole and loudest on the right side of the thorax toward the apex. Heart failure follows this vascular accident. Occasionally a dissecting aneurysm forms along the wall of the aorta. Similar distress is evident at the time the lesion develops although no murmur is evident and the condition is not associated with arrhythmias. Rupture of the aneurysm and sudden death are the usual outcomes.

Rupture of the uterine and occasionally the cecal or colic artery occurs in the brood mare as a sequel to foaling, not always in association with dystocia (see p. 544). The animal may appear normal after foaling, only to die suddenly within the next 24 hours. The problem has been associated with low blood copper levels.

Rupture of the pulmonary artery during exercise is occasionally reported as a cause of sudden death, although it is probably very uncommon despite the significant elevation in pulmonary arterial pressure which appears to occur with exercise in the horse.

Parasitic Arteritis. Extensive damage to the cranial mesenteric artery can occur as a result of *S. vulgaris* infestation (see p. 70). The vascular consequences of such parasitism upon the gastrointestinal tract include thromboembolism and colic. Aberrant migration of larvae into the thoracic aorta appears to occur not infrequently and has been associated with episodes of coronary thromboembolism leading to small areas of myocardial infarction. The relationship between these infarcts and arrhythmias has not been determined.

Arterial Obstruction. Interference with arterial supply to a tissue can occur as a complication of a range of traumatic injuries. Examples include intermittent occlusion of the femoral artery at the femoral ring as the wing of the ilium rotates in some cases of pelvic fracture, and occlusion of arteries passing through confined spaces as a result of local inflammation. This may occur for example when the inferior check ligament is blocked during diagnostic procedures for lameness. Careful palpation of the limb to detect temperature and the character of the pulse at every available site will allow a diagnosis of arterial occlusion and will often reveal the approximate level of the obstruction. When necessary arteriography may be employed, although care should be taken that local blood supply is not further compromised as a result. Rapid diagnosis of arterial occlusion is essential if infarction and necrosis are to be avoided.

Arteriovenous Fistula. Arteriovenous fistulas may be congenital or acquired. Congenital lesions can arise anywhere in the body and are usually incidental findings. Acquired lesions are usually associated with trauma, including traumatic intravenous technique. Clinical manifestations include fremitus over the site and possibly swelling. Fremitus may vary with position of an extremity. In the case of a fistula in a superficial site, the distal vein may be distended. If necessary, diagnosis can be confirmed by arteriography, although this is rarely necessary with superficial lesions.

The clinical significance of an arteriovenous fistula is slight in most cases. Venous rupture is not a likely sequel. However, these fistulas promote a high cardiac output as a result of reduced afterload augmented by increased venous return. Large fistulas can cause heart failure.

Surgical correction should be approached with caution. The fistula may not be a discrete channel but a complex network of vessels and may defy simple closure. When collateral circulation is adequate, the artery supplying the fistula should be ligated.

AORTIC-ILIAC THROMBOSIS

Aortic-iliac thrombosis (AIT) is an acquired, progressive vascular disease of unknown etiology involving the terminal aorta, aortic quadrifurcation, internal and external iliac arteries, and their major branches down to the level of the major muscular arteries. The pathogenesis of the condition was discussed extensively on page 153 of the first edition of this book.

Clinical Signs. Affected animals are most often male, intact or recently castrated, are usually young, and have exhibited promising performance. They present with vague hind-end lameness or suboptimal performance of several weeks to months' duration. Horses tend to move roughly or stiffly behind after fast work and may appear restless immediately after exercise. A range of treatments have often been applied before signs become sufficiently distinct for the diagnosis to suggest itself. Worsening of the condition may be apparent over a period of months, although when horses are kept in training

there may be sufficient stimulation of collateral circulation for signs and performance to stabilize.

The condition most often becomes evident after affected animals have been given a period off work. In these cases the collateral circulation probably becomes reduced and lameness occurs at much slower rates of working. Affected animals appear grossly normal at rest and during light exercise. As exercise intensity increases, stiffness in one or both hind limbs and later a tendency to knuckle over on the fetlock is seen. In severe cases, or if the animal is forced to work further, the hind limbs become almost rigid, the back arched, and the horse walks on its toes and may go down. Anxiety may be evident and the animal may sweat over its body out of proportion to the amount of work performed, while sweating is absent over the hind end. The severity of signs is proportional to the extent of the vascular lesion and the intensity of the work.

Palpation of the limbs immediately after exercise reveals coldness, most commonly from the midgaskin distally, and an absence of pulse in the digital artery. This latter finding should be checked again after recovery since the digital pulse is naturally reduced immediately after intense exercise. If the saphenous veins are examined immediately upon halting they will take considerably longer than the normal 10 seconds to fill. The horse will tend to stamp its hind limbs as circulation returns and to kick out for no apparent reason. Clinical signs subside rapidly, so that by as little as 15 minutes after exercise the animal appears clinically normal. In some cases muscle wasting over the hindquarters may be evident, although this is not a prominent sign.

Definitive diagnosis is achieved by careful palpation of the contour of the peripheral pulses at all available sites, the pulse in the affected limb being flat and prolonged, by careful examination of the temperature of the distal limb, and by rectal palpation of the aortic quadrifurcation and its intrapelvic branches. Rectal examination should be performed very carefully so as to avoid a false-negative result. The pulse wave in the abdominal aorta will be accentuated by the obstruction and will be passed along the wall of the affected vessels even though they are obstructed. Not all branches will be obstructed in every case, while in some cases there may be partial thrombosis of the quadrifurcation and total obstruction distally in the femoral vessel but patency of the external iliac artery, which thus pulsates normally.

A thrombus can often be palpated in the aorta and just ahead of the quadrifurcation by lightly compressing the vessel between pulse waves. Loss of local pulse and/or enlargement of the internal or external iliac arteries or their palpable branches, firmness of vessels, abnormal changes in diameter, and asymmetry also confirm the diagnosis. In very early cases the thrombus in the aorta may be relatively small and difficult to palpate, with clinical signs being related to obstruction of extrapelvic vessels, such as the popliteal at its bifurcation into the cranial and caudal tibial arteries. With practice the diagnosis in such cases can be confidently arrived at by palpation of peripheral pulses and observation of the characteristic clinical signs. Confirmation of diagnosis by arteriography is recommended. Adequate access to the vascular tree of the hind limb can be gained by catheterization of the saphenous artery, which lies on the medial aspect of the limb beneath the leading edge of the saphenous vein.

The condition is distinguished from acute thromboembolism or "saddle thrombus" by the absence of acute signs in the majority of cases. However, in occasional animals a piece of the thrombus at the aortic quadrifurcation may detach. This may cause an acute ischemic episode but may also go unnoticed if the thrombus is small.

Treatment. Although reports will be found in the literature concerning the use of sodium gluconate in cases of AIT, there is little evidence that this treatment is effective. In view of the nature of the lesion, a therapeutic response would not be expected. Since neither the pathogenesis nor the natural history of the disease is established, and since by the time diagnosis is achieved the lesion consists largely of mature fibrous tissue, anticoagulation is not rational and is unlikely to be effective. The use of anticoagulation in acute thromboembolic episodes secondary to thrombosis of the aortic quadrifurcation is unlikely to have any long-lasting effect since massive muscle infarction has probably occurred before drug therapy could be effective.

The most effective approach to management is to maintain the horse in work since this supports the collateral circulation. This should be done only if the horse is able to work at the required level without obvious discomfort, since to do otherwise would cause the horse distress and would also be dangerous under race conditions.

Supplemental Readings

Cranley, J. J., and McCullogh, K. G.: Ischemic myocardial fibrosis and aortic strongylosis in the horse. Equine Vet. J., 13:35, 1981.

Maxie, M. G.: The Vascular System. In Jubb, K.V.F., Kennedy, P. C., and Palmer, N. (eds.): Pathology of Domestic Animals, 3rd ed. New York, Academic Press, pp. 34–69, 1985.

Maxie, M. G., and Physick-Sheard, P. W.: Aortic-iliac thrombosis in horses. Vet. Pathol., 22:238, 1985.

Rooney, J. R., Prickett, M. E., and Crowe, M. W.: Aortic ring rupture in stallions. Pathol. Vet., 4:268, 1967.

Scott, E. A., Byars, T. D., and Lamar, A. M.: Warfarin anticoagulation in the horse. J. Am. Vet. Med. Assoc., 177:1146, 1980.

Stowe, H. D.: Effects of age and impending parturition upon serum copper of Thoroughbred mares. J. Nutrition, 95:179, 1968.

Exercise-Related Cardiovascular Problems

Alexander Littlejohn, NEWMARKET, ENGLAND

CARDIOVASCULAR RESPONSES TO EXERCISE

When the motor cortex of the brain commands a horse to move, a complex series of responses occur in the heart and vascular system. These responses provide oxygen-rich blood to the musculoskeletal system by boosting both cardiac output and the oxygen-carrying capacity of the blood, and they divert blood from organs not involved in locomotion to the musculoskeletal system, the thorax, and the skin.

Cardiac output (CO) increases in a linear fashion between speeds of 3 and 14 m per second. There is a six- to sevenfold increase in CO from rest to maximum effort. In terms of body mass this represents an increase from 80 ml per kg per minute to more than 500 ml per kg per minute. A cardiac output of more than 250 L per minute has been recorded during tethered swimming, and it is possible that even higher levels could occur during flat races or steeplechases. The increase in cardiac output is caused by increases in both heart rate and stroke volume.

Heart rate is not a linear function of speed of travel. Between rest and 3 m per second, heart rate increases most rapidly. Between 3 m per second and 14 m per second, heart rate increases linearly, while at greater speeds, the increase in heart rate with increasing speeds tends to become asymptotic.

Heart rates in excess of 240 per minute have been recorded during maximal exercise, a near sevenfold increase from the average resting value. However, there is little information available at present about the relative contributions of heart rate and stroke volume to the cardiac output at heart rates greater than 200 per minute. At such high heart rates, the time available for ventricular filling is less than 80 msec, a time interval that doubtless becomes increasingly inadequate as the heart rate approaches 250 per minute.

The stroke volume (SV) also increases with exercise, but to a smaller extent than the heart rate. The increase in SV is 20 to 30 per cent in average horses, but a considerably greater increase occurs in trained subjects, perhaps as much as 50 per cent in top performers at peak fitness. The increase in stroke volume is related directly to myocardial contractility and power of ventricular muscle, which are greatly strengthened by training. This effect of training is responsible for the lower heart rate of fit racehorses compared with those unfit, both at rest and during work. In fit horses, the SV contributes a greater proportion of the cardiac output at any given work rate than it contributes in untrained horses, thus allowing for a lower heart rate, lower energy cost, a longer diastolic filling time, and a greater cardiac reserve. The end result of these adaptations to training is thus an increase in the cardiac reserve. Since the heart derives its energy almost wholly from oxidative reactions in the myocardium, the cardiac reserve may be defined as the difference between myocardial oxygen uptake at rest and at maximal exercise.

In addition to and parallel with the cardiac response, the vascular system is stimulated by neural, hormonal, and other stimuli. Red cells are mobilized primarily from the spleen but also from the gastrointestinal tract, including the liver. Blood is diverted away from the spleen, liver, gastrointestinal tract, and urogenital system toward the musculoskeletal system, the thoracic organs, the skin, and the central nervous system. These adaptations are mediated neurally and humorally by the autonomic nervous system and the adrenal gland, and by autoregulation.

The result of strenuous muscle activity is a 20-fold increase in the blood flow through skeletal muscle and an increase in ventricular myocardial blood flow directly proportional to the cardiac output. However, while the ventricular muscle as a whole receives the same percentage of cardiac output during exercise as it does at rest, the left ventricle receives a smaller fraction than the right ventricle at maximal exercise.

One of the end results of the surge of cardiovascular activity with exercise is an increase in both systemic and pulmonary circulatory pressures. Mean carotid pressure exceeds 30 kPa (225 mm Hg), and mean pulmonary arterial pressure is in excess of 6 kPa (45 mm Hg) during maximal exercise.

Training diminishes the rise in systemic blood pressure with exercise but increases the rise in right atrial pressure. The rise in right atrial pressure facilitates rapid filling of the right ventricle during the short diastolic interval when 1 kg of blood must fill the ventricle in 60 to 80 msec.

Since left ventricular end-diastolic pressure increases more than threefold and right ventricular twofold, the transseptal pressures during diastole may limit septal blood flow during that phase of the cardiac cycle when myocardial blood flow should be at its highest. Although myocardial blood flow has been shown to be adequate in the ventricle of ponies running on a treadmill at a speed of 8.89 meters per second, it may not be adequate in the ventricular myocardium of Thoroughbred racehorses carrying weight at heavy work rates. Since hypoxemia is a feature of maximum work rates in many if not all horses, the ventricular myocardium may suffer from continuous hypoxia during sustained severe exertion. The heart of a galloping horse carrying a rider is thus subjected to mechanical stresses imposed by the inflow and outflow of blood, and biochemical stresses caused by lack of oxygen.

CARDIAC CONDITIONS

Arrhythmias. There is a considerable body of circumstantial, pathologic, and experimental evidence that points to myocardial hypoxia during exercise as a major factor contributing to the development of some cardiac arrhythmias. Several investigations have described fibrotic degenerative lesions and microvascular changes in the myocardium of horses with arrhythmias such as wandering pacemaker, partial atrioventricular block, extrasystole, and atrial fibrillation. Such lesions are not present in the myocardium of clinically normal horses with no arrhythmias. It is, therefore, possible that such lesions may develop as a result of severe hypoxic episodes, and be directly responsible for the actual arrhythmias.

While exercise-induced myocardial hypoxia is probably an important factor in the genesis of arrhythmias, any condition that causes anemia or hypoxemia, e.g., bacterial, viral or protozoal infections and pulmonary disease, makes the myocardium more susceptible to exercise-induced hypoxia. Both valvular endocarditis and viral myocarditis have been associated with arrhythmias in horses, and significant changes have also been demonstrated in electrocardiograms of horses with chronic lung disease. Arrhythmias that are provoked by exercise include atrial extrasystole (synonym: supraventricular or atrial ectopic beat), atrial tachycardia and atrial fibrillation, ventricular extrasystole, ventricular tachycardia, and ventricular fibrillation. Atrial fibrillation is a well-known cause of diminished cardiac output and performance, and extrasystole and tachycardias are also associated with reduced performance. Sinoatrial block is of interest in that it is a relatively uncommon arrhythmia and has been recorded in both poorly and normally performing horses. Most authors consider that sinoatrial block is associated with diminished performance, and the occurrence of this arrhythmia in an electrocardiographic tracing at more than isolated intervals may signal the presence of myocardial abnormalities involving the sinoatrial node or its junctional fibres.

Both intra-atrial block and intraventricular block are known to be associated with diminished performance. The pathogenesis of these conditions is unknown, with myocardial hypoxia a prime suspect.

Changes in the form and polarity of the T waves in certain electrocardiographic lead tracings are considered to be evidence of severe hypoxic episodes in myocardium. Such changes can be elicited by many diseases (such as pneumonia and respiratory viral infections) and certain drugs, as well as by severe exercise stress. It may be that T-wave changes during training herald imminent development of the microscopic myocardial lesions that have been noted in horses with various arrhythmias. T-wave changes have been observed to appear concurrently with the arterial hypoxemia of African horse sickness, without any appearance of myocarditis in histopathologic sections at autopsy. According to some workers, horses with repolarization disturbances have diminished aerobic capacity.

Valvular Diseases. To what extent exercise stress is responsible for diseases of heart valves is not known. Of five cases of rupture of mitral chordae tendinae reported in recent years, only one was associated with strenuous exercise. Two cases occurred after light work; one subject had chronic pulmonary disease and one was not directly associated with work. It is, however, possible that the valve cusp lesions that have been described by many authors are associated with the rapid and turbulent blood flow that accompanies exercise.

Thus, while the role of exercise in the development of valvular abnormalities is not proved, there is little doubt that when valvular insufficiencies do exist, the great increases in pressure that occur during exercise will tend to exacerbate jet lesions of the endocardium and subendothelial tissues.

VASCULAR CONDITIONS

One of the factors considered to be responsible for the development of arterial thrombi in humans and animals is the physical damage to the intima caused by the combined effects of pressure, flow, and turbulence at sites where large arteries branch. During exercise, both pressure and flow rates in the arterial tree increase dramatically, conceivably altering the flow characteristics at arterial branching sites in potentially damaging ways.

Predilection sites for thrombus formation in the horse are the cranial mesenteric, the internal, and external iliac arteries. Thrombi at these and other sites in the circulatory system are often associated with larvae of *S. vulgaris*, but physical damage to the intima may precede parasitic attachments.

The great increases in systemic and pulmonary arterial pressures that occur during exercise are undoubtedly important factors in the etiology of numerous cases of ruptured blood vessels that have been recorded during exercise, including exercise-induced pulmonary hemorrhage. The latter is, in my opinion, caused by pulmonary hypertension resulting in part from the hypoxemia of strenuous exercise and in part from the presence of lung disease.

DIAGNOSIS

The importance of a detailed record of history, management, training schedule, signs and athletic performance—particularly the rider's and trainer's assessments thereof—cannot be overemphasized. This should be followed by a careful clinical examination in a true resting state. Auscultation is the most valuable method of evaluation of heart function. A written record of the heart sounds at each valve site is essential for each examination. An ECG is recorded. The horse is then subjected to its normal work and observed closely. The type of work should always be that for which the horse is intended. Immediately after the workout, auscultation of the heart is performed and repeated at regular intervals for several minutes thereafter.

Such a schedule is designed to reveal what, if any, special diagnostic investigations may be necessary, such as an ECG during and immediately after exercise, cardiac and intravascular hemodynamic measurements, and echocardiography.

With all the findings and data at hand and the diagnosis made, the question that the veterinarian should attempt to answer is: To what degree, if any, does this particular cardiovascular condition diminish cardiovascular function, performance, and safety?

RELATIONSHIPS BETWEEN CARDIAC ARRYTHMIAS AND EXERCISE

The prognosis for horses with cardiovascular conditions obviously depends on the nature of the abnormality, its severity, the extent to which cardiovascular function is compromised, and whether optimal function can be fully or partly restored. Bearing in mind the principles outlined previously, the value of exercise as an aid to reaching an informed decision about cardiovascular conditions should not be underestimated.

Exercise abolishes wandering pacemaker, and provided there are no other arrhythmias present and no other signs of cardiac disease, it should be regarded simply as an electrocardiographic variant with no measurable effect on cardiac function. No therapy is indicated.

Second-degree partial atrioventricular block is a very common arrhythmia that almost invariably disappears with exercise or mild excitement. Occasionally it is noted during early cardiac deceleration after mild exercise; doubtless it is a result of unstable vagal activity. At such transient and isolated frequencies, this arrhythmia can be ignored provided no other arrhythmias are present and there are no signs of cardiac disease.

Extrasystoles (ectopic beats) may be noted after exercise but not at rest—or the frequency may increase after exercise. Infrequent isolated ectopic beats, the frequency of which does not increase during or after exercise and that are not accompanied by any signs of cardiac disease, are of no clinical significance. Frequent extrasystoles either at rest or after exercise have a guarded prognosis and may indicate myocarditis. Here the medical and athletic history, the presence of other clinical signs, and the use for which the horse is intended should be assessed. In general, the more frequently they occur the more they should be viewed with suspicion as a signal of diminished cardiac efficiency, diminished performance, or myocardial pathology. Thus, atrial or ventricular ectopic beats in bigeminal or trigeminal rhythm are of far greater significance than one isolated extrasystole observed in a 10-minute tracing.

Atrial and ventricular tachycardia are often associated with myocardial or valvular disease and thus have a poor prognosis. If they occur in short bursts from ectopic foci in atria or ventricles, they are termed paroxysmal. They may be induced by exercise, hence the necessity for exercise tests with direct or telemetric recording of the electrocardiogram. Paroxysmal tachycardias in humans, paradoxically, cause an immediate decrease in cardiac output that persists while the arrhythmia is present. The same is probably true in the horse.

Paroxysmal atrial fibrillation has been diagnosed during the running of races. The onset is sudden, occurs during the last few hundred meters of the race, and causes an immediate drop in running speed, many affected horses finishing last. Like the preceding arrhythmia, atrial fibrillation causes an immediate decrease in cardiac output. Nevertheless, some show-jumpers with atrial fibrillation can compensate for the dysfunction sufficiently well to compete in graded events for many years. Presumably myocardial changes are minimal in such cases.

Intra-atrial and intraventricular block do not disappear with exercise, do not respond to rest or treatment, and are responsible for poor performance in racehorses. However, while racehorses do not perform well, the performance of show jumpers with intra-atrial or intraventricular block does not appear to be affected. One would prefer not to see either of these two electrocardiograhic abnormalities in an eventer. Ability to carry weight at speed may be compromised.

LIFE-THREATENING CARDIOVASCULAR CONDITIONS

Any cardiovascular condition that increases the possibility of cardiac arrest during exercise is patently life-threatening. Diseases of the valves, gross myocardial lesions including generalized myocarditis, and cardiac tamponade obviously fall into this category. Similarly, any circulatory condition that predisposes to a vascular catastrophe such as rupture of a major blood vessel or embolism of a vital organ is included in the list. Unfortunately, there are no statistics available to help us predict the possibility of sudden death or the life expectancy for each and every condition encountered.

In each individual case, therefore, the findings of clinical examinations and exercise tests, the medical and athletic history, the results of special diagnostic procedures, and the purposes for which the horse may be used all have to be taken into account when giving a prognosis. Conditions in which the threat to the life of the subject is potentially high are the following:

1. Frequent extrasystoles; paroxysmal tachycardia; atrial fibrillation; bradycardia with arrhythmia; generalized myocarditis.

2. Pansystolic and pandiastolic murmurs, particularly if loud and harsh.

3. Thrombosis of major vessels; severe systemic and pulmonary hypertension.

Contrary to commonly held belief, horses with cardiovascular abnormalities rarely "drop dead" under the rider. Even horses that suffer a cardiovascular collapse during the running of a race or other sporting event give several seconds' warning of imminent collapse and usually can be pulled up in time for the rider to dismount. This is because cerebral anoxia takes some seconds to develop after cardiac arrest. Locomotor system breakdowns such as limb bone fractures offer far greater chances of a dangerous fall, since the horse may plunge instantaneously and moreover may do so in the middle of the field of horses. Nonetheless, the safety of the rider must always be taken into account. In general, any condition whose rapid deterioration could lead to syncope should be regarded as potentially unsafe and the rider warned accordingly. Needless to state, the more demanding the exercise task, the greater this possibility of syncope will be.

ENDOCRINE DISEASES

Edited by C. L. Chen

Diabetes Mellitus

Alfred M. Merritt, GAINESVILLE, FLORIDA

Practically every published case of "diabetes mellitus" in the horse has been the result of a pituitary tumor. Thus, by strict definition, these horses do not have diabetes mellitus, which is glucosuria resulting from hyperglycemia caused by pancreatic islet beta cell deficiency. Instead, their hyperglycemia is due most probably to excess endogenous ACTH or growth hormone (GH) release.

It appears that true diabetes mellitus in the horse is an extremely rare condition; two published cases seem to qualify. The first animal described was a seven-year-old pony that was underweight, polydipsic, and emitted "a strange urine odor." Clinical laboratory analysis revealed a persistent hyperglycemia, with daily values ranging between 300 and 500 mg per dl, 4+ glucosuria, and 2+ ketonuria. The hyperglycemia was insulin-responsive, although a very large dose of 8 units per kg of regular insulin intravenously could not cause the blood sugar concentration to drop into the normal range. Protamine zinc insulin, at doses of 0.5 and 1.0 units per kg, was much more effective in combatting the hyperglycemia. In contrast, horses with hyperglycemia secondary to pituitary tumor seem to be totally insulin-resistant. Pathologically, the pony with the apparent true diabetes mellitus had a chronic pancreatitis, with islets present but surrounded by fibrosis.

The second case was also a pony, a 12-year-old

TABLE 1. PERTINENT CLINICAL FEATURES OF TRUE DIABETES MELLITUS VS. TUMOR OF THE PARS INTERMEDIA OF THE PITUITARY GLAND IN HORSES

Clinical Features	Diabetes Mellitus	Pituitary Tumor
Hirsutism	No	Yes
Hyperhydrosis	No	Yes
Polydipsia and polyuria	Yes	Usually
Hypothalamic dysfunction*	No	Often
Glucosuria	Yes	Usually
Ketonuria	Yes	No
Fasting blood glucose (mg/dl)	300–500	80–300
Insulin-responsive hyperglycemia	Yes	No

*Includes wildly fluctuating appetite and body temperature. Occasionally seizures are seen.

Shetland, with a history of weight loss and anorexia of three months' duration. Polyphagia, along with polydipsia and polyuria, was seen when the animal was hospitalized. Pertinent clinical laboratory values included hyperglycemia (468 to 551 mg per dl in four different samples), and hyperglobulinemia, notable glucosuria (2 gm per dl) with a normal urine specific gravity, and mild hypoalbuminemia and azotemia. No indications of hyperketonemia were found, however. Unfortunately, no insulin-response studies could be done and the pony was euthanized. Significant necropsy findings were a severe chronic abscess of the pancreas such that only about 5 per cent of normal pancreatic tissue could be found on representative histologic sections, and some sclerosing glomerulonephritis that might have explained the normal urine specific gravity in spite of the glucosuria.

In contrast, the pancreas of horses with pituitary tumor is grossly and histologically normal. Table 1 lists the most important clinical features that differentiate hyperglycemia due to insulin deficiency (diabetes mellitus) from hyperglycemia due to pituitary tumor.

Supplemental Readings

Jeffrey, J. R.: Diabetes mellitus secondary to chronic pancreatitis in a pony. J. Am. Vet. Med. Assoc., *153*:1168, 1968.

King, J. M., Kavanaugh, J. F., and Bentinck-Smith, J.: Diabetes mellitus with pituitary neoplasms in a horse and dog. Cornell Vet., *52*:133, 1962.

Riggs, W. L.: Diabetes mellitus secondary to chronic necrotizing pancreatitis in a pony. Southwest. Vet., *25*:149, 1972

Tasker, J. B., Whiteman, C. E., and Martin, B. R.: Diabetes mellitus in the horse. J. Am. Vet. Med. Assoc., *149*:393, 1966.

Tumors of the Pituitary Gland (Pars Intermedia)

Jill Beech, KENNETT SQUARE, PENNSYLVANIA

Adenomas of the pars intermedia of the pituitary gland occur primarily in aged horses and are more common in females than males. There is no breed predilection. The tumor may be an incidental necropsy finding or may cause clinical signs.

In humans neoplasia of the pituitary occur mainly in the pars distalis but in horses tumors are in the pars intermedia. Because adrenocorticotropic hormone (ACTH) secretion from the pars intermedia is under inhibitory dopaminergic control, horses with pars intermedia tumors lack normal glucocorticoid feedback on ACTH secretion.

CLINICAL SIGNS

Affected horses are usually presented with polyuria and polydipsia (PUPD), hirsutism, and failure to shed. Polyuria and polydipsia are usually first noticed when horses are stabled; some may drink more than 80 L of water per day instead of the normal 20 to 30 L. The hair coat is often coarse, brittle, long, and shaggy and may become wavy or curly and matted with sweat. The long hair may be diffuse or limited to the limbs, withers, and over the thorax and croup. The mane and tail are normal. The skin may be dry and scaly or greasy. Animals frequently appear "swaybacked" and "potbellied" with loss of muscle, especially the dorsal epaxial and gluteal muscles; the tuber coxae and tuber sacrale appear prominent. Condition is lost despite a normal or increased appetite. Horses are more susceptible to concurrent diseases such as skin infections, respiratory disease, infections of tendon sheaths and joints, buccal ulcers, laminitis, and foot abscesses. Intramuscular and intravenous injection sites are prone to infections, and wound healing is delayed. Weakness may cause an ataxic appearance. Occasionally, affected horses have dilated pupils, abnormal pupillary light responses, and visual defects. Episodes of tachypnea, and profound bradycardia have also been observed. When horses are turned out, many of these signs are missed. In mares, estrus cycles may be suppressed or abnormal and at least one mare presented had galactorrhea despite her nongravid nonpostparturient status.

When a horse is presented with the aforementioned history, careful physical examination and clinical laboratory tests are necessary for diagnosis. Chronic debilitation due to poor management and nutrition, ill-kept teeth, parasitism, and other systemic diseases such as neoplasia, internal abscesses, and intestinal malabsorption must be eliminated from consideration. PUPD of unknown etiology may occasionally be seen in otherwise healthy horses and it may also accompany chronic renal failure. Spontaneous diabetes mellitus that could cause PUPD and weight loss has rarely been documented in horses (see p. 181). Pheochromocytomas may cause bouts of hyperhidrosis, hyperthermia, tachycardia, and tachypnea as well as weight loss.

CLINICAL LABORATORY TESTS

Laboratory testing initially should include a complete blood count, chemistry screen (including glucose, creatinine, and electrolytes) and a urinalysis. A gray or bluish hue to the plasma indicates gross lipemia, which may occur in affected ponies. Unless there is an infection causing leukocytosis, the white blood cell count will be normal or even low. Typically there is absolute or relative neutrophilia and lymphopenia and eosinophilia. The hematocrit and red blood cell count are often normal, although some patients may have a mild normocytic normochromic anemia. Anemia of chronic disease may exist if the animal has concurrent infection(s). Affected horses are usually, but not consistently, hyperglycemic; blood glucose values often exceed 150 mg per dl and are sometimes even greater than 300 mg per dl. If a normal value is obtained from an animal with a suspected case, additional samples should be obtained. Electrolyte values and creatinine are usually normal. Urine specific gravity may be low or within normal range. There is glucosuria and sometimes ketonuria when the animal is in a negative energy balance.

These findings are sufficient to warrant the following additional tests: plasma hydrocortisone (cortisol) or total corticoids; insulin levels at rest and in response to intravenous glucose, cortisol concentration following ACTH stimulation and dexamethasone suppression, and TSH-releasing hormone (TRH) stimulation tests (Table 1). Separate dexamethasone suppression and ACTH stimulation tests are more helpful than the combined test, as the latter does not allow evaluation of the rebound of cortisol seen in affected horses 24 hours after dexamethasone administration. An intravenous insulin tolerance test can be performed if diabetes is strongly suspected.

Blood samples for hydrocortisone (cortisol) should be kept cool and centrifuged as soon as possible to allow freezing of the plasma. Plasma hydrocortisone levels vary somewhat among the different laboratories. If no normal values are available from the laboratory, control samples should be submitted. Preferably the samples should be sent to a laboratory specializing in hormonal assays. Evening levels (6 to 10 P.M.) are said to be of two thirds of the morning values (6 to 10 A.M.) However, levels fluctuate and secretion appears to be episodic. In horses with pituitary adenoma, plasma cortisol or corticoid levels are frequently increased. Diurnal rhythm is usually lost.

Even when baseline concentrations of corticoids are only minimally elevated, adrenal hyperplasia results in an exaggerated increase in cortisol levels in response to ACTH. In normal horses, 1 unit per kg ACTH gel causes a two- to threefold increase in

cortisol within four to eight hours. The same dose of ACTH given to horses with pituitary tumors increases cortisol fourfold. Response to ACTH indicates that the adrenal glands remain under pituitary control. Dexamethasone suppresses plasma cortisol in normal horses because of negative feedback on ACTH release. Cortisol levels are not suppressed by dexamethasone in horses with pituitary tumors. While neither the dexamethasone suppression test nor ACTH stimulation test is specific for diagnosis of pituitary tumors, an exaggerated response to ACTH and decreased response to dexamethasone would be highly suggestive of pituitary adenoma. Likewise, an increase in cortisol following TRH administration appears characteristic of horses with a pituitary tumor.

Assays for equine ACTH, melanocyte-stimulating hormone (MSH), and other proopiolipomelanocortin (POLMC) peptides would provide the diagnosis, as the tumors have been shown to produce and secrete high levels of these hormones. As of this writing, none of these assays are readily or cheaply available to practitioners. If hormonal assays are unavailable, an intravenous glucose tolerance test (0.5 gm per kg of 50 per cent glucose intravenously) may be helpful for diagnosis. Horses with pituitary adenomas have a different response curve compared with normal horses, showing less rise and then a more gradual decline in blood glucose. Simultaneous measurements of insulin concentrations show a relative lack of insulin response, and horses with pituitary tumors usually have a highly elevated baseline insulin value.

PATHOLOGY

Necropsy examination reveals a tumor of the pars intermedia, the size of which is variable and does not necessarily correlate with clinical signs. Tumors are nonencapsulated but sharply delineated. There is prominent vascularization, minimal necrosis, and a low mitotic rate. The neoplastic spindle-shaped cells have well-developed rough endoplasmic reticulum and secretory granules and a small Golgi apparatus. The tumor usually expands dorsally and causes pressure on the posterior lobe of the pituitary and the hypothalamus. The posterior lobe and infundibular stalk may be infiltrated peripherally but there is no metastasis. The tumor may cause pressure on the optic chiasm. The adrenal cortex is usually hypertrophied and multiple sites of infection are frequently found.

TREATMENT

Few horses with pituitary tumors are treated because of the nature of the disease and general severity of clinical signs. Mild cases may merit treatment. Cyproheptadine has been used for ther-

TABLE 1. SUMMARY OF ENDOCRINE FUNCTION TESTS USED IN DIAGNOSIS OF TUMORS OF THE PARS INTERMEDIA OF THE PITUITARY GLAND

Hormone Test	Normal Value	Reference
Hydrocortisone (cortisol)	3–7 µg/100 ml	Garcia, unpublished
	≤13 µg/100 ml	James et al., 1970
	2.67 µg/100 ml	Bottoms et al., 1972
	8.6 and 11 µg/100 ml	Eiler et al., 1979
	7 µg/100 ml	Gribble, 1972
Total corticoids (resting horse)	5.1 µg/100 ml	Hoffsis et al., 1970
(Standardbred racehorse)	8.2 µg/100 ml	Hoffsis et al., 1970
ACTH stimulation (rise in cortisol)		
1 unit/kg ACTH gel IM	2–3 times increased by 8 hours	James et al., 1970
Pre and 8-hour sample		Hoffsis et al., 1970
		Gribble, 1972
200 IU corticotropin gel* IM	100% increased by 1 hour and persisting at least 4 hours	Eiler et al., 1979
100 IU cosyntropin† IV	80% increased by 2 hours	Eiler et al., 1979
Pre and 2-hour sample		
1 unit/kg ACTH IV	2–3 times increased by 2 hours	Gribble, 1972
Combined test with dexamethasone (DXM)		Eiler et al., 1979
10 mg DXM IM; pre- and 3-hour sample; then 100 IU cosyntropin† IV and sample 2 hours later	Decrease to ⅓ baseline and then approximately 2 times increase of baseline by cosyntropin†	
Dexamethasone suppression (decrease in cortisol)		
40 µg/kg IM	66% decrease by 12 hours	Gribble, 1972
20 mg IM	50% decrease at 2 hours	Eiler, 1979
	70% decrease by 4 hours	
	80% decrease at 6 hours	
	Still decreased to 31% baseline value at 24 hours	
Insulin tolerance (decrease in glucose)		
0.4 units/kg insulin BP	76% decrease at 2 hours	James et al., 1970
0.05 units/kg crystallin insulin IV	30–45% decrease at 15 min, 60% decrease at 30 min, and normal at 2 hours	Beech and Garcia, unpublished
Glucose tolerance (IV)		
0.5 g/kg 50% glucose	600–700% increase in insulin at 15 and 30 min, then decrease	Beech and Garcia, 1985
	>300% increase in glucose at 15 min, then rapid decrease	
ACTH level	0800 hours—35 ± 11.8 pg/ml	Orth, 1981
	2200 hours—21.4 ± 9.6 pg/ml	
T_3	.09 ± .02 µg/100 ml	Garcia, 1981
T_4	1.8 ± .8 µg/100 ml	Garcia, 1981
TRH response test		
Plasma cortisol before and 15, 30, 60, 120, and 180 min after 1 mg TRH IV	No change in baseline cortisol	Beech and Garcia, 1985

*Adrenomone, Burns Biotec Laboratory, Oakland, CA
†Cortrosyn, Organon, Inc., West Orange, NJ

apy. Treatment is initiated at a dose of 0.6 mg per $kg^{3/4}$ (58 mg for a 450-kg horse) with an increase over several weeks to 1.2 mg per $kg^{3/4}$ (117 mg for a 450-kg horse) given orally in the morning. (For reference, 200 $kg^{3/4}$ = 53.2 kg; 300 $kg^{3/4}$ = 72.1 kg; 500 $kg^{3/4}$ = 105.7 kg.) The drug may be given twice daily. Responsive horses usually improve in six to eight weeks. Alternate-day dosing may be necessary after the initial three-month treatment period. Pergolide and bromocriptine (dopaminergic agonists) have been used experimentally for treatment of pituitary adenomas in a small number of horses, and both drugs caused a clinical improvement. Pergolide is usually administered at a dose of 0.01 mg per kg orally once daily and bromocriptine has been administered at a dose of 0.02 mg per kg intramuscularly twice daily.

If the owner elects to maintain a horse with a pituitary tumor for a period of time, a high plane of nutrition and attempts to minimize infections will be necessary. Any infections should be treated, but wounds will be slow to heal, and these animals are probably more susceptible to stress and disease than are normal animals.

Supplemental Readings

Beech, J.: Tumors of the pituitary gland (pars intermedia). *In* Robinson, N. E. (ed.), Current Therapy in Equine Medicine. Philadelphia, W. B. Saunders Company, 1983, pp. 164–168.

Eiler, H., Goble, D., and Oliver, J.: Adrenal gland function in the horse: Effects of cosyntropin (synthetic) and corticotropin (natural) stimulation. Am. J. Vet. Res., 40:724, 1979.

Eiler, H., Oliver, J., and Goble, D.: Adrenal gland function in the horse: Effect of dexamethasone on hydrocortisone secretion and blood cellularity and plasma electrolyte concentrations. Am. J. Vet. Res., 40:727, 1979.

Evans, D. R.: The recognition and diagnosis of a pituitary tumor in the horse. Proc. 18th Annu. Conv. Am. Assoc. Eq. Pract., 1972, p. 417.

Gribble, D. H.: The endocrine system. *In* Catcott, E. J. and Smithcors, J. F. (eds.): Equine Medicine and Surgery, 2nd ed. Wheaton, IL, American Veterinary Publications, 1972.

Moore, J., Steiss, J., Nicholson, W. E., and Orth, D. N.: A case of pituitary adrenocorticotropin-dependent Cushing's syndrome in the horse. Endocrinology 104:576, 1979.

Orth, D. N., Holscher, M. A., Wilson, M. G., Nicholson, W. E., Pleui, R. E., and Mount, C. D.: Equine Cushing's disease: Plasma immunoreactive proopiolipomelanocortin peptide and cortisol levels basally and in response to diagnostic tests. Endocrinology 110:1430, 1982.

Hypothyroidism

David C. L. Chen, GAINESVILLE, FLORIDA

Oliver W. I. Li, GAINESVILLE, FLORIDA

Thyroid hormones, thyroxine (T_4), and triiodothyronine (T_3) affect virtually every organ system by assisting in the regulation of growth, cell differentiation, and oxidative metabolism. The mechanism of the peripheral action of thyroid hormone is not completely understood. A current hypothesis is that after thyroid hormones enter the cell, T_4 is converted to biologically active T_3 by 5' monodeiodination. T_3 then binds to specific receptor proteins in the cell nucleus and activates DNA-dependent RNA polymerase, resulting in the formation of new mRNA and eventually of new protein in the cell. T_3 also binds to receptors on membranes and mitochondria, and thus may have multiple sites of action.

After administration of T_4 or T_3, oxygen consumption is increased in heart, liver, muscle, kidney, and white blood cells. Thyroid hormones also cause increases in heat production, metabolism of carbohydrates, fats, and proteins, cardiac output, and irritability of the nervous system. It has been suggested that the metabolic rate is increased by the action of thyroid hormones on the cytochrome oxidase enzyme.

HYPOTHYROIDISM

The clinical state of hypothyroidism has not been readily recognized. However, with the advent of radioimmunoassay for thyroid hormones, there have been more reports on thyroid function in horses. The frequency of thyroid disease in horses may be quite high in the United States, and it is especially prevalent in young horses and older mares. Hypothyroidism in equine fetuses and neonates has been linked to clinical signs of prematurity and defective ossification. Lack of adequate T_4 levels causes a specific epiphyseal dysgenesis. Abnormal hormone values lead to either rapid or delayed growth, which may result in permanent disproportion in the skeleton or in permanent tendon contracture. Foals with hypothyroidism exhibit osseous degenerative changes involving the tarsal bones of the hock. Collapse of the central and third tarsal bones can occur. When hypothyroidism begins early in fetal development, the neonate fails to establish normal respiration at birth, whereas onset in late pregnancy or after birth causes lethargy and an inability to stand and suckle. Several reports indicate that foals of dams fed excess iodine have a variety of signs, including long hair, general physical weakness, contracted tendons, marked limb abnormalities, and limb weaknesses. Hypothyroidism also has been associated with myopathy in racing Thoroughbreds and Standardbreds. Clinical signs include erratic appetite, decreased endurance, dullness, and stiffness of gait. Secondary hypothyroidism was diagnosed in one case based on histologic findings and lack of response to administration of thyroid-stimulating hormone (TSH).

DIAGNOSTIC STUDIES

Hormone Assay. Many veterinary diagnostic laboratories and human clinical laboratories have adapted a radioimmunoassay procedure to measure equine serum thyroid hormones. Care should be

TABLE 1. SERUM T_4 AND T_3 CONCENTRATIONS IN HORSES

Age	No. of Animals	T_4 (μg/dl)		T_3 (ng/dl)	
		Mean ± SEM	Min–Max	Mean ± SEM	Min–Max
1.5 to 4 months	14	4.02 ± 0.19	2.9–5.25	192.86 ± 8.54	135–270
2 to 5 years	15	1.94 ± 0.13	1.2–2.9	120.27 ± 8.66	72–180
6 to 10 years	12	1.73 ± 0.07	1.3–2.2	85.58 ± 7.46	48–118
11 to 25 years	11	1.55 ± 0.13	0.9–2.2	83.54 ± 9.03 '	47–145

From Chen, C. L., and Riley, A. M.: Serum thyroxine and triiodothyronine concentrations in neonatal foals and mature horses. Am. J. Vet. Res., 42:1415–1417, 1981.

taken to inform the personnel of human clinical laboratories that the equine species has a much lower (one fourth) serum level of T_4 than the human species and that the assay procedure for human samples needs to be modified in order to assay equine T_4 with any degree of reliability. Most laboratories prefer serum samples for hormone assays. Serum samples should be submitted as soon as possible, although it has been reported that serum levels of thyroid hormones are relatively stable for up to two days.

Normal Serum Levels of Thyroid Hormones. Although T_3 is the more active hormone, many scientists believe that emphasis should be placed on interpreting serum levels of T_4 because of the variability of the T_3 radioimmunoassay. Horse serum thyroid hormone levels decrease with age, foals having twice the T_4 values of 2- to 25-year-old horses (Table 1). There are also differences in thyroid hormone levels among stallions, mares, and geldings (Table 2). There appear to be no breed differences in serum levels of thyroid hormones.

TSH Stimulation Test. Administration of exogenous (bovine) TSH followed by measurement of serum levels of T_4 provides reliable information for the diagnosis of hypothyroidism. Five to 10 IU of bovine TSH administered intravenously should elicit a sufficient increase in T_4 and T_3 in four to eight hours. Increases in thyroid hormone levels can vary but a normal thyroid gland should produce a two- to fourfold increase in serum levels of T_4 and T_3.

TRH Stimulation Test. A hypothalamic hormone, TSH-releasing hormone (TRH), can be used as a stimulation test and/or for the differential diagnosis of primary and secondary hypothyroidism. Three to five mg of TRH is administered intravenously after an initial blood sample is taken. A second blood sample taken four to eight hours later should show two to threefold increase in T_4 (unpublished observations). TRH elicits the secretion of endogenous TSH and is readily available through human pharmacies.

TREATMENT

Ten mg of powdered sodium levothyroxine in 70 ml of corn syrup administered orally increases the blood levels of thyroid hormones in most horses for approximately 24 hours. Therefore, daily medication with 10 mg of sodium levothyroxine is sufficient to alleviate hypothyroidism. It is advisable to monitor serum levels of T_4 following one week of medication. A blood sample should be taken before dosing and another sample should be taken in two to three hours following medication. Adjustment of dosage should be made according to the serum levels of T_4.

Oral medication with iodinated casein (5 gm) has been recommended for treating hypothyroidism in horses. Since iodinated casein contains 1 per cent of T_4, 5 gm of iodinated casein contains 50 mg of thyroxine. This is five times the recommended dosage of sodium levothyroxine. It is therefore advisable to monitor serum levels of T_4 following casein medication and to adjust the dosage accordingly.

TABLE 2. SERUM T_4 AND T_3 CONCENTRATIONS IN FOALS, MARES, STALLIONS, AND GELDINGS

Age	Sex	No. of Animals	T_4 (μg/dl)		T_3 (ng/dl)	
			Mean ± SEM	Min–Max	Mean ± SEM	Min–Max
1.5–3.0 months	Female	9	3.82 ± 0.18*	2.9–4.6	198.33 ± 12.5	135–270
	Male	5	4.38 ± 0.38†	3.3–5.25	197.00 ± 10.07	165–220
2–25 years	Mare	18	1.70 ± 0.10	0.9–2.4	89.83 ± 7.92	48–180
	Gelding	11	1.69 ± 0.14	1.0–2.7	92.90 ± 9.73	50–150
	Stallion	9	1.97 ± 0.16	1.6–2.9	123.44 ± 9.71	84–165

*Significantly different from 2- to 25-year-old horses (P < 0.001).
†Significantly different from mare and gelding (P < 0.05).
From Chen, C. L., and Riley, A. M.: Serum thyroxine and triiodothyronine concentrations in neonatal foals and mature horses. Am. J. Vet. Res., 42:1415–1417, 1981.

Supplemental Readings

Chen, C. L., McNulty, M. E., McNulty, P. K., and Asbury, A. C.: Serum levels of thyroxine and triiodothyronine in mature horses following oral administration of synthetic thyroxine (Synthroid). J. Equine Vet. Sci., 4:5, 1984.

Chen, C. L., and Riley, A. M.: Serum thyroxine and triiodothyronine concentrations in neonatal foals and mature horses. Am. J. Vet. Res., 42:1415, 1981.

Drew, B., Barber, W. P., and Williams, D. G.: The effect of excess dietary iodine on pregnant mares and foals. Vet. Rec. 97:93, 1975.

Gribble, D. H.: The endocrine system. In Equine Medicine and Surgery, 2nd ed. Catcott, E. J. and Smithcors, J. F. (eds.): Wheaton, I1, American Veterinary Publications Inc., 1972, pp. 433–457.

Held, J. P., and Oliver, J. W.: A sampling protocol for the thyrotropin-stimulation test in the horse. J. Am. Vet. Med. Assoc., 184:326, 1984.

Irvine, C. H. G., and Evans, M. J.: Hypothyroidism in foals. N.Z. Vet. J., 25:354, 1977.

Schlotthauer, C. F.: The incidence and types of disease of the thyroid gland of adult horses. J. Am. Vet. Med. Assoc., 78:211, 1931.

Shaver, J. R., Fretz, P. B., Doige, C. E., and Williams, D. M.: Skeletal manifestations of suspected hypothyroidism in two foals. J. Equine Med. Surg., 3:269, 1979.

Waldron-Mease, E.: Hypothyroidism and myopathy in racing thoroughbreds and standardbreds. J. Equine Med. Surg., 3:124, 1979.

Anhidrosis

Angeline Warner, BOSTON, MASSACHUSETTS

Anhidrosis, the inability to sweat in response to an adequate stimulus, is a problem affecting many horses in the Gulf Coast states today. It is seen most often in hot, humid climates. Historically, the disorder crippled the athletic performance of many English Thoroughbreds taken to the tropical colonies. Sweating is the major heat dissipation mechanism of the horse, and affected horses are unable to thermoregulate in extreme heat. Rectal temperature may reach 41.7 to 42.2° C, resulting in collapse if exertion is continued. Thus, competition performance is often severely compromised.

A survey of contemporary cases in Florida shows that anhidrosis affects horses of all ages, breeds, colors, and horses native to hot, humid climates as well as those undergoing acclimatization. Horses in rigorous training for racing, polo, or showing, and those on a high-concentrate diet have been reported as more commonly affected, but recent data show that brood mares and idle pleasure horses are affected with equal frequency. No particular diet, vitamin or mineral supplement, or lack thereof can be incriminated in the etiology. Hereditary predisposition appears unlikely, considering evidence to date. Etiology is as yet uncertain, and no consistently effective therapy has emerged.

CLINICAL SIGNS

Signs commonly noted at the onset are tachypnea, poor exercise tolerance, and alopecia, especially of the face. Profuse sweating before onset of anhidrosis is part of the classical description in the unacclimatized horse but is not seen frequently in contemporary cases. Decreased appetite, changes in water consumption, and loss of body condition are occasionally seen. Onset is usually during the spring or summer and may be abrupt or gradual. Cessation of sweating may be partial or complete. Many horses will maintain residual sweat production under the mane and over the brisket and perineum, but sweat is scant, with little or no lather production. Partial anhidrosis may incompletely resolve (i.e., more normal sweating occurs) during winter.

The diagnosis is made on the basis of inadequate sweat production after appropriate stimulation. Affected horses uniformly display blowing, rapid respiration during hot weather in their attempt to thermoregulate. Rectal temperatures may be markedly elevated. Laboratory values for hematology, electrolytes, and serum enzymes are frequently unremarkable in the anhidrotic horse. Skin biopsies are not diagnostic. Inadequate gland response may be confirmed by intradermal epinephrine challenge. The equine sweat gland is apocrine and responds to postganglionic adrenergic stimulation and circulating catecholamines. Intradermal injection of 0.5 ml of 1:1000 epinephrine will cause sweating over the bleb and in tracks radiating outward in normal skin within an hour, and usually much less. The response will be decreased or absent and may be delayed up to four to five hours in affected horses. The area under the mane (if that skin has been observed to sweat) or a normal horse should be used as a positive control. Total lack of sweat production at the site of epinephrine injection in the affected skin is considered a poor prognostic sign, as the concentration of transmitter is locally very high. Intravenous challenge should be avoided, since although the whole body sweating pattern may be demonstrated, a prolonged refractory period may follow.

POSSIBLE PATHOGENESIS OF ANHIDROSIS

Onset of anhidrosis may not be secondary to poor acclimatization, as once thought, but it does appear to be precipated by heat stress in a humid environment whether or not the individual has previously experienced such conditions. Equine anhidrosis could be accounted for by changes in sweat gland stimulation, gland function, or impaired extrusion of sweat onto the skin surface. Down regulation of sweat gland beta$_2$ receptors in response to higher than normal concentrations of circulating epinephrine secondary to heat stress has been suggested as a cause of anhidrosis, and recently horses with anhidrosis have been shown to have higher levels of circulating epinephrine than normal horses. It is also feasible that the process of sweat gland secretion could be fatigued after prolonged demand, and there is evidence of degenerative changes in normal equine sweat glands after repeated epinephrine injection. Obstruction of the sweat duct can occur in people due to hydration and swelling of keratin after prolonged sweating, and anhidrosis may persist until the obstructing keratin layer undergoes normal sloughing with epidermal turnover. The equine apocrine duct empties into the hair follicle above the sebaceous gland duct, and interference with delivery of sebaceous secretion might contribute to the poor coat condition and alopecia seen in many cases.

The dry skin, alopecia, and decreased exercise tolerance in hot weather seen with anhidrosis have led to the suggestion of hypothyroidism as a contributing factor. Serum T$_3$ and T$_4$ are reported to be low in some anhidrotic horses, but there are no data available on changes in thyroid secretion in normal horses during heat stress, and experimentally thyroidectomized horses sweat normally. Empirically, some nonsweating horses have improved after administration of sodium iodide, potassium iodide, iodinated casein, or thyroid hormone replacement, but presently no experimental evidence exists suggesting hypothyroidsim as an etiology.

THERAPY

A variety of empiric approaches have been tried with variable to poor success to induce sweating in affected horses. These include intravenous and oral electrolytes, oral vitamin E and iodinated casein supplements, dietary change to minimize concentrates, and ACTH injection. Oral supplementation of electrolytes is the most common therapy used today, and some horses do appear to improve. A number of commercial electrolyte supplements have been used,* and there appear to be no differences among them. There is to date no consistently effective therapy to induce sweating. Symptomatic efforts should be aimed at providing a cooler environment via fans or shade, clipping the body, and wetting the horse down with water to provide for evaporative cooling. Many anhidrotic horses are maintained using such measures and judicious exercise during cooler hours of the day. Moving the horse to a temperate climate or providing air-conditioned quarters during the summer will obviously make the animal more comfortable, and frequently the decreased heat stress is associated with more normal sweating.

---

*Electrofin, Haver-Lockhart, Shawnee, KS

Supplemental Reading

Beadle, R. E., Norwood, G. L., and Brencick, V. A.: Summertime plasma catecholamine concentration in healthy and anhidrotic horses in Louisiana. Am. J. Vet. Res., *43*:1446, 1982.

Carlson, G. P., and Ocen, P. O.: Composition of equine sweat following exercise in high environmental temperatures and in response to intravenous epinephrine administration. J. Equine Med. Surg., 3:27, 1979.

Evans, C. L., Smith, D. F. G., Ross, K. A., et al.: Physiologic factors on the condition of "dry coat" in horses. Vet. Rec., 69:1, 1957.

Warner, A. E.: Equine anhidrosis. Compend. Cont. Ed. Pract. Vet., 4:S434, 1982.

Warner, A. E., and Mayhew, I. G.: Equine anhidrosis: A survey of affected horses in Florida. J. Am. Vet. Med. Assoc., *180*:627, 1982.

Warner, A. , and Mayhew, I. G.: Equine anhidrosis: A review of pathophysiologic mechanisms. Vet. Res. Comm., 6:249, 1983.

Disorders of Calcium Metabolism

Barbara D. Brewer, GAINESVILLE, FLORIDA

Calcium plays an integral role in many physiologic phenomena including neuronal excitability, muscle contraction, cell membrane structural integrity and permeability, bone formation, enzyme activity, hormone release, and blood coagulation. Total serum calcium, as measured in the laboratory, includes ionized, chelated, and protein-bound calcium in the extracellular fluid compartment. The amount of intracellular calcium is minute. Both chelated and protein-bound calcium are biologically inactive; ionized calcium is the fraction of the most physiologic importance.

Calcium homeostasis is finely controlled by parathyroid hormone (PTH), calcitonin, and vitamin D. Parathyroid hormone is produced by the chief cells of the parathyroid glands. The horse has two pair of parathyroid glands. The upper pair is located dorsolaterally to the trachea, near the thyroid gland. The larger, lower parathyroids are located on the ventral or ventrolateral surface of the trachea near the level of the first rib. Calcitonin is produced by the thyroid C cells. Vitamin D, whether ingested or produced endogenously, is converted to 25-hydroxycholecalciferol (25 [OH]D$_3$) in the liver and further dehydroxylated to 1,25-dihydroxycholecalciferol (1-25 [OH]$_2$D$_3$) in the kidney. The major physiologic actions of these hormones are listed in Table 1. The plasma calcium pool is in a constant state of flux with calcium homeostasis being achieved by the actions of these hormones on their target cells in the intestine, in the kidney, and on bone. Other hormones (estrogen, adrenal corticosteroids, glucagon, and thyroxine) as well as the patient's serum phosphorus and magnesium levels, may contribute to the maintenance of calcium homeostasis.

An alkaline blood pH favors protein binding and an acid pH favors ionization of calcium. Thus, a horse could have a normal total calcium value and be exhibiting signs of hypocalcemia when alkalotic. Likewise, when a patient is hypoproteinemic, total calcium levels may be low, but if ionized calcium levels remain normal, no signs of tetany will be noted.

HYPOCALCEMIA

Lactation Tetany and Idiopathic Hypocalcemia. Lactation tetany and acute idiopathic hypocalcemia are uncommon problems with identical presenta-

TABLE 1. THE MAJOR EFFECTS OF CALCIUM REGULATING HORMONES ON BONE, KIDNEY, AND INTESTINE

1. Parathyroid hormone (PTH)
   a. *Bone*–Enhances synthesis and lysis of bone mineral with a net release of calcium and phosphorus into the extracellular fluid
   b. *Kidney*–Increases tubular resorption of calcium; decreases tubular resorption of phosphorus; increases renal metabolism of 25 (OH)D$_3$ to 1–25 (OH)$_2$ D$_3$
   c. *Intestine*–Increases calcium absorption via vitamin D
   d. *Net effect*–Increases calcium and decreases phosphorus in serum
   e. *Stimulus for Secretion*–Decreased ionized calcium, (increased serum phosphorus will decrease serum calcium and therefore secondarily cause PTH secretion,) adrenergic stimulation, and decreased magnesium
2. Calcitonin
   a. *Bone*–Inhibits resorption and stimulates formation causing decreased entry of calcium and phosphorus into the blood
   b. *Kidney*–Decreases renal absorption of phosphorus
   c. *Intestine*–No direct effect
   d. *Net effect*–Decreases calcium and phosphorus in serum
   e. *Stimulus for Secretion*–Increased ionized calcium
3. Vitamin D
   a. *Bone*–Conflicting evidence exists
   b. *Kidney*–Enhances tubular resorption of phosphorus and calcium
   c. *Intestine*–Increases calcium and phosphorus absorption
   d. *Net effect*–Increases calcium and phosphorus in serum

tions. The clinical signs include depression, tachypnea with flared nostrils, a stiff stilted gait or rear limb ataxia, muscle fasciculations (particularly of the temporal, masseter, and triceps muscles), trismus, inability to chew and swallow, profuse sweating, normal to very high temperatures, tachycardia, cardiac arrhythmias, synchronous diaphragmatic flutter, recumbency, convulsions, and death. Table 2 presents the differential diagnosis of lactation tetany.

Treatment of the horse with lactation tetany or idiopathic hypocalcemia requires 250 ml per 450 kg

TABLE 2. DISEASE CONDITIONS WITH CLINICAL SIGNS RESEMBLING THOSE IN LACTATION TETANY

Tetanus
Laminitis
Myositis
Seizures
Other severe electrolyte imbalances
Colic
Botulism
Other diseases with associated hypocalcemia

of a standard commercially available solution* containing calcium, magnesium, and phosphorus given *slowly* intravenously while the heart is carefully auscultated. The expected cardiovascular response is an increase in the intensity of the heart sounds. An infrequent extrasystole may be expected, but a pronounced change in rate or rhythm is an indication to suspend intravenous treatment at once. After 10 minutes, if no improvement is noted, a second infusion should be administered. Complete recovery may require several hours or days, and retreatment may be necessary as relapses do occur. Calcium solution containing dextrose should be used with caution because perivascular leakage may cause phlebitis.

The role of magnesium in the disease is unclear. Lactating ponies developing tetany following transport can have both low and high serum magnesium levels. Thus, horses that are unresponsive to calcium therapy may respond to treatment with magnesium.

Synchronous Diaphragmatic Flutter. Synchronous diaphragmatic flutter (SDF, "thumps") is a clinical sign in which a flutter or contraction of one or both flanks is observed coincident with the heartbeat. Electrolyte abnormalities in cases of SDF include hypocalcemia, hypokalemia, hypochloremia, and alkalosis. Hypocalcemia seems to be the most consistent of these abnormalities. The diagnosis and therapy of SDF is discussed on p. 485.

Blister Beetle Toxicosis. Blister beetle poisoning (see p. 120) is an acute and often rapidly fatal toxicosis of horses that have eaten beetles (Epicauta spp.) contained in alfalfa hay. Hypocalcemia is a frequent complication of this problem. The clinical signs are variable but may include colic, depression, fever, shock, sweating, seizures, collapse, frequent, often bloody, urination, and synchronous diaphragmatic flutter. The reason why some horses with this condition become hypocalcemic is unknown, but the hypocalcemia may be associated with a poorer prognosis for survival.

Pancreatic Disease. Pancreatic disease (see p. 46) is a rarely *recognized* clinical entity in the horse, and the diagnosis of this problem would be difficult to confirm in the laboratory owing to the paucity of data on the subject. Hypocalcemia is a common clinicopathologic finding in dogs and humans with acute pancreatitis.

Horses in which the only abnormality found at necropsy was pancreatic atrophy have been treated for signs of generalized muscular tremors, synchronous diaphragmatic flutter, and tetany. The signs abated temporarily with administration of calcium but were recurrent, ultimately necessitating eutha-

nasia (A. M. Merritt, University of Florida and C. W. Kohn, Ohio State University, personal communication, 1982). Thus, pancreatic disease, although rarely diagnosed in horses, should be considered in the differential diagnosis of horses experiencing hypocalcemia.

Other Conditions. Hypocalcemia has been associated with malignant hyperthermia, acute experimental oxalate toxicity (chronic oxalate toxicity has been reported to lead to nephrocalcinosis), renal disease, exertional rhabdomyolysis, and postoperative myopathy in the horse. Diseases causing hypoalbuminemia (e.g., chronic liver disease, malabsorption) may be associated with a fall in the level of total serum calcium, but the concentration of ionized calcium is usually not reduced and the patient rarely suffers from signs of hypocalcemia.

HYPERCALCEMIA

Renal Disease. Equine renal disease is discussed in detail in the section on Urinary Tract Diseases. Normal, low, or high serum calcium levels can be a feature of acute *or* chronic renal failure in horses. While dogs and humans occasionally develop hypercalcemia in association with renal disease, this phenomenon seems to be far more common in the horse. Primary hyperparathyroidism does not appear to be the cause of hypercalcemia.

Horses and ponies absorb more calcium from their diets and excrete a much larger proportion of absorbed calcium in the urine than do other species. Moreover, the proportion of absorbed calcium excreted by the kidney of the horse increases as calcium absorption increases, again in contrast to other species. The presence or absence of hypercalcemia in horses with renal failure may be related also to calcium intake and/or loss of albumin coupled with peculiarities of renal function. Nephrectomized ponies fed alfalfa hay develop hypercalcemia while those fed grass hay do not. Ionized calcium levels do increase, however.*

Neoplasia. Neoplastic disease resulting in pseudohyperparathyroidism is second only to primary hyperparathyroidism in producing hypercalcemia in humans. In the horse, gastric squamous cell carcinoma and lymphosarcoma are associated with hypercalcemia.

Primary Hyperparathyroidism. Primary hyperparathyroidism may be a result of parathyroid adenoma, parathyroid hyperplasia, or carcinoma. Only four cases of parathyroid adenoma in old horses have been reported. This general lack of recognition may stem from the fact that the two (and occasion-

---

*Forcal, Bio-Ceutic Laboratories, St. Joseph, MO

*T. J. Divers, University of Pennsylvania, personal communication.

ally more than two) pairs of equine parathyroid glands are widely separated and often difficult to identify. This differential diagnosis should be considered in cases in which unexplained hypercalcemia exists in the horse.

Hypervitaminosis D. Hypervitaminosis D is a relatively rare condition of horses that may result in hypercalcemia. The etiology of the problem is oversupplementation with parenteral vitamin D preparations, inadvertent mixture of excessive amounts of vitamin D in horse feed, or ingestion of plants containing potent vitamin D-like substances. In the United States, two such plants, *Cestrum diurnum* (day blooming jessamine, wild jasmin) in south Florida and Texas and *Solanum sodomaeum* in Hawaii, cause the disease. Horses that have been overdosed with vitamin preparations and those exhibiting *Cestrum diurnum* toxicosis experience similar clinical signs, including depression, weight loss, anorexia, limb stiffness, painful flexor tendons and suspensory ligaments, tachycardia, and often polyuria with compensatory polydipsia.

Laboratory findings may include hypercalcemia, with calcium levels fluctuating between high and normal during the early course of the disease. Hyperphosphatemia occurs with vitamin oversupplementation but may be absent in the plant toxicosis. Urine specific gravity is low and blood urea nitrogen is normal unless massive kidney mineralization has occurred. Creatine phosphokinase and sorbitol dehydrogenase values are low. Hematology is unremarkable. Necropsy findings are very suggestive of the disease with widespread soft tissue mineralization, particularly in the cardiovascular system.

Treatment is supportive with immediate removal of all sources of vitamin D, calcium, and phosphorus. The prognosis is poor for horses exhibiting signs of cardiovascular disease or those with elevated BUN or creatinine. In less severe cases, recovery may require six months or more, and some horses will never return to normal.

Nutritional Secondary Hyperparathyroidism. Nutritional secondary hyperparathyroidism (NSH) is one of the oldest known diseases of the horse. It has been termed "big head," "bran disease," and "Miller's disease." This skeletal disease is seen in horses fed rations containing an excess of phosphorus relative to the amount of calcium. The total calcium content of the diet may actually be marginally adequate.

Young, growing horses are most commonly affected, but pregnancy may also induce the disease. Intermittent, shifting lameness is usually the first clinical sign. Lameness is due to focal periosteal avulsion, torn or detached ligaments or tendons, or subepiphyseal microfractures. Joint pain may occur as a result of erosions of the articular cartilage

TABLE 3. NORMAL LABORATORY VALUES USED IN DIAGNOSIS OF NUTRITIONAL SECONDARY HYPERPARATHYROIDISM

Laboratory Parameter	Normal Range
Serum calcium mg/dl	10.5–13.0
Serum phosphorus mg/dl	2–5
Fractional excretion of phosphorus	0–0.5%
Fractional excretion of calcium	2.5%
Ca excretion* μmole/mosmole	15
P excretion* μmole/mosmole	15

$$*\text{Urine concentration (mM)} \times .04$$
$$\text{specific gravity} - .997$$

apparently due to loss of the underlying trabeculae. Classically, the horses have stiff, stilted gaits. Difficulty masticating develops as the laminae durae are resorbed, bilaterally symmetrical facial swellings occur, and the horse may become cachectic as mastication becomes difficult or locomotion (and grazing) too painful. The maxillae and rami of the mandibles are progressively and irregularly thickened due to hyperostotic fibrous osteodystrophy, resulting from osteoid and fibrous connective tissue deposition in excess of the volume of bone resorbed.

NSH is caused by excessive phosphorus ingestion with elevation of serum phosphorus levels. Hyperphosphatemia lowers the blood calcium level, which then stimulates the parathyroid glands to increase the secretion of PTH, which returns blood calcium levels to near normal. Continued ingestion of the imbalanced ration causes parathyroid gland hypertrophy followed by the development of metabolic bone disease.

The diagnosis is made on the basis of clinical signs and feed analysis. Any supplemental use of bran must be terminated because bran has quite high phosphorus levels. While alfalfa hay is an excellent source of calcium, grass hays are not. Both have similar amounts of phosphorus, usually not enough for the growing horse. Grains are poor sources of calcium and moderate to good sources of phosphorus (see p. 395).

Radiographic loss of the laminae durae is said to be an early pathognomonic change. Serum calcium is usually in the low-normal range by the time the disease is diagnosed (hypocalcemia and hyperphosphatemia occur very early).

There is general agreement that the fractional renal excretion of phosphorus (see Section 18) as determined by calculations utilizing a one-time measurement of urine and serum phosphorus and creatinine is a useful means of detecting mineral imbalances in horses. The ratio of the urine phosphorus concentration to total urine solute concentration requires only a urine specimen and is also useful.

Disagreement exists about the usefulness of similar one-time determination of calcium excretion. Fractional renal excretion of calcium may be difficult to interpret because excreted calcium precipitates as calcium carbonate in the urinary bladder. Several investigators believe, however, that meaningful information can be obtained from the determination and that both calcium and phosphorus determinations in fact should be made since excretion of both minerals in the urine may be affected by the intake of either one. See Table 3 for suggested normal values. Horses with NSH have low normal serum calcium values, normal serum phosphorus values, decreased urinary calcium excretion, decreased fractional excretion of calcium (Ca per cent Cr), and increased urinary phosphorus excretion and fractional excretion of phosphorus (P per cent Cr). Serum alkaline phosphatase levels often are in the high normal range or elevated reflecting increased osteoblastic and osteoclastic activity.

Treatment consists of correcting dietary imbalances and supplementing the diet with calcium carbonate (limestone). Phosphorus-containing supplements such as bone meal should be avoided. The lameness usually improves within two months, but the facial swellings are not likely to regress.

Horses in Australia and Florida grazing improved pastures rich in oxalates develop signs of ill thrift, lameness, and fibrous facial swelling. Calcium and phosphorus levels of the pastures are normal. The combination of calcium and oxalate in the diet may render dietary calcium insoluble in the alimentary tract and thus unavailable for absorption. This situation differs from the classic equine nutritional secondary hyperparathyroidism in that these horses are not fed diets rich in cereal grains, but the resulting syndrome appears to be the same.

Supplemental Readings

Brobst, D. F., Bayly, W. M., Reed, S. M., Howard, G. A., and Torbeck, R. L.: Parathyroid hormone evaluation in normal horses and horses with renal failure. Equine Vet. Sci., 2:150, 1982.

Capen, C.: The calcium regulating hormones: Parathyroid hormone, calcitonin and cholecalciferol. *In* MacDonald, L. (ed.): Veterinary Endocrinology and Reproduction, 3rd ed. Philadelphia, Lea & Febiger, 1980.

Caple, I. W., Doake, P. A., and Ellis, P. G.: Assessment of the calcium and phosphorus, nutrition in horses by analysis of urine. Aust. Vet. J., 58:125, 1982.

Coffman, J. R.: Equine Clinical Chemistry and Pathophysiology. Bonner Springs, KS, Veterinary Medicine Pub. Co., 1981.

Divers, T. J.: Chronic renal failure in horses. Compend. Contin. Educ. Pract. Vet., 5:S310, 1983.

Popovtzer, M. M., and Knochel, J. P.: Disorders of calcium, phosphorus, vitamin D, and parathyroid hormone activity. *In* Schrier, R. W. (ed.): Renal and Electrolyte Disorders. Boston, Little, Brown, 1980.

Tennant, B., Lowe, J., and Tasker, J.: Hypercalcemia and hypophosphatemia in ponies following bilateral nephrectomy. Expl. Biol. Med., 167:365, 1981.

FOAL DISEASES

Edited by C. Hillidge

Identification, Diagnosis, and Treatment of the High-Risk Newborn Foal

Anne M. Koterba, GAINESVILLE, FLORIDA

A healthy and functional fetoplacental unit and uterine environment are crucial for normal fetal development, tolerance of the birth process, and a smooth adaptation to independent life after birth. There are a number of adverse pre- and perinatal conditions that can alter this environment and compromise the well-being of the newborn foal. The extent to which the fetus or newborn is affected depends on a number of factors, including the type and duration of the dysfunction and the stage of fetal development at which it occurs. It is clear that at least some of these abnormal foals, even those seriously ill from adverse peripartum events, can make dramatic recoveries and develop into normal adults if proper supportive techniques are employed to help them through the initial days of adjustment. In order to achieve the most favorable results, however, the situation must be recognized early in the course of the disease process, and rational diagnostic and therapeutic procedures must be instituted without delay.

CAUSES OF FETAL ENVIRONMENTAL DERANGEMENT

In many cases, conditions predisposing to neonatal problems are present before birth, and acquisition of a detailed history to identify any prenatal problems is essential. Some of the more common conditions associated with the abnormal newborn foal are listed in Table 1. Foalings that are associated with one or more of these conditions should be considered at high risk, and the animal should be treated appropriately (see section on Clinical Diagnosis).

Placental insufficiency is a well-established cause of fetal distress. The term describes a pathologic condition in which the efficiency of placental exchange is reduced; the dysfunction may be acute or chronic, infectious or noninfectious in nature (see p. 528).

Chronic, noninfectious causes of placental insufficiency include twinning, body pregnancies, and hypoplasia of the chorionic villi.

Infectious lesions are probably the most common causes of chronic placental insufficiency, fetal stress, and disease. Further information on fetal infection may be found in the chapter on Neonatal Septicemia, p. 222.

The correlation between the severity of gross placental lesions and the degree of compromise to the fetus is not particularly close. For example, serious fetal infection, growth retardation, or both have been observed in the absence of gross placental

TABLE 1. CONDITIONS ASSOCIATED WITH A HIGH-RISK NEWBORN FOAL

I. Maternal conditions
   A. Purulent vaginal discharge
   B. Fever
   C. Hydrops allantois
   D. General anesthesia
   E. Colic surgery
   F. Endotoxemia
   G. Excessive medication administration
   H. Past history of foal with isoerythrolysis, neonatal maladjustment syndrome, congenital anomalies
   I. Excessive colostral leakage before parturition
   J. Poor nutritional status
II. Conditions of labor or delivery
   A. Premature parturition
   B. Abnormally long gestation
   C. Prolonged labor
   D. Induction of labor
   E. Dystocia
   F. Early umbilical cord rupture
   G. Cesarean section
III. Neonatal Conditions
   A. Meconium-stained fluid or foal
   B. Placental abnormalities, premature placental separation
   C. Placentitis—fungal or bacterial
   D. Twins
   E. Orphan
   F. Delayed or lack of intake of colostrum
   G. Immaturity or prematurity
   H. Exposure to infectious diseases
   I. Trauma by birth or predators

pathology, while some foals exposed to what appeared to be extensive placental disease have remained relatively normal. If obvious placental disease is present, however, neonatal compromise must be considered a strong possibility until proved otherwise.

Peripartum events such as dystocia, cesarean section, strangulation of the umbilical cord, and premature placental separation can cause acute placental insufficiency, resulting in a disrupted blood flow to the fetus. Premature placental separation is characterized by the appearance of the bright red unruptured chorioallantois protruding from the vulva prior to delivery of the foal. In order for the foal to survive, the foaling attendant must rupture this membrane. Acute placental insufficiency may be accompanied by an edematous, heavy (more than 15 lb) placenta. In many other cases, no abnormalities are noted either in the placenta or in the events of delivery, yet the clinical signs and postmortem findings of the foal are highly suggestive of asphyxiation.

Other than placental pathology, a number of conditions can result in a weak or abnormal newborn foal. The role of the fetus itself should not be ignored. Structural deformities can result in abnor

mal growth in the uterus or can predispose to dystocia or weakness after delivery. Abnormalities in maternal body systems other than the reproductive tract may also exert a profound influence on development of the fetus. For example, both poor maternal nutritional status and excessive intake of medication are potentially detrimental to the health of the fetus. At this point, however, little is known about the placental transfer of drugs commonly administered to the mare during pregnancy, or their effects on the fetus. With the exception of Equine Herpesvirus type 1, very few congenital viral infections have been associated with neonatal equine illness. In other animal species and in humans, however, a number of chronic viral fetal infections are responsible for both developmental malformations and disease during the neonatal period. The possibility of the involvement of additional viral infections in neonatal equine disease should not be overlooked.

EFFECTS OF UTERINE ENVIRONMENTAL DERANGEMENT ON THE NEWBORN FOAL

GESTATIONAL AGE AND MATURITY

A fetus that has been subjected to an abnormal in utero environment may be born prematurely, at term, or post-term. A term pregnancy has a broad definition; 320 to 360 days, with a mean of 340 days, has been considered to represent the 95 per cent confidence limits for gestational length in Thoroughbreds. Prematurity has been defined as a gestational length of less than 320 days. It is important to remember that there is considerable individual variation in the development of maturity and "readiness for birth." One foal of gestational age of 320 days may appear totally normal, while another of 340 days may appear very immature. Whenever possible, it is useful to compare the true gestational age as calculated from breeding dates with an estimate of gestational age as determined from physical examination. This comparison can help to identify the small for gestational age (SGA) foal, which previously might have been labeled as immature or dysmature. Small for gestational age implies that some type of chronic derangement during gestation, such as malnutrition, placental insufficiency, infection, and congenital defects, interrupted normal growth processes. The small for gestational age animal often has difficulty in adapting to the extrauterine environment and may well be in need of special care during this transition period.

The premature foal potentially has many imma

ture organ systems. This immaturity places it at much higher risk than the term foal for developing a variety of respiratory, metabolic, thermoregulatory, hormonal, and infectious problems after birth. Rarely, however, is the foal *only* premature; there is generally a major underlying problem causing the premature delivery in the first place. The most commonly diagnosed pre-existing condition is probably fetal or placental infection. In these cases, the effects of sepsis become superimposed on those of prematurity, and further complicate the clinical course.

Placental insufficiency, intrauterine growth retardation, and increased perinatal mortality can also be associated with abnormally long gestations. It is thought that the respiratory and nutritive functions of the placenta are reduced as gestational length is prolonged. In humans, fetal distress is noted in one third of post-term pregnancies. Although the post-term foal is in many cases perfectly normal, the possibility that it may be suffering from malnutrition or chronic hypoxia or both should be kept in mind. In the future, diagnostic ultrasound may be able to detect those fetuses that are distressed or growth-retarded in utero, and allow more rational management.

BODY SYSTEM DYSFUNCTION

There is great potential for even the normal foal to become severely asphyxiated during the birth process. Indeed, in most normal births, some degree of hypoxemia and respiratory acidosis is observed transiently. Although the normal newborn animal generally tolerates asphyxia better than the adult, severe or prolonged hypoxemia may well overcome any protective mechanisms in operation. In addition, those animals that were exposed to adverse in utero conditions are frequently impaired in their ability to tolerate the birth process and other peripartum events. One factor that is considered important in the ability of the newborn to maintain its circulation in the face of asphyxia is a high fetal cardiac glycogen level. During asphyxia, the arterial PO_2 falls rapidly; within about two minutes, the oxygen content of the blood is exhausted. At this time, the ability of the heart to continue to pump blood depends on energy production via anaerobic glycolysis of the cardiac glycogen stores. The cost of this process, however, is elevated tissue and blood lactate levels, with resulting metabolic acidosis. It is thought that repeated episodes of hypoxia during gestation slowly deplete cardiac glycogen stores, impairing the ability of the heart to pump blood in the face of hypoxia. Thus, the already compromised animal becomes

more susceptible to tissue damage secondary to acute hypoxemia.

Cells may be deprived of oxygen by either of two major mechanisms: hypoxemia, a decreased amount of oxygen in the blood, or ischemia, a decreased amount of blood perfusing the tissues. Although the physiologic response to the two conditions is similar in some ways, there are important distinctions. In general, there is good evidence to support the idea that an ischemic insult is more damaging to an organism than is hypoxia. Metabolites of anaerobic metabolism cannot be removed from the tissues until the blood supply is restored, and tissue lactate levels become markedly elevated during ischemia. Severe intracellular acidosis frequently results, and markedly interferes with cellular functions. In addition, the integrity of the circulation may be severely compromised following ischemic injury. It is suspected that oxygen-derived free radicals are responsible, at least in part, for the enhanced capillary permeability, edema formation, and tissue damage that commonly follows reperfusion.

Hypovolemia secondary to peripartum hemorrhage or blood deprivation such as occurs following premature rupture of umbilical cord may not be obvious until several hours after the birth. Blood pressure may actually be normal initially because of constriction of numerous vascular capacitance beds by catecholamines, alpha-adrenergic stimulation, and other hormonal influences. With time, however, the acute peripartum stresses lessen, circulating hormonal levels fall, and progressive systemic hypotension and acidosis may develop. The pulmonary circulation may reflexly constrict secondary to the acidosis or hypoxemia or both, pulmonary arterial pressure may exceed the decreasing systemic pressure, and right to left shunting away from the lungs through the ductus may result. Thus, the fetal circulation is re-established and interferes with blood oxygenation. Intervention at this late stage is often futile because irreversible cellular damage has usually already occurred. The outcome can be much better if hypovolemia is recognized and corrected earlier in the clinical course.

A good understanding of these concepts is useful when evaluating the asphyxiated or the abnormal newborn foal. Virtually any organ system can be adversely affected, and multisystem dysfunction is the rule rather than the exception. Table 2 lists some of the more common potential sequelae to chronic and/or acute hypoxia and ischemia; many of these will be described in more detail in the following sections. It should be kept in mind that while in some circumstances asphyxiation or hemorrhage is easily recognized, in many others the event is entirely overlooked.

TABLE 2. POSSIBLE SEQUELAE TO ASPHYXIATION IN THE NEWBORN FOAL

Organ System/Disease	Clinical Signs/Laboratory Data	Pathology
RESPIRATORY SYSTEM		
Meconium aspiration	Meconium-covered foal; respiratory distress	Pneumonia, meconium in lung
Surfactant dysfunction	Respiratory distress	Atelectasis, edema
Pulmonary hypertension	Hypoxemia	Persistent fetal circulation
NERVOUS SYSTEM		
Brain	Seizures, abnormal behavior, depression	Hemorrhage, ischemic necrosis, edema
Spinal cord	Weakness, abnormal limb reflexes	Same as above
CARDIOVASCULAR		
Heart	Low cardiac output, arrhythmias	Myocardial infarcts
Circulation	Generalized edema, low effective circulating volume, poor pulses	Generalized edema
LIVER	Increased liver enzymes; nonspecific signs	Hepatic necrosis
KIDNEY	Oliguria, acute renal failure	Acute tubular necrosis, infarcts
GASTROINTESTINAL	Poor gut motility, constipation, gastric reflux	Gastrointestinal hemorrhage, ulceration
ADRENAL GLAND	Vague, nonlocalizing, low cortisol (?)	Hemorrhage, necrosis, congestion
METABOLIC		
Hypoglycemia	Weakness, collapse	Nonspecific
Acidosis	Same; respiratory rate sometimes increased	Same as above
Disseminated intravascular coagulation	Petechiation, hemorrhage; low platelets, fibrin split products	Petechiation, hemorrhage

CLINICAL DIAGNOSIS IN THE ABNORMAL NEWBORN FOAL

Every attempt should be made to define the extent of the compromise to homeostatic mechanisms as precisely as possible and to establish the presence or absence of infection. It must be emphasized that not all signs of organ dysfunction will be apparent immediately after birth; over 24 hours may elapse before specific manifestations of adverse peripartum events will be noted. For example, obvious signs of respiratory disease secondary to asphyxia or in utero sepsis may not be obvious until well after birth. Yet, if appropriate treatment is withheld until clinical signs are severe, a poor outcome often results. Therefore, in the high-risk individual, a complete work-up (Table 3), *not* mere observation, is highly recommended as soon as possible after the high-risk animal is identified. After the initial work-up, the foal should be closely monitored for changes in condition and for the development of new problems.

PHYSICAL EXAMINATION

An accurate examination depends on familiarity with what constitutes normal behavior and physical findings in the newborn foal. Any foal that fails to stand and nurse within two hours of birth should be considered potentially abnormal. Regardless of the problem, the most common signs of abnormality are vague and nonspecific: delay in standing, weakness, poor suck reflex, and lack of affinity for the

TABLE 3. PROTOCOL FOR RECEIVING SICK NEONATAL FOALS UNIVERSITY OF FLORIDA, 1985

1. Assess immediate needs. Evaluate *breathing pattern, respiratory rate, heart rate,* and *mucous membrane perfusion.* Perform **resuscitation** procedures or begin **oxygen** therapy **before** proceeding with further diagnostic tests.
2. If body temperature is less than 37.7°C (100°F), apply heat lamps and heating blankets.
3. Assess **fluid balance** and insert IV catheter if fluid therapy is indicated.
4. Draw EDTA and clot blood tubes to:
   a. Perform whole blood glucose determination. If less than 40 mg/dl, infuse 10% solution to give 8–12 mg/kg/min of glucose. Provide continuous infusion.
   b. Perform complete and differential cell count and fibrinogen level.
   c. Measure serum Na, K, Cl, Ca, P, creatinine, blood urea nitrogen, liver enzymes, albumin, and zinc sulfate turbidity test and set up radial immunodiffusion test for IgG.
5. Draw aerobic and anaerobic **blood cultures.**
6. In any recumbent or dehydrated foal, take indirect **blood pressure** and record.
7. Attempt to acquire arterial **blood gas** sample. If pulse quality is very poor, obtain venous sample for metabolic evaluation.
8. When condition is stabilized, **x-ray** thorax and, if indicated, abdomen.
9. Assess probability of sepsis *as soon as* lab data are available.
10. Weigh foal.
11. Evaluate lab data and physical exam results and decide on appropriate antibiotic, plasma, fluid therapy, tetanus prophylaxis, and umbilical care.
    a. In premature foal, **IV plasma** as well as **colostrum** should be administered during first 24 hours of life. One liter of plasma can be expected to raise IgG levels 100–250 mg/dl. We want a final IgG level of 800 mg/dl or greater.

mare are some of the more common signs reported. The animal should be closely examined for congenital defects, signs of immaturity, or outward indications of birth trauma. Fractured ribs are easily overlooked on routine physical but often become clinically important. Difficulty in body temperature regulation, with a tendency for hypothermia, is common in the abnormal newborn. The adequacy of circulating volume should be assessed frequently; marked changes can occur in a very short period of time. As dysfunction of the pulmonary system is common, careful attention should be paid to evaluation of respiratory rate, character of breathing, and lung auscultation. On the basis of physical examination alone, however, accurate evaluation of specific organ systems can be difficult. For example, although severe pathology may be present, lung auscultation, respiratory rate, and mucous membrane color may be well within the normal range. More specialized tests, such as arterial blood gas analysis and chest radiology, are often essential to identify and treat certain conditions.

The identification of prenatally acquired infections is frequently a diagnostic challenge as well. These types of infections can be manifested in a variety of ways in the newborn. In some animals, localizing signs such as uveitis, pneumonia, and diarrhea are present from delivery and indicate the strong likelihood of infection. In most cases, however, only vague signs of weakness and lethargy are seen. The absence of fever is *not* sufficient evidence to rule out infection; in fact, in one survey of in utero acquired infections, none of the foals displayed a temperature higher than 39° C during the early stages of infection. Because diagnosis of infection is difficult in many individuals, hematology and blood cultures are recommended in every abnormal foal (see p. 223).

HEMATOLOGY

A complete blood count (CBC), differential blood count and plasma fibrinogen determination may provide useful information. Neutropenia, neutrophilia, an increased number of band neutrophils, and toxic changes in the neutrophils have been identified as the most common hematologic alterations in the septicemic foal. These abnormalities, however, are not only observed in infectious conditions. The same changes have been detected in many asphyxiated or severely hypothermic foals in which infection could not be confirmed. The emergence of band cells has also been associated with asphyxia in human neonates. If any of the aforementioned white blood cell (WBC) abnormalities are present, however, sepsis should be considered high on the list of differential diagnoses until ruled out. Although the presence of a completely normal WBC and differential cell count does not eliminate the possibility of sepsis, the diagnosis is considered

less likely. In the high-risk animal, serial CBC measurements, once or twice per day, are indicated both for early detection of infection and to monitor the patient's progress once sepsis is diagnosed.

On the basis of studies of premature foals acquired by early induction of labor, Jeffcott et al. suggested that persistent leukopenia and a narrow neutrophil:lymphocyte ratio indicated a lack of readiness for birth and a poor chance for survival. At the University of Florida, however, no correlation has been found between WBC count and survival in foals that were spontaneously delivered prematurely because of prenatal infection or placentitis. Some infected foals with very low WBC counts (1500 per μl) with severe toxicity did survive. In a group of noninfected foals that were delivered by cesarean section or by induced labor because of maternal illness, however, the same parameters were associated with a poor prognosis.

Elevation of plasma fibrinogen concentration has been associated with in utero infections in foals. A normal value of less than 400 mg per dl, however, does not rule out the possibility of infection.

CLINICAL CHEMISTRY AND SERUM ELECTROLYTES

These tests can provide both a crude estimate of liver and renal function and critical information regarding electrolyte status. Electrolyte balance may be normal or markedly deranged secondary to asphyxia, dehydration, sepsis, or blood volume depletion. Without actual performance of the appropriate tests, it is difficult to predict which parameters will be abnormal in an individual animal. One metabolic abnormality that is consistently seen in abnormal or septic foals less than 24 hours of age is hypoglycemia. Blood glucose levels may be life-threateningly low; if irreversible cell damage is to be avoided, therapy must be instituted promptly. Whole-blood glucose levels can be rapidly and satisfactorily determined at the farm by several types of reagent strips.

BLOOD CULTURES

The importance of identification of the bacteria responsible for neonatal disease cannot be overestimated. Blood cultures have been found to be surprisingly effective in identification of neonatal septicemia. Further details concerning blood culture technique and interpretation can be found in the chapter on Neonatal Septicemia (p. 222).

ASSESSMENT OF PASSIVE IMMUNITY

In providing intensive care to an abnormal foal, one of the most important goals is provision of *normal* immunoglobulin levels greater than 800 mg per dl. Although previous reports have considered values of 400 mg per dl or more to indicate adequate passive transfer of immunity, we believe strongly that the already compromised foal with an IgG level in the gray zone between 400 and 800 mg per dl is still at high risk of acquiring a severe bacterial infection after birth, and we prefer to see higher levels. A quantitative test for assessing adequacy of transfer of passive immunity is recommended (see p. 213).

PRINCIPLES OF THERAPY IN THE HIGH-RISK NEWBORN FOAL

Treatment of the abnormal neonatal foal is frequently a very challenging proposition. It is characteristic of the sick foal to have a number of problems; for example, signs of prematurity, asphyxia, and sepsis are often superimposed in one animal. A successful outcome ultimately depends on the *commitment* of the veterinarian, owner, and foal attendants to intensive nursing care and support of the animal. Once this commitment has been made, the basic aim is to maintain homeostasis during the period that the animal is adjusting to life outside the uterus and repairing any damage to its organ systems. In addition, every attempt must be made to avoid adding iatrogenic problems to the pre-existing ones. Frequently the animal dies of a problem caused by inappropriate treatment rather than the initial insult. As the most frequent complication of intensive care is secondary infection, it is important that aseptic technique be maintained and good passive immunity be provided. A problem-oriented approach, in which each problem is listed and addressed separately, allows a better grasp of a complicated case and helps to prevent the tendency to overlook a major but less obvious problem that is not the primary diagnosis.

Techniques of therapy and support of specific organ systems may be found in the chapters that follow. This discussion will be limited to general support of the abnormal newborn animal.

Although good nursing care is a time-consuming proposition, its value cannot be overestimated. The area in which the foal is treated should be warm and easily cleaned and disinfected; soft bedding that cannot be inhaled or ingested should be provided. Unfortunately, in many cases fulfillment of these requirements necessitates removal of the foal from the mother. A thermoneutral environment minimizes energy requirements and helps to prevent hypothermia. Although hypothermia is most commonly observed, certain poorly adapted foals may also develop hyperthermia when placed in a very warm environment. The environment of the neonatal foal should be designed to minimize the potential for self-inflicted injury. Decubital and corneal ulcers are common complications. Use of a twin-sized heated waterbed, effective seizure control, prompt correction of entropion, careful manual restraint, and frequent change of position can minimize these problems.

In order for growth to continue and reparative mechanisms to function optimally, adequate nutritional intake must be maintained (see p. 205). In the collapsed foal with no suck reflex, provision of even maintenance requirements can be difficult. Although some "down" foals can tolerate a milk diet supplied via nasogastric tube, in a number of premature or very ill animals, any sort of enteral alimentation is contraindicated because of poor gut motility and subsequent gastric reflux, bloating, or colic. In these patients, total parenteral alimentation presents a viable alternative. Glucose solutions, at gradually increasing concentrations, are useful for maintaining serum glucose concentrations in foals that have a tendency for hypoglycemia and for supply of a part of the caloric requirement. If oral alimentation is not reinstituted within one to two days, however, a source of amino acids should be given intravenously along with the glucose solution. Unfortunately, equine neonatal nutrition is at a very early stage of development. Because knowledge of equine neonatal nutrition is limited, almost nothing is known about any special nutritional requirements of the premature or growth-retarded foal.

Knowledge concerning optimal physical therapy of the premature or recumbent foal is also rudimentary. How best to manage the foal with immature bones or connective tissue or both and the resulting angular limb deformities is unclear. As increasing numbers of immature foals survive the early neonatal period, these questions will need to be answered.

Effective treatment of primary prenatal infections and prevention of secondary infections are important considerations. Delay in recognition and treatment of septicemia almost invariably results in a poor outcome. If any suspicion of infection exists, broad-spectrum antibiotics should be given immediately following acquisition of appropriate bacterial cultures. As essential as appropriate antibiotic therapy can be, however, it is only one aspect in the approach to infection. Generally, the best outcome is observed in the foal that has acquired a good level of immunoglobulin early in life; the incidence of additional infections and serious complications such as osteomyelitis is much reduced. As a group, premature or immature stressed foals tend to acquire poor serum immunoglobulin levels even after ingestion of what appears to be good-quality colostrum. It is therefore recommended that, in addition to any colostrum given per os, plasma be routinely supplemented intravenously at a rate of 40 ml per kg during the first 24 hours of life. Immunoglobulin levels should then be checked at 18 to 24 hours to ensure that normal levels of at least 800 mg per dl are achieved.

The question of hormonal supplementation in the premature or immature foal has not been resolved. Rossdale and his colleagues, in their model of equine prematurity, have suggested that "unreadiness for birth" in the equine is associated with an inability of the adrenal cortex to respond to endogenous or exogenous ACTH. This is not a common feature of human prematurity. As plasma cortisol levels remain low in these foals, a rational therapy would appear to consist of physiologic doses of corticosteroids; an optimal dosage regimen, however, has not been established. There is little information regarding the incidence of adrenal insufficiency in the spontaneously delivered, abnormal premature foal or the potential complications of excessive corticosteroid administration.

Supplemental Readings

Dorand, R. D.: Neonatal assphyxia. An approach to physiology and management. Pediatr. Clin. North Am., *24*:455, 1977.

Jeffcott, L. B., Rossdale, P. D., and Leadon, D. P.: Hematological changes in the neonatal period of normal and induced premature foals. J. Reprod. Fert. (Suppl.), *32*:537, 1982.

Koterba, A. M., Brewer, B. D., and Tarplee, F. A.: Clinical and clinicopathological characteristics of the septicemic neonatal foal: A review of 38 cases. Equine Vet. J., *16*:376, 1984.

Koterba, A. M.: Prenatal influences on neonatal survival in the foal. Proc. 29th Annu. Meet. Am. Assoc. Eq. Prac., 1983, pp. 139–151.

Manroe, B. L., Weinberg, A. G., Rosenfeld, C. R., and Browne, R.: The neonatal blood count in health and disease. Reference values for neutrophilic cells. J. Pediatr., *95*:89, 1979.

McCord, J. M.: Oxygen-derived free radicals in postischemic tissue injury. N. Engl. J. Med., *312*:159, 1985.

Prickett, M. E.: The pathology of the equine placenta and its effects on the fetus. Proc. 13th Annu. Meet. Am. Assoc. Eq. Prac., 1967, pp. 201–206.

Rose, R. J., Rossdale, P. D., and Leadon, D. P.: Blood gas and acid-base status in spontaneously delivered, term-induced, and induced premature foals. J. Reprod. Fert. (Suppl.), *32*:521, 1982.

Rossdale, P. D., Silver, M., Ellis, L., and Frauenfelder, H.: Response of the adrenal cortex to tetracosactrin ($ACTH_{1-24}$) in the premature and full-term foal. J. Reprod. Fert. (Suppl.), *27*:545, 1982.

Rossdale, P. D.: Prematurity, dysmaturity and the concept of readiness for birth. Proc. 29th Annu. Meet. Am. Assoc. Eq. Prac., 1983, pp. 127–138.

Rossdale, P. D., and Ricketts, S. W.: The Practice of Equine Stud Medicine. Baltimore, Williams & Wilkins, 1974.

Stewart, J. H., Rose, R. J., and Barko, A. M.: Respiratory studies in foals from birth to seven days old. Equine Vet. J., *16*:323, 1984.

Neurologic Examination of the Newborn Foal

Ragan Adams, GAINESVILLE, FLORIDA

Compromised newborn foals often show clinical signs that indicate dysfunction in their nervous systems. A complete neurologic examination should be performed on these patients to decide if neurologic disease exists and, if so, to locate the damage in the nervous system.

Preliminary observation indicates that the appropriate format for examination of, and the responses expected from, newborn foals differ from those of adult horses. The purpose of this chapter is to briefly explain the format used at the University of Florida Neonatal Intensive Care Unit and to review considerations to keep in mind when evaluating foals suspected of having nervous system disease.

PROTOCOL FOR TESTING THE NERVOUS SYSTEM

An examination protocol has been devised on the basis of techniques used to evaluate adult horses and those used to examine human neonates (Fig. 1). Thus, this protocol records observations and elicits responses not used in the examination of adult patients.

When considering the behavior of the foal, it is important to note the degree of affinity for the mare. Loss of or failure to develop the maternal bond may be an early sign of abnormal behavior. When a foal is held firmly with one arm around the buttocks and one arm around the chest, it alternates vigorously struggling with relaxing into an almost catatonic state called *flopping*. Also, when restrained firmly foals often show submissive behavior, which consists of teeth snapping, flehmen, and odontoprisis. Only when these gestures are performed excessively are they considered abnormal. Foals spend much of their time sleeping. This should not be considered a sign of mental dullness, unless they cannot be aroused easily.

Examination of cranial nerve function in foals is

similar to the procedure used for adult horses (p. 339). However, along with the local cranial nerve response, foals usually attempt to pull away or move their heads vigorously when the reflex is tested. This is considered a sign of cerebral recognition. It is not clear if newborn foals respond to the "slap test" for laryngeal adductory function, but since this response can be assessed by palpating the larynx externally it should be evaluated in neonatal foals routinely.

Limb reflexes that are elicited in the foal in the same manner as in other species are an important part of the examination. When foals are too vigorous to be forcefully placed in lateral recumbency, they will often tolerate examination if they are caught while recumbent. The recumbent extensor thrust reflex is elicited by extending all limb joints and putting sudden pressure on the sole of the hoof to extend the toe further. The response is to extend the entire limb with a jerk and is most prominent in the pelvic limbs. The pathway for this reflex is uncertain but is postulated to involve tendon stretch receptors and the pathways that integrate the flexors and extensors of the limb.

The category of passive range of motion of the limbs is included to assess the rapid change in flexibility noted in the newborn foal. This is determined by the inherent elasticity of the soft tissue of the limb as well as the neural activity that controls muscular contraction. Shortly after birth it is possible to flex the forelimb sufficiently for the toe to touch the dorsal aspect of the scapula. In the hindlimb the third metatarsus can easily be made to appose the tibial tuberosity when the limb is flexed. Within the first few days of life this apparent flexibility or range of motion of the limb decreases rapidly in foals that exercise vigorously. In human neonates a similar decrease in passive range of motion is noted during postnatal development and appears to parallel the development of extensor dominance, which enables the child to sit and later stand.

Limb position and pastern axis are recorded. Traditionally, the abnormal pastern axes that occur in both clinically ill and apparently healthy newborn foals are considered to be caused by muscle, skeletal, or joint lesions. However, given the rapid change in passive tone of an individual foal's limbs in the first few days after birth, the developing nervous system may play a role in the expression of abnormal limb positions and pastern axis.

The gait of the neonatal foal is best observed while the foal is following the mare. The foal is usually not cooperative when forced to lead, circle, hemiwalk, or back. The foal's strength that may be evaluated by pushing down on the back or pulling the tail to one side may be underestimated simply because of the foal's smaller size.

RESPONSE TO TESTING

The type of behavior and the response to testing observed in newborn foals differ from the responses seen in apparently healthy adult horses. Of course, some variation exists between apparently healthy newborn individuals of the same age. Because of the inherently subjective nature of neurologic testing, subtle differences are also observed when different clinicians examine the same foal. Finally, the responses of an individual foal will change with time from birth throughout the neonatal period until that foal's responses resemble those of the adult.

The most striking differences between the adult horse and the newborn foal are summarized in Table 1. This preliminary information is based on the examination of 29 apparently healthy newborn foals born near full term of gestation. As experience with newborn foals increases, the data base should be expanded.

One of the greatest gaps in our knowledge concerns the neurologic examination of the premature foal. Physicians caring for human infants have established a set of behavior and response characteristics considered appropriate for infants of various gestational ages. There is no such data base for the equine neonate. When evaluating a premature foal, it is difficult to discern whether the abnormal responses are caused by neurologic dysfunction or merely by the stage of maturity of the nervous system.

The clinical expression of damage within the nervous system will depend on the stage of its maturation when the insult occurs. Without a data base for foals of various gestational ages, the early diagnosis of disease is difficult. For example, recognition of certain seizure activity in the newborn is confusing. Subtle signs of seizure activity include salivation, lip smacking, excessive blinking, jerky eye movements, tremors, and irregular breathing patterns. In contrast, overt signs of seizure are more obvious and include spontaneous nystagmus, odontoprisis, "chewing gum fits," paddling of the limbs, and opisthotonos. It is not known if the resulting insult to the nervous system from more subtle types of seizure is as severe as that of the overt seizure activity. In fact, the relationship between any form of seizure activity and brain lesions identified at postmortem in newborn foals is not clear.

At this time, we believe the menace reflex should be completely present within seven days of age, though ventromedial strabismus may persist for two weeks. The extensor recumbent thrust reflex disappears by 18 hours of age; the limb reflexes remain exaggerated for at least two weeks and the crossed extensor reflex may be present to some degree for a month. The limb reflexes of the foal can change rapidly and thus appear to depend on the amount

**VETERINARY MEDICAL TEACHING HOSPITAL
UNIVERSITY OF FLORIDA**

LARGE ANIMAL NEONATAL NEUROLOGICAL EXAMINATION

Physical Examination: _____

Temperature: _____
Pulse: _____
Respirations: _____

EVALUATION OF THE HEAD
BEHAVIOR:

Affinity for the mare: ____
Flopping: _____ Shivering _____
Flegmen: _____ Odontoprisis: _____ Salivation: _____ Snapping: _____

MENTAL STATUS: _____
HEAD POSTURE AND COORDINATION: _____
CRANIAL NERVES:

	RIGHT	LEFT
Ophthalmic Examination:		
Vision (II):		
Menace (II-VII, Cerebellum):		
Pupil Size (II, III, Symp.):		
Pupil Symmetry (II, III, Symp.):		
PLR (II, III):		
Blink to Bright Light (II, VII):		
Strabismus (III, IV, VI, VIII):		
Nystagmus, vestibular (III, IV, VI, VIII):		
Nystagmus, spontaneous (III, IV, VI, VIII):		
Corneal Reflex (V, VII):		
Ear, Eye, & Lip (V, VII):		
Muscle Mass & Jaw Tone (V):		
Smile (V, VII):		
Swallow (IX, X):		
Voice (IX, X):		
Tongue (XIII):		
Endoscopy:		
Slap Test:		

FORELIMBS AND NECK

	RIGHT	LEFT
Cervical-local:		
Cervical-face:		
Muscle Mass:		
Sweating:		
Triceps Reflex:		
Biceps Reflex:		
Ex. Ca. Ra. Reflex:		
Flexor Reflex:		
Crossed Extensor Reflex:		
Babinski Sign:		
Extensor Strength:		
Proprioception:		
Recumbent Extensor Thrust:		

REARLIMBS, TAIL AND ANUS

	RIGHT	LEFT
Panniculus:		
Muscle Mass:		
Sweating:		
Patellar Reflex:		
Cr. Tibial Reflex:		
Gastrocnemius Reflex:		
Flexor Reflex:		
Crossed Extensor Reflex:		
Babinski Sign:		
Extensor Strength:		
Proprioception:		
Recumbent Extensor Thrust:		
Tail:		
Anus:		

PASSIVE TONE: FLEXOR VERSUS EXTENSOR STRENGTH
Forelimb: Heel to elbow, acromion, mid-scapular spine, dorsal scapula.
Hindlimb: Minimum distance between Tibial Tuberosity and Third Metatarsus. _____

Neck Movement: _____
Trunk Movement: _____

LIMB POSITION AND PASTERN AXIS:

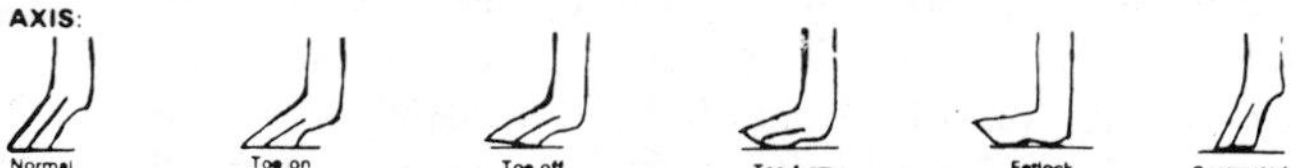

Normal ≅ 50° | Toe on Ground ≈ 50° | Toe off Ground 30° | Toe 1 cm off Ground < 30° | Fetlock on Ground | Contracted > 50°

EVALUATION OF GAIT AND STRENGTH:

_____

Lesion site(s): _____
Possible etiology: _____
Plan: _____

Signature _____ Date _____

WHITE-Medical Records; GREEN-Clinician; PINK-Billing Tracer   VMTH-N3B 7/83

Figure 1. Protocol for examination of the nervous system of the newborn foal.

of exercise the foal has had, and the degree of relaxation ("flopping") during evaluation.

The significance of the timing of the onset of reflexes resembling those in the adult is not clear. The progressive change in passive range of motion and spinal reflexes appears to parallel the change in gait characteristics and limb positions.

ANCILLARY AIDS

When neurologic disease is suspected and an anatomic lesion proposed, the mechanisms causing disease—be they congenital, metabolic, traumatic, infectious, vascular, or idiopathic—are considered. By the use of ancillary aids and laboratory tests, a differential diagnosis can be formulated.

The complete data base includes a blood count, biochemistry panel, blood gas analysis, measurement of serum immunoglobulins, urine and cerebrospinal fluid (CSF) analyses, and culture of body fluids. The total protein level in the CSF of apparently healthy newborn foals is consistently higher than levels measured in adult horses, averaging 138 mg per dl in 21 pony foals tested during the first

TABLE 1. DIFFERENCES IN RESPONSE TO NEUROLOGIC TESTING
BETWEEN ADULT HORSES AND NEONATAL FOALS

Reflex	Response
Head posture	Foal's head more flexed than dam's.
Head movement	Foal moves head jerkily. Some almost have intention movements resembling those in adults with cerebellar disease.
Cranial nerves	Local response often accompanied by a head movement suggestive of cerebral perception.
Menace response	Incomplete or absent at birth but should be present by 7 days of age.
Pupillary light reflex	Usually present but may not be obvious in an excited or stressed foal.
Strabismus	Angle of pupil slightly ventromedial to the palpebral fissure compared to the slight dorsomedial angle of adult.
Sensory V and motor VII reflex arc	Presence of this response must be differentiated from its strength. Foals with soft lips and ears may have the response but appear weak.
Limb reflexes	Generally, exaggerated compared to adult. Patellar reflex may even exhibit clonus.
Withdrawal	Reflex strong with marked extension of contralateral limb, "crossed extensor" reflex.
Gait	Initially, has short, choppy strides with exaggerated extensor tone.

40 hours postpartum. However, values for adults and neonates should be established for each laboratory because variation exists even when the same technique and same sample are employed. The immaturity of the blood-brain barrier is postulated as the reason for the elevated protein content in the CSF of apparently healthy newborn foals.

Radiology. Interpretation of plain radiographs of the skeletal system of newborns is difficult because of breed differences and open physeal lines. Skeletal lesions can only be incriminated as the cause of the neurologic signs if the results of the neurologic examination locate the neural lesion at the site of the skeletal lesion.

Ultrasonography. Sonography is used in human medicine to evaluate the neonatal brain for swelling, hemorrhage, and hydrocephalus. Although this non-invasive technique has potential in equine neonatal medicine, visualization of the brain is limited because the fontanelles are usually closed at birth.

Electrodiagnostics. Needle electromyography (EMG) can be used to assess the integrity of the lower motor neurons (LMN) and muscle. Most likely, the waves of fibrillations, positive sharp waves, and bizarre high-frequency waves are indicative of disease in the neonate as it is in the adult horse. Age-related references for nerve conduction velocities (NCV) are needed before this technique can be used clinically. Reference values for electroencephalographic patterns of clinically normal, sedated, and tranquilized foals (day 3 to day 200) using disc electrodes have been documented. Near birth the electroencephalogram (EEG) has low-frequency and high-voltage characteristics. As the foal matures the low-voltage, faster activity typical of the adult horse develops. At 100 to 200 days of age the EEG of the foal resembles that of the adult.

Supplemental Readings

Adams, R., and Mayhew, I. G.: Neurologic examination of newborn foals. Equine Vet. J., *16*:306, 1984.

Adams, R., and Mayhew, I. G.: Neurologic diseases. Vet. Clin. North Am. (Equine Pract.), *1*:209, 1985.

Amiel-Tison, C.: Evaluation of the neuromuscular system of the infant. Pediatrics, *60*:155, 1977.

Greet, T. R. C., Jeffcott, L. B., Whitwell, K. E., and Cook, W. R.: The slap test for laryngeal adductory function in horses with suspected cervical spinal cord damage. Equine Vet. J., *12*:127, 1980.

Mayhew, I. G., and MacKay, R. J.: The nervous system. *In* Mansmann, R. A., McAllister, E. S., and Pratt, P. W. (eds.): Equine Medicine and Surgery, 3rd ed. Santa Barbara, CA, American Veterinary Publications, 1982.

Mysinger, P. W., Redding, R. W., Vaughan, J. T., Purohit, R. C., and Holladay, J. A.: Electroencephalographic patterns of clinically normal, sedated, and tranquilized newborn foals and adult horses. Am. J. Vet. Res., *46*:36, 1985.

Rossdale, P. D., Cash, R. S. G., and Leadon, D. P.: Biochemical constituents of cerebrospinal fluid in premature and full term foals. Equine Vet. J., *14*:134, 1982.

Volpe, J. J.: Neurology of the Newborn. Philadelphia, W. B. Saunders Company, 1981.

Restraint and Anesthesia of the Foal

Alistair I. Webb, GAINESVILLE, FLORIDA

Anesthetizing a foal is a task involving parameters and guidelines that change as the foal grows and matures. It is convenient to consider foals at two levels of development: neonate and juvenile. The foals in each stage tend to require anesthesia for differing reasons; therefore, different anesthetic techniques are indicated. Yet these boundaries are arbitrary and can obscure the similarities while highlighting the differences. Another problem in discussing the topic of foal anesthesia is that so little is known of anesthesia in the foal per se. Because there are few studies reported in the literature, we still anesthetize foals using extrapolation from neonates of other species and from anesthetic methods used in adult horses.

In approaching each administration of anesthesia, it is important first to delineate the problems involved, then to develop a plan of achieving anesthesia that allows for the problems presented. Finally, the plan has to be executed in the context of clinical realities and patient responses.

BASIC PROBLEMS

The principal problems, in addition to the condition initiating the requirement for anesthesia, relate to the foal's size, immaturity, bonding with its dam, disease immune status, and special equipment requirements.

The problems of size change as the foal grows. Initially the foal is the size of a small human and the solution is to use equipment designed for humans. When the foal is in lateral recumbency its legs need support. An anesthetic breathing circle made for human use (a double carbon dioxide absorber canister is essential) will suffice for foals up to 100 kg when purpose-designed adult equine systems can be used. The basic anesthetic machine, compressed gas source, pressure regulators, flow meters, and vaporizer are universal to all species. Only minor "plumbing alterations" are required to divert the fresh gas flow to the desired breathing circuit. As the foal grows the operating table and handling equipment that were formerly adequate become too small. However, the foal is often not yet large enough for conventional equine equipment and techniques. This requires improvisation and compromise for both foal and practitioner.

The true extent of the normal foal's immaturity is an area of uncertainty. The ability to handle exogenous compounds appears impaired but not to the extent predicted in the literature. The foal appears sensitive to parenteral central nervous system depressants such as diazepam and xylazine. Xylazine has been associated with collapse and apnea in foals and should be used with caution. However, diazepam has been widely used to provide deep and safe sedation to the point of recumbency for 15 to 20 minutes after slow intravenous injections of 0.1 to 0.3 mg per kg. Immature drug handling capability indicates that inhalant anesthesia could be the method of choice for routine production of general anesthesia. Other aspects of the foal's immaturity are the ease of compromise of homeostatic mechanisms with subsequent risk of hypoglycemia, hypothermia, and exhausted stress reserves.

The cardiovascular system is in a state of flux in the first days of life. The onset of anesthesia may be speeded by persistent fetal circulatory patterns, and anesthesia may adversely affect the compensatory heart rate mechanisms involved in cardiovascular homeostasis. These facts dictate that anesthesia be induced slowly and that the depth of anesthesia be maintained as light as is practicable. In the period immediately after birth, the ventilation control is similarly immature and fatigues easily. For that reason, neonatal foals may require ventilatory support during anesthesia (see p. 247).

When dealing with the foal it is necessary to consider the dam also. She can be protective and anxious to the point of being obstructive, but usually her presence soothes the foal and makes moving it easier. The mare can become agitated when parted from her foal and at these times some sedation is advisable. Acepromazine, xylazine, and chloral hydrate are suitable agents. The dam's presence at induction of anesthesia is a big advantage and, with sedation, it is easy to return her to the stall once the foal becomes unconscious. Likewise, upon recovery from anesthesia the foal should be reunited with its dam as soon as possible. Often recovery is faster when the foal is stimulated by the dam's attention and vocalization.

Immunity to disease is often poor. Foals may be considered at risk from cross infection, in view of the immune depression that accompanies surgery and anesthesia. It is important to check histories for such diseases and take adequate precautions when indicated. It is also vital that the anesthetic breathing apparatus and accessories be cleaned after each patient use so they do not act as fomites.

The anesthetic equipment requirements are simple. The clinician needs a sufficient variety of foal tubes to cover neonates through to weanling stages (9 to 18 mm internal diameter). If nasotracheal intubation is practiced the tubes need to be longer than conventional tubes, 55 cm is preferable, and of silicone rubber rather than the older red rubber type. As alluded to already, human-orientated anesthetic breathing circle circuits are suitable until the foal is big enough to be placed on adult equine systems. Induction with inhalant agents is best performed using a large T-Piece system such as Mapleson D with a five-liter open-ended bag on the expiratory limb. A Magill (Mapleson A) system is more economical as regards gas flows but is not easily found in North America. Either system delivers gases directly from the machine at the concentration of the vaporizer's setting. The fresh gas line can be of any desired length so the machine can be kept out of the immediate induction area. Operating tables and transport carts have to be adapted or manufactured as the foal grows. No special monitoring equipment is required above that used in equine critical care.

NEONATAL FOAL ANESTHESIA

The neonatal foal requires anesthesia for two types of problems. Anesthesia in the first 48 hours of life almost invariably is for exploratory abdominal surgery, whereas after five days of age the purpose tends to be mainly orthopedic in nature. The abdominal crisis patient, while representing an emergency, still needs careful evaluation and preparation if anesthesia is to be optimal. Attention to fluid and electrolyte balance before surgery is rewarding in terms of stability under anesthesia.

Neonatal foals should not be fasted before anesthesia because of their inability to maintain normoglycemia. The foal and dam are brought to the induction area, which should be free of noise and nonessential personnel. The foal is not usually premedicated, but if it is very fractious a small dose of diazepam (0.05 to 0.1 mg per kg) can be given intravenously. The nose is cleaned and the nasal passage lubricated with lidocaine ointment before the endotracheal tube is passed into the trachea using the nasotracheal approach. To use this technique successfully, the foal's nose should be elevated so that the frontal bones are nearly horizontal and the neck is extended. A well-lubricated 8- or 9-mm internal diameter tube is passed along the floor of the ventral meatus through the pharynx into the larynx. The endotracheal tube cuff is inflated

and a T-Piece anesthetic breathing system connected to the endotracheal tube and anesthesia induction commenced.

Alternatively, the foal can be masked down with the inhalant agent, but this involves more struggling and is less satisfactory than the nasal intubation technique. The use of parenteral agents to induce anesthesia is largely ignored. If it should be required, ketamine (1 to 2 mg per kg intravenously) preceded by diazepam is my choice. The fresh-gas flows have to be fairly high during anesthesia induction, greater than 75 ml per kg, with inhalant anesthetic vaporizer settings on fully. The choice of inhalant agent is probably limited to what the practice has; this is usually halothane in equine practice. Enflurane and isoflurane are excellent but more expensive alternatives. Methoxyflurane, with its high solubility, produces too slow an induction and recovery to be recommended.

Regardless of choice, it should be noted that, although foals are more resistant to anesthetics than are adult horses, the inspired concentrations should be kept as low as possible, because the cardiopulmonary and other depressive effects of anesthetics are all dose-related. Nitrous oxide can be helpful in the induction period but it must be used with caution in cases of gastrointestinal tympany, as it will enhance the accumulation of gas. Nitrous oxide may also be contraindicated in foals with respiratory dysfunction, because its use lowers inspired oxygen concentrations.

Under quiet conditions and gentle restraint, the foal at induction of anesthesia should slowly subside to the floor and can be then lifted onto a transport cart or operating table. The foal should then be reconnected to a circle anesthetic breathing system and the fresh-gas flow and vaporizer settings reduced to maintenance levels. The nasal tube can also be replaced with an oral tube at this time if it is thought advisable to use a larger size tube. Caution must be exercised when placing the foal in dorsal recumbency, as this is often physiologically resented and can precipitate cardiovascular collapse. In the immediate postpartum period the foal may not be able to respond well to stress because of adrenal exhaustion. Compensation may be made by the judicious use of corticosteroids before anesthesia and surgery.

Monitoring during anesthesia has to be thorough, with emphasis on the cardiopulmonary systems including blood pressure, heart and respiratory rates, mucous membrane color and capillary refill time, ECG, and arterial blood gases. The foal must be kept warm and its eyes protected during anesthesia. Fluid therapy is important and the inclusion of glucose in any regimen is mandatory. The rate of fluid administration usually varies between 5 and 10 ml per kg per hour, but the hemodilution response should be evaluated by periodic measurements of hematocrit and total plasma protein concentration. The foal maintains adequate ventilation by means of a high respiratory rate. Because this can be fatiguing, it is desirable to assist or even control ventilation during anesthesia. If manpower or mechanical ventilators permit, muscle relaxants such as pancuronium (0.05 mg per kg) may be used to considerable advantage in critical cases when anesthesia must be kept as light as possible. The most common problem in these critically ill patients is hypotension. This can usually be managed merely by lightening anesthesia and increasing fluid administration to a more adequate rate. In recalcitrant cases, the judicious infusion of inotropic agents such as dobutamine or dopamine may be needed.

The foal's core body temperature should be monitored. This can be done using an esophageal temperature probe. Hypothermia during any long anesthetic period is inevitable unless aggressive methods are used to warm the foal. Circulating hot water blankets and heat lamps seem the best methods in situations when environmental temperature cannot be manipulated. This warming should continue into the recovery phase until the foal is able to stabilize its own temperature.

At the completion of anesthesia the foal is put into sternal recumbency and awakened while initially breathing 100 per cent oxygen. Extubation can be carried out when there are vigorous swallowing reflexes. The foal should be kept stimulated in this period to keep ventilation up to speed recovery. If recovery is prolonged the foal should receive nasal oxygen insufflation until recovery is complete.

JUVENILE FOAL ANESTHESIA

As the foal ages, and anesthesia becomes more difficult to induce with inhaled agents, parenteral induction agents are utilized. Xylazine (0.25 to 0.75 mg per kg intravenously) followed by ketamine (1.0 to 2.0 mg per kg) are commonly used as is guaifenesin (5 per cent infused to effect) followed by either ketamine or thiobarbiturate (5 to 10 mg per kg). Because the foal can be manipulated onto a transport cart as it loses consciousness, special induction protocols such as those used in the adult horse are not needed. Maintenance and monitoring do not require any special effort or equipment additional to that used in neonates. Unfortunately, as the foal grows its response to controlled ventilation becomes more like that of an adult—namely, a higher incidence of lowered arterial oxygen tensions that do not respond readily to positive-pressure ventilation.

RECOVERY

It is vital that care of the foal continues unabated in the immediate postanesthetic period. The foal must be kept warm and receive oxygen supplementation until ventilation returns to normal. When significant postoperative discomfort and pain are expected, analgesics should be administered. Depending on the degree of sedation considered acceptable in individual patients, drugs such as butorphanol, meperidine, pentazocine, and xylazine would be commonly used. As soon as practical the foal should be returned to its dam and helped, if necessary, to suckle. If still unable to suckle, it should be given dextrose intravenously or fed by stomach tube if hypoglycemia is to be avoided.

Supplemental Readings

Hall, L. W.: The anaesthesia and euthanasia of neonatal and juvenile dogs and cats. Vet. Rec., 90:303, 1972.
Jones, R. S.: Anaesthesia in the foal. Proc. Assoc. Vet. Anaesth. Gt. Britain and Ireland 10:96, 1982.
Waugh, R., and Johnson, G. G.: Current considerations in neonatal anaesthesia. Can. Anaesth. Soc. J., 31:700–709, 1984.
Webb, A. I.: Nasotracheal intubation in the foal. J. Am. Vet. Med. Assoc., 185:48, 1984.

Feeding the Sick or Orphaned Foal

Jonathan M. Naylor, SASKATOON, SASKATCHEWAN, CANADA

R. J. Bell, SASKATOON, SASKATCHEWAN, CANADA

There are many similarities in the care of sick foals and of orphans. The most important ingredient is sound nutritional management. The newborn foal possesses very little energy stores and may quickly become hypoglycemic if undernourished—particularly if it is also septic or immature. Sound nutritional management involves several factors. The foal should get an adequate amount of colostrum early in life. Later, mare's milk or a milk substitute should be fed depending on the circumstances. Foals that are too sick to nurse are usually hand fed their dams' milk. Orphan foals are best fostered onto a lactating mare. Mare's milk substitutes can be used to hand rear sick or orphaned foals if a lactating mare is not available.

NORMAL PERINATAL BEHAVIOR

The mare is usually recumbent when the foal is born. As the foal moves and tries to stand she may nuzzle it and vigorously lick it. This period of vigorous licking establishes the bond between foal and dam. The mare may also show interest in objects coated with birth fluids. Once the foal stands the mare may assist suckling by stepping forward to bring her udder to the foal's head, standing still and flexing the hindlimb on the side away from the foal to point the teat toward the foal. Suckling may be further encouraged by the mare's nuzzling and licking the foal's hindquarters.

Mares initially recognize their foals by smell. The appearance and sounds of the foal are also important in recognition of foals at a distance. Mares reject foreign foals by threatening behavior, biting, and kicking. A mare may also end a nursing bout by her own foal by moving away from it, pushing it away with her hind leg, lashing her tail, pawing the ground, or kicking or biting the foal.

Although mares and foals have innate mothering and suckling drives at parturition, these are further refined by experience. Foals nurse better as they locate the teat and are rewarded by milk. An active foal stimulates mothering, which is rewarded in part by relief of the discomfort arising from the distended udder.

COLOSTRUM

An adequate intake of colostrum is critical to the health of the newborn foal. Septicemia, diarrhea, omphalophlebitis, and arthritis are all seen in colostrum-deprived foals. Immunoglobulin is concentrated in the mare's udder during the last weeks of pregnancy, and first milking colostrum has a high immunoglobulin content. Once nursing commences immunoglobulin concentrations drop rapidly as milk replaces colostrum. Milk samples collected four to eight hours after birth have 15 per cent of the immunoglobulin concentration of colostrum samples collected in the first three hours postpartum.

A colostrum bank can be established for colostrum-deficient foals. Colostrum should be collected hygienically soon after parturition. About 250 ml of colostrum can be milked from a brood mare after her own foal has suckled. Samples should be dated and stored deep frozen at -15 to -20° C. Colostrum is stable for a year at these temperatures.

Foals should receive 250 ml of colostrum every hour for the first six hours of life. A bottle with a lamb's nipple can be used to feed the colostrum. Foals without a sucking reflex should be intubated. To facilitate repeated feedings, a small stomach tube (or No. 28 French catheter) may be sutured into the foal's nostril using adhesive tape and nonabsorbable suture. Foals absorb colostrum best in the first hours of life. Because absorption ceases by 24 hours of age, it is important to ensure that they receive adequate amounts (at least 1.5 L) during this time period.

THE SICK FOAL

Foals that are too sick or weak to nurse are usually hand fed milk obtained from their own dams. It is important to keep the foal and mare fairly close to each other, so that olfactory and visual contact are maintained. A low partition can be constructed out of plywood panels or straw bales to restrain the foal in a corner of a large box stall in which the mare is housed. This contact, along with frequent milking, helps to maintain the mare's milk production. Cooperative mares are quite easy to milk by application of moderate pressure between the thumb and forefinger of one hand to the base of either teat. A very cooperative mare will begin to run milk from all four teat orifices shortly after the start of this procedure. Mares with small teats or edematous or tightly stretched udders may be more easily milked using a human milking apparatus.

As a guide to the number of times a day the mare should be milked and the foal fed, the feeding schedule for hand feeding fortified cow's milk can be used (Table 1). If the mare's milk production is much less than the amount recommended in the table, supplementary cow's milk or mare's milk replacer should also be fed.

Sick foals are often dehydrated when presented to the veterinarian. If intravenous electrolyte solutions are given it is a good idea to add 2.5 per cent dextrose to protect against hypoglycemia. Oral feeding may be impractical if ileus or physical obstruction prevents passage of feed. Oral feeding may also be of limited benefit if severe intestinal damage results in maldigestion or malabsorption of food. These foals are best supported by intravenous nutrition (p. 424).

TABLE 1. SUGGESTED COW'S MILK FEEDING REGIMEN FOR A FOAL (50 kg BIRTH WEIGHT)

Days of age	1	2	3	4	5	6	7	8	9	10	11	12	13	Over 14
Number of feedings per day	16	14	12	12	12	10	10	10	9	8	7	6	6	4
Intervals between feedings (in hours)														
Day	1.5	1.5	2	2	2	2	2	2	2	2.5	3	4	4	5
Night	1.5	2	2	2	2	3	3	3	4	4	4	4	4	9
Amount of milk per feeding (in L)	0.3	0.4	0.5	0.6	0.7	0.9	1.0	1.1	1.3	1.5	1.8	2.1	2.1	3.0
Daily milk intake* (in L)	4.8	5.6	6.0	7.2	8.4	9.0	10	11	11.7	12	12.6	12.6	12.6	12.0

*2% fat cow's milk fortified with dextrose at the rate of 20 gm per L.
1 L equals approximately 1 U.S. quart.

FOSTERING THE ORPHAN FOAL

Orphan foals require care and attention best provided by a foster mare. Fostering can be time consuming and there is a risk of trauma to the foal. Hand rearing can be successful but stunted growth and abnormal behavior patterns can be a problem.

Foals are opportunistic nursers and will try to nurse any mare. The mare, in contrast, usually only allows her own foal to suckle. Antagonistic behavior by the mare is overcome by keeping the foal and mare together for several hours in an environment in which aggressive behavior by the mare is discouraged. In general, fostering is easiest if the foal has not been trained to a bottle and if the mare has recently foaled. The disposition of the mare is the greatest determinant of the ease of fostering.

Foster mares can be obtained from a number of sources. It may be possible to obtain a mare who has lost her foal, a near-term pregnant mare can be purchased and induced to foal (the natural foal being reared on milk replacer), or agencies specializing in foster mares can be contacted. Occasionally an agreeable mare producing plenty of milk may accept an additional foal. The growth rate and condition of one of the two foals (not necessarily the orphan) may be compromised slightly but this disadvantage can be mitigated by providing a balanced and concentrated grain supplement free choice to foals.

Healthy foals of various ages, and even foals that have been fed from a bottle while a foster mare is located, will readily approach and attempt to suckle a strange mare. Sometimes suckling can be further encouraged by gently rubbing the back and perineal region of the foal. It may be useful to mask the foster mare's sense of smell with oil of wintergreen or Vicks VapoRub. The same fragrances may be applied to the head, mane, and hindquarters of the foal. If the mare's own foal has recently died, the scraped hide from her foal may be rubbed all over and then tied onto the orphan foal. With a small percentage of mares, these techniques plus a minimum of hand restraint may suffice to allow acceptance of the new foal. More often, however, additional physical and often chemical restraint is required. Often a full-time watch must be kept for several hours before it is safe to leave the foal with its new dam.

The simplest restraint is the application of a twitch or a lipchain. Breeding hobbles that do not interfere with the accessibility of the udder are useful to prevent kicking. These may be left in place overnight with the mare tied to allow her some mobility while the majority of a large box stall acts as "safe" territory for the foal. A handler's appearance every one to two hours will allow the foal to nurse at these intervals. Foals quickly associate human presence with a "safe" time for nursing. An alternative procedure is to separate the mare and foal by a partition low enough to allow communication but high enough to prevent the mare from kicking or the foal jumping out. A handler must put the two together and restrain the mare at feeding times. Many mares require tranquilization in addition to physical restraint, especially when the foal is first being introduced. Combinations of xylazine* and acepromazine,† pentazocine‡ or both are administered intravenously initially; the dosage sometimes must be repeated intramuscularly at two- to three-hour intervals several times before the mare is comfortable with the new foal.

Fostering is very successful with a wide variety of mares. If a mare will not accept the surrogate offspring, she may cease to lactate within a few days. The foal may then be fostered onto another mare, or hand reared successfully thereafter.

REARING ON MARE'S MILK SUBSTITUTES

If the foal's dam is not available and it is impracticable to obtain a foster mother the foal can be reared on a milk substitute. Fortified cow's milk and commercial foal milk replacers are commonly used, although foals have been raised on evaporated milk (Table 2). Milk replacer should be introduced gradually. Feeding regimens should try to mimic

*Rompun, Haver-Lockhart, Shawnee, KS
†Atravet, Ayerst, New York, NY
‡Talwin, Winthrop-Breon Laboratories, New York, NY

TABLE 2. COMPOSITION OF MARE'S MILK (11 DAYS POSTPARTUM) AND VARIOUS SUBSTITUTES

| Item | Mare's Milk | Milk Replacers | | | Milk | | | |
		Foal-Lac†	Nutrequin‡	Wet Nurses§	Cow‖	Goat‖	Ewe‖	Sow‖
Fat, % of DM	15*	14.4	16	12–15	29	34	38	42
Protein, % of DM	22.8*	20.2	22	18	27	25	32	29
Sugar, % of DM	58.8*	52.6			38	31	25	24
Fiber, % of DM	0	0.2 (up to 0.5%)	0.25	<0.25	0	0	0	0
Total solids, as fed, %	11.6*	20	20		12.3	13.2	19.3	20.1
Minerals, % of DM								
Calcium	1.11	0.9	1.0	0.9	1.06	0.98		0.12
Phosphorus	0.38** and 0.69††	0.8	0.75	0.7	0.73	0.83		0.84
Sodium	0.21	0.6	0.98					
Ash	4.8	7.2		<10				

*From Oftedal, O. T., Hintz, H. F., and Schryver, H. F.: Lactation in the horse: Milk composition and intake by foals. J. Nutr., *113*:2096–2106, 1983.

†Borden, Inc., Pet-Ag Division, Pet/Vet Products, Hampshire, IL

‡Vetrepharm Inc., London, Ontario, Canada

§Prairie Microtech Inc., Regina, Saskatchewan, Canada

‖From McDonald, P., Edwards, R. A., and Greenhalgh, J. F. D.: Animal Nutrition, 2nd ed. Edinburg, Oliver and Boyd, 1973, p. 314.

**From Ullrey, D. E., Struthers, R. D., Hendricks, D. G., et al.: Composition of mare's milk. J. Anim. Sci., 25:217–222, 1966, for milk samples collected 8 days postpartum.

††From Bouwman, H., and Van Der Schee, W.: Composition and production of milk from Dutch warmblooded saddle horse mares. Z. Tierphysiol. Tiernahr., *40*:39–53, 1978, for milk samples collected 10 days postpartum.

the pattern of milk intake obtained by natural rearing. The following sections deal with selection and feeding of milk replacer and management of hand-reared foals.

The *amount* of milk produced by the mare is very large, peaking at a daily production of about 3 per cent of the mare's weight. A 600-kg mare produces 1600 kg of milk in the first 100 days of lactation. As a result, foals drink much larger volumes of milk than are used in the hand feeding of calves. Suckling foals consume about 25 per cent of body weight daily as milk compared with the 10 per cent of body weight that is usually fed to calves.

A feeding regimen for fortified cow's milk can be started at 10 per cent of body weight a day at day 1 of age and then slowly increased to 25 per cent of body weight at 10 days of age. This amount should then be held constant until weaning (see Table 1).

Manufacturer's recommendations for milk replacer feeding vary greatly and do not mimic the intake of a sucking foal (Table 3). Some foals get fat on milk replacer but often growth rates are slower than for foals reared by their dams. Weaning foals are able to compensate for periods of poor growth—particularly when fed liberal amounts of a high-protein, high-energy diet. However, in other species growth retardation in early life has permanent consequences, and poor milk replacer intake by nursing foals may contribute to stunting. Because of these potential problems we recommend feeding a 12.5 per cent solution of milk replacer starting at 10 per cent of the foal's body weight at day 1 and slowly building up to 20 per cent of body weight at day 10. Although this feeding regimen has not been extensively tested, it more closely mimics intakes obtained by mothered foals.

Frequency of feeding is important. Foals nurse their dams seven times an hour at one week of age; however, this declines rapidly to three times an hour at 24 weeks of age. Many manufacturers have simplified feeding by recommending four times a day feeding. A more natural regimen would be many small feedings of milk. This will also decrease the risk of digestive upsets and diarrhea. Recommendations on frequency, amount, and dilution for feeding milk replacers are summarized in Table 4.

Feeding methods involve either nipple or bucket feeding. Colostrum is best fed from a bottle using a lamb's nipple. As the foal gets stronger it can be taught to drink from a bucket. The foal's muzzle is

TABLE 3. MILK INTAKE (kg OF DRY MATTER PER DAY) OF THOROUGHBRED AND STANDARDBRED FOALS SUCKLING THE MARE OR HAND FED ACCORDING TO MANUFACTURER'S INSTRUCTIONS

| Milk Source | Days Post Partum | | |
	11	25	39
Mare*	1.86	1.58	1.85
Foal-Lac†	0.91	0.91	1.36
Nutrequin‡	1.5	2.25	3.5
Wet Nurse§	0.9	1.00	1.25

*Oftedal, O. T., Hintz, H. F., and Schryver, H. F.: Lactation in the horse: Milk composition and intake by foals. J. Nutr., *113*:2096–2106, 1983.

†Borden, Inc., Pet-Ag Division, Pet/Vet Products, Hampshire, IL

‡Vetrepharm Inc., London, Ontario, Canada

§Prairie Microtech Inc., Regina, Saskatchewan, Canada

TABLE 4. SUGGESTED FEEDING REGIMEN FOR A FOAL (50 kg BIRTH WEIGHT) REARED ON MILK REPLACER

Days of age	1	2	3–5	6–8	9–11	12–14	15 on
Number of feedings per day	16	14	12	10	8	7	5
Interval between feedings (in hours)							
Day	1.5	1.5	2	2	3	3	4
Night	1.5	2	2	3	3	4	6
Amount of powder per feeding (in gm)	30	45	75	120	180	250	310
Volume of each feeding (in L*)	0.25	0.40	0.6	1.0	1.5	2.0	2.5
Daily powder intake (in kg†)	0.48	0.63	0.9	1.2	1.44	1.75	1.55

*Place powder in graduated measuring container and add water to this volume.

†If foal will not drink all the milk in one feed, increase number of feeds so total daily milk intake is maintained. If foal is bucket-trained, milk can be left in front of the foal.

placed on the surface of the milk and a finger wetted with milk is placed in its mouth. With persistence the foal will learn to drink. Foals have been reared on automated feeding systems. A mixing and heating unit prepares the milk replacer as needed and supplies a nipple mounted horizontally on the wall of the foal's stall. The nipple should be firmly attached to the hose using a hose clamp (jubilee clip).

Hygiene should be stressed when instructing the feeding personnel. Nipples and buckets should be thoroughly cleaned between feedings. Automated systems should be stripped and cleaned daily. Store-bought cow's milk can contain a surprising number of bacteria, and it may be worthwhile to pasteurize it by heating to 70° C for 15 seconds. The milk is then cooled and dextrose (20 gm per L) added before feeding.

Solid food should be introduced at two weeks of age. Fresh water, hay, and a good-quality "creep" feed with at least 18 per cent crude protein and a balanced mineral content should be offered. Foals can be weaned at 8 to 12 weeks of age if they are eating solid food. Weaning is best done by gradually decreasing the number of milk feedings.

Behavioral problems such as excessive attachment to the handler and failure to socialize with horses may arise in orphan foals, particularly if they are isolated from other horses. Foals kept in small loose boxes may not get enough exercise for muscle and bone development. Healthy neonatal foals can be kept in small groups in scrupulously clean pens. Normally developed foals can be led out starting at a few days of age. They should be allowed to see horses. Foals over a month of age can be turned out to pasture daily—a quiet pony can be turned out with the foals to act as a role model.

The human factor in foal rearing should not be overlooked. Hand rearing a foal is neither easy nor inexpensive. Personnel should be prepared to commit their time and resources; they need to thoroughly understand the objectives of the nutritional and management program. The best time to read instructions is before starting, and requirements change rapidly as the foal develops. Experienced, conscientious personnel are essential in hand rearing a foal.

Supplemental Readings

Bouwman, H., and Van Der Schee, W.: Composition and production of milk from Dutch warmblooded saddle horse mares. Z. Tierphysiol. Tiernahr. Futtermittelkd., *40*:39, 1978.

Carson, K., and Wood-Gush, D. G. M.: Behavior of thoroughbred foals during nursing. Equine Vet. J., *15*:257, 1983.

Glendinning, A. S.: A system of rearing foals on an automatic calf feeding machine. Equine Vet. J., *6*:12, 1974.

Naylor, J. M.: Colostral immunity in the calf and the foal. Vet. Clin. North Am. (Large Anim. Pract.), *1*:331, 1979.

Oftedal, O. T., Hintz, H. F., and Schryver, H. F.: Lactation in the horse: Milk composition and intake by foals. J. Nutr., *113*:2096, 1983.

Rossdale, P. D., and Ricketts, S. W.: Equine Stud Farm Medicine, 2nd ed. Philadelphia, Lea and Febiger, 1980, pp. 372–378.

Passive Transfer of Immunity to Foals

Leo B. Jeffcott, MELBOURNE, AUSTRALIA

Apart from low levels of IgM the foal is essentially agammaglobulinemic at birth. This is because the mare's diffuse epitheliochorial placenta prevents in utero transfer of circulating maternal antibody [IgG and IgG(T)] to the fetus and so this must be provided postnatally via the colostrum. The newly born foal's immune system is capable of responding to pathogenic challenge, but in the neonatal period it is sluggish or ineffective, presumably because of the lack of antigenic stimulation during gestation. Therefore it is vital to provide some temporary protection against the many virulent or opportunist microorganisms with which the foal is bombarded on its emergence into the world. Any delay or fault in this complicated mechanism of immunoglobulin transmission will predispose the foal to infection or septicemia.

The objective of this chapter is to consider the salient points of the method of transfer of immunity, its efficiency and duration, as well as the reasons that it may fail and which tests to use to diagnose the problem. Finally, some consideration is given to the current techniques available to remedy the situation of partial or complete failure of passive transfer (FPT).

MECHANISM OF TRANSMISSION OF PASSIVE IMMUNITY

Colostrum Production. Although the essential significance of colostral-derived immunoglobulins has been recognized for over 60 years, the exact mechanism of their production and the controlling hormonal factors have not been conclusively reported. Presuckling equine colostrum contains predominantly (i.e., >80 per cent) IgG and IgG(T) with much lower levels of IgA and aggregating immunoglobulin (AI). The content of secretory IgA rises during lactation while that of the others rapidly declines after parturition. The volume of colostrum ingested by newly born foals is not accurately known. For pony foals this is approximately 160 ml per hour for the first 24 hours. This means approximately 2 liters in the first 12 hours of life with protein values of milk being 20 to 25 gm per L immediately after birth and declining to 5 gm per L by 12 hours. Colostrum, as well as supplying a source of immune proteins, contains substances capable of enhancing the efficacy of absorption of macromolecules. These substances appear to be of low molecular weight and do not actually affect uptake, but are important in assisting transfer from the intestinal cell into the villus lacteal.

The mammary gland does not synthesize any immune proteins, apart from IgA; however, it selectively concentrates immunoglobulins from the blood before foaling. This can be seen as a drop in circulating serum protein and gamma globulin levels before parturition. Colostrum formation is thought to be triggered by changing hormone levels around the time of parturition. If the trigger mechanism occurs before term, resulting in premature lactation, colostrum may be lost and no more is produced at parturition.

Uptake of Macromolecules. A simplified theoretical representation of the method of uptake and transcellular absorption is given in Figure 1. The absorption of colostral proteins is carried out by specialized cells of the small intestine. These cells have a rapid turnover rate after birth and are replaced by more mature-looking cells within 38 hours of life. The uptake of macromolecules occurs uniformly throughout the small intestine. The larger macromolecules (i.e., immunoglobulins) are taken up into the absorptive cells by pinocytosis so that protein is absorbed in a finely divided form. The resulting microglobules then pass to the base of the cell where they merge into one or more large globules. The cells appear to absorb protein maximally before discharging it into the intercellular space. The material then passes into the local lacteals before reaching the blood. Peak absorption is reached about six hours after administration into the stomach. It seems likely that smaller molecules (i.e., milk protein) may pass directly into the intestinal capillaries or via the duodenal cells and thence to the portal circulation (Fig. 1).

The absorptive cells are apparently nonselective in their uptake of macromolecules as the selection of suitable immune proteins takes place in the mammary gland. Colostral gamma globulin, a variety of specific antibodies, and the synthetic polymer with the same molecular size as gamma globulin, polyvinyl pyrrolidone (PVP K.60), are all readily absorbed.

Efficiency of Absorption. The absorptive efficiency of the small intestine is maximal immediately after birth and declines progressively over the first 24 hours of life. The apparent efficiency of absorp-

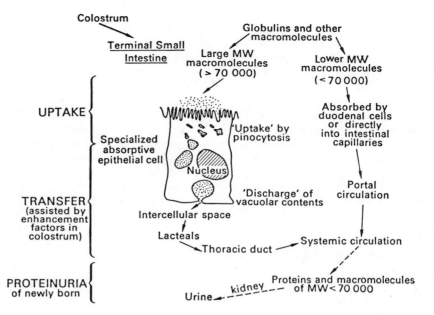

Figure 1. Schematic representation of absorption of globulins and other macromolecules from the small intestine of ungulates. (From Jeffcott, L. B.: Passive immunity and its transfer with special reference to the horse. Biol. Rev., 47:439–464, 1972.)

tion of I^{125} labeled PVP, with a mean molecular weight of 160,000, is 22 per cent and declines linearly to less than 1 per cent by 24 hours of life. If equilibration of material into the extravascular pool is also considered, the absorptive efficiency is doubled, because there is an extravascular:intravascular ratio of 1:1 for IgG.

Absorption is reduced by 10 per cent when foals are deprived of colostrum, presumably because of the absence of absorption enhancement factors in colostrum.

Termination of Absorption or "Closure." Intestinal permeability to macromolecules can persist for up to 14 hours in normally suckled foals and no appreciable difference is noted in colostrum-deprived foals. Complete starvation may lengthen the absorptive period. Immediately after birth the specialized epithelial cells are rapidly replaced by more mature-looking cells, which are unable to absorb macromolecules. This explains why absorption is maximal immediately after birth, falling off in a linear fashion to complete cessation.

The mechanism increasing the turnover rate of intestinal cells may be the high levels of adrenal corticoids present at parturition, and these hormones may also influence the postnatal change in permeability of the intestinal cells. The situation is further complicated because essentially two mechanisms are involved in absorption. Although the uptake of macromolecules into the intestinal cells may occur beyond 24 hours, the cells are no longer able to transfer molecules into the bloodstream.

Neonatal Proteinuria. A marked, transient proteinuria occurs in foals that receive colostrum during the period of intestinal permeability. Urinary protein levels initially rise rapidly to a peak by 6 to 12 hours and then decline between 24 and 38 hours. The urinary protein is devoid of gamma globulin and consists almost exclusively of small molecular weight milk proteins, probably alpha-lactalbumin and beta-lactoglobulin. These small proteins are absorbed by the intestine together with the larger molecules (Fig. 1), but are selectively excreted in the urine because of their small size. The cessation of proteinuria is therefore judged to be a reflection of cessation of macromolecular absorption and not any renal or metabolic dysfunction.

DURATION OF PASSIVE IMMUNITY AND ONSET OF ACTIVE IMMUNITY

Passive antibody levels reach their maximum within 24 hours but fall progressively thereafter. This is due not only to the catabolism of antibody but also to dilution caused by the increasing plasma volume in the growing foal. The half-time for disappearance of maternally derived immunoglobulin is approximately 21 days. There does seem to be some variation when specific antibodies are examined, but levels will always be minimal by five to six months of age. As a rough guide the useful protective value of passive antibodies persists for only the first month of life. This should provide sufficient time for the effective maturation of the foal's own active immune system.

The ability to synthesize gamma globulin is first recognized from two weeks of life. Assuming a lag period for production of 7 to 15 days, this indicates that immunologic competence is acquired very soon after birth. Although peak levels of the different immunoglobulin systems vary, adequate protective levels should be attained by about four months. Foals that are deliberately deprived of colostrum show evidence of an earlier and more rapid rise of autogenous gamma globulin than foals with normal passive immune status.

In optimal circumstances there is an overlap of passive and active immune systems, providing a transitional period from about two weeks to four months of age. However, if passive transfer is less than adequate there will be a particularly dangerous period about four weeks after birth.

FAILURE OF PASSIVE TRANSFER

Incidence. Failure of passive transfer (FPT) is considered to occur if the foal's IgG level does not rise above 4 gm per L. Levels below 2 gm per L are designated as failure and those between 2 and 4 gm per L are partial failure. There is a higher prevalence of septicemia and foalhood infections in foals with IgG levels of less than 4 gm per L than in foals with levels of more than 4 gm per L. However, relatively few surveys have been carried out to establish the exact incidence of FPT on stud farms. Those performed in the United States and in Australia (Table 1) show 10 to 24 per cent of normal foals with some degree of FPT; in foals that are clinically abnormal after birth the incidence is dramatically increased. Many of these foals were known to have received less than adequate amounts of colostrum in the first 12 hours of life.

Causes

FPT may result from problems (Table 2) associated with the secretion of colostrum (i.e., maternal factors) or some impediment in the absorption of immunoglobulins (i.e., foal factors).

MATERNAL FACTORS. Some mares produce colostrum with inadequate levels of immunoglobulins, less than 10 gm IgG per L. The prevalence of this situation has not been accurately documented. It is presumably associated with a failure of the selective transfer mechanism in the mammary gland to concentrate immune proteins from the blood before parturition. In stud farm management little emphasis has been placed on assessment of presuckling colostral immunoglobulin status. It is conceivable that poor colostrum quality in mares is not so much caused by a failure of production but by the premature onset of lactation so that the immunoglobulin-rich secretion is lost before the foal sucks. This condition is one of the most important causes of FPT. It is relatively common for lactation to commence before parturition, particularly in older multiparous mares. They may start to run milk a few hours to a few days before foaling. The exact cause is obscure, but it is presumably initiated by changing hormone levels. In cases in which a degree of placentitis or placental separation or both exist, premature lactation frequently occurs. This is commonly seen with fungal or bacterial placentitis and in twin pregnancy when lactation can start several weeks before parturition. Since colostrum is secreted only once, a steady drip from the udder over a few days will materially reduce the amount of immunoglobulin available to the foal.

A failure of milk let-down occurs occasionally in mares that may not be sufficiently responsive to endogenous oxytocin release. This may be associated with nervous temperament in maiden mares or pain from an engorged udder. The delay in let-down means the foal is unable to suck and is temporarily deprived of maternal immunoglobulins. Careful manual stripping of the udder or small doses of intravenous oxytocin (1 to 3 IU) will usually overcome this problem.

If a mare is known to be isosensitized (i.e., carrying a foal with neonatal isoerythrolysis) the foal must be prevented access to her colostrum as it contains harmful isoantibodies. The udder must be regularly stripped over the first 24 hours and the colostrum discarded. The foal must be supplied with passive immunity by some alternative means.

FOAL FACTORS. FPT is a common problem in premature foals having a gestation length less than 320 days. However, prematurity itself should not affect the ability of the neonatal intestine to absorb

TABLE 1. RESULTS OF SURVEYS ASSESSING INCIDENCE OF FAILURE OF PASSIVE TRANSFER IN FOALS

Surveys Performed	Foals Examined	No.	IgG levels		
			0–2 gm/L	2–4 gm/L	0–4 gm/L
McGuire et al., 1977	Normal TB	87	9	12	21 (24%)
McGuire et al., 1977	Abnormal mixed breeds	11	6	4	10 (91%)
McGuire et al., 1975	Normal Arab	46	9	—	9 (20%)
Pemberton et al., 1980	Normal TB	70	4	3	7 (10%)
Pemberton et al., 1980	Abnormal TB	12	7	5	12 (100%)

TB, Thoroughbred.

TABLE 2. MAJOR CAUSES OF FAILURE OF PASSIVE TRANSFER IN FOALS

Maternal Factors
Inadequate concentration of IgG in colostrum
Premature onset of lactation
Inadequate let-down of colostrum
Serious parturient condition (e.g., rupture of cecum or utero-ovarian artery) or death of dam
Known isosensitization of mare

Foal Factors
Prematurity/dysmaturity
Delayed ingestion of colostrum:
  a. Congenital anomalies (wry nose, cleft palate)
  b. Delayed or impaired suck reflex
  c. Inability to stand (weakness, severe limb contractures)
Intestinal malabsorption of immunoglobulins

immune proteins, because the intestines of fetal animals are quite capable of macromolecular uptake. Premature foals have deficient transfer of immunity for either of two reasons: failure of the mare to produce adequate colostrum or delayed ingestion due to weakness or impaired suck reflex.

The most important cause of FPT in foals is delay in the ingestion of colostrum for reasons that prevent or delay sucking (see Table 2). A syndrome of malabsorption of immunoglobulins has been alluded to, but not confirmed. The condition occurs in foals that apparently ingest an adequate volume of immunoglobulin-rich colostrum but fail to show satisfactory blood levels. Stress at or around the time of parturition may hasten the time of closure of the bowel to immunoglobulins.

Methods of Assessing Failure of Passive Transfer

An extensive range of techniques is available to evaluate passive immune status and specific immunoglobulin levels in plasma, serum, whole blood, and colostrum samples (Table 3). Some are simple and can be carried out directly on the stud farm or in the practice laboratory while others take longer and require more sophisticated equipment.

NONSPECIFIC METHODS. Detailed observation of

the mare and foal in the perinatal period can identify foals at risk for FPT. Visual inspection of the character and consistency of early colostrum and an estimate of the time the foal first sucks are useful predictors of FPT.

Recently a simple hydrometer (colostrometer)* has been developed that measures the specific gravity of colostrum. There is an excellent correlation between specific gravity and immunoglobulin content. The determination of total solids in foal plasma by use of a simple refractometer will provide a crude estimate of whether immunoglobulin absorption has taken place. Presuckling values are approximately 4.3 gm per L and should increase by 2 to 4 gm per L.

PROTEIN FRACTIONATION. Total serum protein is usually determined by the biuret reaction. The individual protein fractions (alpha, beta, and gamma) can be separated by electrophoresis, visualized with a standard protein stain, and if the total protein is known quantitated using a densitometer. This is a useful method but is time-consuming and requires special equipment and considerable expertise to perform well.

PROTEIN PRECIPITATION (NEPHELOMETRY). The method of choice is the zinc sulfate turbidity test, which involves preparing a solution of 250 mg per L zinc sulfate ($ZnSO_4$ $7H_2O$) in freshly boiled water to drive off all carbon dioxide. This solution is stored in airtight containers such as vacutainers or in a bottle with an autopipetting device and an air inlet with a soda lime trap for carbon dioxide. The test is performed with 0.1 ml serum in 6.0 ml zinc sulfate solution. In the presence of immunoglobulin a precipitate makes the solution opaque. The result can be appraised visually immediately or can be quantitated after 60 minutes at room temperature by comparison of the optical density against a standard dilution curve of IgG or barium sulfate. The major difficulty is hemolysis in the sample, although

*Lane Manufacturing Inc., Denver, CO

TABLE 3. METHODS OF TESTING FOR FAILURE OF PASSIVE TRANSFER IN FOALS

Method of Assessment	Comments
Stud farm husbandry	Nonspecific, rule of thumb only but useful evaluation of colostrum quality and assessment of sucking, neonatal behavior, etc.
Colostral specific gravity	Simple, quick, and effective
Refractometry for total solids determination	Simple, quick, but nonspecific; low levels assumes FPT
Protein fractionation by electrophoresis	Quantitates α-globulin from total protein but time consuming and requires special equipment
Protein tests:	
1. Zinc sulfate turbidity	Simple, quick, effective, and cheap except for hemolysed samples
2. Sodium sulfite turbidity	Simple, but too unpredictable
Specific immunoglobulin in assay (single radial immunodiffusion)	Good kits available, but time-consuming (>24 h) and expensive
Latex agglutination	Quick, simple kits available, can use on whole blood and colostrum, but expensive

it is possible to make a correction for this if it is not too severe.

The sodium sulfite turbidity test is unreliable in diagnosing FPT.

SPECIFIC IMMUNOGLOBULIN ASSAY. There are several immunoglobulin assays available, although IgG alone is generally accepted as being a satisfactory index of total immunoglobulin. The usual method involves single radial immunodiffusion (SRID) in agarose plates impregnated with monospecifc antiserum. The resultant antigen-antibody reaction is seen as a precipitin ring, the diameter of which can be measured to quantitate the assay. Results obtainable with commercial kits are satisfactory provided testing is performed strictly according to the manufacturer's instructions. The disadvantages of SRID to the practitioner are the time taken to perform the test, more than 24 hours, and the expense.

LATEX AGGLUTINATION TESTS. The use of polystyrene particles (latex beads) to visualize the reaction between a protein and its antibody is a recent innovation. Specific immunoglobulin antiserum is coated onto a latex reagent and mixed with the sample under test. Positive agglutination occurs within 15 minutes and the end point can be roughly quantitated. There are a number of commercial kits on the market, some for use only on plasma and serum and some for use on plasma and serum, whole blood, and colostrum. This is a test that can easily be carried out on the stud farm or in the practice laboratory, but further field trials may be necessary on some of the kits. They are also expensive.

Management of Failure of Passive Transfer

STUD FARM MANAGEMENT. It is an advantage for mares to foal at home or to arrive at stud at least two weeks before foaling to allow sufficient time to produce antibodies to microorganisms in the new environment. Observation at foaling provides a chance to note early behavioral patterns and the timing of onset of suckling. It also gives an opportunity to evaluate the quality of presuckling colostrum.

On some stud farms, which have a perennial problem with neonatal septicemia due to *Actinobacillus equuli*, a short course of antibiotic immediately after birth is a standard practice. Foals that are muzzled to prevent neonatal isoerythrolysis or are known to have FPT also require antibiotic cover for four to five days and careful surveillance to detect early signs of infection or diarrhea.

TREATMENT OF FOALS UNDER 12 HOURS OLD. Foals with suspected FPT can be given colostrum or some other source of IgG while the small intestine is permeable to immunoglobulins. The maintenance of a bank of deep-frozen colostrum is a simple, cheap, and convenient source of additional IgG. It is usually quite safe to collect 180 to 250 ml of colostrum from normal healthy mares. This is best collected into plastic containers after the mare's own foal has sucked. The quality of the sample should be assessed and labeled accordingly, with the date of collection. It should be quickly transferred to a deep freeze and maintained at $-15°$ to $-20°$ C. Under these conditions it will last for at least a year. Thawing and refreezing will denature the protein, making the colostrum useless.

The volume of colostrum given by nasogastric tube depends on the size of the foal, the time of administration after birth, and the severity of FPT. The following calculations may be of some assistance:

Plasma volume of 50-kg foal (60 ml per kg) = 3 L
Total quantity of IgG to provide 6 gm per L = 18 gm IgG
Assume efficiency of absorption of colostral IgG at 25% = 72 gm IgG
Colostrum with IgG content of 36 gm per L = 2 L dosage of colostrum
To achieve minimal acceptable value of 4 gm per L IgG requires 1.3 L colostrum

Instead of feeding colostrum it is possible to administer plasma or serum orally with approximately 15 gm IgG per L, but to provide the foal with the same level as the example (i.e., 6 gm IgG per L) would require 4.8 L of plasma. However, if the serum is lyophilized it can be reconstituted to 20 per cent of the original volume, a more practical volume for dosing.

TREATMENT OF FOALS OVER 12 HOURS OLD. Additional immunoglobulin administration must be given parenterally to foals in which the small intestine is rapidly becoming impermeable or has already closed. The usual procedure is to collect donor plasma and transfer by slow intravenous injection.

Plasma volume of 50-kg foal (60 ml per kg) = 3 L
Total quantity of IgG to provide 6 gm per L = 18 gm IgG
Assume equilibration of IgG from intravascular to extravascular component 1:1 = 36 gm IgG
Using plasma of 15 gm IgG per L = 2.4 L dosage required

There is a simple and practical method of reducing the volume to be administered by concentrating the plasma with a freeze-thaw technique. Six hundred ml frozen plasma is exposed to a higher temperature and the initial 250 ml that thaws is collected. This volume contains 85 per cent of the total immunoglobulin at about double the original plasma concentration.

Finally, there are some commercial preparations of gamma globulin on the market. However, their concentration and the recommended dosage are unlikely to increase the IgG levels satisfactorily in foals with complete FPT.

HAZARDS OF TRANSMISSION OF PASSIVE IMMUNITY. There are two potentially deleterious effects of passive transmission of immunity. Absorption of colostral antibody may precipitate neonatal isoerythrolysis. Fortunately this condition is uncommon (see p. 244).

Active immunization of the young foal may be hampered if specific maternal antibodies are still present. Live virus vaccines such as African horse sickness and equine viral arteritis may become inactivated by circulating antibody before the viruses have had a chance to multiply and exert their full antigenic effect. These vaccines should not be given until three to four months of age. The problem is less likely to arise with killed vaccines such as strangles and influenza or with toxoid such as tetanus. Therefore they can be usefully given from one month of age.

In conclusion, the deleterious effects of passive transfer are of little consequence in comparison with the overall importance of ensuring adequate immune status during the neonatal period and for the first month of life.

Supplemental Readings

Burton, S. C., Hintz, H. F., Kemen, M. J., and Holmes, D. F.: Lyophilized hyperimmune serum as a source of antibodies for neonatal foals. Am. J. Vet. Res., 42:308, 1981.

Crawford, T. B., and Perryman, L. E.: Diagnosis and treatment of failure of passive transfer in the foal. Equine Pract., 2:17, 1980.

Jeffcott, L. B.: Passive immunity and its transfer with special reference to the horse. Biol. Rev., 47:439, 1972.

Jeffcott, L. B.: The mechanism of transfer of maternal immunity to the foal. Proc. 3rd Int. Conf. Eq. Infect. Dis., Paris, Karger, Basel, p. 419, 1973.

Kent, J. E., and Blackmore, D. K.: The measurement of IgG in equine blood by immunoturbidimetry and latex agglutination. Equine Vet. J., 17:125, 1985.

LeBlanc, M. M., McLauren, B. I., and Baswell, R.: Evaluation of colostral immunoglobulin transfer in the foal using a hydrometer. Proc. 31st Ann. Conv. Am. Assoc. Eq. Pract., 1985.

McGuire, T. C., Poppie, M. J., and Banks, K. L.: Hypogammaglobulinemia predisposing to infection in foals. J. Am. Vet. Med. Assoc., 166:71, 1975.

McGuire, T. C., Crawford, T. B., Hallowell, A. L., and Macomber, L. E.: Failure of colostral immunoglobulin transfer as an explanation for most infections and deaths of neonatal foals. J. Am. Vet. Med. Assoc., 170:1302, 1977.

Pemberton, D. H., Thomas, K. W., and Terry, M. J.: Hypogammaglobulinaemia in foals: Prevalence on Victorian studs and simple methods for detection and correction in the field. Aust. Vet. J., 56:469, 1980.

Rumbaugh, G. E., Ardans, A. A., Ginno, D., and Trommershausen-Smith, A.: Measurement of neonatal equine immunoglobulins for assessment of colostral immunoglobulin transfer: Comparison of single radial immunodiffusion with the zinc sulfate turbidity test, serum electrophoresis, refractometry for total serum protein, and the sodium sulfite precipitation test. J. Am. Vet. Med. Assoc., 172:321, 1978.

Simpson-Morgan, M. W., and Smeaton, T. C.: The transfer of antibodies by neonates and adults. Adv. Vet. Sci. Comp. Med., 16:355, 1972.

Thomas, K. W., and Pemberton, D. H.: Freeze-thaw method for concentrating plasma and serum for treatment of hypogammaglobulinaemia. Aust. J. Exp. Biol. Med. Sci., 58:133, 1980.

Watson, D. L., Bennett, M. A., and Griffiths, J. R.: A rapid, specific test for detecting absorption of colostral IgG by the neonatal foal. Aust. Vet. J., 56:513, 1980.

Immune Deficiency Syndromes

Lance E. Perryman, PULLMAN, WASHINGTON

Mark V. Crisman, PULLMAN, WASHINGTON

It has been well documented that normal foals are immunocompetent at birth. There are, however, several disorders that compromise the equine immune system. Foals with these disorders are very susceptible to infection and are generally refractory to conventional therapy. Annual monetary losses as a result of inadequate colostral immunoglobulin transfer and combined immunodeficiency (CID) have been conservatively estimated at $5,000,000 in the United States. Because of the clinical and financial impact of immunodeficiency diseases, it is important that clinicians be cognizant of the currently recognized immunologic disorders and include them in the differential diagnosis for any sick foal that does not respond to therapy.

ORGANIZATION OF THE IMMUNE SYSTEM

Immunologic responses are mediated by two distinct lymphocyte populations. T lymphocytes are required for cell-mediated immune responses, which protect against fungal, protozoal, intracellular bacterial, and many viral infections. T lymphocytes are also responsible for regulating the immune response through the action of helper T cells and suppressor T cells, which augment and depress immune responses, respectively. The second major class of lymphocytes, B lymphocytes, are the precursors of specific antibody-producing cells. These cells produce IgM, IgA, IgG, and IgG(T); these provide defense against extracellular bacterial and certain viral infections. A deficiency of functional T cells, B cells, or both will predispose animals to infections that may result in death (Fig. 1).

EVALUATION OF THE EQUINE IMMUNE SYSTEM

Recurrent episodes of infection by low-grade pathogens are often observed in horses with immune system defects. Evaluation of the numbers and functional activities of B and T lymphocytes is recommended in those horses with histories suggestive of immunodeficiency disorders. There are several sophisticated tests to evaluate the equine immune system. Most require specialized reagents, expensive equipment, and technical expertise to perform. These tests will not be described here. Instead, a diagnostic strategy, utilizing tests that may be performed on site without reliance on sophisticated laboratory facilities, will be presented.

Complete Blood Count. The first step in the evaluation of the equine immune system is to quantitate peripheral blood lymphocytes. Persistent lymphopenia of less than 1000 cells per μl is typical of some immunodeficiency disorders and indicates the need for additional assessment of B and T lymphocyte activity.

Evaluation of B Lymphocyte Activity. Since immunoglobulins are produced by B cells, quantitation of immunoglobulins is a useful approach to assess B lymphocyte activity. The standard procedure for immunoglobulin quantitation is single radial immunodiffusion (SRID), in which a measured volume of equine serum is applied to the well of an agar-coated slide. The agar contains monospecific anti-body reactive with the class of immunoglobulin to be quantitated. As the serum diffuses out of the well and into the agar, a circle of precipitation is formed, the diameter of which is proportional to the concentration of the immunoglobulin class recognized by the antiserum in the agar. Single radial immunodiffusion kits for the quantitation of equine IgM and IgG are commercially available,* making it possible to perform the test on site. Normal values for equine immunoglobulins are age-dependent. Therefore, normal and abnormal values will be presented for each immune disorder described below.

Evaluation of T Lymphocyte Activity. A simple method for determining T cell function involves intradermal injection of phytohemagglutinin (PHA), and measurement of the increase in skin thickness caused by the infiltration of T lymphocytes and other cells. Following surgical preparation of the injection site and a preinjection measurement of skin thickness, 50 μg PHA† in phosphate-buffered saline (PBS) is injected intradermally. The same volume of PBS is injected at a control site. After 24 hours, the skin thickness is again measured with constant-tension calipers, and the change in skin thickness determined. The increase in skin thickness for normal foals and adult horses is approximately 1 to 3 mm. A defect in cell-mediated immunity is indicated by a lack of response to PHA (increased skin thickness of 0.6 mm or less). The advantages of this in vivo test are simplicity, speed (no previous sensitization is required), and its ability to identify deficient T cell activity.

Most immunodeficiencies can be diagnosed from the results of the tests just described. Definitive diagnosis of some disorders may require more specialized procedures, including in vitro lymphocyte cultures, analysis of lymphocyte surface markers

---

*Veterinary Medical Research and Development, P.O. Box 502, Pullman, WA
†Phytohemagglutinin P, Difco Labs, Detroit, MI

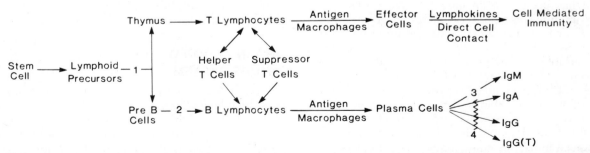

Figure 1. Schematic overview of the equine immune system. Impaired lymphocyte development results in the following immunodeficiency disorders: (1) combined immunodeficiency; (2) agammaglobulinemia; (3) selective IgM deficiency; and (4) transient hypogammaglobulinemia.

with monoclonal antibodies, and histologic evaluation of lymphoid tissues. These tests are mentioned for those disorders that require them.

INADEQUATE PASSIVE TRANSFER OF COLOSTRAL IMMUNOGLOBULINS

This disorder occurs commonly in foals, and is the single most important predisposing factor to neonatal infections and deaths. The diagnosis is established by demonstrating a serum IgG concentration of less than 400 mg per dl in foals over 24 hours of age (Table 1). Proper management of affected foals is described on p. 214.

COMBINED IMMUNODEFICIENCY (CID)

CID is a genetic disorder of foals that is inherited as an autosomal recessive trait. Prior to 1984, this disorder was considered to be limited to Arabian foals, but the report of CID in an Appaloosa foal raised the possibility that at least one additional breed is involved. Affected foals appear normal at birth and will remain free of clinical signs until maternal immunoglobulins are catabolized to non-protective concentrations. Foals then develop infections, usually of the respiratory tract. The major pathogens include adenovirus, the protozoan *Pneumocystis carinii*, and a variety of bacteria.

The pathogenesis of CID involves the inability of affected foals to produce lymphocytes required for normal immune responses. Therefore, a consistent feature of CID is profound lymphopenia, as evidenced by lymphocyte counts below 1000 per μl, and often less than 500 per μl. The few lymphocytes that are produced are nonfunctional in standard laboratory assays. Affected foals are unable to produce immunoglobulins, and their lymphocytes do not respond normally to PHA stimulation. Such foals are highly susceptible to infections, with death occurring before five months of age.

Three criteria are utilized to establish a diagnosis of CID. They are: (1) lymphopenia with less than 1000 lymphocytes per μl, (2) absence of serum IgM, and (3) hypoplasia of lymphoid tissues, determined by microscopic examination of spleen and thymus after death of the foal. No single criterion is sufficient to establish the diagnosis. We require that two criteria be fulfilled before classifying a foal as a CID *suspect*. All three criteria must be fulfilled before giving a definitive diagnosis. This conservative approach to diagnosis is necessary because of the genetic basis of the disease and the implications of a positive diagnosis for the dam and sire. Since the disorder is inherited as an autosomal recessive trait, the dam and sire of an affected foal are obligate heterozygotes for the CID gene. The identification of horses as heterozygotes for the CID trait profoundly diminishes their value in breeding programs. Therefore, accuracy of the diagnosis is essential.

Because of its high prevalence, CID should be considered in the differential diagnosis of any Arabian or part-Arabian foal presented with signs of infection. Identification of a foal as a CID suspect can be readily achieved through quantitation of

TABLE 1. DIFFERENTIAL DIAGNOSIS OF IMMUNE DEFICIENCY DISORDERS

Disorder	Breeds Affected	Age	Absolute Lymphocyte Count (cells/μl)	Immunoglobulins (mg/dl)		Intradermal PHA Test
				IgM	*IgG*	
Normal	All	Newborn, presuckle	750–2000	5–15	1–10	NR*
	All	>24 hours, postsuckle	1000–2000	10–45	>400	+
Insufficient passive immunity	All	>24 hours	1000–2000	5–15	<400	+
Combined immunodeficiency (CID)	Arabian	Newborn, presuckle	<1000	Undetectable	0	NR
	Appaloosa	1–15 days	<1000	0–15	>400	−
Transient hypo-gammaglobulinemia	Arabian	2 months	>1000	30	30	NR
		3–4 months	>1000	25	100–250	+
Agammaglobulinemia	Thoroughbred	2 months	>1000	Undetectable	300	+
	Standardbred Quarterhorse	16 months	>1000	Undetectable	10–200	+
Selective IgM deficiency	Arabian	4 months	>1000	0–15 ⎫		+
	Quarterhorse	8 months	>1000	0–15 ⎬ 500–3000		+
	Thoroughbred Paso Fino	>2 years†	>1000	0–25 ⎭		+

*NR, Not reported.
†Adult horses with selective IgM deficiency often have concomitant lymphosarcoma.

IgM, IgG, and the absolute lymphocyte count. Interpretation of the results depends on the age of the foal at the time of testing (Table 1). Note that newborn, normal, presuckle foals may have lymphocyte counts of less than 1000 per μl, but always have detectable IgM. By 24 hours of age, the absolute lymphocyte count in normal foals increases to more than 1000 per μl. In contrast, the lymphocyte count is persistently low in foals with CID, and IgM is never detected in the serum of a *presuckle* CID foal. After nursing, CID foals usually absorb maternal IgM from colostrum, which is then detected by SRID. The maternal IgM is catabolically eliminated, usually by the time the CID foal is two weeks old; however, we have documented cases in which CID foals retained maternal IgM for as long as 30 days before it declined to undetectable concentrations. Therefore, it may be necessary to repeat the IgM quantitation if an Arabian foal is lymphopenic but has nursed and has detectable IgM.

Once a foal is identified as a CID suspect, the management strategy involves client education, and confirmation of the diagnosis. The disorder is invariably fatal, even with the best of symptomatic and antimicrobial treatment. It is important to explain the genetic basis of CID, and to emphasize the implications of continued use of heterozygous horses in breeding programs. Prompt diagnosis of CID reduces the financial and emotional frustrations of treating a hopeless case, and allows owners to make rational changes in breeding programs. Presented with this information, owners may ask if euthanasia is justified. In all cases in which we have examined lymphoid tissues from foals in which lymphopenia and absence of IgM were demonstrated, the lesions confirmed the diagnosis. Therefore, it is reasonable to honor an owner's request for euthanasia of Arabian foals that are lymphopenic and lack IgM.

TRANSIENT HYPOGAMMAGLOBULINEMIA

This rare disorder has been diagnosed in two Arabian foals and is characterized by a delayed onset of immunoglobulin synthesis. Affected foals are protected by maternal immunoglobulins until specific antibodies derived from colostrum are catabolized to nonprotective concentrations. Foals are then susceptible to infections and experience repeated episodes of disease until they are able to synthesize adequate quantities of specific antibodies, which may require as long as six months. During that time, clinical management involves supportive therapy, antimicrobial treatment, and transfusion of serum or plasma from a suitably matched donor to provide protective immunoglobulins.

Diagnosis of transient hypogammaglobulinemia requires quantitation of serum immunoglobulins. Absolute lymphocyte counts are normal, as is the response of lymphocytes to PHA stimulation. IgM and IgA concentrations are at the low end of the normal range, while IgG and IgG(T) are significantly below normal.

AGAMMAGLOBULINEMIA

This uncommon immunodeficiency has been diagnosed in four males of Standardbred, Thoroughbred, and Quarterhorse breeds. Affected horses lack detectable B lymphocytes and are unable to synthesize immunoglobulins. They produce normal numbers of lymphocytes and retain full T lymphocyte activity. Presence of T lymphocytes is biologically significant, since it permits survival of affected horses up to 18 months of age, far longer than CID foals lacking both B cells and T cells. Clinical signs of pneumonia, enteritis, dermatitis, arthritis, and laminitis are noted at two to six months of age following catabolic elimination of maternally derived immunoglobulins. Death occurs from 2 to 18 months of age.

A tentative diagnosis is indicated in male horses with normal lymphocyte counts, absence of IgM, low and declining concentrations of IgG, and normal response to PHA stimulation. The diagnosis is confirmed by specialized laboratory assays that reveal an absence of B lymphocytes, undetectable quantities of IgA, low and declining concentrations of IgG(T), and hypoplasia of B lymphocyte–dependent regions of spleen and lymph nodes.

Clinical management consists of symptomatic and antimicrobial therapy, as well as provision of antibodies through transfusion of suitably matched serum or plasma. Treatment of established cases is of value for preserving the animals for study but is not practical from the standpoint of maintaining the horse as an athlete or herd sire.

An interesting feature of this disease is its occurrence in males. Agammaglobulinemia is an X-linked genetic disorder in people. Thus, mothers of affected boys carry the trait on one X chromosome. Irrespective of the father, half the daughters of carrier mothers will be carriers of the trait, and half the sons of carrier mothers will be affected. The occurrence of agammaglobulinemia in male horses suggests, but does not prove, that this disorder is X-linked in horses. Nevertheless, owners of dams producing affected foals should be informed of the possible genetic implications, and all future offspring should be evaluated at an early age for evidence of B lymphocyte abnormalities.

SELECTIVE IgM DEFICIENCY

Selective IgM deficiency is a clinically significant immune disorder affecting both males and females. Most diagnoses have been made in Arabians and Quarterhorses, although other breeds are affected. Three clinical manifestations have been observed. The most common presentation involves foals with severe pneumonia, arthritis, or enteritis resulting in death before 10 months of age. Some of these foals have significant enlargement of peripheral lymph nodes. The second presentation involves foals with a history of repeated episodes of infections that respond to antimicrobial therapy but that recur when treatment is stopped. Slow growth rates are characteristic of this group. These foals survive for one to two years before death from infections or euthanasia. Recovery has been noted only in a single case. The third presentation involves horses two to five years old at the time of initial diagnosis. Approximately half of the horses in this group have, or ultimately develop, lymphosarcoma. In one case, the neoplastic cells had suppressor activity, suggesting this is one mechanism for deficiency of IgM production.

Diagnosis depends on immunoglobulin quantitation data (see Table 1). Affected horses have normal lymphocyte counts and adequate lymphocyte responses to PHA stimulation. IgG concentrations are normal or elevated, but IgM is either undetectable or more than two standard deviations below the mean for age-matched controls. Additional laboratory tests reveal normal concentrations of IgA, IgG(T), and the third component of complement (C3). B lymphocytes are present in normal numbers, and the B cells do express surface IgM. When IgM is deficient in adult horses, careful examination is recommended to determine if lymphosarcoma is present.

Management of these cases is usually frustrating.

Response to therapy is often noted, but infections recur when treatment is stopped. Owners become discouraged with failure of horses to thrive, even when free of clinical signs of infection. Specific protocols to replace IgM or stimulate its production are not available.

The pathogenesis of this disorder is unknown. Some cases may have a genetic basis, as observed in primary selective IgM deficiency in man. The occurrence of multiple cases within groups of related horses supports this hypothesis. However, no firm genetic data are available. Many of the cases are secondary to other disorders (lymphosarcoma) and are not genetically defined. Further studies are required to determine if any cases are genetically defined and to delineate the mode of transmission in those which prove to be inherited. Until such data exist, it is advisable to quantitate lymphocytes and immunoglobulin concentrations in subsequent foals from mares that have produced affected offspring.

Supplemental Readings

Hodgin, E. C., McGuire, T. C., Perryman, L. E., and Grant, B. D.: Evaluation of delayed hypersensitivity responses in normal and immunodeficient foals. Am. J. Vet. Res., 39:1161, 1978.

McGuire, T. C., and Perryman, L. E.: Combined immunodeficiency of Arabian foals. In Gershwin, M. E., and Merchant, B. (eds.): Immunologic Defects in Laboratory Animals, vol. 2. New York, Plenum Publishing Corp., 1981, pp. 185–203.

Perryman, L. E., and McGuire, T. C.: Evaluation for immune system failures in horses and ponies. J. Am. Vet. Med. Assoc., 176:1374, 1980.

Perryman, L. E., Boreson, C. R., Conaway, M. W., and Bartsch, R. C.: Combined immunodeficiency in an Appaloosa foal. Vet. Pathol., 21:547, 1984.

Perryman, L. E., Wyatt, C. R., and Magnuson, N. S.: Biochemical and functional characterization of lymphocytes from a horse with lymphosarcoma and IgM deficiency. Comp. Immun. Microbiol. Infect. Dis., 7:53, 1984.

Studdert, M. J.: Primary, severe, combined immunodeficiency disease of Arabian foals. Aust. Vet. J., 54:411, 1978.

Neonatal Maladjustment Syndrome

Peter D. Rossdale, NEWMARKET, ENGLAND

The neonatal maladjustment syndrome (NMS) describes foals suffering from gross behavioral disturbances in the first week after birth, the disturbances having a noninfective cause. The term was first used to describe foals suffering from convulsions and other neurologic disturbances including loss of sucking and righting reflexes. It is therefore considered appropriate for animals previously designated "barkers," "wanderers," "dummies," and "convulsives."

CLINICAL SIGNS

The neurologic signs of NMS include convulsions, disorientation, and incoordination, and loss of the suck reflex. Convulsions take the form of myoclonic jerking, especially of the facial, neck, and shoulder muscles. This phase may be followed by violent activity in which the foal makes galloping movements with its limbs and emits high-pitched, frantic whinnying, or "barking," sounds.

Loss of righting reflexes is the most obvious indication of disorientation and incoordination. The foal may thrash with its legs as if convulsing because it is unable to use the normal sequence of raising the head and flexing the limbs in a manner necessary to turn onto its brisket. This activity is, therefore, sometimes erroneously described as convulsing. If the foal is turned onto its brisket, it may become calm. However, these individuals also lose the coordinated reflexes required to stand so that, once on its brisket, the next phase may be that the foal moves uncontrollably in an unavailing effort to stand.

Loss of the sucking reflex is a pathognomonic sign of NMS but not of prematurity. The foal is also unable to respond to environmental stimuli and is apparently blind and loses affinity for its dam.

Secondary signs include loss of thermoregulation, gastrointestinal, respiratory, and cardiovascular problems, and fluid and electrolyte imbalance. Rectal temperature may increase during convulsions and fall, unchecked, toward room temperature during periods of quiescence and coma. Alimentary disturbances arise partly from the need for artificial feeding and consequent impairment of motility and digestion. Flatus of the stomach and small intestines may lead to colic. Feces become "doughy" and sticky, making it difficult for the foal to evacuate colonic and rectal contents. Foals suffering convulsions are acidemic. Electrolyte and fluid balance disturbances depend on the severity of the convulsions and the extent to which renal and hepatic function is impaired by hypoxia and acidemia. Hematocrit rises, partly because of catecholamine release and partly from dehydration or shift of fluid from the vascular to other compartments of the extra- or intracellular spaces.

In the initial stages of convulsive activity, respiratory function appears normal with Pa_{O_2} maintained within normal limits. However, as the convulsions develop, lactacidemia, decreasing Pa_{O_2}, and metabolic and/or respiratory acidosis occur. Pulmonary function deteriorates, tidal volume (V_T) and maximal tidal volume ($MaxV_T$ or "vital capacity") decreases and respiratory rate increases. Radiographically, lung areas become opaque as alveolar atelectasis develops. This dysfunction is partly the result of decreasing functional residual capacity. The lungs lose air because the chest wall is relatively compliant. Hypoxia and hypercapnia result from the mismatching of ventilation and perfusion, which is accentuated by the foal remaining recumbent for long periods.

Cardiovascular disturbances are evidenced by bradycardia and tachycardia, depending on whether the foal is convulsing or in a coma. A hammer type of pulse may be recognizable with increased blood pressure, and the jugular vein may become engorged and a pulse wave may be present.

THERAPY

CONVULSIONS

Control of convulsions is an urgent necessity to reduce energy demands and thus to avoid cardiac and circulatory failure.

Drugs. Primary agents useful in anticonvulsant therapy are hydantoins, benzodiazepines, and barbiturates. Other therapy includes the use of dexamethasone and mannitol.

Barbiturates reduce nervous excitability. Phenobarbitone sodium may be administered at a dosage rate of up to 20 mg per kg body weight followed by a maintenance dose of up to 9 mg per kg body weight every eight hours. In pony foals these dosage rates achieve serum levels of 11.6 to 53 μg per ml, which is considered to be in the therapeutic range. Convulsing foals have alterations of metabolic activity; they may be receiving other drugs that affect the metabolism of barbiturates. Also, they may have cerebral edema and/or hemorrhage that might affect the pharmacokinetics of the drug within the nervous system. In my experience, the optimal approach is to administer pentobarbitone sodium *slowly* in a diluted form, for example 300 mg in 20 ml sterile water given to effect, and to repeat the dose according to response every three to six hours for 24 to 48 hours. The side effects of barbiturates are apnea, hypertension, ataxia, and hypothermia. Individuals vary widely as to the required dose for a given effect. It is important to have a respiratory stimulant available. Doxapram hydrochloride at a dosage rate of 0.5 to 1.0 mg per kg intravenously at five-minute intervals to total dose of 2 mg per kg is recommended. However, it is preferable to have some means of assisted ventilation available through an endotracheal nasal tube (see p. 247).

Primidone, the active metabolites of which are phenobarbital and phenylmethyl malanamide, may be used per os at a dosage rate of 500 mg to 2 gm repeated as required, up to four times daily. The side effects are minimal but the drug is not as useful for controlling severe convulsions as is phenobarbitone or pentobarbitone sodium.

Of the hydantoins, phenytoin is that most usually employed. Hydantoins stabilize membranes rather than elevating the seizure threshold. The dose recommended for a foal is 5 mg per kg intravenously, repeated to the desired effect. Maintenance doses of 125 mg intravenously, intramuscularly, or per os three times a day are recommended for a 50-kg foal. Side effects include thrombophlebitis and there are wide variations in metabolism, especially if other drugs are being administered.

Diazepam is a tranquilizer, anticonvulsant sedative, and muscle relaxant. It is useful at a dosage rate of 10 to 20 mg according to signs with a maximum of 30 mg administered to a 50-kg foal over eight hours (0.6 mg per kg body weight). The drug is administered intravenously and should be given slowly to avoid apnea. It is more useful for maintenance of a sedative state than for controlling acute convulsions.

Dexamethasone is the corticosteroid usually employed for anticonvulsive therapy. It has a biologic half-life in plasma of about 190 minutes and it is used to reduce cerebral edema. A dose of 4 mg intravenously followed by 4 mg twice or three times a day for a 50-kg foal is useful. Side effects include inhibition of secretion of corticotropin, increased liability to infection, possible inhibition of intestinal absorption of immunoglobulins, and retention of sodium. Continued therapy should be accompanied by the administration of depot ACTH 0.4 mg for a 50-kg foal per day.

Cerebral decompression may be attempted by the administration of up to 200 gm mannitol by slow intravenous infusion with a single dose of up to 50 gm in a 20 per cent solution. Side effects include thrombophlebitis and acute hypervolemia.

Thermoregulatory Support. Foals unable to maintain their body temperatures require elevated ambient temperatures and measures to reduce heat loss. Because about 70 per cent of heat is lost from the body through radiation, applying blankets or clothing, placing the foal in a well-insulated building, and using a source of radiant heat are among the most helpful measures. The application of rugs heated by electricity or hot water is another means of reducing heat loss.

Assistance. Careful and sympathetic handling, on suitable bedding, forms an integral part of therapy. Foals are motivated by the need to stand in order to suckle and swallow milk. This motivation is satisfied by the use of righting reflexes by which the foal turns from the recumbent position onto its brisket and then stands. If part or all of this reflex behavior is deranged, assistance may be helpful and therefore have a "sedative" effect. For example, if a foal is in full lateral recumbency and cannot coordinate the raising of its head and the extension of forelimbs and withdrawal of hindlimbs involved

in turning onto its brisket, support of the foal to bring it into this position may quiet it. Similarly, raising it to its feet so that it can stand with support for short periods may be beneficial.

A reasonably soft surface, made of absorbant material, is useful to avoid bedsores and contamination with urine and feces. I have found that a Vetbed* placed on straw is an improvement over the use of rugs. Special beds made of plastic or other material are particularly useful because contact of the foal with straw is avoided. Convulsive foals often suffer periods of persistent chewing and may take straw into their mouths, and swallow it, thus traumatizing the gastrointestinal lining.

Respiratory Support. Low Pa_{O_2} may be treated by raising the inspired oxygen fraction (FI_{O_2}) to greater than 22 per cent oxygen. However, raising alveolar PO_2 does not increase arterial PO_2 if there are substantial right-to-left shunts through unventilated areas of lung or through a right-to-left shunting ductus arteriosus. The administration of oxygen at a flow rate of about 10 liters per minute through a tube inserted in the nasal meatus is sufficient to provide oxygen therapy. The countering of physiologic shunt may require intermittent positive-pressure ventilation or positive end-expiratory pressure. For these purposes, an intranasal endotracheal tube is particularly useful. If therapy is continued over prolonged periods, measures should be taken to humidify the inspired gas to prevent excessive drying of the airways (see p. 247).

PREMATURE AND DYSMATURE FOALS

More recently, the term NMS has been taken to include prematurity, dysmaturity, and other states of neurologic deficit not associated directly with infection. Prematurity and dysmaturity are conditions of hypoadrenocortical activity. This may be diagnosed by the administration of about 0.0025 mg short-acting synthetic ACTH† per kg and observing the response of the neutrophil:lymphocyte ratio 120 minutes later. A normal full-term foal has a neutrophil:lymphocyte ratio of about 2:1, which widens significantly 120 minutes after administration of ACTH. The ratio in premature foals is nearer 1:1 and there is little or no widening following ACTH challenge.

Therapy for affected foals should consist of administering depot ACTH (0.4 mg twice a day for two or three days depending on response). Once the short-acting test proves positive, the dosage may be reduced or therapy discontinued. On the first day, before the depot ACTH has had time to

---

*Veterinary Drug Company PLC, London, UK
†Cortrosyn, Organon Pharmaceuticals, West Orange, NJ

take effect, cortisol may be administered intravenously at a bolus dose of 50 mg or, preferably, by intravenous infusion over a 12-hour period or in repeated fractional bolus doses. Antibiotic or chemotherapeutic preventive therapy should accompany this therapy. Trimethoprim and sulphadiazine or an aminoglycoside such as amikacin is a suitable chemotherapeutic agent.

Supplemental Readings

Adams, R., and Mayhew, I. G.: Neurologic diseases. Vet. Clin. North Am. (Equine Pract.), *1*:209, 1985.

Kosch, P. C., Koterba, A. M., Koons, T. J., and Webb, A. I.: Developments in management of the newborn foal in respiratory distress 1: Evaluation. Equine Vet. J., *16*:312, 1984.

Rossdale, P. D.: Sir Frederick Hobday Memorial Lecture. Part I: Practice, teaching and research—a common philosophy. Part II: Concepts of critical care in the newborn foal. Equine Vet. J., *17*:343, 1985.

Rossdale, P. D., and Ricketts S. W.: Equine Stud Farm Medicine, 2nd ed. London, Bailliere Tindall, 1980, pp. 314–335.

Webb, A. I., Coons, T. J., Koterba, A. M., and Kosch, P. C.: Developments in management of the newborn foal in respiratory distress 2: Treatment. Equine Vet. J., *16*:319, 1984.

Neonatal Septicemia

Barbara D. Brewer, GAINESVILLE, FLORIDA
Anne M. Koterba, GAINESVILLE, FLORIDA

Although the incidence of neonatal septicemia on well-managed farms is quite low, this problem remains a common cause of mortality of neonatal foals. Even with intensive supportive care, the survival rate can be as low as 26 per cent. Recovery is frequently complicated by osteomyelitis, suppurative arthritis, or severe pneumonia. Management is best directed at prevention; however, when infection is not prevented, early detection and appropriate treatment are essential.

ETIOLOGY

Neonatal infections can be acquired either in utero or postnatally. Bacteria can enter the uterine environment via the maternal bloodstream, from the local spread of endometritis, and from the posterior genital tract through the cervix. Most infections in the pregnant mare occur via the last route, placental lesions being most severe and chronic adjacent to the internal os of the cervix. Spread of infection from the chorion can then occur through either the umbilical vein or the allantoic and amnionic sacs to the stomach or lungs.

While severe fetal infections can occur with no obvious placental abnormalities and foals with very abnormal placentas may be nonseptic, placentas should be examined for abnormal thickening, plaques, discoloration, denuded villi, and ulcerations whenever possible. These abnormalities signal the need for careful evaluation of the neonate. Table 1 lists other conditions that have been associated with either in utero or postnatally acquired infections.

Failure to acquire sufficient colostral immuno-

TABLE 1. CONDITIONS ASSOCIATED WITH SEPTICEMIA IN FOALS

Maternal Problems
  Placentitis
  Vaginal discharge prior to foaling
  Endotoxemia
  Colic prior to foaling
  Fever
  Shipping long distances immediately prior to foaling
  Dripping significant amounts of colostrum prior to foaling
  Previous history of abnormal foals
  Poor nutritional status

Problems at Foaling
  Dystocia
  Induced parturition

Foal Problems
  Prematurity
  Neonatal maladjustment syndrome
  Prolonged gestation
  Delayed or feeble suck reflex
  Deformities of limb or mouth preventing nursing

Environmental Factors
  Unsanitary foaling conditions
  Overcrowding
  Poor ventilation
  Continued use of same foaling area

globulins is probably the *leading* contributory cause of neonatal infection (see p. 210). In two random surveys of neonatal foals, failure or partial failure of passive transfer of immunoglobulins was diagnosed in 19.7 per cent and 24 per cent of the foals. Colostral deprivation may be deliberate to prevent illness in foals known to be at risk for neonatal isoerythrolysis or can be the result of sudden death of the mare. The mare may drip milk before parturition and lose colostrum or she may have inadequate colostral immunoglobulin levels. Finally, the foal may not ingest colostrum during the period available for antibody absorption. This may result from a delayed or feeble suck reflex or deformities of the limb or mouth making normal nursing difficult or impossible. Some foals, particularly those that are premature or stressed, have failed to achieve normal immunoglobulin levels in spite of ingestion of good-quality colostrum. The reasons for this phenomenon are unknown.

Most neonatal infections are caused by opportunistic organisms that live in the genital tract of the mare, on the skin of normal horses, and in the environment. Portals of entry include the respiratory or gastrointestinal tracts, the umbilicus, and the placenta. Although the offending organisms vary throughout the world, gram-negative infections predominate. Gram-negative infections with *E. coli* and Klebsiella are common in Florida. Other gram-negative etiologic agents include Actinobacillus, Pseudomonas, Enterobacter, Salmonella, Pasteurella, Listeria, Serratia, and Proteus species. Gram-positive organisms observed less frequently include beta-hemolytic and alpha-hemolytic Streptococcus, Corynebacterium, Staphylococcus, and Clostridium species.

CLINICAL SIGNS

The early diagnosis of neonatal sepsis can be difficult because there is no single pathognomonic clinical sign. Earliest signs such as decreased appetite, weakening suck reflex, mild dehydration, and slight lethargy are often subtle and are missed by all but the most astute of observers. Fever or hypothermia may be present but normothermia is equally likely. Convulsions or coma due to meningitis, diarrhea, abdominal pain, pneumonia (rarely pleuritis), lameness associated with joint distention or osteomyelitis, omphalophlebitis, and uveitis are frequent signs associated with septicemia. Unfortunately by the time these signs are obvious, the animal's prognosis for survival is far poorer than if treatment had been undertaken earlier. The veterinarian's main objectives must include identifying the foal at risk, working the case up promptly and

appropriately, following it closely, and instituting treatment early in the disease.

DIAGNOSIS

A definitive diagnosis of septicemia is made antemortem by a positive blood culture. Blood culturing is easily performed. The venipuncture site is surgically prepared and 10 ml of blood is withdrawn aseptically and deposited into aerobic and anaerobic blood culture bottles, which are then incubated. A positive culture is characterized by marked turbidity in the media. Further plating for organism identification and sensitivity patterns is then done. Bacterial cultures of specimens of urine, joint fluid, feces, cerebrospinal fluid, and body cavity exudates may be helpful as well. Results of cultures are not available for 24 to 72 hours, and cultures can be falsely negative, particularly if the animal has already been treated with antibiotics. Nonetheless, the yield of positive blood cultures can be surprisingly high, and blood cultures should be an integral part of the work-up of *all* abnormal neonatal foals.

Since the early clinical signs and laboratory changes associated with neonatal septicemia are variable, inconsistent, and common to multiple disorders, various parameters have been identified that when viewed as a whole should lead to a strong suspicion of sepsis. These indices can be checked with little difficulty within an hour or so of the foal's presentation.

Historical Data. Placentitis, vulvar discharge prior to foaling, maternal illness or fever, dystocia, prematurity, and low birth weight have strong associations with neonatal septicemia.

Clinical Examination. Petechiation, scleral injection, dehydration, the presence of diarrhea, respiratory distress, hypotonia, coma, and convulsions may signal the presence of sepsis. More subtle signs such as mild depression or weakening suck reflex may be the only notable early signs. Swollen joints, painful bones, lameness, anterior uveitis, obviously infected wounds, pneumonia, and umbilical abscesses are obvious indications of infection. Pneumonia can be difficult to diagnose by auscultation, and thus many sick neonates should undergo thoracic radiography. Internal umbilical abscesses can be confirmed with ultrasound. Although fever or hypothermia can be seen in septic foals, a normal body temperature is equally likely. In summary, the early signs of sepsis can be very subtle. All too often, a swollen joint or lameness problem is dismissed as caused by trauma, a weakening neonate with a normal temperature is not regarded as infected, a diagnosis of pneumonia is not entertained because lung sounds are normal, and diarrhea in a three-day-old foal is attributed to milk intolerance rather than septicemia. Obviously, these may be correct explanations in many cases. Since delay in therapy for as few as 24 hours can lead to rapid fatality, a thorough work-up (including serial complete blood counts) should be performed on any foal with such signs.

Complete Blood Count. Almost 40 per cent of septicemic foals have white blood cell counts within the normal range of 6,000 to 12,000 per μl at the time of initial positive blood cultures. Differential cell counts may provide more useful information. Typical hematologic abnormalities are neutropenia with less than 4000 per μl segmented neutrophils, neutrophilia with over 8000 per μl segmented neutrophils, and increased number of band neutrophils (over 50 per μl), and the presence of toxic changes such as Döhle bodies, basophilic cytoplasm, and cytoplasmic vacuolization. These changes, although not diagnostic, are not usually observed in the hemograms of normal foals. Serum fibrinogen levels are often elevated in association with infections acquired in utero, but are usually near normal when measured at the onset of infection. Serial complete blood counts should be performed in at-risk foals, as major changes can occur in 12 hours or less.

Other Laboratory Data. The importance of assessment of passive transfer of immunity has already been discussed. It is frequently stated that an IgG level of 400 mg per dl is adequate for the normal foal. However, infected foals or foals at risk for infection such as hospitalized foals or foals with open wounds, maladjustment syndrome, or prematurity fare much better when their IgG levels are greater than 800 mg per dl. Hypoglycemia, metabolic acidosis, and low arterial oxygen levels are common findings in septicemic neonates. It must be reiterated that neither the presence of any one of these indices nor the absence of any is sufficient evidence to rule out infection. However, when these parameters are all considered immediately at the onset of any potential problem and are then checked often, neonatal septicemia can be suspected at an early stage and treatment initiated immediately.

TREATMENT

Antibiotics. Prompt and aggressive antibiotic and plasma therapy is essential to eradication of neonatal septicemia. Treatment should begin immediately after cultures have been obtained. Foals with suspected septicemia should be placed on potent broad-spectrum antibiotics such as a combination of a penicillin plus an aminoglycoside. Dosages are listed in Table 2. Sensitivity results are at times crucial. For example, 81 per cent of the blood cultures of foals admitted to the neonatal intensive care unit of the University of Florida had gram-negative isolates that were resistant to ampicillin, neomycin, and kanamycin. Several gram-negative isolates were also resistant to gentamicin. After culture results and susceptibility studies are completed, the safest, most effective, and most economical antibiotics should be used. The duration of therapy depends on the severity and location of the infection and the clinical response. If the patient ceases to respond or its condition deteriorates, cultures should be repeated in case an organism has developed resistance or a different organism has become involved. Minimal duration of therapy for documented septicemia without focal infection should be two weeks. In persistent infection such as septic arthritis, pneumonia, osteomyelitis, and meningitis, long-term therapy for more than one month is often critical. Few pharmacokinetic studies have been done in neonatal foals to enable rational usage of specific dosage schedules. Furthermore, physiologic factors affecting drug metabolism probably change during the first month of life.

Immunoglobulins. Since most septicemic foals have less than optimal IgG levels, plasma transfusion is frequently a necessity. The most commonly recommended dosage of plasma for treatment of failure of passive transfer of immunoglobulins is 20 ml per kg or approximately 1 L for a 45-kg foal. This volume of plasma however raises foals' IgG levels only 200 to 300 mg per dl. To produce an IgG of greater than 800 mg per dl in a foal that has ingested little or no colostrum, 2 to 4 L of plasma must be infused.

Theoretically, more effective treatment for septicemic foals would involve provision of specific antibodies to the disease-causing organism. A hyperimmune serum of this type has been reported to be effective in the treatment of adult human septicemia. Clinical trials utilizing hyperimmune serum in foals are currently underway at several veterinary schools.

Supportive Intensive Care. Good nursing care is essential in the treatment of the septicemic foal. It is usually a tedious, time-consuming, and often frustrating undertaking, but the survival of many foals depends on this round-the-clock attention.

The foal, particularly if it is hypothermic, must be kept warm, clean, and dry. Respiratory and nutritional support may be needed (see p. 247 and p. 205). A good restraint is critical if the foal is convulsing, thrashing, or unable to walk. Care must be taken that the foal does not injure itself and that the mare does not injure the foal. Recumbent foals are often removed from the mare and placed on a thermoregulated water bed, mat, or sheepskins to prevent the development of pressure sores. These foals should be turned every hour, or preferably maintained in a sternal position.

TABLE 2. ANTIMICROBIAL DOSAGES SUGGESTED FOR FOAL SEPTICEMIA

Drug	Route	Dosage	Interval
Sodium penicillin	IV	20,000–50,000 IU/kg	QID
Potassium penicillin	IV	20,000–50,000 IU/kg	QID
Procaine penicillin	IM	20,000 IU/kg	BID
Ampicillin	IV	20 mg/kg	QID
Chloramphenicol succinate	IV	25 mg/kg	QID or Q 4 h
Trimethoprim-sulfadiazine	IV	15 mg/kg	BID
Gentamicin	IV or IM	2 mg/kg	TID
Amikacin	IV or IM	7 mg/kg	TID

Corneal ulcerations, secondary to trauma or entropion, are common. The eyes should be checked frequently and treatment instituted promptly. Another common complication in the recumbent or debilitated foal is the development of a patent urachus. Careful cauterization with silver nitrate sticks three times daily results in closure and no further complication in almost all cases, negating the need for surgery.

PREVENTION

Advanced life support techniques and more potent antibiotics are not the total solution to septicemia. Veterinarians teaching good management techniques and stressing the importance of documenting colostrum ingestion will do more to help the equine industry than all the intensive care units in the world. However, even under the best of conditions, some foals will develop infection. Early recognition and appropriate therapy of adequate duration are the best defenses against this devastating problem.

Supplemental Readings

Brewer, B., and Koterba, A.: Preliminary report on the utilization of a score system as an aid to the diagnosis of sepsis in the equine neonate. Proc. 3rd Annu. Eq. Neonatol. Res. Conf., 1984 (Abstract).

Harris, M. C., and Polin, R. A.: Neonatal septicemia. Pediatr. Clin. North Am., 30:243, 1983.

Koterba, A., Brewer, B., and Tarplee, F.: Clinical and clinicopathological characteristics of the septicemic neonatal foal. Review of 38 cases. Equine Vet. J., 16:376, 1984.

McGuire, T., Crawford, T., Hallowell, A., and Macomber, E.: Failure of colostral immunoglobulin transfer as an explanation for most infections and neonatal deaths in foals. J. Am. Vet. Med. Assoc., 170:1302, 1977.

Perryman, L., and McGuire, T.: Evaluation for immune system failures in horses and ponies. J. Am. Vet. Med. Assoc., 176:1374, 1980.

Rumbaugh, G., Ardans, A., Ginno, D., et al.: Identification and treatment of colostrum deficient foals. J. Am. Vet. Med. Assoc., 174:274, 1979.

Ziegler, E., McCutchan, J., Fierer, J., et al.: Treatment of gram-negative bacteremia and shock with human antiserum to a mutant Escherichia coli. N. Engl. J. Med., 307:1225, 1982.

Septic Arthritis and Osteomyelitis

Ronald J. Martens, COLLEGE STATION, TEXAS

G. Kent Carter, COLLEGE STATION, TEXAS

The septic arthritis and osteomyelitis syndrome has plagued the equine industry for many years. Common names for this complex are joint-ill, navel-ill, septic polyarthritis, septic epiphysitis, and septic physitis. These infections, which involve the synovial membrane or periarticular bone or both, frequently occur simultaneously, usually in foals less than 60 days of age. More than one joint is commonly involved, and generally a primary site of sepsis exists elsewhere in the body, causing bacteremia.

CLINICAL SIGNS

The infectious arthritis and osteomyelitis syndrome has been classified as the presence of a serofibrinous or fibrinopurulent arthritis accompanied by one of the following: synovitis with no macroscopic evidence of osteomyelitis at necropsy (S type), osteomyelitis of the epiphysis at the subchondral bone and cartilage junction (E type), or osteomyelitis directly adjacent to the physis (P type).

Foals with synovial (S type) arthritis may be only a few days old, and may have systemic illness, and one or more distended, warm and painful joints. The purulent synovial fluid is characterized by a predominance of neutrophils. Epiphyseal (E type) osteomyelitis is usually seen in foals older than those with S type lesions, and presents as severe lameness with or without synovial distention. Differentiation from S type is based upon the presence of radiolucent lesions in the epiphysis of affected joints. The most commonly affected sites, in order of incidence, are the medial femoral condyle, the lateral femoral condyle, the tibial tarsal condyles, the lateral styloid process of the distal radius, the distal tibia, and the patella. Foals with P type osteomyelitis are usually older than those with S or E type lesions and may range to three months of age. Physeal (P type) osteomyelitis usually presents as severe lameness with or without swelling in or around one or more joints. Frequently there is minimal swelling but pronounced sensitivity to palpation of the affected physeal area. As the disease progresses there may be extensive edematous swelling around the joint, synovial distention or subcutaneous or subfacial abscesses, or all three. Diagnosis of P type osteomyelitis is confirmed by the presence of radiolucent lesions in the metaphysis, physis, or epiphysis, or all of these.

The early manifestations of septic arthritis and osteomyelitis may be nonspecific. Although there is usually a concurrent septicemia, there may be no apparent systemic involvement. A traumatic etiology, "stepped on or kicked by the mare," is frequently assumed in affected foals. This assumption, which is often based on the rapid onset of lameness and the lack of other systemic signs of disease, may cause a delay in the initiation of therapy. Therefore, any young foal that suddenly becomes lame, has periarticular edema or pain or both, or a distended joint capsule should be suspected of having septic arthritis or osteomyelitis or both. If one joint is obviously affected the other articulations should be carefully examined. Involvement of the shoulder, elbow, and hip joints is difficult to assess. However, diagnostic attempts such as observation, manipulation, arthrocentesis, and radiography should be made to rule out their involvement.

PATHOPHYSIOLOGY

Host-microbial interactions are important in understanding why bacterial arthritis and osteomyelitis develop in certain foals, whereas most septicemias do not result in an infected joint. Host factors may predispose an animal to recurrent septicemia or may interfere with the ability to eradicate a deepseated infection. Such factors may include rare conditions such as phagocytic cell defects or complement deficiencies, or more common conditions involving a generalized deficient defense mechanism. The most common immunodeficiency in foals is hypogammaglobulinemia caused by inadequate transfer of colostral immunoglobulins. The systemic administration of corticosteroids, with or without antibiotics, suppresses the immune system, which permits extension of an infectious process.

In septic arthritis, regardless of the cause, there is ultimately synovitis. Infection may occur as an extension from the adjacent tissues, whereby the organisms directly invade the synovium or extend via transphyseal vessels to the highly vascular synovial membrane. The organisms pass through the synovial membrane capillary walls and subsequently colonize the synovium. Any articulation may be involved; however, the larger joints such as the stifle, hock, and carpus are most frequently affected. The organisms multiply within the synovium, causing the primary lesions, and the secondary appearance of bacteria within the synovial fluid is variable. It is often difficult or impossible to isolate the etiologic agent from the synovial fluid until late in disease progression or when there is direct extension from infected bone. This is an enigma that has complicated the understanding and consequently the therapy of infectious arthritis in the past.

The inflammatory alterations that occur in the synovial membrane are reflected in the synovial fluid. Inflammation produces thrombosis of the synovial vascular bed and alters the synovial cells themselves. This interferes with the synovial membrane's ability to dialyse plasma efficiently and thereby produce normal synovial fluid. A synovial effusion develops, the synovial fluid becomes more acidic, leukocytes are attracted, and proteolytic enzymes are activated. Hyaluronic acid or mucin, which is responsible for synovial membrane lubrication, decreases in quantity because of dilution, degradation by lysozymes, and reduced production by the damaged synovium. There is an increase in the number of leukocytes with a shift in predominance from mononuclear to polymorphonuclear, and an increase in the protein constituents.

The hyaline cartilage of the articular surfaces is avascular. Consequently, its nutritional requirements depend on the diffusion of nutritional substances from the synovial fluid. The nutritional capacity of the synovial fluid may be diminished by qualitative changes, by interference with the cartilage-synovial fluid interface by exudate, or later in the degenerative process by pannus or granulation tissue. Because of these changes the articular cartilage undergoes degeneration as a result of inadequate nutrition and enzymatic degradation. These degradation products of the articular cartilage also cause a synovitis and a vicious cycle develops. The end result of unchecked septic arthritis is cartilage erosion and the clinical syndrome of degenerative joint disease, which is often too far advanced for therapy to be effective (Fig. 1).

DIAGNOSIS

The key to the diagnosis of infectious arthritis and osteomyelitis is an awareness of the possibility of a joint infection, with immediate aspiration and analysis of the synovial fluid. Analysis of the synovial fluid is based on color and clarity, viscosity, white blood cell (WBC) count, red blood cell (RBC) count, Gram stain and microbiological cultures (Table 1). Normal saline is the preferred diluent when total WBC and RBC counts are determined, since the acidic nature of some WBC diluents may produce coagulation of the hyaluronic acid. This causes clumping of the cells and results in inaccurate counts. As discussed previously, the predominant cell type changes from mononuclear to segmented neutrophils, which is a diagnostic hallmark of septic arthritis. The bacterial agents most commonly associated with septic arthritis and osteomyelitis are Salmonella sp., *Escherichia coli* and *Actinobacillus equuli*. Also, *Corynebacterium equi*, Streptococcus sp., *Staphylococcus aureus*, Klebsiella sp., and Bacteroides sp. have been isolated from affected joints.

Although the results of synovial fluid cultures are frequently inconclusive in the evaluation of a presumed septic joint, both aerobic and anaerobic samples should be submitted. Blood agar is routinely used for aerobic cultures. The infusion of several milliliters of synovial fluid into thioglycolate broth, a blood culture medium, will enhance the recovery of many aerobic, microaerophilic and anaerobic bacteria. A Gram stain should also be performed on the synovial fluid because it may yield results more rapidly than a culture, and bacterial growth may be inhibited by previous antibiotic therapy.

When surgical intervention is incorporated in the therapeutic regimen a synovial membrane biopsy should be obtained for bacterial culture in the case of septic arthritis, or purulent exudate and necrotic debris in cases of osteomyelitis. The increased use of diagnostic arthroscopy may promote the use of synovial membrane biopsies in septic arthritis, as well as provide valuable information about joint damage. Since microorganisms colonize within the synovium or bone, and may or may not enter the synovial fluid, these tissue cultures are usually more rewarding. When other systems are involved and an etiologic agent has not been identified, it is advisable to obtain bacterial cultures from other tissues such as blood, cerebrospinal fluid, urine, and tracheobronchial fluid. These cultures are not always productive; however, if a systemic infective agent is identified more definitive therapy can be instituted.

Radiographic examination for the presence of osteomyelitis or articular fractures should be included in the initial examination. When osteomyelitis is suspected and no evidence of osteolysis exists on the initial radiographic examination, a re-examination should be performed in several days. In the young foal significant osteolysis may occur within three days. Although periosteal proliferation and a decreased joint space (which are frequently associated with septic arthritis) may not be evident until at least 14 to 21 days after infection, radiography is an important diagnostic and prognostic aid.

TREATMENT

Optimal therapy of septic arthritis and osteomyelitis includes antibiotics, drainage, and articular rest. In selection of a therapeutic regimen many factors must be considered, such as the type and virulence of the infecting organism, local and general host defense capabilities, the clinical course of the infection, and economic feasibility. Delay in the onset of treatment, for whatever reason, significantly alters the therapeutic approach and worsens the prognosis. As mentioned previously, more than one joint is frequently involved, and there is an inverse relationship between the number affected and the probability of complete recovery. Although young animals can regenerate damaged articular cartilage more efficiently than adults, a guarded

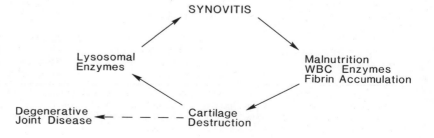

Figure 1. The destructive cycle initiated by synovitis that culminates in degenerative joint disease.

TABLE 1. SYNOVIAL FLUID ANALYSIS

Parameter	Normal	Septic
Color	Yellow-amber	Amber, bloody
Clarity	Clear	Turbid
Viscosity	High	Low
RBC/mm^3	Rare	Few or many
WBC/mm^3	800 ±	50,000 ±
Neutrophils	8%	90%
Mononuclear	92%	10%
Gram stain (bacteria)	−	±
Culture (bacteria)	−	±

prognosis is usually indicated even if appropriate therapy is initiated promptly. This is of particular importance in the foal that is expected to achieve athletic prowess.

Antibiotics. The therapeutic regimen should include systemic antibiotics, adequate serum immunoglobulin levels, and maintenance of homeostasis, nutrition, acid-base balance, fluids, and electrolytes. In the absence of an etiologic diagnosis and with the likelihood of a concurrent systemic infection, vigorous broad-spectrum bactericidal antibiotic therapy should be used initially. The initial regimen may require modification on the basis of bacterial cultures and sensitivities. Systemic antimicrobial therapy should be continued for at least two weeks following the cessation of clinical signs (Table 2). Permeability of the inflamed synovial membrane to most antibiotics has been well documented; consequently, it is not considered necessary to instill antibiotics directly into the joint. This reduces the risk of introducing additional infectious agents and causing chemical synovitis. The repeated use of systemic corticosteroids, which is encouraged by the availability of various antibiotic-corticosteroid combination products, is contraindicated in the treatment of systemic infections and consequently in septic arthritis and osteomyelitis.

Joint Irrigation. The principle of drainage and removal of debris from the joint and adjacent tissues is of paramount importance in septic arthritis, as in any closed space infection. In very early cases, systemic antibiotics and synovial aspiration alone may be adequate. However, since lysosomal enzymes are the major cause of cartilage destruction, their elimination is extremely important. If within 24 to 48 hours no clinical response to drainage and systemic antibiotics is evident or if exacerbations require repeated drainage, synovial distention and irrigation and/or joint lavage are indicated.

Distention and irrigation is accomplished by inserting a 14- to 16-gauge needle or polyvinyl catheter into the most ventral aspect of the joint capsule and alternately infusing and aspirating an irrigating solution. The synovium should be distended to facilitate cleansing of all surfaces and dissipation of fibrin clots and debris. Strict asepsis must be maintained and the procedure repeated until the aspirated fluid is clear. Most joints require flushing with 1 to 2 L of fluid. The foal should be sedated and physically restrained during this procedure, since excessive movement may result in additional damage to the synovium or cartilage or both. A local anesthetic agent such as lidocaine or carbocaine may be instilled into the joint before irrigation to minimize the discomfort associated with joint distention. This procedure should be repeated daily or every other day depending upon the severity of the condition.

Irrigation with a balanced buffered polyionic so-

TABLE 2. SUGGESTED ANTIMICROBIAL DOSAGES

Drug	Dosage		
	Intravenous	Intramuscular	Oral
Amikacin sulfate	7 mg/kg, BID	Same as IV	Not used
Ampicillin, sodium	11–44 mg/kg, QID	Same as IV	Not used
Ampicillin, trihydrate*	Not used	5 mg/kg, BID	Not used
Cefazolin, sodium	11 mg/kg, QID	Same as IV	Not used
Cephalothin, sodium	18 mg/kg, QID	Same as IV	Not used
Chloramphenicol	18 mg/kg, q2h	Not used	50 mg/kg, QID
Dihydrostreptomycin	Not used	11 mg/kg, TID	Not used
Gentamicin sulfate	1.75 mg/kg, TID	Same as IV	Not used
Kanamycin sulfate	Not used	11 mg/kg, BID or TID	Not used
Oxytetracycline	3.5–6.5 mg/kg, BID	Not used	Not used
Penicillin G			
Procaine	Not used	22,000–44,000 U/kg, BID	Not used
Sodium or potassium	11,000–44,000 U/kg, BID	Same as IV	Not used
Potentiated sulfa†	15 mg/kg, BID‡	Not used	15 mg/kg, BID
Ticarcillin	44 mg/kg, q5h	44 mg/kg, TID	Not used

*Not recommended because of low blood levels, unless used in conjunction with sodium ampicillin.
†Dosage determined by adding milligrams of both sulfa and trimethoprim.
‡Tribrissen injectable (Wellcome Animal Health Div., Kansas City, MO) is approved for subcutaneous use in dogs; however, subcutaneous use in the horse causes a severe local reaction.

lution* is preferred since it more closely approximates the pH of normal synovial fluid; however, lactated Ringer's solution (pH 6.7) or physiologic saline (pH 5.7) may be used. The addition of antibiotics to the lavage solution remains a controversial topic, as does the use of drugs with detergent and mucolytic actions, or the fibrinolytics, which have been advocated to eliminate accumulations of fibrin in the synovial exudate. Many of these drugs are irritating and may cause a chemical synovitis, which in itself is potentially detrimental to the cartilage. Although antibiotics are frequently infused into the joint following irrigation, these intermittent local infusions are of questionable value since more consistent levels are maintained in the synovium following systemic administration.

Through-and-through joint lavage is an alternate approach to distention and irrigation, and can be accomplished by inserting two needles or catheters into the synovial cavity. Maximal separation of the inflow and outflow tracts provides the best opportunity for irrigation of the entire cavity and distention can be produced by periodic occlusion of the outflow tract. Through-and-through lavage can also be accomplished very effectively via an arthroscope.

Surgical Drainage. Distention-irrigation and through-and-through lavage are rarely effective if the inflammatory process is advanced and debris is too large or too viscous to be aspirated. When fibrin clots have organized to this extent, usually within 7 to 10 days, or the animal has not responded to conservative therapy, it is necessary to perform open surgical drainage, debride adherent exudate and synovial tags, perform extensive lavage, and establish adequate drainage. Simple arthrotomy may be performed at the distal limit of the joint capsule to establish drainage and permit irrigation. However, this does not facilitate optimal through-and-through irrigation and the arthrotomy incision usually heals prematurely and may have to be repeated. The use of a continuous suction apparatus and indwelling surgical drains has been described. The most beneficial aspect of local therapy is probably mechanical lavage and removal of debris.

When osteomyelitis is diagnosed early, specific systemic antimicrobial therapy alone may be effective. However, it must be kept in mind that ischemia is an important aspect of osteomyelitis and that microorganisms thrive in avascular bone. Therefore, when there is evidence of abscessation, bone sequestration, or severe lysis, it is important to surgically decompress the abscess and excise all dead bone, scar and infected tissue. Following surgical debridement, under general anesthesia, a surgical drain and polyvinyl or Silastic infusion catheter should be inserted into the wound to ensure and maintain adequate drainage. A Robert Jones splint bandage is applied when appropriate and the wound flushed daily with irrigating solutions similar to those used in the therapy of septic arthritis. Successful therapy may result in premature closure of the affected physis and an angular limb deformity. Consequently, the patient should be monitored for several months. If a deformity begins to develop, periosteal transection or growth retardation of the physis or both may be necessary. The prognosis for septic osteomyelitis is guarded to poor. It may be necessary to maintain the patient on antimicrobial therapy for two to three months because bacteria can survive in the bone and epiphyseal cartilage for long periods of time. It is not uncommon for the infection to recur when antimicrobial therapy is stopped. The existence of osteomyelitis in conjunction with septic synovitis indicates a poorer prognosis.

Other Therapy. Failure of passive transfer of colostral immunoglobulins is the most common predisposing factor to the acquisition of infections in the neonate. Its diagnosis and therapy are described on p. 210.

The adjunctive use of anti-inflammatory drugs is indicated because chronically inflamed synovial tissue and its associated byproducts can perpetuate cartilage destruction, even in the absence of sepsis. Prostaglandins, which are released from inflamed tissues, cause erythema and edema, and accentuate the response to pain. The systemic administration of nonsteroidal anti-inflammatory drugs, which are prostaglandin synthetase inhibitors, is beneficial in relieving pain and diminishing the adverse effects of inflammation. Nonsteroidal anti-inflammatory drugs have been incriminated as a contributing factor in the gastric ulcer syndrome of foals. Therefore, long-term therapy at high doses should be avoided.

Even if the infection is treated successfully and further cartilage degeneration arrested, the clinician still must deal with the damage that has already occurred to the articular cartilage—that is the degenerative joint disease. Polysulfated glycosaminoglycan (PSGAG)*, a highly sulfated polysaccharide with alternating units of glucuronic acid and galactosamine, is used in the treatment of degenerative joint disease. PSGAG stimulates the metabolic repair of cartilage, inhibits enzymatic processes that cause cartilage degeneration, suppresses prostaglandin formation, and inhibits glycoside degrading enzymes including hyaluronidase, which depletes endogenous hyaluronic acid. Although definitive studies with PSGAG have not been conducted in

---

*Normosol R, pH 7.4, Abbott Laboratories, North Chicago, IL

---

*Adequan, Luitpold Pharmaceuticals, Inc., Shirley, NY

horses with septic arthritis, it has been successfully after the infectious process has been resolved. The recommended regimen is 250 mg intra-articularly once a week for five weeks.

Supplemental Readings

Auer, J. A., Martens, R. J., and Morris, E. L.: Angular limb deformities in foals: Developmental factors. Comp. Cont. Ed. Pract. Vet., 5:S27, 1983.

Firth, E. C.: Current concepts of infectious polyarthritis in foals. Equine Vet. J., 15:5, 1983.

Firth, E. C., and Poulos, P. W.: Microangiographic studies of metaphyseal vessels in young foals. Res. Vet. Sci., 34:231, 1983.

Koch, D. B.: Management of infectious arthritis in the horse. Comp. Cont. Ed. Pract. Vet., 1:S45, 1979.

Leitch, M.: Diagnosis and treatment of septic arthritis in the horse. J. Am. Vet. Med. Assoc., 175:701, 1979.

Morris, P. G.: The clinical management of septic arthritis in the horse. Compend. Cont. Ed. Pract. Vet., 2:S207, 1980.

Martens, R. J.: Pathogenesis, diagnosis, and therapy of septic arthritis in foals. J. Vet. Orthoped., 2:49, 1981.

Martens, R. J.: Pediatrics, In Mansmann, R. A., McAllister, E. S., and Pratt, P. W. (eds.): Equine Medicine Surgery, 3rd ed. Santa Barbara, CA, American Veterinary Publications, 1982.

Corynebacterium equi Lung Abscesses in Foals

Christopher J. Hillidge, GAINESVILLE, FLORIDA

Juan-Manuel L. Zertuche, GAINESVILLE, FLORIDA

Corynebacterium (Rhodococcus) equi is gaining increasing significance as a cause of suppurative bronchopneumonia and lung abscess in foals. Morbidity rates of 5 to 17 per cent worldwide, with mortality rates of up to 80 per cent, have recently been reported. Foals between two and four months of age are particularly vulnerable to infection, owing to waning maternally derived antibody levels and incompletely developed immune responses of their own. Animals over six months of age rarely show clinical signs of disease unless other immunocompromising factors coexist.

PATHOGENESIS

The primary route of natural *C. equi* infection remains controversial. However, an aerosol spread is suggested by the presence of the bacterium in soil isolates, the increased prevalence of the disease during the dry season in dusty environments, and the fact that the lesions are usually more extensive in the right lung than in the left. *Corynebacterium equi* is a gram-positive pleomorphic rod, with a polysaccharide capsule that is believed to enable the bacterium to adhere to cells, and to inhibit both antibody production and digestion within phagocytes. The mechanism of pathogenicity is unknown at present; *C. equi* is nonhemolytic and nonmotile, and it does not form spores. Although no toxin formation has been demonstrated, phospholipase and cholesterol oxidase enzymes are produced by *C. equi* organisms and these may have pathogenic significance.

Histologically, the lung lesions caused by *C. equi* are granulomatous in appearance and contain thick caseous material. Numerous macrophages and neutrophils are present throughout the necrotic areas, and these cells are frequently seen to contain intact bacteria. This suggests that the *C. equi* organism is a facultative intracellular parasite, capable of survival within phagocytes and thus able to escape not only the normal pulmonary defense mechanisms, particularly in animals with impaired cellular immunity, but also most bactericidal substances. It is possible that much of the tissue destruction associated with *C. equi* lesions is caused by lysosomal enzymes and free oxygen radicals released from intact and degenerating neutrophils and macrophages.

DIAGNOSIS

The optimal method of clinical diagnosis as of this writing is by microbial culture of transtracheal aspirates; however, false-negative results may occur because the bacteria are often intracellular. Similarly, thoracic auscultation is an unreliable test early in the course of the disease, as airway involvement may not be evident at this time. Radiographic evidence of lung abscesses in a young foal is highly suggestive of *C. equi* infection, and advanced pulmonary disease may be present before onset of clinical signs. At the University of Florida, we are confident to initiate therapy on radiographic evidence alone, pending transtracheal aspirate culture results.

Serologic tests have been considered of little value in the diagnosis of *C. equi* infection. However, it has been shown that antibody to *C. equi factors* (the enzymes produced by *C. equi* organisms) can be used to diagnose naturally occurring corynebacterial pneumonia in foals, at least in its later stages. A lymphocyte stimulation test can also be used to identify diseased foals if they are over two months of age.

Nonspecific signs usually exhibited by foals with *C. equi* pneumonia and lung abscessation include neutrophilic leukocytosis, fever, tachycardia, tachypnea, and a markedly elevated plasma fibrinogen concentration.

THERAPY

Early treatment of *C. equi* pneumonia with high doses of penicillin and gentamicin has been recommended, but results have generally been disappointing owing to the presence of lung abscesses. It is often assumed that irreversible lung damage exists by the time that the disease is diagnosed, but our experience suggests that this usually is not the case. Low success rates mainly result from inappropriate antimicrobial therapy.

It is frequently emphasized that the selection of antibiotics should be made on the basis of results of in vitro sensitivity tests, but this is not the only relevant consideration. The antibiotic of choice should have good distribution and activity within the affected tissue in vivo. It must be administered at an adequate dosage, by an appropriate route, and for a sufficient length of time.

It is generally accepted that rifampin, erythromycin, neomycin, and gentamicin are all effective against *C. equi* organisms in vitro, and that penicillin is relatively ineffective. In terms of minimal inhibitory concentrations, rifampin is 90 times as potent as penicillin and five times as potent as gentamicin, while erythromycin is 30 times as potent as penicillin and almost twice as potent as gentamicin. Furthermore, by combining rifampin and erythromycin a synergistic effect against *C. equi* is produced.

In order to treat *C. equi* infections successfully in vivo, the antibiotic of choice should have good distribution and activity in the lungs, the capability of penetrating thick caseous abscesses, and the ability to kill bacteria within macrophages and neutrophils. Penicillin and erythromycin become widely distributed throughout the body, achieving high levels in lung tissue and bronchial secretions, while rifampin effectively penetrates almost all body tissues and achieves lung concentrations that exceed peak serum levels. Gentamicin, on the other hand, as with all aminoglycosides, does not readily achieve high concentrations in the lungs or in any other tissue except the renal cortex. Rifampin, and to a lesser extent erythromycin, is highly lipid soluble and able to penetrate and sterilize caseous material. Penicillin and gentamicin, both highly polar compounds insoluble in lipids, are unable to do so. For this reason, concentrations of rifampin and erythromycin within *C. equi* abscesses are likely to be far higher than those of either penicillin or gentamicin. Finally, both rifampin and erythromycin, by virtue of their lipid solubility, are able to enter and become concentrated within macrophages and neutrophils and to kill intracellular bacteria. In common with all other antibiotics currently available, penicillin and gentamicin do not have this ability, even when present in amounts many hundreds of times greater than their minimal inhibitory concentration. For these reasons, rifampin and erythromycin should be regarded as the drugs of choice for treatment of *C. equi* bronchopneumonia and lung abscessation in foals. Using this antibiotic combination therapeutically for periods of four to nine weeks, our success rate at the University of Florida has exceeded 80 per cent.

It has been suggested that, with the exception of the aminoglycosides, all antibiotics to which *C. equi* is sensitive are bacteriostatic, and thus unsuitable for animals with an already compromised immune system. In fact, rifampin is bactericidal, as is erythromycin at high dose levels. We routinely administer 25 mg per kg of the acid-stable erythromycin estolate* or ethylsuccinate* esters orally three times daily, in combination with rifampin. Both are absorbed well from the gastrointestinal tract. Ethylsuccinate may be preferable because its absorption is enhanced in the presence of food. Erythromycin is directly irritating to tissues, and may cause gastritis if given on an empty stomach. Intramuscular injection causes pain and inflammation, and there is no major advantage to be gained by using the far more expensive lactobionate salt intravenously. Erythromycin has caused reversible hepatotoxicosis and icterus when used in humans for prolonged periods, and its use in adult horses has been associated with severe diarrhea. We have not encountered either of these adverse side effects in foals, other than a mild self-limiting diarrhea in some animals, which has not necessitated termination of the therapy. Similarly, rifampin† appears to be a very safe antibiotic for use in foals. Initially, extrapolating from human practice, we used a twice-daily

---

*Henry Schein Inc., Port Washington, NY
†Rifamate, Merrell Dow Pharmaceuticals, Cincinnati, OH

oral rifampin dosage of 7.5 mg per kg. Subsequently, on the basis of a study of rifampin pharmacokinetics in horses, this was reduced to 5.0 mg per kg twice daily. We have not encountered any adverse side effects of daily rifampin therapy in foals for up to nine weeks at this dosage rate, although, as in humans, it may cause the urine to become red. Although rifampin is extremely potent against *C. equi* both in vitro and in vivo, it is important that it be used in combination with erythromycin and not on its own, as bacterial resistance to it can develop rapidly in this situation. Furthermore, a continuous course of rifampin should be administered, as allergic reactions in humans have been associated with its intermittent use.

Expense is the only major disadvantage of using rifampin and erythromycin in combination for the treatment of *C. equi* pneumonia and lung abscesses in foals. However, using chest radiographs and plasma fibrinogen concentrations as prognostic indicators, it is possible to identify within the first week those animals that will respond to therapy. If no improvement is evident in these parameters, the prognosis is poor. It is essential to continue treatment until both the chest radiographs and the plasma fibrinogen concentration have returned to normal. On one occasion, we terminated therapy when the plasma fibrinogen concentration was still elevated. The foal developed peritonitis associated with *C. equi* abscessation of the mesenteric lymph nodes some six months later. The lungs, however, were grossly and microscopically normal at necropsy, demonstrating that even multiple severe *C. equi* lung abscesses in foals can resolve completely.

IMMUNITY

It has already been mentioned that horses over six months of age are resistant to *C. equi* infection, and intradermal tests have indicated that cell-mediated immunity may be more important than humoral immunity in determining the outcome of natural infection. The demonstration of serum antibody probably indicates mainly that the animal has been exposed to *C. equi*, although recent studies suggest that it may give some protection. No commercial vaccines are currently available. A formalinized *C. equi* bacterin has been found to cause lymphocyte transformation in foals, but it was unable to confer any significant immunity. Clearly, further investigations into the stimulation of cell-mediated immunity to this disease are indicated.

Supplemental Readings

Barton, M. C., and Hughes, K. L.: *Corynebacterium equi*: a review. Vet. Bull., *50*:65, 1980.
Burrows, G. E., MacAllister, C. G., Beckstrom, D. A., and Nick, J. T.: Rifampin in the horse: Comparison of intravenous, intramuscular, and oral administrations. Am. J. Vet. Res., *46*:442, 1985.
Elissalde, G. S., Renshaw, H. W., and Walberg, J. A.: *Corynebacterium equi*: An interhost review with emphasis on the foal. Comp. Immun. Microbiol. Infect. Dis., *3*:433, 1980.
Martens, R. J., Fiske, R. A., and Renshaw, H. W.: Experimental subacute foal pneumonia induced by aerosol administration of *Corynebacterium equi*. Equine Vet. J., *14*:111, 1982.
Prescott, J. F.: The susceptibility of isolates of *Corynebacterium equi* to antimicrobial drugs. J. Vet. Pharmacol. Ther., *4*:27, 1981.
Prescott, J. F., and Nicholson, V. M.: The effects of combinations of selected antibiotics on the growth of *Corynebacterium equi*. J. Vet. Pharmacol. Ther., *7*:61, 1984.

Gastrointestinal Problems in Foals

Julia H. Wilson, GAINESVILLE, FLORIDA

The gastrointestinal tract is a frequent problem source in foals, as it is in adult horses. In addition to the wide range of colic, parasitic, and diarrheal syndromes seen in mature horses, congenital defects, meconium impaction, foal heat diarrhea, and gastroduodenal ulcers must be considered. The clinical approach to diagnosis of gastrointestinal disorders in foals should include a complete history and a thorough physical examination, including abdominal palpation and ancillary tests as indicated. Therapy must be instituted rapidly, often before an etiologic diagnosis is reached, particularly in young foals, which are less able to withstand the stress of colic, hypovolemia, hypoglycemia, and electrolyte imbalances.

NEONATAL INTESTINAL OBSTRUCTION

A variety of problems can cause distention of the abdomen in the neonatal foal. The most common cause is retention of meconium, which must be distinguished from congenital defects of the intestinal tract, intestinal accidents such as intussusception, volvulus, torsion, and internal hernias, as well as functional obstruction due to ileus.

Meconium is the dark green-brown firm, sticky fecal material formed in utero from digested amniotic fluid, intestinal and glandular secretions, and cellular debris. Normally, a foal passes all its meconium in the first few hours of life. Meconium retention requiring veterinary attention develops in approximately 1.5 per cent of foals. Male foals, prolonged-gestation foals, foals born to stall-fed dams, and weak foals seem to have a higher incidence of meconium problems. Meconium is most frequently retained in the rectum but may cause obstruction in the small colon or less commonly in the large intestine.

Congenital defects of the intestinal tract may occur at any level. The lethal white syndrome of intestinal obstruction is seen in Overo Paint foals as an autosomal recessive trait in white or predominantly white foals. Typically, large multiple areas of hypoplastic or atretic bowel result from the defective development of myenteric and submucosal neuronal plexuses throughout the intestinal tract. Congenital atresia of the anus or colon infrequently occurs in many breeds and has not been associated with teratogenic or hereditary causes. Functional intestinal obstruction with abdominal distention due to gas accumulation is a frequent complication in severely ill neonatal foals. Weak, recumbent foals that are not nursing and require bottle or tube feeding may develop progressive distention and gas accumulation, particularly in the small intestine. This is presumably due to fermentation of milk or aerophagia combined with decreased peristalsis. Diminished intestinal motor activity may result from altered autonomic nervous system input such as in maladjusted foals or those with severe thoracic disease affecting the vagus, or from electrolyte imbalances (particularly potassium and calcium). Regional inflammation caused by enteritis or peritonitis may also affect intestinal motility.

Definitive causes of intestinal accidents in foals have not been ascertained. Altered motility caused by regional inflammatory lesions has been hypothesized to be a factor in some cases.

CLINICAL SIGNS

Obstruction of the rectum in the first 24 hours of life usually produces signs of straining, tail flagging and pollakiuria, similar to those in foals with ruptured bladder. If the obstruction is not relieved the foal may begin to show colic signs such as kicking at the abdomen, looking at the flanks, rolling, lying in dorsal recumbency, and gradually increasing abdominal distention. Some foals may stop nursing. If the small colon is obstructed, similar signs will be seen; however, the foal may not strain to defecate.

Meconium impaction of the small colon may be palpable through the abdominal wall.

Obstruction produced by large intestinal torsion usually does not cause straining, and abdominal distention may develop more rapidly. "Pings" may be elicited by simultaneous auscultation and percussion in the paralumbar fossas. Colic signs may range from minimal to quite violent. Severe bowel distention may push the diaphragm cranially and compromise respiration.

Small intestinal obstruction rapidly results in abdominal enlargement, particularly in the cranial and midabdomen. Fluid and gas may accumulate in the stomach. Colic signs progress in severity and the foal usually stops nursing.

Prolonged intestinal obstruction may lead to cardiovascular collapse, shock, and respiratory distress, gastric or intestinal rupture, peritonitis, or death.

DIAGNOSIS

Meconium retention is the most common cause of obstruction in the neonate and produces clinical signs within the first 24 hours. A history of complete or partial failure of meconium passage is very suggestive, especially if accompanied by signs of straining and tail swishing. A digital rectal examination and enema are indicated. If no obstructing fecal material is encountered, abdominal palpation should be performed and may reveal meconium in the small colon as a firm movable mass in the caudal abdomen. A well-lubricated soft rubber stallion urinary catheter or foal nasogastric tube may be gently passed proximally into the rectum until resistance is encountered to estimate the location of the obstruction. Lack of fecal staining on the tube and the presence of mucus is highly suggestive of atresia coli. Abdominocentesis may be useful in differentiating uncomplicated meconium retention from ruptured bladder, in which the peritoneal fluid will produce an ammonia odor when heated. Alternatively, solutions such as dilute sterile methylene blue may be instilled in the bladder via a urethral catheter followed 30 minutes later by abdominocentesis to check for dye-stained peritoneal fluid. Also, peritoneal fluid creatinine content will be higher than serum creatinine in ruptured-bladder foals. In hospital settings, lateral abdominal radiographs may indicate the site and nature of obstruction, particularly if a barium enema is performed first.

Intestinal accidents such as intussusception, torsion, volvulus, and internal hernias can occur at any age, often have a more rapidly progressive clinical course, and may be clinically indistinguishable until an exploratory laparotomy is performed. Intussusceptions may occasionally be detected by abdominal palpation. Gastric reflux on passage of a nasogastric tube suggests a pyloric or small intestinal obstruction, whereas "pings" over large areas of the flanks suggest distention of the large intestine. Inguinal and umbilical hernias with bowel entrapment are diagnosed on physical examination. Diaphragmatic hernias may be asymptomatic if bowel is not entrapped. Elevated respiratory rates without abnormal lung sounds plus abnormal dullness on thoracic percussion should increase the clinical index of suspicion. Abdominal radiography may allow differentiation of intussusception and diaphragmatic hernia from large bowel problems and can be readily performed using conventional small animal radiographic equipment. Analysis of peritoneal fluid obtained by abdominocentesis may aid in the differentiation of strangulated bowel, peritonitis secondary to bowel inflammation, and bowel rupture.

Functional intestinal obstruction is diagnosed on the basis of history and clinical signs, following the ruling out of other forms of obstruction. Greatly diminished or absent intestinal sounds, gradually increasing abdominal distention, and mild colic signs are characteristic. Acid base and electrolyte imbalances are often present as contributing factors.

THERAPY

Intestinal obstruction, regardless of etiology, should be approached as a clinical emergency in the neonatal foal. Intravenous analgesic agents such as dipyrone (22 mg per kg) or flunixin meglumine (0.5 to 1.0 mg per kg) at minimum effective dosages should be used judiciously to prevent self-trauma and to allow complete physical examination of the colicky foal. Xylazine and acepromazine should be avoided because of their vasoactive effects. If signs of hypovolemic shock are present, fluid therapy with balanced electrolyte solutions should be instituted via an aseptically placed intravenous catheter. Commercially available reagent strips for blood glucose can be utilized to determine if dextrose should be added to fluids.

In retained meconium cases, a dilute mild soapy warm water enema should be administered with a lubricated soft rubber tube. Solutions containing mineral oil or glycerine can also be used. Mild enemas may be repeated several times if not initially successful. Use of hygroscopic agents such as the radiographic contrast medium, meglumine diatrizoate* has also been recommended but these are potentially dehydrating. If initial enemas are not completely successful, dioctyl sodium sulfosuccinate (20 ml of 5 per cent solution in 100 ml H_2O) or mineral oil (100 to 150 ml) administered via nasogastric tube may be of some benefit in softening the impaction. If multiple enemas have already been given, irritation and edema of the rectal mucosa may develop. This precludes further enemas and

requires local administration of corticosteroid creams. If the impaction is resistant to therapy and the foal continues to have colic and bloat, surgical intervention is indicated.

Intestinal obstruction due to volvulus, torsion, strangulation, intussusception, or congenital defects such as atresia coli should be managed surgically as soon as possible if economically warranted. If time permits, abnormalities of hydration, acid-base, electrolyte, and glucose status should be addressed with fluid therapy before surgery. Functional obstruction due to ileus should be initially medically approached in the neonate. A nasogastric tube should be utilized to relieve gas and fluid accumulation in the stomach. If the tube is left in place, the distal end should be occluded to prevent air aspiration and accumulation in the stomach. If the foal is ambulatory and not in shock, short walks will encourage gas expulsion. No feeding should be allowed until the ileus is relieved. (The foal's dam must be milked every one to two hours to maintain milk production.) The foal's energy, fluid, and electrolyte needs should be met with intravenous multielectrolyte solutions with added glucose (5 to 10 per cent). Underlying causes such as enteritis, uroperitonitis, and neurologic disease should be sought and treated accordingly. If distention of the abdomen continues to increase and/or colic pain becomes uncontrollable, exploratory laparotomy and bowel decompression should be considered. As ileus and distention resolve, feeding should be gradually reintroduced. Frequent administration of small amounts of warm dilute electrolyte solution and gradual reintroduction of milk over a 24- to 48-hour period usually allows for a smooth transition back to full feeding with the dam. If gas distention recurs with reintroduction of milk, a lactase deficiency may have resulted from damage to the small intestinal villi. Premixing the mare's milk with commercial lactase preparations* may alleviate the problem until the intestine recovers. Alternatively, goat's milk may be fed because clinical impressions suggest that some foals have less difficulty digesting it.

FOAL DIARRHEA

A multiplicity of agents and conditions have been associated with diarrhea in foals. Serious fluid, acid-base, and electrolyte deficits may develop rapidly, particularly in neonates. Therapy is therefore often instituted on a symptomatic basis, because a definitive etiologic diagnosis may not be made for several days if made at all. Diarrheal syndromes in foals may be caused by intestinal parasites, diet, me-

---

*Gastrografin, E. R. Squibb, Princeton, NJ

*Lact-Aid, Lactaid Inc., Pleasantville, NJ

chanical irritation, physiologic changes, and infectious agents such as bacteria, viruses, and protozoans. Mechanisms producing increased fecal water content include hypersecretion, malabsorption, maldigestion, and increased permeability. Hypersecretion results from stimulation of the small intestinal crypts by enterotoxins produced by some strains of *E. coli*. The enterotoxin increases the mucosal levels of cyclic adenosine monophosphate (cAMP), inducing hypersecretion of a magnitude that exceeds the villous absorptive capacity. Particularly in young foals, rotavirus selectively invades the intestinal epithelium of the tips of the villi, diminishing absorptive capacity while leaving secretion intact. Damage to the brush border also impairs disaccharidase activity, including lactase. The undigested, nonabsorbed sugars and fats osmotically draw more fluid into the lumen. Additionally, the sugars may be fermented to short-chain fatty acids by bacteria in the large intestine, further increasing osmolarity and interfering with absorption. Mechanical irritation of the bowel by ingested sand or dirt and parasite migration as well as mucosal invasion by bacteria such as Salmonella cause inflammation of the mucosa. The inflammatory process increases hydrostatic pressure in the bowel wall and increases pore size. This allows fluid to move down the pressure gradient from blood to lumen. Tissue destruction results in even larger pores and exudation of protein, blood, and fibrin.

Foal heat diarrhea occurs in virtually all foals beginning at 6 to 14 days of age, often coincident with the onset of estrus in the mare. Multiple etiologies have been suggested, but recent studies indicate that physiologic changes in the large intestine are responsible. The sum of fecal electrolytes (sodium, chloride, potassium) doubles at the onset of diarrhea while fecal osmolarity decreases, indicating a net secretion of electrolytes by the small intestine. Also, protozoa first appear in the feces after the onset of the diarrhea at this time. The diarrhea usually resolves uneventfully in three to five days. No therapy other than cleaning of the perineum and application of petroleum jelly to the area is routinely required.

CLINICAL SIGNS

A wet or caked perineum or fecal material matted on the tail is usually the first sign of diarrhea. Intestinal sounds are often increased in frequency and suggest the presence of liquids. Signs of systemic illness such as fever, depression, and variable appetite often accompany enteritis produced by invasive or toxin-producing infectious agents such as Salmonella, Clostridia, Actinobacillus, and *E. coli*. Dehydration may develop rapidly. If the foal is septicemic, joint infections, meningitis, or pneumonia may be evident. Bowel that becomes severely

inflamed may be instrumental in development of peritonitis and signs of abdominal tenderness. Ileus, abdominal distention, and colic may also develop. Severe bowel damage may lead to hypoproteinemia and ventral edema. Highly pathogenic strains of bacteria can produce severe dehydration, hypovolemic shock, and even death before diarrhea becomes evident. Marked leukopenia and toxic neutrophil changes are characteristic of Salmonella infections but may also result from septicemia with *E. coli*, *Actinobacillus equuli*, or *Clostridium perfringens*. *Clostridium perfringens* has been specifically associated with bloody diarrhea in the neonate.

Although rotaviral infection in older foals may be asymptomatic, in foals less than a month old it can produce a watery greenish-yellow to gray stool. Fever accompanied by depression may be evident in the initial stages and followed by dehydration and diarrhea. Hematologic findings are variable and may reflect concurrent infection with bacterial pathogens. Several foals are often affected.

Chronic diarrhea accompanied by fever, nasal discharge, cough, and weight loss is suggestive of *Corynebacterium equi* infection, although gastrointestinal signs are far less common than pneumonia.

Intermittent diarrhea, colic, and fever may be produced by migrating *Strongylus vulgaris* or *Strongylus edentatus*. Mild anemia, leukocytosis with or without eosinophilia, and elevated globulins are characteristic. Clinical signs associated with these and other causes of diarrhea are presented in Table 1.

DIAGNOSIS

Signalment, history, and physical findings are often sufficient for diagnosis of uncomplicated diarrhea cases such as foal heat diarrhea, overeating, and sand enteritis. Acid fecal pH and the presence of reducing sugars in the stool* support a diagnosis of overeating. Carbohydrate intolerance can be documented using the lactose tolerance test or by response to treatment with lactase preparations.† In sand enteritis, sand may be grossly visible or evident when feces are mixed with water in a plastic cup or sleeve and allowed to settle.

In neonatal foals with signs of systemic illness, the data base should include fecal and blood cultures, complete blood count (CBC), and if available results on electrolytes, zinc sulfate turbidity or IgG quantitation, BUN or creatinine, and blood gases (see p. 248). Fecal cultures for Salmonella spp. and fecal examination for parasites should be considered, especially in febrile foals. Conventionally, five

---

*Clinitest, Ames Co., Division Miles Laboratories, Elkhart, IN

†Lact-Aid, Lactaid Inc., Pleasantville, NJ

TABLE 1. DIFFERENTIAL DIAGNOSIS OF DIARRHEA IN FOALS

Condition	Age Group	Predominant Clinical Signs	Diagnostics	Therapy
Infectious Diseases				
Salmonellosis	Any; most severe in neonates; stress associated	Watery, foul-smelling diarrhea may contain fibrin and blood; occasional colic, fever, depression, dehydration, and variable appetite. In neonatal septic joints, osteomyelitis, pneumonia, meningitis; may occur as outbreak	Multiple fecal cultures, culture of rectal biopsy in older foals, blood cultures if signs of septicemia. Complete blood count: leukopenia	Fluid therapy, oral electrolytes. Oral bismuth subsalicylate (0.5 ml/kg q 4–6 h). Activated charcoal if signs of toxemia (1 oz/50 kg BID). Parenteral antibiotics (gentamicin 2 mg/kg TID) (trimethroprim sulfa 15 mg/kg BID) (chloramphenicol 25–50 mg/kg IV or PO q8H) Plasma if total plasma proteins <5.0.
Escherichia coli	Primarily neonates	Watery diarrhea, evidence of sepsis, fever, depression, and dehydration; failure of passive transfer common	Blood cultures, fecal cultures (*E. coli* is a normal bowel inhabitant; tests to demonstrate enteropathogenicity are lacking in foals.)	As for *Salmonella*; plasma transfusion if failure of passive transfer.
Clostridium perfringens Types A, B, or C	Primarily neonates	Severe diarrhea, often bloody, marked dehydration, depression	Quantitative anaerobic fecal cultures, mouse inoculations, blood cultures	Fluid therapy, bismuth subsalicylate, charcoal as for Salmonella. High levels of penicillin (50,000 IU/kg IV QID); *Clostridium perfringens* antitoxin*
Actinobacillus equuli	Neonatal foals	Failure of passive transfer; signs of septicemia and severe enteritis	Blood and joint fluid cultures	Fluid therapy, gentamicin 2.0 mg/kg TID; plasma transfusion; joint flushes.
Corynebacterium equi	Foals 1 month old	Loose to watery stools; weight loss, fever, variable cough, nasal discharge, peritonitis	Abdominocentesis—culture and cytology: thoracic radiographs; transtracheal wash; complete blood count—elevated fibrinogen	Bismuth subsalicylate. Antibiotics (erythromycin estolate 25 mg/kg PO QID) or gentamicin (2 mg/kg TID).
Rotavirus	Predominately foals 1 month of age or less	Yellowish-green to gray diarrhea, preceded by fever and depression; rapid onset of dehydration; outbreaks typical	Rotazyme-ELISA on stool. Direct scanning electron microscopy on stool in first days post-infection Lactose tolerance test if secondary carbohydrate intolerance is suspected	Oral electrolytes plus glucose. Intravenous fluid therapy. Decreased milk intake for 36–48 hours. Supplemental lactase. Antibiotic therapy if secondary bacterial infection develops.
Cryptosporidia	Arabian foals less than one month old with combined immunodeficiency	Acute onset; diarrhea, fever, dehydration, rapid death	Direct smear-carbofuchsin or safranin stain, acid fast stain on tissues. Sucrose centrifugation and stain as above	Fluid therapy.

Noninfectious Conditions

Condition	Age	Clinical Signs	Diagnosis	Treatment
Foal heat diarrhea	Onset at 6–14 days of age	Pasty yellow to watery greenish brown diarrhea	None. If prolonged, rule out infectious causes	Clean tail and perineum. If prolonged, bismuth subsalicylate or transfaunation may help.
Overeating	Any age	Variable consistency, diarrhea with flatus; signs of dehydration, shock, toxemia, laminitis if excessive grain consumption	Acid pH of stool; presence of reducing sugars; undigested grain in stool	Oral electrolytes. Decrease feed intake. Milk mare before foal nurses.
Strongyloides westeri	2–4 weeks	Watery diarrhea; very rarely, fever	Fecal flotation of fresh stool; rule out infectious causes	Thiabendazole (44 mg/kg), cambendazole (20 mg/kg), oxibendazole (10 mg/kg).
Strongylus vulgaris	1 month of age or older	Diarrhea (may be intermittent) fever up to 41°C, depression, colic, rapid weight loss	History of poor parasite control. Leukocytosis ± eosinophilia, mild anemia. Fecal flotation may be negative in foals under 6 months (prepatent phase). Increased serum alpha and beta globulins.	Ivermectin (0.2 mg/kg), fenbendazole (10 mg/kg × 5 days).
Strongylus edentatus	2 months and older	Intermittent diarrhea, colic and inappetance, undulating low-grade fever, depression	As for *Strongylus vulgaris*	As for *Strongylus vulgaris*

*Bio-Ceutic Laboratories, St. Joseph, MO

negative consecutive daily fecal cultures are required to rule out Salmonella infection.

A history of poor parasite control should be considered strong evidence for implicating *Strongylus vulgaris* or *edentatus* in foals older than one month even if fecal flotation is negative because of the long prepatent phase. Elevated eosinophil numbers in the blood and peritoneal fluid, mild anemia, and elevated globulins are supportive evidence. A new serologic test* detects IgG (T) levels reflecting a strongyle problem and may prove useful as a diagnostic aid.

As *Corynebacterium equi* is a normal fecal inhabitant, isolation of the organism from transtracheal wash or peritoneal fluid is required for definitive diagnosis. Fecal rotaviral antigen can be detected by enzyme immunoassay available as a kit.† It should be remembered that many foals without diarrhea also have rotavirus, so a history of herd outbreak and exclusion of other causes are important in making this diagnosis.

Cryptosporidia, associated to date only with diarrhea in combined immunodeficiency foals, can be detected in direct fecal smears using safranin or carbofuchsin as a negative stain or in fecal material concentrated by a sucrose centrifugation technique and then stained similarly. Serologic evidence suggests normal foals may be asymptomatically infected.

THERAPY

Replacement of fluid losses with oral electrolytes or intravenous balanced multielectrolyte solutions is the most important facet of therapy. Peripheral perfusion, capillary refill time, and skin turgor should be used to clinically estimate the degree of dehydration. If the foal will drink water freely, commercial preparations with sodium, potassium, chloride, and glucose can be used.‡ Nasogastric intubation with such solutions is an alternative that must be weighed against the stress of passing a nasogastric tube, particularly if the latter is necessary repeatedly. Moderate or severe dehydration is better treated with intravenous fluids via an aseptically placed jugular catheter. One half of the estimated fluid deficit can be given over the first two hours and the rest replaced more slowly. If signs of hypovolemic shock and a rapid respiratory rate are present, a significant metabolic acidosis is likely. An approximation of the blood bicarbonate concentration can be made by measuring the total carbon dioxide with the Harleco CO_2 Apparatus. If not available, a clinical thumb rule can be employed: mild, moderate, or severe dehydration will produce approximate base excesses (BE) of minus 3, minus 6, and minus 9, respectively. The formula for calculating the milliequivalents of bicarbonate needed, BE × body weight (kg) × 0.3 can be used; however, it may be more accurate to use 0.5 rather than 0.3 in the neonatal foal. It should be remembered that 5 per cent bicarbonate is hypertonic and must be given slowly. Patients with persistent diarrhea will likely need supplemental potassium in the fluids. Neonates may also require extra glucose, especially in the initial stages of therapy.

Bismuth subsalicylate preparations, which act as protectants and neutralize bacterial toxins,* are efficacious in the majority of foal diarrheas. Empirical dosages of 0.5 ml per kg orally every four to six hours have been clinically beneficial. A response is usually evident within 48 hours. A slight change in fecal color may be noted. Once the diarrhea resolves, the drug dosage should be gradually reduced, because abrupt discontinuation has been associated with relapses in fecal consistency.

The decision to begin antimicrobial therapy is more readily reached in the neonate in which diarrhea is often a manifestation of septicemia. In the older foal the dangers of further disruption of the enteric flora and development of resistant strains of enteropathogens must be considered. Fever, leukopenia, and signs of toxemia suggest possible septicemia and may justify the use of parenteral broad-spectrum antibiotics. Aminoglycosides such as gentamicin, kanamycin, and amikacin are often effective against gram-negative enteropathogens, but they are nephrotoxic and a degree of renal impairment secondary to dehydration may already be present. Creatinine or blood urea nitrogen or both should therefore be monitored if aminoglycosides are used. Trimethoprim sulfa is a reasonable alternative but is also excreted through the kidney. Chloramphenicol has been recommended for salmonellosis; however, it is expensive and perhaps should be reserved for use in humans to reduce the likelihood of development of bacterial resistance.

Activated charcoal may be of benefit in enteritis produced by toxin-producing organisms such as *E. coli*, Salmonella, and Clostridium spp. Likewise, the nonsteroidal anti-inflammatory drugs (NSAID) such as flunixin meglumine† may diminish the inflammatory effects of toxin. The renal and gastric side effects of NSAID must be considered. If its use is elected, the minimum effective dosage should be used.

Mineral oil and cathartics have been recom-

---

*McCullough Cartwright Pharmaceutical Corp., Barrington, IL
†Rotazyme-Abbott, Abbott Laboratories, North Chicago, IL
‡Eltrad-4000, Haver-Lockhart, Shawnee, KS

*Corrective Mixture, Beecham Laboratories, Bristol, TN or Pepto-Bismol, Norwich-Eaton Pharmaceuticals, Inc., Norwich, NY
†Banamine, Schering Corp., Kenilworth, NJ

mended in treatment of overeating-induced enteritis and sand enteritis. Bulk laxatives may be safer for use in foals with sand enteritis than are cathartics. Hemicellulose flakes* and bran mashes are most commonly employed and may be repeated for several days if necessary.

Foals two weeks old or older that have had persistent diarrhea may have significant derangement of the intestinal flora. If no active protozoa are observed in a fresh fecal sample, transfaunation with fresh fecal contents from a healthy horse or cecal contents from an elective euthanasia case may be of benefit. The fecal or cecal contents can be strained through stockinette or cheesecloth and administered via nasogastric tube. A slight risk of Salmonella transmission exists with this technique. If no protozoa are evident in the recipient's feces in 36 hours the transfaunation should be repeated. Intestinal inoculants may also be used with a similar goal in mind.

Hypoproteinemia may develop if there is significant protein leakage through inflamed bowel wall, or in chronic diarrhea cases with malabsorption and severe weight loss. These patients may temporarily improve if a plasma transfusion is given. With the advent of commercially available plasma† this therapeutic modality may be practical if economically feasible, and may support the foal until the intestinal mucosa can heal.

In all instances, it is advisable to keep the foal's perineum clean and dry. Water repellant ointments applied after cleaning will help minimize hair loss and protect the skin from scalding.

CONTROL

A foal with diarrhea should always be considered a potential danger to other foals and horses on the premises if salmonellosis is at all likely. In neonatal foals, highly pathogenic enteropathogens, particularly *E. coli*, may colonize foaling areas and present a threat to all subsequent foals. Foals with diarrhea should therefore be isolated if possible, fed last, and their stalls should be cleaned with separate utensils. Traffic in and out of the stall should be kept to a minimum and a disinfectant footbath should be used. Once the stall becomes vacant it should be completely stripped and disinfected. If a diagnosis of Salmonella was made, steam cleaning and digging out of a dirt stall floor are necessary. Should salmonellosis become a chronic problem on a farm, the use of Salmonella bacterins as a prophylactic measure should be considered.

*Mucilose, Winthrop-Breon Laboratories, New York, NY
†Plasmate, Application Technologies and Pharmaceuticals, Inc., Atlanta, GA

GASTRODUODENAL ULCERS

Ulceration of the gastric or duodenal mucosa may occur any time the mucus-glycoprotein barrier and the integrity of the epithelial cells are disrupted, allowing gastric acid and pepsin to "autodigest" the mucosa. Ulcers in foals most commonly occur at the junction of the squamous and glandular mucosa of the stomach and in the proximal duodenum at the level of the common bile duct. Ulcers may also occur in the glandular mucosa or less commonly the squamous (nonglandular) portion of the stomach. Foals of any age may be affected, although the disease is most prevalent in suckling foals under four months of age.

In recent years, gastric and duodenal ulcers have emerged as an increasing problem. Epidemics of ulcers in foals have occurred on farms in Kentucky and Florida. Multiple causes have been suggested but no single one has been responsible for the farm outbreaks. Stress is virtually always evident in the history. Antecedent diarrhea occasionally accompanied by fever in several foals suggests an infectious agent. Rotavirus, Salmonella, and Candida have been isolated from some but not all foals with the syndrome. As mentioned in the previous section, rotavirus can be isolated from healthy foals as well. Campylobacter infection was reported in five foals with enteritis, three of which showed signs of ulcer disease. Dietary factors have also been suggested, as overly nutritious rations fed to the mare may increase the plant steroids and toxins in the milk, particularly if the milk has a high fat content. These steroids are believed to have an irritating effect on the foal's gastric mucosa and lead to gastritis and ulceration or colonization by the botulism organism. The source of this hypothesis is that if the farm's brood mare ration is changed from alfalfa hay and sweet feed to grass hay and oats, the incidence of clinical ulcers declines. Parasite damage to the stomach has also been hypothesized. Foals may secondarily develop ulcers if another serious problem is present; stress is believed to cause increased endogenous steroid production. If nonsteroidal anti-inflammatory drugs are given, these can cause ulceration of the glandular mucosa of the stomach even in the recommended dosage range. (See p. 118). Environmental stresses such as very hot weather or a sudden drop in barometric pressure are also implicated factors.

In children, stress ulcers are more common in those less than four years of age and are precipitated by conditions leading to shock. Primary ulcers are more common in older children who have symptoms of abdominal pain and gastrointestinal bleeding.

CLINICAL SIGNS

Depressed appetite, depression, bruxism, occasional colic, excessive salivation, retching-like motions, and diarrhea have been associated with gastric and duodenal ulcers. Excessive salivation and retching are specifically associated with duodenal ulcers or subsequent scars that affect pyloric outflow from the stomach. These signs are caused by reflux of stomach contents into the esophagus, which often produces severe ulceration and necrosis of the distal esophagus. A tendency to lie in dorsal recumbency has been associated with esophagitis. Aspiration pneumonia may also develop. If either a duodenal or a gastric ulcer perforates, signs of peritonitis may be apparent, such as abdominal tenderness, fever, and ileus. Unfortunately, many ulcers will produce few if any clinical signs and will be incidental findings at necropsy or produce sudden death in foals, particularly neonates. Gross evidence of blood in the feces is seldom observed.

DIAGNOSIS

The clinical signs of bruxism in combination with diarrhea are often the basis for suspecting ulcers, particularly if other foals on the farm are affected. Excessive salivation and retching movements suggest obstruction of gastric outflow and esophagitis. Diagnostic aids that may be utilized include examination of the upper gastrointestinal tract with a fiberoptic endoscope, determination of occult blood status of the gastric contents and feces, serum pepsinogen levels, abdominocentesis, and abdominal radiography. Endoscopy is useful in foals that are not so compromised that nasogastric passage of the endoscope is dangerous. An endoscope with a minimum length of 180 cm is necessary to reach the stomach in most foals; however, the external diameter must be 9 mm or less to readily pass through the turbinates. Otherwise, a short-acting general anesthetic is necessary followed by oral passage of the endoscope, an additional stress on the foal. For optimal visibility, the stomach should be empty, requiring fasting for at least four hours, yet even then suction capability of the endoscope is needed.

Nasogastric intubation to relieve gastric fluid build-up may yield several liters of fluid if gastric outflow is obstructed. The presence of a strongly positive occult blood reaction* should be considered supportive evidence only, as blood in the fluid may be a consequence of tube passage. Likewise, strongly positive occult blood reactions in the feces should be interpreted in light of the difficulty in obtaining the sample if digital extraction was used.

By no means do negative occult blood reactions indicate the absence of ulcers.

Serum pepsinogen determinations are a relatively new diagnostic aid in ulcer diagnosis in foals. Pepsinogen is secreted by chief cells in the gastric glands in amounts proportional to hydrochloride secretion. If the gastric mucosa is damaged, pepsinogen will back diffuse into the circulation in increased amounts. Levels higher than 240 ng per ml are significant in foals older than two weeks of age.

Abdominocentesis should be performed if ulcer perforation is a possibility. Elevated protein and white blood cell counts plus the presence of bacteria and feed material are consistent with a ruptured viscus. However, the omentum may effectively wall off small perforations in either the stomach or the duodenum and few pathologic changes will be evident in the peritoneal fluid.

Abdominal radiography may be rewarding in young foals. Distention and gas accumulation in the stomach are visible on plain lateral films of the abdomen, as may be free gas in the peritoneal cavity. Double-contrast radiography using barium sulfate and air can delineate ulcers in the gastric wall and duodenal strictures.

THERAPY

The foal with mild signs of gastric or duodenal ulcer disease may be successfully managed by minimizing stress and using drugs developed for ulcer therapy in man. These drugs are not approved by the Food and Drug Administration for use in the horse. Histamine (H_2) receptors on the hydrochloride-producing parietal cells stimulate acid secretion. Cimetidine and ranitidine are both H_2-receptor blockers that decrease gastric acid output in the foal for several hours after administration. Cimetidine is available in injectable and oral forms* and as of this writing has not been associated with adverse effects in the foal at a dose rate of 2 mg per kg four times a day intravenously, intramuscularly, or orally. Ranitidine is available in oral form† and appears to be as clinically efficacious in the foal at a dosage of 0.5 mg per kg twice a day orally. Gastric protectants have also been utilized in the foals but should not be given within an hour of oral H_2-receptor blockers. Sucralfate‡ is a sulfated sugar compound that binds to damaged mucosa, forming a protective barrier. This prevents further damage by gastric acid. The dose of sucralfate is 2 mg per kg three times a day orally. Bismuth subcitrate also acts as a protectant and has been efficacious in human studies in Europe. Although antacids have

---

*Hematest, Ames Co., Division of Miles Laboratories, Elkhart, IN

*Tagamet, Smith, Kline and French Laboratories, Philadelphia, PA
†Zantac, Glaxo, Inc., Research Triangle Park, NC
‡Carafate, Marion Laboratories, Inc., Kansas City, MO

been similarly utilized in foals with apparent efficacy, they must be given often; this may additionally stress the foal. If excessive amounts are given, diarrhea may result and antacids containing magnesium hydroxide may produce hypermagnesemia. Antacids should not be administered at the same time as H_2-receptor blockers. In the future prostaglandin E_2 or synthetic derivatives that increase gastric mucus production and inhibit acid and pepsin secretion may become available.

The more severely affected foal that has not been eating may develop serious dehydration, requiring fluid and electrolyte therapy. If colic signs are present, some form of analgesia is needed. The nonsteroidal anti-inflammatory drugs may damage the gastroduodenal mucosa and should therefore only be used if absolutely necessary. Xylazine alone or in conjunction with butorphanol may provide temporary pain relief. Gastric decompression via nasogastric tube may also relieve abdominal pain. Metaclopramide hydrochloride,* a drug that facilitates gastric emptying, may be of benefit (10 mg per kg intravenously). If signs of gastric distention or esophagitis are present or pain persists or recurs frequently, a gastrojejunostomy should be strongly considered before the foal becomes weak and debilitated, making it a poor surgical risk. The gastrojejunostomy procedure provides a second outlet for the stomach, relieving pain and pressure. At the same time, ulcers that have perforated or that are close to perforating can be oversewn. If peritonitis has developed the abdomen can be lavaged. Foals that underwent this procedure relatively early in the course of their ulcer disease showed marked improvement postoperatively and did well over subsequent months. However, those that were symptomatic for more than several days did not grow as well as their herdmates, or died of ulcer-related complications. This suggests that this procedure is useful when economically warranted and if utilized early in the course of the disease.

CONTROL

If there is a high incidence of ulcers on a farm, several steps can be taken to minimize the likelihood of further cases. Management practices should be examined to check for possible stress sources such as overcrowding, excessive handling, overmedication, and overfeeding. Weaning should be de-

---

*Reglan, A. H. Robins Co., Inc., Richmond, VA

layed if there is any question of the foal's health. Affected foals with diarrhea should be isolated from other foals and the potential role of Salmonella in the farm's problem should be investigated. If parasites potentially play a role, anthelmintic schedules should be modified. Foals at risk should be watched closely for early signs of diarrhea, fever, or anorexia. The recent practice of putting all sick foals, regardless of malady, on prophylactic antiulcer therapy such as antacids, sucralfate, and/or H_2-receptor blockers is not only expensive but perhaps unnecessary if conscientious farm staff are aware of clinical signs suggestive of gastroduodenal ulceration and can notify the veterinarian at their first appearance.

Supplemental Readings

Atherton, J. G., and Ricketts, S. W.: Campylobacter infection from foals. Correspondence. Vet. Record, *107*:264, 1980.

Barton, M. D., and Hughes, K. L.: *Corynebacterium equi*: A review. Vet. Bull. *50*:65, 1980.

Becht, J. L., Hendricks, J. B., and Merritt, A. M.: Current concepts of the foal ulcer syndrome. Proc. 30th Annu. Conv. Am. Assoc. Eq. Pract., 1984, p. 419.

Bergman, R.V.: Retained meconium. *In* Current Therapy in Equine Medicine, Robinson, N. E. (ed.); Philadelphia, W. B. Saunders Company, 1983, pp. 260–263.

Campbell, M. L., Ackerman, N., and Peyton L. S.: Radiographic gastrointestinal anatomy of the foal. Vet. Radio., *25*:194, 1984.

Campbell, M. L., Brown, M. P., Merritt, A. M., and Levy, M.: Evaluation of gastrojejunostomy in 8 foals with gastroduodenal ulcer disease. J. Vet. Surg. *14*:50, 1985.

Dickie, C. W., Klinkerman, D. L., and Petrie, R. J.: Enterotoxemia in two foals. J. Am. Vet. Med. Assoc., *173*:306, 1978.

Lewis, J. H.: Treatment of gastric ulcer: What is old and what is new. Arch. Int. Med. *143*:264, 1983.

Martens, R. J., and Scrutchfield, W. L.: Foal diarrhea: Pathogenesis, etiology, and therapy. Compend. Cont. Educ. Pract. Vet., *4*:S175, 1982.

Masri, M., Merritt, A. M., Gronwall, R., and Burrows, C. F.: Fecal composition in foal heat diarrhea. *In* Proceedings Equine Neonatology Research Conference, Gainesville, FL, 1984 p. 16.

Reed, S. L. Traub, J., Everman, J., Bayly, W., Penney, R., Simon, B., and Ward, A.: Foal enteritis. Equine Pract. 5:19, 1983.

Rossdale, P. D., and Ricketts, S. W.: The Practice of Equine Stud Farm Medicine. London, Balliere Tindall, 1980, p. 335.

Soule, C., Plateau, E., Perret, C., Chermette, R., and Feton, M. M.: Observation de cryptosporidies chez le poulain. Rec. Med. Vet., *159*:719, 1983.

Swerczek, T. W.: Foal ills linked to diet. DVM *15*:40, 1984.

Tolia, V., and Dubois, R. S.: Peptic ulcer disease in children and adolescents. Clin. Pediatr., 22:665, 1983.

Traub, J. L., Galhra, A. M., Grant, B. D., Reed, S. M., Gavin, P. R., and Paulsen, L. M.: Phenylbutazone toxicosis in the foal. Am. J. Vet. Res., *44*:1410, 1983.

Wilson, J. H., and Malone, M.: Serum pepsinogen levels in foals with gastroduodenal ulcers. *In* Proc. Eq. Neonatol. Res. Conf. Gainesville, FL, 1984, p. 15.

Hepatic Disease in Foals

Thomas J. Divers, KENNETT SQUARE, PENNSYLVANIA

Hepatic disease in foals may result from infectious agents, toxic causes, and mechanical obstruction of the biliary system. At least one half to three fourths of the liver must be damaged before clinical signs of hepatic disease are evident. Therefore, most hepatic disease in the foal does not progress to hepatic failure. This chapter will discuss causes, diagnosis, and therapy in foals with hepatic disease.

ETIOLOGY

Equine rhinopneumonitis and *Tyzzer's disease* are the two most common infectious causes of hepatic disease in foals. Equine herpesvirus I (rhinopneumonitis) is a sporadic cause of hepatic disease and interstitial pneumonia in newborn foals. The infection is believed to be acquired in utero. Affected foals are therefore weak at birth and usually die within the first week of life. The concomitant pneumonia may cause the most pronounced clinical signs, although icterus and severe depression, suggestive of hepatic failure, are also frequently seen. Within livers of affected foals are multifocal discolored areas of necrosis. Intranuclear inclusion bodies can be observed in the liver, and fluorescent antibody for equine herpesvirus in the lung or liver confirms the diagnosis.

Tyzzer's disease caused by *Bacillus piliformis*, a gram-negative sporulating organism, has been reported in foals 9 to 42 days of age. The incidence is usually sporadic in foals and because of the apparent peracute nature of the disease, clinical signs may not be observed before death. If clinical signs are observed, they include high heart rate and peripheral vascular collapse indicative of septicemia and icterus with neurologic disturbances reflecting hepatic failure. Icterus may not be observed because of the peracute nature of the disease. The predominant lesion in foals is in the liver; the organ is swollen and has widespread focal necrosis. Necrosis may also be observed in the distal bowel or heart or both. The organism cannot be cultured in cell-free media, but can be seen on microscopic examination of silver-stained sections of the liver. Foals are thought to develop the infection after ingesting the sporulating organism, but other information on epidemiology is lacking.

Other bacteria such as Salmonella and Actinobacillus may occasionally invade the liver of bacteremic foals resulting in liver disease. A more chronic abscessation infrequently found as an extension of an umbilical vein infection may be seen by ultra-sonic examination. Parasitic migration by *Ascaris equorum* or strongyle may cause liver disease in foals with heavy parasite burdens.

The liver is usually the first organ exposed to substances given by the oral route. It also has a major role in the metabolism or detoxification or both of foreign substances, suggesting that it would be particularly susceptible to chemical injury. Zimmerman has established a listing of potential hepatotoxins and their site of injury (cytotoxic, cholestatic, or mixed).

A syndrome causing toxic hepatopathy in newborn foals occurred during 1980 to 1983, as a result of oral administration of a nutritive supplement composed of microorganisms, vitamins, and minerals to newborn foals. The toxic principle of this paste was ferrous fumarate. The product was apparently innocuous when given to older foals and horses, but caused both cytotoxic and cholestatic injury and hepatic failure in many foals given the product at birth. The newborn foal's liver might have been more susceptible to this orally administered product because of the nonselectively enhanced permeability of its intestine. A relative deficiency of protective hepatic enzymes in the newborn foal might also have enhanced the toxic effect. This product has been withdrawn from the market.

An apparent steroid hepatopathy was observed in one foal that had received high levels of corticosteroids for several days. There are no documented reports of antimicrobials causing hepatic failure in foals, although a few are considered potential hepatotoxins. Isoerythrolysis or other hemolytic diseases may cause hypoxic (centrilobular) and cholestatic hepatic disease. An elevation in hepatic enzymes and conjugated bilirubin suggesting liver dysfunction may be found with severe hemolysis. Obstructive hepatic failure has been reported in a foal due to congenital biliary atresia. Duodenal ulceration may also obstruct the biliary tract via cicatrix formation at the common bile duct opening or from ingesta moving by reflux up the bile ducts.

DIAGNOSIS

The diagnosis of liver disease in the foal is usually based on an abnormally high serum concentration of hepatic enzymes or microscopic examination of the liver. The serum level of aspartate aminotransferase (SGOT, AST) is most consistently elevated in foals with hepatic disease. The level of this enzyme may also be abnormally elevated with muscle disease. Sorbitol dehydrogenase (SDH) and ornithine carbamyl transferase (OCT) are considered hepatic-specific enzymes. Serum levels of these two enzymes are usually elevated in foals with hepatic disease. However, because of their short serum half-life and instability in stored serum, the tests are not valuable in many clinical situations. Elevation of serum levels of gamma glutamyl transferase (GGT) is a consistent finding in foals with hepatic disease. The measurement of serum GGT offers two advantages to the equine practitioner: (1) elevations in the serum can be assumed to be of hepatic origin and (2) the enzyme remains stable in frozen serum for up to 30 days. Mild (twofold) elevations should not be overemphasized in the foal since many septic or premature foals, and some apparently normal foals, develop these elevations within the first week of life. The measurement of serum alkaline phosphatase is of minimal benefit in the foal.

Ultrasonic or radiographic examination of the anterior abdomen may assist in the diagnosis of hepatic masses, abscesses, biliary obstruction, and hepatic enlargement. Abdominal radiographs taken after oral barium administration may confirm reflux of intestinal contents into the biliary system in foals with duodenal ulceration and elevated biliary enzymes.

The laboratory diagnosis of hepatic failure cannot be determined by the measurement of serum enzymes but requires tests of hepatic function similar to those used in the adult horse. Increases in both total and direct serum bilirubin concentrations are usually found with hepatic failure, although the most marked increase is usually in the indirect concentration. Prothrombin time (PT) and partial thromboplastin time (PTT) are usually increased in foals with hepatic failure. The half-life of these clotting proteins is short (hours), and once 70 per cent or more of hepatic function is lost, PT and PTT may become elevated. Hypoglycemia is present and usually marked in foals with hepatic failure but may also occur with many foal diseases involving other organs. Blood ammonia concentrations are usually abnormally elevated and blood urea concentrations decreased in foals with hepatic failure. Blood urea concentrations normally decline within the first week of life in the young foal and a low blood urea (less than 10 mg per dl) should not be considered abnormal in the young foal. Plasma concentrations of aromatic amino acids are usually increased in foals with hepatic failure, and acidosis is often marked. Sulfobromophthalein clearance may be used to help confirm liver failure in foals without hyperbilirubinemia. The excretion rate can be determined at veterinary laboratories on three to five plasma samples collected at different times and within 15 minutes after the intravenous administration of the substance at 2 to 4 mg per kg.

The results of a liver biopsy might prove useful in determining the etiology and duration of hepatic disease or failure, but the interpretation of the biopsy rarely has an effect on treatment of the foal. One unusual finding in horses is the prominent biliary hyperplasia that may be found within three days after a hepatic insult. Liver biopsy may be performed in the standing or laterally recumbent foal after 5 to 15 mg of diazepam are given intravenously. The biopsy is performed at the right 12th intercostal space just above a line drawn from the olecranon to the tuber coxae and with the biopsy needle directed toward the opposite chest wall. The biopsy can be performed either from the right side or from the lower left if the liver is viewed first by ultrasound.

TREATMENT

When specific therapy for the primary cause of liver disease is provided, metabolism must be supported while the liver regenerates. The initial therapy should include a slow intravenous infusion of 5 per cent dextrose and isotonic sodium bicarbonate, along with more rapid correction of volume deficit by isotonic electrolytes. If after correction of the hypoglycemia and acidosis the neurologic status is not improved, a plasma exchange transfusion may be attempted in the hope of decreasing blood ammonia and false neurotransmitters. A solution of branched-chain amino acids is available for intravenous administration, but its safety or efficacy in foals with hepatic failure has not been determined. If sedation is needed in cases of hepatoencephalopathy, 5 to 10 mg diazepam may be given initially and the dosage decreased thereafter. Laxatives such as mineral oil should be administered to promote intestinal content movement. Bleeding tendencies, although rare, may be corrected with 1 to 2 or more L of fresh plasma.

Bactericidal broad-spectrum antibiotics are recommended for suspected cholangiohepatitis, focal liver abscess, salmonellosis, Tyzzer's disease, and cases in which bacteremia and liver disease coexist. Intravenously administered aqueous penicillin, along with an aminoglycoside, would be recommended as initial therapy. Antimicrobial therapy for salmonellosis may then need to be adjusted on the basis of sensitivity results and the ability of the selected drug to penetrate intracellularly. Intravenous fluid and acid-base deficits should also be corrected in bacteremic foals. Duodenal strictures as a result of ulceration require surgical correction. Foals with both duodenal and bile duct obstruction do not have as good a prognosis as those with duodenal strictures alone.

Supplemental Readings

Cornelius, C. E.: *In* Kaneko J. J., and Cornelius, C. E. (eds.): Clinical Biochemistry of Domestic Animals, 2nd ed. New York, Academic Press, 1971.

Crossley, I. R., Wardle, E. N., and Williams, R.: Biochemical mechanisms of hepatic encephalopathy. Clin. Sci., *64*:247, 1983.

Divers, T. J., Warner, A., Vaala, W. E., Whitlock, R. H., et al.: Toxic hepatic failure in newborn foals. J. Am. Vet. Med. Assoc., *183*:1407, 1983.

Hall, W. C., and Van Kruiningen, H. J.: Tyzzer's disease in a horse. J. Am. Vet. Med. Assoc., *164*:1187, 1974.

Hartley, W. J., and Dixon, R. J.: An outbreak of foal perinatal mortality due to equid herpesvirus type I: Pathological observations. Equine Vet. J., *11*:215, 1979.

Noonan, N. E.: Variations of plasma enzymes in the pony and the dog after carbon tetrachloride administration. Am. J. Vet. Res., *42*:674, 1981.

Rico, A. G., Braun, J. P., Bernard, P., et al.: Tissue distribution and blood levels of gamma glutamyl transferase in the horse. Equine Vet. J., *9*:100, 1977.

VanDerLuer, R. J. T., and Kroneman, J.: Biliary atresia in a foal. Aust. Vet. J., *14*:91, 1982.

Whitwell, K. E.: Four cases of Tyzzer's disease in foals in England. Equine Vet. J., *8*:118, 1976.

Zimmerman, H. J.: Hepatotoxic evaluation methodology. *In* Diagnostic Procedures in the Evaluation of Hepatic Diseases. New York, Alan R. Liss, Inc., 1983.

Neonatal Isoerythrolysis

James L. Becht, ATHENS, GEORGIA

Neonatal isoerythrolysis (NI) or hemolytic anemia of the newborn, although not commonly encountered in equine practice, is an important immunologic disease of foals that often results in a fatal hemolytic crisis. Erythrocytes of affected foals are destroyed by alloantibodies produced by the mare as a result of alloimmunization by erythrocyte antigens foreign to her but possessed by the stallion and inherited by the foal. Alloantibodies are concentrated in the colostrum and initiate intra- and extravascular hemolysis when absorbed into the foal's circulation following successful passage of colostral antibodies.

Foals that develop NI are normal at birth, ingest colostrum uneventfully, and exhibit normal behavior until erythrolysis precipitates anemia and resulting clinical signs. Since colostral proteins, including antibodies, can be demonstrated in the foal's serum as early as six hours after first suckling, signs of NI in severely affected foals may occur shortly after this time. More commonly, affected foals begin to exhibit signs between 12 hours and 5 days of age. Generally, the younger the foal when signs are observed, the poorer the prognosis for life, and the greater the need for therapy and supportive management.

DIAGNOSIS

Two of the most important clinical signs of NI are icterus and hemoglobinuria. Although not pathognomonic for NI, these signs suggest NI in a weak, depressed foal born to a multiparous mare. Icterus rarely occurs before the second day of the disease, and increases in intensity during the following days. Thus, a foal can die of NI before developing obvious icterus. Icterus seen in foals with NI is associated with an increase in predominantly unconjugated bilirubin, which may reach levels of 20 to 40 mg per dl. The presence of icterus can best be determined by examination of the foal's sclerae in natural sunlight. It is noteworthy to remember that neonatal foals with septicemia or meconium impactions frequently exhibit varying degrees of icterus.

Hemoglobinuria, although not commonly present, may be seen in peracute cases and may be the first clinical sign observed. Its presence suggests profound intravascular hemolysis with release of hemoglobin into the bloodstream. This free hemoglobin overwhelms the binding capacity of plasma haptoglobin and is passed in the urine.

Progressive weakness is commonly observed in foals with NI. Foals may be found in lateral recumbency or in sternal recumbency, resting the chin on the ground. A mare with an udder full of milk should alert the practitioner that the foal may be spending less time than normal nursing. Rectal temperature is usually within normal limits or slightly elevated owing to the accompanying hemolysis. The pulse and respiratory rates are usually elevated because of the hemolytic anemia and the foal's tissue oxygen debt. With progression of the anemia, respirations become rapid and shallow, and shortly before death they become labored as the foal exhibits periods of gasping. During terminal stages, the foal may convulse and become comatose. Postmortem findings suggestive of NI include splenomegaly, pale and/or icteric body tissues, and hemoglobinuria.

Laboratory support greatly facilitates the clinical diagnosis of NI. It provides valuable information regarding the severity of the disease and the approach to therapy indicated. The blood erythrocyte count and packed cell volume (PCV) should be assessed to determine the severity of the anemia. Anemia is present in a neonatal foal when the erythrocyte count is less than 6×10^6 per cu mm or the PCV is less than 25 per cent. Foals with severe NI usually have a rapidly progressive anemia with a PCV of 6 to 10 per cent and erythrocyte count of less than 3×10^6 per cu mm. In most clinical cases, the severity of clinical signs is directly related to the degree of the anemia. Generally, foals with NI that have an erythrocyte count of 4×10^6 per cu mm nurse frequently for short periods, whereas foals with less than 3×10^6 per cu mm rarely nurse.

Despite a history compatible with NI, laboratory confirmation of anemia, and clinical signs of weakness, icterus, hemoglobinuria, and increased vital parameters, a definitive diagnosis of NI can be made only when alloantibodies are demonstrated on the foal's erythrocytes. Basically, serodiagnostic testing for NI demonstrates either agglutination or hemolysis of sensitized foal erythrocytes. Since alloantibodies responsible for NI act stronger as hemolysins that cause hemolysis than as agglutinins that cause agglutination, preferred tests should detect hemolysis of the foal's erythrocytes. Even though the hemolytic test has been established as a superior test when compared with tests detecting agglutination such as the conventional cross-match and the antiglobulin or Coombs' test, it is rather impractical for use in the field. The test requires an exogenous complement source that is furnished in commercially available pooled rabbit sera.* Since rabbits have naturally occurring antiequine antibodies, rabbit sera must be processed with erythrocytes of healthy horses to remove these antibodies. The rabbit sera is best preserved by freezing at extremely low temperatures, which adds to its impracticality for the equine practitioner. A major advantage of the hemolytic test when compared with tests that demonstrate agglutination is the ease of test interpretation. Hemolysis is quickly identified grossly as a winelike discoloration of the supernatant in a tube containing sensitized erythrocytes whereas rouleaux formation of equine erythrocytes often interferes with microscopic assessment of agglutination.

Several laboratories presently perform the hemolytic test for NI in foals. Even though with this approach the diagnosis is delayed by mailing of samples to the laboratory, a confirmation of the disease can be obtained. Two laboratories that provide excellent testing services are the Serology Laboratory at the University of California and Stormont Laboratories at Woodland, California. Addresses are given in the discussion of blood transfusions (see p. 320).

Tests that demonstrate agglutination of sensitized erythrocytes are more available to the practicing veterinarian and can be helpful in the diagnosis of NI. Agglutination of washed foal erythrocytes resuspended in saline or following the addition of Coombs' sera containing antiequine IgG confirm the diagnosis of NI. Before use, the Coombs' serum must also be processed to remove antiequine antibodies possessed by rabbits used to prepare the reagent. Generally, a foal with NI will not exhibit autoagglutination—that is, erythrocytes will not agglutinate in saline following washing, until the disease is severe and life-threatening. Even though these procedures may confirm the diagnosis, it should be remembered that alloantibodies react primarily as hemolysins, and may therefore not be detected by tests that detect agglutination.

In summary, in vitro agglutination and hemolysis are dependent upon the relative amounts of alloantigen or erythrocytes and alloantibody or serum. Therefore simple tests in which blood of the foal is mixed with serum or colostrum from the mare are inaccurate and often misleading. Furthermore, serodiagnostic tests for NI are rather laborious and difficult to perform in the practice setting for several reasons. First, erythrocytes must be washed free of serum proteins, other blood cell types, and platelets, which may interfere with results. Second, incubation for at least 30 minutes is usually required before any meaningful results can be obtained. Third, special reagents are required, which include pooled rabbit sera for the hemolytic test and antiglobulin serum for the Coombs' test. And finally, these reagents require special storage and processing before use in the diagnostic tests. The tests required for accurate NI diagnosis are not too sophisticated for the practicing veterinarian to perform. However, if the tests are to be worthwhile and the results reliable, dedication to the steps involved and a sound basic understanding of the testing procedures are mandatory.

THERAPY AND MANAGEMENT

General approaches to management of foals with NI include prevention of further ingestion of alloantibodies, adequate nutrition, consideration of corticosteroid therapy, protection against opportunistic infections, and replacement of plasma volume and

---

*Pel-Freez Biologicals, P. O. Box 68, Rogers, AK

erythrocytes until the bone marrow responds to the anemia. If the foal is less than 24 hours old when NI is diagnosed, it should be muzzled and fed supplemental milk or a commercially available milk preparation.* Since the foal's intestine becomes impermeable to colostral antibodies by 24 hours of age, prevention of nursing until the foal is 30 hours old should be adequate. During this period, the mare should be milked at approximately two-hour intervals to ensure continued milk production. Separation of the foal and mare is not recommended, as it tends to unnecessarily stress the already compromised foal. Testing the mare's milk for alloantibody levels and not allowing the foal to return to nursing until alloantibodies are no longer detectable is probably not worthwhile. Even if the antibody levels are detectable, the foal's intestine should be unable to absorb them into circulation after 24 hours of age.

The question of corticosteroid therapy in foals with NI has not been adequately addressed. Although infections by opportunistic organisms are of concern in foals with NI, one administration of corticosteroids may be helpful in diminishing the hemolytic process. An intravenous injection of dexamethasone (5 to 20 mg) appears to have some clinical benefit in severe NI cases. As mentioned previously, antibiotic coverage with such preparations as trimethoprim-sulfa or ampicillin also aids in prevention of secondary bacterial infections.

Erythrocyte supplementation is an important adjunct to the successful management of foals with NI. However, it is important to remember that a decrease in circulating blood volume also occurs and should be addressed while supplemental blood is being obtained. Administration of plasma from an acceptable donor or sodium-containing isotonic fluid replacement is helpful in the immediate management of a foal with NI. The PCV should be monitored during such therapy because further hemodilution will occur.

The need for supplemental erythrocytes should be based on the erythrocyte count or the PCV or both. Not only is the absolute value important, but also important is the rapidity with which these parameters are declining. Foals with NI warrant PCV determinations at least twice daily until the progression of anemia can be characterized. Irrespective of the rapidity of the declining PCV, a transfusion is indicated when the PCV and erythrocyte count fall to less than 12 per cent and 3×10^6 per cu mm, respectively. Clinical appearance of the affected foal should also be taken into consideration when the need for supplemental erythrocytes is considered, as several foals have spontaneously recovered from NI following anemia with a PCV as low as 12 per cent.

The best donor of erythrocytes for a foal with NI is the mare, but this means that the serum containing the offending alloantibodies must be removed. Allowing whole anticoagulated blood collected from the mare to settle followed by siphoning of the serum is acceptable, but the settled-erythrocyte preparation contains alloantibodies. Washing mare erythrocytes by mixing with saline and repeated centrifugation is the preferred method, but rather impractical unless the practitioner has access to a large refrigerated centrifuge.

Administration of the sire's erythrocytes will result in destruction of his erythrocytes until the alloantibodies are consumed. This adds further insult to the foal's reticuloendothelial system and is not advisable. If washed erythrocytes of the mare are not available, erythrocytes from an "acceptable blood-typed donor horse" are recommended. An acceptable blood-typed donor horse is one whose blood has been characterized by one of the two serology laboratories already mentioned, and found to be free of significant alloantibodies in the serum and Aa and Qa surface antigens on the erythrocytes (see p. 317). Alloantibodies against these antigens are most often responsible for field cases of NI. Transfusion of 1 to 2 liters of whole blood usually has a dramatically favorable effect on the foal's clinical appearance. Since transfused equine erythrocytes have a short half-life, the transfusion may need to be repeated if the anemia is progressive. The PCV should be determined after each transfusion to serve as a baseline, which will enable detection of the need for repeat transfusions. Exchange transfusion whereby blood is withdrawn from one vein while it is supplemented through another vein may benefit severely affected foals. However, the need for increased manipulation of the foal and possible sedation make this procedure less attractive as a useful adjunct to therapy.

PREVENTION

Neonatal isoerythrolysis can be effectively prevented by withholding the offending colostrum and providing colostrum from a nonsensitized mare. It is important to test supplemental colostrum, as NI can be induced with supplemental colostrum that contains alloantibodies. An aliquot of stored colostrum should be analyzed by one of the laboratories mentioned previously to ensure it is free of alloantibodies, especially anti-Aa and anti-Qa.

A common question by concerned horseowners regarding NI is: "I'm afraid that my mare is carrying a foal that might develop NI. What should I do?" The best approach to this question is to acquire

---

*Foal Lac, Borden, Inc., Pet-Ag Division, Pet/Vet Products, Hampshire, IL

serum from the mare during late pregnancy, preferably during the last two to three weeks, and mail the sample to one of the serologic laboratories to determine if the mare has a significant titer to erythrocyte alloantigens. If a high titer to one or more alloantibodies is detected, recommendations should include withholding the mare's colostrum from the foal and provision for supplemental colostrum. Such results do not mean that the foal will definitely develop NI, because the foal may not inherit the offending alloantigen types from the stallion, and therefore the foal's erythrocytes would not be affected by alloantibodies in the colostrum.

Supplemental Readings

Becht, J. L., and Semrad, S. D.: Hematology, blood typing, and immunology of the neonatal foal. Vet. Clin. North Am. (Equine Pract.), *1*:91, 1985.

Becht, J. L.: Neonatal isoerythrolysis in the foal, Part I. Background, blood group antigens, and pathogenesis. Compend. Cont. Ed., 5:S5591, 1983.

Stormont, C.: Neonatal isoerythrolysis in domestic animals: A comparative review. Adv. Vet. Sci. Comp. Med., *19*:23, 1975.

Suzuki, Y., Stormont, C., and Trommershausen-Smith, A.: Alloantibodies: The blood groups they define. Proc. First Internat. Symp. Eq. Hematol., 1975, pp. 34–41.

Trommershausen-Smith, A., Stormont, C., and Suzuki, Y.: Alloantibodies: Their role in equine neonatal isoerythrolysis. Proc. First Internat. Symp. Eq. Hematol., 1975, pp. 349–354.

Respiratory Support for the Newborn Foal

Philip C. Kosch, GAINESVILLE, FLORIDA

Anne M. Koterba, GAINESVILLE, FLORIDA

Diseases associated with the respiratory tract are common in the neonatal foal, occurring both as primary conditions and secondary to other disease processes. In many foals, abnormalities result from failure of the lungs to make a complete transition from a collapsed, liquid-filled, relatively inactive organ to an air-filled structure responsible for acquiring sufficient oxygen for the entire body. Even if the lungs are reasonably normal at birth, lung pathology often develops during the course of a neonate's illness and is often overlooked clinically. Therefore, a careful and thorough work-up of the abnormal neonatal foal is paramount in order to recognize any respiratory abnormalities, to find the cause, and to carefully determine the foal's need for respiratory support.

DETERMINATION OF THERAPEUTIC NEEDS

In evaluation of the respiratory system, respiratory rate, pattern and effort of breathing, and mucous membrane color should be observed and recorded at frequent intervals. Vital signs charted frequently are often useful for spotting trends, such as a progressive rise of respiratory rate over six to eight hours. The normal respiratory rate of the neonatal foal is 30 to 40 breaths per minute. Many factors that are nonrespiratory in nature—excite-

ment, pain, high environmental temperatures, fever, metabolic acidosis, systemic hypotension, and neurologic disease—may also elevate respiratory rate. In some cases, an elevation in respiratory rate does correspond closely with a worsening pulmonary condition; however, a normal respiratory rate and pattern may be present in spite of severe lung pathology. Although auscultation of the lung fields is often essential in order to identify respiratory abnormalities, lung sounds do not always correlate well with disease severity. Foals with few or no audible thoracic abnormalities may have severe pulmonary pathology, especially interstitial lung involvement and atelectasis. Increasingly obvious adventitial lung sounds may be associated with recovery rather than deterioration in condition. Mucous membrane color is not a reliable indicator of the adequacy of oxygenation of the neonatal foal. Cyanotic mucous membranes are usually not observed until the partial pressure of arterial oxygen (Pa_{O_2}) reaches very low levels, less than 40 mm Hg. A cough is usually not present.

In many foals, data from clinical pathology and chest radiography are necessary for accurate diagnosis and to adequately define the foal's need for respiratory support. Chest radiographs and arterial blood gas analyses are potentially very useful as sensitive and specific indicators of subtle respiratory disease.

In a large group of septicemic foals in our hospital, pulmonary involvement was frequently not even suspected until routine chest radiographs and arterial blood gas values were evaluated. Gas exchange abnormalities were detected in several cases.

THORACIC RADIOLOGY

Thoracic radiology is often necessary to firmly establish that a respiratory problem exists and to determine the extent of pulmonary involvement. Radiology is also useful to monitor the progress of a respiratory condition. It must be kept in mind that radiographic changes may follow or precede changes in clinical condition and that major changes can occur surprisingly rapidly. Unfortunately, at this time, gaps still exist in our knowledge of even the normal radiographic appearance of the foal's thorax at different gestational ages. In the past, thoracic films have not been easily available to the veterinary practitioner in the field, but with the development of rare earth screens, chest radiography is possible using portable x-ray units.

ARTERIAL BLOOD GAS ANALYSIS

Arterial blood gas analysis has been traditionally avoided by veterinarians for a variety of reasons. Blood gas analysis is often expensive, and laboratories with the necessary equipment are not always conveniently located. Arterial blood samples can be quite difficult to obtain, and many veterinarians are uncertain about interpreting the resulting values. However, it is difficult to safely and effectively administer respiratory support to neonates without a means to monitor Pa_{O_2}. Arterial blood gas data are important to define the severity of respiratory compromise, the type of therapy indicated, and the response to therapy.

Arterial blood gases can be obtained by direct puncture from several sites. Although the carotid is the largest artery, hematomas commonly form after a few samplings. More peripheral arteries, such as the brachial as it crosses the medial aspect of the foreleg, the great metatarsal, and the facial, are readily palpable if blood pressure is adequate. The brachial vein may be inadvertently sampled fairly easily. However, the likelihood of mistakenly acquiring venous blood in the area of the great metatarsal artery is much less, for in most foals the vein is absent or is very small. A small bleb of local anesthetic (lidocaine 2 per cent, without epinephrine) can greatly facilitate proper collection and minimize needless struggling and subsequent hyperventilation. A 25-gauge, five eights inch needle attached to a 3-ml syringe with the hub filled with heparin is recommended for arterial sampling. Any air bubbles should be removed. The syringe should be sealed with a rubber cork and placed in ice slush until analysis is carried out. A sample handled in this manner may be stored for six hours without major changes in Pa_{O_2}. Pressure should be applied

to the arterial puncture site for at least two minutes after needle withdrawal to avoid formation of a hematoma.

Problems caused by poor patient compliance and vessel trauma after multiple punctures can be serious limitations to adequate blood gas monitoring. Percutaneous placement of an indwelling arterial catheter in the great metatarsal artery is not difficult if pulse quality is adequate, but maintenance of catheter position and patency can be difficult in all but the most depressed patients. The catheter must be firmly sutured to the skin and bandaged carefully to limit motion and maintain sterility. A slow constant saline infusion system is safer and more effective than intermittent heparin flushes in maintaining patency. Other options for catheter insertion include surgical cutdown on the great metatarsal artery or, if the birth of a high-risk foal is attended, insertion of an umbilical arterial catheter. In each case, the advantages of continuous access to an artery must be carefully weighed against the disadvantages, including the potential for introduction of serious systemic and local infection and hemorrhage.

Valid interpretation depends not only on correct sampling and measurement techniques but also involves weighing the circumstances present at the time of sampling. These include the position of the foal, degree and duration of struggling, inspired oxygen concentration, and gestational age of the foal. In certain foals, particularly those with immature or diseased lungs, a significant decrease in Pa_{O_2} is caused by repositioning from sternal to lateral recumbency. This observation also becomes important in treatment consideration. Struggling and subsequent hyperventilation will usually result in a temporary decrease in Pa_{CO_2}. With supplemental oxygen, Pa_{O_2} will be increased variably, depending on the amount of right to left shunting present. For example, Pa_{O_2} of 85 torr would be considered normal in a foal breathing room air, but it would be abnormal if the animal was breathing 100 per cent oxygen. Finally, "normal" blood gas values are influenced by both gestational and postnatal age of the foal. A summary of previously reported normal blood gas values is presented in Table 1. Interpretation of blood gas values of venous blood are notoriously deceptive and are properly restricted to evaluation of metabolic status. In the absence of arterial blood gas values, venous values from a free-flowing jugular vein may be used to provide guidance as to the importance of obtaining an arterial sample—for example, to determine if a cut-down is justified. If the jugular venous P_{CO_2} is greater than 60 mm Hg arterial hypercapnia should be considered likely and if jugular venous PO_2 is less than 20 mm Hg, either arterial hypoxemia or cardiac failure should be suspected.

TABLE 1. ARTERIAL BLOOD GAS VALUES REPORTED FOR NORMAL TERM AND PREMATURE FOALS*

Foal			PaO$_2$ (mmHg)		PaCO$_2$ (mmHg)		pHa	
Gestational Status	Age Postpartum (Hours)	Number	Mean ± SEM	95% Confidence Limits	Mean ± SEM	95% Confidence Limits	Mean ± SEM	95% Confidence Limits
Normal	3–168	10	80.1 ± 3.8	56–104	47.5 ± 2.6	31–62	7.354 ± 0.011	7.28–7.42
Normal	1–12	6	77.4 ± 3.1	60–92	42.2 ± 1.8	34–50	7.378 ± 0.015	7.34–7.41
Normal	12–48	6	83.2 ± 3.1	68–98	44.5 ± 1.2	38–50	7.374 ± 0.004	7.35–7.39
Normal	48–168	5	88.2 ± 5.9	61–114	42.4 ± 1.0	37–47	7.384 ± 0.014	7.32–7.45
Normal	4–11	5	83.8 ± 6.3	55–111	39.5 ± 1.8	31–47	7.367 ± 0.010	7.32–7.41
Premature	0.5–11	7	53.7 ± 1.5	45–62	55.3 ± 3.6	36–74	7.208 ± 0.048	6.95–7.46

*From Kosch, P. C., Koterba, A. M., Coons, T. J., et al.: Developments in management of the newborn foal in respiratory distress. 1. Evaluation. Equine Vet. J., *16*:312–318, 1984.

One of two patterns of blood gas derangements is generally encountered: hypoxemia, Pa$_{O_2}$ less than 70 mm Hg, with normal or low Pa$_{CO_2}$, and hypoxemia with hypercapnia. If there is hypercapnia and resulting respiratory acidosis, hypoventilation is diagnosed. Hypoventilation usually results from the inability or unwillingness of the animal to breathe hard enough to compensate for the lung pathology present. Clinical signs must be evaluated in addition to blood gas analysis in order to choose the appropriate therapy. Certain hypoxic foals do not display signs of respiratory distress, whereas others with the same blood gas picture may be markedly distressed; the reasons for these discrepancies are not well understood but may include rapidity of development of the problem, developmental or pathologic variations in chemoreceptor function, and type of lung pathology present.

The goal of the evaluation process is to correctly identify the type and severity of respiratory compromise in order to best determine the appropriate course of action. If treatment is desired, appropriate therapy should be instituted *without delay* if the outcome is to be successful. The choice of therapeutic strategy to support respiratory function depends on the veterinarian's ability to assess the foal's need for oxygen therapy or ventilatory support or both. Likewise, making appropriate changes in therapy depends on ability to monitor the adequacy of the foal's oxygenation and alveolar ventilation by repeating many of the aforementioned evaluation procedures.

THERAPEUTIC STRATEGY

The priorities in respiratory therapy are based on preservation of the foal's life by supporting respiratory function—namely, maintenance of a patent airway, provision of humidified oxygen to raise inspired oxygen tension sufficiently to avoid hypoxemia, and provision of ventilatory support when hypercapnia becomes critical. Secondary techniques include airway hygiene and use of suction, chest coupage, maintenance of an upright body position, drug therapy, and stress management. These support techniques will be presented in order from the most simple to more complex.

Oxygen Therapy. The most common therapeutic need in many foals is supplemental oxygen therapy. The correction of hypoxia involves optimization of breathing efforts by ensuring a patent airway and by upright positioning of the foal, and increasing the fractional inspired concentration of oxygen (FI$_{O_2}$) to provide adequate arterial oxygenation. The possibility of inadvertent inspiration of dirt or bedding should be minimized. Excessive secretions or foreign substances should be suctioned from the airways. When foals with pulmonary immaturity or pathology are repositioned from lateral to sternal recumbency, rapid and consistent improvement in arterial oxygen partial pressure (Pa$_{O_2}$) and less labored breathing have been noted. In light of this, a concerted effort should be made to maintain respiratory-distressed foals propped up in a sternal body position. If the sternal position is not possible, foals should be turned often in an attempt to avoid progressive atelectasis and subsequent formation of intrapulmonary right-to-left shunts. Every effort should be made to have foals stand and walk as frequently as possible, but unfortunately many critically ill foals are not able to stand without assistance during the early stages of illness.

Inspired oxygen concentration is most easily increased by insufflation using a bias flow of 100 per cent oxygen. Nonirritating, flexible plastic tubing may be introduced into the nasopharynx via the ventral meatus and sutured or taped to the nose. Oxygen should initially be delivered at a flow rate between 5 to 10 L per minute. In order to prevent drying of the airways, it is important that the gas be humidified. The catheters, humidifiers, and tubing should be replaced daily, and the nose examined for erosions. Most foals tolerate the tubing very well; the major complication is a mucopurulent nasal discharge that spontaneously resolves. The actual oxygen concentration delivered by this method to the lungs is not easily determined. It depends on several factors, including the position of the tube and depth of breathing. Oxygen therapy should be directed at maintaining a Pa_{O_2} of 70 to 100 mm Hg, and the flow rate should be adjusted according to blood gas results. If severe intrapulmonary or cardiac shunts are present, even high flow rates may raise Pa_{O_2} very little. Weaning from oxygen therapy should be done gradually, with frequent blood gas reassessments to ensure that the foal's condition remains stable. It should be kept in mind that the exact Pa_{O_2} that produces tissue hypoxia in a particular neonatal foal cannot be predicted.

The decision on when to institute oxygen therapy is somewhat subjective and should be based on clinical signs and blood gas analysis. An elevated respiratory rate, labored respirations with excessive intercostal and abdominal muscle activity, cyanotic mucous membranes, and restlessness should be considered indications for a trial of oxygen administration. The diagnosis is often confirmed by a marked improvement in attitude or breathing pattern concurrent with oxygen delivery. Absence of response may indicate either a nonrespiratory origin of the clinical signs or severe lung pathology with shunting. If blood gases are analyzed, we consider a Pa_{O_2} of less than 60 mm Hg in lateral recumbency an objective indication for oxygen therapy. Excessively elevated oxygen tensions may result in pulmonary oxygen toxicity, so when Pa_{O_2} rises above 90 to 100 mm Hg, some reduction in FI_{O_2} or oxygen flow rates is indicated. Cessation of oxygen therapy is indicated when Pa_{O_2} is sustained within normal limits and the foal's clinical condition is either stable or continuing to improve. Such withdrawal of therapy should be done gradually with reassurances that the foal's condition remains stable with no recurrence of distressed respirations and no deterioration in blood gases.

Clearing Secretions. In the foal with pneumonia, routine chest coupage to loosen adherent secretions in lower airways is highly recommended. While the foal is in a sternal or standing position, both sides of the chest are rapped firmly and repeatedly with a cupped hand. A cough is usually elicited and secretions are effectively moved out of the lower airways. Foals usually tolerate this procedure well and it can be carried out several times a day. Some clinicians advocate the use of bronchodilators to aid in breathing and airway clearance; however, their efficacy has not been adequately studied in newborn foals. Nebulization of water and drugs is reputed to be a useful technique to place these materials into the foal's respiratory tract. It is doubtful that drug deposition reaches substantially beyond the upper airway passages unless a direct tracheal inhalation technique is utilized. Nevertheless, the added moisture may serve to help mobilize accumulated upper airway secretions and make the foal more comfort-

able. Routine cleaning and suction of the oropharynx and trachea should be performed about every four hours in foals unable to clear their own airway. Suction should be performed with a 56 cm, 10 to 15 French gauge suction catheter. Suction is applied as the catheter is withdrawn from the airway. Best results are obtained if the catheter is rotated as it is withdrawn in order to clear the walls. Care should be taken to avoid long periods of suction that can promote lung collapse and transient but substantial falls in arterial oxygenation.

Nursing Care. A weak premature foal unable to stand that has respiratory compromise cannot tolerate unnecessary stress. If possible, the foal should be kept comfortable and free from excessive viewing and handling. Frequent feedings and treatment procedures, although essential, make stress management difficult. Removal of the newborn from the mother for treatment is necessary in many cases to provide quality care in a controlled environment. If separation only lasts a day or two, mares usually reaccept their foals; however, the client should be prepared to hand-raise the foal if maternal rejection does occur.

Resuscitation. In the case of a collapsed foal that may be hypothermic, hypotensive, and/or unresponsive, immediate resuscitative procedures are required to avoid irreversible cardiopulmonary failure. Guidelines for resuscitation are outlined in Figure 1 and emergency drug doses are listed in Table 2. The sequence of resuscitative efforts must be determined by the condition of the animal. Reevaluation of efficacy of efforts should be made frequently. The veterinarian must always take care not to be too aggressive in intervening when the animal is making adequate progress.

The natural history of asphyxia has been experimentally reproduced in several species and is divided into four stages. Rapid gasps occurring shortly after the onset of asphyxia cease after about one minute, beginning the period of primary apnea. This apnea lasts about a minute and is followed by a series of spontaneous deep gasps lasting for four to five minutes, which weaken and then end after about eight minutes of total anoxia. This final period, called secondary apnea, is followed by death if no ventilatory support is given. A major difference between primary and secondary apnea is that, in the latter, the respiratory center is no longer responsive to sensory or chemical stimuli. Therefore, there is no indication for use of analeptic drugs such as doxapram during this final stage of apnea; they may be of benefit only during primary apnea. Once secondary apnea occurs, it can be reversed only by assisted ventilation and circulatory support. As it is usually difficult to determine whether primary or secondary apnea is present, the latter should be assumed.

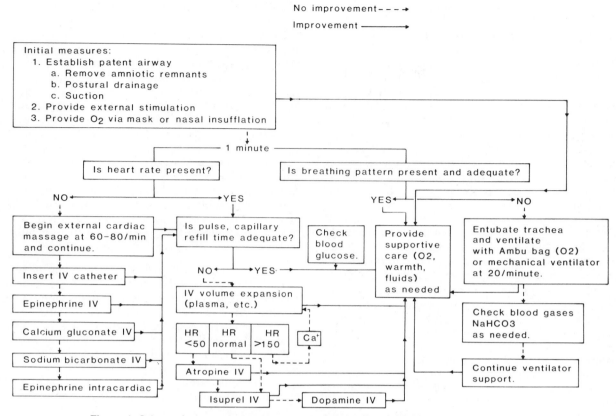

Figure 1. Schema for resuscitation of the newborn foal. (Drug dosages are given in Table 2.)

Although the newborn mammal generally tolerates asphyxia better than the adult, severe hypoxia may well overcome any protective mechanisms in operation. Acid-base parameters change dramatically during total asphyxia. The pH drops sharply as the Pa_{CO_2} rises, and severe respiratory acidosis and severe hypoxia result. Blood lactate levels also rise, reflecting a switch to anaerobic metabolism and accumulation of excess acid. Therefore, when asphyxia is prolonged, metabolic acidosis as well as the primary respiratory acidosis may result. The appropriate treatment for respiratory acidosis is adequate ventilation. Any attempt to correct the condition with $NaHCO_3$ without ample ventilation may serve to worsen the acidosis because $NaHCO_3$ is converted to carbon dioxide and is retained. The use of hypertonic $NaHCO_3$ solutions has also been associated with both severe hyperosmolarity and an increased incidence of cerebral vascular accidents, especially in newborn premature human infants. Because of these potential complications, $NaHCO_3$ solutions should be administered with caution. Metabolic acidosis can often be completely corrected with appropriate ventilation and by improving circulation volume, thus eliminating the need for alkali therapy. However, if a foal's clinical condition does not improve after adequate ventilation has been instituted, and blood gas analysis is not available, $NaHCO_3$ may be used empirically at a dose of 2 mEq per kg intravenously (0.5 mEq per L) for treatment of suspected metabolic acidosis.

Ventilation. In an emergency situation, adequate ventilation can usually be achieved by mouth-to-nose resuscitation. The neck should be extended, the nostrils cleared, the down nostril occluded, and a breath delivered to the up nostril approximately 20 to 30 times per minute. The size of the breaths delivered should be sufficient to cause reasonably prominent thoracic excursions. Ventilation can be

TABLE 2. EMERGENCY DRUGS AND THEIR DOSES FOR NEONATAL RESUSCITATION

Drug	Dosage	Route
Epinephrine	0.1 ml/kg, 1:10,000 solution	IV
Calcium gluconate	1–2 ml/kg, 10% solution	IV
Sodium bicarbonate	2 mEq/kg (.5 mEq/ml)	IV
Atropine	0.02 mg/kg	SQ, IV
Isoproterenol	0.05–1.0 μg/kg/min	IV
Dopamine	2–5 μg/kg/min	IV
Dobutamine	2–10 μg/kg/min	IV
Doxapram	0.02–0.05 mg/kg/min	IV

provided more efficiently via an endotracheal tube, but the necessary equipment—an endotracheal tube, syringe for cuff inflation, and lubrication—must be at hand. Silicone rubber endotracheal tubes* 8 to 10 mm in internal diameter and 45 to 55 cm in length are recommended for foals up to one month of age; these may be passed into the trachea from the mouth or the nose. Ventilation can be delivered with a one-L self-inflating, nonrebreathing bag† that delivers oxygen-enriched room air.

A mild build-up of Pa_{CO_2} is not necessarily harmful because the associated release of catecholamines may stimulate cardiac function beneficially. However, secondary acid-base derangements may depress vital organs such as the brain and myocardium. Elevated carbon dioxide levels between 50 and 60 mm Hg, if stable, may not automatically necessitate mechanical ventilation. However, if the increases in Pa_{CO_2} are rapid or are continuing to rise above 60 mm Hg, respiratory failure is often imminent. Intervention to increase ventilation is necessary, if aggressive therapy is desired. Hypercapnia indicates either a primary depression of central respiratory drive or decompensation during the latter stages of a severe restrictive or obstructive respiratory disorder. When the mechanical load to breathing is sufficiently high, compared with the metabolic resources of a sick foal, respiratory failure will ensue and can only be dealt with by increasing ventilation either chemically or by positive-pressure ventilation (PPV).

The use of doxapram hydrochloride, a respiratory stimulant that affects both peripheral chemoreceptors and medullary respiratory neurons, should be restricted to cases of central nervous system depression and/or circumstances when equipment to provide PPV is not available. Although ventilation is usually increased by this stimulant, it does not benefit collapsed airways or alveoli. It also has the undesirable property of increasing myocardial work and oxygen requirements at a time when oxygenation is impaired. As mentioned earlier, doxapram will not stimulate ventilation if used during secondary apnea in asphyxiated foals because their central nervous system is nonresponsive. Theophylline (or aminophylline) is used conventionally as a bronchodilator, but has also been shown in humans and dogs to improve the contractibility of the fatigued diaphragm. Should this effect also occur in foals it would effectively assist their breathing efforts. Any improvement in respiratory muscle strength and endurance may allow time for pulmonary function to improve with treatment (e.g., antibiotics), possibly avoiding the need for mechanical intervention.

Most foals in respiratory failure with severe carbon dioxide retention require PPV to survive. Unfortunately, there are few procedures in equine neonatal intensive care that are as time-consuming and involved as long-term mechanical ventilation. Provisions must be made for nutritional support, blood gas monitoring, long-term sedation, or paralysis as well as continuous surveillance of the equipment and patient. At this time, although experience with ventilation of foals is still quite limited, some neonates with severely compromised lungs have been maintained on a ventilator from 12 hours to 5 days and then successfully weaned from it. They are developing normally and show no clinical evidence of residual lung damage at the present time.

It is not possible to describe here all of the details of ventilating a foal, and the reader is referred to the supplemental reading sources for further information. A few generalities are presented.

1. Candidates selected for ventilation ideally should have pulmonary disorders that are potentially readily reversible, such as hyaline membrane disease and congenital or aspiration pneumonias. For example, the colostrum-deprived foal in septic shock with joint and other organ involvement would not be considered an ideal candidate with our present state of knowledge.

2. Administration of PPV is most easily achieved by use of intermittent mandatory ventilation (IMV). This provides a certain number of mandatory breaths around which the foal can breathe spontaneously. The suitability of high-frequency ventilation for use in the foal is under investigation.

3. In foals, administration of PPV is probably best accomplished after nasal-endotracheal intubation. This technique has an advantage over oral-tracheal intubation in that the tube can be placed and maintained in the awake foal with surprisingly little difficulty.

4. A volume-cycled ventilator* appears preferable to pressure-cycled ventilators for delivery of IMV to the spontaneously breathing foal, in terms of patient compliance and ease of operation. This type of ventilator also has the capacity to deliver humidified and heated gases and provide positive end-expiratory pressure (PEEP) and continuous positive airway pressure (CPAP).

5. The optimal ventilator settings are extremely individual. In the volume-cycled ventilator, tidal volume, frequency, and $F_{I_{O_2}}$ are set and a peak inspiratory pressure (PIP) is generated. In the normal 40-kg foal, a tidal volume of 500 ml (12 ml per kg) with a frequency of 20 breaths per minute might be expected to generate a peak inspiratory pressure of around 20 cm H_2O and maintain normal blood

---

*Bivona Surgical, Inc., Gary, IN
†Ambu Bag, North American Drager, Telford, PA

*Ventilator Model 3-AVM, J. H. Emerson Co., Cambridge, MA

gases. However, in the diseased lung, a higher tidal volume and PIP may be required to maintain even marginally adequate blood gases. As PIP is increased, the risk of pneumothorax and cardiovascular compromise is also increased. Ideally, $F_{I_{O_2}}$ should be adjusted to maintain Pa_{O_2} between 70 and 100 mm Hg.

6. In some foals, improved gas exchange may be achieved by use of PEEP or CPAP, both of which maintain airway pressure above atmospheric pressure during expiration. This acts to prevent closure of small airways at end-expiration, to decrease the inspiratory pressure necessary to reopen closed airways, and thus to reduce the work of breathing. These techniques have been extremely useful in improving survival rates of premature human infants with hyaline membrane disease and may be of use in the foal as well. However, their effects need to be more thoroughly studied in the foal.

7. Assisted ventilation, in which the animal initiates inspiration and then the breath is completed with positive pressure, may be delivered with a demand valve* on a temporary basis to a foal in respiratory distress.

8. A nasogastric tube should be left in place during positive-pressure ventilation to allow evacuation of any gas that inadvertently collects in the stomach. Oral feeding may also be done through this tube if the gastrointestinal tract will tolerate this form of nutrition. However, in many of these foals, gastrointestinal function is not normal and the animals are best fed by parenteral alimentation.

9. Maintenance of hygiene is of utmost importance in any animal receiving ventilatory support. Many of the normal defense mechanisms of the respiratory system are bypassed or altered by endotracheal intubation, increasing the risk of bacterial invasion and colonization. Tubes should be kept clean and free of secretions by suction with sterile catheters every three to four hours or as needed. If pneumonia develops, antibiotics should be administered according to culture and sensitivity results.

Pa_{CO_2} is the definitive guide to the efficacy of mechanical ventilation; therefore, decisions on ventilator adjustments and weaning are best made by observations of the foal together with evaluation of blood gases. If ventilator therapy is successfully instituted and blood gases are normalized, one should attempt to adjust the $F_{I_{O_2}}$ and PPV to minimum maintenance levels. Usually, because PPV is the most difficult to provide, it is convenient for mechanical ventilation to be the first to be reduced and, if possible, discontinued. For maintenance, $F_{I_{O_2}}$ is maintained at sufficiently high yet safe levels by nasal insufflation as described earlier.

Foal restraint, at our present state of knowledge, is a major limiting factor in the provision of respiratory therapy. The severely depressed or comatose foal is the exception. Most foals are likely to struggle from anxiety, pain, or hypoxia. Hypoxic foals usually calm down and often fall asleep once Pa_{O_2} is normalized. Unfortunately not all foals are so cooperative, and restraint is often necessary to prevent self-trauma. Sedation, anesthesia, or neuromuscular paralysis may become necessary if ventilatory support is to be maintained. In skilled hands this is practicable, but it is difficult to maintain this quality of care on a continual basis in veterinary practice.

A distinctive characteristic of neonates that one must always keep in mind is the tendency of their condition to undergo dramatic changes. These changes occur often within a short period of time with little advance notice. Under these circumstances there is usually little time for leisurely contemplation of case management, as is often possible with medical problems of adults. Careful and close observation of the foal is essential so that subtle abnormalities or changes in behavior can be quickly detected and treated. Without means to monitor arterial blood gas tensions, it is often difficult to effectively and safely administer respiratory support to neonates.

Good basic nursing care and the use of elementary respiratory therapy techniques can markedly improve survival rates of many foals presenting with respiratory disease. Some foals may require only brief assistance to overcome a transient respiratory problem. Others necessitate continual support of respiratory function for several hours to a few days until other treatments such as antibodies and antibiotics can reverse the existing pathophysiology. The decision to use state of the art support techniques to aggressively treat a critically ill foal must take into account the worth of the animal, prognosis, manpower available, and client desires.

Supplemental Readings

Beech, J.: Respiratory problems in foals. Vet. Clin. North Am. (Equine Pract.), *1*:131, 1985.

Kosch, P. C., Koterba, A. M., Webb, A. I., and Hillidge, C. J.: Methods of respiratory support in the newborn foal. Proc. 29th Annu. Conv. Am. Assoc. Eq. Pract., 1983, pp. 193–203.

Kosch, P. C., Koterba, A. M., Coons, T. J., and Webb, A. I.: Developments in management of the newborn foal in respiratory distress. 1. Evaluation. Equine Vet. J., *16*:312, 1984.

Koterba, A. M., Drummond, W. H., and Kosch, P. C.: Intensive care of the neonatal foal. Vet. Clin. North Am. (Equine Pract.), *1*:3, 1985.

Webb, A. I., Coons, T. J., Koterba, A. M., and Kosch, P. C.: Developments in management of the newborn foal in respiratory distress 2: Treatment. Equine Vet. J., *16*:319, 1984.

---

*Hudson Oxygen Therapy Sales Co., Orange Park, FL

FOOT DISEASES

Edited by J. A. Stick

Anatomy of the Foot

Charles D. Diesem, COLUMBUS, OHIO

The term "foot" is used here in the popular sense, to designate the pastern joint, the coffin joint, the hoof, and all structures that lie within the hoof (Figs. 1 and 2). The bones in this region include the proximal phalanx (os compedale), the middle phalanx (os coronale) and the distal phalanx (os ungulare). The tendons in the distal portion of the limb are the terminal portion of the extensor tendon (Fig. 2B), which terminates on the extensor process of the first phalanx, the deep flexor tendon (Figs. 1L and 2L), which terminates on the solar surface of the distal phalanx, and the distal portion of the superficial flexor tendon (Figs. 1F and 2F), which terminates on the palmar surface of the middle phalanx and proximal phalanx of the thoracic limb and the plantar surface of the middle phalanx and proximal phalanx of the pelvic limb.

The joints within the equine foot are the proximal interphalangeal joint (pastern joint) and the distal interphalangeal joint (coffin joint). The coffin joint, which also includes the articulation between the distal sesamoid bone and the distal and middle phalanx, is entirely enclosed by the keratinized hoof. The hair may be quite long on the distal portion of the limb of some breeds of horses and may obscure the anatomic structures.

The proximal interphalangeal joint is formed by the distal extremity of the proximal phalanx and the proximal extremity of the middle phalanx. The distal portion of the proximal phalanx consists of a middle sagittal groove separating two condyles. Two

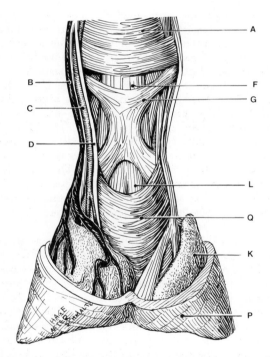

Figure 1. Palmar surface of the foot. *A,* Superficial transverse metacarpal ligament (palmar annular ligament); *B,* Medial digital vein; *C,* Medial digital artery; *D,* Medial digital nerve; *F,* Superficial digital flexor tendon; *G,* Proximal digital annular ligament (vaginal ligament); *K,* Lateral cartilage of distal phalanx; *L,* Deep digital flexor tendon; *P,* Heel of hoof; *Q,* Distal digital annular ligament.

255

depressions are found on the medial and lateral sides of the distal articular surface of the proximal phalanx, which serve as the site of origin for the collateral ligaments of the pastern joint. Palmar to the attachment of the collateral ligaments of the pastern joint is found a medial and lateral tubercle for attachment of the superficial flexor tendon. Similar arrangements for the tendons and ligaments also exist in the distal rear limb.

The proximal extremity of the middle phalanx has two articular depressions separated by a low ridge. The dorsal surface of this extremity is roughened to provide attachment for the common digital extensor tendon (Fig. 2B). The medial and lateral surfaces of the proximal extremity provide a tubercle for the attachment of the collateral ligaments and the superficial flexor tendon. The joint capsule is close fitting dorsally, and on the sides the joint capsule is restricted by the collateral ligaments. The joint capsule extends proximally on the palmar surface of the articular cartilage of the proximal phalanx. The palmar portion of the joint capsule is restricted by the straight sesamoidean ligament and the flexor tendons.

On the palmar surface of the joint, the palmar ligaments consist of the axial pair and the abaxial pair, which lie lateral or medial to the superficial sesamoidean ligament (Fig. 2H) and in addition the central pair of palmar ligaments may partially overlie the oblique sesamoidean ligaments. The palmar ligaments extend from the midportion of the palmar surface of the proximal phalanx to the proximal extremity of the middle phalanx (Fig. 2H). The palmar ligaments assist the superficial sesamoidean ligament and the collateral ligaments in preventing overextension of the pastern joint. The superficial sesamoidean ligament is indicated dorsal to F in Figure 2. The superficial sesamoidean ligament arises from the proximal sesamoid bones and extends to the middle phalanx.

The distal interphalangeal joint (coffin joint) is a ginglymus or hinge type of joint formed by the middle and distal phalanges and the distal sesamoid bone. The distal articular surface of the middle phalanx is convex in a sagittal direction but slightly concave in a transverse direction. The articular surface of the distal extremity of the middle phalanx encroaches upon the dorsal and palmar surface of the bone. The distal end of the middle phalanx fits into the concave surface of the proximal articular area of the distal phalanx. The palmar borders of the distal phalanx and the middle phalanx are slightly flattened to accommodate the distal sesamoid bone. The outer margin of the distal phalanx forms a modified semicircle, and the bone is entirely obscured by the keratinized portion of the hoof.

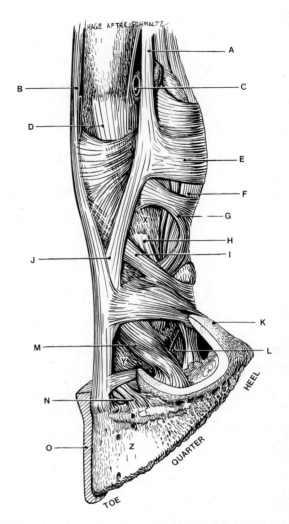

Figure 2. Lateral view of the foot. *A,* Tendon of interosseous muscle; *B,* Tendon of common digital extensor muscle; *C,* Sectioned portion of fetlock joint capsule; *D,* Collateral ligament of the fetlock joint; *E,* Collateral sesamoidean ligament of proximal sesamoid (ligament passes deep to proximal digital annular ligament); *F,* Superficial flexor tendon; *G,* Proximal digital annular ligament; *H,* Medial palmar ligament; *I,* Proximal portion of distal digital annular ligament; *J,* Dorsal branch of interosseous muscle to the extensor tendon; *K,* Cartilage of distal phalanx (cut to reveal deep structures); *L,* Tendon of deep digital flexor; *M,* Collateral sesamoidean ligament; *N,* Collateral ligament (ligg. chondroungularia collateralia) from middle phalanx to distal phalanx and lateral cartilage; *O,* Sectioned hoof wall; *X,* Proximal phalanx.

Only the rhomboid-shaped lateral cartilages that attach to the angles of the distal phalanx extend above the coronary border of the hoof wall, making it possible to palpate their flexibility in the living animal (Fig. 1K). The coronary border of the distal

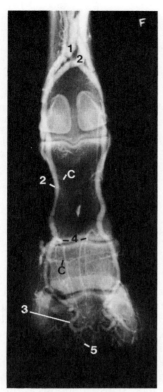

Figure 3. Angiograph of the right front foot—palmar to dorsal view. *1,* Digital vein; *2,* Digital artery; *3,* Terminal arch of digital arteries; *4,* Branch of digital arteries passing to digital cushion; *5,* Artery radiating from terminal arch in distal phalanx; *C,* Collateral branch of digital arteries; *F,* Indicates right front limb.

phalanx has a central eminence for the attachment of the common digital extensor tendon. Palmar-medial or palmar-lateral to this extensor eminence is found a depression for the attachment of the collateral ligaments of the coffin joint (Fig. 2N).

The dorsal surface of the distal phalanx is sloped away from the central axis of the limb and foot. The slope of the toe makes an angle of approximately 45 degrees with the plane of support. The slope angle is usually greater on the medial side of the distal phalanx than on the lateral side of the bone.

If one examines the angle of slope for the toe on the pelvic limb, it will usually be found to be 50 to 60 degrees with reference to the plane of support—that is, steeper than on the front limb. The dorsal surface of the distal phalanx is porous to allow vessels to pass from the interior of the bone to the vascular corium that covers the exterior of the distal phalanx (Fig. 3, No. 5).

The palmar processes (angles) of the distal phalanx support the lateral cartilages. The angular processes are partially divided into proximal and distal por-

tions by a notch or foramen, which gives passage to a vessel that enters a parietal sulcus on each side of the phalanx.

The distal sesamoid bone lies on the palmar aspect of the coffin joint and it articulates with the middle and distal phalanges. It is attached to the middle phalanx by the collateral sesamoidean ligaments (Fig. 2M) and to the distal phalanx by the distal ligament of the distal sesamoid (sesamoid impar ligament). The deep flexor tendon passes over the distal sesamoid and attaches to the solar surface of the distal phalanx. The tendon is inserted into the semilunar line and the central rough area palmar to it.

The joint capsule for the coffin joint lies in front of the distal sesamoid bone and the deep flexor tendon. It extends proximal to the articular surface of the bones forming the joint. The *bursa podotrochlearis* lies between the distal sesamoid bone and the deep flexor tendon. The lateral and medial movement of the distal sesamoid bones is limited by the lateral cartilages of the distal phalanx and the collateral ligaments.

The hoof is the epidermal structure that surrounds the distal joints of the equine limb and is in immediate contact with the plane of support. The hoof wall is the portion seen when the horse is in the standing position. The wall is reflected to the palmar and then to the ventral surface of the foot to form the bars. The bars are two ridges that converge to delineate the solar surface of the foot into the sole and frog.

The periople (stratum tectorium) covers the wall and arises from the perioplic corium. This layer is only a few cells thick over the toe and quarters of the hoof but it thickens in the vicinity of the heel and fuses with the dermis of the wall. The stratum medium forms the bulk of the wall since it is composed of tubular and intertubular horn (Fig. 4, No. 2). The wall may exhibit parallel ridges and depressions that extend from the plane of support to the coronary band. Apparently, variation in the state of nutrition to the coronary corium and the germinal cells of the hoof may affect height of these ridges or depth of the depressions.

The deeper portion of the wall is referred to as the stratum lamellatum and it is formed by approximately 600 nonsensitive laminae that are parallel to one another and extend in a vertical direction from the proximal portion of the hoof wall to the point of junction between the hoof wall and the sole. These laminae interdigitate with the sensitive laminae of the laminar corium or dermis. Microscopic examination reveals that these primary laminae, whether a part of the hoof wall or the corium, give rise to secondary laminae that allow much

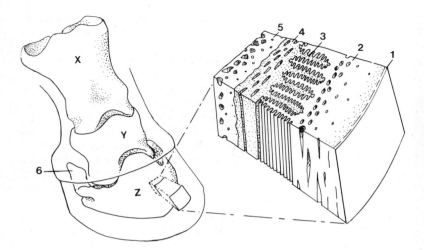

Figure 4. Structure of the hoof wall. *1*, Stratum tectorium; *2*, Stratum medium; *3*, Stratum lamellatum; *4*, Laminar corium; *5*, Bone of distal phalanx; *6*, Cartilage of distal phalanx; *X*, Proximal phalanx; *Y*, Middle phalanx; *Z*, Distal phalanx.

greater areas of contact to exist between the sensitive and nonsensitive portions of the hoof wall (Fig. 4, Nos. 3 and 4).

The sole of the hoof occupies the space between the frog and wall on the solar surface of the foot. The sole is slightly concave when viewed from the exterior of the hoof; however, if the hoof is removed from the distal phalanx, the dorsal surface of the sole and the frog are convex. The dorsal surface of the sole contacts the corium of the sole. When pulled away from the corium layer, it reveals innumerable small holes that accommodate the papillae of the sole corium. This is the origin of the keratinized portion of the sole.

The linear junction formed by the periphery of the sole with the laminae of the hoof wall is relatively free of pigment and is referred to as the linea alba (white line). When the sole is well trimmed, this line may be seen on the solar surface of the foot; it delineates the sensitive from the nonsensitive portion of the foot. Farriers use this line as an indication as to where a nail should be inserted when placing a shoe. If a nail is placed peripheral to the "white line" there is little possibility of injuring the sensitive tissue that underlies the keratinized tissue of the hoof wall or sole.

The frog is the third structure that contacts the plane of support. This is the triangular-shaped area extending forward from the bulbs of the heel to the sole. It is delineated from the bars of the hoof by two sulci that extend forward to form its apex. It is partially divided into right and left portions by a ventral groove. On the dorsal surface, the frog exhibits a ridge opposite this ventral groove, which is termed the frog stay (spina cunei). The frog is formed by the corium, which lies between the keratinized tissue and the palmar portion of the distal phalanx.

Corium or dermis occupies the space between the keratinized portion of the hoof and the underlying bony structures. This soft tissue is a continuous covering for the distal phalanx. The shape of the dermis coincides with the portion of the hoof with which it maintains contact. The corium of the hoof is composed of elastic and collagenous tissue and it contains the nerves and the nutritional vascular supply of the foot. It also functions as the attachment between the hoof and the bone of the distal limb. The entire corium is covered with germinal epithelium, which gives origin to the various portions of the hoof. Changes in blood flow can have a direct effect on germinal epithelium and an indirect effect on hoof growth. Laminitis is one example of a condition in which cellular chemistry of germinal epithelium is modified.

Blood supply and nerve supply to the front and the rear foot are similar, thus the vascular and nerve pattern of distribution for the distal forelimb only will be presented. The *medial and lateral digital arteries* (Fig. 5C) supply the equine foot and they arise from the medial and lateral palmar arteries and the palmar arch that lies between the suspensory ligament and the third metacarpal bone. The palmar arch receives some blood from the palmar metacarpal vessels and dorsal metacarpal vessels. As the digital arteries course down the limb, they give off collateral branches to each phalangeal joint and then form a terminal arch (Fig. 3, No. 3). As the paired arteries approach the lateral cartilages of the distal phalanx, they divide. A dorsal branch passes medial to each lateral cartilage and continues in the dorsal parietal sulci on each side of the distal phalanx and then continues into the foramina on the dorsal surface of the bone (Fig. 6, No. 3). The palmar branch of each digital artery passes medial to the cartilage on each side of the foot and proceeds to a solar foramen on the solar surface of the distal phalanx and terminates by forming an arch within

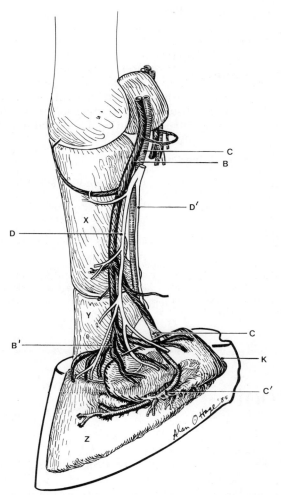

Figure 5. Blood vessels and nerves of the foot. *B*, Digital vein (medial); *B'*, Digital vein at level of hoof; *C*, Digital artery (medial); *C'*, Dorsal branch of digital artery; *D*, Dorsal branch of medial digital nerve; *D'*, Palmar branch of medial digital nerve; *K*, Cartilage of distal phalanx (shown as being transparent to reveal digital vessels); *X*, Proximal phalanx; *Y*, Middle phalanx; *Z*, Distal phalanx.

the semicircular canal which is embedded within this phalanx (Fig. 3, No. 3). Arteries radiate from the terminal arch to the surface of the bone to supply the corium of the hoof. The other major division of the digital artery passes to the tissue in the digital cushion (Fig. 3, No. 4) (Fig. 6, No. 4). This branch varies in size and may not arise in the same manner from the right and left digital artery.

Digital nerves provide the major innervation to the equine foot. Sack reported that the dorsal ulnar innervation does not extend distal to the fetlock joint and palmar metacarpal nerves usually do not innervate structures distal to the pastern joint.

The palmar branch of the medial digital nerve (excluding the dorsal branch) has superficial and deep portions. Its innervation is considerably more

complicated than previously described (Fig. 5*D'*). Proximal to the pastern, the medial digital nerve has a superficial portion that gives off four cutaneous branches. Distal to the pastern joint, the superficial portion gives off an additional six branches that supply the digital cushion, the palmar skin above the hoof, the corium of the frog, and the skin at the caudal border of the cartilage of the hoof; at the level of the distal sesamoid, the superficial portion supplies the laminar corium of the heel and the quarter. Before the digital nerve enters the parietal groove of the distal phalanx with a branch of the digital artery, it supplies branches to the corium of the sole and the frog.

The deeper portion of the medial digital nerve (excluding the dorsal branch) has approximately 10 collateral branches. These deeper nerves are supplied at different levels: two at the fetlock supply the palmar pouch, another supplies the digital sheath, two other branches pass below the interosseous muscle to supply the fetlock joint capsule and the straight and oblique sesamoidean ligaments. At

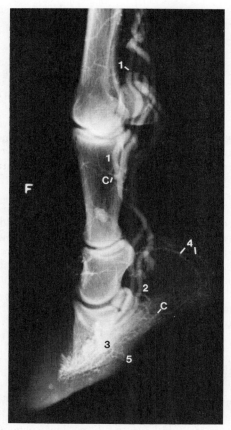

Figure 6. Angiograph of the foot—Medial to lateral view. *1*, Digital vein; *2*, Digital artery; *3*, Digital artery passing into solar foramen to form terminal arch; *4*, Branch of medial digital artery passing to digital cushion; *5*, Branch radiating from terminal arch; *C*, Collateral branch of digital artery; *F*, Indicates front limb.

the pastern joint, fifth and sixth branches supply the palmar pouch and digital sheath. The seventh branch passes to the middle phalanx and continues to supply the coffin joint; the eighth branch passes to the distal sesamoidean ligament; the ninth branch supplies the navicular bursa. The tenth or last branch arises just before the caudal branch of the medial digital nerve enters the parietal groove and ramifies in the digital cushion. The branches arising from the medial digital nerve after it enters the parietal groove supply the laminar corium and the corium of the sole. The dorsal branches of the medial and lateral digital nerves or their plexuses are cutaneous and supply the sides of the fetlock and dorsal surfaces of the pastern joint (Fig. 5D). Distal portions of the dorsal digital nerve branches are found subcutaneously or superficial to the lateral cartilages and descend into laminar corium of the heels and quarters or innervate the coronary corium.

When comparing the lateral digital nerve (excluding its dorsal branch) with the medial digital nerve,

Sack pointed out the branching and distribution of fibers of a medial nerve may not be a mirror image of the branching noted for a lateral digital nerve or vice versa. The deeper branch of the lateral digital nerve gives off fewer collateral branches than does the medial digital nerve. The lateral nerve supplies a thin branch that enters the semicircular canal in the sole of the distal phalanx, thus following the digital artery as is true for the medial digital nerve.

Supplemental Readings

Banks, W. J.: Applied Veterinary Histology. Baltimore, Waverly Press, 1981.

Dellmann, H., and Brown, E. M.: Textbook of Veterinary Histology, 2nd Ed., Philadelphia, Lea and Febiger, 1981.

Getty, R.: Sisson and Grossman's The Anatomy of the Domestic Animals, 5th ed. Philadelphia, W. B. Saunders Company, 1975.

Sack, W. O.: Nerve distribution in the metacarpus and front digit of the horse. J. Am. Vet. Med. Assoc., 167:298, 1975.

Stump, J. E.: Anatomy of the normal equine foot, including microscopic features of the laminar region. J. Am. Vet. Med. Assoc., 151:1588, 1967.

Radiology of the Foot

Russ L. Stickle, EAST LANSING, MICHIGAN

This chapter describes the positioning, normal radiographic anatomy, and indications for routine views of the equine foot. Current nomenclature is used, with old or common terms in parentheses. The nomenclature is for the front limb.

For optimal film quality, the foot should be cleaned, trimmed if necessary, and shoes and pads removed. Packing the bottom of the foot with a water-dense material (such as petrolatum) to remove air from the sulci and other deep irregularities is especially valuable for evaluation of the distal sesamoid but may also be useful for other views. Submerging the foot in a plastic tub of water will serve the same purpose.

LATEROMEDIAL (LATERAL) VIEW

Positioning is illustrated in Figure 1A. The foot is usually placed on a block so that its entire subsolar region is included on the film. The distal (third) phalanx and joint spaces are best evaluated on a true lateral view, since any obliqueness of the x-ray beam will produce some distortion of the anatomic relationships and overlap of structures. The major

anatomic features are illustrated in Figures 1B and C. The dorsal margin of the distal phalanx should be parallel with the hoof wall on a true lateral view. The soft tissues of the hoof should have a relatively uniform density similar to water.

The lateromedial view is a routine view in almost all radiographic studies of the equine foot and is usually combined with one or more other views. When horses with laminitis are evaluated for distal phalanx rotation and/or laminar gas pockets, the lateromedial view is of major importance and is sometimes used alone for this purpose.

DORSOPALMAR (ANTERIOPOSTERIOR) VIEW

Positioning is illustrated in Figure 2A. The foot is set on a block so that the entire foot is on the film. Major anatomic features are illustrated in Figures 2B and C. This view is not commonly used but may be useful in evaluation of the subsolar region of the hoof for gas density in suspected abscesses. The interphalangeal joint spaces and

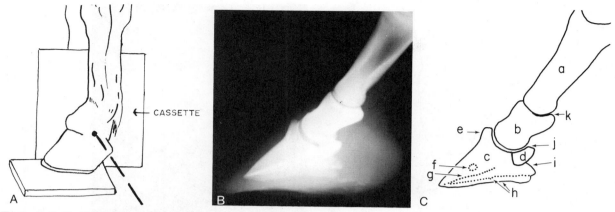

Figure 1. *A,* Positioning for the lateromedial view of the foot and pastern. The broken line represents the central ray of the x-ray beam. *B,* Lateromedial radiograph. *C,* a – proximal phalanx, b – middle phalanx, c – distal phalanx, d – distal sesamoid, e – extensor process, f – solar canal, g – solar margin in the central area of the bone, h – solar margins of the medial and lateral edges, i – palmar processes, j – distal interphalangeal joint, k – proximal interphalangeal joint.

abaxial margins of the distal sesamoid are seen reasonably well on this view.

DORSOPROXIMAL-PALMARODISTAL (DORSOVENTRAL) VIEW FOR THE DORSAL SESAMOID

This is for the distal (third) phalanx. Positioning is illustrated in Figure 3A. The foot is placed on the cassette, which is protected by a sheet of sturdy radiolucent material such as Plexiglas placed above the cassette to support the weight of the foot. The central ray of the x-ray beam should be at an angle of approximately 65 degrees to the floor. The major anatomic features are illustrated in Figures 3B and C. The distal phalanx may appear somewhat elongated depending on the angle of the central ray of the x-ray beam.

This view is used commonly with a lateromedial view for routine studies of the foot. It is useful in evaluating the distal phalanx for sepsis, fracture, and pedal osteitis. Subsolar gas pockets may be seen, particularly if the gas is not superimposed over the distal phalanx. Fractures of the palmar processes (wings) of the distal phalanx may be difficult to see on this view. The distal sesamoid may be evaluated on this view but will require a darker exposure than is used for examination of the distal phalanx. The distal sesamoid can be projected more uniformly using another view described later in this chapter.

DORSOPROXIMAL-PALMARODISTAL OBLIQUE (DORSOVENTRAL OBLIQUE) VIEW

This view is for the palmar processes (wings) of the distal phalanx. Positioning is similar to that for the view previously described except that the cen-

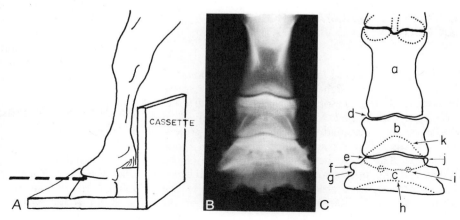

Figure 2. *A,* Positioning for the dorsopalmar view. *B,* Dorsopalmar radiograph. *C,* a – proximal phalanx, b – middle phalanx, c – distal phalanx, d – proximal interphalangeal joint, e – distal interphalangeal joint, f – palmar process, g – parietal groove, h – solar margin in the central area of the bone, i – solar foramen, j – distal sesamoid, k – extensor process.

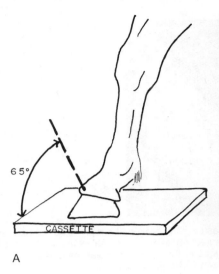

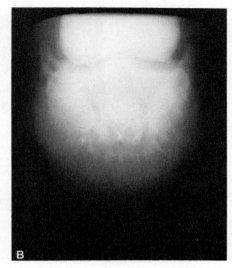

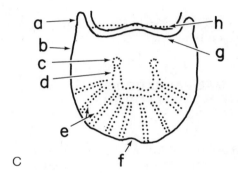

Figure 3. *A,* Positioning for the dorsoproximal-palmarodistal view. *B,* Dorsoproximal-palmarodistal radiograph. *C,* a – palmar process, b – solar margin, c – solar foramen, d – solar (semicircular) canal, e – vascular channels, f – crena, g – distal interphalangeal joint, h – palmar edge of the distal phalanx.

tral ray of the x-ray beam is not in the midsagittal plane of the limb but is angled from either the lateral or the medial side to project the palmar process on the same side (Fig. 4A–C).

This view is commonly used to evaluate fractures and other lesions involving the palmar processes of the distal phalanx. In some cases it may be the only view that positively demonstrates the lesion. The abaxial margin of the distal sesamoid is also seen.

DORSOPROXIMAL-PALMARODISTAL (DORSOVENTRAL) VIEW FOR THE DISTAL SESAMOID

The distal sesamoid (navicular) bone is evaluated by this view. Although the distal sesamoid can be evaluated on the dorsoproximal-palmarodistal view previously described for the distal phalanx if a darker exposure is made, a more consistent projection can usually be made utilizing a special block (Fig. 5A). The angle between the long face of the block and the floor should be at least 50 degrees but less than 60 degrees. The central ray of the x-ray beam is parallel with the floor. It is important

that the foot be well cleaned and packed to eliminate superimposed shadows. Shoes should be pulled. Additional procedures to increase detail include coning down the beam to the area of interest as much as possible and using a grid.

The major anatomic features are illustrated in Fig. 5B and C. The distal margin of the bone is usually the major area of interest. This should not be superimposed over the distal interphalangeal joint space. Use of the positioning described earlier will usually ensure that the entire distal sesamoid is projected proximal to the joint space. The palmar processes (wings) of the distal phalanx are prominent on this view and should not be misdiagnosed as ossification of the collateral cartilages (sidebone).

PALMAROPROXIMAL-PALMARODISTAL (SKYLINE) VIEW

The distal sesamoid (navicular) bone is evaluated with this view. For it, the foot is typically positioned caudal to the normal standing position, which straightens the pastern and fetlock, and the foot is

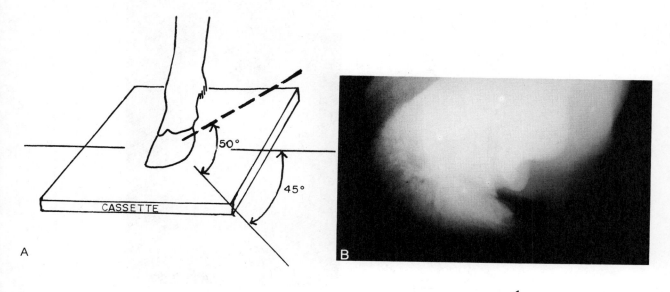

A

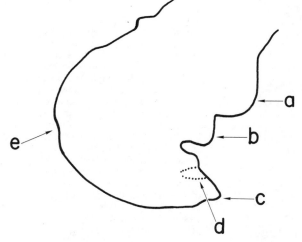

B

C

Figure 4. *A,* Positioning for the dorsoproximal-palmarodistal oblique view. Angles are approximations. The broken line represents the central ray of the x-ray beam. *B,* Dorsoproximal-palmarodistal oblique radiograph. Note the numerous vascular channels that radiate from the central portion of the distal phalanx. *C,* a – middle phalanx, b – distal sesamoid, c – palmar process of distal phalanx, d – parietal groove, e – crena.

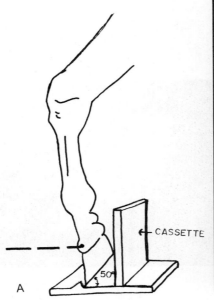

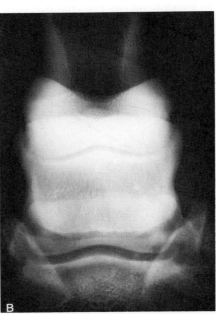

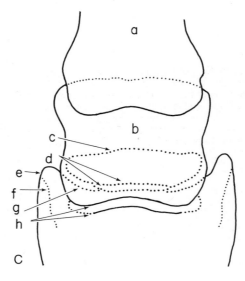

Figure 5. *A,* Positioning for the dorsoproximal-palmarodistal view for the distal sesamoid. The central ray is in the midsagittal plane of the limb. The angle indicated for the block should be between 50 and 60 degrees. *B,* Dorsoproximal-palmarodistal radiograph for the distal sesamoid. The exposure may be "coned down" more to the specific area of interest. *C,* a – proximal phalanx, b – middle phalanx, c – proximal border of the distal sesamoid, d – distal border of the sesamoid (two lines are seen radiographically due to the shape of the distal border), e – palmar process of the distal phalanx, f – abaxial border of the palmar process, g – palmar edge of the distal phalanx, h – distal interphalangeal joint.

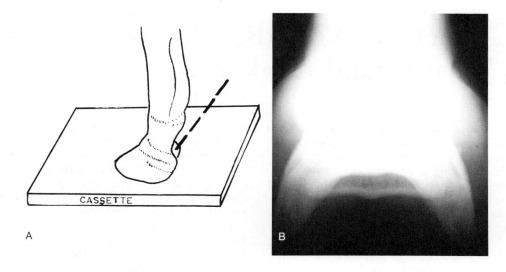

A

B

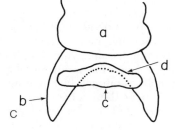

C

Figure 6. *A,* Positioning for the palmaroproximal-palmaro-distal view of the distal sesamoid. The foot must be placed caudal to the normal standing position. The angle of the central ray is approximately 75 degrees to the floor. *B,* Palmaroproximal-palmarodistal radiograph. The dark area in the central portion of the sesamoid is the medullary cavity. Several foramina in the distal border of the bone can be seen superimposed on the medullary cavity in this view. *C,* a – middle phalanx, b – palmar process of the distal phalanx, c – flexor surface of the distal sesamoid with normal sagittal ridge, d – articular surface of the distal sesamoid.

placed on the cassette (Fig. 6*A*). Some elevation of the heel using a small wedge may be helpful. The angle of the central ray of the x-ray beam to the floor varies but is approximately 75 degrees. Previous considerations on preparation of the foot apply. Positioning requires the x-ray tube to be placed close to the horse; the animal's temperament must be considered. A relatively short focal-film distance must be used. The major anatomic features are illustrated in Fig. 6*B* and *C*.

This view is commonly used in conjunction with other views to evaluate the distal sesamoid. The flexor surface of the distal sesamoid is usually the primary area of interest; however, fractures of the distal sesamoid are usually easily seen on this view. The palmar processes of the distal phalanx are projected well. This view can also be used to demonstrate lesions involving these latter structures.

Supplemental Readings

Adams, O. R.: Lameness in Horses, 3rd ed. Philadelphia, Lea & Febiger, 1974.

Smallwood, J. E., Shively, M. J., Rendano, V. T., and Habel, R. E.: A standardized nomenclature for radiographic projections used in veterinary medicine. Vet. Radiol., *26:*2, 1985.

Ticer, J. W.: Radiographic Technique in Veterinary Practice, 2nd ed. Philadelphia, W. B. Saunders Company, 1986.

Puncture Wounds, Abscesses, Thrush, and Canker

Robert R. Steckel, NORTH GRAFTON, MASSACHUSETTS

A knowledge of the mechanism of hoof horn regeneration after injury, coupled with careful examination of each wound encountered, allows accurate prognostication and forms the basis of a rational approach to treatment. Hoof horn is a modified continuation of skin epidermis. It differs from normal skin because it lacks the stratum granulosum and stratum lucidum, and keratohyalin is not formed. This results in "hard" keratin being produced. Immediately under the thick hard outer layers, which are the stratum medium and lamellatum, lies a thin stratum germinativum. It varies from a few to several cell layers in thickness. The stratum germinativum is subdivided into two layers: the outer stratum spinosum, or keratinizing layer, and the deeper stratum basale, where replication occurs. The germinal layer forms an envelope of keratin-producing cells, completely covering and situated immediately over the hoof corium.

Corium is the homolog of the dermis of skin and forms a continuous layer enclosing all the deeper structures. The corium is divided geographically into five regions—perioplic corium, coronary corium, laminar (wall) corium, solar corium, and frog corium. Corium is dense collagenous connective tissue that, in addition to providing support and attachment for the hard outer shell of horn, contains a rich vascular and nerve supply to nourish the germinal layer. Separation of the nonviable hard horn (stratum lamellatum) due to injury or surgical manipulation usually occurs at the junction of that layer with the stratum germinativum, leaving the germinal layer attached to the corium.

HORN REGENERATION

Repair of a wound in hoof horn depends on the integrity of both the germinal layer and its nourishing dermis. If a horn defect is superficial and does not traverse the germinal layer, proliferation of new tissue and subsequent keratinization of hard replacement horn will be rapid. Conversely, if the wounding results in loss of the germinal layer and its supporting dermis, granulation tissue forms in the wound cavity, as with any other full-thickness epithelial injury that cannot be sutured. Granulation tissue provides a new base of support and a source of nutrition for proliferating epithelial cells from the intact stratum germinativum at the wound margin.

They migrate across the defect and cover it, thus re-establishing epithelial continuity. Initially, this new epithelium is very thin, creamy white, and easily disrupted. With time, it thickens as its keratin content increases. The new epithelium becomes darker and hardens, eventually resembling the surrounding layer of outer horn.

Healing of full-thickness integumentary defects is the result of a combination of two independent processes: (1) epithelial proliferation and migration from the intact germinal layer at the wound margin, and (2) wound contraction. Since the hoof is a semirigid structure, second-intention healing differs from that seen in other body areas in that wound contraction cannot occur. Establishment of epithelial continuity following disruption depends solely on the process of epithelialization. If an area of full-thickness horn loss is large, the clinician should expect the repair process to be comparatively slow. With this slower healing process kept in mind, current recommendations for treatment are designed to allow tissue repair to proceed unimpeded.

Traditional treatments recommended for subsolar abscesses or punctures of the hoof's horny capsule included the use of astringents to dry the wound, frequent soaking, or poultices to help decrease inflammation. These methods of medical therapy are still valuable in some cases but are not universally applicable. Specifically, the use of vesicants or astringents on a raw granulating surface and tender new epithelium retards the overall epithelialization process in open wounds. Any topical compound that is caustic enough to debride necrotic tissue or retard exuberant granulation also damages the immature epithelium and ultimately prolongs wound healing. Soaking or poulticing is beneficial when hoof inflammation is severe and cellulitis extends above the coronet. For a properly drained subsolar abscess, poulticing provides no added advantage over good wound care and a proper bandage. Astringents should be used only when the wound has completely epithelialized. Even then, the advantage of additionally desiccating the new horn is questionable since it will occur naturally through keratinization.

In the special case of canker the information subsequently cited advocates the use of broadspectrum systemic antibiotics. The only other place for these drugs appears to be in the treatment of deep puncture injuries. Clearly, the efficacy of antibiotics in necrotic bone or tendon is nil. However, as will be discussed in a succeeding chapter, the consequences of the spread of infection following injury to deep foot structures are so grave that any treatment modality serving to contain it should be employed. It is emphasized here that in those cases, systemic antibiotic therapy alone is ineffective.

ANAMNESIS

Acute hoof wounds such as subsolar abscesses and solar punctures do not require extensive anamnesis. Identification of the affected foot and determining the duration of the lameness are all that is necessary. With chronic lesions, however, the practitioner should obtain as complete a case history as possible. Special attention should be given to the duration of the condition and the response to any previous treatment. Inappropriate treatment, for example the overuse of harsh caustics or vesicants, might indeed be the main reason for prolongation of wound morbidity.

Immunity against tetanus should always be considered when dealing with injuries of the equine hoof. The risk of that disease is always present because of close constant contact with soil microflora. If an adequate vaccination history within the previous six months cannot be established, standard doses of tetanus toxoid and antitoxin should be given prophylactically.

EXAMINATION OF THE FOOT

Subsolar abscesses can occur in any area of the sole or frog, and puncture wounds can be seen on both the solar and laminar (wall) surfaces. Both of these conditions can vary enough in location and severity to occasionally cause difficulty in diagnosing their exact nature or extent. The affected foot can be identified on the basis of the history and a routine examination of the gait. Careful and systematic examination of the affected foot is the essential element in diagnosing common hoof diseases. The specific sequence of diagnostic methods varies somewhat with the individual case. A reiteration of the individual tests is inappropriate here. Figure 1 reviews the steps routinely employed in diagnosis.

The examination protocol should follow a consistent, logical sequence. Complete examination of the foot, either externally or with radiography, cannot be done with a horseshoe in place. Similarly, unless the entire ground contact surface is pared to expose fresh underlying horn, a solar lesion can be missed. Regional anesthesia should be employed to confirm the diagnosis in the case of occult lesions, and as needed to allow painless completion of the examination.

SUBSOLAR ABSCESS

Subsolar abscess results from injury to the ground contact surface of the hoof. A severe bruise from a stone or other hard object results in hematoma formation at the junction of the stratum corneum with the combined stratum germinativum-corium layers. If the lesion is severe enough, local necrosis of connective tissue results in loss of the attachment of the stratum corneum. Subsequent trauma in the same area leads to the formation of small cracks, which allow bacterial penetration. Alternatively, a small sharp object can penetrate through any region of the hard horn on the ventral hoof surface, cause local hemorrhage in the viable tissue layers, simultaneously leave an inoculum of bacteria, and be quickly withdrawn as the horse moves over the object. A subsolar abscess usually results because the entrance hole in the hard horn closes when the penetrating object is removed. In either case, liquefaction necrosis produces pus that cannot drain because of the rigid encasement of hard horn. Acute pain is manifested as the abscess cavity accumulates pus and/or gas, and pressure under the horn increases. If the cavity is not mechanically evacuated, a necrotic tract develops (Fig. 2), or the liquefaction follows the path of least resistance between the stratum corneum and stratum germinativum, often erupting at the coronary band.

A special form of abscess results when a horseshoe nail is driven deep to the stratum corneum into viable layers of the hoof wall. Migration of microorganisms around the nail results in a small abscess at the sole-wall junction (white line) where the nail has entered viable tissue. Removal of the nail allows exudation of a typical watery black pus from the nail hole. The process may be slow enough to have a lag phase of several weeks between injury (shoeing) and clinical signs (severe lameness).

TREATMENT

Regardless of the cause of subsolar abscessation, the main component of therapy is to allow drainage of the abscess cavity by removing the overlaying layer of detached hard horn (Fig. 3). Opening the cavity relieves the pain caused by pressure. Removal of locally toxic chemicals in the purulent debris augments epithelialization. During debridement, an evaluation of the depth of the wound should be made. Determining which layers of horn have been injured and to what extent are the keys to determining the most successful mode of treatment.

Most subsolar abscesses are superficial and do

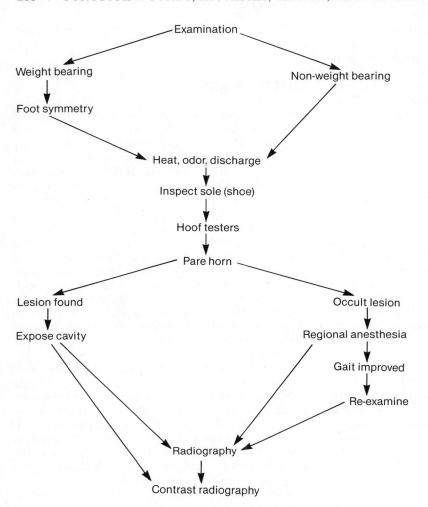

Figure 1. Flow chart of steps in examination and diagnosis of common hoof diseases.

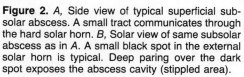
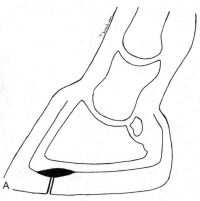
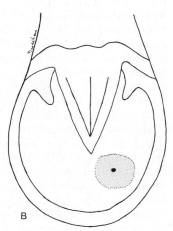

Figure 2. *A,* Side view of typical superficial subsolar abscess. A small tract communicates through the hard solar horn. *B,* Solar view of same subsolar abscess as in *A.* A small black spot in the external solar horn is typical. Deep paring over the dark spot exposes the abscess cavity (stippled area).

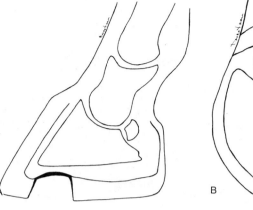

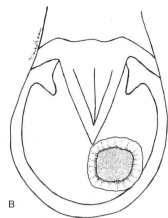

Figure 3. *A,* Side view of proper excavation of subsolar abscess. The margins of the cavity are pared until confluent with the surrounding healthy hard horn. New epithelium (*heavy dark line*) fills the base of the cavity. *B,* Solar view of proper excavation of subsolar abscess. The edges of the surrounding horn are tapered down to the base of the cavity.

not severely damage the stratum germinativum or underlying dermis. In these cases, removal of overlaying separated horn usually reveals that regeneration has already begun. Superficial abscesses need only to be opened for drainage, the entire hoof cleansed thoroughly for bandaging, and a topical antiseptic* or antibiotic† dressing applied locally under a clean, dry bandage. The primary bandage should be waterproofed with tape or a plastic hoof boot. Bandaging is repeated daily until the abscess cavity contains firm, dry horn. Production of replacement horn should be monitored by evaluation at approximately weekly intervals. When sufficient hard horn fills the solar defect, local therapy may be discontinued and maturation of the new epithelium can proceed under a padded horseshoe. Before pad application, the sole should be packed with a bacteriostatic filler.‡ Healing time in most cases will be less than 14 days. With superficial horn loss the deep hoof tissues are never in jeopardy, so the prognosis for prompt and complete restoration of a functional weight-bearing surface is excellent.

Deeper subsolar abscesses, most often resulting from punctures, traverse the stratum germinativum and the underlying dermis. Removal of the detached horn will show early granulation tissue surrounded by a ring of creamy white immature new horn (Fig. 4). Since the epithelialization process in these wounds is slowed, the bandaging period must be more protracted and attention to local wound (foot) hygiene must be meticulous. An absorbent sterile dressing with a local topical antiseptic or antibiotic ointment next to the granulating wound is preferred. Bandaging and hoof hygiene should be continued until the granulating area has been completely covered by replacement epithelium. Again, when the immature horn has proliferated suffi-

*Betadine Ointment, Purdue-Frederick Co., Norwalk, CT
†Furacin Dressing, Norden Laboratories, Inc., Lincoln, NE
‡Oakum, New Pak of New Orleans, Inc., Chicago, IL

ciently, maturation can be completed under a padded horseshoe. Total healing time depends on the size of the lesion. Although slightly longer than that with superficial abscesses, it seldom exceeds four weeks. Again, the prognosis for a complete return to functional weight-bearing is good after healing has been completed.

The practitioner should completely remove devitalized, loose horn from the sole or frog. Incomplete debridement of this overlaying shelf of hard horn (Fig. 5) is the most common reason for inadequate drainage and subsequent failure of normal wound healing. The abscess cavity may even expand, permitting extension of the infection into the deeper tissues of the foot. On occasion I have had to remove the entire sole or frog in cases of long duration, to reveal a complete new layer of epithelium that matured to fully functional, protective horn.

THRUSH

One needs only to observe a horse gallop across a pasture kicking out clods of dirt from the soles of its feet to understand the natural hoof cleaning process. Thrush is a disease of unhygienic practices in stables, poor foot care, and inadequate free exercise at pasture, all of which can lead to accumulation and retention of soil and fecal material. Moisture promotes the proliferation of resident bacteria trapped deep in the crevices.

This disease may also be predisposed to by chronic lameness. Decreased weight-bearing causes poor heel expansion and decreased wear, both of which promote the growth of long, so-called contracted heels, with resultant deep hoof sulci and impairment of the natural hoof-cleaning mechanism.

Thrush is a moist exudative dermatitis that specifically involves the central and lateral sulci of the frog. A commonly isolated organism is *Fusobacte-*

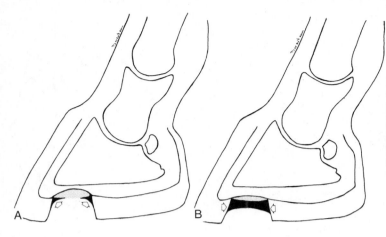

Figure 4. *A,* Side view of early healing in deeper subsolar abscess. Granulation tissue (*stippled area*) fills the wound cavity. Early epithelialization has begun (*arrows*). *B,* Side view of advanced healing of deep subsolar abscess. Granulation tissue (*stippled area*) has decreased in quantity. New horn has thickened and filled the defect (*arrows*).

rium necrophorus, but its role in thrush is unknown. A fetid gray to black exudate and soft, disintegrated frog horn are typical findings. Although a histologic study has not been reported, clinical findings in most cases suggest that the infection is confined to the deep layers of the stratum medium. The existing frog horn is redundant and tends to overlay the sulci. Pain can vary depending on the depth to which the infection has progressed. Lameness is not evident until the infection involves viable tissue under the horn or the sulci progressively deepen, cross the coronet at the bulb of the heels, and develop fissures in the skin above the coronary band. Redness, pain, and swelling are all obvious in the skin surrounding these fissures, which discharge typical malodorous pus.

TREATMENT

By far the most effective treatment is prevention. Improved stable hygiene, daily picking of the feet, regular and accurate hoof trimming, and free exercise on dry pasture should all be used as preventive practices. In cases secondary to chronic lameness, the underlying orthopedic problem should be identified and corrected as an integral part of treatment. The maintenance of correct balance in such shrunken atrophic feet is considerably more challenging to the farrier, but it is of paramount importance to the maintenance of soundness.

If the sensitive tissue of the frog or heels is involved, regional anesthesia or even sedation may be necessary to enable initial treatment. All loose overlaying frog and sole horn that might trap exudative material must be removed. After proper preparation of the rest of the hoof for bandaging, surgical sponges or cotton soaked with antiseptic* are packed into the depths of the debrided sulci and covered with a dry, secure bandage. Bandaging is repeated daily until the purulent discharge ceases and healthy horn re-forms. Thereafter, the preventive measures previously outlined should be employed. The prognosis for complete healing in most cases is good. Healing time is short (10 to 14 days) because severe injury to the germinal tissue layer seldom occurs.

CANKER

Equine canker is infrequently seen in modern veterinary practice. According to reports in the literature, this disease most commonly afflicted draft horses. Perhaps a breed predilection and decreased use of horses for heavy work have resulted in lowered incidence.

This condition should be specifically differentiated from equine thrush. Again, the predisposing causes are unsanitary stabling conditions and neglected routine foot care. A general distinguishing feature is the tendency to see this disease in horses

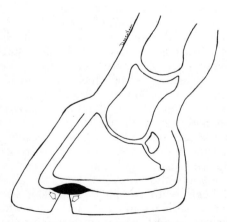

Figure 5. Side view of typical superficial subsolar abscess improperly drained. Shelves of hard horn (*arrows*) retard drainage.

---

*Betadine Solution, Purdue-Frederick Co., Norwalk, CT

living on continuously wet pastureland in year-round warm climates.

Canker is also a moist, exudative dermatitis characterized by a foul-smelling exudate. In contrast to equine thrush, the body of the frog is the most common predilection site. In advanced cases, the infection will spread across the lateral sulci to involve the sole at the heels, or even extend onto the walls at the heel. Another distinguishing feature is that abnormal horn is produced by the germinal layer of the frog. Hypertrophic horn is produced in filamentous fronds instead of a uniform flat elastic layer. Local inflammation, pain, and lameness are the rule rather than the exception, again differentiating this disease from thrush.

Histologically, the lesion is characterized as a chronic pododermatitis. It is caused by a gram-negative coccobacillary microbial infection in the stratum germinativum layer of frog horn. The infectious process appears to alter the keratin-producing ability of this cell layer, a so-called dyskeratosis, resulting in the production of abnormally shaped hypertrophic horn. Although the microorganisms are not yet identified, the most likely bacterial species are *Fusobacterium necrophorum* and *Bacteroides corrodens*. The possibility of a synergism between these two organisms, mimicking the pathogenesis of foot rot in sheep, has been suggested.

TREATMENT

Since canker is a true dermatitis with the causative organism localizing in the viable layers of horn-generating tissue, removal of the dystrophic overlaying frog horn is insufficient. The best results are obtained by performing careful debridement of the hoof with the horse under general anesthesia. Postoperatively, hoof hygiene and bandaging must be meticulous. Systemic chloramphenicol* (25 to 50 mg per kg, orally four times a day) administered for 14 days, will help resolve the dermatitis. Results are uniformly good with this treatment regimen, whereas other local treatments may be ineffective. Other reports in the literature mention good results from treatment with systemic penicillin, topical sulphanilamide, or tetracycline powder, in conjunction with surgical debridement and postoperative bandaging. Preventive husbandry measures outlined for equine thrush are also applicable to this disease.

Depending on the duration of the condition and the amount of scar that forms in the germinal layer of frog corium, abnormal deformation of the frog can result. The replacement horn is functional in terms of its protective ability, however, and once the lesion has healed residual lameness does not

---

*Anacetin, Bio-Ceutic Laboratories, St. Joseph, MO

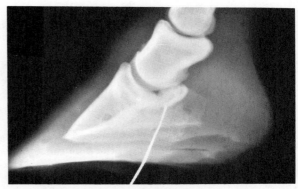

Figure 6. Lateral contrast radiograph of an equine hoof with a deep puncture wound through the frog. A lead probe touches the flexor surface of the distal sesamoid (navicular) bone.

occur. The prognosis for working soundness is fair to good.

DEEP PUNCTURE WOUNDS

In contrast to superficial punctures of the sole resulting in subsolar abscess, this disease of the equine hoof implies wounding through the stratum germinativum and dermis into a deeper structure such as the distal phalanx or navicular bursa. As with superficial puncture, a minimum injury is hemorrhage around the tract and inoculation of organisms causing abscesses. The injury portal through the stratum corneum collapses with retraction of the penetrating object and spontaneous drainage is prevented. An important distinction between this condition and simple subsolar abscessation is that direct injury to deep structures, and/or subsequent infection resulting from the injury, may result in future loss of functional use of the animal. Osteomyelitis, fracture, septic bursitis, and septic

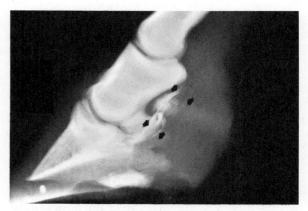

Figure 7. Lateral contrast radiograph of a hoof with a deep puncture wound through the frog. Contrast medium fills the navicular bursa and the distal deep flexor tendon sheath (*arrows*).

tendovaginitis all are possible sequelae to deep penetrations of the hoof. Any one of these conditions not only compromises the future for long-term soundness but may even necessitate euthanasia.

Diagnostic evaluations of deep puncture wounds should have one common goal: to determine the depth of penetration and accurately identify the lesions deep within the hoof. Careful visual inspection follows cleansing and paring of the entire solar surface. If an offending foreign body has been removed, the horn surrounding the puncture should be pared into a cone to allow ventral drainage. Radiography performed with the sole packed to minimize artifacts will help identify fractures. Standard radiographs may not, however, show the depth of a soft tissue tract. For this, two simple contrast radiographic techniques can be used: insertion of a sterile malleable probe (Fig. 6), or injection of a liquid radiopaque contrast medium* (Fig. 7). Both techniques should follow careful aseptic preparation of the foot. Introduction of the contrast solution is facilitated by the use of an 18-gauge, 2-inch Teflon catheter.† Contrast material filling either the navicular bursa or the deep flexor tendon sheath or both is irrefutable evidence of penetration, and the presence of a closed-cavity infection should be presumed.

TREATMENT

Although a retrospective study of a large number of horses with septic navicular bursitis has not yet appeared, clinical experience indicates that the disease is refractory to medical treatment alone and requires radical debridement and drainage through the substance of the frog, the digital cushion, and the deep flexor tendon. Accessibility is limited and even radical surgical intervention can fail. Osteomyelitis of the distal phalanx has a better prognosis

---

*MD-76, Mallinckrodt, Inc., St. Louis, MO
†Abbocath, Abbott Hospitals, Inc., North Chicago, IL

after surgical treatment if it is uncomplicated by septic arthritis of the distal interphalangeal joint. Infected soft tissue structures, such as the digital cushion or the collateral cartilages, usually heal completely following adequate debridement.

Complete debridement and drainage can resolve these sometimes devastating closed-cavity infections, but chronicity may lead to localization of infection in surgically inaccessible areas. Cases referred to surgical centers are commonly several weeks in duration and the animals become candidates for drainage only when response to local therapy and systemic antibiotics has been poor. The limited success of surgical treatment in such cases is not surprising. A positive result depends upon early diagnosis and prompt, aggressive therapy. The examining veterinarian should establish the extent of the penetration in the first 24 to 48 hours. If the diagnosis of a deep penetration is confirmed and facilities are not readily available, the practitioner should recommend immediate referral to a surgical facility. Conservative medical treatment in the field and delay in surgical intervention increases the risk of refractory infection, and markedly decreases the possibility of a favorable outcome.

Supplemental Readings

Adams, O. R.: Lameness in Horses, 3rd ed. Philadelphia, Lea and Febiger, 1974.

Hunt, T. K., and VanWinkle, W.: Normal repair. In Hunt, T. K., and Dunphy, J. E. (eds.): Fundamentals of Wound Management. New York, Appleton-Century-Crofts, 1979.

Johnson, J. H.: The foot. In Mansmann, R. A., McAllister, E. S. and Pratt, P. W. (eds.): Equine Medicine and Surgery, 3rd ed. Santa Barbara, CA, American Veterinary Publications, 1982.

Stump, J. E.: Anatomy of the normal equine foot, including microscopic features of the laminar region. J. Am. Vet. Med. Assoc., 151:1588, 1967.

Wilson, D. G.: Equine canker: A prospective and retrospective study. 20th Annu. Meet. Am. Coll. Vet. Surg., San Diego, 1985.

Hoof Cracks

Frank A. Nickels, EAST LANSING, MICHIGAN

Hoof cracks are an interruption of continuity of the wall extending in the direction of the horn tubules. An interruption of continuity of the wall, at right angles to the direction of the horn tubules, is referred to as a horn cleft. Hoof cracks, according to their location, extent and severity, not only have various names but also have varying significance.

They can commence at either the weight-bearing surface of the hoof, extending up a variable distance, or at the coronary band and extend downward.

Hoof cracks are classified by their position as toe, quarter, and heel cracks; by their length as being complete, extending from one border to the other, or incomplete; and by their severity, as simple when only the horn is involved and complicated or deep when it penetrates through the entire wall to the sensitive tissue. Incomplete cracks that affect the upper borders are referred to as coronary cracks and those limited to the lower border are sometimes designated as low cracks.

There are many causes of hoof cracks. Besides wounds to the coronary band, anything that impairs the elasticity of the hoof, weakens it, or causes an overloading can cause cracks. Faulty conformation, imbalance of the hoof, or improper application of toe or heel calks can lead to overloading portions of the hoof. Dry, brittle hooves and thin walls are predisposing factors for hoof cracks. Excessive growth of the hoof wall from lack of routine trimming is also a common cause of incomplete superficial cracks. Spontaneous complicated or deep cracks can also develop when horses are worked at speed on hard or uneven surfaces.

Hoof cracks have varying morbidity depending on the underlying cause and the function of the horse. Incomplete, low, superficial cracks are of questionable significance, in contrast to complicated or deep cracks originating at the weight-bearing surface. Incomplete coronary cracks are also very troublesome because the underlying cause may be more difficult to correct. Although the treatment of an existing crack may be easily accomplished in most cases, the cause should be determined to avoid recurrence.

TREATMENT

Treatment of hoof cracks involves removing pressure from the free extremity of the crack and immobilizing its edges. Various methods for repair have been reported, including (1) proper balance of the hoof; (2) corrective shoeing; (3) grooving of the hoof wall; (4) use of clamping across the crack with nails, a Vachette clamp, or mechanical clamps; and (5) use of various prosthetic hoof repair materials.

Routine trimming and the use of an open shoe is usually all that is required for incomplete, superficial low cracks. A bar shoe is advised for all other cracks because it will continuously protect the affected area of wall from pressure. The use of shoe "clips" on either side of the crack can further minimize the movements caused by expansion and contraction of the hoof wall. Proper placement of clips for a toe crack is between the first and second nail holes of both branches of the horseshoe. In no case should a "clip" be placed immediately below the crack. "Easing" or removing horn from the bearing surface of the hoof wall (Fig. 1) below the crack reduces the effects of pressure and concussion and is used in conjunction with corrective shoeing. Whenever "easing" of the hoof wall is used, the

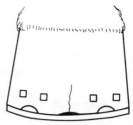

Figure 1. A hoof showing a toe crack. Black area ventral to toe crack represents area of resected wall to "ease" the weight-bearing surface of hoof. Proper placement of clips on the shoe for toe crack is illustrated.

space between the wall and shoe should be cleaned daily with a hacksaw blade to prevent pressure from accumulation of dirt.

Grooving the hoof wall is a successful means of isolating and reducing pressure at the extremity of some cracks and is most applicable for incomplete cracks originating at either the weight-bearing surface or coronary band. The technique may be done in a variety of ways. However, a single horizontal groove at the upper extremity of a low crack or two grooves arranged in the form of a V (Fig. 2) at the distal extremity of coronary cracks is most effective. Whichever method is used, care should be taken to carry the groove deep enough into the horn to be effective but not involve the sensitive structures. Another method of immobilizing the borders of a crack is by clamping the edges of the crack. Various methods have been reported in the literature but are not commonly used. Clamping by any method should be undertaken only if the horn is moderately strong and thick. This practically limits the use of clamps to the toe. With any of the methods of clamping, new cracks occasionally develop at the point of insertion.

Painful, complicated, or deep cracks may require greater stability than provided by methods previously mentioned, especially in the competition horse. Because of the economic demands placed on these horses, it is difficult to prescribe sufficient time to allow the hoof crack to resolve naturally.

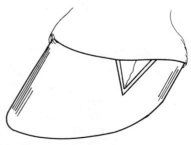

Figure 2. A hoof showing a coronary crack. The V-shaped parallel lines illustrate one method of grooving the hoof to prevent a coronary crack from worsening.

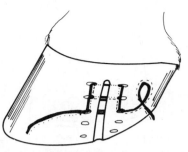

Figure 3. Shoemaker's suture pattern for lacing a hoof crack for acrylic repair.

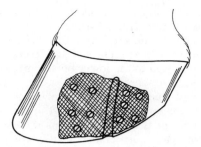

Figure 5. Use of fiber glass cloth and sheet metal screws for repair of a hoof crack.

There are various techniques reported using prosthetic hoof wall material such as acrylics, fiber glass, and epoxy resins in combination with such implants as umbilical tape or wire, sheet metal screws, and other synthetic materials.

Regardless of the technique used for the repair of hoof cracks utilizing prosthetic materials, the hoof must be properly prepared. The hoof should be trimmed and balanced and shod with a bar shoe. The hoof wall should be thoroughly clean and dry. The hoof is scrubbed with a detergent and then cleaned with a solvent (ether or acetone) to remove any oils and dry the hoof wall. The hoof crack is then opened its entire length down to the depth of the crack with a small motorized hand tool* utilizing burrs. The edge of the crack is undermined the entire length, especially for the acrylic repair method. The crack should be free from hemorrhage or sepsis, or in the case of hoof wall loss, completely keratinized and cornified before sealing with prosthetic hoof wall materials. If not, the repair should be delayed until healing has occurred to avoid complication.

A technique of hoof repair with acrylic (Fig. 3) using one eighth–inch umbilical tape to lace the crack and act as scaffold has been reported. This

---

*Dremel, Dremel Manufacturing Co., Racine, WI

technique for repair is effective but difficult to perform. Paired holes are drilled perpendicular to the crack to communicate at its depth. These holes are placed one fourth inch from the edge of the crack and are evenly spaced through its length. Umbilical tape is then laced through the holes in a shoemaker's suture pattern. Diagonal lacing as in a shoe should not be used because it will cause the wall to tear at the holes. Once the acrylic is applied, it hardens in approximately 10 minutes and then can be rasped smooth to provide a strong cosmetic repair. Because the acrylic becomes so hard and brittle, the shoe must be placed on the hoof before the repair. Another technique using this hoof repair material in combination with blunted sheet metal screws (⅜ inch × 8 gauge) and 18-gauge cerclage wire (Fig. 4) also provides a strong repair but has one major disadvantage. The correct depth of the drilled holes for the sheet metal screws can be difficult to obtain, especially in a thin-walled hoof.

A technique utilizing fiber glass and sheet metal screws (⅜ inch × 8 gauge) provides a very strong repair but is technically difficult and requires more expertise than other methods (Fig. 5). Experience with fiber glass materials is necessary before this method can be used to repair hoof cracks. Choice of the correct fiber glass cloth weight (No. 3) is also important to minimize the bulk of the patch while retaining its strength. Approximately 10 layers of

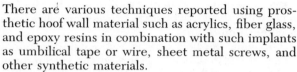

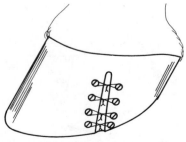

Figure 4. Use of sheet metal screws and 18-gauge cerclage wire to immobilize the edges of a hoof crack for acrylic repair.

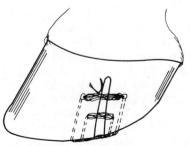

Figure 6. Drilled holes in hoof and a far-near, near-far suture pattern for repair of a hoof crack using a multifibered synthetic material and epoxy.

fiber glass cloth are attached with blunted sheet metal screws to the area of the hoof to be patched and an additional five layers are used to cover this attached patch. The placement of the blunted sheet metal screws at the proper depth in the hoof wall is difficult, especially in a thin-walled hoof.

Another technique utilizing a synthetic, multifiber suture and epoxy* (Fig. 6) has been used successfully in racing Standardbreds. The strength of the repair depends on the bulky, synthetic suture material that is used. Two holes are drilled on either side of the crack, one half inch apart. The drill holes are started through the bottom of the hoof just outside the white line and extend proximally to exit at a point normally achieved when driving horseshoe nails. The suture is then laced through the holes with a far-near, near-far suture pattern. The final step is to saturate the suture material and the

_____

*10x, Farriers, Inc., Wilmington, DE

crack with the epoxy. If the hoof crack is accompanied with a hoof wall loss, a webbing material made · from the same material as the suture is incorporated in the suture pattern to reinforce the patch. This technique is simple and the application is made easy. Kits are available which provide all the necessary materials for the desired application.*

_____

*10x, Farriers, Inc., Wilmington, DE

Supplemental Readings

Adams, O. R.: Lameness, _In_ Lameness in Horses, 2nd ed., Philadelphia, Lea & Febiger, 1973.
Butler, J.: The repair of hoof defects using fiberglass and screws. Proc. 22nd Annu. Meet. Am. Assoc. Eq. Pract., 1976, pp. 235–237.
Evans, L. H., Jenny, J.: The repair of hoof cracks with acrylic. J. Am. Vet. Med. Assoc., _148_:355, 1966.
Moyer, W.: Repairing hoof cracks in the horse: A review and report of a new technique. Comp. Cont. Ed., 5:S495, 1983.
Reeks, H. C.: Diseases arising from faulty conformation. _In_ Diseases of the Horse's Foot. London, England, Bailliere Tindall and Cox, 1906.

Hoof Lacerations and Avulsions

Frank A. Nickels, EAST LANSING, MICHIGAN

Horses frequently sustain minor lacerations and abrasions of the skin of the pastern area, coronary band, and bulbs of the heels. These wounds usually respond to traditional methods of wound management. Deep lacerations of these structures, severe wounds with loss of germinal tissue, and partial or complete avulsion of the hoof are not common injuries. The management of these wounds can be difficult and usually requires extensive treatment.

PRINCIPLES OF WOUND EVALUATION AND MANAGEMENT

Adequate collateral circulation can develop following major insult to the vascular supply to the foot, but ischemia will impair healing. Locally effective blood supply is probably the most important natural defense mechanism against infection. Permanent loss of blood supply leads to more serious complications and necessitates reassessment during the course of treatment. This may not be related to the original traumatic incident but to subsequent development of thrombosis.

Complete denervation of the foot, in addition to trauma, infection, and a compromised blood supply, may result in digital necrosis. One study showed that complete denervation of the foot caused loss of

bone mass and strength. It was proposed that these changes may be associated with spontaneous rupture or avulsion of tendon and ligament attachments. However, the investigator did not propose this as the sole cause of the digital necrosis occasionally seen in neurectomized horses.

If corium of the foot is involved in the wound, it must be examined closely. A thorough knowledge of the physiology and anatomy of the hoof is necessary (see p. 255). The corium is specially modified and a highly vascular part of the common integument that furnishes nutrition. Injury to the coronary band can be serious and usually results in a permanent defect in the hoof wall. If the injury results in avulsion or necrosis of the corium of the hoof, the prognosis for normal hoof growth must be assessed accordingly. However, if there is no loss of the tissues, the integrity of the hoof may be difficult to assess until some regrowth has occurred.

Contraction is minimal in hoof wounds involving horn tissue, and healing occurs by epithelial migration and connective tissue synthesis (see p. 266). All components of the corium can migrate and cover a defect if the granulation bed is healthy. However, epithelialization is practically impossible in the presence of infection. With adequate debridement, proper wound management, and, if possible, precise approximation of tissue margins, a minor defect may result from what appeared to be a major coronary injury. These defects lead to a permanent crack defect in the hoof wall, although not all cause functional impairment or lameness. Preventive measures such as regular trimming and corrective shoeing and acrylic repair may reduce or eliminate the consequences of these problems (see p. 272).

Without proper and immediate care, damage to the periosteum of the second and third phalanx and to the collateral ligaments of the proximal and distal interphalangeal joints may result in chronic lameness. Even with proper care it is difficult to predict the response of these tissues to injury and the effect on the final outcome.

Open joints are a serious problem, but with adequate debridement of the devitalized tissue surrounding the joint, joint lavage, and appropriate parenteral antibiotics, management of this problem can be rewarding. Postoperatively, protection and immobilization of the affected joint is also important. Immobilization of the joint with a cast ensures a more rapid closure of the joint capsule, but requires astute clinical judgment to determine the appropriate time interval for subsequent cast changes and joint lavage. Clinical experience has shown that open contaminated joints can be adequately treated by cast changes to allow cleaning of the wound and joint lavage performed every five to seven days until the joint capsule closes.

In addition to the nature and extent of the injury, there are other factors such as age, value and function of the horse, chronicity of the injury, and concurrent problems that must be considered before care is undertaken. Treatment may be expensive and protracted. If the horse is valuable, has sentimental value, or has an alternative nonathletic function, the owner may request treatment regardless of the possible outcome.

CLINICAL EXAMINATION

A thorough examination of the wound is essential before treatment is begun because of the potential expense and extended convalescence. The foot, like other tissues, has a great capacity to heal but the prognosis for return to full function is unlikely in wounds with severe tissue destruction.

A critical evaluation of the tissues involved is essential. The blood and nerve supply to the foot should be assessed, as well as the integrity of joint capsules. The tendons, ligaments, collateral cartilages, phalanges, and germinal tissue of the hoof should also be assessed. The hair should be clipped to aid in the evaluation and survey radiographs should be taken.

WOUND MANAGEMENT

The preparation of the injured limb is routine as for any aseptic surgery with the exception of a few minor points. The hoof and sole should be trimmed short and the wall of the hoof rasped smooth to remove extraneous debris and reduce the residual contamination in cracks and crevices of the hoof. The hair from the lower limb is clipped liberally to reduce the resident bacterial flora. The hoof is scrubbed thoroughly with povidone-iodine soap. Any exposed tissues are irrigated with warm isotonic solutions such as saline or lactated Ringer's solution. A povidone-iodine solution is applied to the entire hoof and lower limb. Harsh antiseptics should be avoided on exposed tissue. The wound is covered with a nonadherent sterile dressing, and the entire hoof and the lower limb are covered with an impervious bandage to protect the wound and prevent additional contamination until surgery.

Depending on the nature and extent of the wound and the temperament of the patient, the surgery may be performed with sedation and regional local anesthesia. General anesthesia provides optimal conditions to establish and maintain aseptic techniques for surgical care. The principal goal of surgical management of the wound is to create a healthy environment for wound healing and to obtain the most favorable cosmetic and functional results. All traumatic wounds are contaminated and some are infected owing to the natural habitat, amount of tissue trauma, comprised local tissue defenses, and the length of the interval between injury and definitive care. The wound should be cultured and antibiotic sensitivity testing performed, especially when the joint is open.

The most important single factor in the management of contaminated wounds is adequate debridement. Devitalized or severaly damaged tissue and foreign material provide a medium for bacteria and act as physical impediments to healing. Removal of such tissue also reduces the bacterial inoculum within the wound. A specific exception to the general rule of removing all devitalized tissue involves the handling of special tissue such as nerves and tendons that perform important physical functions. Since primary closure of the wounds usually cannot be and should not be contemplated, the viability of these tissues can be evaluated later. Complete wound excision is the most effective method of debridement, but when this is not feasible, simple debridement should be combined with wound irrigation. Pulsating tissue lavage is more effective than low-flow systems in removing tissue fragments and bacteria from contaminated wounds. Clinically, the incidence of wound infection seems to be inversely proportional to the amount of wound irrigation and debridement at the time of injury.

If there is any suspicion that a synovial structure is open, this should be determined at this time. The joint can be injected with sterile isotonic fluid to check for leakage. If a joint is open, it should be lavaged with copious amounts of lactated Ringer's solution through a site distant to the wound.

Adequate hemostasis must be maintained, but because of the dense nature of some tissues, ligation and electrocautery may not be sufficient. A temporary pressure bandage is usually necessary. The final step is to apply a sterile dressing with antimicrobial ointment to the surface of the wound before bandaging.

Postoperatively, immobilization and protection of the wound are paramount to prevent contamination from moisture or fecal material and to ensure a conducive environment for wound healing. This is best accomplished with a cast that encases the hoof. Casts are a convenient method of decreasing postoperative care while still providing better protection and immobilization than with bandaging material. A short cast that comes up only to the fetlock may suffice or a half limb cast may be more appropriate, especially on the hindlimb. The cast is usually changed at two-week intervals unless there is an open synovial structure, in which case more frequent cast changes are necessary. An impervious bandage may be adequate for less severe wounds of the foot.

When the cast is changed, there will be a considerable accumulation of exudative material under the cast. This is to be expected. The decision to apply a second cast or proceed with sterile bandages at this time depends on the progress of wound healing. The type of bandage material is a matter of personal preference, but the wound should be covered with a sterile dressing with a waterproof outer layer.

Prophylactic systemic antibiotics are advocated during the acute phase of wound healing or if a joint is involved. Topical antibacterial preparations are more appropriate for other chronic wounds. Nonsteroidal anti-inflammatory medication is recommended to reduce inflammation and thereby pain and to minimize the adverse consequences of uneven weight-bearing. One of the most important points to ensure a successful outcome is good nursing care during the postoperative period. Bandaging of the hoof is essential until epithelialization is complete and cornification has occurred.

Supplemental Readings

Fessler, J. F.: Surgical management of equine foot injuries. Mod. Vet. Pract., 52:41, 1971.

Hackett, R. P.: Management of traumatic wounds. Proceed. 24th Annu. Meet. Am. Assoc. Eq. Pract., 1978, pp. 363–367.

Peacock, E. E., and VanWinkle, W.: Wound Repair, 2nd ed. Philadelphia, W. B. Saunders Company, 1976, pp. 204–270.

Steckel, R. R.: Surgical management of severe hoof wounds in the horse: A retrospective study of 30 cases. Comp. Cont. Ed., 5:S435, 1983.

Laminitis

John A. Stick, EAST LANSING, MICHIGAN

Acute laminitis in a horse should be treated as an emergency. It produces severe lameness that if untreated or unresponsive to treatment will progress to the chronic form and will probably cause permanent loss of function in the performance horse. Lameness from laminitis may be severe enough to justify euthanasia. Early diagnosis and appropriate therapy can lessen the degree of laminar damage and arrest the disease process.

As a local manifestation of a systemic metabolic disturbance, laminitis is a complex disease and its pathophysiology is not completely understood. It is generally considered an inflammatory condition of the hoof. Congestion, ischemia, and necrosis of the laminae are disturbances that have been related to the acute phase of this disease. Because its pathogenesis is not completely understood, therapeutic approaches are based on previous responses to therapy, as well as on recent findings. Discussed here are the inciting causes, predisposing factors, and clinical signs of laminitis. Also addressed are the therapeutic rationale for the classic forms of this disease: acute, refractory, and chronic.

CAUSES AND PREDISPOSING FACTORS

The incidence of laminitis is highest in ponies, lower in geldings, and least in stallions and mares. Seasonal variation of the disease is seen with early growth of pasture in the spring, and overweight horses and especially ponies on pasture are affected.

A common cause of laminitis is grain overload; in support of this, carbohydrate overload has been a reliable way to reproduce laminitis experimentally. Toxemia secondary to retained placenta and acute gastrointestinal diseases also may cause laminitis. Traumatic laminitis can occur when overweight unfit animals are exercised on a hard surface. A condition referred to as "support laminitis" is frequently seen when one limb, particularly a forelimb, bears excessive weight, as may occur during the recuperative period following certain fractures. Drug-induced laminitis has been observed following the administration of certain corticosteroids. Laminitis has also been related to excessive water consumption immediately after exercise.

Overweight horses frequently have recurrent attacks of acute laminitis whenever their feed is changed. Horses with previous laminar disease resulting from laminitis, severe sole abscesses, and puncture wounds are predisposed to subsequent attacks of acute laminitis.

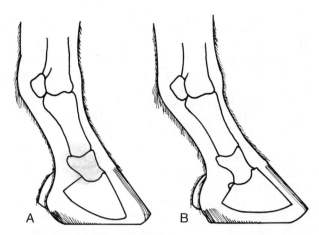

Figure 1. Schematic lateral radiographs of the distal equine limb (*A*) showing rotation of the pedal bone within a laminitic foot and (*B*) showing the normal position of the pedal bone within the hoof.

CLINICAL SIGNS

Acute Form. Laminitis in the horse as an emergency necessitates immediate attention comparable to colic, dystocia, fracture, laceration, and eye injuries. Although front feet are most commonly affected, all four feet may be involved. Lameness develops rapidly in the acute form and affected animals may shift their weight from one foot to another. The stance of a horse with acute laminitis is typical; the horse will rock back on the heels of the front feet and take more weight onto the hind limbs by shifting the hind limbs forward under its body. This stance is exaggerated when the horse is made to walk or turn in a circle or both. Strides are shortened, with each foot placed quickly after leaving the ground. Horses in severe pain will remain recumbent and will rise only when forced. Laminitis is characterized by warmth in the hoof area and exaggerated pulsation of digital vessels. A horse with laminitis in the forefeet is reluctant to stand on one foot while the other is lifted for examination. Pain when pressure is applied over the sole with hoof testers is common.

Radiographic examination of the foot may reveal rotation of the pedal bone (Fig. 1A) from its normal position (Fig. 1B) as early as 24 hours after the onset of clinical signs. Radiographs should be taken initially for two reasons: to rule out previous pedal bone rotation and to establish a baseline position of the pedal bone. Radiographic examination at four- to five-day intervals identifies subsequent changes as they occur. Laminitis can result from systemic disease that is the inciting cause. The diagnosis and management of systemic disease is accomplished by thorough history in conjunction with physical examination and ancillary diagnostic support.

Refractory Form. Acute laminitis treated properly should show progressive daily response to therapy. When exacerbation of the disease occurs, or no improvement is seen following initial therapy, laminitis should be considered refractory. This form (refractory laminitis) has the most serious consequences and carries an unfavorable prognosis. Efforts should be intensified to more accurately define and reverse the inciting disturbance. Aggressive initial medical therapy is indicated as discussed later to combat pedal rotation, which can occur rapidly. Failure to reverse clinical signs in three to four days is an indication that pedal bone rotation has occurred. Penetration of the sole with subsequent development of septic pedal osteitis and abscess of the foot is a grave situation that results from progressive, uncontrolled pedal rotation.

Chronic Form. The chronic form of laminitis causes recurrent lameness aggravated by recent foot trimming, uneven hard ground, and exercise on firm surfaces. This form of laminitis follows the acute and refractory forms of the disease in which pedal bone rotation has occurred. Laminar damage results in abnormal hoof growth seen as diverging rings around the hoof wall, wider at the heel than the toe (Fig. 2). A flattened or convex sole (dropped sole) and an abnormally long toe will occur when trimming is not regular and corrective in nature.

Horses with chronic laminitis usually travel with a two-phase placement of the feet: heel-toe, heel-toe, best observed when the horse is trotting. The foundered foot has increased sensitivity to hoof testers, especially over the sole, midway between the apex of the frog and the toe area of hoof wall. Bruising of the sole in a foundered foot appears as a crescent shaped area of sole hemorrhage, outlining the perimeter of the pedal bone. Separation of wall and sole occurs at the toe in the white line, which is widened. Chronic laminitis predisposes the hoof

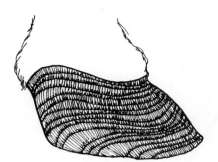

Figure 2. A horse's foot affected by chronic laminitis showing diverging rings around the hoof wall (wider at the heel than the toe).

wall to cracking, and subsolar abscesses are common.

Diagnostic anesthesia should be part of the initial examination if other causes of lameness are suspected. A medial and lateral palmar digital nerve block should alleviate only part of the lameness with laminitis. If the dorsal branches of the digital nerve are anesthetized with a low palmar or basal sesamoid block, alleviation of the greatest portion of the lameness from laminitis will occur. If the lameness is due to sole abscessation, the results would be similar.

If radiographic examination of the foot reveals rotation of the pedal bone with osteolysis and gas in laminar areas, chronic laminitis is the radiographic diagnosis. Measurement of the degree of pedal bone rotation can be used to predict the prognosis for return of function (Fig. 3A and B). Horses with less than 5.5 degrees rotation may return to athletic function with corrective trimming and shoeing. Horses with more than 11.5 degrees rotation are lost as performance animals.

TREATMENT OF LAMINITIS

Acute Form. Prompt correction of physiologic disturbances reduces the severity of damage occurring to laminae, and improves the chance of return to functional soundness. If the cause of laminitis is known, palliative measures should be instituted to reduce the severity of the metabolic disturbance. For example, mineral oil may be given by nasogastric tube to remove or block the uptake of undesirable intestinal contents, intravenous fluids can be provided to correct electrolyte and fluid imbalances, and antibiotics are administered when septicemia is suspected.

Phenylbutazone* (4.4 mg per kg) is the single most important therapeutic agent in treating acute laminitis. Initially it can be given intravenously and

followed with an oral form at 12-hour intervals. This drug reduces inflammation, which is responsible in part for subsequent separation of the laminae in the hoof. The analgesic action reduces pain associated with both acute and chronic laminitis and promotes return of physiologic foot function associated with weight-bearing and walking. The drug should be continued until the signs of inflammation have subsided, heat in the foot is decreased, pain is less, and the "bounding" digital pulse resolves. Phenylbutazone is slowly withdrawn over four to five days, to prevent recurrence of acute signs.

Flunixin meglumine* (1.1 mg per kg) can be given in conjunction with phenylbutazone or in its place if endotoxemia is the suspected cause of laminitis. Grain overload and retained placenta are clinical conditions that cause laminitis, and medical therapy should include flunixin meglumine and antimicrobial drugs.

Because frog pressure is important in moving blood through the foot circulation, it is necessary to restore normal foot function as soon as possible. Frog pressure should be maintained by slight lowering of the heels and padding of the bottom of the hoof. Unvulcanized rubber† (tire retread, die size 62–76–14) or other thick padding material that will conform to the shape of the sole will evenly distribute weight and help alleviate pain, permitting the animal to stand and walk more normally. To facilitate walking, alleviation of lameness by blocking the nerves to the foot may be necessary. Walking should be encouraged three to four times a day to prevent blood stasis, a factor that can lead to thrombus formation within the foot vascular system.

Histamine release into the bloodstream is believed to be partially responsible for circulatory derangement in certain types of laminitis (particularly "grain founder"). Use of an antihistamine‡ (0.55 mg per kg subcutaneously) may be indicated as part of the therapy in these cases. This drug is useful only during the early stages of acute laminitis and should be repeated at frequent intervals (i.e., every four hours for the first 24 hours following onset).

Grain and legume hay should be eliminated from the diet and foundered horses fed only grass hay until the acute signs of laminitis have been alleviated. Thereafter, the diet should not contain high ratios of grain or high protein legumes, and changes in feed should be made gradually. If the foundered horse is obese, the animal's weight should be reduced through dieting.

A case of acute laminitis may require two days to two weeks to completely respond to treatment.

---

*Butazolidin, Burroughs Wellcome Co., Kansas City, MO

*Banamine, Schering Corp., Kenilworth, NJ
†Long Mile Tire Co., Cline Tire Service, Mason, MI
‡A-H Injection, Burroughs Wellcome Co., Kansas City, MO

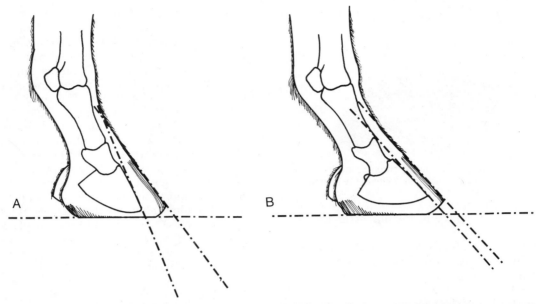

Figure 3. Schematic of lateral radiographs of the distal equine limb demonstrating the measurement of pedal bone rotation. When pedal bone rotation has occurred (*A*), the angle of the hoof wall (formed by the line drawn parallel to the dorsum of the hoof wall and the horizontal line) subtracted from the angle of the pedal bone (formed by the line drawn parallel to the dorsum of the pedal bone and the horizontal line) equals the degree of pedal bone rotation. In a foot unaffected by laminitis (*B*), the amount of rotation is zero.

Successful management should be judged on the basis of progressive daily improvement. If relapse occurs or clinical signs do not improve in the first 48 hours, the case should be considered refractory.

Refractory Form. A number of therapeutic agents are used empirically with clinical success. D-L Methionine* (22 mg per kg per os once daily for the first week, 11 mg per kg once daily for the second week, and 5.5 mg per kg once daily for the third week) has been reported to provide a disulfide bond substrate for maintenance of the hoof-pedal bone bond. To control the hypertension that accompanies laminitis, the sodium intake should be lowered (salt block should be removed) and potassium chloride† (66 mg per kg once daily) should be given orally for a week.

In severe cases, two additional medications may be given and have reversed progressive signs of laminitis in my experience. However, the risks may outweigh the benefits, and owners should be advised of the lack of evaluation of the safety of these drugs. The administration of sodium heparin‡ (44 to 66 IU per kg intravenously every four hours) may benefit acutely affected horses before laminar ischemia has occurred by preventing thrombosis. This treatment should be monitored by partial throm-boplastin times, which should not exceed two times normal values one hour after heparin administration. Horses with compromised coagulation—for example, those with diarrhea or endotoxemia—may require much smaller doses of heparin to produce the same degree of anticoagulation.

Phenoxybenzamine HCl* (0.66 mg per kg in 500 ml saline) given slowly intravenously provides alpha-adrenergic blockade and vasodilation for 12 to 24 hours. This solution may be made by adding the powder of 10 mg capsules to heated saline and passing this solution through a micropore filter before administration. Although the results can be rewarding with great improvement in signs occurring within 24 hours, retreatment is not recommended. Because phenoxybenzamine decreases blood pressure, some horses will become depressed and will need aggressive shock therapy. In systemically ill animals, this therapy should be used with caution or not at all.

Chronic Form. Chronic laminitis results when coffin bone rotation has occurred after the abatement of the acute signs. The greater the degree of rotation, the greater the loss of function. Significant improvement can be made in the return to normal use with corrective trimming and shoeing at this stage of the disease. Frequent trimming and shoeing are vitally important.

*Ammonil Tablets, Daniels Pharmaceuticals, Inc., St. Petersburg, FL
†Mallinckrodt Inc., Paris, KY
‡Lypho Med Inc., Melrose Park, IL

*Dibenzyline Capsules, SmithKline Corp., Philadelphia, PA

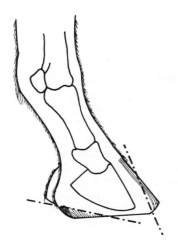

Figure 4. A horse's foot affected by chronic laminitis demonstrating the areas of hoof to be removed during corrective trimming. The vertical line shows the amount of hoof wall to be removed so that it parallels the dorsum of the pedal bone. The horizontal line shows the amount of heel area of hoof to be removed so that the weight bearing surface of the pedal bone is parallel to the ground.

Corrective trimming for chronic laminitis should provide a nonpainful bearing surface, returning the coffin bone to its normal position in relation to the rest of the distal limb and hoof. The heels should be lowered as much as possible or until the ventral surface of the coffin bone is parallel to the bearing surface of the hoof (Fig. 4). This returns the coffin bone to its normal weight-bearing position, while allowing the horse to stand and travel on a "normal" area of hoof at the heels. Removal of the long toe from the face of the hoof returns the shape of the hoof to normal in relation to the coffin bone (Fig. 4). Toe removal eliminates stumbling and reduces the lever-arm effect that eventually causes turning up of the toe.

The principle behind corrective shoeing of the chronic laminitis foot is reduction of contact of the painful area of the sole with the ground. The repair should prevent further damage to the abnormal laminae at the toe of the hoof while providing a more cosmetic appearance to the foot. The dry, abnormal laminae should be removed from the anterior surface of the toe, and a small lip of normal horn should be left in place. A wide-web shoe can be nailed onto the foot, extending forward as if the hoof was normal. This protects the laminae and the sole from ground contact. A full pad could also be used to further protect the sole if necessary.

The defect at the toe can be filled with hoof acrylic if abscessation is absent. The shoe and lip of normal horn at the toe provide stability to the acrylic after it hardens. Nails placed in the remaining holes in the shoe also help in this respect. Aluminum foil is used to mold the hardening acrylic to the contour of the hoof. Filling the defect in this manner provides protection against both moisture loss in the hoof and formation of abscesses. After hardening, the foil is removed and the acrylic smoothed with a hoof rasp, providing a cosmetically acceptable hoof.

This type of trimming and shoeing may have to be repeated several times before an acceptable level of function returns. However, if the coffin bone is returned to a more normal position following correction, acceptable results can be achieved with time. Although the foot will always need some correction, the amount will depend on the frequency of trimming. The absence of proper care will allow the foot to return to its original shape with a resultant loss of function of the animal.

Supplemental Readings

Coffman, J. R., Johnson, J. H., Guffy, M. M., et al.: Hoof circulation in equine laminitis. J. Am. Vet. Med. Assoc., *156*:76, 1970.

Coffman, J. R.: Refractory laminitis. Vet. Clin. North Am. 3:291, 1973.

Johnson, J. H.: The foot. *In* Mansmann, R. A., McAllister, E. S., and Pratt, P.W. (eds.): Equine Medicine and Surgery, 3rd ed. Santa Barbara, CA, American Veterinary Publications, 1982, pp. 1033–1055.

Robinson, N. E., Scott, J. B., Dabney, J. M., et al.: Digital vascular responses and permeability in equine alimentary laminitis. Am. J. Vet. Res. 37:1171, 1976.

Stick, J. A., Jann, H. W., Scott, E. A., et al.: Pedal bone rotation as a prognostic sign in laminitis of horses. J. Am. Vet. Med. Assoc. *180*:251, 1982.

Orthopedic Problems of the Foot

Robert K. Schneider, GILBERT, ARIZONA

Russ L. Stickle, EAST LANSING, MICHIGAN

Diseases that involve the bones or synovial structures or both in the horse's foot are difficult to differentiate by clinical examination. The foot is covered by the epidermal hoof, which makes palpation of internal structures impossible. The examining veterinarian relies largely on hoof testers and diagnostic nerve blocks to localize the problem to specific areas in the foot. For this reason, diseases in this section are divided by their response to nerve blocks.

CONDITIONS THAT IMPROVE WITH PALMAR DIGITAL NERVE BLOCK

A palmar digital nerve (PDN) block is done by injecting 1.5 to 2 ml of local anesthetic subcutaneously over the medial and lateral palmar digital nerves. The anesthetic is injected through a fine-gauge needle placed through the skin caudal to the digital triad and proximal to the cartilage of the distal phalanx on the medial and lateral sides of the pastern. This block desensitizes the caudal half of the foot, including (1) the navicular bursa; (2) the deep digital flexor tendon distal to the proximal interphalangeal joint; (3) palmar portions of the distal interphalangeal joint, proximal interphalangeal joint, and cartilages of the distal phalanx; (4) the laminar corium; (5) the corium of the bars, frog, and sole; (6) the digital cushion; and (7) the skin on the palmar surface of the pastern and digital cushion.

NAVICULAR DISEASE

Navicular disease is a common cause of lameness, especially in older Quarterhorses and Thoroughbreds. The low incidence in Arabians suggests a hereditary predisposition to the disease in other breeds. The etiology and pathogenesis of the disease are still debated. Ischemia due to interruption of the blood supply to the distal sesamoid is one theory. The more traditional view is that the disease results from concussion and "wear and tear" on the distal sesamoid, bursa, and deep flexor tendon, beginning as bursitis and progressing to degeneration of the bone with adhesion to the deep digital flexor (DDF) tendon. Degenerative joint disease and synovitis of the distal interphalangeal joint have been implicated in the pathogenesis of the disease.

Normal age-related radiographic changes occur in the area, making diagnosis difficult. The heel of the foot contains several important structures, and damage to any of these can result in lameness that clinically cannot be differentiated from navicular disease. Further research is necessary to improve our understanding of the pathophysiology involved in navicular disease.

Clinical Signs. The diagnosis of navicular disease is made from clinical findings and response to diagnostic nerve blocks. It is a bilateral chronic forelimb lameness. Horses with navicular disease have a short-strided, choppy gait and may not exhibit obvious lameness when worked in a straight line. Decreased weight-bearing on the inside limb is usually observed when the horse is worked in small circles at a trot. (The horse is lame on the left when circling to the left and lame on the right when circling to the right). The lameness is exacerbated when the horse is worked over a hard or uneven surface. Horses with navicular disease are usually sensitive to hoof tester pressure over the frog and heel of both front feet. The degree of lameness can be increased by application of pressure to the frog for 10 to 15 seconds before jogging the horse. Affected horses may resent manual flexion of the lower limb and will trot off more lame following 15 seconds of flexion. Examination of the shoes usually reveals excessive wear at the toe with very little wear at the heel. These horses frequently have a small foot with contracted heels and/or a long toe, low heel conformation. A PDN block performed on the more lame front limb makes the horse sound on that limb and lame on the opposite limb. This can be dramatic in horses that are equally lame in both forelimbs and do not show an obvious gait deficit until the heel of one foot is anesthetized to produce a sound limb. A PDN block on the other limb will resolve the lameness. It is important to be sure that only the heel is desensitized and not the entire foot to make an accurate diagnosis of navicular disease.

Radiography. Radiographs of both front feet are useful in evaluating horses with navicular disease, but a diagnosis of navicular disease usually cannot be made from the radiographs alone. This is because of the current difficulty in correlating radiographic signs with clinical findings; some horses without radiographic lesions are lame while others with marked radiographic changes in the distal sesamoid are sound. Three views of the foot are routinely taken to evaluate the distal sesamoid: lateromedial, dorsoproximal-palmarodistal, and palmaroproximal-palmarodistal (skyline) projections. Radiographic findings compatible with a diagnosis of navicular disease include spurring and osteophyte formation on the proximal or distal border of the bone, small lytic lesions in the distal border, large areas of lysis in the center of the bone, and loss of cortical bone over the flexor surface (Figs. 1 and 2). Of these changes the latter is the most severe and indicates adhesion formation between the bone and DDF tendon. This is a poor prognostic sign, because little can be done to return these horses to soundness once the bone is adherent to the tendon. Absence of radiographic lesions does not rule out navicular disease because soft tissue structures (proximal and distal suspensory ligaments of the distal sesamoid, DDF tendon, and navicular bursa) may be involved and would not be demonstrated radiographically.

Treatment. Navicular disease is a progressive, degenerative condition for which there is presently no treatment that will return the horse to complete soundness without recurrence of the problem. Current treatments are aimed at protecting the frog and the heel of the foot and reducing inflammation in order to prolong the horse's useful athletic life.

Regardless of other modes of treatment employed, almost all horses with navicular disease require corrective shoeing to protect the frog and heel from pressure and concussion. Two basic shoeing techniques are commonly used: an egg bar shoe or a wedge pad–shoe combination. An egg bar shoe is an oval shoe that extends caudally behind the horse's heel (Fig. 3). It is particularly useful in horses with a long toe-low heel conformation because it moves the weight-bearing surface caudal to the normal position beneath the bulbs of the heel. The shoe is made wider than the foot at the heel and the nails are placed in the cranial half of the shoe; both of these promote expansion of the heel during weight-bearing. A half-round shoe with a wide web is preferred; it provides a "rocker" effect as the foot breaks over the toe. A wedge pad placed between the shoe and the foot provides protection to the bottom of the foot and has been commonly used in horses with navicular disease. It increases the hoof angle and theoretically decreases strain on the DDF tendon and navicular bone. Silicone or okum is used to fill the space between the pad and the foot. Regardless of the shoeing technique employed, there are certain principles that should not be violated. The toe should be maintained as short as possible to allow rapid and easy breakover of the foot. This may mean more frequent trimming and resetting of the shoes than normal. Rounding the toe of the shoe (or using a half-round shoe) also promotes earlier breakover of the foot. The horse's normal angle should be maintained; the slope of the pastern should equal the slope of the hoof wall. This is especially important if a wedge pad is used; it is a mistake to automatically raise a horse's heel and create a broken foot axis. A standard corrective shoeing technique cannot be used on every horse with navicular disease. Each horse's foot, natural

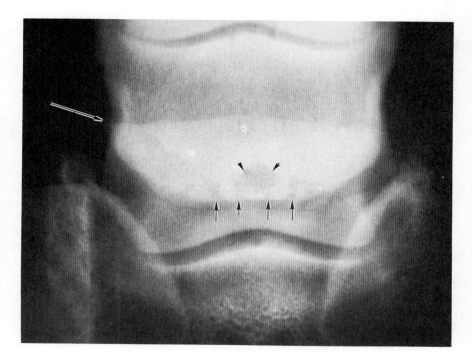

Figure 1. Dorsoproximal-palmarodistal view of the distal sesamoid of a horse with signs of navicular disease. Numerous mushroom-shaped lucencies (*short arrows*) are seen associated with the distal margin of the distal sesamoid. There is a large lucency (*arrowheads*) in the central portion of the bone and spur formation (*long arrow*) on one abaxial margin. The film was made using a stationary grid.

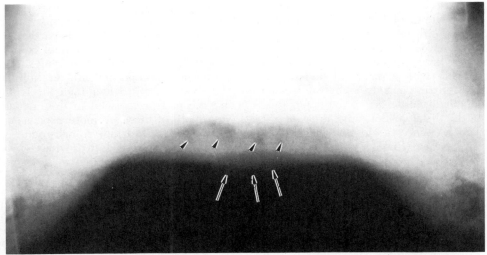

Figure 2. Skyline view of the distal sesamoid. Poorly marginated lucencies (*arrowheads*) in the central portion of the distal sesamoid represent the same lucencies seen associated with the distal margin on the dorsoproximal-palmarodistal view (Fig. 1). This horse also has a large lucency (*arrows*) involving the flexor surface of the distal sesamoid in the region of the sagittal ridge. This is an unfavorable prognostic sign.

angle, and conformation must be analyzed and corrective shoeing adjusted on the basis of the individual case. An egg bar shoe is indicated in

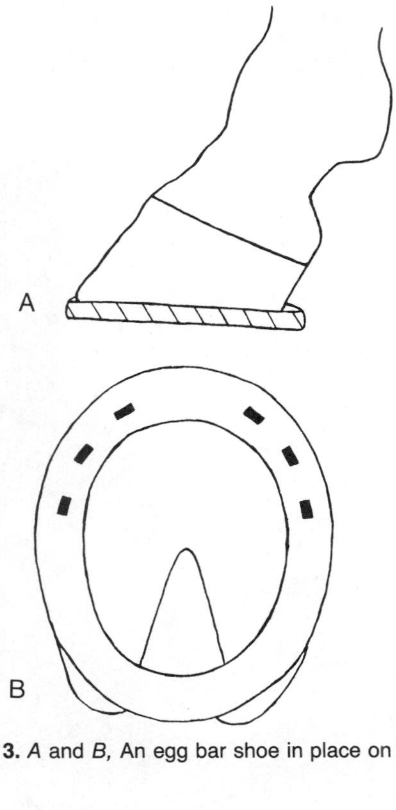

Figure 3. *A* and *B,* An egg bar shoe in place on the hoof.

more horses than is the more traditional wedge pad technique.

Phenylbutazone is effective in horses with navicular disease and when used in appropriate doses can prolong the horse's useful life. It can be given at a dose of 1 to 2 gm a day orally for months at a time or it can be used intermittently for short periods to allow the horse to maximize performance. Phenylbutazone masks the clinical signs and by reducing inflammation relieves pain but does not treat the disease itself.

Isoxuprine is a peripheral vasodilating drug that has been used successfully to treat horses with navicular disease. The recommended dose is 0.6 mg per kg twice a day for periods of 6 to 14 weeks. Although this drug appears to have beneficial effects in some horses, our observed recurrence rate has been fairly high. More research and experience with this drug is necessary before firm conclusions can be made; however, it appears that the drug is less successful than previously reported.

Palmar digital neurectomy is the last consideration in horses that are unresponsive to corrective shoeing and to dosages of phenylbutazone or isoxuprine or both. Each horse must be carefully evaluated as a neurectomy candidate. Horses that remain lame following a bilateral PDN block are not good candidates since lameness will persist after the nerves are severed. It is also important to be sure that just the heels are desensitized when examining these horses. Horses with radiographic evidence of erosion of the flexor surface of the distal sesamoid may have adhesions to the DDF tendon and are not good candidates for neurectomy. A neurectomy should be considered a temporary solution. The nerves can regrow, neuromas can develop, or eventually adhesion to the DDF tendon occurs and the tendon becomes painful above the desensitized area. On the other hand, neurectomy does allow some horses to return to athletic soundness, in some cases for several years.

Although navicular disease is common, it is also excessively diagnosed. There are many causes of heel soreness, such as unbalanced heels, improper shoeing, and stone bruises. As we learn more about navicular disease it appears that currently several diseases we cannot accurately differentiate are lumped together as navicular disease.

DISTAL SESAMOID FRACTURES

Fracture of the distal sesamoid usually results from a trauma to the foot from an uneven surface or a blunt object. Horses with such fractures are quite lame and very sensitive to hoof testers over the frog after the acute injury. If the fracture has been present for some time, lameness and sensitivity to hoof testers may be decreased. A PDN block markedly improves the lameness. The clinician making a diagnosis of a fractured distal sesamoid relies on high-quality radiographs (Fig. 4). Packing the collateral sulci of the foot on either side of the frog with Play-Doh or similar materials eliminates the air pattern on the radiographs (see p. 260). The skyline radiographic projection is also helpful in

evaluating fractures of the navicular bone. Bipartite or tripartite navicular bones result from abnormal ossification of the navicular bone and are present at birth. They are distinguished from fractures by the relative symmetry of the ossification centers and wide lucent lines separating them. These congenital anomalies are usually bilateral. They may predispose to fractures along the cartilage lines.

Treatment. Successful treatment of fractures of the navicular bone is difficult. The navicular bone is slow to heal and healing is further delayed by the flux of synovial fluid between the navicular bursa and distal interphalangeal joint through the fracture line. One treatment is to immobilize the foot with a bar shoe and clips and give the horse eight months of stall rest. Another option is to perform a palmar digital neurectomy, which relieves the pain and permits use of the horse. However, the fracture does communicate with the joint and continued use with an unstable fracture can eventually lead to degenerative joint disease and pain beyond the desensitized area. It is preferable to delay the neurectomy until a fibrous union has occurred at the fracture site. In many cases only a fibrous union will occur and radiographic evidence of bone union should not be expected in distal sesamoid fractures.

Successful repair of a distal sesamoid fracture has been accomplished using a lag screw placed through the hoof wall. The technique employed an aiming device and intraoperative fluoroscopy to align the screw correctly. It is a difficult technique that requires the appropriate equipment and experi-

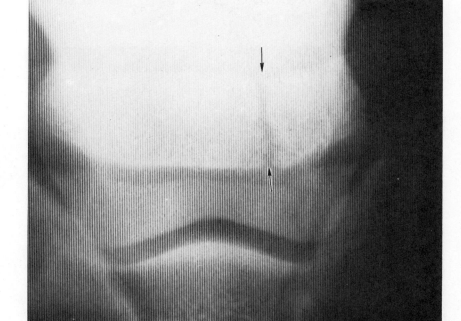

Figure 4. Dorsoproximal-palmarodistal view showing a fracture of the distal sesamoid (*arrows*). The film was made using a stationary grid and the vertical grid lines are seen on this close-up photograph.

ence. The risk of infection exists during the postoperative period while the hoof wall is healing.

SIDEBONES

Sidebones are ossification of the cartilages of the distal phalanx and are usually seen only in the front feet. The specific cause of sidebone formation is unknown but increased concussion in the heel is commonly incriminated. Some horses may have a predisposition to this condition. Regardless of the cause, sidebones rarely result in lameness and are frequently an incidental finding. They are a source of lameness only if fractured or when they are extremely large and interfere with the DDF tendon or middle phalanx. Diagnosing sidebones as a cause of lameness can be done only after a careful clinical examination, radiographs, and diagnostic nerve blocks have been used to rule out other more common causes of lameness.

There is some variation in the degree and rate of ossification of the cartilages. Small sidebones in which the cartilage has just started to ossify are clinically inapparent and found only on radiographs. Large sidebones in which most of the cartilage has turned to bone are easily palpable over the horse's heel. If the sidebones are causing a problem, slight heat and increased sensitivity can be detected over the involved heel. Comparison should be made between the medial and lateral sidebones as well as any on the opposite foot. Radiographs of the foot may confirm a fractured sidebone; however, the separate center of ossification in the cartilage usually results in a division between the sidebone and the distal phalanx. This should not be mistaken for a fracture line (Fig. 5). Diagnosing a large sidebone

as a cause of lameness is more difficult, the clinical findings and response to local anesthesia must be relied upon. These horses become sound when just the suspected side (medial or lateral) of the heel is desensitized with a PDN block; they do not improve when the distal interphalangeal joint or navicular bursa is injected with local anesthetic.

Treatment. Treatment for horses with a fractured sidebone or with an excessively large sidebone involves surgical removal of the ossified cartilage. Horses with fractured sidebones may be treated conservatively with rest. However, the bone is slow to heal and the injury is likely to recur with a return to work and increased concussion.

CONDITIONS THAT IMPROVE WHEN THE ENTIRE FOOT IS DESENSITIZED

The nerves supplying the horse's foot are commonly anesthetized at one of three sites on the lower leg: the dorsal and palmar branches of the medial and lateral digital nerves at the level of the pastern, the same nerves over the abaxial surface of the proximal sesamoid bones, and the traditional "low volar block," in which the medial and lateral digital nerves before they branch proximal to the metacarpophalangeal joint are anesthetized. Of these, the dorsal and palmar (plantar) digital nerve (D & PDN) block is preferred because it is more specific and does not desensitize structures higher on the limb. This nerve block is performed by injecting 2 to 3 ml of local anesthetic through a 22-gauge 1-inch needle, which is initially placed through the skin caudal to the PDN. The needle is

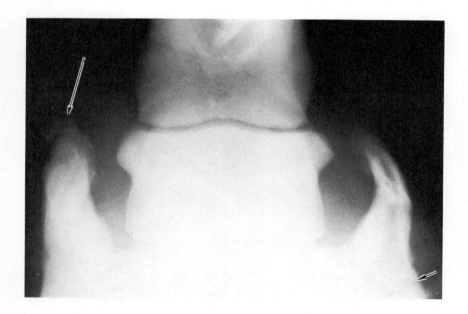

Figure 5. Dorsopalmar view of the hoof of a draft horse with large sidebones. A separate ossification center (*long arrow*) is seen at the tip of one sidebone. A lucent line (*short arrow*) is present where the mineralized cartilage has not united with the distal phalanx. This horse was not lame. The sidebone was presumed to be incidental.

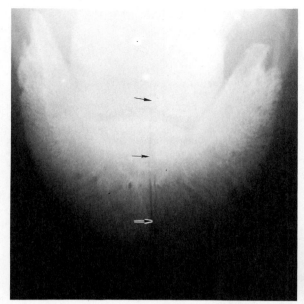

Figure 6. Dorsoproximal-palmarodistal view showing a mid-sagittal distal phalanx fracture (*arrows*). Although the fracture line appears to cross the joint proximally, it actually passes to the palmar margin of the distal phalanx.

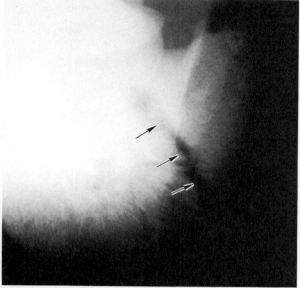

Figure 8. Dorsoproximal-palmarodistal oblique view showing a fracture (*arrows*) of one palmar process of the distal phalanx. This fracture appears to enter the joint.

DISTAL PHALANX FRACTURES

Fractures of the distal phalanx are not an uncommon injury. Although most fractures occur when the horse is working at speed, they also can result from the horse kicking a wall. Acutely, horses with a distal phalanx fracture are quite lame with an increased pulse in the digital arteries and marked sensitivity to hoof testers over the sole. With time the pulse will be less noticeable and the sensitivity to hoof testers will become localized to the area of the fracture. Clinical signs are similar to those displayed by horses with a sole abscess or a severe sole bruise; radiographs of the foot are necessary to confirm a fracture. Distal phalanx fractures tend to occur through only one plane and are not usually comminuted. The fracture line must be distinguished from the vascular channels that radiate from the semicircular (solar) canal to the periphery of the bone. In acute cases the fracture may not be visible. Repeat radiographs may be necessary 7 to 10 days later when bone demineralization has occurred at the site of injury demonstrating the fracture line. Classification and treatment of fractures of the distal phalanx are based on their location in the bone.

Midsagittal fractures (type III) divide the bone in half and enter the joint (Fig. 6). Treatment is aimed at immobilizing the distal phalanx until bone union can occur. A bar shoe with side clips stabilizes the bone within the hoof by preventing normal expansion of the hoof wall during weight-bearing (Fig. 7). The side clips should extend well up the hoof wall and should be placed toward the heel of the foot. A bar shoe with a full rim around its edge serves

then directed dorsally and local anesthetic is infiltrated along a line extending in front of the digital triad. This nerve block desensitizes all of the structures in the foot distal to the coronary band and part or all of the proximal interphalangeal joint. The abaxial nerve block is technically easier because the nerves are readily palpated over the abaxial surface of the proximal sesamoid bones. However, this nerve block desensitizes more of the lower limb and it is possible to confuse a sesamoid lesion (which is anesthetized by local diffusion of the anesthetic) with a problem in the foot. This is also true for the medial and lateral digital nerve block proximal to the metacarpophalangeal joint, which desensitizes even more of the fetlock.

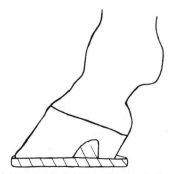

Figure 7. A bar shoe with side clips in place on the hoof.

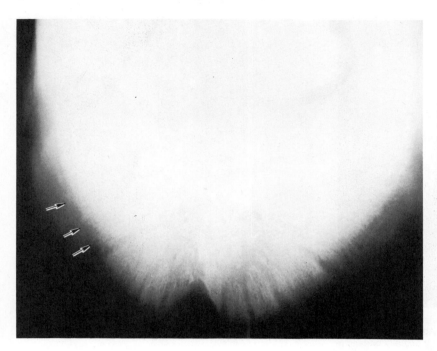

Figure 9. Dorsoproximal-palmarodistal view of a distal phalanx showing pedal osteitis. One solar margin is more irregular (*arrows*) than the opposite side. Some degree of normal variation can be expected and caution should be used in radiographic interpretation of this area. The presence of appropriate clinical signs is significant in the diagnosis. This horse also shows an unusually deep notch (crena) at the tip of the distal phalanx, which may not be significant.

the same purpose but is more difficult to make and requires an exact fit to the foot. A full pad is sometimes used under the shoe to protect the bottom of the foot. Internal fixation of distal phalanx fractures has been accomplished using a lag screw placed through the hoof wall. However, the procedure involves a high risk of infection, the cupped shape of the coffin bone necessitates precise screw placement to achieve accurate alignment, and the porous nature of the bone makes it difficult to maintain interfragmentary compression because of bone lysis around the head of the screw. Regardless of the method of stabilization employed, horses with distal phalanx fractures should be confined to a stall for six to eight months to allow time for adequate healing. Recurrence of the fracture following a return to exercise in some cases suggests that the foot should be kept in a bar shoe with quarter clips even after the fracture has healed. The prognosis for horses with a midsagittal fracture is only fair regardless of the treatment selected. Since lag screw fixation increases the expense and the possibility of complications, corrective shoeing is currently preferred.

Alar fractures or fractures of the palmar process of the distal phalanx may or may not communicate with the joint (Fig. 8). Fractures of the palmar process that enter the joint (type II) are managed similarly to midsagittal fractures. Internal fixation of these fractures with a lag screw is more difficult because the fragment is small, leaving very little bone through which a lag screw can be accurately placed. Therefore, use of a bar shoe and clips is the

preferred method of treatment. Fractures that do not communicate with the joint (type I) should also be correctively shod to minimize motion at the fracture site. However, because these fractures are in the area innervated by the palmar digital nerve, a neurectomy should also be considered. Although it is preferable to allow at least a fibrous union to develop before the neurectomy, a neurectomy performed in the acute case will also return these horses to soundness. Only the PDN to the affected heel needs to be cut to desensitize the fracture. Horses with fractures involving the joint will not become sound following a neurectomy because the entire distal interphalangeal joint is not desensitized by a palmar digital neurectomy. The prognosis for fractures is good for those that do not enter the joint, but only fair for those that involve the joint.

Marginal fractures of the third phalanx are not common. They occur at the periphery of the bone where it is thin and susceptible to trauma. The presence of bone pathology such as osteomyelitis may predispose the horse to fracture but pathologic changes are not necessary for this fracture to occur. Radiographs must be examined carefully to avoid missing these small fragments along the margins of the bone, especially if the radiographic technique used is for the navicular bone and the distal phalanx is overexposed. Treatment is similar to other P3 fractures; the horse is placed in a bar shoe with quarter clips.

Fractures of the extensor process of P3 (type IV) result in swelling dorsal to the coronary band at the front of the foot. They are an avulsion fracture in

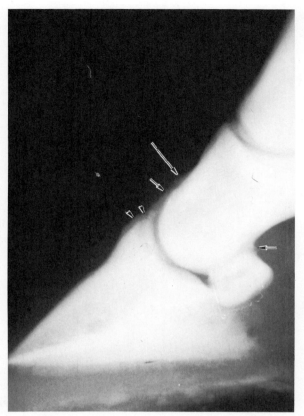

Figure 10. Lateromedial view of a horse with low ringbone. The extensor process has irregular margins (*arrowheads*) and there is osteophyte production (*short arrows*) on the distal margins of the middle phalanx. The periosteal irregularity seen proximal to the joint (*long arrow*) is not articular and probably represents the rough margin of the collateral ligament fossa as it is projected on this view.

the attachment of the common digital extensor tendon. Fractures of the extensor process are variable in size; treatment depends on the size of the fragment. Smaller fragments can be surgically removed and larger fragments can be stabilized with a lag screw. Prolonged rest is a third treatment option. Regardless of how these fractures are managed, the prognosis is poor because of the degenerative joint disease that frequently results.

PEDAL OSTEITIS

Pedal osteitis is a radiographic diagnosis. Reactive changes in and around the margin of the distal phalanx result in rough and irregular borders of the bone, best seen on a dorsoproximal-palmarodistal view (Fig. 9). On the lateromedial projection there is spur formation and remodeling of the tip of the distal phalanx with new bone production. These changes result from inflammation of the sensitive tissue around the bone. Laminitis, subsolar abscess,

and chronic bruising can all cause these changes. Also, horses that are worked on a hard surface can develop these changes in response to chronic increased concussion. Pedal osteitis is not a clinical diagnosis and treatment should be aimed at the primary cause of these changes—for example, laminitis or sole abscess. Horses with sore feet from hard work should be shod with a full pad to protect the foot.

OSTEOARTHRITIS OF THE DISTAL INTERPHALANGEAL JOINT

Another term for osteoarthritis of the distal interphalangeal joint is low ringbone. This is distinguished from pyramidal disease and buttress foot, which refer to bony reaction around the extensor process from pulling of the attachments of the common digital extensor tendon. Osteoarthritis of the distal interphalangeal joint results from repeated wear and tear injury to the joint. Poor hoof care leading to a broken hoof axis or an unbalanced foot (longer on one side than the other) can contribute to the development of degenerative joint disease. Bony reaction of the extensor process may also occur in horses with degenerative joint disease. Horses with low ringbone have a firm swelling just above the coronary band on the front of the foot that is differentiated from the enlargement that occurs with osteoarthritis of the proximal interphalangeal joint by its more distal location on the limb. These horses resent flexion of the lower limb and lameness is increased by this manipulation. The diagnosis of low ringbone is confirmed by radiographs demonstrating osteophyte production, periosteal new bone production around the joint, and thinning of the joint space (Fig. 10). The roughened area of attachment of the collateral ligaments on the lateral and medial surface of the middle phalanx is normal and should not be misdiagnosed as a sign of low ringbone. Pyramidal disease is distinguished from osteoarthritis of the distal interphalangeal joint by the lack of bony reaction on P2, but differentiating between these two problems is not of great importance since the treatment and prognosis is similar for both.

Treatment of horses with low ringbone involves correcting any abnormal hoof-pastern conformation problems, balancing the foot, trimming the toe short, and rolling the toe of the shoe to encourage early breakover of the foot. The prognosis for these horses returning to complete soundness is poor and phenylbutazone is frequently necessary for the horse to function. Some horses will be able to continue for several years on phenylbutazone. Fusion of the distal interphalangeal joint is not a viable alternative because such horses are not sound.

HEMATOPOIETIC DISEASES

Edited by Debra Deem Morris

Evaluation of the Erythron

John C. Bloom, PHILADELPHIA, PENNSYLVANIA

Kate A. W. Roby, KENNETT SQUARE, PENNSYLVANIA

Evaluating the erythron and determining the significance of changes in red cell mass parameters in the horse poses a diagnostic challenge that is unique to this species. In this chapter we will review the circumstances that complicate investigations of pathogenesis and causes of anemia in the horse. Our discussion will focus on the principles and laboratory tests useful in establishing the pathogenesis and causes of these disorders. Subsequent chapters in this section include a more comprehensive discussion of diagnosis and management of specific diseases causing equine anemia.

SPECIAL FEATURES OF THE EQUINE ERYTHRON

Features unique to the equine erythron that profoundly complicate and sometimes confound diagnostic efforts include the wide range of normal erythron values, the role of the spleen in red cell storage and distribution, the dirth of peripheral blood changes reflecting the bone marrow's response to anemia, the characteristics of the red cell itself, and the distribution of hematopoietic cells in the equine bone marrow. In order to interpret hematologic data correctly, the clinician must understand these characteristics, which distinguish the horse from other domestic mammals.

Normal red cell mass values (packed cell volume [PCV], red cell count, and hemoglobin concentration) vary according to age (Table 1), breed (Table 2), type of activity in which the horse is engaged, and level of training. Consequently, the reference range for the PCV in the horse can extend from 23 to 55 per cent, depending on the aforementioned factors. Racing Thoroughbreds in training tend to have the highest erythrocyte parameters. Unconditioned horses have lower PCVs and "cold-blooded" and draft breeds the lowest PCV of all.

Perhaps most unique among the factors important in the hematologic assessment of the horse is the nature of the equine spleen. The extensive muscular, highly innervated red pulp of this organ holds up to one third of the red cell mass. This reserve may be rapidly released into the circulation on adrenergic stimulation, resulting in as much as a 50 per cent increase in PCV during excitement or vigorous exercise. Because individual horses respond differently to stress associated with exercise, shipping, and examination by a veterinarian, red cell distribution is an important variable to consider when assessing red cell mass.

Unlike most other domestic species in which the

TABLE 1. ERYTHROCYTE PARAMETERS IN YOUNG HORSES

	RBC (× 10^6/μl)	Hb (gm/dl)	PCV (%)	MCV (fl)
1 day	10.5 ± 1.4	14.2 ± 1.3	41.7 ± 3.6	40.1 ± 3.8
2–7 days	9.5 ± 0.8	12.7 ± 0.9	37.1 ± 2.8	39.2 ± 2.8
8–14 days	9.0 ± 0.8	11.8 ± 1.2	34.9 ± 3.7	39.1 ± 2.2
21–30 days	11.2 ± 1.3	13.1 ± 1.1	37.8 ± 3.3	34.0 ± 2.4
1–3 months	11.9 ± 1.3	13.4 ± 1.6	38.3 ± 4.1	32.4 ± 1.9
8–18 months	8.6 ± 0.6	11.8 ± 1.6	34.5 ± 3.8	40.1 ± 2.9

Data from Schalm, O. W., Jain, N. C., and Carroll, E. J.: Veterinary Hematology, 3rd ed. Philadelphia, Lea and Febiger, 1975.

red cells are released as reticulocytes into the blood, the equine red cell appears to remain in the bone marrow until fully mature, even when erythropoiesis is intense. Consequently, reticulocytosis, polychromasia, macrocytosis, marked anisocytosis, and metarubricytosis, which reflect the release of less mature red cells into the blood and are useful indications in other animals of a regenerative anemia, are not commonly observed in horses. Howell-Jolly bodies, although present in small numbers in normal horses, may be increased during regenerative anemia. Mild to moderate anisocytosis may also be observed. Occasional reticulocytes may sometimes be seen, appearing in the blood as the PCV falls to 10 per cent or below. These subtle changes are most discernible on smears stained with new methylene blue. The absence of clear indications in the peripheral blood of increased erythropoietic activity in the bone marrow often makes it difficult to adequately assess the erythron of anemic horses using peripheral blood alone.

Red blood cell creatine concentration has been used in the horse to indicate the presence of young red cells in the peripheral blood and therefore a regenerative response. Although this biochemical assay is relatively easy to set up and shows promise as a peripheral reflection of bone marrow erythroid activity, it has yet to be widely employed for this purpose.

The small red cell size and tendency to exhibit rouleaux formation (in which the erythrocytes appear stacked like coins) serve to obscure changes in red cell morphology, thus further complicating the morphologic assessment. Marked rouleaux formation may sometimes be confused with the autoagglutination associated with autoimmune hemolytic anemia. Because rouleaux formation depends on protein concentration, the two may be distinguished by simply diluting the blood with normal saline before examining under the microscope. The tendency of normal horse red cells to exhibit rouleaux formation also causes an increased sedimentation rate, necessitating more thorough mixing of the blood sample before erythron parameters are measured.

Finally, the myeloid:erythroid (M:E) ratio of normal horse bone marrow is usually considerably lower than that of other species. Interpretation of an erythroid response, based on marrow observations, must be made with care. Human pathologists or hematologists assisting the veterinary clinician in the interpretation of such specimens must therefore be reminded of this special feature, as well as the others just described.

DIAGNOSTIC APPROACH TO ANEMIA

Anemia, or decreased oxygen-carrying capacity of the blood, is a common complication of a variety of disorders. As such, it is important that the clinician determine the underlying cause, the extent to which the problem contributes to the clinical signs, and rational therapy for the disease. A thoughtful approach to determining the cause of anemia must include a working understanding of fundamental principles of clinical hematology. Among these is the fact that all anemias occur in one of four ways: (1) loss of red cells, (2) increased red cell destruction, (3) decreased red cell production, or (4) a combination of these three disorders. Anemias due solely to blood loss or hemolysis are regenerative, with increased red cell production (erythroid hyperplasia) in the bone marrow and, in species other than the horse, the appearance of immature red cells in the peripheral blood. Anemias associated with bone marrow depression are nonregenerative and do not show these signs. The judicious use of information derived from the clinical history, physical examination, and laboratory observations allow the clinician to characterize the anemia in one of these two categories and determine which of these pathogeneses are probable. By following a logical sequence of diagnostic steps, while mindful of both

TABLE 2. DIFFERENCE IN ERYTHROCYTE PARAMETERS BETWEEN LIGHT AND HEAVY BREEDS

	Light Breeds		Heavy Breeds	
	Range	*Mean*	*Range*	*Mean*
PCV (%)	32.0–53.0	41.0	24.0–44.0	35.0
RBC (× 10^6/μl)	6.8–12.9	9.0	5.5–9.5	7.5
Hb (gm/dl)	11.0–19.0	14.4	8.0–14.0	11.5

Data from Schalm, O. W., Jain, N. C., and Carroll, E. J.: Veterinary Hematology, 3rd ed. Philadelphia, Lea and Febiger, 1975.)

the special features of the equine erythron and diseases associated with anemia in this species, the veterinary practitioner can arrive at a diagnosis for most anemias that occur in practice.

It is axiomatic that primary hematologic disorders are uncommon, whereas changes in blood parameters secondary to systemic disease or disorders of other organ systems are common. For this reason, a detailed history of the illness, as well as a thorough physical examination, form the indispensable foundation of clinical investigation of anemia and an essential context within which rational interpretation of laboratory data can be made. This information also allows the clinician to begin to narrow the differential for mechanisms of the anemia from the broad categories just outlined.

Of historic importance, in this regard, is the time course of the illness, the drug and deworming history, diet, pasture, or housing conditions, and status of Coggins testing. The horse's travel history may be influential in the consideration of some parasitic or viral disorders that cause anemia and have specific geographic distributions. An alert owner can also be encouraged to recount illnesses or observations in the past suggestive of chronic disease that may now be subclinical and associated with anemia. Clinical or accompanying laboratory data defining the onset and progression of the anemia, although seldom available, are particularly helpful. Rapidly declining red cell mass values indicate blood loss or hemolytic disease, whereas a slowly falling hematocrit is compatible with impaired red cell production.

Clinical signs referable to the anemia itself include exercise intolerance, tachycardia, tachypnea, pale mucous membranes, a low-grade systolic murmur, and depression. Other clinical signs may be useful in helping to determine the mechanism of the anemia. Fever, icterus, and red urine (hemoglobinuria) are signs of acute hemolytic disease. Dark tarry feces, red urine (hematuria), and evidence of epistaxis are among the signs that indicate possible sources of chronic blood loss. The presence of chronic disease in other organ systems—particularly respiratory and gastrointestinal—may be the most important information to consider in the diagnostic work-up for mild to moderate anemia, as chronic inflammatory disease is the most common cause of this condition in the horse. Underlying disorders, such as an abdominal abscess or tumor, may often present a diagnostic problem requiring considerable detective work.

Initial laboratory observations, including a complete blood count, total plasma protein, and plasma fibrinogen concentration, serve to define the severity of the anemia and provide further clues as to the pathogenesis and etiology of the problem. Despite the special features already discussed, which severely limit the sensitivity with which erythroid regenerative and hemolytic processes are reflected peripherally in the horse, a substantial amount of information can be gained through these routine observations. Red cell mass parameters must be interpreted in the context of total plasma protein (or total solids) and the clinical assessment of whether excitement or dehydration was present at the time the sample was collected, as discussed later in this chapter. Red cell morphology, although not as revealing as in species that show regenerative changes peripherally and have larger red cells, will show fragmentation with extensive thrombotic or defibrinating disorders, spherocytosis with immunoinjury, the refractile membrane inclusions associated with oxidative insults and red cell parasites, among other reflections of primary and secondary hematopathology. Red cell indices also lack the sensitivity of those of other species, although a progressively increasing mean corpuscular volume (often remaining within the normal range) can be observed with regenerative anemia. Microcytic, hypochromic, and macrocytic states are otherwise seldom observed in the horse, with the latter seen on rare occasions with severe iron deficiency anemia. The leukogram and plasma fibrinogen concentration are useful barometers for intercurrent inflammatory disease or more specific insults (such as the eosinophilia seen occasionally with parasitic disease). Thus they point to other possible causes of anemia.

In most domestic species the clinician has adequate information at this juncture to prepare a working differential diagnosis. In the horse, however, for reasons already discussed, a bone marrow examination is often necessary to adequately characterize the anemia as regenerative or nonregenerative. This step is therefore required more frequently and earlier in the investigation than in other domestic animals. Bone marrow can be collected under field conditions from the rib, iliac crest, or sternum. A practical method for obtaining a bone marrow sample from the sternum is as follows:

Clip and aseptically scrub a small area of skin just behind the olecranon over the ventral midline or fibrous juncture of the deep pectoral muscles. Swab the area with 70 per cent alcohol. Grasp a three-and-a-half inch, 18-gauge, disposable spinal needle with your gloved hand, holding it between thumb and forefinger approximately one inch from the tip, while anchoring the hub of the needle against your palm. Insert the needle with a rapid thrust perpendicularly through the fibrous midline into the subcutaneous tissue. After rapidly penetrating the skin, advance the needle more slowly until the tip comes to rest on the hard ventral cortex of the sternum. Grasping the hub of the needle, slowly rotate the needle back and forth, working the tip into the bone. As it becomes firmly embedded in the bone (the cortex of the sternum is thin

TABLE 3. ETIOLOGIC CLASSIFICATION
OF ANEMIAS

I. Blood loss
  A. Chronic bleeding
    1. Gastrointestinal (ulcers, neoplasia)
    2. Urinary (urolithiasis)
    3. Hemostatic disorders (immune-mediated thrombocytopenia, chronic liver disease, congenital defect)
    4. Blood-sucking parasites (ascarids, strongyles, ticks, lice)
  B. Acute bleeding
    1. Trauma
    2. Surgery
    3. Dicoumarin poisoning (warfarin, sweet clover)
    4. Thrombocytopenia (drug-induced, myelophthisic, immune-mediated thrombocytopenia)
    5. Other (ruptured abscess, guttural pouch mycosis, hemophilia)
II. Increased red cell destruction
  A. Toxic
    1. Oxidants (drugs, onions, nitrites, red maple leaves)
    2. Bacterial toxins (staphylococcal, clostridial)
    3. Heavy metals (copper, lead, iron?)
    4. Other (snake venom)
  B. Infectious
    1. Red cell parasites (babesia, ehrlichia)
    2. Leptospirosis
    3. Equine infectious anemia
  C. Immune-mediated
    1. Neonatal isoerythrolysis
    2. Autoimmune (idiopathic, poststreptococcal, lymphosarcoma)
    3. Transfusion reactions
  D. Mechanical damage (disseminated intravascular coagulation, vasculitis, endocarditis)
  E. Congenital disorders
III. Decreased red cell production
  A. Anemia of chronic inflammatory disease
  B. Nutritional deficiency (protein, iron, cobalt, iron, copper, B_{12}, folate)
  C. Myelophthisis (lymphosarcoma)
  D. Aplastic anemia (drug-induced, toxic)

and easily penetrated), remove the stylet and connect a 20- or 30-cc syringe. Pull back rapidly and firmly on the plunger and release it immediately. The objective is to exert negative pressure strong enough to break apart the marrow stroma, sucking it into the needle, but not to exert prolonged suction that would allow blood to enter the puncture site and dilute the specimen. Repeat the process twice or until marrow appears from the hub of the needle in the syringe. If no marrow is obtained, replace the stylet, advance the needle slightly, and repeat the aspirate. Occasionally, the needle is positioned in an intersternebral junction, in which case it must be repositioned and the aspirate repeated. As soon as marrow is observed, stop the aspiration and immediately remove the needle and syringe together. Push the contents of the needle onto clean slides, placing one small drop near the frosted end of several slides. Holding the slide with one hand, place another clean slide face down over the drop of marrow so that the drop begins to spread in a thin layer between the slides. Pull the slides apart, sliding one over the other to create a thin smear. Dry the smear

quickly by waving it in the air. In order to have cell morphology adequate for interpretation, the smears must be both thin and rapidly dried to prevent cell distortion. Once dry, the smears may be transported or stored for several weeks. If they are to be stored unstained for longer periods, they should be fixed (about 3 min) in methanol. The marrow smears may be stained routinely, as one would stain peripheral blood smears, or special stains (new methylene blue, Prussian blue, Gram stain) may be applied.

Interpretation of an erythroid response is predicated on an M:E ratio of 0.5:1 or less, in the absence of concurrent inflammation, and in the presence of readily demonstrable marrow reticulocytes or polychromatophilic red cells. The latter observation is required for the interpretation of increased effective erythropoiesis. Obviously, defining the bone marrow response to anemia has prognostic as well as diagnostic implications. On the basis of information derived from the history, physical examination, and initial laboratory observations, and after characterization of the anemia, the differential diagnosis can be narrowed. Helpful in this effort is knowledge of diseases associated with anemia in the horse and their pathogenesis. Some of these disorders are listed in Table 3.

Additional laboratory tests can now be performed that specifically address the causes suspected. For example, an acute onset of depression with fever, icterus, hemoglobinuria, and a rapidly declining hematocrit in a horse that has recently received a sulfa antibiotic should raise the suspicion of drug-induced oxidative hemolytic disease. The clinician may therefore request that a test for Heinz bodies be performed. The practitioner could easily investigate this possibility by staining a peripheral blood smear with new methylene blue and examining the red cells for the small refractile membrane-bound inclusions. A bone marrow examination may not be necessary to reach a diagnosis in this case.

The etiology and even the mechanism of anemia, however, are often less obvious. An animal may be presented with a mild anemia for which the history, physical examination, and initial laboratory data provide no explanation. An erythroid hyperplastic, or regenerative, bone marrow indicates the probability of blood loss or low-grade hemolytic disease. The latter possibility can be investigated by ordering a red cell osmotic fragility test. An abnormally increased osmotic fragility indicates that the red cells are compromised or damaged and is suggestive of hemolytic disease. Conversely, increased resistance to hypotonic lysis suggests a regenerative response with a greater portion of less mature cells in the circulation. Subsequent laboratory investigations—such as serologic tests for antibodies against the equine infectious anemia virus or babesia, an antiglobulin (Coombs') test for the presence of red cell antibodies, or a test for Heinz bodies—may be necessary in order to find the cause and mechanism of the anemia.

Often several mechanisms contribute to the anemia but hold little diagnostic significance and need not be demonstrated in the laboratory. For example, a horse with a history of upper respiratory infection presenting with extensive lesions suggestive of purpura hemorrhagica may show moderate to severe anemia. Chronic inflammation leading to decreased red cell production, blood loss due to the vascular lesions, and fibrin-mediated hemolysis may all contribute significantly to the anemia. The history and physical findings, however, hold far greater diagnostic and therapeutic significance in this case

than laboratory tests documenting these mechanisms.

Supplemental Readings

Archer, R. K., and Jeffcott, L. B.: Comparative Clinical Hematology. London, Blackwell Scientific Publications, 1977.

Gerber, H., Tschudi, P., and Straub, R.: Normal values for different breeds of horses. 1st Int. Symp. Eq. Hematol., Michigan State University, 1975, pp. 266–275.

Osbaldiston, G. W., Coffman, J. R., and Kruckenberg, S. M.: Biochemical differentiation of equine anemias. J. Am. Vet. Med. Assoc., *157*:322, 1970.

Schalm, O. W., Jain, N. C., and Carroll, E. J.: Veterinary Hematology, 3rd ed. Philadelphia, Lea & Febiger, 1975.

Schalm, O. W.: Bone marrow erythroid cytology in anemias of the horse. 1st Int. Symp. Eq. Hematol., Michigan State University, 1985, p. 17.

Hemolytic Anemias

Angeline Warner, BROOKLINE, MASSACHUSETTS
Debra Deem Morris, KENNETT SQUARE, PENNSYLVANIA

Although immune-mediated hemolytic anemia is relatively uncommon in adult horses, neonatal isoerythrolysis (NI), or hemolytic disease of the newborn, affects up to 1 per cent of Thoroughbred foals and is a major concern of the breeding industry. Because of their differences in etiology and therapy, these two entities will be considered separately.

NEONATAL ISOERYTHROLYSIS (HEMOLYTIC DISEASE OF NEWBORN)

Neonatal isoerythrolysis is destruction of erythrocytes in the newborn foal mediated by anti–red cell antibodies produced by the mare and absorbed by the foal from colostrum. The clinical disease has several prerequisites: (1) the mare must have been sensitized to incompatible red cell surface antigen(s) by retroplacental hemorrhage during a previous pregnancy, by previous whole blood or red cell–contaminated plasma transfusion, or by vaccine products contaminated by red cells; (2) the foal must inherit from the sire red cell surface antigens to which the mare has been sensitized; (3) the mare must mount an anamnestic response (usually subsequent to retroplacental hemorrhage) and concentrate anti–red cell IgG in the colostrum; and (4) the foal must suckle colostrum and absorb anti–red cell antibodies during the first 24 hours of life. When these stipulations are met, the foal will develop a peracute, acute, or insidious erythrocyte destruc-

tion depending on the dose of antibody absorbed. The clinical signs, diagnosis, treatment, and prevention of neonatal isoerythrolysis are described on p. 244.

IMMUNE-MEDIATED HEMOLYTIC ANEMIA IN THE ADULT

In contrast to hemolytic disease of the newborn, immune-mediated hemolysis is uncommon in the adult horse. There is acute or chronic red blood cell destruction due to antierythrocyte antibody coating of the red cells and consequent intravascular lysis or phagocytosis by macrophages of the reticuloendothelial system. The source of antibody may be idiopathic, and thus the disease is termed *autoimmune*. Alternatively, red cell cross-reacting antibody may have been formed in response to antigenic determinants in drugs, infectious agents, or neoplastic cells. The resulting anemia may be acute, but it is often chronic and insidious.

Clinical Signs. The patient may be any age or breed, and either sex. Clinical signs include exercise intolerance, weakness, and pale or icteric mucous membranes. Fever may or may not be present. Tachypnea and tachycardia may develop at rest, depending on the severity of anemia. Hemoglobinuria is uncommon.

A complete blood count shows anemia, with PCV often 10 to 20 per cent, and often a neutrophilic leukocytosis. The anemia is regenerative, but this is difficult to assess in the horse without a bone marrow aspirate. The most definitive diagnostic aid is a positive Coombs' (antiglobulin) test, which demonstrates the presence of antibody on red blood cells. At autopsy, horses that succumb have pale or icteric tissues and enlargement of liver and spleen.

The offending antibody is usually of the IgG class, and results in partial red cell phagocytosis, generating spherocytes, and finally hemolytic destruction, primarily in the spleen. Complement activation may or may not be involved but is necessary for significant intravascular hemolysis. Antierythrocyte antibody or immune complexes mediating red cell destruction may follow sensitization to an exogenously administered drug or to antigens from pathogenic microorganisms. Lymphoproliferative neoplasia can result in cross-reacting antibody to tumor antigen, or abnormal antibody production by neoplastic cells.

Therapy. Once the diagnosis is confirmed with the Coombs' test, any exogenous drug therapy should be discontinued. The PCV should be monitored and a transfusion performed (see p. 317) if the PCV drops below 12 per cent. Cross-matched donor blood is of utmost importance to prevent administration of red cells that will be rapidly hemolyzed. In some cases, however, it is difficult to perform the cross-match because of the fragile antibody-coated recipient cells and antierythrocyte antibody in the serum.

Glucocorticoids are important in therapy to decrease production of anti–red cell antibody and to decrease erythrophagocytosis of antibody-coated cells by the reticuloendothelial macrophages of the spleen and liver. Dexamethasone,* 0.1 to 0.2 mg per kg daily in one or two intramuscular or intravenous doses, or 2 to 3 mg per kg prednisolone† divided between two intramuscular doses each day, is recommended. Once the PCV has risen and the patient's condition stabilized, the dose of glucocorticoid should be gradually tapered to the lowest possible maintenance dosage and preferably alternate-day therapy. Oral prednisone‡ may be substituted for prednisolone once the disease is controlled. Splenectomy and cytotoxic drugs, which are therapeutic modalities used in small animals, are generally not economically feasible for horses.

Once the patient's condition is stabilized therapeutically, diagnostic efforts should be turned toward occult sites of infection or neoplasia, because long-term remission will be difficult to achieve if stimulation of antibody production continues.

---

*Azium, Schering Corp., Kenilworth, NJ
†Meticortelone Acetate, Schering Corp., Kenilworth, NJ
‡Deltasone, Upjohn Co., Kalamazoo, MI

OXIDANT-INDUCED HEMOLYTIC ANEMIA

The effects of oxidizing agents on red blood cells include formation of Heinz bodies (precipitated oxidized hemoglobin) or of methemoglobin (oxidation of iron from ferrous to ferric form). Phenothiazine-containing anthelmintics, wild onions, and red maple leaf toxin have been reported to induce Heinz body formation in the horse. Nitrites and red maple leaf toxin have been implicated in methemoglobin formation.

Clinical Signs. The clinical signs of oxidant-induced hemolytic anemia are similar regardless of the agent, and are sequelae of red blood cell destruction and hemoglobin release. Affected horses are weak, often depressed, and may have tachycardia and tachypnea. Mucous membranes and sclera are often icteric, but the color may be modified by cyanosis or the chocolate-brown of methemoglobin, resulting in gray- or bronze-tinged mucosae. Depending on the dose of oxidizing agent, the condition of individuals may deteriorate rapidly and they may be found moribund or dead. The urine is nearly always discolored by pigment and may range from wine-colored to brown or black. Neurologic deficits may be apparent, most likely due to hypoxemia resulting from reduced functional red cell mass.

Diagnosis. Differential diagnoses include the infectious causes of hemolysis discussed later in this article (piroplasmosis, ehrlichiosis, equine infectious anemia EIA) and immune-mediated hemolysis. The possible etiology of an oxidant insult is determined by demonstration of Heinz bodies in red cells or by the presence of methemoglobin. Heinz bodies are refractile precipitates of hemoglobin that attach to and bulge the erythrocyte membrane. They are best demonstrated with new methylene blue staining. The percentage of red cells containing Heinz bodies correlates with the oxidant dose and decreases gradually as the horse recovers. Methemoglobin imparts a chocolate color to blood. The amount can be quantitated spectrophotometrically at 630 nm. A Coombs' test, an examination of a routine blood smear, and a Coggins test can be used to help rule out immune-mediated hemolysis, Babesia infection, and EIA, respectively.

Affected horses show variably severe regenerative anemia, elevated aspartate aminotransferase (AST or SGOT), sorbitol dehydrogenase (SDH), creatine phosphokinase (CPK), and indirect bilirubin. There may be proteinuria and pigment-containing casts in urine sediment. Acute renal failure due to pigment nephropathy may ensue. Gross pathologic findings include generalized icterus, splenic engorgement, and discoloration of the kidneys. Microscopically there is erythrophagocytosis by macrophages of the reticuloendothelial system, pigment casts within renal tubules, some sloughing of renal epithelial cells, and lipid accumulation in hepatocytes.

Oxidation of iron from the ferrous to ferric form is the cause of methemoglobinemia. Oxidation also causes disulfide bond formation in the globin molecule, progressive denaturation, and finally precipitation as refractile Heinz bodies that attach to the cell membrane. The red cell is then rendered more osmotically fragile, less deformable, and more likely to be removed from circulation by reticuloendothelial macrophage phagocytosis. The functional red cell mass is reduced by intravascular hemolysis, erythrophagocytosis, and decreased oxygen-carrying capacity after methemoglobin formation. Red blood cells have several normal defense mechanisms against oxidation of iron and globin, but the equine erythrocyte has a decreased capacity for methemoglobin reduction, and is thus relatively susceptible to oxidant damage.

Differentiation among the various causes of oxidant-induced hemolytic anemia depends on history and potential exposure. Clinical signs of *red maple toxicity* appear within three to four days of ingestion of dried or withered leaves. The tree *(Acer rubrum)* is found in the United States from Texas to the east coast and north to Nova Scotia. There is an apparent seasonal incidence, with reported cases clustered from June to October. Fresh leaves are apparently not hazardous, and the toxic agent in the dried leaves is as yet undetermined. Both *wild and cultivated onions* (Allium sp.) have been reported to cause hemolytic disease in horses, with up to one week intervening between initial exposure and clinical signs. The toxic principle is *n*-propyl disulfide. Phenothiazine disulfide, a metabolite of phenothiazine absorbed from the intestine, can cause oxidant hemolysis in horses within one to two weeks of exposure. Individual susceptibility varies; some horses apparently have an idiosyncratic sensitivity, and debilitated animals may be affected at a dose that is safe for healthy animals. Nitrite toxicity occurs after metabolism of nitrate to nitrite within the cecum and colon.

Therapy. Therapy is independent of the etiologic agent, although determination of the cause is important to terminate exposure and reduce risk to other individuals. Efforts to terminate ongoing oxidant damage are generally not feasible. Methylene blue is relatively ineffective in methemoglobin reduction in equine erythrocytes, and may enhance Heinz body formation. Its use in horses has been disappointing. Corticosteroids may theoretically discourage phagocytosis of damaged erythrocytes by the reticuloendothelial system, but red cells containing Heinz bodies or methemoglobin have decreased oxygen-carrying capacity, and suppression of their phagocytosis does not augment the total functional erythrocyte mass.

Therapy is mainly supportive and is dictated by the degree of anemia. The patient should be kept in warm, comfortable quarters, and should not undergo stress. Supplemental oxygen or a whole blood transfusion (p. 317) may be warranted, depending on the degree of anemia and hypoxia. A cross-match should be performed whenever possible to avoid administration of incompatible blood resulting in additional hemolysis. Most patients experience some degree of dehydration and may require intravenous fluid replacement with a balanced electrolyte solution.

Attention should be paid to renal function because hemoglobin, especially coupled with dehydration and acidosis, may be nephrotoxic. Supplemental fluids to ensure adequate renal perfusion and glomerular filtration will help prevent formation of precipitated hemoglobin casts. Treatment of acidosis by administration of fluids containing isotonic bicarbonate is recommended.

The prognosis depends on the cumulative dose of oxidant and on the resulting degree of anemia. In cases of red maple leaf toxicity, demonstration of Heinz bodies has been associated with survival more often than has methemoglobinemia, but it is impossible to determine the toxic agent or give a definitive prognosis on the basis of which of these two oxidant products is present.

EQUINE INFECTIOUS ANEMIA

Equine infectious anemia (EIA) is a multisystemic disease caused by a retrovirus, which affects only members of the equine family. There is no predilection for age, sex, or breed. EIA occurs in a variety of clinical forms ranging from peracute to chronic, and some horses are inapparently infected. All infected horses, however, remain viremic and are persistent carriers of the virus for life. Blood from infected horses is the major source of virus for transmission of the disease, which occurs mechanically by blood-feeding vectors or through unsanitary veterinary procedures. In nature, the horsefly is by far the most significant vector because of its feeding habits and ability to transfer larger amounts of blood and virus.

The EIA virus multiplies in tissues throughout the body, especially the spleen, liver, kidneys, and cardiovascular system. Viral proteins elaborated in infected cells stimulate both T and B cell responses, with subsequent lymphoid hyperplasia and hypergammaglobulinemia in chronically infected horses. Damage to the vascular intima of small blood vessels leads to inflammatory changes in parenchymatous organs, particularly the liver. The virus persists, despite the presence of a high antibody titer. Signs wane when virus-neutralizing antibodies restrain viral multiplication. Recrudescence of clinical signs is due to the emergence of new antigenic variants of the virus.

Clinical Signs. Acute EIA is usually associated with first exposure to the virus, although inapparent carriers may develop acute clinical disease, especially during periods of stress. Fever, anorexia, and petechial hemorrhages on mucous membranes (especially the tongue and conjunctivae) may be evident 7 to 30 days after initial viral infection. This stage of the disease is generally transient but is often followed by recurring cycles of illness characterized by fever, edema, anemia, icterus, depression, and progressive weight loss. Less common signs include infertility, abortion, colic, and ataxia. The frequency and severity of these clinical episodes in horses with chronic EIA are unpredictable but usually decline with time. Stress, associated with adverse environmental or management conditions, can induce recrudescence of clinical disease in the horse with chronic EIA as well as previously inapparently infected horses. These bouts of illness may last a few days to several months and death may occur during any clinical flare-up.

Many of the clinical signs in chronic EIA are referable to the immune reactions to viral products. Anemia is thought to be immune-mediated, although this is not completely proven. Virus particles attach to erythrocytes, then are subsequently bound by antiviral antibodies that attract complement, and the complex is removed from circulation by the reticuloendothelial system. The bone marrow response to the anemia is inadequate, because of altered iron kinetics and control of erythropoiesis.

Clinical Laboratory Findings. Laboratory abnormalities vary with the stage of disease and none are pathognomonic for EIA. Although a mild thrombocytopenia occurs coincident with fever, it is not associated with excessive hemorrhage. Mild neutropenia, lymphocytosis, and monocytosis accompanies clinical EIA. Anemia of varying severity develops and worsens with each clinical flare-up. Initially the PCV returns to normal in the intervening periods, but the anemia may become unresponsive in horses with chronic EIA, which suffer multiple recurrent episodes of disease. Horses may have hyperbilirubinemia when there is rapid extravascular hemolysis, or significant hepatic involvement. Serum concentrations of biliary epithelial enzymes, gamma glutamyltransferase, and alkaline phosphatase are often elevated. Hypergammaglobulinemia results from the chronic viral antigenic stimulation.

Diagnosis. Chronic EIA can often be tentatively diagnosed on the basis of the history of recurrent bouts of fever, anorexia, icterus, edema, and ane-

mia, associated with chronic weight loss. However, none of the signs are pathognomonic and may individually or collectively be associated with several diseases, including abdominal abscessation, chronic pneumonia, chronic liver disease, internal neoplasia, purpura hemorrhagica, equine viral arteritis, and autoimmune hemolytic anemia. The geographic location can help in the diagnosis, since there is a much higher incidence of EIA in the southern and eastern United States due to the prevalence of insect vectors. The most practical procedure for diagnosis of EIA is the serum agar gel immunodiffusion test, which detects antibodies to the EIA virus (AGID or Coggins test). This test is accurate, sensitive, and positively correlated with viremia. False-positive results occur in noninfected foals that have acquired colostral antibodies from mares infected with EIA virus. False-negatives occur in cases of acute EIA when there has not been sufficient time for antibody production and in about 5 per cent of horses with chronic EIA, which are inapparently infected. Repeated testing can overcome some disadvantages: antibodies are usually detectable within 45 days of infection and are thought to persist for life; passively acquired antibodies are usually lost by six months of age, although some noninfected foals remain AGID-positive for up to nine months. The horse inoculation test is the most sensitive and certain means of detecting EIA virus in the blood of an infected horse. It is the only acceptable alternative diagnostic test for EIA approved by the United States Department of Agriculture. However, this test is expensive, time-consuming, and wasteful of equine resources.

Therapy. There is no known treatment to eliminate EIA virus from an infected horse. Supportive care such as rest, intravenous fluids, and blood transfusion may aid in clinical recovery; however, all horses surviving clinical EIA remain viremic, serve as a source of infection for other horses, and often have relapses.

Prevention. A satisfactory vaccine has not been produced, so the only effective preventive measures are aimed at identification and controlling the movement of infected horses. Precautions during surgical treatment, and injection procedures should be followed to prevent the passage of blood from an infected to a susceptible horse. However, most natural transmission occurs by the interrupted feeding of horseflies. All horses infected with EIA virus remain viremic and are therefore capable of spreading the disease, even though the potential of an inapparent carrier to do so is much smaller than that of the horse with clinical EIA. Frequent testing and removal of all AGID-test positive horses from an area is a successful method of local eradication. The United States Department of Agriculture does not have a program of eradication, but has established a national approved laboratory system for performing the AGID test. The interstate transport of animals with positive test results is prohibited. State regulations for the control of EIA vary considerably. Forty-two states require entering horses to have negative AGID test results, and about half of these require positive horses to be quarantined. Although transmission of EIA virus can be reduced by insect control procedures such as repellents and screening, this is not as effective as geographic isolation of infected horses. Studies on fly behavior indicate that a 200-yard buffer zone is an acceptable quarantine barrier.

EQUINE PIROPLASMOSIS (BABESIOSIS)

Equine piroplasmosis (EP) is caused by the hemoprotozoan parasites *Babesia caballi* or *Babesia equi*. Natural transmission occurs by ticks, although uncommonly the parasites can be mechanically transmitted by unsanitary veterinary practices. The prevalence of EP depends upon the presence of ticks to transmit the protozoa. Presently, only *B. caballi* is endemic in the United States and the tropical horse tick, *Dermacentor nitens*, is considered to be the principal vector. *Dermacentor nitens* is permanently established in areas where the average January temperature is greater than 60° F. The tick which generally infests the ears of equidae has been reported in Florida, Texas, Mexico, Cuba, Puerto Rico, Central and South America, and numerous Caribbean Islands. This tick is a one-host tick and transmits *B. caballi* transovarially. *Babesia equi* is transmitted by numerous species of ticks, and is endemic to Russia, Asia, India, Africa, Germany, France, and Brazil. No American ticks have been established as vectors of *B. equi*; however, *Rhipicephalus sanguineous* is the most likely potential vector.

Horses raised in EP-endemic areas are generally carriers of *Babesia* but rarely show clinical piroplasmosis. Foals are believed to experience subclinical infection once maternal antibodies have waned, then develop strong active immunity that depends upon constant presence of the organism. Stress such as heavy training, transport, and pregnancy may precipitate clinical signs in inapparent carriers.

Clinical Signs. Adult horses, originating from EP-free areas and placed in a pasture in EP-endemic areas, generally develop signs of acute EP in 7 to 21 days. Clinical signs include fever, depression, anorexia, tachypnea, pale or icteric mucous membranes, ecchymosis of the nictitans, and edema of the head, limbs, and ventral abdomen. Hemoglobinuria accompanies the severe anemia that develops due to intravascular destruction of parasitized erythrocytes. Infection by *B. equi* produces more severe clinical disease and some horses die of hypoxia during a hemolytic crisis, 24 to 48 hours after the onset of signs. Necropsy findings may include icterus, excessive fluid in serous cavities, bone marrow hyperplasia, splenomegaly, and hepatic centrilobular necrosis.

Diagnosis. Differential diagnosis of EP includes equine infectious anemia, purpura hemorrhagica, equine viral arteritis, and equine ehrlichiosis. Recent history of travel in tropical or subtropical areas of the world known to be endemic for *D. nitens* and EP is important in consideration of the disease. Evidence of past or present tick infestation also supports the diagnosis. Identification of the parasite by examination of blood smears is a positive method of diagnosis. However, negative results do not exclude the disease since parasitemia is brief and often precedes the onset of obvious clinical signs. The inoculation of susceptible horses with suspected parasitized blood is definitive but expensive and time-consuming. The complement-fixation (CF) test for EP detects antibodies to the protozoa, the presence of which usually indicates ongoing infection. Horses that survive clinical piroplasmosis remain inapparent carriers for several years unless they are treated. Serum (at least 5 ml, chilled) can be submitted to most state diagnostic laboratories, from which it is forwarded to the National Animal Disease Center in Ames, Iowa, for piroplasmosis testing. Since 1970, the United States Department of Agriculture has mandated that horses entering the country be CF test-negative for both *B. caballi* and *B. equi*. The CF test has been calibrated against transmission studies to determine the titer below which EP carrier horses cannot spread the disease.

Therapy. Treatment for EP differs for horses in nonenzootic and enzootic areas. When re-exposure is probable, the use of drugs in dosages that depress parasitemia and effect clinical remission of EP, without clearing the infection and its attendant premunition, is desirable. Imidocarb diproprionate [3.3′-bis-(2-imidazolin-2-yl) carbanilide dihydrochloride]* given once at a dosage of 2.2 mg per kg intramuscularly generally improves the clinical signs of EP. Control of EP in endemic areas is most effectively aimed at tick elimination.

Horses that live in or are being shipped to nonenzootic EP areas should be held in a tick-free environment and receive babesiacidal therapy. Infection with *B. caballi* is generally eliminated by imidocarb at a dosage of 2 mg per kg intramuscularly once daily for two treatments. *B. equi* is more resistant and the recommended dosage of imidocarb, 4 mg per kg intramuscularly every 72 hours

---

*Burroughs Wellcome Co., Research Triangle Park, NC

for four treatments, eliminates the infection from only 50 to 60 per cent of treated horses.

Side effects of imidocarb include colic, salivation, and diarrhea. Horses effectively cleared of *Babesia* remain positive to the CF test for several months.

EQUINE EHRLICHIOSIS

Equine ehrlichiosis is a blood-borne disease of horses caused by the rickettsial agent *Ehrlichia equi*. The disease is thought to be transmitted by ticks and usually occurs in horses maintained in the foothills of California's Sacramento Valley; however, cases have been reported in Florida, Colorado, Illinois, and New Jersey. Although clinically striking in horses, the incidence of equine ehrlichiosis is very low and mortality is rare. Dogs, cats, sheep, goats and nonhuman primates are susceptible to infection, but the natural reservoir of infection is unknown.

Clinical signs include fever, anorexia, depression, edema, mucosal petechiae, and ataxia. The incubation period in experimentally infected horses varies from one to nine days. Edema develops rapidly and may involve only the lower limbs, or include the ventral abdomen and prepuce. Fever usually abates after six days and edema resolves by two weeks. Death is rare. Laboratory abnormalities include leukopenia, thrombocytopenia, and anemia. Equine ehrlichiosis is diagnosed definitively by the presence of characteristic granular inclusion bodies in the cytoplasm of neutrophils and eosinophils on a blood smear stained with Giemsa, Wright-Giemsa, Wright-Leishman, or periodic acid-Schiff stain. The inclusions consist of one or a group of coccobacillary organisms, which vary from 0.2 to 5μ in diameter.

Ehrlichiosis generally runs a benign clinical course and horses recover over a period of two weeks unless there are secondary complications. Therapy with oxytetracycline* (2.4 mg per kg intravenously once or twice daily) will hasten recovery. Since the reservoir is unknown, the only modes of prevention are tick control and sanitary veterinary practices to prevent transfer of blood from infected to susceptible horses.

---

*Biocycline, Upjohn Co., Kalamazoo, MI

Supplemental Readings

Becht, J.: Medical diseases of foals. I. Neonatal isoerythrolysis (hemolytic disease of newborn). Proc. 2nd Annu. Forum Am. Coll. Vet. Int. Med., 1984, pp. 267–270.

Brewer, B. D., Harvey, J. W., Mayhew, I. G., et al.: Ehrlichiosis in a Florida horse. J. Am. Vet. Med. Assoc., 185:446, 1984.

Coggins, L.: Carriers of equine infectious anemia virus. J. Am. Vet. Med. Assoc., 184:279, 1984.

George, L. W., Divers, T. J., Mahaffey, E. A., and Saurez, M. J. H.: Heinz body anemia and methemoglobinemia in ponies given red maple (Acer rubrum) leaves. Vet. Pathol., 190:521, 1982.

Issel, C. J., Coggins, L.: Equine infectious anemia: Current knowledge. J. Am. Vet. Med. Assoc., 174:727, 1979.

Knowles, R. C., and Moulton, W. M.: Exotic Diseases. In Mansmann, R. S., McAlliser, E. S. and Pratt, P. W. (eds.): Equine Medicine and Surgery. 3rd ed., Santa Barbara, CA, American Veterinary Publications, 1982.

Pearson, J. E., and Knowles, R. C.: Standardization of the equine infectious anemia immunodiffusion test and its application to the control of the disease in the United States. J. Am. Vet. Med. Assoc., 184:298, 1984.

Pierce, K. R., Joyce, J. R., England, R. B., and Jones, L. P.: Acute hemolytic anemia caused by wild onion poisoning in horses. J. Am. Vet. Med. Assoc., 160:323, 1972.

Tashjian, R. J.: Transmission and clinical evaluation of an equine infectious anemia herd and their offspring over a 13-year period. J. Am. Vet. Med. Assoc., 184:282, 1984.

Blood Loss Anemia

E. Susan Clark, KENNETT SQUARE, PENNSYLVANIA

Blood loss may be acute and massive with impending cardiovascular collapse, subacute with a duration of a few days, or chronic with a duration of weeks or months. Wounds or hemorrhage from surgical procedures may result in severe blood loss. Lesions of the respiratory tract resulting in epistaxis may cause severe hemorrhage as with guttural pouch mycosis causing erosion of the internal carotid artery. Petechiation, ecchymosis, or frank hemorrhage may occur with thrombocytopenia or other coagulopathies. Gastrointestinal lesions, renal lesions, and hemorrhage into body cavities are causes of occult blood loss.

The therapeutic approach is determined by the rate, severity, and cause of blood loss. The source of the blood loss should be identified and treated when possible and consideration given to the need for correction of fluid and erythrocyte losses.

ACUTE BLOOD LOSS

Clinical Signs. With acute massive blood loss, clinical signs result from hypovolemic shock and include increased heart rate, decreased pulse strength, pale mucous membranes, prolonged capillary refill time, poor jugular distensibility, muscular weakness, depression, and oliguria. Signs vary with the rate of blood loss. Acute loss of 30 per cent or more of blood volume can result in signs of shock. (Blood volume [L] normally equals 7 to 8 per cent of body weight [kg].) Physiologic compensation for shock includes redistribution of interstitial fluid from tissue spaces into capillaries to expand circulating fluid volume. As a result of fluid shifts packed cell volume and total protein are decreased. Redistribution requires 12 to 24 hours and hematologic changes do not correlate with the degree of blood loss during this time. Sympathetic activity subsequent to arterial hypotension causes splenic contraction, which increases PCV. Clinical signs of anemia may not become obvious until PCV is below 15 per cent; these signs represent physiologic compensation for the relative anoxia caused by decreased hemoglobin concentration. Initially there is tachycardia (to increase cardiac output) and pallor (due to vasoconstriction causing blood redistribution) followed by depression, weakness, and tachypnea, which are signs of incipient cardiopulmonary failure.

Causes. There are many causes of blood loss in the horse. Severe lacerations and complications following surgery such as castration may result in blood loss. Acute severe hemorrhage can result from erosion of the wall of the internal carotid artery by guttural pouch mycosis. About 50 per cent of cases of guttural pouch mycosis are presented with epistaxis as the primary complaint. Early differentiation of the cause of epistaxis (including nasal and sinus tumors and polyps, pulmonary hemorrhage, coagulopathies, and guttural pouch mycosis) is important because lethal hemorrhage can occur. Coagulopathies including disseminated intravascular coagulation, hemophilia, warfarin poisoning, and thrombocytopenia may cause blood loss by epistaxis, hematuria, subcutaneous hemorrhage, and gastrointestinal bleeding. Mucosal petechiation and ecchymosis result from thrombocytopenia or vascular disorders. Disseminated intravascular coagulation may cause petechiation from thrombocytopenia.

Laboratory determination of the platelet count, activated partial thromboplastin time, prothrombin time, and concentration of fibrinolytic degradation products may help in detection of these disorders. Intraperitoneal and intrathoracic hemorrhage may rarely accompany hemostatic abnormalities. Hemoperitoneum may occur after (1) trauma (most commonly splenic rupture), (2) rupture of the mesen-teric arteries as a result of intimal damage by strongyle larvae migration, (3) bleeding from mesenteric vessels caused by necrosis of neoplastic lesions or abscesses, or (4) spontaneous rupture of the uterine artery during parturition. Hemothorax may occur with thoracic trauma or bleeding resulting from rupture of a pulmonary abscess. Clinical signs of intraperitoneal hemorrhage may include gastrointestinal ileus and signs of colic. Signs of hemothorax are tachypnea and dyspnea. Hemoperitoneum and hemothorax are definitively diagnosed by paracentesis of the abdomen and thorax, respectively. Blood may be introduced into peritoneal fluid during sampling by aspiration of splenic blood, and both peritoneal and thoracic fluids may be contaminated by laceration of a subcutaneous vessel. If contaminated by blood from a subcutaneous vessel, fluid may be successfully obtained from another site. Cytologic evidence of erythrophagocytosis would suggest that hemorrhage occurred before the paracentesis unless the fluid was not analyzed promptly. Clinically significant anemia is generally not seen with exercise-induced pulmonary hemorrhage; however, rarely a major artery ruptures, resulting in massive hemorrhage followed by cardiovascular collapse.

Therapy. The initial treatment of acute blood loss should be to stop the hemorrhage, if possible using pressure bandages and ligatures. Elaborate surgical intervention is often necessary to prevent hemorrhage due to guttural pouch mycosis. With acute massive hemorrhage (greater than 30 per cent of blood volume), the major clinical problem is hypovolemic shock. This must be treated by prompt intravenous therapy with balanced crystalloid solutions (lactated Ringer's solution) to increase vascular volume. Replacement fluid volume necessary to maintain perfusion in shock is usually two to seven times greater than the actual blood loss, because redistribution within the entire extracellular space occurs. Through monitoring of the clinical response to fluid replacement along with the volume and rate of blood loss, ongoing needs can be assessed. Improvement in jugular distensibility and capillary refill time, increased pulse strength, and decreased heart rate are indications of improved cardiovascular status.

In most instances, acute hemorrhage can be successfully treated with only crystalloid solutions; however, severe cases may require a whole blood transfusion to increase oncotic pressure and oxygen-carrying capacity. Donor selection and blood collection is discussed in the chapter on blood and plasma therapy (see p. 317). The volume of blood transfusion will depend on the rate and quantity of blood loss. Whole blood should be administered at 15 to 25 ml per kg of body weight and repeated if hemorrhage is ongoing or the clinical response is inadequate. Balanced crystalloid solutions should be administered concurrently to maintain perfusion.

When blood loss occurs over a period of a few days, there is minimal hypovolemia because plasma is replaced by extracellular fluid and intravenous fluid replacement may not be necessary. When the packed cell volume is decreased to 15 per cent, the patient's condition should be carefully monitored. However, transfusion is usually not indicated until the PCV is below 10 per cent. Transfused red cells survive only four to six days in the horse, so the increase in PCV is only transient. Also, the increase in PCV will blunt the marrow response to the anemia.

Hematologic abnormalities associated with acute blood loss will be seen after the initial 24 hours and include anemia (a decrease in PCV, erythrocyte count, and hemoglobin concentration) and decreased total plasma protein. The horse does not show evidence of a regenerative response in the peripheral blood. The normal bone marrow will show a proliferative response in about three days and begin to replace the erythrocyte loss in five to seven days if blood loss has been controlled. Sequential measurement of PCV will be helpful in determining whether the blood loss and resulting anemia are progressive or controlled. Consideration should be given to whether or not the blood loss is related to hemostatic abnormalities (such as warfarin poisoning, DIC, and thrombocytopenia).

CHRONIC BLOOD LOSS

Blood loss associated with certain diseases may be slow, with the only physical abnormalities being those related to the primary disease problem. Since there is time for physiologic adaptation to the gradually developing hypoxia, signs of anemia will generally not be apparent until the PCV is less than 12 to 13 per cent. Early in the disease process a bone marrow proliferative response is seen until iron reserves have been depleted by continued blood loss. Iron deficiency anemia (see p. 303) may then intervene, characterized by hypoferremia, increased total iron-binding capacity, absence of marrow iron, and decrease in the marrow's regenerative response. In chronic blood loss anemia, efforts should be directed toward diagnosis and treatment of the primary cause. PCV and total plasma protein should be monitored to follow the progression of the blood loss. Treatment of secondary iron deficiency is rarely necessary as the quantity of iron in the diet usually exceeds actual requirements. Use of a parenteral iron compound should be avoided. Fatal reactions have resulted from use of iron dextran preparations in horses. Oral administration of dietary supplements containing ferrous sulfate at 2 mg per kg daily will provide about twice the daily requirements for a normal 500-kg horse.

Causes of chronic blood loss include gastrointestinal lesions, renal lesions, thrombocytopenia, and other coagulopathies. Chronic gastrointestinal blood loss is usually occult. Blood originating from the small colon or rectum may rarely cause the stool to be red (hematochezia). Bleeding from the proximal gastrointestinal tract or large colon may cause the stool to be black, with a tarry consistency (melena). Small increases in blood content may not alter the appearance of the stool. Fecal occult blood can be detected using chemical tests.* Occult blood testing is usually necessary to detect gastrointestinal bleeding in horses. Bleeding into the digestive tract may result from neoplastic infiltration of the bowel wall, infiltration by parasites, or mucosal ulceration. Anemia of chronic inflammatory disease may complicate intestinal neoplastic disease. Occasionally damage caused by neoplastic infiltration of the intestinal wall and tumor necrosis causing ulceration can result in gastrointestinal blood loss. This has been seen most often with squamous cell carcinoma of the stomach and less frequently with intestinal lymphosarcoma. Significant blood loss resulting in anemia occurs rarely with equine strongylosis. Damage to the intestinal wall and blood ingestion by adult *Strongylus vulgaris* may cause significant gastrointestinal blood loss in severe infections. Rarely, damage to intestinal vessels and the intestinal wall by migration of large numbers of *Strongylus vulgaris* larvae may result in blood loss anemia. Moderate anemia may accompany colonic damage caused by infections with small strongyles. Examination of fecal flotations may help in assessment of the severity of the adult parasite burden; however, severe infection by larval stages may not be reflected by fecal ova counts. Gastrointestinal ulceration is seen in adult horses and foals with phenylbutazone toxicosis, along with depression, colic, weight loss, and hypoproteinemia. Occasionally, gastrointestinal blood loss and anemia result from phenylbutazone toxicosis. Gastric and duodenal ulceration occur in suckling and neonatal foals as a result of phenylbutazone toxicosis, stress, and other unknown causes. Feces are often positive for occult blood but blood loss anemia is rare. Although the alimentary mucosa often is damaged with acute salmonellosis, significant blood loss seldom occurs. Chronic blood loss secondary to renal disease is rare; however, it may accompany renal neoplasia, congenital renal vascular anomalies, or urinary calculi.

---

*Hemoccult test: SmithKline Diagnostics, Sunnyvale, CA.

Supplemental Readings

Carlson, G. P.: Evaluation of responsive anemias in horses. Proceed. 1st Int. Symp. Eq. Hematol., Michigan State University, p. 327, 1975.

Kolata, R. J.: The clinical management of circulatory shock based on pathophysiological patterns. Comp. Cont. Ed. Pract. Vet., 2:314, 1980.

Schalm, O. W. and Carlson, G. P.: The blood and blood forming organs, In Mansmann, R. A., McAllister, E. S., and Pratt, P. W. (eds.): Equine Medicine and Surgery, 3rd ed. Santa Barbara, CA, American Veterinary Publications, 1982.

Anemia Due to Inadequate Erythropoiesis

Wendy E. Vaala, KENNETT SQUARE, PENNSYLVANIA

Depression or nonregenerative anemia due to decreased erythropoiesis is one of the most common and diagnostically frustrating forms of anemia encountered in equine medicine. The causes of nonregenerative anemia include chronic inflammatory disease, iron deficiency, tumor invasion of the bone marrow (myelophthisic disease), and intrinsic bone marrow disorders. These anemias are usually of mild to moderate severity, are only gradually progressive or static, and are associated with decreased or complete suppression of erythropoiesis. Since the normal equine red cell life span is approximately 140 to 155 days, a prolonged time period may be required before clinical signs of anemia develop. The clinical features of the primary disease process frequently overshadow the signs caused by anemia, which is itself only an indication of disease. Often signs of anemia are seen only if the animal is stressed or exercised and may be characterized by poor performance, early fatigue, prolonged recovery following exercise, tachycardia, and pronounced mucosal pallor.

IRON DEFICIENCY ANEMIA

Although iron deficiency anemia is uncommon in horses it is most often seen in association with chronic blood loss. The most common causes of chronic blood loss include ulcerative, invasive gastrointestinal neoplasia, coagulopathies, and severe gastrointestinal parasitism. Young foals suffering from gastrointestinal blood loss (such as that associated with severe gastrointestinal ulcers) may be more susceptible to developing significant anemia because of their iron-deficient milk diet. If the anemia becomes severe, clinical signs of mucosal pallor, weakness, lethargy, exercise intolerance, and tachycardia may develop. Passage of dark, occult blood–positive feces is a sign of significant gastrointestinal bleeding. A depraved appetite (pica) has been described in some horses with iron deficiency anemia. The ingestion of dirt or sand may be related to its iron content.

Dietary iron is in the trivalent (ferric) form and must be reduced to the bivalent (ferrous) form before absorption can occur. Maximal absorption of iron occurs within the duodenum with the degree of absorption varying directly with the rate of erythropoiesis and indirectly with total body iron stores. Uptake of iron by the small intestinal mucosal cells is followed by active transport and release into the plasma. Iron is transported in the plasma bound to the carrier protein transferrin. It is stored as either soluble ferritin or insoluble hemosiderin. Hemosiderin stores can be evaluated using Prussian blue stain to examine a bone marrow aspirate or histologic sections of spleen, kidney, and liver. In humans and in other species iron deficiency has been associated with achlorhydria (absence of gastric secretion of hydrochloride), diets with high levels of phosphorus, and iron-deficient diets. These causes have not been documented in horses.

Iron deficiency anemia in the horse is usually normocytic and normochromic. With moderate to severe iron depletion, microcytic hypochromic red cells may be observed accompanied by a modest thrombocytosis. Serum iron levels are low and total iron-binding capacity (TIBC) is usually elevated. There is a decrease in bone marrow iron stores that can be qualitatively evaluated using the Prussian blue iron stain on a bone marrow smear.

Hemoglobin synthesis is depressed in iron-deficient states, resulting in a late maturation arrest of the erythroid series. While cells in the late rubricyte stage are awaiting hemoglobin synthesis, further cell division may occur, resulting in smaller than normal cells containing a decreased hemoglobin concentration. Maturation of this cell type constitutes a hypochromic microcytic anemia.

Therapy should be directed at the primary disorders. There are many iron-containing hematinics commercially available for oral and parenteral use in the horse. The iron contained in most parenteral preparations is bound to dextran moieties. Anaphylactoid reactions have been reported in horses receiving certain parenteral dextran formulations. Iron cacodylate (1 gram intravenously for an adult horse) is one of the safest preparations available for equine use. Good-quality forage is another source of iron. Overzealous and unnecessary parenteral administration of iron-containing hematinics produces iatrogenic iron overload and should be avoided.

ANEMIA OF CHRONIC DISEASE

The anemia of chronic disease (ACD) is associated with any chronic inflammatory condition such as infection, autoimmunity, and malignancy. Chronic systemic diseases such as pleuritis and pneumonia, internal abscesses, liver and kidney failure, and some forms of neoplasia, are most commonly associated with ACD in the horse. These anemias are usually moderate in severity and rarely attract primary attention because of their subtle clinical signs. The anemia of chronic disorders is characterized by disturbed iron kinetics, inadequate compensatory erythropoiesis, and a shortened red cell life span. Anemia accompanying chronic renal failure may also be complicated by hemolysis and impaired erythropoietin production.

A low serum iron level despite adequate iron stores suggests a significant disruption of iron kinetics. A defect in iron mobilization and release from ferritin and hemosiderin stores has been proposed in patients with chronic disease. There is some evidence that a shift occurs from ferritin- to hemosiderin-stored iron, the latter of which is less easily mobilized. The oxidizing environment associated with inflammation may be responsible for the shift in iron stores. Total iron-binding capacity (TIBC) is normal or decreased in contrast to iron deficiency anemia. ACD is usually normocytic and normochromic initially and only in extreme states may become microcytic and hypochromic.

Inadequate red cell production in response to anemia may result from a relative bone marrow failure that includes decreased marrow responsiveness to circulating erythropoietin and suppressed erythropoiesis associated with hypoferremia. Low serum iron levels may be responsible for suppressed erythroid activity since iron is a crucial constituent of the hemoglobin molecule as well as several enzymes that are essential in the erythropoietic pathway. In this manner horses affected with equine infectious anemia also experience suppressed erythropoiesis, in addition to hemolysis, as a result of iron redistribution within the reticuloendothelial system and temporary decreases in available iron during febrile episodes.

Extracorpuscular factors are believed responsible for the reduced red cell longevity and may include damage to red cells as they pass through injured or inflamed tissues. Hyperplasia of the reticuloendothelial system resulting in increased erythrocyte sequestration and destruction also contributes to premature cell death. In chronic renal failure there is a proven decrease in activity of the sodium-potassium pump and glutathione reduction systems causing osmotic lysis and increased oxidative stress on red blood cells.

Decreased marrow responsiveness, abnormal iron metabolism, and decreased red cell longevity all contribute to the development of ACD. Laboratory tests reveal a normal to decreased TIBC and low serum iron levels accompanying normocytic, normochromic anemia. Prussian blue stains of bone marrow aspirates confirm adequate reticuloendothelial iron stores but decreased amounts of iron within erythrocyte precursors. Therapy must be directed at the primary disorder. The use of iron-containing hematinics is valueless since total body iron stores are adequate but are unable to be mobilized effectively.

MYELOPHTHISIS

Invasion and replacement of normal marrow elements by abnormal cells is termed *myelophthisis* and is confirmed by bone marrow biopsy or aspiration. Although neoplastic invasion and proliferation of the hematopoietic tissues are rare in the horse, lymphoid malignancies and myeloproliferative diseases have been reported to involve equine marrow. Tumor cell proliferation proceeds at the expense of normal hematopoiesis causing a decrease in any or all marrow-derived elements in the peripheral circulation. Myelophthisic anemia may be one result of neoplastic infiltration of the marrow, but leukopenia and thrombocytopenia can also occur. Thrombocytopenia and leukopenia generally are evident before anemia owing to the shorter half-life of platelets and granulocytes. Therefore, the presenting clinical sign of myelophthisic disease is usually abnormal bleeding or excessive infections or both. The clinical features associated with infiltrative marrow disorders may be related to the underlying disease, but usually they include increased bleeding tendency secondary to thrombocytopenia. Signs of infection subsequent to leukopenia, followed by severe refractory anemia late in the disease process, may occur.

Initially, myelophthisic anemia is mild to moderate and may be associated with shortened red cell life span, ineffective erythropoiesis, blood loss, or intrinsic red cell disorders. Bone marrow evaluation is used to confirm neoplastic infiltration of the marrow with a subsequent decrease or absence of erythroid activity. Plasma cell myelomatosis, myelomonocytic myeloproliferative disease, lymphoma, and granulocytic leukemia have been associated with varying degrees of secondary myelophthisic anemia in the horse. Extramedullary erythropoiesis in the liver, spleen, kidney, lymph nodes, and adrenal glands has been observed in cases of severe unresponsive anemia and represents an attempt by the body to compensate for the lack of normal red cell production in the marrow.

There is no specific therapy for myelophthisic anemia since it is generally unresponsive and is usually secondary to a primary neoplastic process. Blood transfusions are only palliative. Hematopoietic neoplasia in the horse is usually considered fatal with only rare and limited success reported with experimental chemotherapy.

INTRINSIC BONE MARROW DISEASE

Intrinsic marrow disease resulting in aplastic pancytopenia is associated with decreased numbers of all hematopoietic precursors. Aplastic anemia is one manifestation of this acquired disorder. Total bone marrow suppression is rare in the horse but may result from exposure to heavy metals, ionizing radiation, insecticides, organic solvents, and trichloroethylene-extracted soybean oil meal. Recent reports have suggested the development of toxic bone marrow suppression and hypoplastic anemia in a horse secondary to phenylbutazone administration. Evaluation of bone marrow aspirates aids in the diagnosis of intrinsic marrow disorders. If exposure to a myelotoxin is suspected, elimination of the offending agent is essential to the therapeutic plan because most instances of marrow suppression are reversible. Total bone marrow aplasia is an irreversible idiosyncratic reaction to some drugs and is usually fatal.

Idiopathic marrow dysplasia has been reported in a horse. This marrow abnormality, characterized by asynchronous maturation and ineffective production of both erythroid and myeloid cells, has been associated with the preleukemic stages of lymphoid neoplasia in humans.

Supplemental Readings

Brumbaugh, G. W., Stitzel, K. A., Zinkl, J. G., and Feldman, B. F.: Myelomonocytic myeloproliferative disease in a horse. J. Am. Vet. Med. Assoc., *180*:313, 1982.

Kitchen, H., and Krehbiel, J. D. (eds.): Proc. 1st Intern. Symp. Eq. Hematol., Michigan State University, 1975.

Rossoff, I. S.: Handbook of Veterinary Drugs: A Compendium for Research and Clinical Use. New York, Springer Publishing Co., 1975.

Schalm, O. W., and Carlson, G. P.: The Blood and Blood-Forming Organs. *In* Mansmann, R. A., McAllister, E. S., and Pratt, P. W.(eds.): Equine Medicine and Surgery, 3rd ed. Santa Barbara, CA, American Veterinary Publications, 1982.

Williams, W. J., Beuther, E., Erslev, A. J., and Lichtman, M. A. (eds.): Hematology, 3rd ed. New York, McGraw-Hill, 1983.

Warfarin Toxicosis

T. D. Byars, LEXINGTON, KENTUCKY

The use of the dicoumarol derivative warfarin as an antithrombotic drug has increased in recent years. It is a therapeutic agent for horses with navicular disease. Toxic exposure can occur in horses exposed either accidentally or deliberately to warfarin as a rodenticide in grains or feedstuffs. Rarely, natural exposure can occur if horses are exposed to certain clovers. The syndrome is termed "moldy sweet clover toxicity."

Warfarin is a vitamin K antagonist, producing abnormal clotting proteins (Factors II, VII, IX, X). The most immediate changes occur in Factor VII (proconvertin), causing a change in the extrinsic clotting system approximately 36 hours after dosing. The intrinsic system (Factors II, IX, and X) subsequently becomes deficient. The one-stage prothrombin time (OSPT), which detects earlier changes occurring in the extrinsic system, is used to monitor the therapeutic use of warfarin.

Therapeutic levels of warfarin can become toxic if a cumulative effect occurs, if the diet is altered and contains fewer vitamin K constituents, or if the concurrent use of protein-bound drugs causes an increase in the free unbound level of warfarin. Drugs enhancing warfarin toxicity by displacement include oxyphenylbutazone, phenylbutazone, and chloral hydrate. Hypoalbuminemic states may cause excessive free warfarin. The simultaneous use of other anticoagulation drugs such as heparin and aspirin may be synergistic and may result in hemorrhage. Drugs that activate the hepatic microsomal enzyme system, such as rifampin and barbiturates, accelerate the breakdown of warfarin; therefore, higher doses are required to achieve a therapeutic effect. If these drugs are withdrawn and the level of warfarin held constant, signs of warfarin toxicity can appear. The use of warfarin in horses with liver disease is contraindicated.

Horses that are presented with anemia and hypoproteinemia, accompanied by a history of lameness or corrective shoeing, can be tentatively suspected of warfarin toxicity resulting from navicular disease therapy. Warfarin-induced hemorrhage usually presents clinically as ecchymotic effusions of the subcutis or mucous membranes, hematoma formation, epistaxis, hematuria, or gastrointestinal bleeding (melena).

Diagnosis of warfarin toxicosis should be confirmed in the laboratory. Prolongation of the OSPT, either singularly or in conjunction with an elevated activated partial thromboplastin time (APTT), is diagnostic whenever other coagulation laboratory findings are normal. Samples should be collected on ice in 1:9 sodium citrate and transported to the laboratory as soon as possible.

Treatment of warfarin toxicity can be accomplished by withdrawal of the drug with an expected return to normal clotting function in three to four days. Vitamin K_1 (500 mg) should be given subcutaneously every four to six hours until the OSPT returns to normal control values. In case of significant hemorrhage, a transfusion of one to two liters of fresh plasma can quickly reverse the bleeding tendency. In severe cases, whole blood in conjunction with vitamin K_1 is indicated (see p. 317). The response to treatment is usually rapid, occurring in one to two hours.

Supplemental Readings

Colles, C. M.: A preliminary report on the use of warfarin in the treatment of navicular disease. Equine Vet. J., *11*:187, 1979.

Mount, M. E.: Vitamin K and its therapeutic importance. J. Am. Vet. Med. Assoc., *180*:1354, 1982.

Scott, E. A., Byars, T. D., and Lamar, A. M.: Warfarin anticoagulation in the horse. J. Am. Vet. Med. Assoc., *177*:1146, 1980.

Scott, E. A., Sandler, G. A., and Byars, T. D.: Warfarin: Effects on anticoagulant, hematologic, and blood enzyme values in normal ponies. Am. J. Vet. Res., *40*:142, 1979.

Disseminated Intravascular Coagulation

T. D. Byars, LEXINGTON, KENTUCKY

Although disseminated intravascular coagulation (DIC) has been adequately documented in the horse, it remains an infrequently diagnosed process occurring in a myriad of equine diseases. The syndrome can be defined as the secondary pathologic acceleration of the clotting system. The horse has a relatively inhibited coagulation mechanism compared with other domestic species and rarely completes the processes of clotting and clot dissolution rapidly enough for a classical clinicopathologic diagnosis of DIC. Horses appear to be particularly prone to low-grade forms of DIC commonly associated with thrombotic and ischemic disorders. Table 1 lists conditions associated with DIC. Its existence should be clinically suspected in all fibrin-forming or thrombotic and hemorrhagic disorders secondary to shock, septicemia, viremia, renal disease, liver disease, peritonitis, necrotic pleuropneumonia, and postoperative hemorrhage.

PATHOPHYSIOLOGY

Disseminated intravascular coagulation refers to an exaggeration of the clotting system with subsequent consumption of the clotting proteins (factors) and platelets. Activation of the clotting system occurs in response to an increase of a systemic procoagulant substance(s) or a loss of the vascular endothelial lining that allows exposure of collagen to platelets. A hypercoagulable state precedes the blood clotting. Intravascular coagulation initially results in fibrin deposition in the general microcirculation, including that of many vital organs and larger vessels. Microthrombi decrease perfusion, and vascular ischemia initiates the enzymatic degradation (secondary fibrinolysis) of fibrinogen and fibrin. Fibrinogen and fibrin degradation products (FDPs) are breakdown products of clot dissolution, which, when they enter the systemic circulation,

TABLE 1. DISEASES ASSOCIATED WITH DISSEMINATED INTRAVASCULAR COAGULATION

Gastrointestinal disorders
    Strangulation/obstruction
    Diarrhea (necrotizing enterocolitis)
    Endotoxemia (Schwartzman phenomenon)
Laminitis
Postoperative hemorrhage
Hemolytic crisis (± microangiopathic hemolytic anemia)
Obstetric complications
Heat stroke
Renal disease (renal corticomedullary necrosis/Schwartzman phenomenon)
Sepsis (viral, bacterial, fungal)
Trauma
Myositis
Burns
Necrosis
Disseminated malignancies
Shock
Toxins (snake bite, spider bite, mold toxins)
Adrenal crisis (Waterhouse-Friderichsen syndrome)

TABLE 2. PRIMARY CAUSES OF DISSEMINATED INTRAVASCULAR COAGULATION

Acidosis
Anoxia
Hypoxia
Collagen exposure
Viremia
Septicemia
Endotoxemia
Reticuloendothelial system failure (e.g., shock)
Thrombin hemoconcentration
Intravascular hemolysis
Necrotic procoagulants (e.g., uterine)
Antigen-antibody complexes (complement activation)

act as potent anticoagulants to prevent ongoing fibrin formation (Fig. 1). DIC is therefore a consumptive coagulopathy that may present clinically as a thrombotic crisis or a hemorrhagic diathesis. The syndrome may occur in a generalized, local, acute, or chronic (low-grade) form. In fulminant disease, DIC should be considered as an integral part of the shock syndrome.

Disseminated intravascular coagulation is always secondary to an underlying primary disease process. Table 2 is a list of DIC-associated disorders that may be considered as probable primary triggering mechanisms or as active parts of the cycle of pathogenesis. Since DIC is difficult to document in the

horse, the precise underlying mechanism is seldom determined and makes the primary entity elusive.

CLINICAL SIGNS

The presentation of profound hemorrhage with DIC is rare in the horse. The clinician should attempt to make a diagnosis on the basis of subtle lesions of thrombosis and hemorrhage in conjunction with a suitable predisposing cause. Petechiation and ecchymosis are most frequently found on the mucous membranes, nictitating membranes, sclerae, and the inner pinna and retinas of foals. Epistaxis and melena can be observed in severe cases. Hematoma formation or oozing after venipuncture occasionally occurs, but more often rapid thrombosis of either veins or arteries follows a perforating procedure. Spontaneous thrombosis is often associated with a severe primary systemic disease. DIC should be suspected in cases of advanced disease whenever the sequelae indicate that microvascular thrombosis is responsible for the deterioration of vital organ function. Laminitis, colic, and dysfunction of the adrenals, kidneys, liver, and reticuloendothelial system can be considered as clinical sequelae to DIC as well as predisposing causes.

DIAGNOSIS

The confirmation of a clinical diagnosis must be made in the laboratory or at necropsy. In order for a precise diagnosis to be made, at least three of the laboratory tests should be abnormal in a hemostatic profile (Table 3). Since changes in coagulation are subtle in the horse, DIC is seldom diagnosed. Tests of clotting function are frequently within normal limits even in the face of a consumptive coagulopathy owing to the hypercoagulable status of the patient. The activated coagulation time (ACT) test will allow for an initial assessment of clotting func-

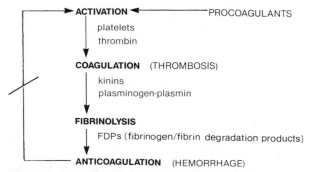

Figure 1. A simplified scheme of the pathophysiologic steps involved in disseminated intravascular coagulation. The process may not always be completed, leading to thrombosis as the major presentation.

TABLE 3. RECOMMENDED HEMOSTATIC PROFILE FOR DIAGNOSIS OF DISSEMINATED INTRAVASCULAR COAGULATION

Prothrombin time (PT)
Partial thromboplastin time (PTT)
Activated coagulation time (ACT)
Fibrinogen/fibrin degradation products (FDPs)
Thrombin time (TT)
Platelet count
Fibrinogen concentration

A control sample must be analyzed with tests of clotting time. Normal values will vary and must be established for each laboratory.

tion under field conditions and serves as an indicator for further testing. Although the ACT may be within normal limits, clot formation with DIC is sluggish. Clots are poorly formed and often show evidence of clot lysis within the tube.

Platelet counts are usually lowered in acute DIC. An absolute platelet count is recommended, although a scan for adequate platelets under a high-powered field usually correlates well with the actual number of platelets. Horses with a thrombocyte count of less than 20,000 per μl are clinically prone to spontaneous hemorrhage because of this defect alone. Although decreases of fibrinogen concentration might be anticipated, hypofibrinogenemia is not common in horses with DIC. In chronic cases the fibrinogen content may be elevated because of overcompensation or the erroneous measurement of substances other than fibrinogen, which may interfere with conventional fibrinogen estimation.

Fibrin degradation products (FDPs) are best detected and quantified using a commercially available standard kit.* Fibrin degradation products are rapidly cleared by an intact reticuloendothelial system and may not be present in detectable quantities in the systemic circulation of low-grade cases of DIC. False-positives can be encountered in normal horses, but rarely above a 1:5 dilution. If FDPs are elevated above the control, the amount of elevation should be considered irrelevant, since their presence ensures that fibrinolysis as a component of DIC has occurred. In order to separate the FDPs generated from fibrinogen (primary fibrinogenolysis) from those of fibrin, the protamine sulfate test can be used to detect the soluble monomers of fibrinogen degradation. Other laboratory tests that offer diagnostic potential include circulating antithrombin III levels, the euglobulin lysis time test, and plasminogen and plasmin quantification.

At postmortem examination, DIC can be suspected whenever diffuse thrombosis and hemor-

rhage are both evident. Histologic confirmation is difficult because fibrinolysis continues in the postmortem state.

THERAPY

DIC therapy involves three basic steps: treatment of (1) the primary disorder, (2) of DIC, and (3) of sequelae. Treatment of the disorder responsible for DIC is essential. An assessment of the inciting cause and evaluation of DIC severity should influence the clinician's decision on treatment. For example, if sepsis due to bacterial infection was the cause of DIC, treatment with the appropriate antibiotic and supportive care might be all that are required to control the syndrome.

Direct treatment of DIC is aimed at inactivation of the procoagulant activity. This can be accomplished by volume expansion to prevent hemoconcentration in the microvasculature, drugs to stabilize the endothelial lining to decrease contact activation and production of inflammatory procoagulants, and anticoagulants to inhibit the consumptive process. Volume dilution is achieved by appropriate balanced fluid therapy to restore cardiovascular integrity and acid-base homeostasis. Restoration of fluid volume will increase perfusion of the microvasculature and will decrease capillary sludging. Drugs that stabilize the endothelium and increase capillary perfusion act as adjuncts to fluid therapy. Steroids, although potent anti-inflammatory compounds, may exacerbate DIC by reducing the procoagulant clearance activity of the reticuloendothelial system.

Use of systemic anticoagulants in a potential bleeding disorder is a paradoxic treatment that is utilized to inhibit the consumptive process. Heparin is the most commonly used anticoagulant. In therapeutic doses, it has varying degrees of success. Since antithrombin III is required for heparin to function as an anticoagulant, failure of heparin can occur in cases of DIC because of decreased levels of antithrombin III. Replacement therapy with antithrombin III concentrates may be indicated if they become available in the future. If heparin therapy is employed, 80 to 100 IU per kg intravenously is recommended every four to six hours, or it can be added to fluids as a continuous drip. The low-grade form of DIC is treated with 25 to 40 IU per kg subcutaneously two or three times daily. Other anticoagulants have not been investigated sufficiently to recommend their use in place of heparin.

Aspirin has been recommended in the treatment of DIC in place of or with heparin. Aspirin is a potent platelet inhibitor and must be given orally. Recent studies suggest that aspirin at 60 grains orally once every other day significantly affects

---

*Thrombo-Wellcotest, Burroughs Wellcome Co., Research Triangle Park, NC

platelet function, although minidoses (2 to 5 mg per kg per day) may theoretically accomplish a similar inhibition.

Use of blood transfusions or plasma platelet concentrates or both is considered controversial without prior heparinization. Although transfusions may provide additional substrate for ongoing DIC, the treatment is considered relatively successful. Since massive hemorrhage due to DIC is rare in the horse, whole blood transfusions are not needed except in cases of fulminant blood loss. Plasma exchange (plasmapheresis) to remove the inciting cause has been suggested in humans, but as of this writing remains a subjective approach to management.

Treatment of sequelae varies according to the organ involvement. Liver and kidney function should be assessed whenever DIC has been diagnosed.

Supplemental Readings

Bick, R. L.: Disseminated Intravascular Coagulation and Related Syndromes, Boca Raton, CRC Press, 1983.

Hood, D. M., Gremmel, S. M., Amoss, M. S., et al.: Equine laminitis III. Coagulation dysfunction in the development of acute disease. J. Equine Med. Surg., 3:355, 1979.

McClure, J. R., McClure, J. J., and Usenik, E. A.: Disseminated intravascular coagulation in ponies with surgically induced strangulation obstruction of the small intestine. Vet. Surg., 8:78, 1979.

Meyers, K., Reed, S., Keck, M., and Bayly, W.: Circulating endotoxin-like substance(s) and altered hemostasis in horses with gastrointestinal disorders: An interim report. Am. J. Vet. Res., 43:2233, 1982.

Morris, D. D., and Beech, J.: Disseminated intravascular coagulation in six horses. J. Am. Vet. Med. Assoc., 183:1067, 1983.

Pablo, L. S., Purohit, R. C., Teer, P. A., et al.: Disseminated intravascular coagulation in experimental intestinal strangulation obstruction in ponies. Am. J. Vet. Res., 44:2115, 1983.

Rawlings, C. A., Byars, T. D., Van Noy, M. K., and Bisgard, G. E.: Activated coagulation test in normal and heparinized ponies and horses. Am. J. Vet. Res., 36:711, 1975.

Hemophilia

T. D. Byars, LEXINGTON, KENTUCKY

Hemophilia presents in different species as either hemophilia A (Factor VIII deficiency), hemophilia B (Factor IX deficiency), or the related syndrome of von Willebrand's disease. Horses have been historically considered a hemophiliod-like species because in vitro clotting time test results are slower than in humans. Results of factor assays, especially of Factors XII and IX, are similarly decreased. Hemophilia A is the only true hemophilia documented in horses as a clinical entity. It is inherited as an X-chromosome homozygous recessive similar to the hereditary pattern seen in humans. It is carried by females and is clinically apparent in males. It has been described in the Thoroughbred, Standardbred, Arabian, and Quarterhorse.

CLINICAL SIGNS

The clinical signs of hemophilia A are usually seen in young colts from a few days of age to weaning. The disease has also been described in a three-year-old gelding. Hemarthrosis is the most common clinical complaint, although any form of excessive hemorrhage can occur. Easy bruising and subsequent hematoma formation usually precede a fatal hemorrhage. Petechial and ecchymotic hemorrhages of the mucous membranes are not expected in hemophilia A unless a concurrent platelet defect is present.

DIAGNOSIS

Diagnostic tests include a prolonged activated partial thromboplastin time (APTT) and a quantitation of Factor VIII expressed as the percentage of normal. Blood samples should be collected both from the patient and a normal control horse in sodium citrate tubes. Ideally, the samples should be placed in chilled plastic tubes, kept on ice, and transported to a laboratory capable of performing the necessary coagulation tests. Similar samples should be submitted from the colt's dam, since carrier females will have Factor VIII concentrations from 40 to 60 per cent of normal while their affected offspring are usually less than 10 per cent.

THERAPY

Treatment is palliative. Plasma transfusions of 40 to 50 ml per kg are recommended as an immediate form of therapy. Any potential for trauma should be avoided. In humans, frozen cryoprecipitates of concentrated Factor VIII are transfused periodically. Even if commercially available concentrates were available for affected foals, their practicality would be primarily for patient maintenance for research purposes. Genetic counseling is important in the overall management of the problem, and would center on the confirmed carrier females from the affected family.

Supplemental Readings

Bell, W. N., Tomlin, S. C., Archer R. K.: The coagulation mechanism of the blood of the horse with particular reference to its "hemophiliod" status. J. Comp. Path. 65:255, 1955.

Dodds, W. J.: Hemophilia in the horse. In Proc. 1st Intern. Eq. Hematol. Symp., Michigan State University, 1975, pp. 206–208.

Feldman, B. F., and Giacopuzzi, R. L.: Hemophilia A (Factor VIII deficiency) in a colt. Equine Pract. 4:24, 1982.

Mills, J. N., and Bolton, J. R.: Haemophilia A in a 3-year-old Thoroughbred horse. Aust. Vet. J., 60:63, 1983.

Immune-Mediated Thrombocytopenia

Debra Deem Morris, KENNETT SQUARE, PENNSYLVANIA

Thrombocytopenia, without disseminated coagulopathy, in horses is usually due to immune-mediated mechanisms, the cause of which is generally unknown. Aside from excessive utilization and immune-mediated destruction, thrombocytopenia may be caused by a bone marrow abnormality resulting in decreased production of platelets. Possible causes for the latter include idiosyncratic drug reactions, cytotoxic agents, radiation damage, and myelophthisic disease; however, decreased megakaryocytic proliferation is only rarely recognized in horses.

PATHOPHYSIOLOGY

Immune-mediated thrombocytopenia (IMTP) in horses may be primary (idiopathic) or secondary to therapy with certain drugs, viral diseases (especially equine infectious anemia), bacterial infections, lymphoproliferative disorders, or rarely neoplastic diseases. The majority of cases of IMTP have no apparent underlying cause. Most evidence suggests that idiopathic thrombocytopenia is caused by IgG autoantibodies produced largely in the spleen and directed against circulating platelets. Platelets that have reacted with antibody have a shortened life span and are destroyed by macrophages, located primarily in the spleen and liver. In secondary thrombocytopenia, platelets undergo destruction in the reticuloendothelial (monocyte-macrophage) system because they have been bound by immune complexes, made up of antibody against a particular drug, viral, bacterial, or neoplastic antigen. Alternatively the platelet membrane may be changed by a primary disease process exposing novel antigens that result in the production of autoantibodies or that are able to cross-react with pre-existing antibodies. Immune destruction of platelets by cell-mediated mechanisms has been implicated but not yet convincingly proved.

Horses of any age may be affected by IMTP, and there is no known sex or breed predisposition. The history depends upon whether disease is primary or secondary, but there are no consistent precipitating events. Current drug history is important because those cases that are drug-induced respond only if the offending drug is discontinued.

CLINICAL AND LABORATORY ABNORMALITIES

Clinical signs usually include manifestations of hemorrhagic diathesis such as epistaxis, melena, hyphema, hematoma formation following minor trauma, and bleeding following injections. Spontaneous hemorrhage rarely occurs unless the platelet count is less than 10,000 per μl. Affected horses are generally bright, alert, and afebrile, with no other obvious signs of illness. Since one of the major functions of platelets is to maintain microvascular integrity, horses with IMTP usually have petechial hemorrhages on the nasal or vaginal mucous membranes, the third eyelid and/or the sclerae. Although mild ventral subcutaneous edema may occur, the absence of hot, painful swellings helps to differentiate IMTP from vasculitis syndromes (such as equine purpura hemorrhagica), which also result in mucosal petechiae.

Consistent laboratory abnormalities include severe thrombocytopenia (usually less than 40,000 per μl) and prolonged bleeding time. Anemia and mild hypoproteinemia may be present if there has been significant ongoing blood loss. The feces and urine are often positive for occult blood. The prothrombin time (PT), activated partial thromboplastin time (APTT), and plasma fibrinogen are normal. Fibrinolytic degradation products (FDPs) measured by the commercial Latex agglutination method* are often 10 to 40 µg per ml, secondary to excessive fibrin formation and subsequent lysis at sites of hemorrhage. Bone marrow aspirates usually show megakaryocytic hyperplasia; however, interpretation may be difficult because sternal marrow samples from thrombocytopenic horses are often hemodiluted.

DIAGNOSIS

Definitive diagnosis of IMTP depends on demonstration of antiplatelet antibody or activity in the plasma. Antiplatelet antibody can be indirectly measured by the platelet factor 3 (PF-3) immunoinjury technique, which has been adapted for equine plasma. PF-3 is a membrane-bound phospholipid that is released when platelets are injured. Plasma that contains antiplatelet antibody can cause accelerated clotting of platelet-rich plasma through the release of PF-3. The antiplatelet activity of PF-3–positive samples can be identified as antibody if there is significant reduction in the plasma procoagulant activity by adsorption with monospecific antisera to homologous immunoglobulin. Despite indirect evidence that most cases of idiopathic or secondary thrombocytopenia in horses are immune-mediated, the PF-3 test is often negative or inconclusive. Antiplatelet antibodies are difficult to detect if immunosuppressive therapy has been instituted. Platelets from different horses may vary in their sensitivity to antiplatelet antibody. Tests to directly measure platelet-bound antibody, using enzyme-linked immunosorbent assay or fluorescent antibody techniques, have been devised for humans and dogs but are not commercially available for horses. Cell-mediated hypersensitivity mechanisms without PF-3 release have been implicated in some cases of idiopathic thrombocytopenia. A diagnosis of IMTP is assumed when the horse has normal coagulation parameters (PT, APTT) and no clinical evidence of consumptive coagulopathy or other diseases. Response to corticosteroid therapy is supportive of the diagnosis.

TREATMENT

The first step in treating a horse with suspected IMTP is the immediate discontinuation of any current medication. Drug-induced thrombocytopenia is difficult to document but only fully responds if the sensitizing drug is withdrawn. If the horse absolutely requires a certain medication, such as an antimicrobial for existing infection, it should be replaced by the most chemically dissimilar pharmacologic substitute. A transfusion of fresh whole blood or platelet-rich plasma may be necessary to arrest acute life-threatening hemorrhage in severely thrombocytopenic horses. Platelet-rich plasma can be prepared by centrifugation of freshly collected blood in acid-citrated dextrose solution for 3 to 5 minutes at 250 × g to remove cells. Contact of blood or plasma with glass should be minimized to prevent adhesion and activation of platelets. Platelets should not be stored more than six hours before use because of rapid in vitro loss of hemostatic activity.

The majority of horses with IMTP improve when treated with corticosteroids. Although the exact mechanism of their action is not known, corticosteroids improve capillary integrity and reduce phagocytic clearance of platelets in reticuloendothelial organs. They may impair antiplatelet antibody production, impede platelet-antibody interaction, and increase platelet production. An initial dosage of dexamethasone* of 0.05 to 0.2 mg per kg intravenously or intramuscularly once in the morning for three to four days is generally sufficient to raise the platelet count to more than 100,000 per µl. Once the platelet count has risen to within the normal range, the dose of dexamethasone should be reduced 5 to 10 mg daily, while the platelet count is monitored at least every two days. Prednisolone† may be substituted for dexamethasone, at an initial dosage of 1 mg per kg intramuscularly twice daily. The dose rate can be decreased to once daily after the platelet count has risen to normal, and subsequently the dosage can be tapered off by 50 to 100 mg each day or two. Corticosteroids can usually be discontinued after a period of 10 to 14 days, provided the platelet count remains normal. If the period of steroid therapy has extended beyond 14 days, a low dosage of dexamethasone (0.01 mg per kg) should be given on alternate mornings for an additional week. Chronic or recurrent IMTP, requiring constant or intermittent corticosteroid therapy, has been reported in horses; however, most cases of IMTP have a good prognosis and completely resolve after 14 to 21 days of treatment.

Since IMTP that is refractory to corticosteroids is rare in horses, alternate methods of therapy are unproved. Splenectomy is suggested for treatment of humans and dogs with IMTP that is unresponsive to corticosteroids. Splenectomy removes a large site for destruction of immunologically damaged platelets, as well as an important source of antiplatelet

---

*Thrombo-Wellcotest, Burroughs Wellcome Co., Research Triangle Park, NC

*Azium, Schering Corp., Kenilworth, NJ
†Meticortelone Acetate, Schering Corp., Kenilworth, NJ

antibody. Although splenectomy has been reported in horses, its benefit for treatment of IMTP is not documented. Various cytotoxic agents have been tried in treatment of chronic IMTP in humans and dogs. Vinca alkaloids, which appear to cause increased platelet production in addition to immunosuppression, have been most useful. Dogs with IMTP that is refractory to corticosteroids alone have been effectively treated with one or two intravenous injections of vincristine* at a dosage of 0.01 to 0.025 mg per kg.

Recently, impressive improvement in people with IMTP has followed therapy with high-dosage intravenous immunoglobulins (1 gm per kg). The IgG molecules are believed to coat Fc receptors on macrophages and interfere with clearance of platelet-antiplatelet antibody complexes. Since there are no commercially available concentrated equine immunoglobulin preparations, the volume of plasma necessary to achieve this dosage in horses is almost prohibitive (approximately 33 liters per 500 kg

*Oncovin, Eli Lilly and Co., Indianapolis, IN

horse). However, high-dose immunoglobulin therapy carries less risk to the patient than splenectomy or cytotoxic chemotherapy and may offer a reasonable alternative for equine cases of IMTP that are refractory to corticosteroids. Plasmapheresis to remove plasma antiplatelet antibodies may be a useful therapeutic approach to IMTP; however, only research or large hospital facilities would likely be equipped to provide this treatment to horses.

Supplemental Readings

Byars, T. D., and Greene, C. E.: Idiopathic thrombocytopenic purpura in the horse. J. Am. Vet. Med. Assoc., 180:1422, 1982.

Carroll, R. R., Noyes, W. D., and Kitchens, C. S.: High-dose intravenous immunoglobulin therapy in patients with immune thrombocytopenic purpura. J. Am. Med. Assoc., 249:1748, 1983.

Karpatkin, S.: Autoimmune thrombocytopenic purpura. Blood, 56:329, 1980.

McMillan, R.: Chronic idiopathic thrombocytopenic purpura. N. Engl. J. Med., 304:1135, 1981.

Morris, D. D., and Whitlock, R. H.: Relapsing idiopathic thrombocytopenia in a horse. Equine Vet. J., 15:73, 1983.

Vasculitis

Virginia B. Reef, KENNETT SQUARE, PENNSYLVANIA

Vasculitis, or inflammation of blood vessels, is an uncommon disorder in horses. The two most common types of equine vasculitis are immune-mediated vasculitis and vasculitis secondary to viral pathogens, specifically equine viral arteritis. Bacterial or fungal pathogens and drugs may also initiate vascular inflammatory disease in horses.

The signs of vasculitis are similar regardless of the mechanism involved. Dependent edema, especially in the distal extremities, is often one of the first clinical signs. Lethargy and reluctance to move are common clinical signs and the affected areas may be painful to palpation. Fever may also be seen with the onset of vasculitis, especially if the vasculitis is initiated by a virus or bacterial pathogen.

PURPURA HEMORRHAGICA

Purpura hemorrhagica is a syndrome primarily seen in young adult horses several weeks after an episode of respiratory disease. The cause of this syndrome is thought to be an immune-mediated vasculitis and represents the most commonly recognized vasculitis in horses. Although most cases occur secondary to an infection with *Streptococcus equi*, the disease may be associated with previous and/or concurrent beta-hemolytic streptococcal infection, influenza, or drug-induced allergies.

Clinical Signs. Affected horses have extensive subcutaneous edema involving the face, muzzle, limbs, ventral abdomen, or other areas. Often the edema is symmetrical but may begin in just one area or distal extremity. It is generally warm and painful to palpation. Petechial and ecchymotic hemorrhages may be seen in the visible mucous membranes. These petechiae and ecchymoses are due to injury to the blood vessel wall and are not associated with thrombocytopenia. Stiffness and reluctance to move are common with this disease; early or mild cases may be mistaken for laminitis. Edema of the upper respiratory tract may cause severe dyspnea. This may result in the need for a tracheostomy to relieve the respiratory distress. Serum will ooze from the severely edematous areas, and skin necrosis and sloughing of the affected skin may be significant secondary problems. Fever may or may not be exhibited by affected horses, while tachycardia and tachypnea are more commonly reported.

Purpura hemorrhagica is a nonthrombocytopenic purpura. Platelet counts performed on affected horses are usually normal. Clotting profiles are also unremarkable. The most consistent hematologic abnormalities are neutrophilic leukocytosis and hyperfibrinogenemia. Many affected horses are anemic, although periodic episodes of hemoconcentration due to loss of plasma constituents into the tissues through damaged vessel walls may occur.

Diagnosis. The diagnosis is based on a history of recent respiratory tract infection, typical clinical signs, and hematologic abnormalities. Confirmation of the diagnosis requires a skin biopsy of the affected areas. This reveals fibrinoid necrosis of the small blood vessels, endothelial swelling, pronounced polymorphonuclear leukocytic infiltration around vessels and in the vessel walls, and extravasation of red blood cells.

Gross necropsy findings include extensive subcutaneous edema and hemorrhage, with necrosis of skeletal muscles. Patchy hemorrhage and necrosis of the intestine resembling the human syndrome of Henoch-Schönlein purpura has been reported in a number of horses as well as petechiae of the heart and spleen. Many horses have an increase in the amount of peritoneal fluid. Areas of internal abscessation, usually caused by beta-hemolytic streptococci, have been found in some cases.

Histologically, the severe aseptic purulent vasculitis is consistent with the findings in an Arthus or type III hypersensitivity reaction. The Arthus reaction is a localized immune complex disease that affects only blood vessel walls. Mural deposits of equine IgA, IgG, and C′3 have been demonstrated. Fragmentation and swelling of muscle fibers with hemorrhages and cellular infiltration are often seen on histologic examination of the muscles.

Therapy. Primary therapy consists of systemic corticosteroids, and systemic antimicrobials should be administered when there is evidence of concurrent bacterial infection. Dexamethasone* (0.05 to 0.2 mg per kg intravenously or intramuscularly, once a day) or prednisolone† (0.5 to 1 mg per kg, intramuscularly, twice a day) should be administered as needed, to result in a significant reduction in edema. The daily dosage should be gradually reduced, over a period of 10 to 21 days. In severe cases it is often necessary to continue dexamethasone or prednisolone therapy in decreasing dosages for two weeks or more. Penicillin is the systemic antimicrobial of choice for streptococcal infection. Minimum dosages are 22,000 units per kg of potassium penicillin intravenously four times daily or 22,000 units per kg of procaine penicillin intramus-

cularly twice daily. Antimicrobial therapy should be continued throughout the period of corticosteroid administration, or until any obvious infection has resolved. Other antimicrobials may be added if gram-negative organisms are suspected or have been identified. Supportive care including hydrotherapy, hand walking (if possible), and support bandages are an important necessary part of the therapy. Extensive skin necrosis of the distal extremities in severe cases may lead to loss of usefulness of the horse because of the need for skin grafting and resultant scar formation. Some horses die in respiratory distress from edema of the airways if corticosteroid therapy is not adequate. Secondary infection (e.g., pneumonia, cellulitis) are common. With early aggressive treatment and good supportive care the mortality rate may be significantly reduced.

EQUINE VIRAL ARTERITIS

Equine viral arteritis should always be considered in the differential diagnosis of purpura hemorrhagica. This viral disease was first recognized in 1953 associated with an outbreak of abortion and influenzalike disease in Bucyrus, Ohio. Serologic studies reveal that the infection is much more common than clinical disease would indicate. Up to 75 per cent of certain equine populations were serologically positive for serum-neutralizing antibody in one study.

Clinical Signs. Clinical signs of equine viral arteritis include fever, lacrimation, dependent limb edema, weakness, diarrhea, and abortion. Fever may persist for up to nine days. Fever and serous nasal discharge occur at the onset of disease with excessive lacrimation and conjunctivitis. Palpebral edema often develops as well as limb edema. Anorexia, depression, dyspnea, colic, and weight loss have been reported in severely affected horses. Abortion often occurs during or immediately after the febrile period.

The most salient laboratory abnormality is leukopenia, primarily due to lymphopenia, which occurs early in the disease course. Hypovolemia and hypotension may be severe because of massive transudation of fluid into the surrounding tissues through damaged blood vessel walls.

The underlying lesion is necrosis of the media of the small muscular arteries, with acute panvasculitis. Edema and congestion of the lymph nodes is followed by necrosis. There is excess pleural and peritoneal fluid and subcutaneous edema. Neutrophilic infiltration and thrombosis of the smaller submucosal vessels in the cecum and colon occurs along with infarction and necrosis of the mucosa. Severe glomerulonephritis has been shown in ex-

---

*Dexamethasone, Beecham Laboratories, Bristol, TN
†Prednisolone Acetate Suspension, Carter-Glogan Laboratories, Inc., Glendale, AR

perimentally infected horses, and the virus persists in the kidneys and may be shed in the urine. Multifocal myometritis is probably responsible for the abortions seen in pregnant mares.

Presumptive diagnosis is based on the characteristic fever, lymphopenia, serous inflammation of the respiratory tract, conjunctivitis, and edema with abortions occurring in pregnant brood mares. Virus can be isolated from nasal swabs of affected febrile horses for up to 14 days. Serum neutralization tests on paired sera collected 10 to 14 days apart will demonstrate at least a fourfold increase in neutralizing antibody.

Therapy. There is no specific treatment for equine viral arteritis. Good supportive care should include three to four weeks of rest, hydrotherapy, and supportive bandaging of the distal extremities.

Systemic antimicrobials are indicated if a secondary bacterial infection is suspected.

Other differential diagnoses that should be ruled out when the clinician is presented with a horse with significant dependent edema are equine infectious anemia, equine ehrlichiosis, congestive heart failure, pleuritis, lymphangitis, and cellulitis.

Supplemental Readings

Gunson, D. E., and Rooney, J. R.: Anaphylactoid purpura in a horse. Vet. Pathol., *14*:325, 1977.

King, A. S.: Studies on equine purpura haemorrhagica. Article No. 3. Morbid Anatomy and Histology. Br. Vet. J., *105*:35, 1949.

Prickett, M. E., McCollum, W. H. and Bryans, J. T.: The gross and microscopic pathology observed in horses experimentally infected with the equine arteritis virus. Proc. 3rd Int. Conf. Eq. Infect. Dis. Paris, 1972, pp. 265–272.

Lymphoproliferative and Myeloproliferative Disorders

Raymond W. Sweeney, KENNETT SQUARE, PENNSYLVANIA

LYMPHOSARCOMA

Although the overall prevalence is not high, lymphosarcoma is one of the more common internal neoplasms affecting the horse. In a recent postmortem survey of 480 horses, 2.5 per cent had lymphosarcoma. Lymphosarcoma accounted for 1 to 3 per cent of all equine tumors in other reports.

Unlike many neoplasms, lymphosarcoma is not restricted to old horses. Fifty per cent of the reported cases of lymphosarcoma occur in horses between four and nine years of age, and it has been seen in several horses less than one year old. There is no reported breed or sex predilection for the disease. The clinical signs of lymphosarcoma vary depending on the organ involvement. The disease may be classified as one of four forms; however, there is considerable overlap between these groups: alimentary, mediastinal, cutaneous, and generalized.

Alimentary Form. In the alimentary form of equine lymphosarcoma, intermittent fever due to necrosis of tumor tissue, mild depression, and decreased appetite are common findings. The fever is typically not responsive to antimicrobial therapy. Neoplastic infiltration of the mesenteric lymph nodes and intestines may cause malabsorption and weight loss. Chronic colic, ascites, and diarrhea are also occasionally seen. Ventral abdominal, pectoral,

and limb edema may result from hypoproteinemia caused by malabsorption or from decreased lymphatic drainage resulting from mechanical obstruction of lymphatics by tumor masses. Frequently there is peripheral lymphadenopathy and occasionally abdominal lymphadenopathy or an abdominal mass may be palpated per rectum. However, the absence of lymphadenopathy or a palpable mass should not discourage the veterinarian from pursuing further diagnostic tests if lymphosarcoma is suspected. In summary, the alimentary form of lymphosarcoma should be suspected in horses of all ages exhibiting chronic fever, weight loss, anorexia, colic, edema, and lymphadenopathy, or with an abdominal mass. It should be noted that horses with lymphosarcoma may have any one or a combination of these signs. In general, however, the clinical signs in affected horses are not pathognomonic, and the diagnosis of lymphosarcoma cannot be made solely on the basis of clinical signs.

Mediastinal Form. Clinical signs associated with the mediastinal (thoracic) form of lymphosarcoma result from enlargement of the mediastinal lymph nodes and also invasion of the lung parenchyma by tumor masses. As in the alimentary form, horses with the thoracic form will frequently have chronic weight loss and anorexia. Pleural effusion is frequently detected on auscultation and percussion or by thoracocentesis. Discernible rales are less commonly found. Fever due to tumor tissue necrosis and peripheral lymphadenopathy are also frequently present.

Generalized Form. The generalized (multicentric) form of lymphosarcoma results from the invasion of multiple organ systems with tumor. The most commonly affected organs (in descending order of frequency) are lymph nodes, liver, spleen, intestines, kidneys, and lung. Lymphosarcoma involving the nasal cavity, larynx, and pharynx may lead to upper respiratory obstruction. Masses involving the heart, brain, ovary, and retrobulbar spaces are reported less commonly. Nonspecific clinical signs as in the other forms of lymphosarcoma include fever, weight loss, and decreased appetite. Other clinical signs depend on the organs involved.

Cutaneous Form. The cutaneous form of lymphosarcoma is characterized by single or multiple nonpainful subcutaneous nodules. Alopecia and skin ulceration usually are not present. If there is no internal involvement, the horse may show no other clinical signs and may survive for several years. However, signs referable to the affected organ system may appear if there is concurrent alimentary or mediastinal involvement.

Diagnosis. The list of diagnoses to rule out is extensive because of the myriad clinical signs that may accompany lymphosarcoma. Common causes of weight loss such as malnutrition, poor dentition, and chronic lameness may be excluded on the basis of a good history and physical examination. Gastrointestinal parasitism must always be considered in horses with weight loss or chronic colic or both. In horses with fever in addition to weight loss and colic, abdominal abscessation and other forms of neoplasia (gastric squamous cell carcinoma) must be ruled out. Granulomatous enteritis can be quite difficult to distinguish from lymphosarcoma, and frequently the two diseases may only be differentiated at postmortem.

If pleural effusion and fever are present, bacterial pleuropneumonia must be ruled out. Dependent edema may result from pleuritis, vasculitis (e.g., purpura hemorrhagica), or hypoproteinemia (granulomatous enteritis) as well as lymphosarcoma. Equine infectious anemia should always be considered in horses with fever of unknown origin or anemia or both.

While a presumptive diagnosis of lymphosarcoma may be suggested on the basis of history and clinical examination findings, confirmation of the diagnosis requires laboratory testing. To make a definitive antemortem diagnosis of lymphosarcoma, neoplastic lymphocytes must be detected in peripheral blood, bone marrow, peritoneal or pleural fluid, or in an aspirate or biopsy sample of a lymph node or tumor mass.

Many horses with lymphosarcoma are anemic, presumably because of the anemia of chronic disease. However, immune-mediated hemolytic anemia occasionally occurs in horses with lymphosarcoma. This may be confirmed by the direct Coombs' test. Hyperproteinemia, hyperfibrinogenemia, and neutrophilia occur in approximately half the horses with lymphosarcoma, but these findings are nonspecific. Hypercalcemia has been reported in one horse with lymphosarcoma possibly because of secretion of parathormonelike substance by tumor cells.

Results of a peripheral blood smear examination are not usually diagnostic for lymphosarcoma. A lymphocytosis is rarely present, but occasionally neoplastic lymphocytes may be detected in the peripheral blood. Circulating neoplastic lymphocytes are usually relatively well differentiated but larger in size than normal lymphocytes. They may have nuclear chromatin clumping, prominent nucleoli, and cytoplasmic basophilia. Lymphocytic infiltration of the bone marrow is rare, but may accompany peripheral lymphocytosis or circulating neoplastic lymphocytes. There is one reported case of primary lymphoid leukemia in which the peripheral blood and bone marrow contained neoplastic lymphocytes and lymphocytic precursor cells, and in which no solid tumor masses were present.

Thoracocentesis and abdominocentesis are frequently helpful in establishing a diagnosis of lymphosarcoma. Pleural and peritoneal fluid should be examined carefully for the presence of neoplastic lymphocytes. In addition to the characteristics just described, mitotic figures and binucleate lymphocytes may be seen. Similar-appearing cells may be present in a lymph node or tumor mass aspirate.

The most reliable method to establish the diagnosis of lymphosarcoma is histopathologic examination of a biopsy specimen from a lymph node or tumor mass. The sample may be obtained with a biopsy needle; however, tissue obtained by surgical excision retains better morphology and improves the chances of a definitive diagnosis. The sample should be fixed in 10 per cent formalin and submitted for histopathologic examination.

Therapy. There is no currently accepted mode of treatment for equine lymphosarcoma and the prognosis is poor. Although there are anecdotal reports of temporary remission induced by glucocorticoid therapy, this has not been documented. Chemotherapy has not been adequately investigated because of the expense associated with its use in the horse.

Pathology. The most common gross necropsy finding is enlargement of the peripheral, mesenteric, or mediastinal lymph nodes. On cut section, there is disruption of the normal lymph node architecture resulting from infiltration by neoplastic cells. Tumor masses vary in size, are tan-white, and may occur as isolated masses or numerous nodules affecting many organs. Tumor masses and affected lymph nodes may have a similar appearance. In alimentary cases, the intestinal wall is diffusely thickened. Samples of lymph nodes and tumor masses should be fixed in 10 per cent formalin and submitted for histopathologic examination to confirm the diagnosis.

PLASMA CELL MYELOMA

Plasma cell myeloma is characterized by the proliferation of neoplastic plasma cells that produce an excessive amount of immunoglobulin. Myeloma cells invade bone marrow, bone (causing lameness and pathologic fractures), and other organs such as liver, spleen, and lymph nodes. A few cases of plasma cell myeloma have been reported in horses. One was a 16-year-old Thoroughbred that had lameness and weakness. Weight loss, edema, and anemia were also present. The white blood cell count was reduced and mature plasma cells were observed in the peripheral blood. Bone marrow aspirates contained a large number of myeloma plasma cells. Serum protein electrophoresis revealed hyperproteinemia (9.7 gm per dl) with hypoalbuminemia. The serum protein elevation was due to a large "spike" (monoclonal elevation) in the beta globulin region. Although Bence Jones proteins (light chains of immunoglobulins) have been detected in the urine of myeloma patients of other species, they were not present in the urine of this horse. Necropsy revealed extensive replacement of normal bone marrow elements by myeloma cells, and osteolysis in the femur, humerus, and thoracic vertebra. Plasma cell myeloma, although obviously quite rare, might be suspected in a horse with lameness, anemia, and marked hyperproteinemia. Serum protein electrophoresis should be performed, and urine should be evaluated for the presence of Bence Jones proteins. The monoclonal hyperglobulinemia in myeloma must be distinguished from the polyclonal gammopathy that occurs in horses with chronic bacterial or viral infections and lymphosarcoma. The presence of typical "punched-out" lesions (well-circumscribed decalcified area) radiographically evident in the long bones supports the diagnosis of myeloma.

GRANULOCYTIC LEUKEMIA

Granulocytic leukemia is a bone marrow dysplasia in which a granulocytic cell line increases in numbers at the expense of the other cell lines. These disorders are extremely rare, with only four cases

reported in the literature. The disease is not restricted to old horses: one case occurred in a 10-month-old colt. Physical findings included depression, weight loss, pale mucous membranes with petechiation, and pitting edema of the limbs. In all cases, the diagnosis of granulocytic leukemia was made on the basis of bizarre granulocytes and granulocyte precursors in the peripheral blood and bone marrow. The granulocytes were eosinophils in two of the horses and not differentiated in the other two. All cases involved myelophthisic anemia and thrombocytopenia. No specific treatment was given and the four horses died or were euthanized shortly after the diagnosis was made. Temporary improvement was afforded by treatment with whole blood transfusions and corticosteroids.

The differential diagnosis for a horse with petechiation, anemia, and limb edema should include purpura hemorrhagica, thrombocytopenia (either immune-mediated or caused by consumptive coagulopathy), and equine infectious anemia. The diagnosis of granulocytic leukemia is confirmed by the results of a complete blood count and examination of the peripheral blood smear and bone marrow aspirate.

ERYTHROCYTOSIS

Erythrocytosis or an increase in packed cell volume (PCV) may be relative (caused by hemoconcentration, or splenic contraction) or pathologic (caused by an increase in red blood cell mass). This last group can be further classified as primary (polycythemia vera) or secondary. Secondary erythrocytosis results from increased erythropoietin, which may be a physiologic response to chronic hypoxemia (heart defects or residence at high altitude) or may be caused by inappropriate erythropoietin release, which occurs in some chronic hepatic and renal disorders, especially neoplasia.

Primary erythrocytosis is a myeloproliferative disease, the cause of which is not understood. It is extremely rare in the horse. Before a diagnosis of primary erythrocytosis can be made, relative erythrocytosis (hemoconcentration, splenic contraction) or a secondary increase in red cell mass as from hypoxemia or renal disease must be ruled out.

Clinical signs in one reported case of primary erythrocytosis were nonspecific: lethargy and weight loss. The packed cell volume was persistently between 60 and 70 per cent. The peripheral red cell morphology, bone marrow aspirates, and serum erythropoietin levels were also normal in this horse.

Erythrocytosis due to hemoconcentration may be ruled out if the horse does not show clinical signs of dehydration or endotoxemia. If the PCV decreases following tranquilization of the horse with xylazine, splenic contraction should be suspected as the cause of the initial erythrocytosis. Chronic hypoxia can be ruled out by the determination of arterial oxygen tension. Since secondary erythrocytosis can occur in animals with chronic hepatic and renal disease, the veterinarian must attempt to exclude these on the basis of biochemical tests such as serum creatinine, Bromsulphalein test, and serum hepatic enzyme concentrations.

Treatment of erythrocytosis consists of periodic phlebotomy to reduce the red blood cell mass. Two to six liters of whole blood may be removed, and an equal volume of balanced electrolyte solution administered intravenously. Packed cell volume should be monitored over subsequent days and phlebotomy repeated as necessary. This is strictly a palliative treatment; the long-term prognosis is guarded.

Supplemental Readings

Neufeld, J. L.: Lymphosarcoma in the horse: A Review. Can. Vet. J., *14*:129, 1973.

Rebhun, W. C., and Bertone, A.: Equine lymphosarcoma. J. Am. Vet. Med. Assoc., *184*:720, 1984.

Schalm, O. W., and Carlson, G. P.: The blood and blood-forming organs. *In* Mansmann, R. A., McAllister, E. S., and Pratt, P. W. (eds.): Equine Medicine and Surgery, 3rd ed. American Veterinary Publications, Santa Barbara, CA, 1982.

Blood and Plasma Therapy

James L. Becht, ATHENS, GEORGIA

Bradley J. Gordon, ATHENS, GEORGIA

OBJECTIVES

The objectives of administration of allogeneic whole blood (donor from same species) are to expand circulatory volume and supplement erythrocytes to improve oxygen delivery to the tissues. The benefits from a whole blood transfusion are temporary, providing supplemental blood until the recipient's bone marrow responds with increased production and release of erythrocytes. Since the need for whole blood supplementation usually arises as an emergency, successful transfusion of blood depends on a basic understanding of the merits and risks involved with the procedure.

When an anemic insult is produced experimentally by removal of approximately two thirds of the blood volume during a three-day period, the equine bone marrow is capable of an energetic regenerative response. Following an acute hemorrhagic episode that is halted, the rate of erythrocyte and hemoglobin replacement increases approximately two- to fourfold. Depending, of course, on the severity of the anemia, this rapid replacement of erythrocytes should lead to resolution of anemia within 20 to 30 days. Of primary importance is the period preceding the increased production and release of erythrocytes into circulation from the bone marrow. While the amount of erythropoiesis may vary among breeds of horses under steady-state conditions, it is likely that the production time for erythroid cells in the horse is approximately four days, which approximates other species. Thus, if transfused erythrocytes remain in the recipient's circulation for at least four days, the benefit of a whole blood transfusion is substantial. Although the mean erythrocyte life span for equine erythrocytes is approximately 150 days, preliminary studies in horses have revealed that allogeneic transfused erythrocytes are lost from the recipient's circulation in two to four days, even when donor selection is based on the conventional cross-matching procedure for compatibility. Following the first transfusion, approximately 60 and 90 per cent of transfused erythrocytes are removed from the recipient's circulation by four and seven days, respectively. After a second transfusion, approximately 80 per cent of erythrocytes are lost by 48 hours post-transfusion. Studies using ponies have revealed that more than 90 per cent of allogeneically transfused erythrocytes are lost from the recipient's circulation within two days, and as much as 50 per cent are lost within four hours after transfusion. Perhaps handling of blood during collection and preparation for administration has an adverse effect on erythrocyte survivability. In the same study using ponies, approximately 20 per cent of the transfused erythrocytes were lost within 24 hours when the transfusion was autogenous (from the same pony). If erythrocytes of the donor and recipient horse have identical or at least similar surface antigens, the survivability of transfused erythocytes should improve. Unfortunately, no such studies have been reported.

Plasma therapy has been used successfully as primary and supportive therapy in several disease conditions of foals and horses. Benefits of plasma administration include maintenance of vascular oncotic pressure and vascular transport capabilities, supplementation of antibodies, addition of enzymes modulating tissue proteases, and supplementation of blood clotting factors. The half-life of plasma proteins varies in the horse. While that of albumin is 18 to 20 days, half-life for the gamma globulins is approximately 11 days. To date, there are no reports addressing plasma protein distribution and half-life in various disease states.

INDICATIONS

Whole blood transfusions are often indicated (1) following acute and severe hemorrhage associated with major surgery of highly vascular tissues, trauma, or parturition, (2) after chronic blood loss, or (3) following erythrocyte destruction during neonatal isoerythrolysis or other hemolytic anemias. When considering the need for whole blood supplementation, several questions must be addressed. How severe is the anemia? How rapidly is the anemia developing? Is there an appreciable erythropoietic response present?

Assessment of the severity of anemia in the horse is often difficult. After acute hemorrhage, usually one to two days are required for splenic erythrocyte depletion and fluid shifts into the vascular space before the extent of blood loss can be assessed. In the case of acute hemorrhage, the erythrocyte content of the spleen serves as a buffer to meet immediate needs for assistance in circulatory volume replacement and oxygen-carrying capacity of the peripheral circulation. Determination of the severity and rapidity of erythrocyte loss or destruction is therefore largely masked by the compensatory function of the spleen. The PCV may actually increase transiently during abrupt hemorrhage due to the release of tremendous numbers of erythrocytes following splenic contraction.

The PCV is the simplest parameter to monitor when evaluating an anemic animal and considering the need for a transfusion. A PCV less than 20 per cent in a horse that was previously healthy and has had an acute hemolytic or hemorrhagic insult indicates that the splenic erythrocyte reservoir is largely depleted. The absolute PCV is not as important an indicator in determination of the need for whole blood supplementation as is the rapidity with which the PCV decreases—hence the importance of PCV monitoring to establish if a decreasing trend is present. A PCV of 12 per cent justifies a blood transfusion if it is suspected that the anemia is progressive.

The loss of blood volume is an often-overlooked factor when deciding if a whole blood transfusion is indicated. Blood volume varies between horses in different breeds and among horses within the same breed managed differently. Thoroughbreds have significantly more and Saddlebreds have significantly less blood in relation to body weight than Standardbreds. Furthermore, "cold-blooded" breeds, such as draft horses, have even less blood volume with respect to body weight than lighter breeds that are considered "hot blooded." Even with acute, severe blood loss, it is the decrease in the circulating blood volume rather than a deficit of erythrocytes that is responsible for the onset of shock. Therefore, if suitable whole blood is unavailable, or during the period when selection of a suitable donor and procurement of blood is under way, administration of plasma or isotonic (sodium-containing) fluid replacement is indicated in the immediate management of a horse with acute blood loss. A further decrease in the PCV will result from hemodilution, but the need for restoration of an adequate blood volume far outweighs the risk of other complications brought on by worsening the anemia.

Plasma contains albumin, immunoglobulins, protease inhibitors, and coagulation factors among other protein fractions. Plasma-addition therapy is indicated in situations in which deficiencies of these factors occur. Hypoproteinemia from such causes as gastrointestinal loss, pleuritis, and abdominal surgery may result in vascular oncotic changes resulting in edema. Plasma administration seems to stabilize these patients. The amount of plasma required varies according to size of the horse, severity of the disease, and magnitude of the protein loss. Plasma supplementation has also been used in foals and horses suffering from clotting factor deficiencies.

Neonatal foals suffering from failure of passive antibody transfer have routinely been given intravenous plasma transfusions. Although some controversy surrounds this practice, plasma has proved beneficial.

SELECTION OF A DONOR

Proper selection of a donor animal for allogeneic blood or plasma is of utmost importance for the successful use of transfusion therapy, and entails a basic understanding of equine immunohematology. Erythrocytes of horses and ponies are covered with numerous membrane antigens, which are termed *alloantigens*. Antibodies produced when foreign alloantigens are introduced into an animal are called *alloantibodies*. Following the first exposure to the foreign alloantigen, alloantibodies are produced and immunologic memory cells are committed to that specific antigen. Upon subsequent exposure to the same alloantigen, an anamnestic response occurs that results in a rapid, profound increase in alloantibodies. Presence of alloantibodies is the basis for compatibility testing of potential donors for a recipient in need of whole blood or plasma supplementation.

More than 30 types of alloantigens that make up eight blood groups or systems have been identified for the horse. Each blood group represents a different location on the chromosomes within the nucleus of erythrocyte stem cells in the bone marrow, which code for erythrocyte alloantigen expression. Each animal has none, one, or two antigenic factors in each blood group, which are reflected as the alloantigen type in each group. Of most importance in blood incompatibilities between horses is alloantigen Aa. This antigen appears to be the most antigenic when injected into recipient horses not possessing it naturally.

Considerable difference in frequencies of erythrocyte alloantigens has been observed among several equine breeds. As an example, alloantigen Aa occurs in approximately 50 per cent of Shetland ponies, 90 per cent of Thoroughbreds, 98 per cent of Arabians, 70 per cent of Quarterhorses, and 80 per cent of Standardbreds. Thus, if a horse that needs a blood transfusion lacks the Aa alloantigen, supplemental blood will probably contain Aa, which will serve to sensitize the recipient. Upon a second transfusion using blood containing the Aa alloantigen, the recipient is at great risk of developing a transfusion reaction. The common occurrence of this alloantigen emphasizes the need for erythrocyte alloantigen determinations in designated donor horses to minimize the risk of serious adverse effects following transfusion.

The presence of naturally occurring alloantibodies in horses has been investigated. A study by Suzuki et al. revealed that of 679 horses, 94 possessed naturally occurring alloantibodies. Analysis of these alloantibodies revealed that their reactivity with equine erythrocytes was very weak, and it was concluded that such alloantibodies are probably insignificant in blood transfusion reactions.

The term "universal blood donor" in its true sense is a misnomer. Although much has been learned about equine blood groups, especially in regard to their application in parentage determination and in the diagnosis of neonatal isoerythrolysis, very little is known about more subtle incompatibilities between erythrocyte alloantigens other than Aa and alloantigens of other blood protein polymorphisms. The number of erythrocyte alloantigen combinations (phenotypes) in horses is estimated at 400,000. Many of these are extremely rare, and some phenotypes are rather common. as evidenced by the common occurrence of alloantigen Aa. Besides erythrocyte surface alloantigens, different phenotypic expression has been demonstrated for

hemoglobin, carbonic anhydrase, phosphogluconate dehydrogenase, phosphoglucomutase, phosphohexose isomerase, catalase, acid phosphatase, and NAD diaphorase in equine erythrocytes. Analysis of serum has likewise revealed numerous alloantigens for equine albumin, transferrin, prealbumin, postalbumin, ceruloplasmin, esterase, and cholinesterase. Thus, it becomes readily apparent that the chances of two horses having exactly the same erythrocyte and serum alloantigen profile is exceedingly small. In fact, there are approximately 125 billion possible alloantigenic combinations in erythrocyte and protein polymorphisms in horses. However, one must keep in mind that the occurrence of each of these possibilities is not equally likely because of patterns of alloantigen frequency. Nevertheless, it is most unlikely in equine blood typing that two horses in 2000 will have identical alloantigen profiles. Therefore, while blood and plasma transfusions have a definite place in equine medicine, the veterinarian must appreciate the tremendous diversity of equine alloantigen types.

Compatibility testing involves procedures that detect agglutination and/or hemolysis of erythrocytes tagged with alloantibodies. The conventional cross-match, wherein washed erythrocytes and serum from the donor and recipient are mixed, incubated, and examined grossly and microscopically, primarily demonstrates the presence of agglutinins. Although the cross-match is the accepted compatibility testing procedure for use in humans and most animals, equine alloantibodies act more strongly as hemolysins rather than agglutinins. Thus, tests used to identify acceptable donors for whole blood and plasma should employ the same type of test used in characterization of equine alloantigens.

In hemolysin testing, an exogenous source of complement is needed for in vitro demonstration of hemolysis by alloantibody-tagged erythrocytes. Pooled serum from rabbits* is utilized for this purpose after naturally occurring anti-horse (Forssman) antibodies possessed by rabbits have been removed by processing with serum from normal horses. The need for exogenous complement and its special handling before use in equine compatibility testing makes this approach difficult in the practice situation. Likewise, the antiglobulin (Coombs) test, which detects agglutinins not detected in the cross-match, may be utilized. However, the expense of the reagent and the laboratory procedure involved makes this test also rather impractical for use by the equine practitioner. As a result, the conventional cross-match is recommended as a general screening test between donor

---

*Pel Freez Biologicals, Rogers, AR

and recipient. However, the results are often not accurate in predicting tolerance or an anaphylactic reaction when whole blood is transfused.

Generally it is safe to give transfusion to a recipient that has not received whole blood or blood components previously. This is primarily due to the low incidence and weak character of naturally occurring alloantibodies in horses. After the first transfusion, alloantibody production may occur and result in an adverse reaction should blood containing the responsible alloantigen be transfused again. Usually it requires at least four to seven days for production of these alloantibodies, so subsequent transfusions during this period should be relatively safe.

A recommended approach to improve service to the horse owner and minimize the possibility of transfusion reactions is to provide a donor horse as part of the veterinary practice. Larger horse farms may also benefit from using a designated animal as an acceptable whole blood or plasma donor. This can be accomplished by having the erythrocyte antigen profile of several potential donors identified and the serum analyzed to ensure that it contains no alloantibodies. Presently there are two laboratories that provide these services:

Serology Laboratory
Department of Veterinary Reproduction
School of Veterinary Medicine
University of California
Davis, CA 95616

Stormont Laboratories, Inc.
1237 E. Beamer St., Suite D
Woodland, CA 95695

Samples required from each animal being tested are serum from a clotted specimen and one sample with acid-citrate-dextrose (ACD) anticoagulant. The ratio of ACD to whole blood is 1.5 ml to 8.5 ml. A letter identifying the samples and describing why tests are desired should accompany each submission. The serum of suitable donors lacks alloantibodies and their erythrocytes lack alloantigen Aa and possibly Qa.

COLLECTION

When there are indications that whole blood supplementation is needed for an anemic horse, four to eight liters is a reasonable quantity to transfuse. Removal of this amount of blood from a healthy donor horse that has not been bled within the last 30 days has minimal adverse effects. The preferred anticoagulant for use in whole blood transfusions is sodium citrate, which acts by chelating calcium. A 4 per cent stock solution can be made (4 gm sodium citrate to 100 ml distilled water) and this stock solution added to an empty blood container at a rate of one part of the solution to nine parts whole blood. The container and anticoagulant solution should be sterilized before use. Heparin is an effective anticoagulant that interferes with the action of thrombin and certain other activated coagulation factors. At five units per ml of whole blood, it exerts an anticoagulant effect, but when more than four liters of heparinized whole blood are transfused, there may be enough heparin present to predispose to hemorrhage in some recipients. Plastic containers are preferable to glass for blood collection and administration, and are commercially available.* An excellent description of the proper use of blood containers was given on page 325 of the first edition of this text. Blood should be collected into sterile containers using aseptic technique. The donor horse should be restrained, and a large-bore (10-gauge) needle or catheter is placed in a jugular vein. The vein is occluded with digital pressure below the venipuncture and blood should flow into the collection apparatus. A slight advantage of glass containers over plastic bags is that it is easier to establish a vacuum in the collection apparatus, which facilitates blood removal.

In the past, plasma harvesting was achieved using manual methods. Whole blood was withdrawn from a donor and the erythrocytes were permitted to settle. Plasma was then withdrawn from the top or the packed red blood cells drained from the bottom of the container. More rapid red cell sedimentation can be achieved by centrifugation of collected blood before removal of the plasma. However, both techniques result in plasma that contains numerous erythrocytes. Recently, essentially erythrocyte-free plasma from donors that lack the Aa and Qa alloantigens and have no serum alloantibodies has become commercially available.†

HANDLING AND ADMINISTRATION

Although it is acceptable to store equine whole blood under refrigeration, there is virtually no information relating to the effects of storage on survival of transfused erythrocytes in the horse. Thus, fresh whole blood should be administered to an animal needing a transfusion. If whole blood is not needed after it is collected, it should be returned to the donor rather than being stored in a refrigerator for several weeks and then being discarded.

Before administration, whole blood or plasma should be gradually warmed to near body temper-

---

*Fenwal System, Division of Travenol Laboratories, Inc., Deerfield, IL

†Application Technologies & Pharmaceuticals, Inc., Atlanta, GA

ature. Incorporation of an in-line filter into the administration system is advised. Since blood compatibility testing results can be misleading, the recipient's tolerance to the transfusion should be assessed before a large amount is administered. This can be accomplished by noting the heart and respiratory rates before the transfusion is begun. After a small amount of blood (20 to 50 ml) is administered slowly, the transfusion is halted for approximately five minutes and the heart and respiratory rates and the recipient's activity are monitored. If these parameters do not change, the transfusion is continued with caution. One liter of whole blood can be safely administered to an adult horse over approximately 10 minutes, whereas one liter should be administered more slowly (preferably over one hour) to a young foal.

Although fresh plasma is preferable to frozen plasma, most proteins survive freezing and thawing before administration. Thawing and subsequent refreezing of unused plasma may result in damage to some plasma components. The routine dosage of plasma to foals with failure of passive antibody transfer is one liter. This usually results in serum IgG levels greater than 400 mg per dl, but follow-up testing of serum IgG concentration is recommended. Immunoglobulin levels do not always increase after plasma transfusion. Although no research has been published, several possible mechanisms may be involved. Laboratory methods utilized to determine concentrations of IgG have inherent variability. Dilution of antibody-rich plasma in a circulating blood volume that is antibody poor or equilibration of IgG between the intravascular and extravascular spaces may account for apparent "loss" of administered antibody. Finally, the time between administration and postadministration evaluations of recipient plasma antibody levels will affect the plasma levels obtained.

COMPLICATIONS

Signs of transfusion reactions include restlessness, respiratory distress, polypnea, tachycardia, defecation, muscle fasciculations, and sudden collapse. The administration of epinephrine, 3 to 5 ml of 1:1000 dilution, may help restore vascular tone and cardiac performance during a transfusion reaction. Corticosteroid therapy may also be beneficial. In any case, epinephrine or similar agents should be available during all transfusions.

Transfusion of whole blood or plasma containing sodium citrate may be associated with sudden hypocalcemia. Signs of citrate toxicity in horses have included apprehension, muscle fasciculations, arrhythmias, and collapse. Affected horses respond to decreases in the infusion rate and administration of calcium gluconate.

Due to the numerous erythrocytes and serum alloantigens, transfusions serve to sensitize the recipient to foreign blood antigens. The administration of plasma containing erythrocytes with the alloantigen Aa to a newborn filly with failure of passive transfer may sensitize her to that alloantigen. As a result, her first foal may be predisposed to develop neonatal isoerythrolysis if the stallion possesses the Aa alloantigen.

ADMINISTRATION OF OTHER BLOOD COMPONENTS

Adaptation of blood component separation devices used in human medicine has permitted successful collection of specific equine blood components.* These devices permit relatively rapid and safe blood component separation and collection with return of unwanted blood fractions to the donor. Consequently, desirable donors may be used more frequently than previously possible using manual methods. These hemapheresis devices produce component separation by centrifugation or hollow fiber filtration of whole blood. They have been used to successfully collect packed erythrocytes, to concentrate leukocytes (neutrophils or lymphocytes), and to concentrate platelets, plasma, and platelet-rich plasma from donor horses.

Plasma exchange, or removal and replacement of a human's plasma, is performed in cases of plasma protein–bound toxins and diseases mediated by antibodies or immune complexes. These procedures have been done only on a limited basis in horses. The eventual beneficial or deleterious effects are presently unknown. Transfusion of packed erythrocytes has been used in cases of hemolytic anemia when volume overload is of concern. Packed erythrocytes can be obtained through collection methods previously described.

Leukocyte transfusions have been beneficial in treating human neonates and laboratory animals that are septic, neutropenic, and nonresponsive to antibiotic therapy. Premature and ill neonates responding most remarkably to these transfusions often possess significant deficiencies in neutrophil functions and storage properties. There are insufficient data at this point to determine the efficacy of leukocyte transfusions in horses. Concentrated platelets or platelet-rich plasma may be beneficial to horses with thrombocytopenia.

---

*Fenwal System, Division of Travenol Laboratories, Inc., Deerfield, IL, or Cobe Laboratories, Lakewood, CA

Supplemental Readings

Gimlette, T. M.: Transfusion of autologous and allogeneic chromium-51 labelled red cells in ponies. J. Roy. Soc. Med. 71:576, 1978.

Jeffcott, L. B.: Clinical hematology of the horse. *In* Archer, R. K., and Jeffcott, L. B. (eds.): Comparative Clinical Hematology. London, Blackwell Scientific Publications, 1977, pp. 162–213.

Kallfelz, F. A., Whitlock, R. H., and Schultz, R. D.: Survival of ^{59}Fe-labeled erythrocytes in cross-transfused equine blood. Am. J. Vet. Res., 39:617, 1978.

Morris, P. G.: Blood Transfusion. *In* Robinson, N. E. (ed.): Current Therapy in Equine Medicine. Philadelphia, W. B. Saunders Co., 1983, pp. 325–328.

Section 8

INTERNAL PARASITES

Edited by R. P. Herd

Diagnosis of Internal Parasites

R. P. Herd, COLUMBUS, OHIO

Internal parasites are one of the greatest limiting factors to successful horse raising throughout the world. All horses at pasture become infected and suffer a wide range of harmful effects ranging from impaired development and performance to death. Despite the availability of a large array of modern anthelmintics, parasite control programs often fail to safeguard horse health. The main reasons for these breakdowns are errors in the choice of anthelmintics and in the timing of treatments. Few people associated with horses understand the prophylactic use of anthelmintics or the epidemiology of worm infection.

In this section, modern epidemiologic approaches to worm control will be discussed. These approaches replace traditional methods that often provide only a few days of protection before horses are reinfected from an environment teeming with infective larvae. In one study in Ohio, it was calculated that over 99 per cent of the worm population was in the pasture, while less than 1 per cent was in untreated horses. Anthelmintic treatment in this situation would remove only a small fraction of the total worm population and horses would be quickly reinfected. Modern epidemiologic control strategies are based on small numbers of prophylactic treatments at key periods of the year or on nonchemical approaches

that ensure a safe pasture. One new program, pasture vacuuming, increases the grazing area by about 50 per cent, in addition to providing excellent parasite control.

It is useful to divide internal parasites into (1) major pathogens that are a constant problem and require continual control strategies and surveillance, and (2) occasional pathogens that require action only when they are perceived to be present in increasing numbers. Major pathogens are large strongyles, cyathostomes, and ascarids; occasional parasites are bots, lungworms, pinworms, stomach worms, tapeworms, and threadworms.

The large strongyles have traditionally been regarded as the most prevalent and pathogenic of worms. Recent studies suggest that the cyathostomes, or small strongyles, have emerged as the major problem in some areas. This may be related to the fact that the most common species of cyathostomes have developed resistance to benzimidazole anthelmintics. By contrast, the benzimidazole drugs have continued to be effective against the large strongyles over a 20-year period. This may account for the low prevalence recently reported in Kentucky, Ohio, and Texas for both intestinal and arterial stages of *S. vulgaris.*

AGE OF HORSE

The age of the horse is an important diagnostic consideration because susceptibility to parasites varies with the horse's age and degree of exposure to worms. Foals are most susceptible to threadworms (*Strongyloides westeri*) in the first few months of life following infection via the mare's milk. They quickly develop a strong immunity so that eggs are rarely seen in their feces after six months of age. Ascarid infection (*Parascaris equorum*) occurs mainly in foals and yearlings but rarely in mature horses. Adult horses that shed ascarid eggs are not likely to harbor many worms, unless immunosuppressed. Ascarids are very prolific egg layers and one female worm can lay 100,000 eggs per day. Consequently, a mature horse with a few worms could still show an appreciable egg count. Tapeworms (*Anoplocephala, Paranoplocephala* spp.) occur in horses of all ages but are more serious in yearlings. Pinworms (*Oxyuris equi*) are more of a problem in stabled horses than in horses at pasture because of the greater exposure to eggs in feeders and water.

Horses of all ages are susceptible to *Strongylus vulgaris* infection. Comparable numbers of adult worms in the gut and migrating larvae in the arteries have been found in naturally infected horses of all age groups. Nevertheless, clear evidence of an acquired immunity has been obtained from studies with experimental infection of worm-free horses. It has also been shown that foals and weanlings are less tolerant of the effects of *S. vulgaris* infection than are older horses and are thus more likely to develop the acute syndrome of anorexia, pyrexia, depression, weight loss, and colic, culminating in death.

The cyathostomes also affect horses of all ages, although clinical signs tend to be more common in horses less than five years old. The disease is most common in northern latitudes in the first five months of the year (winter through spring). This seasonal effect is thought to be related to the emergence of large numbers of cyathostome larvae from the gut wall after they have completed a period of winter hypobiosis, or arrested development, similar to the type II ostertagiasis syndrome of cattle. The emerging cyathostomes also contribute substantially to spring and summer rises in worm egg output. The cyathostomes, normally account for over 95 per cent of the strongyle worm burden and egg output, while the large strongyles account for less than 5 per cent.

HISTORY

A complete history is a vital part of the diagnostic process. Special attention should be given to the grazing history, seasonal conditions, and the choice, timing, and frequency of previous anthelmintic treatments. It is particularly important to know when the horses were at pasture, in which pasture they grazed, which animals contaminated that pasture, when it was contaminated, whether temperature and rainfall conditions were suitable for larval development and migration, which anthelmintics were used, when they were used, and how long the intervals were between treatments. The prevalence of colic in a group of horses is another guide to the effectiveness of the parasite control program.

A good history is often more valuable than fecal or blood tests and can result in an accurate "on the spot" diagnosis without waiting for laboratory results. Nevertheless, fecal egg counts are of value in pinpointing the major groups of parasites involved, the efficacy of recent treatments, and the presence of drug resistance. The value of fecal egg counts in monitoring the efficacy of a control program is discussed on p. 336. Fecal egg counts are of little value in assessing the size of the worm burden and the severity of infection because of the lack of correlation between numbers of eggs and numbers of worms. If horses showing respiratory signs have a history of shared grazing with donkeys, lungworm infection should be suspected and appropriate diagnostic tests performed.

CLINICAL SIGNS

Clinical signs are often variable and nonspecific, with few pathognomonic features.

Large Strongyles (*Strongylus vulgaris, S. edentatus, S. equinus*). It is difficult to attribute specific signs to adult large strongyles in the gut, as they usually occur in mixed infections with other strongylids or nematodes. Nevertheless, adult worms suck in plugs of mucosa and cause considerable erosion and bleeding. They are likely to contribute to poor development and performance, ill-thrift, rough coat, emaciation, weakness, anorexia, anemia, diarrhea, colic, and death. Migrating *S. vulgaris* larvae in the arteries cause arteritis and thromboembolic lesions, which may result in anorexia, pyrexia, depression, weight loss, colic, and death, sometimes associated with intussusception, volvulus, or aneurysms. *S. vulgaris* larvae in the central nervous system have been associated with acute progressive encephalitic disease and with chronic incoordination. Aortic and iliac thrombosis associated with *S. vulgaris* infection has been blamed for hindlimb lameness. Migrating *S. edentatus* larvae occasionally cause massive subperitoneal hemorrhage and death, while *S. equinus* larvae can cause hepatitis and pancreatitis.

Cyathostomes (*Cyathostominae*). These worms are a major problem in most horse-raising areas, but are easily overlooked in diagnosis. They often have been ignored because adult cyathostomes commonly occur in the gut in hundreds of thousands and are relatively nonpathogenic. However, massive numbers of larval cyathostomes emerging from the gut wall can cause the sudden onset of diarrhea with rapid and severe weight loss. Weight loss may occur rapidly despite a reasonably good appetite. Subcutaneous edema is sometimes seen in the muzzle, limbs, ventral abdomen, and sheath. Untreated horses are likely to die.

An important diagnostic feature is the seasonal occurrence in winter and spring (January through May) in northern latitudes, as larvae emerge from winter hypobiosis. In southern latitudes, larval cyathostomiasis can be expected to occur in summer and autumn as larvae emerge from a state of summer hypobiosis. Fecal egg counts are often negative in clinically affected horses. Emerging larvae are too immature to lay eggs, while adult female worms at that time of year have already completed their egg laying.

Ascarids (*Parascaris equorum*). Poor development and performance, ill-thrift, rough coat, pot belly, emaciation, weakness, anorexia, coughing, nasal discharge, depression, diarrhea, colic, intestinal obstruction or rupture, nervous signs, and death can all occur as a result of ascarid infections. Treatment of heavily infected foals sometimes results in a fatal blockage of the small intestine.

Bots (*Gasterophilus* spp.). Annoyance by bot flies, pain on mastication, poor growth, ill-thrift, anorexia, colic, and death due to gastric rupture have been observed.

Lungworms (*Dictyocaulus arnfieldi*). Infected horses may cough, especially during exercise, and show ill-thrift.

Pinworms (*Oxyuris equi*). Anal pruritus, restlessness, and hair loss at the base of the tail are the main signs of pinworm disease.

Stomach worms (*Draschia, Habronema* spp.). There are generally no clinical signs, but death from gastric rupture has been recorded.

Small stomach worms (*Trichostrongylus axei*). The main signs are a capricious appetite, ill-thrift, and emaciation.

Tapeworms (*Anoplocephala, Paranoplacephala* spp.). Tapeworms are occasionally associated with ill-thrift, diarrhea, colic, and death from intestinal obstruction, intussusception, or perforation.

Threadworms (*Strongyloides westeri*). Ill thrift, diarrhea, and colic occur in foals.

DIAGNOSTIC TESTS

Direct Fecal Smear. In this technique, a small amount of feces is mixed with a drop of water on a glass slide and examined microscopically after adding a coverslip. This technique has low accuracy because of the small quantity of feces examined and a negative result is inconclusive. A flotation technique provides more information.

Concentration of Eggs or Oocysts by Flotation. Eggs or oocysts will float when mixed with a flotation solution of specific gravity (SG) higher than that of eggs or oocysts. In this way, eggs or oocysts can be obtained in a relatively clean suspension provided that the SG is not sufficiently high to float up fecal debris. Common flotation solutions include saturated salt (SG 1.2), saturated sodium nitrate (SG 1.4), and Sheather's sugar solution (SG 1.2 to 1.3). Zinc sulphate solution (SG 1.2) has been used for recovery of Giardia cysts, while Sheather's sugar solution (500 gm sucrose, 320 ml water, 6.5 gm melted phenol) is good for the recovery of Cryptosporidium oocysts. The Baermann technique is widely used for the recovery of larvae.

Equine practitioners are strongly urged to do quantitative fecal egg counts using the McMaster technique or modifications of it. This technique is simple and one technician can count about 40 samples per day. McMaster slides at a cost of about $5 each or complete fecal kits* at a cost of about $20 each are available in the United States. It is necessary to weigh out a known quantity of feces such as 4 gm and mix it with a known volume of flotation solution. Using a pipette, the entire area under the counting grids is filled with an aliquot of the fecal suspension. The eggs or oocysts rise and come to rest on the undersurface of the chamber cover and will be found in the same focal plane as air bubbles. All eggs within the counting grid are counted at 100 times magnification. The number of eggs or oocysts counted is multiplied by a dilution factor to give the number of eggs per gram of feces (epg).

The fecal egg count is particularly valuable in practice as it provides an accurate assessment of the degree of pasture contamination. With it, the parasite control program can be evaluated. Pre- and post-treatment egg counts will also help to detect the development of drug resistance. No fecal examination or worm egg count gives a reliable guide to the size or severity of the worm infection, since there is little correlation between fecal egg counts and numbers of worms.

Immature, migrating, or hypobiotic worms do not betray their presence by passage of eggs in the feces. Different worm species lay eggs at different rates and not all female worms are productive at the same time. Female ascarids are very prolific and may lay 100,000 eggs per day, compared to about 5000 for large strongyles and 100 for small strongyles. Worm egg production may also be sup-

---

*Olympic Equine Products, 5004 228th Avenue, S.E., Issaquah, WA 98027, Tel (206) 392-1030.

pressed by host immunity in mature horses. Strongyle eggs in the feces of foals less than six weeks of age are usually the result of coprophagia, as these foals are too young to have acquired a patent infection.

Eggs of the pinworm (*Oxyuris equi*) are rarely seen in the feces, as the female worm deposits most of her eggs on the perineal region. Eggs may be recovered by a simple cellophane tape test. A piece of clear cellophane adhesive tape is pressed against the grayish egg smears around the anus. The tape is then stuck to a glass slide and the characteristic eggs with their flattened side and single operculum can be observed under the microscope. Sedimentation techniques are more sensitive than flotation for recovery of tapeworm eggs.

Larval Cultures. Although strongyle eggs are easily differentiated from those of ascarids, lungworms, pinworms, stomach worms, tapeworms, and threadworms, eggs of the large and small strongyles cannot be differentiated. To do this it is necessary to culture infective third-stage larvae for identification, after incubating horse feces at 26° to 29°C for seven days. Larval development can be accelerated by raising the temperature, but this reduces larval yield. The numbers of larvae of each species recovered do not necessarily reflect the relative proportions of those species because of differential fecundity and larval mortality.

Larval culture techniques vary from laboratory to laboratory. One simple method is to add well-mixed horse feces to a 16 oz jar until it is one third full, then loosely apply the lid. Growth of fungi can be inhibited by stirring the culture daily. After incubation at 26 to 29° C for seven days, away from sunlight, the jar is filled completely with water and inverted over a Petri dish, which is then half filled with water. The infective larvae descend from the fecal mass to the Petri dish and can be recovered in a clean suspension by means of a pipette. Alternatively, infective larvae can be harvested from the incubated feces by the Baermann technique. During incubation, feces should be moistened with water if they become dry; or if they are too wet, charcoal, sphagnum or peat moss, vermiculite, or sterile feces (100° C for 30 minutes) can be added to absorb moisture. Identification of larvae is facilitated if they are killed in an extended state. This can be achieved by gentle heat or by adding a few drops of Lugol's iodine (5 gm iodine, 10 gm potassium iodide, and 100 ml of distilled water).

S. vulgaris infective larvae are large and broad with a mean length of 1010 μm and 28 to 32 gut cells, whereas *S. edentatus* are thin, measure about 790 μm in length, and have 18 to 20 ill-defined gut cells. The small strongyles (cyathostomes) have a mean length of 830 μm but only 8 gut cells. *T. axei*

infective larvae are distinguished by a short tail, a mean length of 650 μm and 16 gut cells.

Baermann Technique. This technique is useful for recovering larvae from fresh feces, incubated feces, pasture, soil, and tissues. It is more sensitive than flotation for recovering lungworm larvae from feces. The Baermann apparatus consists of a large funnel supported by a retort stand. The stem of the funnel is connected to a test tube by a short piece of plastic tubing closed by means of a spring clip. The funnel is filled with enough warm water to cover the sample, which is held in a sieve or tea strainer, or wrapped in cheesecloth. Larvae stimulated by warmth and moisture migrate out of the feces or other material and, unable to swim against gravity, descend to the test tube where they can be recovered in a clean suspension after three to four hours.

Dictyocaulus arnfieldi first-stage larvae are 420 to 480 μm in length and have a small spike at the tip of the tail.

Pasture Larval Counts. Although fecal egg counts provide an accurate assessment of the degree of pasture contamination with worm eggs, they do not give an accurate guide to the degree of pasture infectivity with infective third-stage larvae (L3). This can be assessed only by pasture larval counts. A pasture highly contaminated with eggs may be one of low infectivity with L3, but it has the potential to become highly infective if conditions of temperature and rainfall favor the development and migration of infective L3.

Pasture larval counts are mainly done in parasitology research laboratories and are not feasible in most equine practices. Nevertheless, they provide data of considerable practical importance and might be adopted in practices with plentiful technical assistance. The simplest technique is the Baermann technique and advice on this method can be obtained from most university parasitology laboratories.

Necropsy Examination for Parasites. The size and severity of the gastrointestinal worm burden can be determined only by total worm counts at necropsy. This involves ligation and removal of the stomach, small intestine, cecum, and colon and examination of 10 per cent aliquots of the ingesta as well as digests of the wall of each organ to recover histotropic larvae. The ingesta and washings of each organ are made up to a convenient volume of several liters with water and stirred well before the 10 per cent aliquot is taken.

In many laboratories the worms are washed through course mesh sieves (e.g., 18 mesh:1.00 mm aperture, 35 mesh:0.5 mm aperture) to remove large debris, then washed further and retained in fine mesh sieves (e.g., 325 mesh:45 μm aperture,

400 mesh:38 μm aperture) before transfer to 10 per cent formalin for counting and storage. The aliquot, or subsamples of it, from each organ is examined under an illuminated lens or dissecting microscope. One hundred worms may be randomly selected from each organ for identification using the keys to genera and species devised by Lichtenfels (see Supplemental Readings). Large parasites like *Gasterophilus* larvae or *Parascaris equorum* can be identified and removed manually when the organ is first opened.

Nematode larvae in the gastrointestinal wall are recovered by scraping the mucosa and allowing the scrapings to digest in 1 per cent pepsin and hydrochloric acid at 37° C for two to six hours. This reduces the tissue to the consistency of sand, whereas the worms are little affected because of their tough cuticle. Nevertheless, the shorter the digestion period the better, as overdigestion may damage or destroy larvae. The recovered larvae are counted under a dissecting microscope and species identified when possible. Larvae in the gastrointestinal wall may also be quantitated by transillumination of the wall with a strong light source. This method avoids any loss of worms by digestion; however, tissues must be examined within 24 hours of the horse's death.

The aorta and major branches of the cranial mesenteric artery should be examined for larvae and lesions of *S. vulgaris*. The fourth- and fifth-stage larvae vary in size from 2 mm to 2 cm and can be recovered both by direct examination and by pepsin and hydrochloric acid digestion of arterial scrapings. Larval *S. edentatus* may be recovered by dissection of cysts in the subperitoneal tissues.

Hematology. Hematologic changes are of limited diagnostic value. Anemia has been observed in naturally parasitized horses, but it is not a reliable diagnostic sign. Horses with strongyle infections lose some blood from gastrointestinal hemorrhage, but this does not always result in clinically detectable anemia. Eosinophilia is a frequent but not invariable finding. In some cases, eosinophil counts may be zero or very low, and leukocytosis is associated with a neutrophilia or lymphocytosis.

Serology. Serum protein and IgG(T) concentrations have been used as an aid to the diagnosis of migrating larval *S. vulgaris* and colic due to verminous arteritis. However, these responses are characterized by a lack of specificity and are fraught with numerous difficulties of interpretation. Increases in beta globulin and IgG(T) concentrations are not specific to *S. vulgaris* or to migrating nematodes in general. Increased beta globulin concentrations have been reported in horses experimentally infected with cyathostomes and *S. westeri*. Increased IgG(T) concentrations have been reported in horses with equine infectious anemia, and in horses hyperimmunized with tetanus or diphtheria toxoids. It is likely that any migrating nematode—including large strongyles, cyathostomes, ascarids, lungworms, stomach worms, threadworms, and filarial worms—can induce this type of response.

Problems of interpretation include a time lag of several months between worm infection and serologic response, a slow return to normal values after removal from worm exposure, and a lack of response in some previously sensitized horses. In practice, this means that there could be many false-positives or false-negatives, and horses may die of acute *S. vulgaris* infection before a serum protein response occurs. In one study in which numbers of larval *S. vulgaris* and arterial lesions were scored in 64 naturally infected horses at Cambridge, beta globulin and IgG(T) responses failed to provide a reliable guide to the severity of infection.

Supplemental Readings

Arundel, J. H.: Parasitic Diseases of the Horse. Vet. Rev. No. 18, 83 pp., University of Sydney, The Post-Graduate Foundation in Veterinary Science, Sydney, NSW, Australia, 1978.

Drudge, J. H., and Lyons, E. T.: Ascariasis, Strongylosis, Strongyloidosis, Bots, Cestode infection, Oxyuris infection. *In* Robinson, N. E. (ed.): Current Therapy in Equine Medicine. Philadelphia, W. B. Saunders Company, 1983.

Lichtenfels, J. R.: Helminths of domestic equids. Illustrated keys to genera and species with emphasis on North American forms. Proc. Helminthol. Soc. Wash., 42 (special issue), 92 pp.

Ogbourne, C. P.: Pathogenesis of cyathostome (Trichonema) infections of the horse. A review. Commonwealth Institute of Helminthology, Commonwealth Agricultural Bureaux of The United Kingdom. Misc. Publ. No. 4, 25 pp., 1978.

Ogbourne, C. P., and Duncan, J. L.: *Strongylus vulgaris* in the horse: its biology and veterinary importance. 2nd ed. Commonwealth Institute of Parasitology, Commonwealth Agricultural Bureaux of The United Kingdom. Misc. Publ. No. 9, 68 pp., 1985.

Prophylactic Use of Anthelmintics

R. P. Herd, COLUMBUS, OHIO

The prophylactic use of anthelmintics is based on an understanding of the basic principles of the epidemiology of nematode infection. With this understanding, the practitioner can design effective control strategies to prevent the seasonal build-up of pasture contamination and infectivity. For this reason, the first part of this section is devoted to epidemiologic information of practical use to equine practitioners.

EPIDEMIOLOGY

Although parasite epidemiology is only in its infancy in the United States, enough is known to allow the formulation of some practical control strategies. Different strategies are needed for the northern and the southern United States, because of their different epidemiology and seasonal patterns of pasture contamination and infectivity. Although some concrete recommendations will be made on the basis of present knowledge, it should be kept in mind that this knowledge is incomplete and that improved control programs will evolve in the future as more epidemiologic data become available.

NORTHERN UNITED STATES, UNITED KINGDOM, AND EUROPE

Horses in the northern United States, United Kingdom, and Europe show a seasonal rise in worm egg output with peak egg counts in the spring and summer. This is a seasonal effect in all horses, unrelated to gender, pregnancy, or the date of foaling. It has important epidemiologic implications in that rises in egg counts occur just before the period when climatic conditions favor development of eggs to infective larvae and their migration from fecal reservoirs to pasture.

The cyathostome worms that are mainly responsible for the increased spring and summer egg output appear to be derived largely from larvae ingested in the previous grazing season. They have the ability to remain arrested in the gut wall for long periods, including the adverse northern winters or southern summers. Their emergence from the gut wall poses a double threat to horse health. First, the tissue damage may lead to clinical strongylosis. Second, the emerging worms are ready for final maturation and egg production, resulting in massive contamination of pastures in spring and summer.

Consequently, there is likely to be a potentially dangerous increase in pasture infectivity with third-stage infective larvae in summer or autum or both, depending on the rainfall. A wet summer facilitates the rapid migration of larvae from fecal reservoirs to pasture, while a dry summer may block migration until autumn rains occur. In studies in Ohio, the seasonal summer and autum rise in pasture infectivity persisted until June of the following year before increasing temperatures led to death of larvae. In arid regions survival is shorter, as larvae survive only as long as fecal reservoirs remain moist.

In general, horses in nonarid northern latitudes are likely to be exposed to decreasing strongyle infection in the first half of the year and escalating infection in the second half. Larvae that have overwintered on pastures tend to die off as temperatures rise in spring, and the decrease in numbers is accentuated by the diluting effect of accelerated herbage growth. The spring and summer rises in fecal egg counts subsequently provide a massive pasture contamination, which leads to an explosive summer and autum increase in pasture infectivity with larvae.

A seasonal pattern has also been observed in the migration and maturation of *S. vulgaris*. The risk of thromboembolic colic is greatest during the time of peak larval migration in autumn and winter. As summer progresses and horses are exposed to increasing numbers of infective larvae on pastures, the mean numbers of fourth-stage larvae in the arteries increase to reach a peak in autumn and winter. Since ingested larvae reach the cranial mesenteric artery in two to three weeks and develop there for two to four months, the return migration of fifth-stage larvae occurs predominately in the winter months. As spring approaches, the numbers of larvae in the arteries decline as the larvae mature to adults.

SOUTHERN UNITED STATES

Studies in Texas and Florida indicate that the seasons of greatest worm egg production and pasture infectivity occur later than in the north. A summer and autumn rise in fecal egg counts leading to peak pasture larval counts in autumn and winter has been observed. The increased egg production appears to be derived mainly from maturation of large numbers of larvae acquired in winter and spring. Transmission appears to be minimal in the summer because of high larval mortality. In some of the arid or semiarid regions of the western states, conditions are often unfavorable for development of eggs and larvae, and the transmission period is greatly reduced.

PASTURE LARVAE—DEVELOPMENT, MIGRATION, AND SURVIVAL

Although our knowledge of the development and survival of strongyle larvae on pastures in the United States is incomplete, there is enough information from both here and abroad to make the following general statements. These points should be useful to equine veterinarians when they are assessing the potential dangers of a horse pasture and formulating control strategies.

1. Hatching of strongyle eggs occurs only at temperatures of 7.5° C (45° F) to 38° C (100° F) and is optimal at about 25° C (77° F). Prolonged freezing weather or alternating freezing and thawing results in high mortality of eggs without hatching.

2. Freezing is especially lethal to preinfective larvae (first- and second-stage), larvae being killed faster than eggs. In England, most eggs hatch in the winter, which is less severe than in North America, but few or none of the emerging larvae survive long enough to reach the infective stage.

3. In northern temperate regions, development of infective larvae occurs mainly from April to October, with optimal development in warm, wet summers. Lack of summer rain can inhibit larval development and delay migration of infective larvae from feces to the surrounding pasture.

4. In northern temperate regions, the rate of development of freshly deposited eggs increases as temperatures rise in the spring. During the optimal summer period, infective larvae may develop within a week after feces are passed. The rate of larval development then slows again as temperatures fall in late autumn and may cease entirely in a severe winter.

5. In southern temperate or subtropical zones, development of infective larvae may occur all the year round, but larval mortality is likely to be high, with minimal transmission of infection in the summer. Larvae do not survive well on pasture during the long, hot summers of the humid subtropics.

6. High temperatures and dryness are lethal to both eggs and larvae, especially if feces are broken up and dispersed. In arid regions, feces may dry up before larvae have completed their development to the infective stage. One week of hot dry weather can result in the complete desiccation of a compact heap of horse feces.

7. Moist feces act as a protective reservoir from which the pasture larval population is periodically replenished. The migration of infective larvae from fecal mass to herbage can occur only under moist conditions, and is likely to occur in waves coincident with falls of rain, even after as little rain fall as 2.5 cm.

8. The distance of active larval migration is generally assumed to be limited to less than 30 cm horizontally and 10 cm vertically from the soil surface, but more studies are needed on this point. Larvae may be spread over a wider area by temporary localized flooding, hooves, farm equipment, and other agents.

9. Infective larvae (in contrast to preinfective larvae) survive for long periods at low temperatures, even at many degrees below freezing. A persistent covering of snow may greatly enhance larval survival. Consequently, infective larvae developing in the northern summer may survive on pastures through winter until the following spring when rising temperatures cause their death.

10. The life span of infective larvae on pastures depends mainly on how active they are and on how quickly they use up their food reserves. The higher the temperature, the greater is their activity so they soon exhaust their food reserves and die.

ANTHELMINTIC PROPHYLAXIS

An overall prophylactic control program should be aimed at reducing pasture contamination with worm eggs. A program of this type prevents horses from being exposed to serious infection and removes the need for larvicidal drugs after the damage is done. Great care is needed in (1) choice of anthelmintic, (2) timing of treatments, and (3) monitoring fecal egg counts to check the efficiency of the control program and to detect drug resistance. All horses on a farm should be included in the program and different programs will be required on farms with or without a drug resistance problem.

In recent years it has been widely recommended that horses be treated with anthelmintics every six to eight weeks in order to reduce pasture contamination. Unfortunately, most anthelmintics do not adequately suppress egg counts for the full interval between treatments, and this results in pasture contamination. Ivermectin paste is a notable exception to this rule, as it has the ability to suppress fecal egg counts for 6 to 10 weeks, and this gives it an epidemiologic edge over other anthelmintics. Year-round treatment often has resulted in a serious drug resistance problem. The more frequent the use of an anthelmintic, the greater is selection for the development of drug resistance. On some farms in which anthelmintic treatments are given every month, there is a tremendous selection pressure for drug resistance. Clearly, there is a need for control programs that will safeguard horse health without selecting for drug resistance.

Recent studies in Ohio indicate that as few as two prophylactic treatments a year with ivermectin can have a marked effect if given at key periods of the year. The timing of the treatments is of vital importance and must be tailored to seasonal activities of the worms. Once these types of data are obtained they can be used to formulate rational control programs in any part of the world. A program based on a small number of strategic treatments each year is likely to be less costly, less time-consuming, and more readily adopted by horse owners.

NORTHERN UNITED STATES, UNITED KINGDOM, AND EUROPE

A rational approach to the epidemiologic pattern in the northern United States, the United Kingdom, and Europe is to treat horses in the spring and summer to block the spring and summer rises in fecal egg counts. This prevents the escalation of pasture infectivity in summer and autumn. With most anthelmintics it is necessary to treat horses monthly during spring and summer (April through August), as egg counts are suppressed for only four to five weeks. However, ivermectin paste can be given at eight-week intervals because of its prolonged suppression of egg counts. In one study in Ohio, foaling mares were given two prophylactic treatments with ivermectin, once in early May and again in early June. This suppressed the spring and summer rises in fecal egg output and resulted in a sixfold reduction in pasture infectivity. The effect persisted until early in the next year, even though no further treatments were given, except for a bot treatment in the fall.

If the spring and summer rise in fecal egg counts is not blocked by treatments early in the year, no number of treatments later will stop the summer and autumn rise in pasture infectivity. Consequently, horses will be at high risk if left to graze those pastures, even if treated with larvicidal drugs. This will not stop the constant daily exposure to large numbers of infective larvae. Horses treated in spring and summer may eventually show increased egg counts late in the year. In northern latitudes, this may be of little epidemiologic significance. Few of these eggs are likely to complete their development to infective larvae at a time of year when temperatures fall below 10° C.

SOUTHERN UNITED STATES

Studies in central Texas and Florida have pinpointed summer and autumn rises in fecal egg counts followed by an autumn and winter build-up of infective larvae on pastures. A rational approach to strongyle control would be to initiate strategic treaments in late summer to kill cyathostome worms emerging from the gut wall before they mature and contaminate pastures. This is also the period of minimal reinfection because of high larval mortality on pastures. Consequently, if horses are treated with an effective anthelmintic at a time of minimal reinfection, they will be protected for several months instead of just a few days in a situation of heavy reinfection.

BREEDING FARMS

An effective control program for a breeding farm is designed to keep pasture infectivity at safe levels. It must also overcome problems associated with the constant movement of horses between farms and between paddocks. The greater susceptibility of weanlings and yearlings to ascarids and strongyles must also be taken into account. Recent studies indicate that this group does not respond as well to anthelmintic strategies as do older horses. The following control program, based on epidemiologic principles, has been designed to overcome these problems, and to conserve anthelmintic efficacy by delaying the evolution of drug resistance.

1. Treat all new arrivals or returning mares with a nonbenzimidazole drug, or oxibendazole, and isolate in stalls for 48 hours before going to pasture to ensure that pastures are not contaminated with the progeny of newly introduced benzimidazole-resistant worms.

2. Treat foaling mares within a few days after foaling before they join other mares and foals at pasture. Start treatment of foals at eight weeks of age.

3. Treat mares and foals in the northern United States through spring and summer (April through August) with ivermectin at eight-week intervals or other anthelmintics at four-week intervals.

4. Treat mares and foals in the southern United States from late summer with ivermectin at eight-week intervals or other anthelmintics at four-week intervals.

5. Use anthelmintics in a slow rotation, using each drug for one to two years. If a benzimidazole-resistance problem exists, use only dichlorvos, ivermectin, oxibendazole, or pyrantel pamoate.

6. Treat weanlings before they enter weanling paddocks and keep pastures safe by twice-weekly fecal collection (see p. 334) or by frequent anthelmintic treatments.

7. Treat all horses with a boticide such as dichlorvos, ivermectin, or trichlorfon in the autumn and winter.

8. Monitor the control program several times a year by fecal egg counts of at least six horses from each group to check the degree of pasture contamination and development of drug resistance.

Supplemental Readings

Courtney, C. H., and Asquith, R. L.: Seasonal changes in pasture infectivity by equine cyathostomes in north central Florida. Equine Vet. J., *17*:240, 1985.

Craig, T. M., Bowen, J. M., and Ludwig, K. G.: Transmission of equine cyathostomes (Strongylidae) in central Texas. Am. J. Vet. Res., *44*:1867, 1983.

Herd, R. P., Williardson, K. L., and Gabel, A. A.: Epidemiologic approach to the control of horse strongyles. Equine Vet. J., *17*:202, 1985.

Ogbourne, C. P., and Duncan, J. L.: *Strongylus vulgaris* in the horse: Its biology and veterinary importance. 2nd ed. Commonwealth Institute of Parasitology, Commonwealth Agricultural Bureaux of The United Kingdom. Misc. Publ. No. 9, 68 pp., 1985.

Chemotherapy of Migrating Strongyles

R. P. Herd, COLUMBUS, OHIO

As indicated earlier, a prophylactic approach to worm control is preferable to taking curative action after the damage is done. Nevertheless, equine practitioners often face the latter situation and require a drug effective against migrating large strongyle or cyathostome larvae.

Although several drugs with larvicidal action are now on the market, their use in clinical cases of colic remains to be fully evaluated. The most outstanding drug to date is ivermectin; a single dosage of 0.2 mg per kg is highly effective against migrating *S. vulgaris* and *S. edentatus*. Other drugs depend on elevated dosages, often repeated over several days, to achieve a larvicidal effect. The effects of modern anthelmintics against the cyathostomes, which may also cause colic during their emergence from the gut wall, is less clear. Studies on larvicidal action have yielded conflicting results.

LARGE STRONGYLES

Thiabendazole was the first drug to show larvicidal action against *S. vulgaris*, but it had to be used at 440 mg per kg (10 times the normal dosage) on two consecutive days. Even then it was mainly effective against the early intestinal migration phase that occurs immediately after infection. There was less effect against *S. vulgaris* larvae once they had reached the cranial mesenteric artery. Consequently, thiabendazole at massive dosages was effective in some cases of recurrent colic but not in others.

Conflicting results have also been obtained with the use of fenbendazole at single dosages of 30 to 60 mg per kg against *S. vulgaris*. It appears that better results are obtained by using fenbendazole

at 50 mg per kg for three consecutive days, or at 10 mg per kg for five consecutive days. Albendazole is also larvicidal at multiple high dosages but may be toxic to horses at these dosages. Some larvicidal action has also been exhibited by mebendazole and oxfendazole at high dosages. It appears that repeated high dosages of benzimidazole drugs are needed if sufficient concentrations of drug are to penetrate the thrombotic deposits and reach the arterial worms.

There are now numerous reports to confirm the high larvicidal efficacy of a single recommended dosage of ivermectin (0.2 mg per kg) against arterial stages of *S. vulgaris*. It also appears to be a relatively safe treatment even though dead larvae remain buried within the vessel wall during lesion resolution. There is no evidence that these larvae continue to release antigens or produce lesions. The routine use of ivermectin in prophylactic worm control programs should also help to decrease both total worm populations and the prevalence of verminous arteritis.

CYATHOSTOMES

It appears that ivermectin at normal dosages and benzimidazole drugs at high and repeated dosages have some activity against cyathostome larvae in the gut wall. However, the evidence is conflicting and some of the trial results have been obtained with very small numbers of horses. The variable results may be related to the stage of encystment or emergence of cyathostome larvae at the time of treatment. Horses with severe clinical signs associated with the seasonal emergence of cyathostome larvae have shown clinical responses after a single treatment with ivermectin (0.2 mg per kg) or fenbendazole (60 mg per kg) repeated on three occasions.

Supplemental Readings

Drudge, J. H., and Lyons, E. T.: Strongylosis. In Robinson N. E. (ed.): Current Therapy in Equine Medicine. Philadelphia, W. B. Saunders Company, 1983.

Giles, C. J., Urquhart, K. A., and Longstaff, J. A.: Larval cyathostomiasis (immature trichonema-induced enteropathy): A report of 15 clinical cases. Equine Vet. J., *17*:196, 1985.

Slocombe, J. O. D., McGraw, B. M., Pennock, P. W., and Llewellyn, H. R.: Anthelmintic treatment of migrating stages of *Strongylus vulgaris*. Proc. 26th Annu. Conv. Am. Assoc. Eq. Pract., 1980, pp. 37–44.

Anthelmintics and Drug Resistance

R. P. Herd, COLUMBUS, OHIO

ANTHELMINTICS

In view of the serious and widespread nature of the benzimidazole drug resistance problem in horse-raising areas, it is useful to classify major anthelmintics under the headings of (1) nonbenzimidazole drugs, (2) benzimidazole drugs, and (3) probenzimidazole drugs (Table 1). It is also important to compare drug activity against the prime targets—large strongyles, cyathostomes, and ascarids—and to establish if the farm in question has a drug resistance problem. The nonbenzimidazole drugs include three broad-spectrum anthelmintics that are useful in farms with a drug resistance problem. These are ivermectin, pyrantel pamoate, and dichlorvos. Ivermectin and pyrantel pamoate are widely used, but dichlorvos is less popular because it is unpalatable to some horses.

The benzimidazole and probenzimidazole drugs are of limited usefulness on many farms because of the benzimidazole resistance problem. Side resistance may exist between individual drugs of the benzimidazole family, so that cyathostomes resistant to thiabendazole are also resistant to cambendazole, febantel, fenbendazole, mebendazole, and oxfen-

TABLE 1. MAJOR ANTHELMINTIC DRUGS APPROVED IN THE UNITED STATES

| Anthelmintic | | Dosage | % Efficacy Against Non-migrating Stages of Nematodes | | | | | | Safety* Index |
Generic Name	Trade Name	mg/kg	S. vulgaris	S. edentatus	Cyatho-stomes	Ascarids	Adult Pinworms	Bots	
Nonbenzimidazole drugs									
Ivermectin	Eqvalan	0.2	95–100	95–100	95–100	95–100	95–100	95–100	10X
Pyrantel pamoate	Strongid T								
	Strongid P	6.6	95–100	65–75	90–100	90–100	60–70	0	20X
	Imathal								
Dichlorvos	Equigard	35	95–100	70–80	85–95	95–100	90–100	80–100	3X
	Equigel	10–20†	0–10	0	—	90–100	90–100	90–100	2X
Trichlorfon (TCF)	Combot	40	0	0	0	95–100	90–100	90–100	1X
	Dyrex								
Piperazine (PPZ)	Various	88	40–60	0–10	90–100	95–100	40–60	0	3X
Benzimidazole drugs									
Thiabendazole (TBZ)	Equizole	44–88†	95–100	95–100	90–100‡	10–75	90–100	0	25X
TBZ + PPZ	Equizole A	44/55	95–100	95–100	90–100	95–100	90–100	0	5X
TBZ + TCF	Equizole B	44/40	95–100	95–100	90–100‡	95–100	90–100	95–100	1X
Cambendazole (CBZ)	Camvet	20	95–100	95–100	90–100‡	95–100	90–100	0	30X
Mebendazole (MBZ)	Telmin	8.8	95–100	65–95	80–95‡	95–100	95–100	0	40X
MBZ + TCF	Telmin B	8.8/40	95–100	65–95	80–95‡	95–100	95–100	95–100	1X
Fenbendazole (FBZ)	Panacur	5–10†	95–100	90–100	95–100‡	90–100	95–100	0	100X
Oxfendazole (OFZ)	Benzelmin	10	95–100	95–100	95–100‡	90–100	95–100	0	10X
Oxibendazole (OXB)	Anthelcide	10	95–100	95–100	95–100	90–100	95–100	0	60X
	Equipar								
Probenzimidazole drugs									
Febantel	Rintal	6	95–100	95–100	95–100‡	95–100	95–100	0	40X

*Safety index is the ratio of the maximum tolerated dosage to that recommended.
†Higher dose for ascarids and/or pinworms.
‡Efficacy for susceptible populations, not benzimidazole-resistant strongyles.

dazole. A notable exception is oxibendazole. The reason for the unique performance of oxibendazole is not understood, but from the practical point of view it means that this drug can be used effectively on all farms. The other benzimidazole drugs can be used against resistant worms only if combined with piperazine, since piperazine removes benzimidazole-resistant worms. However, the large volume of the mixture usually necessitates the use of a stomach tube and unnecessary risk to the horse.

Most modern drugs have high efficacy against intestinal ascarids but not migrating stages in the liver and lungs. Consequently, there is always the possibility that these latter stages will mature in the gut soon after treatment. When treating unthrifty and pot-bellied foals suspected of heavy ascarid infections, it is preferable to use low-efficacy drugs such as thiabendazole (44 mg per kg) and fenbendazole (5 mg per kg). This reduces the risk of a fatal blockage with masses of dead worms that might occur following treatment with a high-efficacy drug. A second treatment with a high-efficacy drug will complete the therapy with little risk.

Although large strongyles, cyathostomes, and ascarids should be the prime targets of a control program, it is sometimes necessary to treat diarrheic foals for *Strongyloides westeri* infection in the first few weeks of life. Effective drugs at normal dose rates include thiabendazole (44 mg per kg), cambendazole (20 mg per kg), oxibendazole (10 mg per kg), and ivermectin (0.2 mg per kg). One or two repeat treatments at two-week intervals are usually adequate. A single ivermectin (0.2 mg per kg) treatment of mares on the day of parturition will afford protection to the newborn against early acquisition of *S. westeri* larvae via the milk.

Pyrantel pamoate at twice the normal dosage has high efficacy against the common tapeworm *Anoplocephala perfoliata*. As most anthelmintics used in routine parasite control programs are effective against adult pinworms (*Oxyuris equi*), no specific control program is needed. Ivermectin is especially useful for infestations caused by Draschia, Habronema, Onchocerca, or *Trichostrongylus axei*.

Horses infected with lungworms (*Dictyocaulus arnfieldi*) are commonly, but not always, infected from donkeys. The donkey is regarded as the natural host of the parasite. A large percentage of donkeys are infected and have patent infections for years without showing clinical signs. First-stage larvae can be recovered from rectal fecal samples by the Baermann technique. Horses, by contrast, commonly show clinical signs of infection (ill-thrift, coughing) but embryonated eggs or larvae are less commonly found in their feces. Diagnosis is often based on clinical signs, a history of shared grazing with donkeys, and the finding of worms and eosinophils in centrifuged mucus obtained by a tracheal wash. Horses should be separated from infected donkeys and contaminated pastures and treated with ivermectin at normal dosages or benzimidazole drugs at repeated high dosages (a double dose of mebendazole on five consecutive days has been found effective).

DRUG RESISTANCE

Almost all the common species of cyathostomes have developed resistance to the benzimidazole drugs (except oxibendazole) and there is a recent report from Louisiana of possible resistance of *S. vulgaris* to benzimidazole drugs. Equine practitioners are often unaware that a drug resistance problem exists unless they check pre- and post-treatment fecal egg counts. Many current control programs select strongly for drug resistance, or depend on anthelmintics that have already lost their efficacy. In these circumstances, horses that are regularly treated for worms may suffer chronic parasitism. It is quite common to find high egg counts in horses regularly given probenzimidazole or benzimidazole drugs, without any monitoring of egg counts.

The treatment history on a farm is helpful in determining whether a drug resistance problem exists. There is a direct correlation between the occurrence of resistance and the frequency of use of benzimidazole drugs. If these drugs have been used intensively over a long period, a resistance problem is more likely to have developed. On the other hand, one new horse carrying benzimidazole-resistant worms can introduce a problem to a farm in which anthelmintics have rarely been used. Since drug resistance is genetically inherited, the progeny of resistant worms are also resistant.

In addition to checking the class of anthelmintics and frequency of use, practitioners can get further evidence of drug resistance by monitoring pre- and post-treatment egg counts. This is particulary useful if the suspect anthelmintic is compared with a nonbenzimidazole drug, (ivermectin, pyrantel pamoate, or dichlorvos). It is desirable to treat two groups of at least six horses each and to take fecal samples at the time of treatment and 7 to 14 days later. An effective drug will reduce egg counts from as high as several thousand eggs per gram (epg) of feces to below 50 epg. If there is not a substantial reduction, resistance is the most likely cause. There are several in vitro tests for the detection of drug resistance, but these are not feasible in veterinary practice. Likewise, most practitioners are unable to do total worm counts at necropsy.

At present, drug resistance is the commonest cause of high fecal egg counts after treatment. However, it is not the only cause of a lack of response to treatment. The small stomach worm,

Trichostrongylus axei, is not susceptible to most drugs, and passes eggs that resemble strongyle eggs. *T. axei* eggs are twice as long as broad, with a slight flattening on one side, one pole more pointed than the other, and a morula of 16 to 32 blastomeres. Migrating large strongyle or cyathostome larvae, unaffected by most anthelmintics at normal dosages, may return to the gut lumen and begin laying eggs soon after treatment. A poor response to treatment may also be associated with low dosage, faulty administration, inadequate nutriton, concurrent disease, or rapid reinfection from contaminated pastures. I have also observed individual horses that do not respond to certain anthelmintics, when all others in the group show a marked response. It is possible that metabolism of the drug is in some way altered in these horses.

ROTATION OF ANTHELMINTICS

Much conflicting advice is given on the alternation or rotation of anthelmintics; more research is needed on this question. In the past, most parasitologists recommended the frequent rotation of anthelmintics every few months, but there is no evidence that this delays the development of resistance. It may even accelerate the development of resistance, since each generation of worms is exposed to drugs of several different families. The recommendation to alternate benzimidazole and nonbenzimidazole drugs is valueless once resistance has developed. Each time the benzimidazole drug (except oxibendazole) is reintroduced, the egg counts and pasture contamination rise sharply, thus defeating the whole object of the control program. Once resistance develops to benzimidazole drugs it may be many years before worms revert to susceptibility and the drugs are again effective. Resistance is likely to return quickly once a benzimidazole drug is reintroduced.

As of this writing, it appears rational to rotate anthelmintics in a slow rotation at intervals of one or two years, so that each worm generation is exposed to no more than one class of drug. The generation time, including preparasitic and parasitic development and survival, can be taken as roughly one year. On a farm with a drug resistance problem it would be possible to alternate ivermectin, pyrantel pamoate, oxibendazole, and dichlorvos in a slow rotation. Each of these drugs belongs to a different family with a different mechanism of action. If rotated at yearly intervals, it would be three years before worms were again exposed to the same mechanism of action, and this would provide little pressure for the development of drug resistance.

Supplemental Readings

Bennett, D. G.: Drug resistance and the control of equine strongyles. Compend. Cont. Ed. Pract. Vet., 5:S343, 1983.

Drudge, J. H., Lyons, E. T., and Tolliver, S. C.: Parasite control in horses: A summary of contemporary drugs. Vet. Med. Small Anim. Clin., 76:1479, 1981.

French, D. D., and Klei, T. R.: Benzimidazole-resistant strongyle infections: A review of significance, occurrence, diagnosis and control. Proc. 29th Annu. Conv. Am. Assoc. Eq. Pract., 1983, pp. 313–317.

Pasture Hygiene

R. P. Herd, COLUMBUS, OHIO

It is widely believed that equine strongyles can be controlled only by the regular use of anthelmintics. Much can be achieved, however, by grazing management and pasture hygiene. The regular collection of feces from pasture has been long recommended, but little practiced. Although it is not feasible under conditions of extensive grazing on a big acreage, it can be of great value when horses are restricted in small paddocks. Not only does it provide excellent parasite control, it also increases the grazing area by about 50 per cent by eliminating the characteristic separation of horse pastures into roughs and lawns.

ROUGHS AND LAWNS

It has been observed that stallions defecate an average of 12.8 times in a 24-hour period, mares 6.5 times, and foals 10.3 times daily. A mare with an average strongyle infection producing 1000 epg in a daily total of 15 kg of feces contaminates the pasture with 15 million eggs per day. Fortunately, horses appear to have developed an abhorrence of feces as part of their adaptation to life in a wormy world. They commonly defecate more in certain poorly grazed areas than in areas heavily grazed. Pastures thus develop a characteristic separation into areas of short grazed grass (lawns) and high ungrazed grass around feces (roughs). Adult horses spend most of their time in the lawns. Before defecation, they proceed to a nearby rough, defecate, then return to grazing in the lawns. There is no regularity in the shape, position, or size of the roughs and lawns, but 50 per cent or more of a pasture can be lost to grazing.

Studies in Ohio have shown that the concentrations of strongyle larvae in the roughs may be 15 times higher than in the lawns. Nevertheless, similar seasonal patterns of a late season rise in larval concentrations occurred in both the roughs and lawns, with a 144-fold increase in the lawns after autumn rains. Thus, the protection afforded horses by their aversion to grazing near feces is transient and may break down once conditions favor larval migration and dispersal. Although horses may not be at serious risk from high infectivity of the lawns until the latter part of the grazing season, problems are likely to occur earlier if horses are forced by overcrowding to graze the roughs in spite of their natural aversion. Children's ponies are often kept in restricted areas that force them to graze both roughs and lawns.

COLLECTION OF FECES

My recent studies at The Animal Health Trust Equine Research Station in Newmarket, England showed that a nonchemical approach of pasture cleaning twice a week resulted in better parasite control than that achieved by modern anthelmintics. A nonchemical approach to equine parasite control based on twice weekly removal of feces was evaluated at Newmarket in 1984. The rationale of this approach is that feces are removed from pasture before there is time for dispersal of ascarid eggs or development of strongyle eggs to infective larvae and migration to herbage. On some Thoroughbred farms of several hundred acres at Newmarket, feces are regularly collected by a mechanized vacuum cleaner. A minitractor pulls a collection unit consisting of a trailer fitted with a vacuum unit powered by the tractor or by a small engine. It is coupled to a length of hose for manure pick-up and controlled from a tractor seat. As of this writing studies are in progress in Ohio; in these, various vacuum units and sweepers available in the United States are being tested for their effectiveness in manure collection. Owners with a few horses on a small acreage can keep pastures clean manually with a wheelbarrow and shovel.

The twice-weekly collection of feces in the Newmarket study provided highly effective parasite control, superior to that achieved by anthelmintic treatments with ivermectin at eight-week intervals or oxibendazole at four-week intervals. Concentrations of infective strongyle larvae on cleaned pasture reached a maximum of 1,000 L3 per kg, compared with 18,486 L3 per kg for control pastures and 4,850 to 10,210 L3 per kg for anthelmintic treatment groups. Counts of larvae on the cleaned pasture were low even though the ponies in this group received no anthelmintic treatments and had the highest mean fecal egg counts of all groups (peak 1,722 epg). The removal of feces also increased the grazing area by about 50 per cent through elimination of ungrazed roughs. This is a very significant factor when the high cost of land, fencing, and fertilizer is considered.

OTHER STRATEGIES

Other pasture hygiene and grazing management practices include pasture harrowing, pasture clipping, pasture destocking, biological control, chemical control, and alternate grazing with cattle or sheep. All of these approaches are fraught with dangers, and they do not always provide good parasite control. If pasture harrowing is done in hot dry weather it will effectively break up feces and expose larvae to death by desiccation. If it is done in damp or wet conditions, it may simply disperse viable larvae over a greater area of lawns. Pasture clipping may remove some protective covering for larvae, but horses are likely to ingest more larvae per mouthful because of the greater concentration of infective larvae closer to the soil surface. Pasture destocking will allow larvae to die out, but it may be necessary to remove horses for up to one year to achieve this. Biological control with dung beetles is theoretically feasible, but to date it has been of little practical benefit. Chemical control with larvicidal chemicals shows little promise because of the high cost and damage to pasture.

The parasitologic benefits to be gained from mixed grazing of horses and ruminants is questionable. Cattle initially eat only the upper layers of vegetation where very few horses larvae reside. This could result in an actual increase in the number of horse parasite larvae per unit weight of herbage in the remaining layers of pasture. However, if cattle or sheep grazed horse pastures for the first half of the year in northern latitudes, all horse larvae that had overwintered would have died off by the time of a changeover in July. Horses moved on to that pasture would then be exposed to cattle parasite larvae instead of horse larvae. In southern latitudes, heavy larval mortality occurs on summer pastures. Grazing ruminants in autumn and winter could prevent the usual build-up of horse parasite larvae. Although it is usually assumed that there is little cross-infection between horses and ruminants, one exception is the small stomach worm, *Trichostrongylus axei,* which infects horses, cattle, sheep, goats, and rabbits. This parasite is readily transmitted to horses and may cause marked gastric pathology.

Supplemental Readings

Herd, R. P.: Epidemiology and control of equine strongylosis at Newmarket. Equine Vet. J., In press, 1986.
Herd R. P.: Serum pepsinogen concentrations of ponies naturally infected with *Trichostrongylus axei*. Equine Vet. J., In press, 1986.
Herd, R. P., and Willardson, K. L.: Seasonal distribution of infective strongyle larvae on horse pastures. Equine Vet. J., 17:235, 1985.
Odberg, F. O., and Francis-Smith, K.: A study on eliminative and grazing behaviour—the use of the field by captive horses. Equine Vet. J., 8:147, 1976.
Taylor, E. L.: Grazing behaviour and helminthic disease. Br. J. Anim. Behav., 2:61, 1954.

Monitoring Control Programs

R. P. Herd, COLUMBUS, OHIO

As indicated earlier, there are three essentials to an anthelmintic control program: (1) choice of anthelmintic, (2) timing of treatments, and (3) monitoring of the control program by fecal egg counts. The third component is just as important as the first two, as it enables the veterinarian to compare the efficacy of different anthelmintics, to detect the development of drug resistance, and to assess the effectiveness of the program in reducing pasture contamination.

FECAL EGG COUNTS

It is desirable to do a quantitative fecal egg count using a counting chamber like the McMaster slide, rather than a simple flotation. Although fecal egg counts give little indication of the severity of the worm infection, they do provide an accurate assessment of the degree of pasture contamination. This is vitally important information as the whole object of the control program is to reduce pasture contamination to safe levels. If egg counts are high, then pasture contamination is high and there is a need to change the control program.

If egg counts are kept below 50 epg, pasture infectivity is not likely to rise to dangerous levels. Complete elimination of contamination is undesirable, as this could lead to lack of immunity in foals and disastrous consequences when they are later exposed to serious parasitism. It is preferable that they be exposed to low levels of infection sufficient to induce some immunity, but not sufficient to cause ill health. When egg counts are done at the time of treatment and 7 to 14 days later, drug resistance can be quickly recognized, and use of the offending drug discontinued. It is always desirable to check individual fecal samples from at least six horses of each group, because of the wide variation in egg counts between horses in the same environment. There appear to be marked genetic differences, so that horses from some families are more resistant to worms than horses from other families.

Strongyle and ascarid control should be given top priority in the parasite control program. They are the most common and important everyday threat to horse health throughout the world. It is normal to do separate egg counts for strongyles and ascarids and to try to keep each of them below 50 epg. Strongyle eggs are found in horses of all ages, although the presence of eggs in the feces of foals less than six weeks of age is usually due to coprophagia. Ascarid eggs will be found mainly in the feces of foals and weanlings. The occasional finding of ascarid eggs in the feces of immune adult horses is usually of little concern.

It should be routine practice on all horse farms to set up prophylactic control programs early in the year to block the seasonal rise in pasture contamination and infectivity. Otherwise, horses in northern latitudes will be exposed to serious parasitism at pasture in summer and autumn, while horses in southern latitudes will be exposed to serious infection in autumn and winter. This decision can be made on the basis of general epidemiologic principles and does not require any laboratory tests. If a farm has a history of irregular worm control, there is an obvious need for immediate action to eliminate existing worm burdens, to move horses to safe pastures, and to initiate prophylactic measures to prevent serious worm exposure in the future. Once the prophylactic control program is initiated, it should be carefully monitored by fecal egg counts several times a year.

If horses are stabled, control programs can be relaxed a little, since horses in stalls are not exposed to worms as much as horses at pasture, with the exception of pinworms. It appears that conditions within stalls are inimical for the development of eggs to infective larvae. However, it should be remembered that both large and small strongyles can mature in the intestine up to two years after horses are first infected at pasture. In addition, horses allowed to graze contaminated pastures close to stables can pick up large numbers of larvae within a few hours. Problems are often created when the stable manager does not have control over the worming program, and some horses are treated while others are not. Under training conditions, even a moderate worm infection is likely to have an adverse effect on the horse's performance. It is desirable to treat all horses at the same time, and for the veterinarian to run fecal egg counts. The practice of spreading noncomposted manure from horse stalls to pasture represents a serious danger to grazing horses.

NEUROLOGIC DISEASES

Edited by J. Beech

Neurologic Examination

Raymond W. Sweeney, KENNETT SQUARE, PENNSYLVANIA

The objective of the neurologic examination is to localize the site of the lesion in the nervous system and then decide on possible etiologies.

SIGNALMENT AND HISTORY

Because certain neurologic diseases in horses have breed and age predilections, an accurate signalment is important. Frequently the presumptive diagnosis will be based on information in the history such as the duration and progression of signs, observed changes in behavior, and whether or not trauma was observed. Previous disease history of the herd may provide important clues such as in herpes myelitis and botulism. In addition to a complete history a general physical examination is important so that concurrent and possibly related problems are not overlooked.

NEUROLOGIC EXAMINATION

CEREBRAL DYSFUNCTION

Signs of cerebral disease include blindness (with normal pupillary light reflex), depression, seizures, and behavior changes such as mania, head pressing, and aimless wandering. The gait is usually normal although mild ataxia may be seen. In cases of unilateral central blindness the lesion is contralateral to the blind eye.

CEREBELLAR DYSFUNCTION

The most consistent signs of cerebellar disease are intention tremor of the head and ataxia. The intention tremors may be very fine and sometimes missed. They are often most easily detected when the horse moves its head toward food or water. Cerebellar ataxia is characterized by jerking, exaggerated limb movements (hypermetria) and no loss of strength. The menace response is frequently absent. If the gait abnormalities are unilateral, a lesion in the ipsilateral cerebellum is indicated.

BRAIN STEM AND CRANIAL NERVE DYSFUNCTION

Brain stem lesions result in depression if the reticular activating system, which is in this region, is affected. Because the nuclei of cranial nerves are also located here, brain stem lesions can result in cranial nerve abnormalities. If only one cranial nerve is abnormal (unilateral) and no depression exists, a peripheral cranial nerve lesion should be suspected. If there are multiple cranial nerves involved, if the abnormalities are bilateral, or if the horse is depressed, a brainstem lesion should be suspected. Signs of cranial nerve abnormalities are as follows:

1. *Olfactory.* Not usually assessed.
2. *Optic.* Blindness; loss of menace with retention of ability to blink; loss of pupillary light response. The optic nerve may be examined with the ophthalmoscope.
3. *Oculomotor.* Ventral and lateral deviation of the eye position (strabismus). Loss of pupillary light response because the parasympathetic innervation of the constrictor muscle of the pupil travels with the oculomotor nerve.
4. *Trochlear.* Dorsal and medial strabismus.
5. *Trigeminal.* Loss of sensation to cornea, face, and nasal mucosa. Poor jaw muscle tone or atrophy of muscles of mastication.
6. *Abducens.* Medial strabismus. Loss of globe retraction when cornea is touched.
7. *Facial.* Paralysis of muscles of facial expression, ptosis, loss of ability to blink, ear droop, lip droop, muzzle deviation away from affected side.
8. *Vestibulocochlear.* Deafness, head tilt, nystagmus, ataxia without loss of strength.
9–11. *Glossopharyngeal, Vagus, Spinal Accessory.* Dysphagia, abnormal phonation, laryngeal paralysis.
12. *Hypoglossal.* Paralysis of the tongue. Unilateral lesion causes muscle atrophy of ipsilateral half of tongue without complete loss of function.

SPINAL CORD

Lesions of the spinal cord may be reflected in the horse's gait and spinal reflexes. The patellar reflex and flexor (withdrawal) reflexes usually may be evaluated only in the recumbent horse. The cutaneous and perineal reflexes may be evaluated in the standing horse.

Perineal Reflex. Stimulation of the skin of the perineum elicits puckering of the anus and tail flexion. Lack of this reflex indicates a lesion in the last three sacral segments of the cord. Bladder distention with urinary incontinence provides further evidence of a caudal sacral lesion.

Cutaneous Reflex. Stimulation of the skin along the body wall elicits contraction of the cutaneous trunci muscle and "flicking" of the skin. The afferent portion of the reflex arc involves the segmental spinal nerves at the level of the stimulus and the ascending white matter of the thoracolumbar cord. The motor portion requires the neurons of the ventral gray matter of the last cervical and first thoracic segments to be intact.

Patellar Reflex. With the horse in lateral recumbency the uper pelvic limb is held in a partially flexed position. Striking the patellar tendon with a heavy object such as hoof testers or a pair of pliers should elicit stifle extension. (A reflex hammer may not be heavy enough to elicit the reflex.) This reflex requires an intact femoral nerve and spinal cord segments L4 and L5. Hyper-reflexia is a sign of upper motor neuron disease (lesion above L4). Because the reflex cannot be evaluated in the limb on which the horse is lying, the horse must be rolled over to test the opposite limb.

Triceps Reflex. With the horse in lateral recumbency the front limb is held in flexion. When the elbow is tapped, the elbow joint should extend slightly. This reflex tests the integrity of radial nerve and spinal cord segments C7 to T1.

Flexor (Withdrawal) Reflex. Pinching the skin of the distal limb with a hemostat or similar implement should stimulate flexion of the leg. This response requires intact spinal cord segments L6, S1, and S2 for the pelvic limb reflex and cord segments C6 to T2 for the thoracic limb reflex. In addition to the limb withdrawal reflex, the animal should also have a cerebral response to the painful stimulus. This usually takes the form of kicking, turning the head, or objecting in some way to the stimulus. Absence of this response without loss of the withdrawal reflex is evidence of a lesion involving ascending spinal cord tracts.

The gait should be evaluated for evidence of motor or sensory ataxia and limb weakness. The animal should be walked and, if possible, trotted in a straight line. It should also be walked in a serpentine or figure-eight and walked on an incline. If the horse is not too ataxic, observation of cantering may be helpful. The horse should be turned in a tight circle and also pushed sideways, both while walking in a straight line and when standing still. Backing the horse is also helpful. Blindfolding the horse will not usually exacerbate the ataxia if it is due to a spinal cord lesion.

Signs of ataxia include swaying or incoordination while walking, circumduction of the outside hindlimbs while circling, crossing of the limbs or stepping on the opposite foot, and scuffing or dragging of the toes. At rest the animal may assume a "base-wide" stance, and if the legs are positioned abnormally (e.g., crossed) by the examiner, the horse may not correct their position. Musculoskeletal lameness may mimic ataxia. The use of diagnostic nerve blocks and analgesic medication may aid the clinician in differentiating between these conditions.

The clinician should determine which limbs are affected by the ataxia and whether there is symmetrical or asymmetrical involvement (left versus right). If both pelvic and thoracic limbs are equally affected, or if the pelvic limbs are more severely affected, a cervical lesion should be suspected. If the thoracic limbs are much more severely affected than the pelvic limbs a multifocal lesion should be suspected, because focal cervical lesions usually cause more severe ataxia in the pelvic limbs. Absence of the spinal reflexes and muscle atrophy in the thoracic or pelvic limbs would indicate a lesion in C6 to T2 or L4 to S2 respectively.

PERIPHERAL NERVES

Peripheral nerve lesions (see p. 380) usually manifest as localized areas of cutaneous hypoalgesia or unilateral muscle atrophy and loss of function. Signs of dysfunction of major peripheral nerves are as follows:

Suprascapular Nerve. Atrophy of supraspinatus and infraspinatus muscle and a prominent scapular spine. Colloquially, the signs of suprascapular nerve paralysis are known as "Sweeny."

Radial Nerve. Inability to extend elbow, carpus, and digit. Atrophy of triceps muscles. "Dropped elbow" or knuckling. Hypoalgesia on the dorsum of the distal limb.

Sciatic Nerve. Paralysis and atrophy of the semimembranosus and semitendinosus muscles. Dragging of the foot, loss of sensation to the plantar metatarsal region.

Femoral Nerve. Inability to extend stifle and hock and bear weight. Atrophy of quadriceps muscles. Loss of sensation on medial side of limb.

Peroneal Nerve. Knuckling, inability to extend digit. Loss of sensation to the dorsal metatarsal region.

ANCILLARY TESTS

These tests may be used to aid in further localizing the lesion or determining the nature of the lesion once it has been localized. Analysis of cerebrospinal fluid (CSF) may be useful in documenting an inflammatory lesion (p. 341). Its usefulness is limited, however, because many horses with neurologic disease have normal CSF. Radiographs of the skull and spinal column are employed in an attempt to diagnose skeletal trauma or congenital malformations and stenosis of the spinal canal. Unfortunately, general anesthesia and sophisticated equipment may be required to obtain diagnostic radiographs in the adult horse. Contrast myelography may further aid in delineating a compressive lesion of the cervical spinal cord. Electromyography may be used to document denervation or to aid in the differentiation between neurologic disease and primary muscular disease. Nerve conduction velocity, brain stem auditory evoked responses, and cervical spinal cord electrical conduction studies are now being perfected to aid in the evaluation of the central nervous system. These tests also require somewhat sophisticated equipment and are of limited value to the practicing veterinarian at this time.

Supplemental Readings

deLahunta, A.: Veterinary Neuroanatomy and Clinical Neurology, 2nd ed. Philadelphia, W. B. Saunders Company, 1983.
Mayhew, I. G., deLahunta, A., Whitlock, R. H., Krook, L., and Tasker, J. B.: Spinal cord disease in the horse. Cornell Vet., 68:13, 1978.

Cerebrospinal Fluid Collection

Raymond W. Sweeney, KENNETT SQUARE, PENNSYLVANIA

Cerebrospinal fluid (CSF) analysis is occasionally indicated as a diagnostic aid in horses with neurologic disease. Cerebrospinal fluid may be collected by needle puncture of the subarachnoid space at the lumbosacral (LS) or atlanto-occipital (AO) sites. The LS location is preferred in the standing horse, whereas the AO site usually requires general anesthesia. The LS location is the safer of the two because the conus medullaris can be penetrated without complication, whereas accidental penetration of the brain stem that can occur at the AO site could lead to neurologic dysfunction or death. If a spinal cord lesion is suspected, the lumbosacral site is preferred because of caudal direction of flow of CSF in the subarachnoid space.

COLLECTION FROM THE ATLANTO-OCCIPITAL SITE

The horse is placed under general anesthesia in lateral recumbency with the head flexed so that the median axis of the head is at a right angle to the median axis of the cervical vertebrae. The hair and mane are clipped from the poll and neck (8 cm either side of the midline extending from between the ears 20 cm caudally). The area is prepared aseptically, and sterile gloves should be worn. An 18- or 20-gauge, 9-cm spinal needle* is used. The stilette should remain in place any time the needle

*Becton-Dickinson Co., Rutherford, NJ

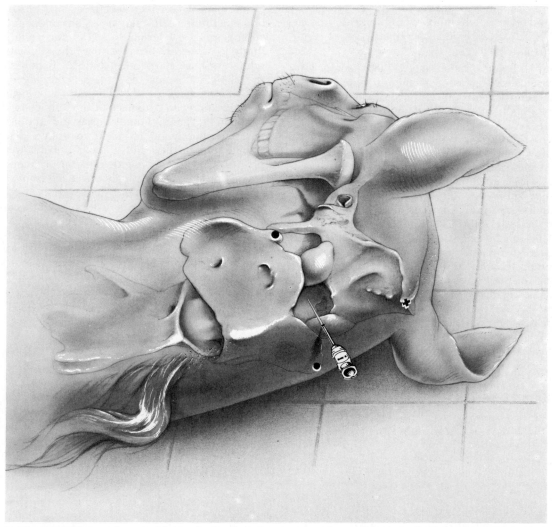

Figure 1. Atlanto-occipital cerebrospinal fluid collection from the recumbent horse. Spinal needle in position with stilette removed. Palpable landmarks are the cranial borders of the atlas (● —— ●) and the median eminence of the nuchal crest (+) on the dorsal median plane. (From deLahunta, A.: Veterinary Neuroanatomy and Clinical Neurology, 2nd ed. Philadelphia, W. B. Saunders Company, 1983, p. 44.)

is advanced to prevent its becoming plugged with tissue. Figure 1 demonstrates the site of skin penetration at the point where a line between the cranial borders of the axis intersects the dorsal midline. The hand holding the needle is rested on the dorsum of the neck to allow steady and slow advancement of the needle. The needle is aimed toward the lower jaw and advanced slowly until a "popping" sensation (sudden decrease in resistance) is detected. The subarachnoid space is usually reached at a depth of 5 to 7 cm. The stilette is withdrawn and the CSF collected by gravity flow or by gentle aspiration with a syringe. If no CSF is obtained the needle may be rotated, or it may be necessary to replace the stilette and advance the needle further. The stilette is then removed and

the hub of the needle is checked again for the appearance of CSF. After the sample is obtained the needle is withdrawn.

Occasionally, frank blood may be obtained if the needle penetrates the epidural venous sinuses that are lateral to the midline. If this occurs the needle should be removed and the attempt repeated with a new needle. Care should be taken to ensure that the needle penetrates along the dorsal midline.

LUMBOSACRAL SITE

The horse is restrained in the standing position with equal weight distribution between the hind limbs. Tranquilization is usually not necessary except with extremely fractious horses and is to be avoided if possible since it may cause the horse to bear weight unevenly. The lumbosacral CSF collection may also be attempted in recumbent horses but can be quite difficult due to displacement of the bony landmarks.

The site of skin penetration is illustrated in Figures 2 and 3. This site is located on the dorsal midline in the depression caudal to the dorsal spine of L6 and cranial to the spine of S2. The spine of S1 is not palpable. The spine of L6 is shorter than that of L5, and the slight depression caudal to L5 may be confused with the proper site. The penetration site is usually directly between the tubera sacrale (Fig. 2), which are usually more easily palpated in mares. A 15-cm square area is clipped and prepared aseptically and surgical gloves should be worn. A small volume (2 to 3ml) of local anesthetic is injected subcutaneously at the penetration site, and a small stab incision through the skin is made. A 15-cm, 18-gauge spinal needle is required

in most adult horses, but an 18-gauge, 9-cm needle is adequate in ponies and foals. The person performing the procedure stands beside the horse, with the hand steadying the needle resting on the dorsal midline of the horse just cranial to the site of penetration. An assistant may stand behind the horse and give directions to ensure that the needle penetrates at a perpendicular angle. The needle is advanced slowly along the median plane until a sudden loss of resistance is detected, usually at a depth of approximately 13 cm. Occasionally bone is struck before this depth is reached, and the needle must be withdrawn to the skin and redirected. Penetration of the subarachnoid space is often accompanied by a local response such as twitching of the tail or flexion of the hind limbs. The stilette is withdrawn and if the needle is correctly placed, gentle aspiration with a 10-ml syringe should be sufficient to withdraw the sample. Excessive suction should not be applied as this can cause hemorrhage. The yield of CSF may be improved by having an

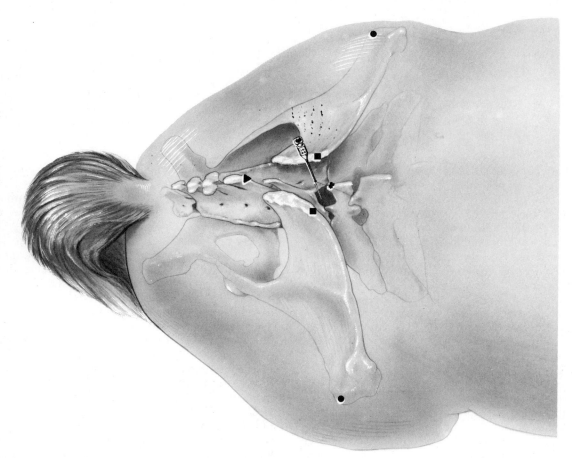

Figure 2. Lumbosacral cerebrospinal fluid collection from the standing horse. Spinal needle in position with stilette removed. Palpable landmarks are the caudal borders of each tuber coxae (● —— ●), the caudal edge of the spine of L6 (+), the cranial edge of the second sacral spine (▲), and the cranial edge of each tuber sacrale (■ —— ■). (From deLahunta, A.: Veterinary Neuroanatomy and Clinical Neurology, 2nd ed. Philadelphia, W. B. Saunders Company, 1983, p. 42.)

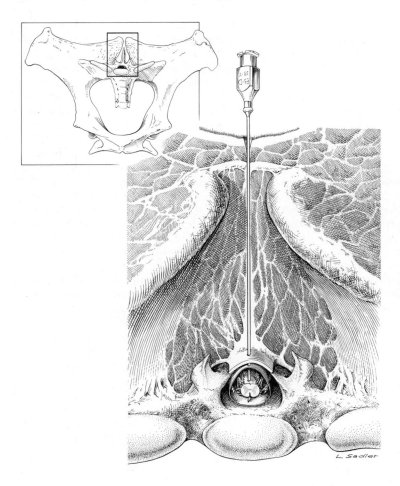

Figure 3. Lumbosacral spinal fluid collection from the horse. Transverse dissection through lumbosacral articulation, cranial view. Spinal needle passes through the skin, thoracolumbar fascia adjacent to the interspinous ligaments, interarcuate ligament, dorsal dura mater and arachnoid, dorsal subarachnoid space, and conus medullaris. Needle point is in ventral subarachnoid space. Cranial view of pelvis, sacrum, and area of dissection (insert). (From deLahunta, A.: Veterinary Neuroanatomy and Clinical Neurology, 2nd ed. Philadelphia, W. B. Saunders Company, 1983, p. 43.)

assistant compress both jugular veins, increasing intraspinal pressure; also, the needle may be rotated to alleviate its plugging with tissue. If no sample is obtained the stilette is replaced and the needle advanced a few millimeters and rechecked. This is repeated until a sample is obtained or until the point of the needle rests against the ventral floor of the spinal canal. If several attempts to reposition the needle are unsuccessful, the needle should then be withdrawn nearly to the skin and redirected. Several attempts may be necessary before a sample is successfully obtained.

ANALYSIS

An aliquot of CSF should be saved in a sterile container in case a future bacterial culture is indicated. The remaining sample should be placed in a blood collection tube containing EDTA for cytologic analysis, and a heparin-containing tube for biochemical analysis. Because of the low number of nucleated cells in most CSF samples, cytocentrifugation is required for cytologic examination.

The CSF should be examined for color and clarity, normal CSF being clear and colorless. Xanthochromia (yellow color) is caused by bilirubin in the CSF from previous hemorrhage such as may result from trauma or vasculitis of herpes myelitis. A red tinge may be caused by hemorrhage from trauma, or by iatrogenic hemorrhage at the time of the CSF collection. If hemorrhage occurs during the collection procedure the color should clear as further CSF is withdrawn, unless, as previously mentioned, a venous sinus is entered.

Cerebrospinal fluid should be analyzed for red blood cell count, nucleated cell count, differential white cell count, and total protein content. Normal CSF should contain less than 6 nucleated cells per μl and these should be primarily lymphocytes and monocytes. Some authors have stated that the nucleated cell count can be adjusted for peripheral blood contamination by subtracting one nucleated cell for every 500 red blood cells present in the CSF, although many believe that such calculations are generally not reliable.

The normal CSF protein content is less than 70 mg per dl (100 mg per dl according to some authors).

CSF glucose concentration should be greater than 80 per cent of the blood glucose value. In general, creatine phosphokinase (CPK) and other enzyme levels in CSF do not provide diagnostic benefit.

INTERPRETATION

Simultaneous elevations in CSF nucleated cell count and total protein content with an increase in the percentage of neutrophils suggest a bacterial meningitis or encephalitis. In these horses the CSF glucose concentration is often less than 80 per cent of the blood value due to bacterial consumption of CSF glucose. A mild mononuclear pleocytosis, a mild protein elevation, and xanthochromia or hemorrhage may occasionally be found in horses with equine protozoal myeloencephalitis, but more frequently the CSF is normal. Similarly, a mild elevation of total protein content with a normal nucleated cell count is occasionally seen in horses with spinal cord compression. However, a normal result is more frequently the case in those horses. A significant protein content increase with little or no pleocytosis (referred to as albuminocytologic dissociation) usually results from the vasculitis associated with herpes myelitis, in which case xanthochromia is frequently present.

Supplemental Reading

Beech, J.: Cytology of equine cerebrospinal fluid. Vet. Pathol., *20*:553, 1983.

deLahunta, A.: Veterinary Neuroanatomy and Clinical Neurology, 2nd ed. Philadelphia, W. B. Saunders Company, 1983.

Mayhew, I. G.: Collection of cerebrospinal fluid from the horse. Cornell Vet., *65*:500, 1975.

Mayhew, I. G., Whitlock, R. H., and Tasker, J. B.: Equine cerebrospinal fluid: Reference values for normal horses. Am. J. Vet. Res., *38*:1271, 1977.

Eastern Equine Encephalomyelitis

Julia H. Wilson, GAINESVILLE, FLORIDA

Eastern equine encephalomyelitis (EEE) is an acute, often fatal disease of horses, humans, pheasants, and Chukar partridges. It has also been reported in two calves. The causative agent is an RNA virus classified as an alphavirus within the Togaviridae family. The disease incidence is sporadic and seasonal except in Florida, where clinical cases are reported year around. The viral life cycle is sylvatic, involving bird and rodent reservoirs and insect vectors. The disease is transmitted to horses by mosquitoes, probably *Coquilettidia perturbans* and Aedes species. The horse is considered a "dead-end" host owing to the low level of viremia in the disease. Epizootics of EEE have been reported in the United States primarily along the Eastern seaboard, Gulf coast, and Great Lakes, and in Alberta, the Caribbean, and Central and South America. North American and South American viral strains are antigenically distinct.

PATHOGENESIS AND CLINICAL SIGNS

After an infective mosquito bites a susceptible horse, proliferation of the virus in regional lymph nodes is followed by viremia. This may result in one of the following syndromes: (1) mild fever, lymphopenia, and neutropenia that often are subclinical; (2) generalized febrile illness with anorexia, depression, tachycardia, high fever (up to 41° C), lymphopenia, and neutropenia; or (3) encephalomyelitis. The clinical signs of the classic encephalitic form typically begin as changes in behavior with loss of appetite and fever several days after viremia, progressing in 12 to 24 hours to dementia with head pressing, teeth grinding, circling, and often blindness. Intense pruritus and hyperexcitability have also been reported. Cranial nerve dysfunctions may produce nystagmus, facial paralysis, and dysphagia. Progressive ataxia and weakness from brain stem and spinal cord involvement result in an inability to stand. Seizures may occur and progress in severity. Respiratory arrest two to three days after the onset of clinical signs is the usual terminal event. Signs may progress more rapidly if brain herniation occurs secondary to edema. Mortality rate varies from 75 to 98 per cent; therefore, a grave prognosis must be given. Surviving horses may have residual central nervous system (CNS) damage such as visual deficits and behavioral and learning disabilities, and frequently are referred to as "dummies" or "sleepers."

Peripheral blood analysis frequently reveals lymphopenia and neutropenia. Cerebrospinal fluid (CSF) may have increased protein content and white cell counts. Neutrophils are often found in CSF in the acute disease; mononuclear cells predominate in later stages.

At necropsy the gross lesions mimic those of brain trauma with patchy discoloration of the brain and spinal cord, edema, and hemorrhage. A diffuse meningoencephalomyelitis is seen histologically. Primarily it affects gray matter, with neuronal degeneration, gliosis, and perivascular infiltrates. These perivascular cuffs consist of neutrophils in the acute stage; later they consist of neutrophils and large and small mononuclear cells.

DIAGNOSIS

Clinical diagnosis of EEE is based on the season, locale, clinical signs and their progression, and ancillary aids. Clinical differentiation from western encephalomyelitis (WEE) or Venezuelan equine encephalomyelitis (VEE) is difficult and usually is done on the basis of the outcome of the case. Identical signs were reported in a California horse from which Main Drain virus was isolated. Confirmation by serologic testing, utilizing either hemagglutination inhibition (HI) or complement fixation (CF) titers, requires demonstration of at least a fourfold rise in antibody titer in samples taken 7 to 10 days apart, or a very high single titer without concurrent elevations of WEE or VEE titers. Definition of a single high titer is controversial. Eastern equine encephalomyelitis titers at least four times greater than WEE and VEE titers are considered diagnostic in Florida.

At postmortem examination, virus isolation from fresh, refrigerated, or deep-frozen portions of the brain should be attempted if facilities are available. Routine histology will define the presence or absence of meningoencephalomyelitis. Immunofluorescent staining of brain tissue (pons and thalamus) may be useful in laboratories not equipped for virus isolation. Other conditions causing diffuse or multifocal neurologic deficits that should be considered in the differential diagnosis include WEE, VEE, head trauma, hepatoencephalopathy, rabies, leukoencephalomalacia, bacterial meningoencephalitis, protozoal myeloencephalitis, and verminous encephalitis.

TREATMENT

If EEE is strongly suspected and the horse is recumbent, any attempts at therapy should be tempered by the bad prognosis for survival and the risk of residual signs. No specific antiviral agents are available currently, hence supportive measures and symptomatic therapy are essential.

In early or mild cases the mode of therapy is identical to that for WEE. Adequate food and water intake should be ensured. Nasogastric tube feeding can be employed to maintain hydration and provide energy if the horse cannot eat or drink. If tube feeding is for more than a few days, rhinitis and pharyngitis may develop, in which case an esophagostomy can be utilized (see p. 426). Intravenous fluids, although more costly, can also be used. Hydration and electrolyte levels should be monitored if inanition lasts for more than a few days.

To minimize the complications of recumbency and self-induced trauma, a well-bedded area should be provided and the horse should be kept as clean and dry as possible. The recumbent horse should be turned several times a day and maintained in a sternal position if possible to minimize pulmonary congestion and prolonged weight-bearing on skin surfaces over bony prominences. Slinging should be attempted if feasible to decrease muscle damage, increase limb use and circulation, and decrease the likelihood of development of decubitus ulcers. Any skin sores or abrasions should be treated meticulously with antiseptic or antibiotic ointments to avoid secondary infections. Topical magnesium and aluminum hydroxide preparations* may help prevent further progression of decubital sores. If spontaneous urination is not observed, the bladder should be manually expressed per rectum or catheterized aseptically. An indwelling urinary catheter may be advisable if prolonged recumbency is anticipated, in which event prophylactic antimicrobials should be considered because of the high risk of ascending infection. Urine scald should be prevented by application of petrolatum or other water-repellent ointments to areas likely to become wet with urine. Manual evacuation of feces several times a day may also be necessary.

Signs of progressing depression and, particularly, dilated pupils that become unresponsive to light suggest potentially fatal cerebral edema. Intravenous dimethylsulfoxide (DMSO), although not approved for this use, has both a diuretic and an anti-inflammatory effect. Medical-grade DMSO† should be given at a dose of 1 gm per kg as a 20 to 40 per cent solution in 5 per cent dextrose over a 30-minute period once a day for up to three days. Intravascular hemolysis and subsequent hemoglobinuria are commonly observed after DMSO therapy but seldom cause clinical problems. However, because of its potential for causing hemoglobinuric nephrosis, DMSO should not be used in patients

---

*Maalox, William H. Rorer, Inc., Fort Washington, PA
†Domoso, 90% solution, Diamond Laboratories, Inc., Des Moines, IA

with compromised renal function or significant dehydration. Alternatively, intravenous mannitol* (20 per cent) may be given by slow intravenous infusion at 0.25 to 0.5 gm per kg. Mannitol is usually not repeated unless after an initial clinical response a relapse occurs in 6 to 24 hours. Furosemide† at 0.5 to 1.0 mg per kg intravenously can be used although this drug is perhaps less effective for such purposes. Furosemide can be repeated at six- to eight-hour intervals with close monitoring of hydration and serum potassium levels.

Anti-inflammatory drugs such as dexamethasone‡ at levels of 0.1 to 0.2 mg per kg four times a day may be indicated to reduce the inflammatory component of the central nervous system tissue damage. Their use is controversial but accepted as current practice, particularly in the face of clinical deterioration. If elected, this therapy should be continued at tapering dosages for several days, and the animal should be monitored closely for signs of laminitis.

High fevers can be treated with antipyretics such as dipyrone§ (11 to 22 mg per kg intravenously) and phenylbutazone‖ (4 to 6 mg per kg intravenously), although these sometimes are ineffective. Alcohol baths usually will reduce fevers, and can be repeated as necessary.

Seizures should be controlled with barbiturates (pentobarbital or phenobarbital), diazepam, chloral hydrate, or guaifenesin to prevent self-trauma and myositis (see p. 352 for dosage). Head padding with foam helmets is advisable to minimize risks of corneal abrasions and skull fractures.

The duration of immunity following natural infection is unknown; therefore, recovered animals should be vaccinated in a routine manner.

PREVENTION

In the face of an EEE outbreak, vaccination may be beneficial, because protective levels of antibody have been demonstrated as early as three days after vaccination in VEE studies. Strict mosquito control measures should be instituted. Current recommendations for routine EEE vaccinations are two injections three to four weeks apart with inactivated EEE + WEE (+VEE) vaccine one month before the mosquito season followed by yearly revaccinations. Clinical experience in areas with long mosquito seasons strongly suggests that semiannual revaccination is necessary. Both intradermal and intramuscular vaccines are available, some in combination with tetanus toxoid and influenza. The inactivated vaccines are safe for use in pregnant mares. Serum antibody levels in foals that have absorbed colostral immunoglobulins are similar to those of the dam. The half-life of maternally derived antibodies in the foal is 20 days and antibody levels usually decline significantly at two months. However, maternal antibodies may persist for variable lengths of time and block active immunization in foals. Consequently, foals of mares vaccinated against EEE should be given a series of two to three monthly vaccinations beginning at two to four months of age. Colostrum-deprived foals should be vaccinated earlier or given plasma transfusions from vaccinated donors. Foals should be revaccinated at 6 and 12 months, particularly in endemic areas.

PUBLIC HEALTH SIGNIFICANCE

Equine cases of EEE do not pose a threat to humans, because circulating virus levels are very rarely high enough to transmit the disease via mosquitoes. Notwithstanding, sufficient viral titers may be present in infected tissues, especially central nervous system tissues; therefore, appropriate precautions should be undertaken at the time of necropsy examination of EEE cases. In humans, the EEE virus causes an acute encephalitis with a mortality rate of approximately 50 per cent. Outbreaks of human cases often coincide with or are preceded by equine epizootics, hence strict mosquito control in affected areas is necessary to prevent both human and equine cases. All equine cases should be reported to state health officials.

Supplemental Readings

Eisner, R. J., and Nusbaum, S. R.: A study to determine the optimum time for vaccination of foals against eastern western encephalitis viruses. Proc. 22nd Annu. Mtg. Assoc. Vet. Lab. Diag., 1979, pp. 435–448.

Emmons, R. W., Woodie, J. D., Lamb, R. L., and Oshiro, L. S.: Main Drain virus as a cause of equine encephalomyelitis. J. Am. Vet. Med. Assoc., *183*:555, 1983.

Ferguson, J. A., Reeves, W. C., and Hardy, J. L.: Studies on immunity to alpha-viruses in foals. Am. J. Vet. Res., *40*:5, 1979.

Gibbs, E. P. J.: Equine viral encephalitis. Equine Vet. J., 8:66, 1976.

Maness, K. S. C., and Calisher, C. H.: Eastern equine encephalitis in the United States, 1971: past and prologue. Curr. Microbiol., 5:311, 1981.

Monath, T. P., McLean, R. G., Cropp, C. B., Parham, G. L., Lazuick, J. S., and Calisher, C. H.: Diagnosis of eastern equine encephalomyelitis by immunofluorescent staining of brain tissue. Am. J. Vet. Res., 42:1418, 1981.

Pursell, A. R., Mitchell, F. E., and Seibold, H. R.: Naturally occurring and experimentally induced eastern encephalomyelitis in calves. J. Am. Vet. Med. Assoc., *169*:1101, 1976.

Walton, T. E.: Venezuelan, Eastern, and Western Equine Encephalomyelitis. *In* Gibbs, E. P. J. (ed.): Virus Diseases of Food Animals—A World Geography, Vol. 2. New York, Academic Press, 1981, pp. 587–625.

*Manni-ject, Hart-Delta, Inc., Baton Rouge, LA
†Lasix, American Hoechst Corp., Somerville, NJ
‡Azium, Schering Corp., Kenilworth, NJ
§Med-Tech Laboratories, Elwood, KS
‖The Butler Co., Columbus, OH

Western Equine Encephalomyelitis

K. C. Kent Lloyd, DAVIS, CALIFORNIA

Western equine encephalomyelitis (WEE) is a potentially fatal disease of horses, mules, donkeys, and humans. It principally occurs west of the Mississippi River Valley and in Western Canada. The disease has a seasonal occurrence that is dependent on the life cycle of its principal vector, the mosquito. Sporadic outbreaks occur during the early summer, with most cases seen during August and September. The incidence declines in the fall, depending on climatic conditions.

The reservoir for the virus is infected wild and domesticated birds, which probably maintain the virus in the environment from year to year. The mosquito (Culex spp.) acquires the virus from infected birds during a blood meal. After a brief life cycle, the virus becomes concentrated in the salivary glands and is shed in the saliva. Spread occurs during feeding by infected mosquitos on horses and humans. Transmission from horses to humans probably does not occur, and both are considered to be dead-end hosts.

Local multiplication of the virus occurs at the site of inoculation. A viremic phase then occurs, at which time the virus can be cleared from the blood by the monocyte and macrophage system of the liver and spleen. If the viremia persists, spread to the central nervous system occurs with penetration of the gray matter of the cerebral cortex, thalamus, and hypothalamus. Infected cells are irreversibly damaged and this damage is the probable cause of the pronounced clinical signs.

CLINICAL SIGNS

A transient fever (39° C to 40.5° C), mild anorexia, and depression may be all the signs observed during the viremic stage. If the virus penetrates the brain and causes infection, neurologic system signs will be seen. Although inconsistently seen in each patient, three phases of neurologic disease are generally recognized. There is an initial period of excitement and mania with hyperreactivity to noise, light, and other environmental stimuli, and apparent blindness. A stage of depression and somnolence rapidly follows. The horse will stand with its head low, and feed may hang from the mouth despite the fact that there is as yet no impairment to swallowing. If allowed freedom of movement, most infected horses will wander aimlessly or head-press into the corner of a stall. They may appear incoordinated and have a tendency to circle or back up. Finally, some horses become obtunded and cannot appropriately respond to external stimuli. They are unable to swallow at this stage. If no longer steady on four legs, animals will become recumbent and may either remain quiet or begin to thrash. If paralyzed, death follows within two to four days from the onset of clinical signs. Most horses recover; however, many of those remain stuporous and demented and are referred to as "dummies."

DIAGNOSIS

Clinical signs, season, the presence of vectors, and inadequate vaccination history provide evidence supporting a presumptive diagnosis of WEE. However, the clinical signs and duration of illness in most terminal cases are sufficiently ambiguous that other diseases, especially rabies, cannot be satisfactorily ruled out prior to death. The diseases caused by the eastern equine encephalomyelitis (EEE) and Venezuelan equine encephalomyelitis (VEE) viruses cannot be clearly differentiated clinically from WEE. In addition, many other diseases should be considered in the differential diagnosis. These include botulism, hepatoencephalopathy, nigropallidal encephalomalacia (yellow star thistle poisoning), abscesses, and trauma to the brain.

Routine clinical pathology data are nondiagnostic for WEE. A transient leukopenia may be seen during the initial viremic stage. An elevated packed cell volume and hyperproteinemia may be evident if the horse is dehydrated. Indirect and total serum bilirubin concentrations may be elevated if the horse has been anorectic for more than a few days. A general serum chemistry panel is usually normal. Analysis of cerebrospinal fluid inconsistently reveals an elevation in total protein and mononuclear leukocytes. However, the horse's incoordinated state or recumbency may significantly endanger the safety of the clinician and patient so as to make collection of CSF fluid inadvisable in some cases.

A fourfold rise in serum-neutralizing or complement-fixing antibody titer is diagnostic for the virus in the horse. Acute and convalescent sera taken two to four weeks apart should be submitted on horses suspected of infection. Histologic examination of the cerebral cortex at necropsy reveals perivascular leukocytic cuffing. No inclusion bodies are present.

All or part (cerebral cortex and midbrain) of the brain can be cold-packed and shipped to a local or state diagnostic laboratory for evaluation. The virus can be identified in brain tissue using immunofluorescent techniques.

MANAGEMENT AND PREVENTION

Because the disease can be confused with rabies, strict isolation should be enforced. Rubber gloves should be worn at all times while handling the horse.

Patients with acute disease require extensive supportive and nursing care (see p. 346). The horse should be placed in a heavily bedded and preferably padded stall. Protective leg wraps and a padded helmet should be used to reduce self-inflicted trauma. Intravenous fluid and electrolyte therapy may be required. Roughage should be withheld because the horse will have difficulty swallowing in the later stages of the disease. A combination of alfalfa meal, dried cottage cheese, dextrose, and electrolytes can be administered via nasogastric tube (p. 425). Excessive fever can be reduced using phenylbutazone (1 to 2 gm per 450 kg intravenously) or Dipyrone (22 mg per kg intravenously or intramuscularly).

Vaccines currently in use are inactivated and either bivalent (WEE and EEE) or trivalent (WEE, EEE, and VEE). Some vaccines are also combined with tetanus toxoid or influenza. Horses can be vaccinated beginning at three months of age with a two-dose primary series and should be revaccinated at 12 months. Annual revaccination is recommended, preferably in the spring, but before the beginning of the mosquito season.

In high-risk areas, horses can be housed in stalls screened with mesh sufficient to act as a mosquito barrier. Topical application of insect repellent may also be helpful in outbreaks. Standing water where mosquitos breed should be eliminated.

Because of the risk of human disease from handling infected brain tissue, verified cases of WEE should be reported to public health officials. Persons should contact their physician if exposure is suspected.

Supplemental Readings

Blood, D. C., Radostits, O. M., and Henderson, J. A.: Diseases caused by viruses and chlamydia-II. *In* Veterinary Medicine, 6th ed. London, Bailliere Tindall, 1983.

Gibbs, E. P. J.: Equine viral encephalitis. Eq. Vet. J., 8:66, 1976.

Gillespie, J. H., and Timoney, J. F.: The Family Togaviridae. *In* Hagan and Bruner's Infectious Diseases of Domestic Animals, 7th ed. Ithaca, Cornell University Press, 1981.

Naylor, J. M., Freeman, D. E., and Kronfeld, D. S.: Alimentation of hypophagic horses. Comp. Cont. Educ. Pract. Vet., 6:S93, 1984.

Narcolepsy and Epilepsy

Corinne Raphel Sweeney, KENNETT SQUARE, PENNSYLVANIA

Thomas O. Hansen, KENNETT SQUARE, PENNSYLVANIA

NARCOLEPSY

Narcolepsy is an incurable, nonprogressive central nervous system disorder characterized by abnormal sleep tendency including excessive daytime sleepiness and pathologic manifestations of rapid eye movement (REM) sleep. In narcolepsy muscle relaxation intrudes abruptly into wakefulness. This muscle weakness produces a collapse, or cataplexy, which is the most obvious objective sign of narcolepsy. Narcolepsy was first reported in horses as a fainting condition in three Suffolk foals. Subsequent reports included a Shetland-Welsh crossbred female pony, a male miniature horse, three crossbred ponies, a Morgan filly, and an aged Quarterhorse mare. A familial occurrence has been recognized in man and in dogs, but not horses.

CLINICAL SIGNS AND DIAGNOSIS

The disease is seen in horses of all ages. The most obvious signs of cataplexy (muscular weakness) involve the face and neck muscles. Although com plete collapse is noticed in some ponies, most horses remain standing, with their heads hanging and resting close to or on the ground. During an attack, flexion of the forelimbs may occur, which the horse tries to prevent by locking its forelimbs.

The eyes may be closed and occasional snoring may be heard. When forced to walk, the horse may be incoordinated, "as if asleep." Complete attacks may occur and result in the horse lying on its side with flaccid limbs. These episodes last from a few seconds to 10 minutes. The horse appears completely normal following these "sleep attacks" with no residual neurologic deficits. As in humans and dogs there is probably a range of severity in the equine disease. The stimulation required to induce an attack may vary from leading a horse out of the stall to stroking the horse's back. The trigger for a cataplectic attack tends to be highly reproducible in an individual but varies between individuals.

Diagnosis of narcolepsy in the horse is based on history, clinical signs, and the absence of other diseases, particularly myasthenia gravis, seizures, and syncope. Narcolepsy in man is characterized by a tetrad of signs and symptoms: daytime sleepiness characterized by REM sleep directly following wakefulness, sudden loss of skeletal muscle tone (cataplexy), hallucinations, and sleep paralysis. In the horse, we focus almost exclusively on the observation of cataplexy. Electroencephalographic monitoring in a horse is not a practical procedure for diagnosis. Laboratory evaluations of horses with narcolepsy including hemogram, serum chemistry profile, and cerebrospinal fluid analysis have been normal.

Pharmacologic testing is a useful adjunct to diagnosis. Several cholinergic and anticholinergic drugs (Table 1) can be administered to test the presumptive diagnosis of narcolepsy-cataplexy. Past studies have shown that the results of these tests are consistent with those seen in dogs. The anticholinesterase physostigmine salicylate, which crosses the blood-brain barrier, significantly increases the severity of cataplexy. When administered intravenously, it induces cataplexy or sleep attack within minutes. On several occasions one horse showed signs of abdominal discomfort following its administration. Although the colic signs were

responsive to a single treatment with an analgesic (flunixin meglumine), this is an undesirable side effect of the test. Because of the effect on gastrointestinal motility, horses may defecate several piles of loose feces within minutes of administration of the drug.

The muscarinic blocker atropine sulfate is effective in reducing the severity of cataplexy. It crosses the blood-brain barrier and eliminates the "sleep attacks" within minutes following intravenous administration. A dose of 0.04 to 0.08 mg per kg prevents the narcoleptic attacks for 3½ to 30 hours after administration.

Neostigmine is a related compound that does not cross the blood-brain barrier effectively and therefore should have no significant effect on the cataplexy because the dysfunction is central. It should be administered at a dose of 0.005 mg per kg intravenously to determine that muscle weakness is not caused by a peripheral dysfunction such as myasthenia gravis.

Tricyclic antidepressants such as imipramine hydrochloride significantly reduce the amount of cataplexy in horses. These compounds are potent suppressors of REM sleep. Imipramine's effects become apparent within several minutes of administration.

THERAPY

Imipramine is used most commonly for the control of cataplexy. It is a tricyclic, antidepressant drug that blocks the uptake of serotonin and norepinephrine and suppresses only REM sleep. Imipramine is effective following intravenous or intramuscular administration (Table 2). Oral administration of imipramine gives inconsistent results. A parenteral dose of 0.55 mg per kg relieves cataplexy for five hours, and longer relief can be obtained with higher dosages. None of the undesirable side effects associated with the use of imipramine in humans, such as dryness of the mouth, sweating, digestive problems, muscle twitches, and intolerance, were seen.

Central nervous system stimulants have been used to treat excessive daytime sleepiness in man. Currently, no narcoleptic horses are known to have been treated with this class of drugs.

TABLE 1. DIAGNOSTIC PHARMACOLOGIC TESTING FOR NARCOLEPSY

Drug	Dose	Route	Effects on Narcoleptic Horse
Physostigmine salicylate*	0.06 to 0.08 mg/kg	IV	Induces narcoleptic/cataleptic attack in 3 to 10 minutes†
Atropine sulfate	0.08 mg/kg	IV	Eliminates sleep attacks within minutes and prevents their occurrence from 3.5 to 30 hours after administration

*Antilirium, O'Neal, Jones, and Feldman, Inc., St. Louis, MO
†Abdominal discomfort may occur.

TABLE 2. PHARMACOLOGIC TREATMENT OF NARCOLEPSY

Drug	Dose	Route	Onset of Effect (min)	Duration of Effect (hr)
Imipramine hydrochloride*	0.55 mg/kg	IV	~ 1	2 to 3
		IM	5 to 10	5 to 10

*Tofranil, Geigy Pharmaceutical, Ardsley, N.Y.

EPILEPSY

The term *epilepsy* implies recurring or repeated seizures in which the primary defect is in the brain. The most remarkable clinical characteristic of epilepsy is the variability of signs with widely varying intervals between attacks. These intervals may be measured in minutes, hours, days, weeks, months, or even years. The fundamental concept of epilepsy is that it is a neural process, a state of nervous discharge occurring excessively and abnormally.

The transient modifications in brain function that mark the seizure can include some, but not necessarily all, of the following: loss of consciousness, tonic and clonic muscular movements, abnormal movements of the head and eyeballs, jaw clamping, opisthotonus, paddling actions, and changes in visceral function (urination, defecation, sweating, and salivation).

Irrespective of whether the primary insult to the brain is ischemic, traumatic, infectious, or associated with neoplasm, seizures are most likely to occur if several sets of criteria are met. First is the location of the lesion. Lesions in acquired epilepsy are mainly found in the cerebral cortex. Lesions confined to subcortical areas, brain stem, or cerebellum rarely cause seizures. Second, epileptogenesis is time related. This is demonstrated in post-traumatic seizures and in the development of brain scars, in which there is a delay from the time of the injury to the establishment of recurring seizures. This delay may be months or years. The third feature is that epileptogenic foci develop in damaged brain and not in areas of total brain destruction. Thus, in destructive processes, foci develop in zones in which morphologic alterations may or may not be observable.

IDIOPATHIC EPILEPSY

Epilepsy is frequently described as being idiopathic, which implies that epilepsy is the disease—with an unknown cause—and the seizure is the clinical sign. Unfortunately, this may be the most common classification encountered in horses until we learn more about seizure disorders. Idiopathic epilepsy has been observed in mares associated with estrus, when estrogen levels are increased. Therefore, reproductive and hormonal analysis in association with seizure episodes in mares should be considered. Ovariectomy, proges-

terone therapy, or anticonvulsant therapy may prove beneficial for these animals.

Horses with recurrent seizures should be thoroughly evaluated by physical examination, neurologic examination, cerebrospinal fluid analysis, skull radiography, and blood chemistry. Cases presented to our hospital with recurrent seizures of an unknown cause have been symptomatically treated with diphenylhydantoin* either orally or intravenously (Table 3). In several horses seizures reportedly ceased only to recur following discontinuation of the diphenylhydantoin.

Epilepsy Following Brain Trauma

Head trauma is not uncommon in horses and may or may not be accompanied by skull fractures. Contusions, lacerations, and hemorrhages can all be a result of a traumatic insult. The most common site for intracranial hemorrhage in the horse is subarachnoid, thereby resulting in meningitis. Early-onset seizures after trauma have a better prognosis than those occurring after a delay or epileptogenic "ripening." Spontaneous improvement can occur and leave an animal seizure-free in spite of withdrawal of anticonvulsant medication. The brain lesion that may result from trauma includes meningocerebral cicatrix or patchy areas of cortical atrophy or both. It is unlikely that radiographs and cerebrospinal fluid analysis will be helpful because of the delay in onset from the time of trauma.

CONVULSIVE FOALS

An idiopathic convulsive syndrome that occurs in foals from several weeks to several months of age has been reported. The syndrome may be more common in weanling foals of the Arabian breed. It is characterized by a sudden onset of recurrent seizures that may increase in frequency over a period of days to weeks so that the foal is convulsing many times a day. Although the seizures reportedly respond well to anticonvulsant therapy, this syndrome appears to be self-limiting, with the foals "growing out" of the disorder. The etiology is unknown.

DIAGNOSIS

Hepatoencephalopathy, rabies, and cardiac arrhythmias can all present with a history compatible

---

*Phenytoin, Dilantin, Parke-Davis & Co., Morris Plains, NJ

TABLE 3. THERAPY FOR SEIZURES

Stage of Treatment	Drug	Foal	Adult
Initial therapy	diazepam*	0.05–0.4 mg/kg IV	25–50 mg IV
	xylazine†	0.4–1.0 mg/kg IV or IM	0.4–1.0 mg/kg IV or IM
	pentobarbital‡	4–6 mg/kg IV to effect	6 mg/kg IV
	phenytoin§	5–10 mg/kg IV or PO	—
	primidone‖	2 gm PO	—
	chloral hydrate**	0.06 gm/kg–0.2 gm/kg IV to effect	15–60 gm IV to effect
Maintenance therapy	phenobarbital††	0.5 mg/kg–1 mg/kg PO twice daily or to effect	0.5–2 mg/kg PO twice daily or to effect
	phenytoin§	1–5 mg/kg PO every 2–4 hr	5–15 mg/kg PO every 8 hrs

*Valium, 5 mg/ml, 10 ml vials. Roche Laboratories, Division of Hoffman-LaRoche, Inc., Nutley, NJ. *Note:* Diazepam is denatured by contact with plastic for more than a few minutes.
†Rompun, 100 mg/ml vials, Haver-Lockhart, Shawnee, KS
‡Sodium pentobarbital injection, 65 mg/ml, 100 ml vials. The Butler Co., Columbus, OH
§Dilantin, 100 mg capsules and 250 mg injection vials. Parke-Davis, Morris Plains, NJ
‖Mysoline, 250 mg tablets. Ayerst Laboratories, Inc., New York, NY
**Chloral-thesia, 30%, 250 ml vials. Veterinary Laboratories, Inc., Lenexa, KS
††30 mg tablets, Rugby Laboratories, Inc., Rockville Centre, NY

with epilepsy. Liver necrosis of Theiler's disease (see p. 110) may produce recurring seizures along with other signs of acute hepatitis. Icterus and elevated liver enzymes should be present in horses with seizures associated with liver disease. Confirmation of hepatitis through a percutaneous liver biopsy may be advocated.

The incidence of rabies (see p. 364) in horses is relatively low and signs are highly variable but may include hyperesthesia, abnormal behavior, and convulsions. Because of the variability of clinical presentations associated with rabies, attending veterinarians should consider rabies as a cause for recurrent seizures of short duration. The average life expectancy for a rabid horse is three to five days.

Cardiac disease does not cause true epilepsy. However, several cases presented to our hospital with a history of recurrent seizures actually involved cardiac arrhythmias including atrial fibrillation, third-degree atrioventricular block, ventricular tachycardia, and advanced second-degree atrioventricular block (see p. 154).

Diagnosis in epilepsy involves a series of interconnected steps. First, it should be determined whether the episodic symptom of which the client complains is caused by epilepsy or by another disorder characterized by "spells." (We would encourage the reader to consult Seizure Disorders on page 344 of Current Therapy in Equine Medicine, 1st Edition, for an excellent review.) Second, an adequate description of the fit should be recorded, along with any provoking or precipitating circumstances. Noise, lights, feeding, or sexual activity may trigger a convulsive episode. Third, a logical attempt should be made to determine the cause. This may require additional diagnostic tests, but emphasis should be placed on history and the clinical examination and its evaluation. The diagnosis of epilepsy should not be static; conclusions

reached at one stage may be subsequently altered during the course of the work-up. It is important to note any changes during the passage of time. An etiologic diagnosis may not be made conclusively in many patients.

Ancillary diagnostic aids may include a complete hemogram, blood chemistry analysis, cerebrospinal fluid analysis, oral or intravenous glucose tolerance to evaluate insulin response, and radiographic studies. Spinal fluid studies or radiographs may be most helpful when there is evidence of an intracranial process. These tests should be run only after a thorough history and physical examination.

TREATMENT

If the frequency of seizures is decreasing over time, it is probable that this trend will continue. The clinician may elect not to treat this animal provided it is not being injured while convulsing, or could alternatively provide a short course of anticonvulsant therapy to abate the convulsive episodes. If the seizures are increasing in frequency, they may continue to do so.

It is usually unsafe to approach a convulsing adult, but if it is deemed necessary, undue restraint should be avoided. If anticonvulsant therapy is required because of repeated frequent seizures, pentobarbital* at 6 mg per kg intravenously or diazepam† at 25 to 50 mg per dose could be given, repeated in 30 minutes if necessary. It is easier to restrain foals for administration of anticonvulsive drugs. Diazepam at 0.05 to 0.4 mg per kg intravenously per dose (usually 10 to 20 mg per dose) repeated at 30-minute intervals as necessary is very effective. Follow-up with oral phenytoin has been recommended both in foals and adults. In all cases the minimum

*The Butler Co., Columbus, OH
†Roche Laboratories, Division of Hoffman-LaRoche, Inc., Nutley, NJ

quantity of anticonvulsant drug required to control the seizures is recommended because of other drug-related effects. For example, pentobarbital also depresses the cardiopulmonary system and may initiate some struggling during the drug elimination period.

Chronic anticonvulsant therapy in horses is rare; however, while treating an epileptic it is necessary to slowly decrease the dosage of the anticonvulsant drug to determine if continuous therapy is still required. For continuous anticonvulsant therapy some guidelines are presented in Table 3.

Supplemental Readings

Narcolepsy

Foutz, A. S., Mitter, M. M., Dement, W. C.: Narcolepsy. Vet. Clin. North Am.: Small Anim. Pract., *10*:65, 1980.

Katherman, A. E.: A comparative review of canine and human narcolepsy. Comp. Cont. Educ., *11*:818, 1980.

Sweeney, C. R., Hendricks, J. C., Beech, J., and Morrison, A.: Narcolepsy in a horse. J. Am. Vet. Med. Assoc., *183*:126, 1983.

Epilepsy

deLahunta, A.: Veterinary Neuroanatomy and Clinical Neurology, 2nd ed. Philadelphia, W. B. Saunders Company, 1983, pp. 326–339.

Evans, J. H.: Post-traumatic epilepsy. Neurology, *13*:207, 1963.

Mayhew, I. G.: Seizure disorders. *In* Robinson, N. E. (ed.): Current Therapy in Equine Medicine, 1st Ed., Philadelphia, W. B. Saunders Company, 1983, pp. 344–349.

Rossdale, P. D.: Differential diagnosis and treatment of equine neonatal disease. Vet. Rec., *91*:581, 1972.

Schmidt, R. P., and Wilder, B. J.: Epilepsy. Contemporary Neurology Series, Philadelphia, F. A. Davis Company, 1968, pp. 43–59.

Equine Degenerative Myeloencephalopathy

Jill Beech, KENNETT SQUARE, PENNSYLVANIA

Equine degenerative myeloencephalopathy (EDM) is a progressive degenerative disorder of the central nervous system. It may affect only a single horse on a farm or it may appear in multiple animals that frequently are related. Currently the cause and pathogenesis are unknown and there is no treatment. Although the disease is seen more frequently in the eastern United States, it has also been reported in the western part of the country. Cases may occur in other regions; however, because of the relative paucity of information on the disease, they may be undetected or the animals may be labeled "wobblers" without further differentiation. There is no sex predilection but EDM appears to be seen more frequently in some breeds than others. Although neurologic disorders are not common in the Arabian, Quarterhorse, Morgan, and Appaloosa breeds within the northeastern United States, EDM has been one of their most frequent neurologic diseases over the past few years. It has also been described in zebras and Mongolian wild horses (*Equus przewalskii*) in captivity. A similar less diffuse degenerative neuroaxonal dystrophy that appears to be familial has been seen in Morgan horses.

HISTORY AND CLINICAL SIGNS

Clinical signs, primarily hindlimb dysmetria, appear between birth and three years of age. Some of this wide age range for onset of signs is probably related to variations in observer astuteness. Animals with subtle cases may not be identified until they are grossly abnormal and then are presented with histories incorrectly reporting recent acute onset of signs. Animals with severe cases tend to show signs at an earlier age, frequently between two and six months of age, whereas those with milder cases may not display overt signs until one and a half to two years of age or older. Rate of progression of signs varies and is more likely to be rapid in those horses that are moderately to severely affected at a young age. The condition in some horses continues to worsen, whereas that in others may stabilize. There is no significant improvement or remission with age. Although the disease is not associated with any systemic illness or muscle wasting, horses with severe cases may lose weight if fed with other horses because their neurologic deficits relegate them to a low position in the "pecking order."

Even when several horses have been affected on one farm, either simultaneously or at different times, no common etiologic agent has been discovered. Husbandry, including deworming and vaccination, has usually been adequate and there is no history of illness or drug administration in an affected animal or its dam during the latter's pregnancy. No causative dietary factors have been identified, although vitamin E deficiency can be associated with similar pathologic lesions in other species and is known to occur in the northeastern United States in animals fed locally grown feeds. Deficiency of vitamin E in serum was associated with EDM in six interrelated Mongolian wild horses receiving a commercial grain concentrate. After a prolonged period of vitamin E supplementation no further cases have been reported. Although this does not prove vitamin E deficiency is the cause, it is implicated as a possible factor. Some zebras developed EDM despite apparently adequate diets including vitamin E and selenium supplementation. However, as neither serum nor tissue levels of vitamin E and selenium were assayed it is not known if supplementation was adequate. Serum levels of vitamin E in several affected domestic horses have been normal. The familial clusters of some cases suggest that inheritance may also be an important factor in the syndrome's pathogenesis. It is possible that a genetic predisposition and nutritional factors both contribute to the disease.

Mildly affected animals have a symmetrical dysmetric hind leg gait. They move dysrhythmically with a jerking, stabbing short-striding gait, sometimes showing hindlimb interference. Signs are often most noticeable at a walk or trot. The canter is often stiff and lacking impulsion. When stopping, horses are often imprecise and stab the hind feet down with excessive force. When circling they tend to sit back on their haunches, pivot on the inside hind foot and sometimes abduct the outside hindlimb. When backed they tend to leave their feet on the ground too long before picking them up, and when swayed sideways they have jerking hind foot movement and may strike the opposite limb and/or step on the anterior aspect of the opposite foot and pastern. In my experience, except in severe cases, forelimb involvement is usually mild or equivocal, although others report it may equal the hindlimb gait disability. When forelimb deficits are seen, the stride is shortened and spastic; normal smooth joint movements are lacking. There are no signs referable to a brain lesion and no changes in skin sensation, tail tone, limb reflexes, or muscle mass.

Severely affected animals show frequent interferences between the hindlimbs and obvious ataxia. They frequently scuff their hind toes and even the dorsal aspect of the hoof in the initial stages of protraction. Their hindquarters often sway markedly from side to side and paresis may cause falling or excessive scrambling when rising. The frequent interference often leads to sores on the medial aspect of the fetlocks. When backed, these horses sit back and may actually dog sit and lose balance if maneuvered too rapidly. If slowly backed they leave their hind feet on the ground, rocking back on their heels and then dragging the hooves before jerking them up, only to replace them still inappropriately too far under the body. The pivoting on the inner hindlimbs and jerking hindlimb movement are very marked when these horses are circled. They may cross one foot over very close to or on the dorsum of the other. These horses also tend to throw their forelimbs out spastically with loss of coordination at all gaits and when circled. They may almost fall if pushed sideways and can easily be displaced from following a straight line by pulling on the tail. When exercised, they are reluctant to move faster than a walk and will often slow down and stop. The canter is ataxic, asynchronous, and bouncy and weak. Stopping with difficulty, these horses frequently step on themselves and may dog sit.

DIAGNOSIS

Diagnosis is based on clinical signs and ruling out other neurologic and neuromuscular syndromes. EDM may be indistinguishable from cervical spinal cord compression (see p. 355) because both syndromes occur in young horses and are characterized by hindlimb ataxia, spasticity, and dysmetria. Horses with cervical cord compression usually markedly circumduct the outside hindlimb when circled, whereas those with EDM tend to show relatively more exaggerated vertical flexion of the outer limb and pivoting on the inside hindlimb. Whereas some horses with low cervical cord compression may show marked asymmetric forelimb proprioceptive and motor deficits if the compression is more severe on one side than the other, forelimb signs are symmetric in horses with EDM. Horses with cervical cord compression are more likely to have hindlimb deficits whereas those with EDM may show equally severe signs in both forelimbs and hindlimbs. Age and breed incidence may also help differentiate the two conditions, but radiographs and myelography may be needed for definitive differentiation. Cerebrospinal fluid (CSF) analysis for cell count and protein is of little value as it is usually normal in both syndromes.

EDM is differentiated from equine protozoal myeloencephalitis (EPM) (see p. 359) and cerebrospinal nematodiasis, because the latter usually cause asymmetric signs and have a more rapid progression. CSF may be abnormal in EPM and cerebrospinal nematodiasis with an increase in both cells and protein. Likewise, herpesvirus I myelopathy (see p. 365) can be differentiated clinically by its acute progressive paresis and ataxia, usually affecting primarily the hindlimbs but sometimes manifested by acute tetraparesis, loss of anal, tail, and bladder tone, and perineal skin sensory alterations. CSF is often xanthochromic with an increased protein content; sequential serum antibody titers are diagnostic. Signs of cerebellar abiotrophy are often manifested at the same age as EDM. Head tremor combined with hypermetria and ataxia serves to differentiate it; also, the former has been described only in the Arabian and Oldenberg breeds.

There are no laboratory tests diagnostic or characteristic of the disease. Although the condition has been associated with low serum vitamin E levels in Mongolian wild horses, the measurement's relevance to the disease has yet to be determined. When interpreting serum levels, one must remember that a normal level does not rule out the possibility of an earlier deficiency resulting in the central nervous system lesions and neither does detection of a low level prove that deficiency is the cause.

PATHOLOGY

There are no gross lesions. The disease is characterized microscopically by diffuse neuraxonal degeneration in many nuclei in the brain stem and the spinal cord, especially in the cranial cervical and midthoracic segments with axonal degeneration and some demyelination in the white matter. Peripheral nerves and other tissues are normal.

TREATMENT AND PREVENTION

To date there is no treatment or known preventive measures. Even in other species in cases of neuraxonal degeneration known to be caused by vitamin E deficiency, administration of vitamin E after signs have developed has had inconsistent or negligible effect on signs. Short-term administration had no obvious benefit in several horses with EDM. On farms with a high incidence, it may be useful to assay and monitor all the horses' serum vitamin E levels so that supplements could be administered if indicated. Because of a possible familial incidence, the presence of the disorder within a family should be considered when breeding stock are selected.

Supplemental Readings

Beech, J.: Neuraxonal dystrophy of the accessory cuneate nucleus in horses. Vet. Pathol., 21:384, 1984.
Lui, S. K., Dolensek, E. P., Adams, C. R., and Tappe, J. P.: Myelopathy and vitamin E deficiency in six Mongolian wild horses. J. Am. Vet. Med. Assoc., 183:1266, 1983.
Mayhew, I. G., deLahunta, A., Whitlock, R. H., Krook, L., and Tasker, J. B.: Spinal cord disease in the horse. Cornell Vet., 68(suppl 6):106, 1978.
Mayhew, I. G., and MacKay, R. J.: The nervous system. In Mansmann, R. A., McAllister, E. S., and Pratt, P. W. (eds.): Equine Medicine and Surgery, 3rd ed. Santa Barbara, CA, American Veterinary Publications, 1982.

Cervical Vertebral Malformation

Pamela C. Wagner, CORVALLIS, OREGON

Cervical vertebral malformation (CVM) refers to abnormalities in the vertebral bodies, articular processes, and vertebral foramina that ultimately result in functional or anatomic stenosis of the vertebral canal. Such abnormalities are not uncommon, the estimated incidence being 10 per cent in the Thoroughbred population. The condition often goes unrecognized unless impingement of the vertebrae on the spinal cord causes focal compression and neurologic signs. Focal spinal cord compression results in gait abnormalities described as part of the wobbler syndrome. The condition has also been referred to as equine sensory ataxia and equine incoordination.

Several types of osseous malformations may be responsible for stenosis of the vertebral canal and pressure-induced lesions of the spinal cord. For the purpose of a therapeutic approach, they may be loosely grouped as follows:

Functional Stenosis. When the neck is flexed or hyperextended, the vertebrae move so as to cause compression of the spinal cord. This has been referred to as spondylolisthesis. Seen most frequently in weanlings and yearlings, the abnormal angulation is often accompanied by articular process changes as well as remodeling of the caudal vertebral epiphyses. With the neck in a neutral position, compression of the spinal cord is reduced; however, the vertebral canal may still be narrowed owing to the remodeling changes. The junction of cervical vertebrae 3 and 4 is most often affected.

Absolute Stenosis. Osseous changes in the vertebrae that cause spinal cord compression not altered by neck positioning have been described.

These include stenosis of the cranial vertebral foramina, medial ingrowth of the cranial articular processes, and arthropathy of the cranial and caudal articular processes. This type of stenosis usually affects horses from one to three years of age, and often is diagnosed while the horse is in training. Cervical vertebrae 5 through 7 are most often affected.

CLINICAL SIGNS

Most horses are affected in the first two years of life, usually as weanlings or yearlings. Onset of signs may be sudden and related to a traumatic incident or insidious with slowly progressive and debilitating incoordination. Several authors have noted a sexual predisposition, with colts being affected more often than fillies. Most affected horses are in good flesh and have had excellent nutrition.

The presenting clinical signs are those of a focal pressure–induced lesion of the cervical spinal cord. Damage to the ascending spinal cord tracts results in proprioceptive deficits of all four limbs that manifest clinically as ataxia and occasionally hypermetria. Damage to the descending spinal cord tracts is evidenced by tetraparesis and degrees of stiffness or hypometria. If the malformation exerts pressure on the cranial cervical spinal cord, the proprioceptive deficits will be more severe in the pelvic limbs than the thoracic limbs. The ataxia is most noticeable at a walk or when the horse is turned in small circles. If the animal is able to gallop, it does so with a characteristic "bunny hop." The rear legs will circumduct, and the toes may drag. The hocks have little flexion, and the stride appears to be prolonged. In general, the hindquarters of the horse seem stiff and unbalanced. If the horse is turned sharply, it may pivot on the inside leg, while a normal horse steps around briskly. While the pelvic limbs appear most involved, subtle signs of foreleg involvement may be noted on close examination. The front legs may be more obviously affected if the vertebral malformation occurs at C5 to C7. The horse may step abnormally wide and cross its forelegs while moving. If the legs are placed in abnormal postures, the horse may not correct its stance.

These signs can be exaggerated by leading the horse downhill or with the head elevated. In general, focal cervical spinal cord compression will result in a horse that has more pronounced signs of ataxia in the pelvic limbs than in the thoracic limbs. Backing the horse may elicit signs of ataxia; however, this is variable. When led over obstacles, the horse may drag its feet and stumble. Usually the proprioceptive signs are bilateral and symmetrical; however, one pelvic limb may appear more affected than the other.

Signs of paresis are elicited by pressure over the withers and loins and by sway tests. If pressure is exerted over the withers or loins, the horse may move downward and may fall if paresis is severe. The sway test should be performed while the horse is moving. The handler pulls the tail firmly to one side as the horse is walked away. A weak horse will be readily pulled to the side, and the severely affected horse may stumble and fall down. Paresis reflects damage to the descending tracts of the upper motor neuron pathways. A sway test may be performed on the forelimbs by grasping the mane with one hand and pushing over the scapula with the other as the horse is moved forward. The affected horse will stumble sideways on its forelimbs.

Some horses show rapid onset of signs with stabilization at variable levels of disability. Signs in some horses never stabilize and slowly get progressively worse, while in others signs may be present for some time and then may appear to improve. Reports of spontaneous full recoveries of confirmed cases of CVM are uncommon.

DIAGNOSIS

Other causes of ataxia such as vertebral trauma, equine degenerative myelopathy, equine protozoal myeloencephalitis, and equine herpesvirus 1 infection must be ruled out. Definitive diagnosis is accomplished by obtaining radiographs and myelograms of the cervical vertebrae to demonstrate focal spinal cord compression. Radiographs should be made with the horse under general anesthesia in lateral recumbency. The cervical spine should be visualized from the base of the skull to the intervertebral space of C7 to T1. After radiographs are made of the neck in the neutral position, the neck should be flexed by gently pulling the horse's muzzle toward the carpus and securing it in this position. This provides adequate flexion of all articulations of the cervical vertebral column. Care should be taken not to overflex the neck, as further damage to the cord may occur if there is a severe subluxation. Areas of apparent stenosis may be confirmed with myelography. The use of metrizamide* as a myelographic agent has made the procedure safe and accurate.

Functional stenosis can be diagnosed with myelography by demonstrating dynamic spinal cord compression. With this type of lesion contrast media is visible in both dorsal and ventral columns when the neck is in a neutral position, but both columns narrow or disappear with neck flexion (Fig. 1).

---

*Accurate Chemical Co., Hicksville, NY

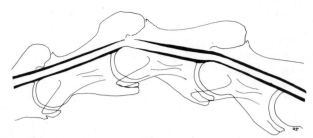

Figure 1. Diagram of a cervical myelographic study of a horse with CVM and functional stenosis. There is dramatic attenuation of the ventral dye column and obliteration of the dorsal dye column at the level of the C3 and C4 vertebral articulation when the neck is in a flexed position.

In many cases of functional stenosis, the vertebrae may also show some degree of absolute narrowing. This narrowing may not, in itself, result in spinal cord compression. The abnormalities leading to narrowing of the canal include dorsal protrusion of the caudal vertebral epiphyses, remodeling of the articular processes, and bony proliferation at the pedicles and facets. The degree to which these changes contribute to the production of a functional stenosis is unknown.

Absolute stenosis causes a static compression of the spinal cord that can be noted on the myelogram when the cervical vertebrae are in extended, neutral, and flexed positions. Compression is due to bony changes of the vertebrae that include absolute stenosis of the cranial or the caudal orifice of the vertebral foramina, remodeling of the articular processes, and exostoses and degeneration of the articular surfaces indicative of degenerative joint disease. An example is shown in the diagram of a myelogram in Figure 2. While the compression may be exaggerated by flexion or hyperextension, it is present at all times.

Cerebrospinal fluid (CSF) analysis has been useful in ruling out other causes of ataxia and paresis. Cerebrospinal fluid from the horse with CVM is usually normal. Electromyography (EMG) is used to differentiate lower motor neuron (LMN) disease from upper motor neuron (UMN) disease. Most

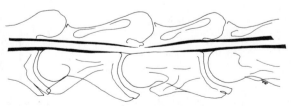

Figure 2. Absolute stenosis of the vertebral canal at the caudal orifice of C5 and the cranial orifice of C6 is evident in this line drawing of a myelogram of a horse with CVM. Many horses with functional stenosis, as depicted in Figure 1, have some degree of absolute vertebral canal stenosis at the site of spinal cord compression.

stenotic cervical lesions result in compression of myelinated fibers, including those in the descending tracts, i.e, UMN damage. The EMG in UMN disease is essentially normal, and thus an EMG of the cervical muscles of horses with stenotic lesions is usually within normal limits. In some cases of absolute stenosis with static cord compression at C5 to C7, some EMG changes have been noted. This has been attributed to pressure on the ventral roots as they leave the vertebral canal.

PATHOGENESIS OF BONY LESIONS

The cause of cervical vertebral malformation is unknown but is probably a result of a combination of factors. The heritability of the condition is in dispute. In most cases, the articular processes and vertebral foramina are malformed, causing cord compression directly or allowing malarticulation that causes compression of the cord during movement that some authorities have interpreted as evidence of instability.

Osteochondrosis-like lesions have been seen in the articular surfaces as well as in the vertebral body growth plates in some horses affected with CVM. It has been reported that the primary etiologic factors causing osteochondrosis are a genetic predisposition for rapid growth combined with a large intake of high-energy food. One recent report indicates that osteochondrosis was diagnosed as the cause of ataxia in four Standardbred horses. The effect of hormonal factors has not been analyzed; however, a reported sex predilection indicates such studies may be helpful.

In all probability, many factors are involved. A horse selected for rapid growth and being fed on a high plane of nutrition is certainly the most likely candidate for this syndrome.

TREATMENT

Cervical spinal cord compression carries a guarded prognosis. Because the course of the clinical syndrome is variable, some treatment may appear to be successful for a period of time and then fail.

MEDICAL MANAGEMENT

Medical treatment is aimed at reducing inflammation at the site of compression. Dexamethasone* at a dosage of 0.1 mg per kg has been used, and some improvement of clinical signs has been noted for the duration of the therapy. Phenylbutazone† at

---

*Dexasone, Med-Tech, Inc., Elwood, KS
†Westazon, Western Medical Supply, Inc., Arcadia, CA

a dosage of 8 to 10 mg per kg also has been used. Some veterinarians have obtained good results using 1 ml per kg of 50 per cent dimethylsulfoxide* in 1 liter of saline intravenously every other day until improvement is noted. With all of these medical treatments, stall rest and feeding and watering the horse from an elevated position to discourage extensive neck movement are recommended. The severely affected horse will be prone to lacerations of the bulbs of the heels of the forelimbs due to overreaching, as well as cuts of the head and body due to hitting objects and falling. Good nursing care is imperative; however, the outcome is usually not rewarding. Some horses will stabilize enough to be used as breeding animals, but many improved horses will worsen when medical therapy is discontinued.

SURGICAL MANAGEMENT

Arthrodesis of the Cervical Spine. The surgical approach to relieve cord compression depends on the nature of the lesion. Functional stenosis that results in maximal cord compression during flexion may be treated by fusion of the affected vertebrae to prevent movement at that site. The Cloward technique of cervical fusion as used in humans has been modified for horses to achieve osseous bridging between two vertebrae, maintaining the vertebrae in the extended position. This technique entails drilling out the intervertebral space and using a bone dowel or cancellous bone screw supported by a metal basket to stabilize and fuse the vertebrae in extension.

In my experience, the majority of improvement is seen in the first year postoperatively. In most cases clinical improvement is seen; however, the degree of improvement depends on several factors: (1) The duration of time the horse has shown signs before surgery. Most surgical cases are not identified and scheduled for surgery less than one month following the onset of signs, and in many the time elapsed is much greater. In general, horses operated upon early after the onset of signs do improve to a greater extent than those that show signs for months before surgery. (2) The severity of signs before surgery. While horses with very severe signs will respond to surgery, the residual level of ataxia still remaining may be greater than that present in the horse with milder signs presurgically. (3) The age of the horse. In general, younger horses appear to improve the most. This may, in fact, reflect the duration of time that signs have existed. Ataxia may be overlooked until the horse is required to work.

Complications of this surgical procedure include

---

*Domoso, Diamond Laboratories, Des Moines, IA

spinal cord trauma, hemorrhage, and damage to the recurrent laryngeal nerve, all of which may be avoided by careful surgical technique. Postsurgical complications include trauma during recovery, as well as failure of the dowel after implantation.

Dorsal Decompressive Laminectomy. Absolute stenosis causing a static compression of the spinal cord in both the extended and flexed positions may be treated by a subtotal dorsal decompressive laminectomy. The surgery requires proper equipment for positioning and operation. The procedure has several complications related to the surgical approach and the postanesthetic recovery and should not be undertaken without considerable preparation and practice. More recently, cervical fusion has been used to treat horses with absolute stenosis. By immobilizing the affected intervertebral space, regression of the proliferative lesions has been demonstrated. Decompression, as evidenced by myelograms made six months after surgery, may be achieved.

The prognosis for return to usefulness of horses with CVM is guarded. Most surgically treated horses with functional stenoses are able to be used for breeding animals, and some can be used in hard work such as racing, show, and pleasure. Those horses with anatomic stenoses requiring dorsal decompressions have a much more guarded prognosis. Much of the return to function depends on the degree of spinal cord damage, and the extent of improvement cannot be evaluated realistically for many months after surgery.

Supplemented Readings

Alitalo, D., and Karkkainen, M.: Osteochondrotic changes in the vertebrae of four ataxic horses suffering from cervical vertebral malformation. Nord. Vet. Med., 35:468, 1983.
DeBowes, R. M, Grant, B. D., Bagby, G. W., Gallina, A. M., Sande, R. D., and Ratzlaff, M. H.: Cervical vertebral interbody fusion in the horse: A comparative study of bovine xenografts and autografts supported by stainless steel baskets. Am. J. Vet. Res., 45:191, 1984.
Dimock, W.: "Wobbles"—an hereditary disease in horses. J. Hered., 41:319, 1950.
Falco, M. J., Whitwell, K., and Palmer, A. C.: An investigation into the genetics of "wobbler disease" in Thoroughbred horses in Britain. Equine Vet. J., 8:165, 1976.
Mayhew, I. G., deLahunta, A., Whitlock, R. H., Krook, L., and Tasker, J. B.: Spinal cord disease in the horse. Cornell Vet., 68(Suppl. 6):1, 1978.
Nixon, A. J., and Stashak, T. S.: Surgical management of cervical vertebral malformation in the horse. Proc. 28th Annu. Meet. Am. Assoc. Eq. Pract., 1982, pp. 267–277.
Nixon, A. J., and Stashak, T. S.: Dorsal laminectomy in the horse. I. Review of the literature and description of a new procedures. Vet. Surgery, 12:172, 1983.
Rantanen, N. W., Gavin, P. R., Barkee, D. D., and Sande, R. D.: Ataxia and paresis in horses. Part II. Radiographic and

myelographic examination of the cervical vertebral column. Comp. Cont. Ed. Prac. Vet., 3:S161, 1981.

Rooney, J. R.: Biomechanics of Lameness in Horses. Baltimore, Williams & Wilkins, 1969, p. 222.

Wagner, P. C., Grant, B. D., Gallina, A., and Bagby, G. W.: Ataxia and paresis in horses. Part III. Surgical treatment of cervical spinal cord compression. Comp. Cont. Ed. Prac. Vet., 3:S192, 1981.

Whitwell, K. E.: Causes of ataxia in horses. In Practice, 2:17, 1980.

Equine Protozoal Myeloencephalitis

Barbara D. Brewer, GAINESVILLE, FLORIDA

Equine protozoal myeloencephalitis (EPM) (previously referred to as focal myelitis-encephalitis, equine toxoplasmosis, or toxoplasma-like encephalomyelitis) is becoming a more frequently diagnosed neurologic disease in the United States and Canada, although its cause and pathogenesis remain obscure. Recent work suggests that the agent is a coccidian parasite similar to the *Sarcocystis* genus, which may have a hematogenous phase of infection. The disease does not appear to be contagious from horse to horse, but since particular farms or race tracks experience multiple cases over the course of several years, a common environmental source of contamination is a possibility. Whether the horse is an intermediate or aberrant host for this coccidian and whether any other animal such as a rodent, bird, cow, dog, or cat is a host is unknown.

Equine protozoal myeloencephalitis has been diagnosed in most areas of the United States (including California, where it had not been found until recently) and Canada, although more frequently in the eastern states. Seen more commonly in one- to four-year-old Thoroughbreds and Standardbreds, it has been reported in most light-breed horses ranging in age from two months to 14 years. The disease may occur more frequently during the warmer months of the year.

HISTORY AND CLINICAL SIGNS

The history is as variable as the disease process itself. Frequently an obscure lameness is first noted. This is unresponsive to anti-inflammatory drugs and is not easily localized or eliminated with local nerve blocks. The "lameness" may rapidly progress to ataxia or remain static (or even improve) for quite some time. Physical examination is unremarkable in acute disease, but in cases of more than two weeks' duration, a careful examination of the animal for signs of muscle atrophy should be performed. Most frequently, the atrophy is asymmetric and often involves the gluteal or longissimus lumborum muscles.

Neurologic signs vary with the site or sites of the lesion. The organism is capable of invading exceedingly specific focal areas such as gray matter supplying one peripheral nerve, or a single brain stem nucleus, but may also be multifocal in distribution. While it is more likely to cause signs of spinal cord disease, it can produce specific cranial or peripheral nerve dysfunction, brain stem signs, or even cerebral signs. Unlike many other neurologic diseases, both white and gray matter can be involved.

Early signs may include symmetrical ataxia and paresis, but with the eventual progression of the disease process (which may occur over hours, days, or months), the signs often become asymmetric, with evidence of multifocal gray matter involvement such as various cranial nerve deficits, muscle atrophy, focal patchy sweating, and loss of reflexes. When the rear limbs are profoundly affected and the forelimbs only mildly affected, multifocal disease is suspected.

In summary, equine protozoal myelitis can mimic almost any neurologic disease. It should be considered foremost when a progressive, asymmetric, multifocal disease process with signs of gray matter involvement is detected, especially if the patient is a young adult Thoroughbred or Standardbred race horse, or a breeding animal.

DIAGNOSIS

There is no means of antemortem confirmation of the disease; the diagnosis is one of exclusion (Table 1). When the clinical signs are compatible with a focal cervical lesion, radiography and myelography can be helpful in ruling out cervical vertebral malformation, neck fractures, or osteomyelitis.

Unfortunately, results of cerebrospinal fluid analysis are within normal limits much of the time. When it is abnormal (in the acute or rapidly pro-

TABLE 1. DIFFERENTIAL DIAGNOSIS OF CONDITIONS RESEMBLING PROTOZOAL MYELITIS

Disease	Frequency	Age, Sex, Breed Predilection	Associated History	Progression	Signs of Gray Matter Involvement	Symmetry	Focal, Multifocal, Diffuse	CSF	Other Diagnostic Aids
A. *Equine Protozoal Myelitis*	Very common	All ages, sexes, breeds; especially 1–4 yr thoroughbred, standardbred, (rarely in foals); has not been diagnosed in ponies or draft breeds	Vague lameness or fulminant neurologic signs	Usually progresses	Frequent	Usually asymmetric	Focal, multifocal, above or below foramen magnum	Mononuclear pleocytosis; usually <50 WBCs; ± slight increased protein ± slight xanthochromia	EMG to confirm lower motor neuron disease
B. *Disease with predominantly cerebral signs*									
1. Idiopathic epilepsy	Uncommon	All; esp. mares in estrus or Arabian foals	Animal totally normal between seizures	No	No	—	—	Normal	EEG
2. Eastern and western equine encephalomyelitis	EEE common in south	All	Usually has poor vaccination history; rarely begins as ataxia, vestibular, or cerebellar syndrome	Yes	Ultimately signs are diffuse	Usually symmetric; may begin as asymmetric	Ultimately signs are diffuse	Usually grossly abnormal; high white cell count, neutrophils, or mono-nuclear cells; protein elevation inconsistent	Serology, EEG, viral isolation
3. Hepatoencephalopathy	Common	All	Possible exposure to hepatotoxin	Not always		Usually symmetric	Diffuse	Normal	Bromsulphalein test; blood ammonia, liver enzymes, liver biopsy
4. Migrating parasites; *S. vulgaris*, Hypoderma, Micronema, Habronema, Draschia	Rare	All	May be febrile; may be signs of colic	Yes	Likely	No	Mainly focal	Varies with parasite (eosinophilis, neutrophils, xanthochromia)	None

Disease	Incidence	Age	History	Progressive?	Painful?	Symmetry	Focal/Diffuse	CSF	Other diagnostic aids
C. Diseases with predominantly vestibular signs									
1. Idiopathic vestibular syndrome	Rare	All	Acute onset	No	No	No	Focal	Normal	Rule out fracture
2. Otitis media interna	Uncommon	All	Pain at base of ear; head shaking	No		Asymmetric	Focal	Normal	Ventrodorsal x-rays
3. Trauma	Common	All; especially young, fractious animals	Trauma	No		Symmetric or asymmetric	Focal	Normal or RBCs present	X-rays
4. Neuritis of cauda equina and polyneuritis equi (NCE and PNE)	Uncommon	Not reported in foals or very old horses	Depression, head or tail rubbing, difficulty urinating	Yes	Yes	Symmetric or asymmetric	Focal or multifocal	Abnormal after several weeks; xanthochromia, pleocytosis prominent; protein elevation	EMG
D. Diseases with predominantly spinal cord signs									
1. Cervical vertebral malformation (CVM)	Very common	6 mo–10 yr but especially 6 mo–3 yr male thoroughbreds, rapidly growing and large	Acute onset esp. noticed when weanlings brought into barn off pasture or yearlings put into training	Yes	Usually not	Usually symmetrical	Focal	Usually normal or mild protein elevation	Standing lateral cervical x-rays, myelography
2. Equid herpesvirus I (EHV-1)	Uncommon	Usually adults, esp. brood mares	Acute onset; often assoc. w/abortion, fever, respiratory disease on farm	No; stable after 1st day	No—except bladder paralysis, sensory deficit in perineum	Usually symmetric; often only involves rear limbs	Diffuse	Xanthochromia, increased protein few cells	Serology viral isolation from nasal swab and buffy coat
3. NCE and PNE	See C-4 above	—	—	No	—	—	—	—	—
4. Equine degenerative myelopathy (EDM)	Uncommon	Many breeds; *usually* signs begin before 6 mo; always before 3 yr	Nothing pertinent; insidious onset	Yes; slowly, but may stabilize	No	Symmetric; fore limbs often as severe as rear limbs	Diffuse; can appear focal	Normal	None; rule out other diseases
5. Migrating parasite: Setaria, *S. vulgaris*	Rare	All	May be associated with pain (colic) or fever	Yes; can stabilize and improve	Yes	Symmetrical	Focal, multifocal, diffuse	Setaria—normal; *S. vulgaris*—may be mildly abnormal or have prominent neutrophilia	None

Table continued on following page

TABLE 1. DIFFERENTIAL DIAGNOSIS OF CONDITIONS RESEMBLING PROTOZOAL MYELITIS *Continued*

Disease	Frequency	Age, Sex, Breed Predilection	Associated History	Progression	Signs of Gray Matter Involvement	Symmetry	Focal, Multifocal, Diffuse	CSF	Other Diagnostic Aids
6. Trauma, especially cervical or sacral	Common	All	History of trauma	No; signs remain stable or improve (unless lesion is unstable or later callus formation impinges on cord)	Yes	Either	Focal	Normal or xanthochromia	X-rays, EMG
7. Vertebral osteomyelitis, discospondylitis	Uncommon in foals; rare in adults	All	Acute onset with pain or stiffness; may be associated with diarrhea or other sites of sepsis; may be focal pain, heat, swelling	Yes	Possibly	Usually symmetric	Focal	Normal; occasionally neutrophils present; occasionally evidence of compression (slight amount mononuclear cells, xanthochromia, protein)	X-rays, EMG
8. Atlantooccipital malformation	Uncommon	Usually Arabian or Arabian crosses	Often signs begin at birth; always within 1st year; palpable deformity; audible clicks sometimes	Yes	No	Usually symmetric	Focal	Normal	X-rays

Peripheral neuropathies are impossible to distinguish from EPM unless there is a history of associated trauma (suggestive of neuropathy) or a history of slow progression with no history of trauma (which is more likely to indicate equine protozoal myeloencephalitis).

gressing stages) there is usually a slight mononuclear pleocytosis, and normal or mildly elevated protein levels with or without xanthochromia. An electromyogram can confirm the presence of lower motor neuron disease and hence is useful in differentiating disuse atrophy from neurogenic atrophy. Aberrantly migrating parasites can be the most difficult differential diagnosis to rule out.

TREATMENT

Treatment is aimed primarily at stopping the progression of the disease. Improvement must depend on resolution of edema and hemorrhage, remyelination of intact axons, and compensation by other areas of the central nervous system. The use of folic acid antagonists in EPM has been based on their successful use in the therapy of various protozoal diseases in humans and experimental animals. Pyrimethamine* and sulfonamides both readily cross the blood-brain barrier. They interfere with the sequential steps of the microbe's biosynthetic pathway, synergistically inhibiting the proliferation of the protozoa. The major side effects of this combination (which have been observed in horses as well as other species) include leukopenia, thrombocytopenia, and anemia. These adverse effects are antagonized by folinic acid and baker's yeast, which mammals can utilize but toxoplasma cannot. Trimethoprim has been shown to have a significant sulfonamide-potentiating effect in the treatment of experimental toxoplasmosis in mice, but it should *not* be considered a substitute for pyrimethamine, because it has no significant activity against toxoplasma.

Pyrimethamine and trimethoprim sulfadiazine combinations have shown potential for the therapy of EPM, particularly when treatment is begun early in the course of the disease. Oral pyrimethamine (0.1 to 0.2 mg per kg once daily) and oral trimethoprim-sulfadiazine† (15 mg per kg twice a day) (neither of which is approved for use in the horse) are used routinely at the University of Florida and have arrested the progress of signs in some cases but have been ineffective in others. Some animals have recovered nearly completely and others have recovered only to relapse within months of cessation of the therapy. (Because these drugs are continued for up to two months, immediate improvement is not to be expected) and therapy is reinstituted if the patient is to be stressed. Long-term intermittent-dosage prophylactic therapy with pyrimethamine may be rational. Since it is impossible to diagnose EPM antemortem, controlled studies of the efficacy of the therapy cannot be done; obviously, caution is in order in the interpretation of apparent successes.

Glucocorticosteroids are contraindicated in most cases of EPM. They suppress immunity to toxoplasma in humans, allowing for relapse in patients with chronically encysted organisms. If the disease is recognized acutely and is rapidly progressing, dimethylsulfoxide (DMSO)* at 1 gm per kg diluted to a 20 to 40 per cent concentration in 5 per cent dextrose may be given intravenously once or twice daily. In suspected cases that continue to progress to the point at which the animal is recumbent in spite of DMSO, pyrimethamine, and trimethoprim-sulfadiazine, a short course of glucocorticoid therapy should be considered. The prognosis for life for any animal with clinical signs compatible with EPM must remain guarded at best, even if there is a positive response to therapy, since relapses are not uncommon.

PATHOLOGY

To date, a definitive diagnosis can only be made postmortem with histologic observation of the parasite, an unidentified protozoan most resembling a Sarcocystis species. Very frequently, only typical lesions (a necrotizing nonsuppurative encephalomyelitis with a proliferative inflammation of gray or white matter or both, and a variable degree of necrosis of myelin and axons), will be seen with no organisms to be found, particularly if the animal has been treated with pyrimethamine and trimethoprim-sulfadiazine. Organisms are found more readily in animals that have been treated with glucocorticosteroids.

---

*Domoso, Diamond Laboratories, Des Moines, IA

Supplemental Readings

Beech, J., and Dodd, D. C.: Toxoplasma-like encephalomyelitis in the horse. Vet. Path., *11*:87, 1974.

Cusick, P., Sells, D., Hamilton, D., and Hardenbrook H.: Toxoplasmosis in two horses. J. Am. Vet. Med. Assoc., *164*:77, 1974.

deLahunta, A.: Veterinary Neuroanatomy and Clinical Neurology, 2nd ed. Philadelphia, W. B. Saunders Company, 1983.

Dorr, T., Higgins, J., Dangler, C., Madigan, J., and Witham, C.: Protozoal myeloencephalitis in horses in California. J. Am. Vet. Med. Assoc., *185*:801, 1984.

Mayhew, I. G., deLahunta, A., Whitlock, R. H., and Pollock, R.V.H.: Equine protozoal myeloencephalitis. Proc. 22nd Annu. Conv. Am. Assoc. Eq. Pract., 1976, pp. 107–114.

Simpson, C. F., and Mayhew, I. G.: Evidence for Sarcocystis as the etiologic agent of equine protozoal myeloencephalitis. J. Protozool., *27*:288, 1980.

---

*Daraprim, Burroughs Wellcome Co., Research Triangle Park, NC

†Tribrissen, Burroughs Wellcome Co., Research Triangle Park, NC

Rabies

K. C. Kent Lloyd, DAVIS, CALIFORNIA

Equine rabies can present with many different clinical manifestations and few typical classical signs. It is therefore one of the most clinically difficult diseases to diagnose in the horse. There are no antemortem laboratory tests currently available that can provide a definitive diagnosis. Many more horses are thus clinically suspect than are actually infected with rabies.

The infectious agent is a rhabdovirus. The viral envelope, capsid proteins, and RNA genome are susceptible to lipid solvents, heat, and radiation. Strong acids and alkalis, 70 per cent alcohol, quaternary ammonium, povidone-iodine, and anionic detergents are effective viricidal chemicals.

Rabies is transmitted to the horse by a bite from a wild carnivore (skunk, raccoon, fox) or insectivorous bat that harbors the virus. Rabid domestic dogs and other horses can also be sources of infection. Not all bites from rabid carriers will necessarily result in transmission. Infection depends on the concentration of virus in salivary secretion. The virus may gain access to the host via contamination of an open wound with saliva. The virus multiplies around the site of inoculation for a variable period before migrating retrograde within the cytoplasm of peripheral and cranial nerves to the spinal cord and brain. The length of the incubation period before onset of clinical signs is likely related to the proximity of the site of inoculation to the central nervous system, i.e., virus deposited in wounds to the head and neck probably reaches the central nervous system sooner than virus deposited in distal regions of a limb.

CLINICAL SIGNS

Classical signs of rabies do not occur reliably enough to permit the disease to be reasonably ruled out in most suspect cases. Horses can be presented with a variety of signs, including colic, lameness, ataxia, paresis, incontinence, dysuria, muscle spasms, dysphagia, uncharacteristic vocalizations, peripheral nerve deficits such as radial nerve paralysis, and hyperesthesia at the site of inoculation.

Infected horses exhibit obvious behavioral changes, the majority showing signs of dullness and depression more often than excitement or mania. They may appear obtunded and nonresponsive to environmental stimulation. Frequently, animals become recumbent and wildly scramble and thrash or appear paralyzed. Death rapidly follows within three to five days of the onset of clinical signs. The rapid progression of the disease to a terminal stage is supporting evidence for a clinical suspicion of rabies. In a very few cases, however, clinical signs can be protracted for up to two weeks before death.

DIAGNOSIS

Rabies should be considered high on a list of differential diagnoses for any horse exhibiting obscure and indistinct neurologic signs of short duration. Other differential diagnoses to be considered include the various causes of encephalitis or encephalomyelitis: viral (western (p. 348), eastern (p. 345), Venezuelan, Main Drain, equine herpesvirus (p. 365), verminous and protozoal myelitis; hepatoencephalopathy (p. 112); nigropallidal encephalomalacia (yellow star thistle poisoning); lead poisoning; botulism; choke; and trauma to the brain or spinal cord (p. 374). Since some of the potential diagnoses may be associated with a successful prognosis, reasonable attempts should be made to examine the patient, characterize the clinical signs, and observe the progression of the disease before a premature decision is made to perform euthanasia.

Clinical laboratory data are nonspecific for rabies. A stress leukogram, elevated packed cell volume, and total protein reflecting dehydration and hypovolemia are inconsistently noted on a complete blood count. Muscle enzymes (SGOT, CPK) may be elevated if the horse has been recumbent or thrashing. Cerebrospinal fluid analysis is nondiagnostic. Obtaining cerebrospinal fluid may actually be an unwarranted risk in terms of the potential exposure and physical danger to the collector.

The postmortem interval probably does not affect the outcome of the specific tests needed to obtain a definitive diagnosis. Only the brain is removed during an abbreviated necropsy. The carcass can be kept refrigerated in isolation for a more complete necropsy if a negative rabies diagnosis is made. Commonly, the whole brain is cold packed (not frozen) and shipped to a public health diagnostic laboratory. Each laboratory has specific requirements for shipping and handling of specimens. Virus antigen can usually be identified by a fluorescent antibody technique that can be performed in less than 24 hours. Intracerebral inoculation of test mice with brain tissue can be used to confirm a diagnosis but several days to a few weeks are required to obtain a result. Negri bodies are intracytoplasmic inclusions found within neurons and can be easily overlooked on histologic section but are pathognomonic if seen. Immunofluorescent examination of the skin as a means of antemortem diagnosis of rabies has been described for horses and may become a diagnostic aid in the future.

MANAGEMENT AND PREVENTION

Because of the serious threat to human life from exposure to rabies virus, suspect horses should be handled as little as possible and contact limited to a minimum of qualified individuals who, preferably, are vaccinated against rabies. An attempt should be made to obtain the names of all persons recently in contact with the horse. Veterinarians should communicate clearly the potential dangers of rabies exposure to clients. Clients can be reassured, however, that transmission of the virus from a rabid horse to another animal or person has not been reported.

Strict isolation protocol must be observed. Rubber gloves should be worn by everyone handling the horse. Any wounds on the horse should be treated with copious lavage and bandaged if necessary. If the horse is recumbent and intractable, sedation (xylazine, 0.5 to 1 mg per kg intravenously) may be required to place it in a heavily bedded stall. Protective leg wraps help to minimize the horse's self-induced trauma.

The National Association of State Public Health Veterinarians annually reviews and revises recommendations for immunization procedures and principles of rabies control. Horses are at risk in areas where rabies is epizootic in wild carnivores. The only vaccine recognized for use in the horse contains inactivated virus of hamster cell line origin.* Two milliliters are injected intramuscularly in one site in the semimembranosus and semitendinosus muscle groups. The vaccine is never administered in the neck. Inoculation can begin when horses are over three months of age; horses should be revaccinated annually.

An unvaccinated horse known to have been bitten by a rabid animal should either be destroyed immediately or observed closely for six months. A vaccinated horse should be observed. No official recommendations are available for postexposure vaccination of previously vaccinated horses but this is probably justifiable. Unvaccinated horses must not receive postexposure prophylaxis until after the six-month observation period.

For the protection of people and livestock, a positive diagnosis of rabies is reportable to public health officials. Persons exposed to rabid horses should see their physician or public health officer.

---

*IMRAB, Pitman-Moore, Washington Crossing, NJ

Supplemental Readings

Blenden, D. C., Bell, J. F., Tsao, A. T., and Umoh, J. U.: Immunofluorescent examination of the skin of rabies-infected animals as a means of early detection of rabies virus antigen. J. Clin. Microb., 18:631, 1983.

Blood, D. C., Radostits, O. M., and Henderson, J. A.: Diseases caused by viruses and chlamydia II. In Veterinary Medicine, 6th ed. London, Bailliere Tindall, 1983.

Gillespie, J. H., and Timoney, J. F.: The Rhabdoviridae. In Hagan and Bruner's Infectious Diseases of Domestic Animals, 7th ed. Ithaca, Cornell University Press, 1981.

Joyce, J. R., and Russell, L. H.: Clinical signs of rabies in horses. Comp. Cont. Ed. 3:S56, 1981.

Martin, M. L., and Sedmak, P. A.: Rabies. Part I. Epidemiology, pathogenesis, and diagnosis. Comp. Cont. Ed. Prac. Vet., 5:521, 1983.

Sedmak, P. A., and Martin, M. L.: Rabies. Part II. Prophylaxis and control. Comp. Cont. Ed. Prac. Vet., 6:49, 1984.

Equine Herpesvirus Type 1 Myeloencephalopathy

Angeline Warner, BROOKLINE, MASSACHUSETTS

Neurologic disease characterized by variably severe ataxia occasionally occurs with equine herpesvirus type 1 (EHV-1) infection. Although this neurologic form is generally sporadic, outbreaks have occurred at breeding farms and race tracks. Neurologic signs may develop in some horses concurrently with the typical upper respiratory form of EHV-1 infection, or with late-gestation abortions among in-contact horses. Pregnant or nonpregnant mares and stallions or geldings may be affected.

Recently neurologic signs associated with EHV-1 infection have been reported in foals.

CLINICAL FINDINGS

Affected horses acutely develop ataxia of the hind or all four limbs. Ataxia may be very mild or the horse may be unable to rise. A fever of 39° to 40° C may have been noted two to three days previously. The incubation period is seven days, and exposure to horses with fever, upper respiratory infection, or abortion one week previously may be reported in the history. The affected horse may demonstrate cough and nasal discharge, or rarely abort, during the course of the neurologic disease. Occasionally subcutaneous edema of the limbs accompanies the onset of ataxia. Neurologic signs often progress rapidly over the first 24 to 48 hours and then stabilize. Ataxia is generally symmetric and most severe in the pelvic limbs. The cranial nerves are generally unaffected. The urinary bladder is often atonic, with urine retention and incontinence. Additional signs that are variably present include an atonic anal sphincter, hypalgesia or analgesia of the perineum, and a flaccid vulva or penis.

LABORATORY AND PATHOLOGIC FINDINGS

The white blood cell count may be subnormal, with lymphopenia during the febrile period. When fever subsides, the white blood cell count returns to normal. Cerebrospinal fluid is often xanthochromic, and characteristically the protein is elevated to more than 80 mg per dl, but cellularity is not increased. Since most horses have a demonstrable serum titer to EHV-1 because of vaccination or previous exposure, paired serum samples two to three weeks apart showing a three- to fourfold increase in serum-neutralizing or complement-fixing antibody titer may be the most reliable diagnostic aid.

Lesions in the neurologic form of EHV-1 are most remarkable in central nervous tissue and are characterized by vasculitis, especially of medium-sized and small arteries. Necrosis of the vessel walls with perivascular cuffing is present. Focal areas of necrosis and malacia in the parenchyma are seen, usually in association with vascular lesions. Hyaline thrombi within affected vessels suggest that the necrotic areas may be secondary to ischemia or hypoxia caused by the vasculitis. Although most severe in the central nervous system, vasculitis is diffuse and can be demonstrated in other tissues. In contrast to neurologic herpesvirus infections of humans, swine, and cattle, the equine type 1 virus does not appear to be neurotropic, and intranuclear inclusions or neuronophagia are absent. Neurologic deficits have been attributed to the effects of local ischemia and metabolic changes on neurons.

PATHOPHYSIOLOGY

The lack of neurotropism and difficulty in isolation of virus from nervous tissue of affected horses has led to the suggestion that the vascular lesions may be immunologically mediated through antibodies or activated host T lymphocytes. Some investigators have suggested that reinfection or recurrent infection in antibody-positive horses may play a role in development of the neurologic form of the disease. The predilection of an immunologically mediated inflammatory response for the central nervous system vasculature remains unexplained, but a neurologic strain of the virus does not appear to be responsible for the predominance of neurologic signs in certain horses.

THERAPY AND PREVENTION

Treatment of EHV-1 myeloencephalopathy is largely supportive and is dictated by the severity of neurologic signs. Mildly affected horses usually continue to eat and drink normally, and frequently recover completely within three weeks to two months. Severely ataxic horses should be confined with easy access to food and water, and ample bedding, in case their condition should deteriorate and they should become recumbent. Those horses that do become recumbent have a less favorable prognosis, but some have recovered with excellent nursing care such as is described on page 348.

Antibiotic therapy is generally not necessary unless the horse becomes recumbent or develops secondary infection. Predisposition to pneumonia and development of abrasions and deep pressure sores in recumbent horses necessitates use of a broad-spectrum antibiotic. Corticosteriod therapy has been advocated because of the evidence that the vasculitis is immunologically mediated rather than a cytopathic effect of the virus on endothelial cells. A single dose of dexamethasone* (0.1 to 0.2 mg per kg intravenously or intramuscularly) given as soon as possible after the onset of signs may be efficacious. The dose may be repeated if neurologic signs worsen or a relapse occurs. Since the condition in many animals stabilizes and improves, response

---

*Azium, Schering Corp., Kenilworth, NJ

to therapy is difficult to judge objectively. Corticosteroids must be used with caution, as they are immunosuppressive and can exacerbate either viral or secondary bacterial infection. Antibiotic therapy should be instituted if pneumonia or other infection is suspected.

The role of vaccination with either the modified live or killed vaccine products currently available* in prevention of the neurologic form of EHV-1 infection is unclear. Since the disease may be immunologically mediated, vaccination may not be protective, and the neurologic form of EHV-1 has been reported in vaccinated individuals. There is no indication that current vaccine products can directly cause the neurologic disease, but vaccination in the face of an outbreak cannot be advocated. When several cases develop, which usually occurs at breeding establishments or race tracks, precautions to prevent spread of disease include strict

---

*Pneumabort-K, Fort Dodge Laboratories, Fort Dodge, IA or Rhinomune, Norden Laboratories, Lincoln, NE

isolation of affected and in-contact individuals, and prevention of exposure of additional horses by limitations on traffic and use of common equipment. Stalls or equipment used by horses with fever, cough, or nasal discharge should be disinfected, and aborted fetuses should be removed and the area thoroughly disinfected.

Supplemental Readings

Campbell, T. M., and Studdert, M. J.: Equine herpesvirus type 1 (EHV-1). Vet. Bull., 53:135, 1983.

Greenwood, R.E.S., and Simson, A. R. B.: Clinical report of a paralytic syndrome affecting stallions, mares, and foals on a Thoroughbred stud farm. Equine Vet. J., 12:113, 1980.

Platt, H., Singh, H., and Whitwell, K. E.: Pathological observations on an outbreak of paralysis in brood mares. Equine Vet. J., 12:118, 1980.

Pursell, A. R., Sangster, L. T., Byars, T. D., Divers, T. J., and Cole, J. R.: Neurologic disease induced by equine herpesvirus 1. J. Am. Vet. Med. Assoc., 175:473, 1979.

Thomson, G. W., McCready, R., Sanford, E., and Gagnon, A.: An outbreak of herpesvirus myeloencephalitis in vaccinated horses. Can. Vet. J., 20:22, 1979.

Botulism

Janet Johnston, KENNETT SQUARE, PENNSYLVANIA

Robert H. Whitlock, KENNETT SQUARE, PENNSYLVANIA

Botulism, a flaccid neuromuscular paralysis, is caused by one of the most potent toxins known. The toxin is produced by the gram-positive bacterium *Clostridium botulinum* and interferes with the release and/or binding of acetylcholine at the neuromuscular junction. All mammals may be affected; however, horses are one of the most susceptible species. The adult form of equine botulism has classically been termed "forage poisoning." The disease in foals is termed "shaker foal syndrome."

ETIOLOGY

Cl. botulinum grows in anaerobic conditions and produces several different toxin types (types A, B, C, C_a, C_b, D, E, and F) all with similar pharmacologic activity. While *Cl. botulinum* spores are found in 18.5 per cent of the soil samples tested in the United States, the distribution of the toxin types is variable. Type A, often implicated in human infant botulism, is most commonly found west of the Rocky Mountains. Type B is also associated with infant botulism, but most commonly affects horses throughout Kentucky and along the mid-Atlantic seaboard. The large population of susceptible foals in Kentucky, coupled with the high concentration *Cl. botulinum* type B in soil, accounts for the prevalence of the shaker foal syndrome in this region. Type C botulinum toxin causes botulism in horses in Europe. In the United States, type C botulism in horses is less commonly reported, although the organism occurs in high concentration in the soils of Florida.

There are three major routes of infection. Ingestion of preformed toxin is probably the most important route in adult animals. Wound botulism probably occurs in horses but has yet to be documented. Toxicoinfectious botulism occurs when the animal ingests the spores, which then vegetate and produce toxin within the gastrointestinal tract. Inflammatory lesions such as gastric ulcers may be potential sites of toxin production. The shaker foal syndrome and some adult equine cases are thought to be toxicoinfectious botulism.

CLINICAL SIGNS

Foals. Affected foals are typically less than eight months and often less than eight weeks old. The foals often have a normal appetite but dribble milk from the mouth and nostrils because of inability to swallow. Suckling may be impaired by decreased tongue tone. Eyelid and tail tone may also be decreased. The pupils may be dilated and slowly responsive to light. Muscle weakness of varying severity is a consistent finding causing the foal to lie down frequently and tire easily. Muscle fasciculations may develop after only a few minutes of standing or walking. In the severely affected foal, as the muscle tremors become more marked, the foal collapses and may be unable to rise. Aspiration pneumonia can result from failure to swallow. Paralysis of intercostal muscles causes difficult breathing and may lead to death from respiratory failure.

Adult Horses. Botulism may occur in any age horse. Loss of tongue and tail tone are the first clinical signs but are difficult to assess and are frequently not observed by owners. Dysphagia, characterized by salivation, spilling of food and water from the commissures of the mouth, and the presence of feed material at the nostrils is often the first noticeable sign. Appetite is normal but because they cannot masticate and swallow, horses "play" in feed and water buckets. Endoscopic examination may reveal dorsal displacement of the soft palate, which contributes to dysphagia and can cause inspiratory stridor. A weakened, shuffling gait may be present and the horse may take stiff, short steps as if "walking on eggs." Walking and muscle activity can exacerbate the weakness and muscle tremors so that horses tire and lie down. If more strenuous exercise is attempted, the horse may refuse to move or may collapse. Following the exercise, muscular tremors, especially of the triceps and flank area, and progressive weakness characterize the symmetrical motor paralysis. The progression and severity of clinical signs can range from a mild motor weakness to nearly total paralysis. Ileus, constipation, and bladder distention are common problems, especially in the advanced stages of the disease when the horse is often recumbent. Respiration becomes labored with an increased abdominal component and decreased thoracic expansion. Death may occur due to paralysis of the respiratory muscles.

Horses and foals that have a rapid (12 to 36 hours) onset of clinical signs usually suffer more severe disease with a worse prognosis than those that have a more gradual onset (2 to 4 days) and progression of signs. The acutely affected individual may succumb to respiratory paralysis within 12 to 48 hours while other animals develop weakness and dysphagia over several days and never suffer obvious respiratory compromise. The rapidity of onset as well as severity of clinical signs is toxin dose related.

DIAGNOSIS

At present, diagnosis of equine botulism is based primarily on history and clinical signs. There are minimal primary clinicopathologic abnormalities, and detection of toxin in the serum is rarely possible. Because the horse is extremely susceptible to the botulism toxin, the amount that kills an adult horse is difficult to detect using the mouse detection test system. Also, only a minute amount of circulating toxin may be present in the affected horse since the majority of toxin is bound to the neuromuscular junctions soon after it enters the circulation. Electromyographic evaluation with repetitive nerve stimulation has been useful in diagnosing human botulism but is difficult to perform in horses.

Cl. botulinum spores can be isolated from the feces of approximately 20 per cent of affected adult horses. Rarely can spores be found in the intestinal contents of normal, healthy adult horses not at risk for botulism. Spores can be found in approximately 80 per cent of affected foals and are present in some animals from farms with a history of clinical botulism. Toxin has yet to be isolated from feces of an adult animal antemortem, but has been identified in the intestinal contents of about 10 per cent of shaker foals.

Necropsy findings are usually unremarkable. Gastric ulcers and necrotic foci in the liver have been demonstrated in shaker foals, and are suspected to be potential sites for infection by *Cl. botulinum.* The ulcers may be due to stress, diet, or a combination of factors.

Initial differential diagnoses of dysphagia include esophageal or pharyngeal obstruction or ulceration, equine protozoal encephalomyelitis, guttural pouch disease, leukoencephalomalacia, yellow star thistle poisoning, and rabies. Other causes of neuromuscular weakness include tick paralysis, organophosphate toxicity, white snake root poisoning, and hypocalcemia. Shaker foals must be differentiated from individuals with white muscle disease, hypoglycemia, and septicemia. A cerebrospinal fluid (CSF) sample may be helpful in differentiating botulism from a central nervous system disease as horses with botulism have normal CSF. However, although abnormal CSF is evidence for lesions in the CNS, normal CSF does not eliminate the latter from consideration. Clinical signs and their progression usually serve to differentiate the conditions.

PROGNOSIS AND TREATMENT

Before the availability of polyvalent equine antitoxin the mortality rate in equine botulism approached 90 per cent. With the use of antitoxin early in the disease the prognosis for survival is good, approaching greater than 70 per cent. However, if the animal is recumbent or has had a rapid onset of clinical signs or both, the prognosis is poor, even with the use of antitoxin. Antitoxin produced by hyperimmunizing horses with *Cl. botulinum* toxoid is expensive, limiting its availability to some patients. The recommended dose is 200 ml for a foal and 500 ml for an adult greater than 400 lb (180 kg). The use of antitoxin is of the utmost importance in the severely affected animal. However, some mildly affected ones that have slowly progressive cases can survive without antitoxin.

In conjunction with the use of antitoxin, optimal nursing care and nutrition are critical. Since affected horses are intermittently or constantly recumbent, adequate bedding to prevent decubitus formation is required. If ulcers occur, thorough daily cleansing is important. A WaterPik* with a dilute antiseptic solution may be useful in cleaning deep wounds. Soft cotton leg wraps are necessary to prevent lower limb abrasions, especially in patients that resist recumbency. Stockinettes rolled in "doughnut" fashion are helpful in preventing decubitus of the tuber coxae, elbows, and shoulders. Lasers have been useful in treating decubital ulcers, as their use seems to dry the wounds and toughen the skin in these areas. Frequent turning from side to side is necessary to minimize decubitus formation as well as hypostatic congestion of the lungs. Supporting the horse in sternal recumbency helps to normalize pulmonary ventilation and perfusion, but it is usually impossible to maintain them in this position for long periods.

Since the majority of patients cannot swallow, supportive alimentation is required. A high-protein, low-residue slurry of alfalfa meal, dextrose, cottage cheese, and electrolytes given via a nasogastric tube has been used for up to a month (see p. 425). The tube may be sutured in place at the nares or passed three to four times daily. If the horse is recumbent, it should be fed in a sternal position and supported during gastric emptying. Administration of mineral oil may be needed to help prevent constipation. This may not be necessary if the aforementioned mixture is used, as the latter usually results in soft manure. Because most horses continue to try to eat, muzzling is necessary to prevent aspiration of food or bedding. It should be remembered that these animals, especially foals, may develop an ileus and may accumulate a large amount of fluid in their stomachs; this must be relieved by nasogastric intubation.

To provide adequate nutrition to a foal, more frequent feeding of a small volume of milk may be necessary because a foal's stomach may not comfortably hold the required amount if the daily requirement is divided into only four to six meals (see p. 205). Extreme caution should be exercised when passing a nasogastric tube in a foal. Death can occur secondary to aspiration or if the stomach has become overdistended secondary to ileus. The distended stomach may cause respiratory compromise or rupture resulting in a fatal peritonitis.

Intravenous total parenteral nutrition may be necessary if animals cannot tolerate oral alimentation. Those with severe cases may become dehydrated due to thrashing and sweating and may require sedation and intravenous fluids. Care of the intravenous catheter in the recumbent horse is extremely important (see p. 174). To avoid catheter-associated sepsis or thrombophlebitis, the catheter should be covered with a sterile dressing that is changed as necessary to keep it dry. Extensions and injection ports should be changed frequently and catheters should be changed at least every 72 hours, preferably using the opposite jugular vein each time.

Since the source of equine botulism is rarely known, penicillin is administered to eliminate any proliferating *Cl. botulinum* organisms. Potassium or sodium penicillin (22,000 to 44,000 IU per kg four times a day) intravenously is preferred. Oral penicillin therapy is contraindicated because it may result in a rapid release of toxin when the vegetative form of the bacterium in the gastrointestinal tract dies. Procaine penicillin, aminoglycosides, and tetracyclines are contraindicated because of their potential neuromuscular blockade effect. If complications such as pneumonia occur, broad-spectrum antibiotics may be needed. Trimethoprim sulfa combinations may be useful in these cases. Oral antibiotics should be avoided since they may alter the gastrointestinal flora and allow overgrowth of the *Cl. botulinum* organism.

Drugs such as neostigmine, guanidine hydrochloride, 3-aminopyridine, and 3,4-diaminopyridine have been used to potentiate neuromuscular transmission. These drugs have only a transient beneficial effect and are contraindicated because they deplete acetylcholine from the neuromuscular junction. Physical exertion in any form should be minimized in horses with botulism in order to conserve acetylcholine. Xylazine or other sedatives may be required to calm patients that violently resist recumbency.

Ventilator support of an adult horse with respiratory paralysis is usually not successful. Ventilatory support of foals has met with variable results. High-frequency ventilation appears promising as a means of long-term ventilation, at least in foals.

---

*Teledyne WaterPik, Fort Collins, CO

PREVENTION

Effective protection by vaccination with *Cl. botulinum* toxoid is possible. At present, *Cl. botulinum* type C toxoid is commercially available, and a limited supply of type B toxoid is available for horses. Maximum protection of foals involves vaccinating the mare three times before foaling. The first dose should be administered approximately three months before parturition followed by a second dose two to four weeks later. The third dose should be administered two to three weeks before foaling. This maximizes the antibody concentration in the colostrum and protects the foal against shaker foal syndrome. Yearly vaccination of adult animals with toxoid will most likely result in effective protection. Unless more than one animal on a farm is affected or there are repeated outbreaks, vaccination of a herd following a single incident is probably not required.

Supplemental Readings

MacKay, R. J., and Berkhoff, G. A.: Type C toxicoinfectious botulism in a foal. J. Am. Vet. Med. Assoc., *180*:163, 1982.

Mayhew, I. G., and MacKay, R. J.: Nervous System. *In* Mansmann, R. A., McAllister, E. S., and Pratt, P. W. (eds.): Equine Medicine and Surgery, 3rd ed. Santa Barbara, CA, American Veterinary Publications, 1972, pp. 1159–1252.

Ricketts, S. W., Greet, T. R. C., Glyn, P. J., Ginett, C. D. R., et al.: Thirteen cases of botulism in horses fed big bale silage. Equine Vet. J. *16*:515, 1984.

Swerczek, T. W.: Experimentally induced toxicoinfectious botulism in horses and foals. Am. J. Vet. Res., *41*:348, 1980.

Swerczek, T. W.: Toxicoinfectious botulism in foals and adult horses. J. Am. Vet. Med. Assoc., *176*:217, 1980.

Tetanus

Janet Johnston, KENNETT SQUARE, PENNSYLVANIA

Tetanus is one of the oldest diseases known to man. It is most common in underdeveloped countries where prophylactic immunization programs are inadequate. No animal is immune to the disease and horses are the most susceptible animal species. The disease usually occurs after a penetrating wound but has also been associated with compound fractures, obstetric complications such as metritis and retained placenta, postcastration infections, severe skin ulcerations, and umbilical infections. A puncture wound in the hoof resulting from a nail or other penetrating foreign body is a frequent cause of tetanus in the horse. If the conditions are right, even the smallest of wounds may provide a nidus of infection. The bacterium is unable to survive in normal tissue and devitalized tissue is a prerequisite for the development of tetanus.

ETIOLOGY

Clostridium tetani is a large gram-positive, spore-forming bacillus that requires an anaerobic environment for survival. It is a normal inhabitant of the gastrointestinal tract and has worldwide distribution. Isolation of the pathogen requires strict attention to anaerobic conditions because as little as 20 minutes of exposure to oxygen may be bactericidal. The best samples for bacterial isolation are biopsy tissues or fluid aspirates, which should be kept at room temperature in an anaerobic environment. Since the best medium for spore isolation is fresh meat, culture media must include fresh blood agar and thioglycolate. The vegetative form is highly susceptible to heat, while the spores are resistant and can survive boiling for 15 minutes.

Laboratory animal inoculation with suspensions of suspected tissue is optimal for demonstration of the bacteria. One group of mice is given the tissue suspension while another group receives the suspension plus tetanus antitoxin. If *Cl. tetani* is present, the unprotected mice will develop clinical signs of tetanus. *Cl. tetani* produces a potent exotoxin that acts primarily on the central nervous system. The toxin is released at the site of infection and is transported by blood as well as by retrograde axonal migration to the central nervous system, where it binds irreversibly to gangliosides in the ventral horn of the gray matter.

The exotoxin is composed of tetanospasmin, tetanolysin, and nonspasmogenic toxin. Tetanospasmin, which is responsible for most of the clinical signs, prevents release of the inhibitory transmitter glycine at the spinal motor neuron and may also inhibit protein synthesis in the brain. Tetanolysin is antiphagocytic and enhances local tissue necrosis. Nonspasmogenic toxin, although poorly understood, is thought to cause paralysis of the peripheral nervous system.

Experimentally, the toxin's effects on the peripheral nervous system include sympathetic nervous system stimulation, neuromuscular blockade during the later stages of the disease, and changes in adrenocorticoid and catecholamine metabolism.

CLINICAL SIGNS

The incubation period, which may vary from days to several months, depends upon factors such as species susceptibility, the number of bacteria present, the local wound environment, and the wound's proximity to the central nervous system. Infrequently the incubation period may be long, and in those cases, unless a previous injury or wound can be recalled by the owner, the initial diagnosis may be difficult. Horses most commonly suffer from the generalized form of tetanus, which usually begins with a wound and is followed in a few days by spasms and paralysis of the voluntary muscles. The clinical signs of tetanus are due to spastic contractions of the striated muscles. Localized tetanus involving only the muscle groups closest to the site of the injury is relatively uncommon.

Classically, spasms of the masseter muscles occur early in the disease, giving rise to the term "lockjaw." These spasms prevent normal prehension, mastication, and swallowing. Attempts to eat and drink may result in excessive salivation seen at the commissures of the mouth, and regurgitation of food and water from the nares. If paralysis of the pharyngeal and laryngeal muscles has occurred, aspiration pneumonia may result. Prolapse of the third eyelid, or "flick of the haw" as it has been described in earlier literature, is characteristic and may be elicited by raising the head or making a gentle tap on the face below the eye. The eyelids may be retracted, the nostrils flared, and the ears held in a rigid upright position as a result of facial muscle spasms giving the animal an anxious or frightened expression.

A stiff "sawhorse" stance and straddling gait are commonly observed. Increased extensor tone results in rigid extension of the extremities. Urine and fecal retention may occur as the animal's stiffness prevents normal voiding posture. Walking can be difficult and if startled, the animal may fall into lateral recumbency and be unable to rise due to the rigidity of the limb musculature. Progressive stiffness of the neck and back may lead to opisthotonus. The tail may also be held in rigid extension. In the recumbent animal, struggling further exacerbates the tonic-clonic spasms and distress. Even minimal stimulation or excitation can result in prolonged generalized muscle spasms. Unexpected loud noises or stimuli may elicit convulsions in hyperesthetic individuals. Although spontaneous convulsions are less common, they can occur late in the disease course. Excessive sweating, cardiac arrhythmias, tachycardia, hypertension, vasoconstriction, and ab-

dominal discomfort are thought to be a result of excessive stimulation of the sympathetic nervous system. The profuse sweating and energy expenditure associated with convulsions can lead to dehydration and metabolic acidosis.

Death may occur secondary to respiratory paralysis or to complications such as aspiration pneumonia, laryngospasm, dehydration, and malnutrition. Complications of recumbency and continual muscle spasms include decubital ulcers. These may lead to severe cellulitis, osteomyelitis, or septicemia, and to rhabdomyolysis, which could cause permanent muscle damage. Affected animals can survive if appropriate therapeutic and supportive care is given, but complete resolution may require a recovery period of weeks to several months. Acute onset of clinical signs indicates a poorer prognosis for survival than when the onset is slower. If the animal does not die in five to seven days the clinical signs usually stabilize, and provided that serious complications do not occur, it gradually recovers. Recovered animals are not immune to further episodes of tetanus because the amount of toxin required to cause disease is less than the antigenic threshold.

DIAGNOSIS

Diagnosis is based primarily on the classic clinical signs and history, which may include an inappropriate immunizatiion program and recollection of a recent wound or injury. Differential diagnoses include eclampsia in lactating mares, hypomagnesemia, cerebrospinal meningitis, strychnine poisoning, acute laminitis, and acute rhabdomyolysis. Eclampsia, although uncommon in mares, can result in increased muscle tension and tremors, anxiety, flaring of the nostrils, and excessive salivation. Synchronous diaphragmatic flutter may be present. Usually the serum calcium level in affected individuals is 4 to 6 mg per dl. Hypomagnesemia results in central nervous system irritability leading to nervousness, muscle tremors, ataxia, and convulsive seizures. The serum magnesium level is usually less than 1 mg per dl. Both hypocalcemia and hypomagnesemia should respond to intravenous supplementation of the deficient mineral. Meningitis may result in multiple clinical signs, but those closely resembling tetanus include rigid extension of the head and neck, opisthotonus, extensor rigidity and seizures. The diagnosis of meningitis is confirmed by an elevated white blood cell count, especially neutrophils, and protein in the cerebrospinal fluid. Bacteria may also be observed. The cerebrospinal fluid in horses with tetanus is normal. Strychnine is used as a rodenticide and a single oral dose may poison a horse. It acts to antagonize inhibitory spinal cord neurons, thereby resulting in convulsions and seizures. The animal is hyperexcitable and hyper-reflexic and only minimal stimulation is required to cause seizures or tetanic convulsions. Although acute laminitis does not result in seizure activity, the affected individual may be in so much pain that it may refuse to walk, sweat profusely, tremble, have elevated respiratory and heart rates, and be extremely anxious. Horses suffering from rhabdomyolysis may also suffer extreme pain with rigidly contracted muscle groups and refuse to walk. The serum concentration of the muscle-specific enzyme, creatine phosphokinase is elevated, and myoglobinuria may be present.

The strict anaerobic conditions required for growth may prevent isolation of *Clostridium tetani* from infected tissues. A Gram stain of the tissue may show gram-positive rods with a characteristic drumstick appearance. Postmortem isolation of *Cl. tetani* may not be significant, since the organism rapidly migrates from the gastrointestinal tract soon after death.

TREATMENT

Tetanus can be a life-threatening disease. Therefore, prompt recognition of the clinical signs and initiation of proper therapy is paramount. Therapy should be aimed at prevention of further toxin absorption by wound care, neutralization of circulating toxin, control of muscle spasms, and supportive care to prevent complications.

The offending wound should be located and meticulously debrided. If the site of infection is not obvious, careful inspection of the feet and distal limbs may reveal the wound. If the animal has recently been castrated, the surgical site should be evaluated. In the postparturient mare the urogenital tract should be carefully examined. Debridement of necrotic tissue, removal of foreign bodies, and thorough cleansing with hydrogen peroxide or other antiseptic solutions is important. It has been suggested that tetanus antitoxin be administered before debridement to neutralize any toxin that may be released during cleaning.

The administration of tetanus antitoxin will not reverse the clinical signs. It is unable to cross the blood-stain barrier or penetrate nervous tissue to combine with toxin that may be in transit to the central nervous system via retrograde axonal migration. Its main purpose when administered intravenously or intramuscularly is to neutralize circulating toxin outside the nervous system. The dosages suggested range from as low as approximately 10 IU per kg to 220 IU per kg. Probably 5,000 to 10,000 IU administered either intravenously or intramuscularly to an adult horse is adequate. As the toxin is quickly bound to the central nervous system and therefore has a short circulating half-life prolonged administration of high doses is probably not necessary and is an unwarranted expense. Tetanus toxoid should be administered, because the natural disease does not induce humoral immunity.

Controversy surrounds the use of intrathecal tetanus antitoxin, as it has met with variable results. In one study, the authors reported a 77.5 per cent recovery rate with the use of intrathecal antitoxin as opposed to a 50 per cent recovery rate when antitoxin was administered intravenously, intramuscularly, or in the epidural space. The improved recovery rate was thought to be caused by the immediate stabilization of clinical signs after the injection. In those horses, the signs remained approximately the same and then gradually improved. Caution should be used when the antitoxin is administered via the intrathecal route as it has been reported to cause convulsions in humans and animal species. The preservative is a phenol that in a 0.25 to 0.50 per cent solution can cause convulsions. This route of antitoxin administration would most likely be beneficial early in the disease course before recumbency or severe muscular rigidity occurs. Reversal of the clinical signs is not likely with the use of intrathecal antitoxin. If antitoxin is administered intrathecally, it should be done aseptically with the horse under general anesthesia. The complete technique is described elsewhere (see p. 341).

Penicillin therapy is recommended to help eradicate any vegetative *Cl. tetani* that might be present. Initially, intravenous potassium or sodium penicillin (22,000 IU per kg to 44,000 IU per kg four times a day) should be used to ensure adequate tissue levels of antibiotic. After several days, intramuscular procaine penicillin may be used; however, one should be aware that the agitation caused by intramuscular administration may incite tetanic spasms in hyperesthetic individuals.

Muscular spasms are best controlled by keeping the animal in a quiet, dark environment with minimal distractions or unexpected noise. If possible it is best to treat the horse in familiar surroundings, as referral centers may be noisy and not designed to provide satisfactory seclusion for optimal treatment. The owner should be made aware of the importance of providing minimal distractions, and establish a safe, efficient routine for feeding, cleaning, and handling the patient to minimize stress.

Control of anxiety, muscle spasms, and convulsions by tranquilizers, sedatives, and/or muscle relaxants may be necessary. Acepromazine, promazine, and xylazine are often useful, although their duration of action is limited. Promazine (0.5 to 1 mg per kg), given intramuscularly, often provides four to eight hours of relaxation, provided that environmental stimuli are minimized. Centrally act ing muscle relaxants such as guaifenesin in a 5 per cent solution may be administered to effect in the standing animal without causing recumbency. Methocarbamol (10 to 20 mg per kg every eight hours) may relieve some muscle rigidity and is safe, but has no tranquilizing activity to minimize the horse's response to stimuli. Diazepam (0.05 to 0.4 mg per kg) has been shown to relieve muscular spasm and anxiety in horses with tetanus; however, its use is expensive in the adult animal. It is relatively safe and, when combined with other drugs such as xylazine, the dosage can be reduced. Xylazine alone has too short a duration of action for maintenance but may be helpful when potentially stressful procedures such as nasogastric intubation or intravenous catheter placement are performed.

D-tubocurare chloride can prevent severe muscular spasm but its use necessitates prolonged positive-pressure ventilation, which is not feasible in the adult. Foals may better tolerate curarization and can be maintained on a ventilator if needed.

Recovery is a gradual process and may take several months; therefore, good supportive care and attention to detail are essential. Cotton may be placed in the patient's ears to decrease audible stimuli. Manipulations should be limited to those essential to the horse's care. The stress associated with repeated venipuncture should be minimized by placing an intravenous catheter for repeated blood sampling and for administration of drugs and fluids. Nonsteroidal anti-inflammatory drugs such as phenylbutazone may be useful for control of pain and pyrexia.

Many animals are dysphagic, requiring passage of a nasogastric tube or feeding via an esophagostomy. If the animal is able to eat and drink without danger of aspiration pneumonia, soft, palatable feeds and water should be provided. Many individuals are unable to eat or drink from the ground; therefore, buckets should be elevated to a comfortable level. Sedation before handling may be necessary and a tracheostomy tube should be available in the event of laryngospasm. A body sling for support may be necessary in some animals.

Regular monitoring of serum electrolytes, renal function, and acid-base status is advisable because animals frequently become dehydrated, azotemic, and acidotic, requiring intravenous fluid and electrolyte therapy. The white blood cell count and fibrinogen may be monitored to assess infectious complications such as pneumonia or decubital ulcers.

If the patient is recumbent a poor prognosis must be given for recovery. Essential to the care of the recumbent individual is prevention of decubital ulcers by use of adequate bedding, bandaging of the distal limbs, and padding over bony protuberances. Frequent alterations of the animal's position are necessary to prevent permanent muscle damage and pneumonia. Manual evacuation of the rectum and catheterization of the bladder may be required, because most horses fail to void while recumbent. In the recumbent tetanic patient, it is difficult to accomplish the required supportive and nursing care without exacerbating severe muscle spasms.

Complications can be fatal. Aspiration pneumonia secondary to dysphagia should be treated with appropriate antibiotics. The accumulation of secretions in the airways may precipitate laryngospasm, necessitating the availability of a tracheostomy set and suction unit for emergency use. Renal failure should be prevented by providing adequate oral or intravenous fluid supplementation as needed. Although the tetanus toxin exerts a nephrotoxic effect on the proximal renal tubules, the damage is reversible with adequate hydration.

IMMUNIZATION AND PREVENTION

If the vaccination history of any injured horse is unknown or nonexistent, 1500 units of equine origin tetanus antitoxin should be administered subcutaneously or intramuscularly. Clients should be advised of the small potential risk of serum-associated hepatopathy with the use of antitoxin. Tetanus toxoid should be administered simultaneously at a separate site, followed by a booster three to four weeks later and annual revaccinations.

Mares should receive a tetanus toxoid booster one month before parturition to ensure colostral antibody protection against tetanus in the newborn foal. The foal should then be vaccinated with tetanus toxoid at approximately two, three, and six months of age. Annual boosters with tetanus toxoid should follow.

Supplemental Readings

Ansari, M. M.: Tetanus. Comp. Cont. Ed., *4*:473, 1982.
Beroza, G. E.: Tetanus in the horse. J. Am. Vet. Med. Assoc., *177*:1152, 1980.
Cohen, M.: Tetanus. *In* Robinson, N. E. (ed.): Current Therapy in Equine Medicine, 1st ed. Philadelphia, W. B. Saunders Company, 1983, pp. 27–29.
Liu, I. K. M., Brown, S., et al.: Duration of maternally derived immunity to tetanus and response in newborn foals given tetanus antitoxin. Am. J. Vet. Res., *43*:2019, 1982.
Mayhew, I. G., MacKay, R. J.: Tetanus. *In* Mansmann, R. A., and McAllister, E. S. (eds.): Equine Medicine and Surgery, 3rd ed. Santa Barbara, CA, American Veterinary Publications, 1982.
Muylle, E., Oyaert, W., Ooms, L., and Decraeemere, H.: Treatment of tetanus in the horse by injections of tetanus antitoxin into the subarachnoid space. J. Am. Vet. Med. Assoc., *167*:47, 1975.

Spinal Cord Trauma

Stephen M. Reed, COLUMBUS, OHIO

One of the most incapacitating injuries of the horse is spinal cord trauma, which may or may not be accompanied by fractures of the vertebral column and lesions of the ligaments. Prevention of further damage to neural tissue is the major aim of both medical and surgical management. One must also be aware of accompanying life-threatening injuries to the head, thorax, or abdomen. Early rehabilitation with a more favorable prognosis depends on correct management at the time of injury and during preparation shipment to the veterinary hospital for further diagnostic evaluation. It also depends on prevention of complications.

TYPES OF VERTEBRAL TRAUMA

Vertebral trauma most commonly occurs as a result of a horse falling or colliding with a relatively immovable object, considerable force being necessary for vertebral displacement. The age of the animal may contribute to the location of spinal cord trauma; foals appear to be more susceptible to vertebral trauma than adults and frequently suffer fractures of the cranial cervical (C), and caudal thoracic (T) regions. Adult horses are more susceptible to injury of the caudal (fifth [C5] through seventh [C7]) cervical vertebrae, and caudal thoracic vertebrae. The higher incidence of luxations, subluxations, and epiphyseal separations in young animals may be because closure of the cervical vertebral (C2 to C6) epiphyseal growth plates occurs around four to five years of age.

A summary of the common types of vertebral injuries, their locations, and the resulting clinical syndromes is given in Table 1. The types of injuries include hyperextension, hyperflexion, dislocation, and compression and result in syndromes varying from tetraplegia to no neurologic deficit. Hyperextension injuries often affect the cervical vertebrae; they may result from a failure to negotiate a jump with the horse landing on the chest and ventrum of the neck. Hyperflexion injuries of the neck may result from a horse stumbling and falling in a somersault fashion. These injuries often result in vertebral fractures with impact to the spinal cord by dislocated osseous fragments. With very severe injury, soft tissue structures supporting the vertebral column may be disrupted, resulting in dislocation of the cervical vertebrae. When dislocations occur, the spinal cord may be seriously damaged. Notwithstanding this, it should be remembered that the vertebral canal is of larger diameter than the spinal cord itself, which undoubtedly accounts for sparing of the spinal cord with some severe vertebral injuries. Luxations of the vertebra frequently occur between the atlas and axis and atlas and occiput as well as in the thoracolumbar region. Subluxations have been recognized as a part of the cervical vertebral malformation syndrome and may result in weakness, ataxia, and spasticity. Compression injuries are associated with a shortening of the vertebral body and usually result from a head-on collision with an immovable object or another horse.

PATHOPHYSIOLOGY OF SPINAL CORD TRAUMA

Following spinal cord injury, deterioration is worse in large, heavily myelinated fibers compared with that in the lightly or nonmyelinated fibers that are important for pain sensation. Thus compression injuries initially lead to loss of proprioception and motor function, followed later by loss of pain.

Impact injuries appear to be most damaging to the gray matter and central white matter. With moderate impact, microvascular tears coupled with hemorrhage and edema occur in the gray matter. When impact is intense, a more severe and wider distribution of lesions is seen, sometimes causing cavitation of the gray and much of the white matter. The release of biogenic amines may result in vasospasm and hypoxia, subsequently leading to tissue necrosis. In addition, prostaglandins appear to play a role in the propagation of spinal cord trauma. The effect appears to be related to the development of ischemia, which further complicates the structural and functional alterations. Rapid decompression is needed to successfully prevent continuing damage.

NEUROLOGIC EXAMINATION

Initial evaluation of any patient suspected of receiving spinal cord injury must be directed toward the most life-threatening factors: these may include obstruction of the airway, cardiovascular collapse, potentially fatal hemorrhage, and concurrent head injuries. Following stabilization of these, the veterinarian should seek an accurate account of the injury, as this may help localize the injured site.

A systematic evaluation should proceed from the head to the tail (see p. 339). After the head is examined for signs of trauma, attention is directed to evaluation of the gait and posture, neck and

TABLE 1. COMMON TYPES OF VERTEBRAL TRAUMA

Level of Injury	Age	Type of Vertebral Trauma	Common Traumatic Incident	Syndrome
Cervical	Foal to yearling	Fracture of dens, luxation C1-C2	Hyperflexion (e.g., somersault)	Tetraparesis, respiratory depression, death
Cervical	Young adult	Epiphyseal fracture	Hyperextension	Tetraparesis to tetraplegia
Cervical	Adult	Compression fracture	Head-on collision	Tetraparesis to tetraplegia
Cranial thoracic	Usually young	Fracture of dorsal spinous process	Flipping over backward	Often none
T2-S1	Any	Transverse fracture of vertebral arch, with dislocation	Somersaulting or falls	Paraparesis
Sacroiliac subluxation	Adult	Subluxation	Falls or slipping on ice	None
Sacral fracture	Any	Compression	Fall over backward or dog-sitting when backed	Urinary and fecal incontinence with or without posterior paresis; paralysis of the tail and anus

forelimbs, trunk and hindlimbs, and tail and anus. A recumbent patient should be observed for the ability to rise. If only the head can be raised, there is probably a cranial cervical lesion (C1 to C3). If the horse is able to raise the head and neck off the ground but is unable to use the thoracic limbs, it is likely the lesion is more caudal, such as C4 to T2. Animals so affected may be able to maintain sternal recumbency but are unable to rise. A horse that can achieve a dog-sitting posture and use the thoracic limbs fairly well probably has a lesion caudal to T2.

Flaccid paralysis with hypo- or areflexia, muscular hypotonia, and neurogenic muscle atrophy are characteristic of a lower motor neuron lesion. Evaluation of these lesions may be assisted by reflex testing. One sign resulting from an upper motor neuron lesion in the cervical region is loss of voluntary motor function, while muscle tone may be increased and spinal reflexes may be normal to hyperactive. Spinal reflexes of the thoracic limbs may be evaluated by pinching the distal extremity and observing for flexion of the joints of the forelimb. This tests the integrity of the peripheral sensory nerve, spinal cord segments C6 to T2, and the motor fibers of the peripheral nerves. If the patient also demonstrates a cerebral response, one can assume that the sensory pathways to the forebrain are intact. A lesion cranial to C6 may result in a loss of the upper motor neuron influences, and the patient should show a hyperactive reflex.

Localization of a lesion caudal to T2 may be aided by identification of a loss of sensation over the trunk or hindlimbs at the level of the lesion. In addition, diffuse sweating may be seen as a result of a lesion in the descending sympathetic tracts of the spinal cord, while patchy sweating may be seen with damage to specific preganglionic or postganglionic sympathetic nerve fibers. Decreased panniculus response suggests a lesion in the region of C8 to T1

or damage to the lateral thoracic spinal nerve. The use of spinal reflex testing of the hindlimbs in recumbent animals is limited to the patellar and flexor reflexes. These reflexes test the femoral nerve and spinal cord segments L4 to L5 and the sciatic nerve and cord segments L5 to S5, respectively. A release of these reflexes from upper motor neuron modulation results in hyperactive reflexes and suggests a lesion cranial to L4.

The final regions to be examined are the tail and anus. The tone of the tail, as well as the perineal reflex, should be examined. Innervation is from the pudendal and caudal rectal nerves, and the sacrococcygeal spinal cord segments. Abnormalities resulting from lesions in the region of L4 through the caudal sacral segments include ataxia and paresis or paralysis of the hindlimbs, poor tail and pelvic limb tone, hypalgesia to analgesia of the affected area, urinary incontinence, and obstipation.

Ancillary diagnostic aids in evaluation of spinal cord trauma should include radiography and rarely myelography. Some benefit may be derived from cerebrospinal fluid (CSF) analysis and electromyography, if available. On CSF analysis, the most common findings associated with spinal cord trauma are xanthochromia and slight to moderate elevation in protein content. If the injury is severe enough, a bloody sample may be obtained. In some instances with a severe fracture-dislocation, collection of CSF from the lumbosacral space may not be possible because of complete obstruction to flow of CSF (i.e., spinal block).

MEDICAL THERAPY

The management of vertebral injuries in the horse depends on the amount of vertebral displacement and in particular the attending neural damage. Vertebral displacement may be obvious if there is a significant malformation of the neck or back. In cases of damage to the cervical region, radiographs may be helpful to determine if a fracture is present as well as to show the amount of vertebral displacement. Therapy should be governed by the patient's response as determined by serial neurologic examinations. Some horses with few or no neurologic abnormalities may require only stall rest and observation.

The drug of choice for immediate management of acute spinal cord trauma is either dexamethasone or dimethyl sulfoxide. Dexamethasone* is used at a dosage of 0.1 to 0.2 mg per kg body weight intravenously or intramuscularly. Higher doses are administered in other species. Some controversy exists over dosage and also its beneficial effects; in my experience laminitis is not an uncommon complication of steroid therapy. The dosage of dexamethasone may be repeated every six to eight hours for 24 hours with a favorable response expected within four to eight hours. Following initial improvement, the patient may be placed on oral prednisolone.

Failure to achieve a favorable response within four hours or deterioration of signs indicates the need for more aggressive treatment. Osmotic diuretic agents such as mannitol†, at a dose of 2 gm per kg as a 20 per cent solution, may be helpful. In fact, these agents may have beneficial therapeutic effects at dosages as low as 0.25 mg per kg. Intravenous mannitol may be repeated at least two times, although continued use of hypertonic solutions intravenously may be complicated by severe dehydration and hypotension. These complications are monitored by evaluating skin elasticity, packed cell volume, plasma total solids, urine output, and central venous pressure.

A less conventional and somewhat controversial therapy is dimethyl sulfoxide (DMSO).‡ The intravenous dosage I recommend is 1.0 gm per kg body weight diluted in saline at concentrations of 10 to 20 per cent; this concentration has an osmolality greater than plasma. This drug has been reported to decrease edema, prevent platelet aggregation, maintain spinal cord vascular integrity, and increase the availability of oxygen to tissues. Some authors have failed to identify a beneficial effect of the drug either alone or in combination with other drugs in treatment of spinal cord trauma in dogs. I recommend treating once a day for three days, followed by alternate-day administration for three further treatments.

SURGICAL INTERVENTION

The decision for surgical intervention is made when there is a lack of response to medical treatment or when radiographs indicate the need for decompression or stabilization. In many instances, the use of medical treatment is necessary to stabilize the patient before surgery is performed. The technique for decompression of compressive lesions has been described in the dog. The same procedures may be utilized in the horse when a lesion is demonstrated radiographically, when there is failure to respond to medical management, or signs progress, such as a change in the location of a sensory deficit along the axial skeleton or a further loss of motor function.

At the time of decompression, it may be prudent to avoid surgical incision of the dura because of its close adherence to the spinal cord. The use of normothermic saline for irrigation and flushing appears to be a beneficial adjunct to decompression. If the trauma has resulted in loss of stability between vertebrae, the technique of ventral fusion of the vertebrae may be useful, especially for treatment of cervical vertebral injuries (see p. 358).

Paraplegic and tetraplegic patients that have lost all response to deep pain caudal to the spinal cord lesion have a functional or anatomic spinal cord transection and are candidates for euthanasia unless response to medical or surgical therapy is noted within 24 hours.

Supplemental Readings

Ducker, T. B., Kindt, G. W., and Kempe, L. G.: Pathological findings in acute experimental spinal cord trauma. J. Neurosurg., 35:700, 1971.
Jeffcott, L. B.: Disorders of the thoracolumbar spine of the horse—a survey of 443 cases. Equine Vet. J., 12:197, 1980.
Nixon, A. J., and Stashak, T. S.: Dorsal laminectomy in the horse. Vet. Surg., 12:172, 1983.
Osterholm, J. L.: The pathophysiological response to spinal cord injury: the current status of related research. J. Neurosurg. 40:5, 1974.
Wagner, P. C., Grant, B. D., Gallina, A., and Bagby, G. W.: Ataxia and paresis in horses. Part III. Surgical treatment of cervical spinal cord compression. Comp. Cont. Ed. Prac. Vet., 3:S192, 1981.

---

*Azium, Schering Corp., Kenilworth, NJ
†Osmitrol, Travenol Laboratories, Deerfield, IL
‡Domoso, Diamond Laboratories, Des Moines, IA

Intracranial Trauma

Stephen M. Reed, COLUMBUS, OHIO

Head trauma with or without fractures is not uncommon in horses. Commonly recognized injuries include fractures of the mandible, maxilla, and incisive bone. Fractures of the basisphenoid and basioccipital bones are associated with a high morbidity and mortality, and often result from the horse falling over backward, striking the poll.

Fractures of the skull often heal by means of dense connective tissue and are functionally stable and satisfactory even without osseous union. Rarely are the fracture fragments themselves life threatening, although the associated neurologic problems may be fatal. It is essential, therefore, that a rapid diagnosis be made and damage to the central nervous system be accurately assessed in order to initiate early medical or surgical therapy.

PATHOPHYSIOLOGY OF CRANIAL TRAUMA

The types of cranial trauma progressing from least to most severe are concussion, contusion, laceration, and hemorrhage. Concussion is usually associated with a short loss of consciousness but without brain damage and has a favorable prognosis. A contusion of the brain indicates both vascular and nervous tissue damage without a major disruption of architecture. Contusions may be either on the same side or on the side away from the site of the injury and result from sudden acceleration or deceleration injuries or severe blows to the head. These injuries may result in intraparenchymal hemorrhage and subsequent cavitation injury within the brain. Cerebral concussion or contusion may be seen without the presence of skull fractures. The prognosis for cerebral contusions must be guarded and primarily is dependent upon the lesion's location. Cerebral lacerations and hemorrhages may also result from accelerations or deceleration injuries but may be produced by penetrating wounds, such as gunshots or skull fractures. The prognosis with these injuries is governed by the same general rules as for concussions and contusions and is significantly worse only when the lesions are large and situated in the brain stem. Intracranial hemorrhages may occur in epidural, subdural, intracerebral, and subarachnoid sites. However, subdural hematomas (i.e., between the dural and arachnoid membranes), as occur in humans, are uncommon in the horse. The more common hemorrhage in the horse appears to be subarachnoid, which reportedly results in aseptic meningitis rather than compression of brain

tissues and intracerebral bleeding. The presence of diffuse subarachnoid hemorrhage is common over the cerebral cortex in premature foals.

Intracerebral hematoma formation with loss of brain parenchyma may result in focal neurologic signs, although these may be difficult to identify because of signs of diffuse brain disease caused by the commonly associated cerebral edema. The greatest concern with intracranial hematomas is their potential for expansion within the intact skull. With such expansion, as with cerebral edema, the resulting brain swelling causes a redistribution of brain tissue with the calvarium. Herniation of brain tissues can thus occur through natural foramina. Parts of the brain stem can be compressed because of the presence of a rigid calvarium. Profound depression, lethargy or coma with asymmetric pupils, and delayed pupillary light reflexes indicate severe midbrain damage or compression. Signs of vestibular dysfunction may accompany brain herniation and may indicate involvement of the medulla oblongata.

In patients with severe cranial injury the causes of death include cardiac and respiratory arrest, which may result from brain stem damage. Medical complications, including septic and aseptic meningitis, may be seen and warrant consideration when planning or evaluating therapy.

A general scheme of events following traumatic head injury is membrane disruption and ischemia that often leads to cellular swelling (especially glial cells), tissue hypoxia, cerebral edema, and, finally, increased intracranial pressure. As the tissues become hypoxic, further membrane disruption and cellular swelling occur, establishing a vicious cycle. Barbiturates, glucocorticoids, dimethyl sulfoxide, and loop diuretics may have a protective effect against cell disruption. Recent experimental evidence suggests that the use of diuretics, which decrease extracellular water, and barbiturates, which produce vasoconstriction, may reduce intracranial pressure, blocking this vicious cycle.

PHYSICAL EXAMINATION

An accurate account of the accident may help to establish the type of injury and locate a depressed skull fracture. A physical examination will identify injuries such as fractures of the axial or appendicular skeleton, as well as trauma to the abdomen or thorax. The identification of blood from the mouth, nose, ears, or other body orifices may direct therapy to areas in need of immediate attention. Respiratory rate, heart rate, and an estimate of blood pressure (i.e., pulse strength and capillary perfusion) must be monitored in order that cardiovascular collapse and inadequate ventilation may be detected and rapidly corrected. Since overhydration may potentiate cerebral edema, fluid therapy should be closely monitored.

NEUROLOGIC EXAMINATION

Following stabilization of the patient's condition, attention is directed toward the neurologic examination. Serial changes in neurologic status help to predict a prognosis and modify therapy. Performance of the neurologic examination may be limited by the patient's condition, resulting in omission of some parts. When it is safe to do so, neurologic examination should be conducted without the influence of sedative drugs. However, I often use xylazine at a dose of 0.1 to 0.15 mg per kg intravenously and 0.2 to 0.5 mg per kg intramuscularly to achieve a calming effect, even though there is a risk of intracranial hemorrhage from the transient hypertension caused by this drug.

The important features of the neurologic examination in cranial injury are level of consciousness, cranial nerve examination (especially pupil size, symmetry, and response), posture and motor function, and respiratory patterns. The patient's level of consciousness depends on the extent of damage to the cerebrum and the ascending reticular activating system in the brain stem. Further definition of the site of a focal brain stem lesion is possible, and an outline of the clinical findings helpful to achieve this is given in Table 1.

Voluntary movements of the limbs in a recumbent patient should be evaluated along with spinal reflexes. The loss of a reflex may indicate concurrent spinal cord or peripheral nerve damage. Rigid extension of all four limbs with opisthotonos suggests a severe brain stem or cerebellar lesion. Damage in the region of the pons and medulla oblongata may result in a head tilt or abnormal torsion of the neck and body, and nystagmus if the vestibular apparatus is damaged. In ambulatory patients it is difficult to separate paresis and ataxia resulting from caudal brain stem injury from a cervical spinal cord injury unless depression or dysphagia is apparent, in which case the lesion is in the brain.

Severe brain stem injuries may also result in abnormal respiratory patterns. The development of apneustic or erratic breathing indicates a poor prognosis. Brain stem injury can result in bilateral miotic, bilateral mydriatic, or asymmetric pupils (Table 2). Bilaterally dilated pupils unresponsive to light indicate an irreversible midbrain lesion. A change in pupil size from bilateral constriction to bilateral dilation with no pupillary light reflexes indicates the need for prompt medical or surgical treatment to combat a progressive midbrain lesion. Asymmetric or bilaterally miotic pupils in a horse sustaining cranial injury is not uncommon, and such a patient should be observed closely for change in pupil size and responsiveness of pupils to light. The return of normal pupillary size and response improves the prognosis.

If the function of a cranial nerve is deficient, the nerve may have been severed or the cranial nerve nucleus damaged. Progressive loss of cranial nerve function indicates a progressive lesion and a less favorable prognosis.

TREATMENT

Medical Therapy. Initial therapy must be prompt, followed by careful monitoring of clinical signs to evaluate progress and thus the effectiveness of therapy. Table 2 is a guide to therapy based on changes in clinical signs. Serial neurologic examination is an essential tool in decision making. One important group of therapeutic agents are the glucocorticoids. They combat shock and reduce cerebral edema associated with trauma. I use dexamethasone 0.1 to 0.15 mg per kg body weight intravenously every 8 to 12 hours for the first 24 hours. A favorable response should be seen within the first 8 to 12 hours.

Osmotic diuretics such as mannitol (0.25 to 2.0 gm per kg) or glycerol (0.5 to 2.0 gm per kg) are advocated to reduce cerebral edema. One of the major benefits of such compounds is the rapid onset of action (30 to 60 minutes). Caution must be used when administering hypertonic fluids, especially if one is uncertain about the presence of intracranial hemorrhage. A decrease in brain edema allows additional space for further hemorrhage, and leakage of a hypertonic solution into an area accentuates local edema. Overhydration must be avoided because it can result in increased intracranial pressure.

I have found DMSO to be helpful at a dosage of 1.0 gm per kg given intravenously as a 10 to 20 per cent solution in saline once a day for three days, followed by once every other day for three further treatments. While its use in patients suffering from cranial trauma may be considered experimental at this time, it remains my current drug of choice. Additional therapeutic agents that may have beneficial effects in cranial trauma patients include barbiturates and loop diuretics, such as furosemide. The combination of mannitol with furosemide en-

TABLE 1. SIGNS CHARACTERISTIC OF FOCAL BRAIN INJURY

Levels	Consciousness	Motor Function	Pupils	Other Signs
Cerebrum	Behavioral change depression, coma	Circling	Normal	Blindness
Cerebellum		Ataxia and hypermetria, intention tremor		Menace response deficit without blindness
Diencephalon (thalamus)	Depression to stupor	Normal to mild tetraparesis, "aversive syndrome"*	Bilateral, nonreactive pupils with visual deficit	None
Midbrain	Stupor to coma	Hemiparesis, tetraparesis or tetraplegia	Nonreactive pupils, mydriasis, anisocoria	Ventrolateral strabismus
Pons	Depression	Ataxia and tetraparesis, tetraplegia	Normal	Head tilt, abnormal nystagmus, facial paralysis, medial strabismus
Rostral medulla oblongata (including inner ear)	Depression	Ataxia or hemiparesis to tetraplegia	Normal	Same
Caudal medulla oblongata	Depression	Ataxia, hemiparesis to tetraparesis, abnormal respiratory patterns	Normal	Dysphagia, flaccid tongue

*Deviation of the head and eyes with circling all toward the side of a unilateral lesion.

TABLE 2. FLOW CHART FOR MANAGEMENT OF CRANIAL TRAUMA

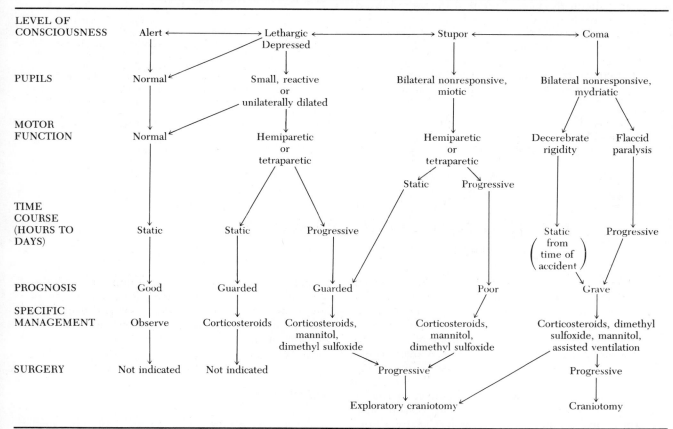

(Modified with permission from Oliver, J. E.: Intracranial injury. *In* Kirk, R. W. (ed.): Current Veterinary Therapy VII: Small Animal Practice. Philadelphia, W. B. Saunders Co., 1980, p. 819.)

hances diuresis and reduces brain bulk but may cause electrolyte imbalances.

Antimicrobial therapy and tetanus prophylaxis are also important when treating head injury. Antimicrobial agents are especially important in conditions such as basilar skull fractures, in which blood and blood-tinged cerebrospinal fluid may be observed in the nasal passages or ear canals. Chloramphenicol at a dose of 25 to 50 mg per kg orally four times a day may be used, although with disruption of the blood-brain barrier, most antimicrobial agents should achieve therapeutic levels at the site of injury. Parenteral administration prevents further trauma caused by manipulation of the head. Currently, trimethoprim-sulfonamide combinations* are my choice for antimicrobial therapy. Initial administration is intravenous, followed later by oral dosing.

Some animals with head trauma have convulsions or become violent. These actions may be controlled with diazepam.† A dose used for foals is 25 mg and for adult horses 100 mg, intravenously, repeated as necessary. Rarely is a total dosage greater than 200 mg necessary for an adult horse.

Surgical Management. Deterioration of neurologic signs in the face of medical therapy indicates progressive cerebral edema or hemorrhage, and an exploratory craniotomy should be considered. The assistance of a human neurosurgeon and a well-equipped equine surgical suite are essential if a craniotomy is considered. Surgical intervention must be undertaken with caution but may provide

---

*Bactrim, Roche Laboratories, Nutley, NJ
†Valium, Roche Laboratories, Nutley, NJ

hemostasis and relief of intracranial hypertension and may allow elevation of depressed bony fragments, evacuation of hematomas, and debridement of contaminated tissue. The evacuation of intracranial hematomas may be accomplished using trephines or twist drill openings, although clotted blood may be difficult to remove through a very small opening and may necessitate larger incisions. Complete surgical debridement is important and may be assisted by flushing with normal saline.

General anesthesia is essential for complete immobility. Inhalation agents such as halothane are the anesthetics of choice. If these agents are not available, then glyceryl guaiacolate or chloral hydrate may be satisfactory. Assisted ventilation is often necessary (see the first edition of this text, p. 475). Possible complications include the formation of brain abscesses or development of meningitis.

Nursing Care. Whenever horses become recumbent as a result of neurological damage, good nursing care is essential to prevent sores and urine and fecal retention. Details of nursing care are provided on p. 346.

Supplemental Readings

Adams, R., and Mayhew, I. G.: Neurological examination of newborn foals. Equine Vet. J., *16*:306, 1984.

Albright, A. L., Latchaw, R. E., Robinson, A. G.: Intracranial and systemic effects of osmotic and oncotic therapy in experimental cerebral edema. J. Neurosurg., *60*:481, 1984.

Fishman, R. A.: Brain edema. N. Engl. J. Med., *293*:706, 1975.

Mayhew, I. G., and Ingram, J. T.: Neurologic evaluation of the horse. Proc. 24th Annu. Conv. Am. Assoc. Eq. Pract., 1978, pp. 525–541.

Raichle, M. E.: The pathophysiology of brain ischemia. Ann. Neurol. *13*:2, 1983.

Peripheral Neuropathies

Stephane Clement, GAINESVILLE, FLORIDA

Dysfunction of the peripheral nervous system may be caused by trauma, malformation, inflammation, infections, or toxic, neoplastic, and idiopathic disorders. There are three types of nerve injury. Neurapraxia is a concussion of the nerve with no disruption of its structures. Axonotmesis is injury with loss of continuity of axons but preservation of the supportive Schwann cells and neural connective tissue. Neurotmesis implies partial or complete severance of a nerve with disruption of axons, myelin sheaths, and connective tissue elements. If separated from the cell body, the distal portion of the axon degenerates (wallerian degeneration). Part of the proximal stump may also degenerate. If the cell body is intact axonal regeneration can take place. Certain toxins and drugs can disrupt the neuromuscular junction and block the release of acetylcholine without causing morphologic changes.

DIAGNOSIS

A careful history including time of onset and progression of signs must precede a thorough physical and neurologic examination. Cranial nerve function and spinal reflexes should receive special attention. Muscle atrophy or sensory deficits or both are warning signs of a peripheral nerve disorder. Cranial nerve involvement causes head signs without other signs of brain stem disease such as depression, weakness, and altered consciousness. A single spinal nerve lesion produces regional muscle weakness, atrophy, and absence of the corresponding spinal reflex. The sensory deficits resulting from specific nerve injuries are poorly defined.

The history may lead to the cause. In infectious or inflammatory diseases the signs may be acute or insidious but usually progress. With trauma there is a sudden onset of signs that quickly stabilize. Secondary clinical signs may result from the effects of inflammation and healing of nervous tissue and surrounding tissues. Toxic, nutritional, and metabolic disease are acute or subacute and then progress or fluctuate. Vascular disorders mimic trauma. Neoplastic disease can produce peracute signs but usually the signs are chronic and progressive.

Hematology, blood chemistry, and enzymes and cerebrospinal fluid analysis may be useful diagnostic aids. Radiology is useful in the diagnosis of fractures and luxations that may result in damage to a nearby peripheral nerve. Electrodiagnostic tests are particularly valuable aids in the diagnosis of peripheral nerve and muscle diseases. Needle electromyography (EMG) is used to assess the function of the motor unit. A needle electrode is inserted into the muscle. The magnified electrical potentials are observed on an oscilloscope and heard on a loudspeaker during insertion of the needle (insertional activity) and with the needle at rest (resting activity). The muscles to be tested are selected on the basis of the postulated clinical diagnosis. The area is screened methodically and may be compared to the opposite side. The needle EMG is an invaluable aid in localizing the lesion; with nerve stimulation it can be used to assess the severity of a neuropathy and to determine the prognosis. Changes in the needle EMG result from denervation and myopathies. Abnormalities appear about 10 to 30 days after denervation. Serial examination executed during the course of the syndrome help to assess disease progression.

Nerve stimulation is performed by stimulating a site on a motor nerve and recording the evoked action potential in the innervated muscle and is used to evaluate the peripheral nerve and neuromuscular junction. Any motor nerve accessible to a needle electrode can be tested. If a nerve is severed, the axon distal to the lesion will not conduct an impulse after a few days. Nerve conduction velocity studies require measurement of two different latencies induced by stimulating two different sites on a nerve. The conduction time along the axon is calculated by the difference between the latencies and used to test the integrity of the efferent (motor) or afferent (sensory) peripheral nervous system.

ETIOLOGY

Trauma can be direct by blunt injury or laceration or indirect by compression of a nerve between bony structures or entrapment in fibrous tissue or against bone. Tumors (lymphosarcomas, melanomas, fibromas) and abscesses may also compress a peripheral nerve and cause nerve conduction dysfunction. Tumors of the peripheral nervous system itself are very rare. Severe myopathies such as those occurring after anesthetic, or with Clostridium sp. infection may result in nerve conduction dysfunction. Severe injury to a peripheral nerve can also be caused by ischemia.

CLINICAL SIGNS

CRANIAL NERVE INJURY

Optic Nerve. The optic nerve is not a peripheral nerve but is a tract of the central nervous system. It does not have the ability to regenerate and in case of severe damage the prognosis for recovery of vision is very poor.

Facial Nerve. The facial nerve divides into the auricular branches to the muscles of the ear, the auriculopalpebral branches to the muscles of the eyelids, and the buccal branches to the muscles of the nares and lips. Causes of facial paralysis include head trauma, fracture of the petrosal bone, otitis media, guttural pouch mycosis, polyneuritis equi, and chronic inflammation of the petrous temporal and stylohyoid bones. The clinical signs depend upon the site of the injury. Damage to the motor fibers of the lacrimal glands may result in keratitis sicca and corneal ulceration. The buccal branches are most commonly affected due to direct trauma to the face or prolonged recumbency. Idiopathic paralysis has been reported, presenting as an acute onset of complete unilateral facial paralysis with no other signs and improvement within days to weeks.

Attempts should be made to diagnose and treat any underlying cause. Nursing care includes daily cleaning of the mouth if the horse stores food in the cheeks. Lubrication of the cornea may be necessary. Some horses learn to retract their ocular globe to allow passive movement of the membrana nictitans and protection of the cornea. The general principles for treatment of peripheral nerve paralysis should be followed (see below). Paralysis of the buccal branches can result in false nostril noise while the horse is exercised. This may require surgical resection of the alar folds and part of the external nares. Bilateral facial paralysis causes dysphagia and the prognosis is poor. In the case of unilateral paralysis due to trauma, the prognosis is good but recovery can take several months. In cases of otitis media the paralysis rarely resolves and it is permanent in polyneuritis equi.

Vestibular Nerve. Signs of peripheral vestibular disease include head tilt toward the affected side, abnormal, vestibular nystagmus, spontaneous nystagmus with the fast phase away from the affected side, exaggerated eye drop on the side of the lesion when the head is elevated, a tendency to circle toward the affected side with asymmetric ataxia, and preservation of strength. The onset of signs is usually acute and unilateral. The horse is deaf if the cochlear branches are paralyzed bilaterally. With central vestibular diseases there are often signs of brain stem involvement, with depression, weakness, and other cranial nerve signs.

Skull trauma is the most common cause of vestibulocochlear disease in the horse. Other causes include otitis media and interna, fracture or inflammation of the petrous temporal bone and surrounding joints, and polyneuritis equi. A vestibular syndrome of unknown etiology can occur with acute onset of unilateral vestibular nerve paralysis resolving within one to three weeks. Treatment should be directed toward the underlying cause if possible. Horses with vestibular disorders can be very dangerous to handle. Left outside they may improve dramatically because they can learn to compensate, presumably by utilizing the visual system and a view of the horizon. The outside area should be made as safe as possible in such cases.

Laryngeal Paralysis. Laryngeal hemiplegia is described on page 611. Toxic neuropathy of the recurrent laryngeal nerves has been reported with administration of haloxon to foals. If the paralysis is bilateral, tracheotomy is necessary.

Horner's Syndrome. Horner's syndrome results from damage to the sympathetic nervous system innervating the head. Injury to the sympathetic supply to the eyeball results in ipsilateral ptosis of the upper eyelid, slight miosis, slight protrusion of the membrane nictitans, and enophthalmos. Other signs include dilation of facial blood vessels, hyperemia of nasal and conjunctival mucosae, increased facial temperature, and facial sweating due to an interruption of the sympathetic innervation to the smooth muscles, glands, and blood vessels of the head. Common causes include cervical trauma, guttural pouch infection, neoplasia, focal infections or foreign bodies ("choke") and periorbital disease. Horner's syndrome can also result from perivascular injection or follow surgery in the region of the carotid artery and vagus nerve.

Dysphagia. The facial, trigeminal, glossopharyngeal, vagus, and hypoglossal nerves are involved in prehension, mastication, and swallowing. While bilateral trigeminal paralysis causes difficulty in mastication, unilateral paralysis does not cause significant dysphagia. Excessive or brutal traction on the tongue can result in temporary tongue paralysis. Hyoid bone fracture can cause unilateral hypoglossal damage. Paralysis of the glossopharyngeal and vagus nerves bilaterally results in pharyngeal paralysis, total inability to swallow, and may cause respiratory noise. With unilateral paralysis swallowing is still possible. Laryngeal paralysis can accompany pharyngeal paralysis.

Guttural pouch mycosis and empyema, ruptured rectus capitis ventralis muscle, and retropharyngeal lymph node abscessation might be accompanied by glossopharyngeal and vagus nerve paralysis plus hypoglossal paralysis. Chronic lead poisoning and botulism also commonly cause dysphagia.

Dysphagic horses are difficult to manage in the short term and almost impossible to manage on a long-term basis. Nasogastric intubation and esophagostomy are possible alternatives for tube feeding. Severe complications can occur, however, and nutritional requirements of an adult horse are difficult to meet with these force-feeding methods (see p. 424). A severe common complication of dysphagia is aspiration pneumonia.

SPINAL NERVE INJURY

Suprascapular Nerve ("Sweeny"). The suprascapular nerve innervates the supraspinatus and infraspinatus muscles. It emerges from the brachial plexus and courses over the cranial border of the scapula before entering the muscles. Damage to the nerve can result from trauma to the shoulder or in draft horses from direct pressure by an ill-fitting collar.

When the horse walks, the shoulder is abducted. This gait is known as "shoulder slip." Supraspinatus and infraspinatus muscle atrophy often appears gradually over one to four weeks, resulting in eventual prominence of the spine of the scapula. Other nerves, muscles, and supporting tissues can be damaged with severe trauma or laceration to the area. This may cause severe laxity and marked gait abnormality. Additional signs of pectoral, subscapular, musculocutaneous, and proximal radial paralyses and avulsion of brachial plexus bundles may be seen. The abduction of the shoulder during weight-bearing has been suggested to cause continued overstretching of the nerve and perpetuation of the paralysis. Surrounding tissue healing may cause entrapment and prevent recovery (see treatment: specific procedures).

Brachial Plexus. Brachial plexus trauma is not common in the horse as this structure is well protected. Severe collision can result in brachial plexus dysfunction, the clinical signs of which resemble those of radial paralysis at the level of the shoulder. Other affected peripheral nerves leaving the brachial plexus will add to the deficit. Examination of the reflexes, the sensory deficit and use of the needle EMG in determining the extent of the damage will help differentiate brachial plexus injury from a single neuropathy (see treatment: specific procedures).

Radial Nerve. The radial nerve innervates the extensor muscles of the elbow, carpal, and digital joints. Depending on the site of the injury the paralysis can be total or partial. When the radial nerve is totally paralyzed, the elbow is dropped and carpus and digit remain flexed. Weight-bearing on the limb is impossible. In the case of partial paralysis the horse stumbles and shows a sliding motion of the foot when the limb is extended. Weight-bearing may be possible. Atrophy of the triceps brachialis, extensor carpi radialis, ulnaris lateralis, and digital extensor is present when the radial paralysis has existed for several weeks.

Trauma from a fractured first rib or humerus or prolonged lateral recumbency resulting in post-anesthetic neuromyopathy are the most common etiologies. The prognosis is grave if nerve regrowth of more than 12 inches is required for recovery. Fibrotic contracture of the muscles is a common complication of prolonged recovery.

Musculocutaneous, Median, and Ulnar Nerves. Traumatic mononeuropathies of these nerves have not been reported. Paralysis of these nerves can be associated with other peripheral nerve dysfunction. With time (two to three months) the horses compensate well for the gait deficit. Therapy may not be indicated.

Femoral Nerve. The quadriceps femoris group of muscles is innervated by the femoral nerve. Inability to extend the stifle results from its paralysis. As a consequence of the stifle flexion, the tarsus and digit are flexed and the horse is unable to bear weight on the limb. The hock can still be flexed to pull the limb forward, but the patellar reflex is depressed or absent. There is hypalgesia of the medial thigh, and the quadriceps muscles atrophy with time. Causes of femoral nerve paralysis include trauma, tumor, abscess, aneurysm, fractured pelvis and femur, and overextension of the limb while in recumbency. The prognosis is guarded if the damage is severe and if the nerve cannot be repaired.

Peroneal Nerve. The peroneal branch of the sciatic nerve innervates the flexor muscles of the tarsus and the extensor muscles of the digit. Paralysis results in knuckling of the fetlock and the interphalangeal joints with extension of the hock. The horse can bear weight on the limb if it is placed under the pelvis. At rest the limb is extended somewhat caudally with the fetlock flexed and the dorsum of the foot on the ground. When the animal walks, the toe is dragged and the leg is thrust caudally in an attempt to bear weight. The nerve is easily injured, because it lies subcutaneously over the lateral condyle of the femur. Trauma by kicks or prolonged lateral recumbency is usually in the history.

Tibial Nerve. The tibial nerve originates from the sciatic nerve and innervates the caudal pelvic limb muscles, which extend the tarsus and flex the digit. When paralysis occurs the resulting gait resembles that of "stringhalt" with overflexion of the hock and dropping of the foot on the ground. Atrophy of the gastrocnemius muscle eventually occurs. Because the nerve is well protected this is a very infrequently seen paralysis.

Sciatic Nerve. Before it branches into the tibial and peroneal nerves the sciatic nerve innervates the extensor muscles of the hip and the flexor muscles of the stifle. Paralysis of all branches proximally results in extension of the stifle and tarsus with flexion of the fetlock and the dorsum of the foot resting on the ground. Severe gait abnormalities result, with the limb being dragged. Hypalgesia to the distal limb may be evident. This nerve is well protected but is closely related to the pelvis. Pelvic fractures and osteomyelitis of the sacrum and pelvis have been associated with sciatic paralysis. Deep intramuscular injection caudal to the proximal femur and deep pelvic abscessation can result in sciatic trauma in foals. The prognosis is always guarded because of the length of the nerve and its branches.

Cranial Gluteal Nerve. Paralysis of this nerve, which causes variable gait deficit and atrophy of the gluteal region (primarily the middle gluteal muscle), can occur with pelvic fracture and prolonged general anesthesia in dorsal recumbency. The most frequent cause of gluteal atrophy in the eastern United States is equine protozoal myelitis (see p. 359); however, the cause of isolated muscle atrophy without development of other signs may remain undetermined without necropsy diagnosis.

Sacral, Coccygeal, and Caudal Nerves. Injury to the sacral and coccygeal vertebrae can cause paralysis of the tail, anus, perineum, bladder, and rectum if the sacral and coccygeal nerves are involved. This syndrome is referred to as the cauda equina syndrome. It also occurs with polyneuritis equi and neoplastic invasion of the sacral-caudal vertebral canal as well as with central nervous system lesions of protozoal myelitis (see p. 359), sorghum cystitis, equine rhinopneumonitis (see p. 365), and rabies (see p. 364). Atrophy of the gluteal region can occur and some horses show subtle gait deficits on the affected side.

NEUROMAS

A neuroma is an abnormal nerve growth that occurs when an injured axon fails to grow in the distal nerve stump. Sensory activity generated in neuromas contributes to the painful sequelae of peripheral nerve injury. When a neurectomy is performed cryoneurectomy and epineurial capping seems to be the most effective method to reduce the incidence of neuromas. Reduced exercise for four weeks postoperatively is recommended.

TREATMENT

NONSURGICAL

The ultimate goal of nonsurgical treatment of peripheral nerve lesions is to allow the nerve to recover its function in the case of neurotmesis. Treatment should ensure that the paralyzed structures are functional if reinnervated. Treatment should decrease the incidence of fibrous tissue and adhesion formation and avoid fibrous degeneration of muscle fibers. Any coexisting injuries should be treated appropriately; if they require surgery, exploration of the nerves involved can be done at that time.

In the case of closed trauma one can assume that the fibrous sheath of nerves is likely to be intact. Suppression of inflammation that could result in further damage is the immediate need after an injury has occurred. Short-term glucocorticoid therapy (e.g., dexamethasone .05 mg per kg intramuscularly twice a day for three days) local application of dimethylsulfoxide (50 per cent solution in water, gel) and ice packs applied to the area might be helpful. For a longer term therapy nonsteroidal anti-inflammatory drugs will help reduce the inflammation and will alleviate the pain (e.g., flunixin meglumine 1 mg per kg intramuscularly, intravenously, or orally once a day or divided twice a day; phenylbutazone 2 to 4 mg per kg orally twice a day).

In the case of neurapraxia, return of function may take days to weeks. If the nerve has been damaged the delay in recovery is a function of the length of regrowth needed; regrowth occurs about one inch per month. Nursing care of the paralyzed structures is vital. Paralyzed limbs should be protected from injuries such as trauma, overstretching, or cold, and adequate circulation should be maintained. Joint deformities should be prevented by maintaining the mobility of joints and tendons. Heavy bandages will protect the paralyzed limb from further trauma. Splinting is often necessary to prevent or correct deformities and to support the joints. Such splinting should ensure a neutral or slightly relaxed position for the paralyzed muscles. Pressure on soft tissue should be avoided and the splints should be easily removed so the affected region can be freed for careful examination and physiotherapy. Plastic pipe or fiber glass casts cut in half make suitable sup-

ports. Compression bandaging, while limiting venous congestion and edema, can have the same supportive role as splinting. Gentle massage and passive movements are essential for maintaining the circulation and the full range of motion of the joints. Electrotherapy does not entirely prevent denervation atrophy but probably slows the process, effectiveness being proportional to the frequency of treatment. Muscle mass once lost cannot be restored by artificial stimulation.

When some motor function is restored, exercise is beneficial for full recovery. Swimming seems to be a good form of exercise because the water supports the paralyzed limb.

In the case of injection injury, 50 to 100 ml of isotonic saline solution should be infiltrated around the injection site. The area should be hot packed to promote vasodilation and rapid absorption of the drug.

SURGICAL

General Procedure. Repair of a severed nerve, exploration of a nerve lesion, and/or freeing an entrapped nerve are the three objectives achieved by surgery. Immediate (primary) nerve repair can be performed in uncomplicated nerve severance when the state of the wound is optimal with little damage to the surrounding tissues and no infection. The procedure should be performed within 12 to 24 hours to avoid tissue retraction and inflammation. If immediate repair is impossible, early secondary suture is indicated three to five weeks after injury. If secondary suturing is elected a few temporary holding sutures should be placed immediately in the nerve ends for attachment to the surrounding tissue to avoid nerve retraction. Radiopaque sutures will also serve as markers for the delayed surgery. In severe injury resulting in bruising of the surrounding tissues and damage to the bones, joints, tendons and/or vessels, nerve repair is greatly delayed by the highly unfavorable conditions. The condition of the wound will then determine the timing of the surgical repair.

In the case of closed trauma or open wounds with no absolute evidence of nerve severance, a conservative approach allowing time for spontaneous recovery is recommended. A delay of three to four months is reasonable. During this time, periodic assessment of the patient's progress is essential. In the case of sudden accentuation of the clinical signs, nerve entrapment is suspected and surgery is indicated.

The exploration and manipulation of a nerve and surrounding tissue should proceed with extreme caution to avoid further damage. The nerve is traced from below or above the site of the lesion and freed from the scar tissue and any adhesions. Scrupulous hemostasis is essential. Electrical stimulation will help determine the condition of the injured segment. Failure to elicit a response after adequate time has been allowed for reinnervation to occur indicates that nerve ressection and repair is justified.

End-to-end anastomosis is the method of choice for repair of a severed nerve providing that it can be done without tension and with an adequate tissue bed and vascularization. A simple interrupted pattern of four to six (5.0 to 7.0 monofilament nylon) sutures should be placed through epineurium only. Return to function should be assessed periodically postoperatively.

SPECIFIC PROCEDURES

"Sweeny." A horse can walk satisfactorily with an uncomplicated suprascapular paralysis. Treatment may be required for performance or cosmetic reasons. If there is no improvement three weeks after the injury, surgical exploration can probably be performed safely. In addition to freeing the nerve from surrounding scar tissue it has been recommended that the operator cut a window (1.5 × 0.5 inches) in the cranial part of the scapula that underlies the nerve. Another option is to perform the surgery on all affected horses at three weeks. This may result in some unnecessary surgeries but it gives the best chances for recovery. Cosmetic treatments such as injecting air or a foreign body under the skin give very unsatisfactory results.

Neuromas. When encountered during nerve exploration, resection of the neuroma and anastomosis of the nerve stumps should be performed only if nerve stimulation fails to induce muscle contractions. In the case of a painful neuroma, that is, a sequela to a palmar digital neurectomy, the prognosis is guarded. Resection of the neuroma, cryoneurectomy, and epineurial capping of the nerve stump can be attempted.

SPECIFIC NEUROPATHIES

POLYNEURITIS EQUI (NEURITIS OF THE CAUDA EQUINA)

Chronic granulomatous inflammation of the extradural spinal nerve roots of the cauda equina can occur in horses and ponies. The name is misleading because other nerves are often affected.

Clinical Signs. Both sexes and mature to older horses are affected. The onset of signs is usually insidious and slowly progressive over several weeks. However, the history can be of an acute onset if the first signs are not noticed. Some horses have a history of previous respiratory infections.

The primary complaints include rubbing of the tail and perineum, colic due to fecal retention, and/or hypersensitivity over the gluteal region.

Some horses presenting with cranial signs of facial, vestibular, and/or trigeminal nerve injury are sensitive around the head. Cranial nerves less commonly involved include the glossopharyngeal, vagus, hypoglossal, oculomotor, and optic nerves. When the horse shows signs of cauda equina involvement, neurologic examination reveals hypalgesia or analgesia of the tail, perineum, penis (not the sheath) or vulva, and gluteal area. Hyperesthesia around the tail head and perineum can occur. There is no tail tone and the urinary bladder, urethral sphincter, rectum, anal sphincter, and penis or vulva are paralyzed. The dribbling of urine causes scalding of the perineum and inner thighs. After a few weeks there is evidence of coccygeal muscle atrophy.

As the disease progresses, pelvic limb weakness and subtle gait abnormalities may be seen. Atrophy of the gluteal, biceps femoris, and other muscles can occur as the inflammation extends cranially. Very rarely, the thoracic limb will show ataxia and weakness.

Diagnosis. Cerebrospinal fluid obtained from the lumbosacral area usually shows elevated protein content and increased numbers of leukocytes (mostly lymphocytes). Circulating antibodies to the neurotigenic bovine myeline protein P2 have been found in a limited number of cases. This finding strengthens the hypothesis that this syndrome is similar to the Guillain-Barré syndrome in humans, an autoimmune disease.

Prognosis and Treatment. Various routines of glucocorticoids and antibiotics have been tried unsuccessfully. The disease is usually progressive and the horses are usually euthanatized. Affected horses can be maintained for long periods with daily nursing care including manual evaluation of the rectum and catheterization of the bladder. Cystitis is a common complication.

Postmortem Findings. Early in the disease there is discoloration and hemorrhage of the cauda equina. Later white and thick fibrous tissue appears that extends extradurally and intradurally along the lumbar, sacral, and coccygeal nerves. Histologically there is proliferation of inflammatory cells with hemorrhage and connective tissue deposition. This is accompanied by degeneration of myelin and axons. Some horses are presented with a polyneuritis identical histologically to polyneuritis equi but the cauda equina is not affected.

CHRONIC LEAD POISONING

This condition is described on page 667.

DISORDERS OF THE NEUROMUSCULAR JUNCTION

Botulism is discussed on page 367.

A myasthenia-like syndrome has been reported

following general anesthesia. All the horses recovered uneventfully within a month with good nursing care. Clinical signs include prolonged recovery, flaccid tongue, dysphagia, mydriasis, and inability to raise the head. Other signs were flaccid tail, reduced patellar reflexes, megaesophagus, and recumbency. The cause of this syndrome is unknown.

OTHER DISORDERS OF PERIPHERAL NERVES

Shivering, tics, and stringhalt are thought to have a neurologic origin. Shivering affects the muscles of the tail and hindlimbs. Affected horses are unable to move backward. When the horse is required to do so the tail is elevated and trembles and the muscles of the hindlimbs are tense and trembling. One hindlimb is often held semiflexed and abducted. Muscle relaxation occurs as the foot is brought back to the ground. Occasionally the muscles of the forelimbs, neck, and face are involved. The disease is usually progressive. There is no known treatment.

Stringhalt is manifested by involuntary hyperflexion of one or both hocks during movement. The intensity of the flexion is variable. The leg is often flexed momentarily before being slammed back to the ground. This can affect each step or be intermittent. The forelimbs may be affected occasionally. The etiology is unknown but the hypothesis of an intoxication has been proposed because outbreaks of stringhalt occur in certain areas of Australia. In the case of Australian stringhalt the horses eventually recover in a period of days to several months. Surgical treatment has been recommended for chronic cases with resection of the tendon and part of the muscle belly of the lateral digital extensor. The success is variable.

Supplemental Readings

Bowen, J. M.: Peripheral nerve electrodiagnostics, electromyography and nerve conduction velocity. *In* Horlein, B. F. (ed.): Canine Neurology, Diagnosis and Treatment, 3rd ed. Philadelphia, W. B. Saunders Company, 1978, pp. 254–279.

deLahunta, A.: Veterinary neuroanatomy and clinical neurology, 2nd ed. Philadelphia, W. B. Saunders Company, 1983.

Mayhew, I. G., and MacKay, R. J.: The nervous system. *In* Mansmann, R. A., McAllister, E. S., and Pratt, P. W. (eds.): Equine Medicine and Surgery, 3rd ed. Santa Barbara, CA, American Veterinary Publications, 1982, pp. 1159–1252.

Mayhew, I. G., and Stashak, T. S.: The nervous system. *In* Jennings, P. B. (ed.): The Practice of Large Animal Surgery. Philadelphia, W. B. Saunders Company, 1984, pp. 983–1041.

Palmer, A. C.: Introduction to animal neurology, 2nd ed. Oxford, Blackwell Scientific Publications, 1976.

Rooney, J. R.: Clinical Neurology of the Horse. Kennett Square, PA, KNA Press, 1971.

NUTRITION

Edited by H. F. Hintz

Energy and Protein

Harold F. Hintz, ITHACA, NEW YORK

Herbert F. Schryver, ITHACA, NEW YORK

ENERGY

Providing an incorrect amount of energy is one of the most common mistakes in the feeding of horses. Acute overfeeding can cause a variety of problems, such as enterotoxemia, colic, and founder. Chronic overfeeding can result in obesity, impaired performance, needless expense, and perhaps skeletal problems. The treatment of overfeeding is simple. The energy intake must be decreased, but the decrease should not be too drastic and abrupt, as metabolic disorders may result (see Hyperlipemia). Unfortunately, some clients do not appreciate the difference in energy concentration among feedstuffs, nor will they accept the fact that under some conditions horses do not need any grain. Furthermore, overfeeding frequently occurs in the preparation of animals for shows and sales. Even though trainers know excess fat is of no value and perhaps harmful, the excess fat makes the animals look better in the eyes of many people and increases sales prices.

Underfeeding can result in loss of weight or reduced weight gain, delay in onset of sexual maturity in young animals, reduced resistance to disease, impaired performance, rough hair coats, and unthrifty appearance.

Inadequate energy can result from several problems other than simply underfeeding. Parasites, dental problems, and malabsorption can all cause decreased utilization of feed. In group feeding situations, some horses may not obtain reasonable access to the feed. Feed intake may be decreased if the water supply is not adequate. Furthermore, many owners fail to recognize chronic weight loss until the situation is severe. They may see the animals every day, but the change is so gradual that they do not realize that the animals are in trouble. For example, a pony was brought to the clinic at Cornell University because the owner thought it had a broken leg. The pony had been housed in a run-in shed with a larger pony. It was winter and the pony had a long hair coat. Upon examination, it was found that the pony did not have a broken leg; rather, it was emaciated and could not walk simply because it was starved. The ponies had been fed together, and apparently the larger pony got most of the feed. The situation was aggravated because the cold weather increased the energy requirement. The long hair coat masked the weight loss. Thus, it is recommended that owners weigh their horses regularly. If scales are not available, measuring tapes placed around the heart girth can be used. Several feed companies supply such tapes, and they are reasonably accurate.

Estimates of energy requirements for various classes of horses are shown in Table 1, but these are only guidelines. If the horse is not in the desired condition and factors such as parasites and dental problems have been corrected, then the amount of grain should be adjusted accordingly.

SOURCES OF ENERGY

Horse owners often feel that energy of one type may be good for certain activities but not for others.

TABLE 1. ENERGY AND PROTEIN REQUIREMENTS OF VARIOUS CLASSES OF HORSES*

| | Expected Mature Weight (kg) | | | | | |
| | 400 | | 500 | | 600 | |
	DE† *Mcal/day*	*Protein* *kg/day*	*DE* *Mcal/day*	*Protein* *kg/day*	*DE* *Mcal/day*	*Protein* *kg/day*
Maintenance, mature	13.86	0.54	16.39	0.63	18.79	0.73
Mares, last 90 days of gestation	15.52	0.64	18.36	0.75	21.04	0.87
Lactating mare, first 3 months	23.36	1.12	28.27	1.36	33.05	1.60
Lactating mare, 3 months to weaning	20.20	0.91	24.31	1.10	28.29	1.29
Weanling	13.03	0.66	15.60	0.79	16.92	0.86
Yearling	13.80	0.60	16.81	0.76	18.85	0.90
Two-year-old	13.89	0.52	16.45	0.63	19.26	0.74

*From the National Research Council. Nutrient Requirements of the Horse. NAS-NRC Publication, Washington, DC, 1978.
†Digestible energy

That is, they want a source of energy that allows the horse to run fast but will not fatten the horse or a source of energy for weight gain but they do not want the horse to get "high." Unfortunately, methods to fraction energy in such divisions have not been developed, and energy must be considered as energy.

Grains

The energy content of some grains is shown in Table 2. Horse owners prefer to feed oats to their horses. Oats are an excellent feed but are often more expensive than other grains. They have the lowest digestible energy (DE) concentration and the lowest weight per volume of most common grains (Table 3). Thus, oats are the safest grain, since owners are much less likely to overfeed oats than other grains. For example, there may be twice as much energy in a quart of shelled corn as there is in a quart of oats. Oats also have a higher protein content than corn, and the protein quality is slightly better than that of corn.

Unfortunately, the quality of oats varies more than the quality of the other grains. The digestible energy content is negatively correlated with the fiber content, and the greater the fiber content the

less weight per bushel. The weight may vary from 25 to 40 lb or more per bushel. The energy content may vary from 2.4 to 3.0 megacalories (Mcal) of DE per kg.

Oats are also frequently dusty and may also contain other excess foreign material unless they are properly cleaned. Thus, care should be taken when purchasing oats.

In parts of the United States, corn is the most economical grain for feeding many horses. However, it has a high DE concentration and, therefore, requires better feeding management than oats.

Although many horse owners feel that corn is a "hot" food and that horses do not perform at their best when fed corn, many experiments have demonstrated that these complaints are incorrect when reasonable feeding care is taken. For example, polo ponies at Cornell performed as well when fed alfalfa and corn as when fed timothy and oats, but the feed intakes were adjusted so that DE intakes were similar. Arabian horses ridden 50 miles in five hours performed satisfactorily when fed alfalfa and corn. As mentioned earlier, corn is much easier to overfeed and, if overfed, produces more heat; when corn and oats are fed to provide the same intake of DE, oats actually provide more heat because of the

TABLE 2. AVERAGE COMPOSITION OF SOME COMMON ENERGY SOURCES*

Grain	DE Mcal/kg	Protein (%)	Fiber (%)	Calcium (%)	Phosphorus (%)
Barley	3.2	11	6	0.08	0.40
Brewers' grains	2.6	27	15	0.27	0.48
Corn (yellow)	3.5	9	2	0.02	0.31
Distillers' grains (corn)	3.2	27	12	0.09	0.37
Oats (high quality)	3.0	13	10	0.10	0.35
Oats (low quality)	2.4	11	13	0.09	0.30
Rye	3.2	12	2	0.06	0.34
Sorghum (milo)	3.4	11	2	0.04	0.29
Wheat	3.5	13	3	0.05	0.36
Molasses, beet	2.6	7	0	0.16	0.01
Molasses, cane	2.4	3	0	0.89	0.04

*From the National Research Council. Nutrient Requirements of the Horse. NAS-NRC Publication, Washington, DC, 1978.

TABLE 3. RELATIVE WEIGHTS OF
SOME COMMON FEEDS*

Feed	Weight of 1 Quart (lb)	Volume of 1 lb (qt)
Alfalfa meal	0.6	1.7
Barley	1.5	0.7
Beet pulp	0.6	1.7
Corn	1.7	0.6
Cottonseed meal	1.5	0.7
Linseed meal	0.9	1.1
Molasses, cane	3.0	0.3
Oats	1.0	1.0
Rye	1.7	0.6
Soybean	1.8	0.6
Wheat	1.9	0.5
Wheat bran	0.5	2.0

*From Morrison, F. B.: Feeds and Feeding. Ithaca, NY, Morrison Publishing Co., 1957.

greater fiber content. Oats or corn can be fed whole, although crimping of oats may improve energy utilization by 7 to 10 per cent.

Unfortunately, several outbreaks of equine leukoencephalomalacia have occurred in recent years. The disease was associated with corn or corn screening contaminated with *Fusarium moniliforme*.

Barley is also excellent for horses and has been used as a horse feed for many years. Barley has a DE content somewhere between that of oats and corn, but the energy concentration is still such that it is relatively easily overfed. Barley may be less palatable than oats or corn. The protein content is similar to that of oats. Some horse owners also consider barley to be a "hot" feed. One owner claimed that barley was a "hot" feed unless you cooked the heat out of it by steaming it. As with corn, it is a matter of feeding the correct amount of DE. Barley should be processed by crimping or rolling. No studies have been conducted on the value of steam-flaking barley for horses, but early studies indicated that cooking provided no benefits above those of crimping or rolling.

Milo has a digestible energy content similar to that of corn. It is an economical grain in the southwestern United States and is a satisfactory grain for horses when properly processed and supplemented. As with corn, if management is not careful, overeating can result in enterotoxemia, colic, or founder.

Rye is seldom fed to horses because of the relatively high price and because horses do not like it. A grain mixture should contain no more than one third rye to avoid decreases in feed intake.

Wheat can sometimes be an economical source of energy. It has a high DE content and must be fed with caution. Milo, rye, and wheat should be processed (cracked, rolled, or steam-rolled) for efficient utilization.

HAYS

Hays contain a lower concentration of energy than grains. Legume hays, such as alfalfa, clover, birdsfoot trefoil, and lespedeza, usually contain a higher amount of digestible energy, calcium, protein, and vitamins than grass hays such as Bermuda,

TABLE 4. ENERGY CONTENT OF HAY AND OTHER NONCONCENTRATE FEEDS*

	Dry Matter (%)	Digestible Energy Mcal/kg	
		1†	2‡
Alfalfa, grazed prebloom	21	0.52	2.51
grazed fullbloom	25	0.57	2.29
hay, earlybloom	90	2.18	2.42
hay, midbloom	89	2.04	2.29
hay, fullbloom	89	1.92	2.16
meal, dehydrated, 17 per cent protein	92	2.26	2.46
Bahiagrass, grazed	30	0.63	2.11
hay	91	1.72	1.89
Barley hay	89	1.68	1.89
straw	90	1.47	1.63
Beet pulp	91	2.60	2.86
Bluegrass, grazed early	31	0.76	2.46
grazed, posthead	35	0.77	2.20
Citrus pulp	90	2.69	2.99
Clover (red), grazed, earlybloom	20	0.50	2.51
hay, late	89	1.92	2.16
Corn cobs	90	1.22	1.36
Cottonseed hulls	91	1.32	1.45
Fescue, hay	88	1.78	2.02
Lespedeza hay	91	1.88	2.07
Timothy, hay, prehead	89	1.96	2.20
head	88	1.74	1.98

*From the National Research Council. Nutrient Requirements of the Horse. NAS-NRC Publication, Washington, DC, 1978.
†As is
‡Dry matter basis

bluegrass, fescue, orchardgrass, reed canary, and timothy (Table 4). The most important criterion to consider when buying hay is not species but rather nutritive value in relation to cost. The primary factor that influences nutritive value is stage of maturity at harvesting.

Young plants contain a greater concentration of DE and nutrients than do old plants. As the plant matures, the amount of lignin and structural components increases. These fractions are not utilized efficiently by horses. The effect of stage of maturity on value is demonstrated in Table 5, and the recommended stage of maturity for harvesting is summarized in Table 6. If the plant is too young when harvested, the nutrient concentration is greatest, but the yield per acre is greatly decreased.

Good-quality hay should be harvested at the proper stage of maturity, should be free from mold, dust, and weeds, and should not be excessively weathered. Weathering can cause loss of leaves and decreased vitamin content. Unless proper harvesting methods are used, legume hay is more likely to be moldy or dusty than grass hay because it has more leaves and drying is more difficult.

Some owners think that the excess protein in alfalfa causes kidney damage. Other owners believe that alfalfa causes horses to sweat more. Neither of these opinions is supported by scientific evidence. Horses fed legumes may urinate more, and there may be a stronger smell of ammonia in the barn because of the higher nitrogen content of alfalfa hay. It is true that alfalfa will usually contain more protein and DE than needed by mature horses. In fact, mature horses fed good-quality legume hay free choice may become overweight.

Alfalfa is used to greatest advantage when fed to growing horses or lactating mares, as these animals have high protein and calcium requirements. Swerczek suggested that the incidence of "shaker foal syndrome" could be reduced by not feeding an excessively nutritious diet such as alfalfa to mares nursing foals. He further suggested that the alfalfa caused an increase in the corticosteroid content of the mare's milk, which in turn made the foal more susceptible to toxicoinfectious botulism and hence

TABLE 6. STAGE OF GROWTH FOR HARVESTING HAY CROPS TO OBTAIN GREATEST AMOUNTS OF DIGESTIBLE NUTRIENTS

Crop	Stage to Harvest
Perennial grasses:	
Coastal Bermudagrass	14–16 in height (maximum 4 weeks' growth)
Common Bermudagrass	Early bloom
Bluestem, introduced and native	Boot—early bloom
Johnsongrass	Boot
Lovegrass	Boot
Timothy	Early head
Smooth bromegrass	Early to medium head
Orchardgrass	Boot to early head
Annual grasses:	
Millet, pearl or cattail	Boot
Sorghum, forage	Bloom-soft dough
Sudan varieties and sudan hybrids	Boot
Oats	Early bloom
Ryegrass	Early bloom
Legumes:	
Alfalfa	Full bud
Clover (crimson, hop, red, white, Persian, and arrowleaf)	¼ to ½ bloom
Birdsfoot trefoil	¼ bloom
Peanut	Harvest to retain maximum leaves
Vetch	Early bloom

shaker foal syndrome. Further studies are needed, however, to establish such relationships.

Blister beetles may be found in alfalfa hay raised in the southwest (see p. 120).

Other Energy Sources

Molasses is an excellent source of energy and is often added to horse rations to reduce dust and increase palatability. However, some horses prefer feeds without molasses; that is, some horses will select the feed without molasses if given a choice. Furthermore, molasses may be an expensive source of energy.

The use of pelleted rations has enabled the use of many feeds that would not normally be consumed by horses. Apple skins, corn cobs, peanut hulls, sunflower hulls, almond hulls, ryegrass straw, corrugated paper boxes, and ammonia-treated straw are examples of unconventional feeds that have been used in horse rations. Many of these feeds provide little nutrition other than DE and fiber, but they are well utilized when properly supplemented. Many of these feeds are not economical at present but are likely to be used in increasing amounts in the future as the prices of primary feedstuffs increase.

PROTEIN

In the evaluation or formulation of rations, protein is usually the next nutrient considered after

TABLE 5. PROTEIN CONTENT OF ALFALFA AND TIMOTHY AT DIFFERENT STAGES OF MATURITY*

	Alfalfa		Timothy	
Date	Stage	Protein	Stage	Protein
May 25	Vegetative	19%	Vegetative	15%
June 5	Bud	16	Boot	12
June 15	Early flower	14	Early head	10
June 20	Flower	11	Heading	9
July 5	Late flower	8	Flower	6
July 25	Green seed	5	Early seed	3

*Dates under New York conditions

energy status has been examined. Theoretically the best measure of protein value for nonruminants is the amount and balance of available essential amino acids. Unfortunately, little information is available on the amino acid requirements of the horse. It has been estimated that weanlings require rations containing about 0.7 per cent lysine, but no values are available for the other amino acids. Generally, therefore, the crude protein content is used to evaluate the ration. Crude protein is estimated by determining the nitrogen content of the feed and multiplying by 6.25 because most proteins contain about 16 per cent nitrogen. This method (Kjeldahl) may overevaluate certain feedstuffs such as silage that contain significant amounts of nonprotein nitrogen, but it is widely used because it is a relatively easy and inexpensive procedure and results in reasonable values for most common feedstuffs.

Knowledge of the digestibility of the feedstuffs would be beneficial. Again data are limited, but fortunately most protein supplements appear to be digested efficiently.

PROTEIN DEFICIENCY

Protein is too ubiquitous a part of the animal to show a specific set of deficiency signs. Deficiency depresses metabolic activities, food intake is decreased, growth is impaired, and reproduction and lactation are suboptimal. Anemia and hypoproteinemia may develop. The animal appears unthrifty, is not alert, and the hair coat is dull. In other species, brain development and learning ability in young animals can be impaired by protein deficiency.

PROTEIN REQUIREMENTS

Requirements can be expressed as daily intakes of protein or as a percentage of the diet. The latter method is probably the one used most commonly. Estimates of the daily crude protein requirements are shown in Table 1. Requirements as a percentage of the diet are shown in Table 7. The daily intake of protein (grams per day) required is constant for a given horse. The percentage of crude protein required in the diet, however, depends on several factors, such as concentration of DE. That is, when significant amounts of grain are fed, the concentration of the DE is greater, and the crude protein content of the total ration should be higher than when only hay is fed, since the horse will need fewer pounds of feed to meet its energy needs. Therefore, the protein concentration must be higher to provide the required protein intake when grain intake is great.

The protein content of the grain mixture needed when feeding grass or legume hay is shown in Table 8. As mentioned earlier, the diet of young growing horses should contain 0.7 per cent lysine, but further studies are needed to determine the requirements for other amino acids.

TABLE 7. ESTIMATES OF PROTEIN REQUIREMENTS EXPRESSED AS PERCENTAGE OF DIET ON 90% DRY MATTER BASIS*

Class	Crude Protein (%)
Mature horse, maintenance	7.7
Mares, last 90 days of gestation	10.0
Lactating mare, first 3 months	12.5
Lactating mare, 3 months to weaning	11.0
Creep feed	16.0
Weanling (6 mos)	14.5
Yearling	12.0
Two-year-old	9.0
Mature working horse	7.7

*From the National Research Council. Nutrient Requirements of the Horse. NAS-NRC Publication, Washington, DC, 1978.

Although protein requirements are listed for several classes of horses, it is obviously not practical to have numerous grain mixtures on the farm. A protein supplement could be added to a basic grain mixture at feeding time according to the horse's needs, but such a practice is often confusing when several horses are involved or when more than one person is doing the feeding. A more practical solution might be to have only four grain mixtures. One mixture would be for creep feed, one for weanlings, one for yearlings and producing mares, and one for mature horses. Of course, if only a few horses are involved, it might be more economical to have only one or two grain mixtures.

SOURCES OF PROTEIN

The composition of some protein sources is shown in Table 9. Legume hay harvested at the proper stage of maturity provides a significant amount of protein. Alfalfa meal is used in many horse rations, particularly the complete pelleted rations, and in addition to protein provides minerals and vitamins.

Good-quality pasture also provides protein. For example, legume pasture such as clover may contain 18 to 20 per cent protein on a dry matter basis. Even grasses such as bluegrass and timothy may

TABLE 8. MINIMUM PROTEIN CONTENT NEEDED IN GRAIN MIXTURES WHEN FEEDING LEGUME HAY OR GRASS HAY

Class of Horse	Legume Hay* (%)	Grass Hay* (%)
Creep feed	16	18
Weanlings	14.5	18
Yearlings: pregnant mares (last 90 days); lactating mares	10–11	15–16
Mature horses	†	8

*Values will depend on protein content of hay. In this example, it was assumed that the legume hay contained 14.5% crude protein and the grass hay contained 8% crude protein.

†In most cases, the legume hay could provide nearly all of the protein needed.

TABLE 9. COMPOSITION OF SOME PROTEIN SOURCES*

	Protein (%)	Lysine (%)	Lysine: Protein (%)	Calcium (%)	Phosphorus (%)
Alfalfa hay—early bloom	16	0.85	5.5	1.58	0.23
—mid bloom	14	0.81	5.6	1.35	0.22
—full bloom	13	0.62	4.6	1.16	0.21
Alfalfa meal—15%	15	0.68	4.5	1.32	0.22
—17%	18	0.88	5.0	1.60	0.23
—20%	21	0.95	4.6	1.70	0.24
Brewers' grains	27	0.90	3.3	0.27	0.48
Cottonseed meal	41	1.76	4.2	0.23	0.90
Distillers' grains, dried	27	0.60	2.2	0.09	0.37
Fish meal (herring)	72	5.70	7.9	2.08	1.55
Linseed meal	33	1.20	3.6	0.39	0.81
Meal and bone meal	50	3.20	6.4	9.42	5.09
Peanut meal	45	1.60	3.6	0.20	0.65
Skim meal (dried)	33	2.60	7.8	1.32	1.05
Soybean meal	45	3.00	6.7	0.25	0.60
Soybean meal, dehulled	48	3.20	6.7	0.25	0.60
Sunflower meal, dehulled	47	1.82	3.9	0.36	0.90

*90% dry matter basis

contain as much as 15 per cent protein during the early growth stages, but the moisture content of pasture is high and may limit intake. The level of protein in the pasture depends greatly on the stage of maturity, fertilizing practices, and weather conditions.

Animal protein supplements such as dried skim milk, fish meal, and meat and bone meal are efficiently utilized, contain a relatively high amount of lysine, and are usually a high-quality protein source. Such sources also provide significant amounts of calcium and phosphorus. However, animal protein supplements are usually much more expensive per unit of protein than vegetable proteins.

Most vegetable protein sources, such as cottonseed meal, have a relatively low content of lysine and a higher content of phosphorus (P) than calcium (Ca) (Table 9). Fortunately, soybean meal has a higher lysine content than most other oil meals. Soybean meal is an excellent protein source for horses, and in most parts of the United States is usually the most economical source. Linseed meal, peanut meal, cottonseed meal, sunflower meal, and brewers' or distillers' grains should not be used as the primary protein source for young horses unless they are fed at higher levels (which is usually uneconomical) or combined with additional lysine sources. The value of the protein sources can be greatly influenced by the method of processing. Untreated legume seeds such as soybeans, raw soybean meal, or kidney beans should not be fed to horses because these feeds contain many factors, such as trypsin inhibitors, that decrease utilization of the feed and decrease feed intake. Heat destroys the deleterious factors, but excess heat decreases the value of the protein because high temperatures cause the protein to bind with carbohydrate fractions. Excessive heat during processing has been reported to decrease the value of soybean meal, alfalfa meal, and brewers' or distillers' grains.

PROTEIN TOXICITY

No studies have demonstrated protein toxicity in horses. Excess protein is broken down, the carbon chain is used for energy, and nitrogen is excreted in the urine. Of course, feeding excess protein is costly because the protein supplement is usually an expensive component of the ration. Furthermore, energy is required to excrete nitrogen.

It has been stated that feeding high levels of protein causes crooked legs and other skeletal deformities in young, fast-growing horses, but it is probably not protein per se that causes the problems. Feeding an unbalanced diet containing high levels of protein results in problems. For example, if protein is added to increase rate of growth without ensuring that necessary amounts of other nutrients such as Ca and P needed for bone formation are present, problems will develop. Studies with rats and humans indicate that high levels of protein cause hypercalciuria, but no such effect was noted in horses fed 22 per cent protein in recent studies.

NONPROTEIN NITROGEN UTILIZATION

Nonprotein nitrogen compounds such as urea are often added to rations for ruminants. The microflora of the rumen use the nitrogen to synthesize protein, which then can be digested and utilized by the host animal. The principal advantages of using nonprotein nitrogen in ruminant rations are reduction of feed costs and utilization of materials that could not be used directly by nonruminants such as humans.

The horse, however, does not appear to be an efficient utilizer of nonprotein nitrogen. Much of the dietary nonprotein nitrogen is absorbed from the small intestine. If the nonprotein nitrogen is urea, most of the absorbed nitrogen is excreted in the urine because mammalian systems do not contain the enzyme urease, which is needed to break down urea into ammonia and carbon dioxide. Some absorbed urea can be secreted into the large intestine, where bacteria can utilize it, and some of the urea reaches the large intestine directly. Unfortunately, quantitative measurements of the amounts of amino acids produced by bacteria and subsequently utilized by the horse are not available. Some studies indicate that amino acids of bacterial origin make significant contributions to the nutritional status of the horse, whereas other studies suggest they do not. However, it appears that the economic advantage of feeding urea to horses is not nearly as great as that of feeding urea to cattle because the horse does not utilize urea as efficiently as cattle. Furthermore, in the classes of horses that require high dietary levels of protein, such as young horses, protein quality of the diet is important.

Nonprotein Nitrogen Toxicity

Ammonia is toxic, but urea per se is not toxic. As mentioned earlier, mammals do not have enzymes to form ammonia from urea. Excessive feeding of urea to cattle can result in ammonia toxicosis because of rapid ammonia release from the rumen by the bacteria. Horses are more tolerant of urea ingestion than cattle because much of the urea is absorbed before it reaches the site of bacterial activity. Ammonia toxicosis was produced in ponies by feeding one pound of urea. Clinical signs were characteristic of severe central nervous system derangement. The earliest signs were aimless wandering and incoordination, followed by head-pressing against fixed objects. Death followed shortly after head-pressing began. Convulsions occasionally occurred as a terminal episode. One pound of urea is much greater than the amount needed to produce ammonia toxicosis in ruminants, and it is highly unlikely that horses will obtain that level of intake under field conditions.

In summary, horse owners should not be concerned about ammonia toxicosis if their horse happens to eat a cattle ration containing urea. If the feed is safe for cattle, it will be safe for horses.

Supplemental Readings

Cunha, T. J.: Horse Feeding and Nutrition. New York, Academic Press, 1980.
Evans, J. W., Borton, A., Hintz, H. F., and Van Vleck, L. D.: The Horse. San Francisco, Freeman, 1977.
National Research Council: Nutrient Requirements of the Horse. NAS-NRC Publication, Washington, DC, 1978.
Roberts, S. J.: Veterinary Obstetrics and Genital Diseases, 2nd ed. Ithaca, NY. Published by author, 1971.
Swerczek, T. W.: Experimentally induced toxicoinfectious botulism in horses and foals. Am. J. Vet. Res., *41*:348, 1980.

MINERALS

H. F. Schryver, ITHACA, NEW YORK

H. F. Hintz, ITHACA, NEW YORK

Minerals comprise about 4 per cent of the weight of the animal body. Among the minerals of concern in equine nutrition are calcium, phosphorus, potassium, sodium, chlorine, magnesium, sulfur, iron, zinc, copper, manganese, iodine, and selenium. These elements are known to perform many vital functions in the structure and metabolism of the body.

Plants, and ultimately the soil in which the plants are grown, are the sources of minerals in the nutrition of the horse. A large number and variety of factors influence the pathway of minerals from soil to plant to animal. The soil may contain too little or too much of essential elements, or alternatively, factors in the soil may reduce the ability of plants to obtain essential elements. These and related factors often result in regional mineral problems in animal agriculture. Some examples of regional problems are the large areas of iodine-deficient soils or regions in which the soil contains an excess or deficiency of selenium. Such areas are often well known and have been mapped (Figs. 1 and 2). Information about regional mineral problems is often available from the local extension service, state college of agriculture, or regional United States Department of Agriculture office.

The soil-plant-animal pathway of minerals is one of changing relationships. The content and availability of minerals in soils and plants may be altered by agricultural techniques, such as fertilizing, spraying, and harvesting. The mineral content and distribution in soils and plants may also be altered by

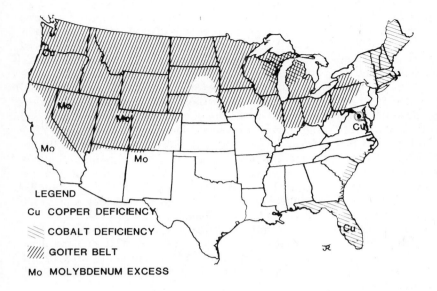

Figure 1. Areas in the United States where mineral deficiency or toxicity is known to occur. (Courtesy of the Plant, Soil, and Nutrition Laboratory of the United States Department of Agriculture, Ithaca, NY.)

LEGEND

Cu COPPER DEFICIENCY

COBALT DEFICIENCY

GOITER BELT

Mo MOLYBDENUM EXCESS

air- or water-borne deposition of elements from industrial pollution and other sources. Acid rain and the consequent changes in pH of soils and water may be an important determinant of mineral availability. For example, decreased soil and water pH leaches copper from soils decreasing its availability to plant and animal but at the same time low soil pH increases the solubility and availability of aluminum. Changing relationships also develop from plant breeding, which introduces new species and varieties that differ in their ability to extract minerals from soils. Animal breeders and husbandmen exert increased pressure on the soil-plant-animal system by demanding more rapid rates of growth from their animals. These and other factors have altered the soil-plant-animal pathway of minerals in the recent past and will continue to do so in the future. Mineral problems that were considered unlikely to occur 25 years ago are now observed frequently in some species of livestock. Similar problems may be expected in horse husbandry in the future.

There are complex interrelationships that exist among minerals themselves. For example, dietary calcium influences phosphorus, magnesium, zinc, copper, and other minerals in the diet, while calcium is itself influenced by phosphorus, magnesium, or iron in the diet. The organic composition

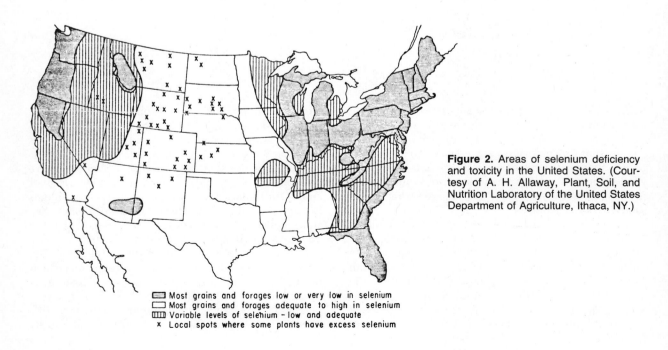

Figure 2. Areas of selenium deficiency and toxicity in the United States. (Courtesy of A. H. Allaway, Plant, Soil, and Nutrition Laboratory of the United States Department of Agriculture, Ithaca, NY.)

▨ Most grains and forages low or very low in selenium
☐ Most grains and forages adequate to high in selenium
▥ Variable levels of selenium – low and adequate
x Local spots where some plants have excess selenium

of a diet also influences mineral nutrition. Calcium absorption is enhanced or inhibited by dietary protein, certain amino acids, some carbohydrates, lipids, and by specific organic substances such as oxalate, phytate, and vitamin D. These relationships determine the availability of minerals in the diet. The presence of natural or synthetic chelating agents also influences the availability of minerals. To be beneficial in nutrition, the chelation or binding of minerals to the chelator must be weaker than the binding capacity of the tissue for the same element. The chelating agent must be able to "deliver" the mineral element of the tissues. Unfortunately, some natural and synthetic chelating agents bind some minerals very strongly and do not release the minerals to the tissues. On the other hand, some chelating agents exchange one mineral for another at the tissue level. Thus, a chelating agent may increase the availability of one mineral but at the expense of creating a deficiency of another. There is no evidence that chelated trace minerals are more effective sources than simple inorganic forms of trace minerals for horses.

Determination of the mineral status of animals suspected of having deficiency, excess, or imbalance of minerals is done most directly and accurately by considering the nutritional history of the animals in question. The nutritional history should include the age and function of the animal and the types and amounts of feeds that have been fed. Soil analysis may provide useful information if home-grown feeds are used. Mineral analysis of feeds is also potentially useful, provided that proper sampling techniques are followed. The feeds sampled must represent feeds that were used during the period of development of the suspected nutritional problem. In agricultural regions, personnel of the extension service or dairy herd improvement services are often equipped with the proper tools and techniques for obtaining useful soil, feed, and water samples.

Determination of the concentration of minerals in blood serum or plasma may be helpful in some cases. However, homeostatic controls and the body stores of minerals may minimize or prevent significant changes in the concentration of some minerals in blood. For example, neither a very low nor a very high calcium diet alters the plasma calcium concentration in horses. A high phosphorus diet may cause plasma calcium to fall, but only to the low normal range. Quite large dietary increases in zinc or copper in horses produce only small increases of the plasma concentration of these elements. On the other hand, severe, prolonged, experimental deficiency of zinc and magnesium causes a marked decrease in concentration of these elements in blood plasma. Blood selenium analysis may be useful in determining selenium status. However, blood analysis should not be the sole criterion

for diagnosis of mineral problems even when blood concentration tends to reflect mineral status. The investigator should seek additional evidence of deficiency or excess.

Blood samples taken for trace element analysis are easily contaminated. Syringes, needles, and evacuated blood sample tubes are common sources of contamination. For example, spuriously high zinc values occur when the freshly drawn blood sample comes in contact with the rubber stoppers of some evacuated blood sample tubes for only a brief period. Special blood sampling tubes are available for obtaining samples for trace element analysis.

Analysis of hair is sometimes suggested as a means of determining the mineral status of horses. A great variety of factors affect the mineral content of hair. These include hair color, rate of hair growth, site on the body, and season of the year. For example, colored hair has three to four times as much calcium, magnesium, and manganese as white hair. The calcium, magnesium, iron, and manganese concentration of hair can vary twofold in different seasons. Contamination of hair by urine, feces, feed, soil, and other environmental sources is a serious and unsolved problem in obtaining hair samples for analysis. The few scientific studies that have been reported indicate that hair analysis is valueless for determining the calcium, phosphorus, copper, or molybdenum status of horses.

CALCIUM AND PHOSPHORUS

Calcium and phosphorus are the most abundant elements in the body, comprising more than 70 per cent of the "ash" of the body. The minerals are commonly considered together because they occur together in bone and because they strongly influence each other in nutrition and metabolism. A deficiency or an excess of one affects the metabolism of the other nutrient.

Greater than 99 per cent of calcium and 80 per cent of the phosphorus of the body occurs in crystalline form in bone as hydroxyapatite, which has the empirical formula $Ca_{10}(PO_4)_6(OH)_2$. The bone crystal, which has a Ca:P ratio of about 2:1, is intimately associated with collagen. Bone also contains carbonate, citrate, and the elements sodium, potassium, fluorine, magnesium, and many other elements. The relationship of these components in the inorganic phase of bone can be influenced in part by diet.

Calcium and phosphorus have a large number of functions in addition to constituting bone crystal. Calcium is necessary in the blood clotting mechanism for the conversion of prothrombin to thrombin. Calcium is involved in transmission of nerve impulses, muscle contraction, and the secretion of many hormones and is necessary for the activation of a number of enzymes. Phosphorus is part of many structural and functional compounds in the body, such as phosphoproteins, phospholipids, and nucleoproteins. Phosphate is an active part of a large number and wide variety of enzyme systems.

Bone acts not only as structural element in the body but also as a store of calcium and phosphorus that can be mobilized and transported by blood to other sites to serve some of the metabolic functions mentioned before. The concentration of calcium in blood plasma is closely regulated by the activities of parathormone, secreted by the parathyroid gland (p. 189), calcitonin, secreted by the C cells of the thyroid gland, and by metabolites of vitamin D. These substances, alone or in combination, influence the intestinal absorption and renal excretion of calcium as well as the mobilization and deposition of calcium in bone. Mobilization of calcium from bone under the influence of parathormone occurs when dietary sources are inadequate for body needs. During mobilization of calcium, both mineral and organic phases are usually removed from bone. Thus, a net loss of bone substance occurs, which may be severe after prolonged calcium mobilization due to dietary deficiency.

CALCIUM AND PHOSPHORUS REQUIREMENTS

The calcium and phosphorus requirement of horses depends on the age and function of the individual. Young, growing horses have high requirements to meet the needs of skeletal development. The requirement of the mare is increased during late pregnancy for bone formation in the developing fetus and during lactation for secretion of calcium and phosphorus in milk. Table 1 shows the estimated dietary requirements of calcium and phosphorus for different classes of horses. Amounts of calcium greatly in excess of the requirement should be avoided. Excess calcium intake appears to inhibit the turnover or remodeling process in bone and interferes with the utilization of phospho-

TABLE 1. APPROXIMATE CALCIUM AND PHOSPHORUS REQUIREMENTS FOR HORSES*

	Percentage in the Diet		Daily Nutrients (gm)	
	Ca	P	Ca	P
Foals, to 6 months	0.80	0.55	33	20
Weanlings	0.60	0.45	34	25
Yearlings	0.50	0.35	31	22
Two-year-olds	0.40	0.30	25	17
Mare, late pregnancy	0.45	0.30	34	23
Mare, lactation	0.45	0.30	50	34
Mature horses, maintenance	0.30	0.20	23	14

*Assuming 500 kg mature weight

TABLE 2. APPROXIMATE MINERAL COMPOSITION OF SOME COMMON FEEDS FOR HORSES

	Ca	P	Mg	K	Zn	Fe	Cu	Mn
	Percentage				Ppm			
Roughages								
Alfalfa	1.3	.25	.29	1.9	17	180	13	30
Bluegrass	.30	.29	.16	1.7	—	260	9	93
Brome grass	.32	.22	.13	2.0	—	100	7	100
Oat hay	.30	.26	.75	1.2	—	400	4	120
Orchard grass	.35	.31	.20	3.0	18	110	14	40
Timothy	.41	.20	.16	1.6	—	140	5	46
Grains								
Barley	.05	.37	.15	.45	17	90	9	19
Corn	.05	.60	.03	.35	21	30	4	6
Oats	.07	.37	.19	.44	33	80	7	43
Wheat	.05	.45	.11	.41	30	40	7	40
Protein Supplements								
Cottonseed meal	.16	1.20	.60	1.50	80	300	20	23
Linseed meal	.43	.90	.67	1.53	—	360	28	42
Skim milk	1.30	1.09	.13	1.66	68	10	1	2
Soybean meal	.31	.70	.30	2.19	48	130	30	48
Miscellaneous								
Beet pulp	.75	.10	.30	.20	10	330	14	38
Molasses, cane	1.05	15	.47	3.80	30	250	80	57
Wheat bran	.12	1.43	.59	1.60	120	190	14	138

The compositions shown in the table are expressed on a dry matter basis and are average compositions for each type of feed. Composition will vary depending on the origin of the feed, stage of maturity at harvest, processing techniques, and many other factors. (Adapted from National Academy of Sciences: Nutrient Requirement of Horses, 4th ed. Washington, DC, National Academy of Sciences–National Research Council, 1978.

rus and other essential minerals. Phosphorus greatly in excess of the requirement and in excess of the calcium intake should also be avoided. Excess phosphorus intake inhibits absorption of calcium and other elements and may alter calcium homeostatic mechanisms and the rate of bone turnover.

The calcium and phosphorus content of some common feeds is shown in Table 2. Cereal grains are poor sources of calcium but moderately good sources of phosphorus. Byproducts of the oil seeds, such as soybean oil meal, contain more calcium and phosphorus than the cereal grains. Hays generally contain considerably more calcium than cereal grains or oil seed products. Legume hays are rich sources of calcium. However, the mineral content of roughage can be very variable depending on the type of roughage, type of soil on which the hay was grown, stage of maturity when hay was cut, handling after harvest, and other factors. The calcium and phosphorus of roughage is highly available to horses. That of cereal grains and oil seed meals is slightly less available, possibly owing to the phytate content of these products (Table 3).

CALCIUM AND PHOSPHORUS SUPPLEMENTS

The calcium and phosphorus content of some common mineral sources is shown in Table 4. The

TABLE 3. AVAILABILITY OF CALCIUM AND PHOSPHORUS IN SOME COMMON HORSE FEEDS AND SUPPLEMENTS

	Ca (Percentage)	P (Percentage)
Corn	—	38
Timothy hay	70	42
Alfalfa hay	77	38
Linseed meal	68	45
Milk products	77	57
Wheat bran	—	34
Limestone	67	—
Dicalcium phosphate	73	44
Bone meal	71	46
Monosodium phosphate	—	47

Availability was determined as the percentage of calcium or phosphorus absorbed by experimental horses when the ingredient listed was the primary source of either calcium or phosphorus in the diet.

minerals in those sources are readily assimilated by horses. The ratio of the minerals in the sources varies so that it is possible to choose a supplement to correct a deficiency or imbalance in a particular diet. Thus, a diet deficient only in calcium can be most easily corrected with limestone, while a diet equally deficient in calcium and phosphorus can be corrected with dicalcium phosphate.

The available experimental evidence indicates that horses, like ruminants, do not have a nutritional sense or nutritional wisdom to select the amount of calcium and/or phosphorus needed from free choice supplements. The horse is not able to balance a ration or to make up a deficit in a ration if offered calcium and phosphorus free choice. This applies even when the free choice minerals contain salt. Free choice calcium and phosphorus give a false sense of security to the horse manager but do little for the horse.

CALCIUM AND PHOSPHORUS DEFICIENCY

Calcium deficiency may be due to simple lack in the diet or may be due to factors that limit calcium utilization in diets in which the calcium level is adequate. Factors that limit dietary calcium utilization include excess dietary phosphate as inorganic phosphate or as phytate phosphate and oxalic acid. Phytate phosphate is a hexaphosphoric acid ester of inositol that occurs in many seed grains and protein supplements. Wheat brain is an especially rich source of phytate. Oxalic acid is found in many species of grasses, particularly those grown in tropical areas. Both of these substances bind dietary calcium (and other divalent cations) and make it less available for absorption from the intestinal tract. Both phytate and oxalate are probably digested in the large intestine of the horse, causing release of the chelated calcium. However, this is of little value to the individual because calcium is poorly absorbed from the large intestine of the horse.

CLINICAL SIGNS OF CALCIUM AND PHOSPHORUS DEFICIENCY

Signs of calcium deficiency are generally seen in the skeletal system. Calcium is mobilized from skeletal stores to maintain other metabolic functions that are calcium-dependent. Thus, deficiency signs relating to calcium-dependent metabolic functions are rare. Skeletal signs depend on the severity and duration of calcium deficiency, on the age, and on the phosphorus or vitamin D status of the affected animals. The net result of calcium deficiency is the formation of too little bone. The cortices of the long bones may be thin-walled, porous, and fragile. The trabeculae of cancellous bone of the axial and appendicular skeleton become thin and sparse. In rickets and ricketslike disorders in which calcium and vitamin D deficiency is combined, mineralization of the organic phase of bone does not take place normally. In nutritional secondary hyperparathyroidism (NSH), a low or marginal intake of calcium is combined with an excessive phosphorus intake. The entire skeleton is affected, but the enlarged facial bones of affected horses have given the name "bighead disease" to the condition.

Calcium deficiency may be undetected for many weeks or months. The skeleton of mature animals contains a very large reserve of calcium that can be called upon to meet other metabolic needs. More than half of the skeletal mineral may be removed before clinical signs appear. Young animals may grow in stature at a normal or only slightly reduced rate while fed a calcium-deficient diet. Bone elongation continues during deficiency because bone is constantly remodeled during growth. Bone mineral removed during remodeling may be deposited at sites of new bone formation. For example, bone mineral removed from an endosteal surface may be reutilized at periosteal surfaces or at the growth plate. The result is that skeletal mass does not keep pace with increasing body size, and the skeleton is more injury-prone.

Phosphorus deficiency affects the skeleton in similar ways. However, young animals fail to grow, probably because they eat poorly and because phosphorus-deficient forage crops are frequently deficient in protein as well. Phosphorus-deficient animals are often lame and walk with a stiff, painful gait. Deficient animals often have a depraved appetite and eat wood, bones, stones, and other objects. Behavioral studies have shown that phosphorus-deficient sheep with depraved appetites do not clearly prefer phosphorus-containing supplements. This indicates that the depravity or pica of phosphorus deficiency is not an example of "nutritional wisdom" or "phosphorus appetite" as commonly thought.

Reproductive inefficiency is a frequent sign of phosphorus deficiency. Affected animals show anestrus or irregular estrus and reduced rate of conception.

Hypophosphatemia is a frequent finding in phosphorus deficiency. In well-documented field cases of phosphorus deficiency in cattle, serum phosphorus may decrease to less than one third of normal levels.

DIAGNOSIS OF CALCIUM AND PHOSPHORUS DEFICIENCY

Diagnosis of suspected calcium and/or phosphorus deficiency may be difficult. Skeletal changes are generally not clinically evident until the disease is well advanced. Conventional radiographic procedures usually are unable to detect loss of skeletal mineral until the losses exceed about 30 per cent. Plasma or serum phosphorus concentration may be decreased in phosphorus deficiency.

Plasma calcium concentration is usually found to be normal in calcium deficiency because the homeostatic mechanisms are effective in maintaining plasma calcium at normal levels. Maintenance of plasma calcium concentration is at the expense of the skeleton. Serum alkaline phosphatase may be intermittently elevated in severe and rapidly developing calcium or phosphorus deficiency. Hair analysis has been suggested as a diagnostic procedure; however, hair does not reflect the calcium or phosphorus status of horses.

The excretion of calcium and phosphorus in urine of horses is generally related directly to the dietary intake of these minerals. This fact has been the basis of urinalysis procedures that have been proposed as a means of assessing the status of calcium or phosphorus nutrition of horses. The procedures compare the urinary excretion of calcium and phosphorus to the excretion of a reference such as creatinine or total urine solids. In practice, the concentration of calcium or phosphorus in a single urine sample is measured and the concentration expressed as a ratio to the creatinine or total solid control of the sample.

Unfortunately, there are few reported applications of these procedures. Those wishing to use this procedure should compare results obtained from suspect animals to results obtained from control horses of similar age, sex, breed and state of training that have been fed adequate levels of calcium and phosphorus. Comparisons should be made on several samples taken on different days and at different times of day.

The most direct and most effective diagnostic procedure is a thorough review of the dietary history of animals suspected of deficiency. If possible, the review should include visual inspection of the feeds used on the farm and should include chemical analysis of the feeds for calcium and phosphorus content.

THERAPY

Calcium or phosphorus deficiency is treated by supplying the deficient nutrients in the diet. This may be done by using feeds that are rich in these nutrients (see Table 2) or by using mineral supplements. Table 4 shows the composition of some commonly used calcium and phosphorus supplements and the grams of element supplied by one tablespoon (about 30 gm) of supplement.

MAGNESIUM

Magnesium is involved with calcium and phosphorus metabolism and is an activator or cofactor of numerous enzymes. Magnesium is particularly important in cellular energy metabolism.

Deficiency of magnesium has been produced experimentally in foals fed purified diets containing only 7 to 8 ppm of magnesium. Some of the deficient foals developed severe signs of central nervous system irritability, including nervousness, muscular tremors, and ataxia. Handling or loud noise caused the foals to develop convulsive seizures with paddling of the legs, hyperpnea, and sweating. Serum

TABLE 4. APPROXIMATE CALCIUM AND PHOSPHORUS CONTENT OF SOME COMMON MINERAL SUPPLEMENTS

	Ca (Percentage)	P (Percentage)	Gm of Element in 30 Gm of Supplement	
			Ca	P
Calcium carbonate	34	0	10	0
Defluorinated phosphate	32	15	10	5
Bone meal	30	14	9	4
Dicalcium phosphate	27	21	8	6
Monocalcium phosphate	17	21	5	6
Monosodium phosphate	0	22	0	7

These are approximate or average values. The calcium content of bone meal, for example, may vary from 27 to 32 per cent.

30 GM is approximately one tablespoon. Thus, one tablespoon of calcium carbonate provides 10 gm of Ca or about one third of the daily requirement of a yearling of 500 kg mature weight (see Table 1).

Limestone or oyster shells are common calcium carbonate sources that are used for mineral supplements for livestock.

magnesium values of deficient foals were less than 1 mg per dl. Serum phosphorus and calcium levels were normal. At postmortem examination of the magnesium-deficient foals, the elastic fibers of the aorta, the pulmonary artery, and other large arteries were found to be mineralized. Mineral deposits were also observed in elastic tissues of the lung and spleen and in the Purkinje fibers in the heart. Degeneration of cardiac and skeletal muscle was observed.

TRANSIT TETANY

Naturally occurring magnesium deficiency has not been described in horses. However, a tetany associated with hypomagnesemia and hypocalcemia has been reported in the midwestern United States and in England. The signs of "equine transit tetany" include sweating, hyperpnea, muscular fibrillation, difficult or uncertain locomotion, incoordination, and collapse with muscular twitching. Death may occur during convulsions. Affected animals respond to intravenous administration of magnesium and calcium salts. The syndrome seems to be brought on by a stressful situation such as shipping. The condition does not appear to be a simple magnesium deficiency; however, tetany-prone animals may be helped by providing additional magnesium in the diet.

Horses require about 0.1 per cent magnesium in the diet or about 4 to 6.5 gm per day for a 1000-pound horse. The magnesium in common feeds and supplements appears to be readily available to horses.

SODIUM AND CHLORIDE

The major functions of sodium and chloride are the regulation of tissue osmotic pressure and acid-base balance. Sodium is important in maintenance of cell membrane potentials and the transmission of nerve impulses. The two elements are usually considered together as sodium chloride and have related functions in tissues.

Horses have a clear salt drive. The needs of the horse can easily be met by providing salt "free choice" either as salt blocks or as loose salt. Salt consumption varies greatly among individual horses. Measurements at Cornell University's Equine Research Park over a 12-month period show consistent daily intakes of salt that vary from as little as 15 gm for some horses to more than 200 gm for others. Most of the horses in the survey consumed 50 to 75 gm of salt per day.

Iodized, trace mineral salt is highly recommended for horses. It provides a simple, safe, dependable means of meeting the requirements for salt and part of the need for iodine and other trace

TABLE 5. MICRONUTRIENT MINERAL ALLOWANCES FOR HORSES

	Mg Element/Kg Diet
Iron	50.0
Zinc	40.0
Manganese	50.0
Copper	9.0
Iodine	0.1
Selenium	0.1
Cobalt	0.1

The amounts given in this table are considered to be adequate for growth and maintenance (National Research Council, 1978).

minerals (Table 5). Table 6 shows the contribution of a commercially available trace mineral salt mixture to the estimated trace mineral requirements of a mature horse, assuming that the horse consumed about 50 gm of salt per day. This is well within the range of salt intake of most horses.

The sodium content of urine and feces has been used in determining sodium status. Sodium levels below 10 mg per dl in urine and 1 to 1.5 gm per kg of dry feces generally indicates an insufficient supply of sodium in the diet.

Salt poisoning can occur in salt-starved horses that are given access to salt without adequate water. Signs of salt poisoning include colic, diarrhea, frequent urination, weakness, staggering, and paralysis of the hindlimbs.

POTASSIUM

Potassium, like sodium and chloride, is important in maintaining tissue osmotic pressure and acid-base equilibrium. It is intimately involved in regulating the passage of nutrients into cells and in water metabolism. Potassium plays an important role in

TABLE 6. CONTRIBUTION OF A TRACE MINERAL SALT MIXTURE TO THE REQUIREMENTS OF A MATURE HORSE FOR TRACE MINERALS

Composition of the Salt Mixture	Mg of Mineral in 50 gm Salt	Multiple of the Requirement
	%	
Cobalt	0.010	5.0	10.0
Copper	0.023	11.5	.2
Iodine	0.007	3.5	7.0
Manganese	0.225	112.5	.6
Zinc	0.200	100.0	.5
Magnesium	0.100	50.0	.002
Iron	0.232	116.0	.6

The salt mixture is typical of an iodized, trace mineralized salt that is commercially available as loose salt or salt blocks. A typical daily consumption by a 1000 lb horse from free choice feeders would be about 50 gm. A daily intake of 50 gm would supply the multiple of the NRC estimated requirements for trace elements as shown.

muscle contraction. Most of the body potassium is intracellular.

Potassium deficiency has been studied experimentally in a number of species. Signs in affected animals include decreased rate of growth, loss of appetite, and decreased serum potassium levels. Naturally occurring or experimental potassium deficiency has not been reported in the horse.

The potassium requirement of the horse is estimated to be about 0.4 to 0.5 per cent of the diet. Most forage crops contain about 1.5 per cent potassium. Thus, dietary potassium deficiency seems unlikely in horses that receive forage as 35 per cent or more of their ration. On the other hand, grains generally contain 0.4 per cent or less of potassium. Thus, rations very high in grains may cause problems as a result of low potassium intake. Increased potassium loss may occur as a result of prolonged hard work as in endurance rides or as a result of diarrhea, acute intestinal obstruction, adrenal cortical dysfunction, and in other pathologic states.

IRON

Iron is an integral part of hemoglobin, the oxygen-carrying protein in red blood cells, of myoglobin in muscle, and of respiratory enzymes such as cytochrome C, peroxidase, and catalase.

Deficiency of iron results in anemia. The red blood cells may be reduced in size, number, and hemoglobin content (p. 303). Anemic animals have pale mucous membranes and are often weak, inactive, and tire easily. The greatest need for iron occurs in the newborn, which has a rapidly expanding red blood cell mass and small iron stores. At the same time, dam's milk is generally a poor source of iron. Thus, iron stores and intake may be insufficient to meet the needs of the newborn, and anemia results. Access to soil and to feeds other than dam's milk provide a source of iron to the newborn and can help prevent anemia.

Under normal circumstances, the body excretes very little iron. The iron stores are reused in hemoglobin synthesis. However, repeated hemorrhage increases iron loss, may deplete iron stores, and may result in anemia. This may occur in certain parasite infections.

The mature horse is estimated to require about 40 ppm of iron and rapidly growing foals about 50 ppm of iron in the diet. Good-quality feeds easily supply this level of iron.

Simple iron deficiency anemia is probably a very rare occurrence in the horse. Anemic horses should be examined carefully, and causes of anemia other than iron deficiency should be sought. Recent work has shown that the concentration of serum ferritin as measured by an enzyme immunoassay is correlated with iron stores in horses. The procedure may be valuable in assessing iron storage in horses suspected of iron deficiency anemia.

Ferrous salts (Fe^{++}) are more efficiently absorbed and are more effective iron supplements than ferric salts (Fe^{+++}). Chelated iron salts do not appear to be more efficiently utilized by horses than simple inorganic iron salts or the iron that is contained in feeds. Injectable iron supplements provide iron immediately to the body, but this is probably of doubtful utility. Some injectable iron dextran supplements that are meant for treating baby pig anemia have produced a severe, shocklike syndrome in horses and should be avoided.

Iron supplements given to normal horses or to horses that do not have simple or induced iron deficiency are of little value. Iron does not stimulate hemoglobin synthesis. Prolonged high iron consumption interferes with phosphorus utilization in ruminants and may do so in horses as well.

COPPER

Copper is important for the utilization of iron in hemoglobin synthesis and in the maturation of red blood cells. Copper is also involved in the function of many enzymes associated with amino acid metabolism and with cellular respiration. Copper is part of the enzyme tyrosinase, which is needed for conversion of tyrosine to melanin in skin. Normal collagen and elastin formation and osteoblast activity are dependent on copper. Copper is an integral part of lysyl oxidase, an enzyme that is responsible for the cross-linking of collagen molecules in the maturation of collagen.

Copper deficiency may be due to simple lack of copper in the diet, or deficiency may be induced by excess molybdenum intake. Horses seem more tolerant of dietary molybdenum than ruminants. Several reports indicate that high molybdenum pastures that have resulted in severe disease in cattle have not affected horses that have also grazed the pastures. Nevertheless, short-term experiments in the horse show that when molybdenum intake exceeds copper intake by several times, copper metabolism may be influenced without producing signs of copper deficiency. The complex interaction of sulfate with molybdenum and copper that has been observed in ruminants has not been studied in horses. Dietary supplements containing copper have been used to counteract excess molybdenum intake in ruminants and presumably would do so in horses.

Copper metabolism may be altered by excessive zinc intake. Cases of osteochondrosis desiccans in foals have been ascribed to zinc contaminated pastures near zinc smelters and to high zinc intake by foals exposed to fresh zinc-based paints on fences.

COPPER REQUIREMENTS

The copper requirement for maintenance of mature ponies has been estimated to be 3.5 ppm of the diet. Young horses probably require 10 ppm in the diet.

Ponies appear to be resistant to chronic copper toxicity and have tolerated up to 80 ppm in the diet for long periods.

CLINICAL SIGNS OF COPPER DEFICIENCY

The signs of copper deficiency are often directly referable to the various functions of copper in the body. Thus, deficient animals may be anemic. The anemia of copper deficiency resembles iron deficiency anemia because iron is poorly utilized in copper deficiency. Copper-deficiency anemic animals do not respond to iron supplements. The hair of deficient animals may become gray owing to the defect of melanin synthesis in the skin.

Affected animals may have bone abnormalities due to defects in collagen maturation and altered osteoblast activity. In dogs and swine, copper deficiency causes a bone disease that resembles rickets. The joints of affected animals are swollen, and the limbs may be deformed. The cortex of the long bones is thin, the trabeculae are few and small, and the growth plates of the bones are widened.

Horses appear to tolerate diets that produce copper deficiency in ruminants. Uncomplicated cases of copper deficiency have not been reported in the horse, but copper deficiency has been implicated in skeletal disease in young horses in copper-deficient areas of Western Australia. In Ireland, copper-responsive osteodystrophies have been described in foals, and a molybdenum-induced copper deficiency has been suggested as a cause of a ricketslike disease. In each of these instances, bone cortices of affected horses have been thin and the joints enlarged, and in some cases there have been limb deformities.

ZINC

Zinc plays an essential role in the function of a large number of enzyme systems that are involved in digestion and metabolism.

CLINICAL SIGNS OF ZINC DEFICIENCY

Naturally occurring zinc deficiency has not been reported in horses, but experimental zinc deficiency has been produced in foals. The deficiency inhibited growth of the foals and caused skin lesions similar to those seen in zinc-deficient pigs. The lesions, called parakeratosis, began on the lower limbs and then extended upward on the body as the deficiency progressed. The first signs were hair loss, followed by scaling of the dried, outer layers of the skin.

Subsequently the affected skin was encrusted by a rough layer of serous exudate and desquamated epithelium. Skin wounds in the affected foals healed poorly. Serum alkaline phosphatase levels were below normal, as were tissue and blood concentrations of zinc. Skeletal abnormalities were not reported in the experimentally deficient foals, but zinc deficiency has resulted in short, thick bones in chickens and in bone deformities in calves. Reproductive and behavioral abnormalities have been observed in zinc-deficient rats, but such findings were not described in experimental zinc deficiency in horses.

ZINC TOXICITY

Excess zinc intake can be toxic. Growing horses fed diets containing 5000 ppm (0.50 per cent) of zinc developed anemia, swelling of the epiphyses of the long bones, stiffness, and lameness. Such a high intake level of zinc may result from contamination of soil and feeds by metal smelters.

Excess zinc is thought to interfere with copper metabolism and produce lesions resembling osteochondrosis in foals.

ZINC REQUIREMENTS

Young horses fed practical rations containing 40 ppm of zinc grew well and maintained their tissue concentrations of zinc, suggesting that this level of zinc is adequate for growth. However, other factors in the diet may affect zinc utilization. For example, high levels of calcium or copper increase the requirements of the pig for zinc. Phytin, a phosphorus-containing chelating agent found in cereal grains and byproducts and in protein supplements such as soybean meal, combines with zinc to decrease its absorption from the digestive tract. Diets high in calcium enhance the detrimental effect of phytin on zinc absorption in pigs. The presence of these factors in horse rations causes some nutritionists to recommend that the horse be given diets containing at least 100 ppm of zinc.

The requirements of the horse for zinc can generally be met from good-quality roughage and from trace mineralized salt. Oral zinc supplements such as zinc oxide, carbonate, and sulfate are effectively utilized.

COBALT

Cobalt occurs in the molecule of vitamin B_{12}. Cobalt may have other functions in the body, but these are not yet well studied. Horses are able to graze pastures that contain levels of cobalt that are deficient for sheep and cattle without ill effects. Cobalt deficiency or toxicity has not been described for horses.

Rations that contain 0.1 ppm of cobalt should be adequate for horses.

IODINE

Much of the body content of iodine is found in the thyroid gland, where the element is incorporated into the thyroid hormone thyroxine. Soils and plants in large areas of the world, including the northern tier of the United States, are iodine-deficient.

Iodine deficiency results in goiter, or enlargement of the thyroid gland. Goiter is also caused by goitrogenic substances found in plants of the cabbage genus Brassica. These include cabbage, Brussels sprouts, kale, and rape. Goitrogens are also found in linseed, peanuts, soybeans, and other legumes. Generally, goiter caused by these goitrogenic plants can be prevented by feeding additional iodine to animals at risk.

Iodine deficiency or the activity of goitrogenic substances results in decreased production of thyroxine. This in turn stimulates production of thyrotropic hormone by the pituitary gland, which causes hyperplasia and enlargement of the thyroid gland. Young animals are most subject to iodine deficiency and goiter. Young born of iodine-deficient dams are often stillborn. Others are weak and unable to nurse. Affected foals have been born with forelimb contracture.

Iodine deficiency affects reproduction in mature animals. Affected mares may exhibit irregular estrus cycles and prolonged gestation.

Thyroid function can be estimated by a competitive protein binding assay for serum levels of thyroxine (T_4 test). The T_4 test has been shown to be more reliable as a test of thyroid function than the protein-bound iodine (PBI) test in thyroidectomized ponies.

IODINE REQUIREMENTS

The horse probably requires about 0.1 ppm of iodine per day. Iodine deficiency is a well-recognized problem, and the use of iodized salt is so widespread and common that iodine deficiency is not encountered often. On the other hand, cases of goiter in foals due to excess iodine intake have been reported several times in Maryland, Virginia, Kentucky, New York, Great Britain, and Japan. The goitrous foals have been born of mares given excess iodine during pregnancy. Excessive iodine intake has come about through the enthusiastic use of iodine supplements or through the use of several iodine supplements simultaneously. Kelp, which is a rich source of iodine, has been an ingredient in each of the cases of iodine-induced goiter.

SULFUR

There appears to be little need for elemental or inorganic forms of sulfur by the animal body. Sulfur is required as organic compounds, such as the sulfur-containing amino acids and vitamins. Excess intake of inorganic forms of sulfur influences the toxicity of molybdenum in ruminants, but its effect in horses is not known.

MANGANESE

Manganese is required in enzymes that are involved in protein metabolism and fatty acid and cholesterol synthesis. Manganese plays a central role in the synthesis of glycosaminoglycans and glycoproteins, which are important constituents of cartilage and bone.

A condition thought to be manganese deficiency has been described in horses in a ranching community where the soils have been heavily limed to combat acidity produced by a nearby zinc smelter. The area soils tend to be marginal or low in manganese, and availability to plants is reduced by soil alkalinity. Samples of alfalfa hay contained as little as 13 ppm of manganese. Mares suffered from reproductive dysfunction that was manifested as delayed estrus, reduced fertility, and spontaneous abortion. Foals were often born with skeletal deformities and muscle contractures. Lesions included asymmetry of the skull, curvature of the vertebral column, shortened limb bones, and enlarged joints. Contracture of neck muscles resulted in a peculiar positioning of the head. Affected foals were often unable to flex their limbs.

The manganese requirements of the horse have not been determined, but estimates place the requirement at about 40 ppm. Some grains such as corn are poor sources of manganese, but roughage tends to be a good source.

SELENIUM

Selenium is a component of glutathione peroxidase, an antioxidant enzyme that catalyzes the conversion of peroxides to alcohols in tissues. Vitamin E and the sulfur-containing amino acids also have antioxidant properties and are able partly to replace one another and selenium in the diet.

Selenium-deficient areas occur in most of the Northeastern United States, the eastern seaboard, the Pacific Northwest, and adjacent areas of Canada (see Fig. 2). Grains and forages grown in these areas tend to be low in selenium. Selenium deficiency results where animals are fed solely on home-grown feeds or on feeds grown in the adjacent selenium-

TABLE 7. SUMMARY OF MINERAL FUNCTIONS, DEFICIENCY SIGNS, AND FEED SOURCES

Mineral	Some Functions	Some Deficiency Signs	Good Feed Sources	Poor Feed Sources
Calcium	Constituent of bone mineral; blood clotting; transmission of nerve impulses; muscle contraction; secretion of hormones; activation of some enzymes	Impaired mineralization of bone and skeletal development: rickets; osteomalacia; nutritional secondary hyper-parathyroidism; osteoporosis; possible bone deformities and/or fracture	Good quality hay, especially legumes; limestone; oyster shells; bone meal; dicalcium phosphate	Most grains; poor quality grass hay
Phosphorus	Constituent of bone mineral; constituent of some structural and functional proteins such as phosphoproteins, phospholipids, nucleoproteins; involved in fat, carbohydrate, and energy metabolism	Impaired mineralization of bone; decreased growth rate; reproductive problems; low blood phosphorus concentration	Most grains; soybean meal; linseed meal; brewers' yeast; bone meal; dicalcium phosphate; monosodium phosphate	Grain straws; beet pulp; citrus pulp; molasses
Magnesium	Constituent of bone mineral; activator or cofactor of numerous enzymes involved in cellular energy metabolism; alkaline and acid phosphatases	Central nervous irritability: nervousness, muscle tremors, ataxia, convulsive seizures; mineralization of elastic tissues of aorta, pulmonary artery, lung, and spleen; serum magnesium less than 1 mg/dl	Good quality hay, especially legumes; protein supplements	Most grains; poor quality grass hay
Sodium, potassium, and chloride	Maintenance of tissue osmotic pressure and acid-base equilibrium; control of water balance and passage of nutrients into cells; involved in transmission of nerve impulses and muscle contraction	Craving for salt; hyperexcitability; decreased growth rate; loss of appetite; decreased serum potassium	Common salt is composed of sodium and chloride; most roughages are good sources of potassium	Most feeds are inadequate sources of sodium and chloride; grains are generally inadequate sources of potassium
Iodine	Component of thyroxine; needed for thyroid functions	Goiter; reduced rate of growth, low body temperature; impaired development of hair and skin; foals weak at birth	Iodized salt	Most animal feeds in iodine deficiency regions
Manganese	Involved in protein, fatty acid, and cholesterol synthesis; synthesis of glucoproteins and glycosaminoglycans necessary in chondrogenesis and osteogenesis	Reproductive dysfunction: delayed estrus, reduced fertility, spontaneous abortion in mares; foals born with skeletal deformities, shortened limb bones, enlarged joints, and contractures	Roughage is generally a good source except on heavily limed soils	Grains; some roughage grown on heavily limed soils; milk and milk products.
Selenium	Constituent of glutathione peroxidase, which catalyzes the removal of peroxides from tissues	Muscular dystrophy: white muscle disease; low serum selenium and serum glutathione peroxidase concentrations; elevated serum glutamic-oxaloacetic transaminase concentration	Depends on soil content	All feeds grown in regions with selenium-deficient soils
Molybdenum	Constituent of xanthine oxidase			
Iron	Constituent of hemoglobin, myoglobin, cytochrome C, peroxidase, catalase; involved in oxygen transport	Anemia: pallor, low endurance; depressed growth	All roughage	Milk and milk products; wheat; corn; sorghum
Copper	Involved in iron absorption and hemoglobin synthesis; involved in melanin synthesis in skin; synthesis and cross-linking of collagen	Anemia; pigment loss in hair; ricketslike disease of bone; swollen joints, deformed long bones with thin cortices	Legume hay; molasses; linseed meal; soybean meal	Milk and milk products
Zinc	Cofactor or activator of large number of enzymes in digestion and metabolism	Parakeratosis: hair loss, scaling of skin, serous exudation and desquamation of skin; poor wound healing; low serum alkaline phosphatase; reproductive, behavioral, and skeletal abnormalities in some species	Insufficient data available	Beet pulp

deficient areas. Animals are often protected against deficiency when part of their ration contains feeds shipped from selenium-adequate areas.

SELENIUM DEFICIENCY (WHITE MUSCLE DISEASE)

Selenium deficiency leads to muscular dystrophy. The severe dystrophy that occurs in young foals is called white muscle disease. This disease has been recognized with increasing frequency in recent years in the eastern United States and Canada. Affected foals are weak, reluctant to move, tremble when standing, and walk with a stiff gait. The muscles are often bilaterally affected and are swollen and hard or rubbery. Inability to eat leads to rapid inanition. There may be fever and increased heart and respiratory rates. Blood serum selenium and glutathione peroxidase concentrations may be low, and serum glutamic-oxaloacetic transaminase (SGOT) levels may be elevated in affected foals. Low serum selenium and glutathione peroxidase levels may be observed in other animals on the premises. There is some uncertainty about the normal concentration of selenium in blood, but horses at selenium-deficient farms where foals or horses have died with lesions of muscular dystrophy have generally had less than 4 μg Se per dl of serum or blood. Glutathione peroxidase activity and blood selenium concentrations are highly correlated in horses. The foal may have myoglobinuria, which colors the urine brown. Foals may die suddenly as a result of cardiac myopathy. Affected muscles are white or gray and may look like fish flesh. Fat deposits are often discolored yellowish brown.

White muscle disease may respond to oral or intramuscular treatment with selenium–vitamin E. Success depends in large part on the extent of lesions at the time of treatment. Commercial injectable preparations of selenium (as sodium selenite) and vitamin E (alpha-tocopherol) are available.*

Rations that meet the estimated selenium requirement of 0.1 ppm should prevent selenium deficiency and white muscle disease on the farm. Pregnant and lactating mares may also be supplemented with selenium at a rate of about 1 mg of selenium per day. However, only small amounts of selenium cross the placenta. Thus, supplementing the pregnant mare may not benefit the foal. Breeders in selenium-deficient areas should try to employ some feeds imported from the selenium-adequate areas of the midwestern United States, between the Mississippi River and the Rocky Mountains. Soybean meal, linseed meal, and alfalfa are generally good sources of readily available selenium.

"Tying-up" disease is an exercise-related myopathy and associated myoglobinuria. Affected horses appear to be "myopathy-prone" rather than selenium-deficient. Nevertheless, "myopathy-prone" horses often appear to respond to selenium-vitamin E administration (p. 487).

SELENIUM TOXICITY

Selenium is toxic. Supplements should be given and recommended with caution. The use of multiple selenium supplements for the same animal or animals should be avoided. Toxicosis also results when animals in areas where the selenium content of the soil is high are supplemented. Soils that contain greater than 0.5 ppm of selenium are considered potentially dangerous. Seleniferous soils are located in the northern Great Plains, parts of Colorado and western Kansas, and northern New Mexico (Figs. 1 and 2). Horses suffering from selenium toxicosis, also called blind staggers or alkali disease, lose the hair from the mane and tail, the hooves may slough, and the affected horse may become blind and paralyzed.

MOLYBDENUM

Molybdenum is a constituent of the enzyme xanthine oxidase and is an essential element in nutrition. The molybdenum requirement for most animals is not known, and molybdenum deficiency disease has not been described. Horses appear to absorb molybdenum readily from the intestinal tract and to excrete excess molybdenum in the urine. Balance studies suggest that horses fed up to 100 ppm of molybdenum in the diet do not store appreciable amounts of the element in their tissues.

Excess molybdenum intake increases the need for dietary copper and can result in a syndrome identical to copper deficiency. Horses appear to be more tolerant of high molybdenum intake than cattle and have successfully grazed pastures that cause overt molybdenum toxicosis in cattle.

FLUORINE

Fluorine is often classified as an essential element because it appears to reduce the incidence of tooth decay and possibly of osteoporosis in humans. There is no direct evidence to indicate that fluorine is essential or beneficial to horses.

FLUORINE TOXICITY

Fluorine is better known in animal nutrition for the harmful effect of chronic excess intake. The resulting toxicosis, known as fluorosis, may result from long-term ingestion of pasture, hay, water, or mineral supplements that have been contaminated

---

*E-SE, Burns-Biotec, Omaha, NB

by certain industrial operations. Fluorosis may also occur from consumption of water or mineral supplements that contain naturally high levels of fluorine. For example, certain rock phosphates contain excessive fluoride and require special treatment before they may safely be used as mineral supplements.

Horses seem less susceptible to fluorosis than sheep or cattle. Excess fluoride accumulates in bones and teeth and damages both structures. Dental lesions occur only when horses ingest excess fluorine during tooth development. Tooth enamel becomes mottled, chalky, and brittle. The defective enamel may chip, exposing the softer, underlying sensitive tooth structures, which wear more readily. Horses with severely affected teeth eat less and slobber poorly masticated food. Affected horses are frequently stiff and lame. The bones of the limbs, skull, mandible, and ribs show periosteal hyperostosis, particularly at tendon and ligament insertions.

The amount of fluoride considered safe for consumption by horses is controversial. The National Research Council Subcommittee on Horse Nutrition (1978) recommends that horse rations contain no more than 50 ppm. Others consider this level to be far in excess of a safe amount.

Supplemental Readings

Cunha, T. J.: Horse Feeding and Nutrition. New York, Academic Press, 1980.

Maynard, L. A., Loosli, J. K., Hintz, H. F., and Warner, R. G.: Animal Nutrition, 7th ed. New York, McGraw-Hill Book Co., 1979.

National Academy of Sciences: Nutrient Requirement of Horses, 4th ed. Washington, DC, National Academy of Sciences–National Research Council, 1978.

Swenson, M. J. (ed.): Dukes' Physiology of Domestic Animals, 9th ed. Ithaca, NY, Comstock Publishing Associates of Cornell University Press, 1977.

Underwood, E. J.: Trace Elements in Human and Animal Nutrition, 4th ed. New York, Academic Press, 1977.

Vitamins

H. F. Schryver, ITHACA, NEW YORK

H. F. Hintz, ITHACA, NEW YORK

Vitamins are a group of unrelated organic compounds that are required in very small amounts in metabolism. Not all vitamins are dietary essentials for the horse. Some vitamins are synthesized in the tissues or by microorganisms in the large intestine. For example, under normal conditions, enough ascorbic acid is produced by the liver of the horse to meet metabolic needs even in the absence of a dietary source of the vitamin. Microorganisms in the cecum and colon of the horse are known to synthesize an abundance of B vitamins. It is not known how efficiently these substances are absorbed and utilized by the horse. The factors that modify the rates of synthesis by microorganisms and of absorption by the horse are also not known.

Vitamins are commonly classified into two groups: the fat-soluble vitamins, A, D, E, and K, and the water-soluble B vitamins and vitamin C. The classification also distinguishes some aspects of the source and metabolism of the vitamins.

Vitamins are frequently used as therapeutic agents for a variety of conditions. The conditions that are treated sometimes bear a superficial clinical or metabolic resemblance to specific signs of vitamin deficiency that have been observed in one or more species. For example, hemorrhage as a deficiency sign of vitamin C or vitamin K would be treated by very high doses of either or both vitamins C and K. There is little clear-cut experimental evidence that indicates conclusively that vitamins or other nutrients are effective therapeutic agents. Provision of vitamins and other nutrients at the required level or slightly in excess will correct or prevent specific deficiency signs. However, "megadose" therapy is without value at best, and since some vitamins and other nutrients are toxic at very high levels, the practice may be dangerous.

VITAMIN A

Vitamin A is important in vision, in development and maintenance of epithelial cells, in bone development, and in reproduction. Many of the functions of vitamin A are related to the stabilizing effect of the vitamin on the membranes of lysosomes—the subcellular particles that contain degradative enzymes. Controlled release of enzymes from lysosomes is necessary for the removal of cells and intercellular substances during the turnover and remodeling of tissues. For example, failure of release of lysosomal enzymes due to vitamin A deficiency results in failure of maturation and removal of epiphyseal cartilage cells and intercellular matrix. As a consequence, endochondral bone growth is affected.

Vitamin A is involved in the formation, development, and differentiation of epithelial cells. In vitamin A deficiency, differentiated epithelial cells are replaced by relatively undifferentiated stratified squamous, keratin-producing cells. These changes are most prominent in the respiratory, reproductive, urinary and digestive tracts. The replacement of one cell type by another alters the function and the resistance to infection of the affected epithelial surfaces.

Bone growth and remodeling are markedly influenced by vitamin A. The vitamin is essential for the normal sequence of growth, maturation, and degeneration of epiphyseal cartilage cells and for normal functioning of osteoblasts and osteoclasts. Deficiency of vitamin A results in decreased rate of endochondral bone growth and a decreased rate of bone resorption at endosteal and other resorption surfaces. Failure of the resorptive process in developing bone results in relative diminution of the internal dimension of certain bones and foramina. In severe cases of vitamin A deficiency in young animals, bony orifices do not enlarge sufficiently to accommodate important structures such as the spinal cord or optic nerve, resulting in severe nervous signs.

SOURCES OF VITAMIN A

Vitamin A occurs in feeds as precursors called provitamin A. The common provitamin A in horse feeds is carotene. Some carotene is metabolized to vitamin A in the wall of the intestine of the horse, but much of the dietary carotene is absorbed and stored in the liver and adipose tissues. The NRC assumes that the horse converts 1 mg of carotene to about 400 IU of vitamin A.

Carotene is most abundant in green feeds. However, the compound is highly unstable and easily oxidized. Large losses of carotene occur during the curing and storage of hay. For example, losses of carotene in field-cured alfalfa hay may be 90 per cent or greater. Half to three quarters of the carotene remaining in the cured hay may be lost during six months' storage of the hay. Thus, field-cured hay stored for six months or longer may contain less than 5 per cent of the carotene content of the original, uncut, fresh green plant. Hay that has been artificially cured in a hay drier has a much higher carotene content than field- or sun-cured hay. Generally, the degree of greenness of stored hay is a fair index of its carotene content. The carotene of alfalfa hay is more available to horses than that of grass hay. Among the grains, only corn contains carotene, but the amounts in corn are only about one tenth that of good roughage.

VITAMIN A REQUIREMENTS

Horses require about 25 IU of vitamin A per kg of body weight for maintenance, and 50 IU per kg for pregnancy and lactation. This translates to about 4 to 5 mg of carotene per kg of feed. The carotene content of some feeds is shown in Table 1.

The NRC presently suggests that young horses require 40 IU of vitamin A per kg of body weight but recent research indicates that two to four times this amount may be needed for growing horses. The authors of the research caution against levels of vitamin A intake over five times the current NRC recommendation.

TABLE 1. VITAMIN CONTENT OF SOME COMMON HORSE FEEDS

	Carotene	Thiamine	Riboflavin	Vitamin E
	mg/kg			
Alfalfa hay	26	3	11	90
Alfalfa meal	131	4	14	135
Barley	1	5	2	18
Red clover hay	20	2	18	60
Corn	3	2	2	26
Linseed meal	0	9	3	18
Oats	0	7	2	18
Oat hay	15	3	5	12
Rye	1	3	2	17
Skimmed milk, dry	0	4	20	10
Soybean meal	0	6	3	2
Timothy hay	9	2	12	63
Wheat bran	3	7	5	13
Brewers yeast	0	100	40	2

These are approximate and average values. Many factors alter the vitamin content of feeds. The hays listed are sun cured. (Adapted from National Academy of Sciences: Nutrient Requirement of Horses, 4th ed. Washington, DC, National Academy of Sciences–National Research Council, 1978.)

VITAMIN A SUPPLEMENTATION

Horses that have not had access to green feeds for four to six months and that have been fed poorly cured or poorly stored hay may benefit from a vitamin A supplement. Feed sources of carotene include almost any green feed such as pasture or alfalfa meal. Supplemental, oral sources of vitamin A include fish liver oils such as shark, halibut, swordfish, and cod liver oils. Unfortunately, these sources vary greatly in stability, quality, and in vitamin A activity. Long-term oral vitamin A supplementation that exceeds the NRC recommendation of 25 IU of vitamin A per kg of body weight for maintenance, 40 IU per kg for growth, and 50 IU per kg for pregnancy and lactation should be avoided. A variety of commercially available parenteral vitamin A preparations are available.

Carotene has been suggested to have a specific function in reproduction. However, at present there is little evidence to support the use of carotene supplements for horses. If a source of vitamin A is needed, vitamin A palmitate is much more economical than carotene.

DIAGNOSIS OF VITAMIN A STATUS

Determination of vitamin A status may be done by measuring the total vitamin A content of blood serum or plasma or by measuring vitamin A alcohol (retinol) and vitamin A esters (retinyl esters) in plasma. A range of 20 to 175 gm of carotene per dl of plasma or serum has been considered normal for horses. Serum vitamin A levels of 8 gm per dl or less have been observed in experimental vitamin A deficiency in young horses. Young ponies fed approximately adequate amounts of vitamin A (12 gm per kg of body weight per day) had 27 ± 2 gm of total vitamin A per dl of plasma. Surveys in Michigan and Great Britain showed normal horses to have about 150 to 300 gm of retinol per dl of plasma. Ponies fed excess vitamin A had greater than 75 gm of total vitamin A per dl of plasma. Hepatic stores of vitamin A may sometimes maintain serum levels until deficiency is far advanced. Thus, serum vitamin A levels may be less reliable than is commonly thought for diagnosis of deficiency. Response of experimentally deficient animals to parenteral vitamin A administration is often prompt. The response may be used as an indication of vitamin A status.

VITAMIN A DEFICIENCY

Conditions resembling vitamin A deficiency have been reported in horses that have been fed poor quality feeds for long periods. In the past, military horses on long campaigns have often been affected owing to the difficulties in obtaining green feeds.

Marginal vitamin A deficiency has been produced in young ponies by diets low in carotene. Growth in height, weight, and heart girth of the ponies was impaired. The deficient ponies had decreased serum concentration of iron, albumin, cholesterol, and vitamin A.

Signs of experimental vitamin A deficiency in mature horses took as long as one to one and a half years to develop. The first signs were night blindness followed by corneal cloudiness and keratinization. Reproductive problems developed in some of the horses when the deficiency disease was far advanced. Problems in mares included inability to conceive and abortion. Stallions experienced loss of libido. The testes of affected stallions were soft and flabby with a decreased number of seminiferous tubules and an increase in interstitial cells. Foals born of vitamin A–deficient mares were weak and unable to nurse.

Signs of experimental vitamin A deficiency developed more rapidly in young horses fed semipurified diets that contained very little vitamin A. Signs included anorexia, lacrimation, polyuria, and convulsive seizures. The seizures were initiated by excitement. The horses in seizure fell and made paddling movements with the legs. Cerebrospinal fluid pressure in affected horses was elevated to 550 mm of saline.

VITAMIN A TOXICOSIS

Excess dietary vitamin A is stored in the liver, and the accumulated excess can be toxic. Prolonged excess intake may cause bone resorption with subsequent bony deformities, fragility, and fractures. Naturally occurring cases of excess vitamin A intake have not been reported in the horse. Experimental vitamin A intoxication has been produced in young ponies by feeding about 1000 times the level of vitamin A that is suggested as the requirement by the National Research Council (NRC). Vitamin A intoxication impaired the growth of the ponies in terms of gains in body weight, height at the withers, and heart girth. Plasma vitamin A was elevated in affected ponies.

TABLE 2. VITAMIN ALLOWANCES FOR HORSES

	Units/kg of Body Weight	Units/kg of Feed
Vitamin A (IU)		
Growth	40	1800
Pregnancy and lactation	50	2500
Maintenance	25	1500
Vitamin D (IU)	6	275
Vitamin E (mg)	0.4	15
Thiamine (mg)	0.04	3
Riboflavin (mg)	0.07	2

These are approximate amounts of vitamins that are thought to be adequate for growth of young horses or maintenance of mature horses. (Adapted from National Academy of Sciences: Nutrient Requirement of Horses, 4th ed. Washington, DC, National Academy of Sciences–National Research Council, 1978.)

VITAMIN D

Vitamin D facilitates the absorption of calcium and phosphorus from the intestine and the utilization of these minerals for bone formation. Metabolites of vitamin D have complex interrelationships with parathormone (p. 189) and calcitonin to regulate the concentration of blood calcium by means of intestinal absorption of calcium, resorption of calcium from bone, and urinary calcium excretion. Vitamin D is converted to 25-hydroxycholecalciferol in the liver. This substance is modified to 1,25-dihydrocholecalciferol—$1,25(OH)_2D_3$—in the kidney under the influence of parathyroid hormone. $1,25(OH)_2D_3$ is the most physiologically active form of vitamin D and acts to facilitate calcium absorption by stimulating the synthesis of intestinal calcium-binding protein (CaBP). CaBP actively transports calcium across the mucosal cells of the intestinal tract.

Sources of Vitamin D

There are two forms and sources of vitamin D. Ergosterol is found in plants and forms ergocalciferol or vitamin D_2 when the plant is cut and subjected to ultraviolet irradiation, as in the sun curing of hay. Growing plants, grains, and grain byproducts do not contain significant amounts of D_2, but sun-cured hay may contain 150 to 3000 IU per kg. Cholecalciferol or vitamin D_3 is found in animals and results from the ultraviolet irradiation of 7-dehydrocholesterol in the skin. Both vitamin D_2 and D_3 have similar value for many mammals and may do so for the horse as well.

Vitamin D Requirements

The current estimate of the dietary vitamin D requirement for horses is 6.6 IU per kg of body weight or about 3000 IU for a 450 kg horse. Horses normally obtain adequate amounts of vitamin D from exposure to sunlight and from sun-cured forages. Under most circumstances, there is little need for vitamin D supplements for horses. Vitamin D supplements that provide more than 6.6 IU of vitamin D per kg of body weight should be recommended with caution because of the danger of vitamin D intoxication. There is no evidence that supplemental vitamin D is of benefit to horses when the level of calcium and phosphorus in the diet is low or the ratio between them is not correct. Fish oils and fish meals are good sources of vitamin D_3. Irradiated yeast is a common and inexpensive source of vitamin D_2.

Vitamin D Deficiency

Deficiency of vitamin D results in rickets in young animals. The disease is basically a defect in the mineralization of newly formed bone. Bone so formed is weak, soft, and easily deformed. The ends of the long bones tend to enlarge, and the shafts of the bones tend to bend, resulting in the characteristically bowed limbs of rickets. Affected animals may have hypocalcemia, hypophosphatemia, and elevated alkaline phosphatase levels in serum. Well-documented cases of rickets in foals under natural conditions have not been described.

Vitamin D Toxicosis

Excess intake of vitamin D is toxic. Experimental work suggests that high intake of cholecalciferol (D_3) is more toxic than an equivalent intake of ergocalciferol (D_2). Horses fed 100 times the NRC recommended level of vitamin D became depressed, anorexic, lame, and developed hypercalcemia, hyperphosphatemia, and hyposthenuria and had elevated levels of vitamin D metabolites in blood serum. Affected horses died as a result of mineralization in the heart, great vessels, lungs, upper digestive tract, and costal musculature. In short-term studies horses fed 50 times the NRC recommended level of vitamin D did not show clinical signs but absorbed more calcium from the intestine than did control horses, suggesting that more serious toxic effects might develop with prolonged feeding of such a high level of vitamin D. Levels of vitamin D fed to pigs at 50 times the NRC recommended level produced detrimental effects on bone cells. The calcium content of the diet, the potency of the vitamin D preparations, age of the animals, and other factors may modify the toxicity of vitamin D.

A condition resembling vitamin D intoxication in horses results from ingestion of plants that contain compounds with potent vitamin D activity. These include *Trisetum flavescens* (yellow oat grass), a plant of the European Alps; *Solanum malocoxylon*, a South American relative of the potato; and *Cestrum diurnum* (day-blooming jessamine), an ornamental plant grown in the West Indies and recently introduced into the Southern United States. Horses intoxicated by ingestion of these plants lose weight, are lame, and have hypercalcemia. Widespread calcinosis is observed at postmortem examination.

VITAMIN E

Vitamin E is an antioxidant. It prevents peroxidation of the lipids of cell membranes and thus preserves the structural integrity of cells.

Signs of vitamin E deficiency vary greatly among species, but reproductive problems and muscular dystrophy are commonly seen. However, not all reproductive problems and muscular dystrophies are vitamin E–responsive. For example, white muscle disease of foals often responds to selenium but does not respond to vitamin E (alpha-tocopherol). There is only contradictory evidence of a relationship between vitamin E and some reproductive problems in the horse.

Sources of Vitamin E

Animal feeds are generally rich in vitamin E. Cereal grains, grain byproducts, green forage, and hay are excellent sources of vitamin E. On the other hand, the oil meals such as linseed or soybean oil meals often have very little vitamin E because the modern oil extraction process removes the vitamin. Because the vitamin is readily oxidized, rancidity, heating, grinding, pelletting, and long storage of feeds decrease the vitamin E content. Among the natural feedstuffs, alfalfa meal is a particularly rich source of vitamin E.

Alpha-tocopherol, which is the most potent form of vitamin E, is readily available as a synthetic product. One mg of alpha-tocopherol equals 1 IU of the vitamin.

Large doses of vitamin E have been used in attempts to treat barren mares, to improve racing performance, and to improve performance in endurance horses in uncontrolled studies. There is no evidence to indicate that large doses of vitamin E have value. Fortunately, vitamin E appears to be relatively nontoxic.

Vitamin E Deficiency

Experimental vitamin E deficiency has been produced in young horses fed a semipurified diet. Serum tocopherol levels in the deficient foals were about 120 µg per dl. The expected values in horses are 300 to 600 µg per dl. Other signs included increased erythrocyte fragility, elevated serum glutamic-oxaloacetic transaminase (SGOT), intermittent leukocytosis, and hemoglobinuria. Postmortem examination of deficient foals showed acute glomerular nephritis and dystrophic changes in the muscles of the right ventricle, the intercostal and other skeletal muscles, and muscles of the tongue. Deficient foals required 27 µg per kg of body weight of parenteral alpha-tocopherol or 233 µg per kg of body weight of oral tocopherol to maintain the stability of erythrocytes.

Degenerative myelopathy in captive Mongolian wild horses (*Equus przewalskii*) was associated with extremely low plasma alpha-tocopherol concentration. The myelopathy was thought to be due to vitamin E deficiency.

VITAMIN K

Vitamin K is involved in synthesis of prothrombin in the liver and thus is important in blood coagulation.

All green, leafy feeds such as hay or pasture are rich sources of vitamin K.

Deficiency of vitamin K occurs in birds and results in hemorrhagic disease. Vitamin K deficiency may result in mammals in cases of biliary dysfunction because bile is necessary for the intestinal absorption of vitamin K and other fat-soluble vitamins. However, vitamin K is synthesized in large amounts by the intestinal microflora of many species. It is assumed that this is so in horses as well. Clear-cut, well-defined cases of deficiency have not been reported in the horse.

Parenteral administration of greater than 2 mg per kg of body weight of synthetic vitamin K_3 (menadione sodium bisulfate) induced renal toxicosis in healthy race horses that had been given vitamin K_3 as empiric therapy for exercise-induced pulmonary hemorrhage. Renal disease was subsequently induced experimentally in horses with similar doses of vitamin K_3. Clinical signs in affected horses include renal colic, hematuria, azotemia, and electrolyte abnormalities.

VITAMIN C

Ascorbic acid or vitamin C is the antiscorbutic factor. All species appear to require vitamin C in metabolism, but only humans, guinea pigs, subhuman primates, and some bats, birds, and fish have a dietary requirement for vitamin C. These species lack the enzyme necessary for the synthesis of vitamin C from simple sugars. The horse is among the species that are able to synthesize ascorbic acid in the liver.

Vitamin C is important in the hydroxylation of proline and lysine to hydroxyproline and hydroxylysine during collagen synthesis. Deficiency of the vitamin impairs the synthesis of collagen. Many of the signs of scurvy are related to this metabolic defect. In humans these include altered capillary integrity, sore, spongy gums, loosening of the teeth, subcutaneous hemorrhages, edema, joint pain, and anorexia. Plasma ascorbic acid values in human scurvy may fall to 0.05 mg per dl from a normal level of 0.5 to 1.2 mg per dl. Horses fed diets that were free of ascorbic acid for up to six months maintained their whole blood and plasma ascorbic acid levels at the same levels as horses fed normal diets. The horses also excreted as much ascorbic acid in urine as horses fed diets containing ascorbic acid. These findings indicate that the horse is able to synthesize ascorbic acid in the dietary absence of the vitamin. The excess that is synthesized in the tissues is excreted in urine. Whole blood ascorbic acid in horses ranged from 0.35 to 0.48 mg per dl and plasma levels from 0.32 to 0.40 mg per dl. Others have found serum ascorbic acid levels in horses to range from 0.5 to 0.7 mg per dl and to be unaffected by time of day, season of the year, or state of training. There was little difference between the sexes.

Large doses of vitamin C have been used in treatment of reproductive problems in the horse. This application needs controlled study.

THIAMINE

Thiamine serves as a coenzyme in the oxidative decarboxylation of pyruvate to acetate in cellular metabolism.

THIAMINE DEFICIENCY

A deficiency of thiamine results in accumulation of pyruvic and lactic acids in tissues. Thiamine deficiency has characteristic signs in some species, and the deficiency has been given special names such as beriberi in humans, Chastek paralysis in foxes, and polyneuritis in birds. Deficiency results in a wide range of signs, including loss of appetite, weight loss, reduced growth rate, peripheral and central nervous system signs, bradycardia, muscular weakness, and twitching.

Thiamine deficiency has been studied experimentally in horses by feeding diets containing little or no thiamine or by inducing the deficiency by means of thiamine antimetabolites. Biochemical changes that can be observed before clinical signs develop include hypoglycemia and elevated blood pyruvic acid concentration. As the deficiency progressed, affected experimental horses showed bradycardia, dropped heartbeats, ataxia, muscular fasciculations, and periodic hypothermia of the hooves, ears, and muzzle. Some horses lost weight, developed diarrhea, or became blind. Gait changes were among the most prominent clinical signs of induced thiamine deficiency. Weakness in the hindquarters caused swaying. A slow, shuffling gait was necessary to maintain balance. The forelegs often crossed when the horse walked in a circle. Backing was difficult and often ended in a dog-sitting position.

Thiamine deficiency results in many changes in clinical biochemistry. Among the more specific changes are increased blood concentration of pyruvate and an increased thiamine pyrophosphate (TPP) effect. Sorbitol dehydrogenase (SDH) and creatine phosphokinase (CPK) are elevated in serum. In addition to these biochemical changes, blood thiamine levels may be useful in estimating thiamine status.

THIAMINE REQUIREMENTS AND SUPPLEMENTATION

The thiamine requirement of the horse has been estimated to be 3 mg per kg of diet or about 15 to 20 mg for the maintenance of a mature horse. Horses working vigorously may require additional thiamine. Most horse feeds contain liberal amounts of thiamine. Grains and grain byproducts are very good sources. Thiamine tends to be lost during the sun curing of hay. Among the natural feedstuffs, brewers' yeast is an exceptionally good source of thiamine.

ANTITHIAMINE FACTORS

There are many antimetabolites of thiamine. These include thiaminase, which occurs in bracken fern (*Pteridium aquilinum*) and horsetail (*Equisetum arvense*). Other antithiamine factors include the coccidiostat amprolium, caffeic acid, and substances in cotton seed. Increased intake of dietary thiamine can often be used to offset the effects of these antithiamine substances.

RIBOFLAVIN

Riboflavin serves as part of many enzyme systems. Some of the prominent and important signs of human riboflavin deficiency include photophobia, corneal vascularization, conjunctivitis, and lacrimation. These signs bear some resemblance to periodic ophthalmia of horses. However, attempts to treat horses affected with periodic ophthalmia with riboflavin supplementation have not been successful.

The riboflavin requirement of horses is estimated to be about 2.2 mg per kg of feed. Leafy feeds such as hay are good sources. Alfalfa is a very good source. Yeast is a very rich source that can be used as a natural supplement. Cereal grains and byproducts are not good sources of riboflavin.

VITAMIN B$_{12}$

Vitamin B$_{12}$ is a generic term used for a group of compounds that have similar functions. The vitamin is a metabolic essential in all species that have been studied. Some species, such as humans, require a dietary source, while others, such as ruminants and probably horses, synthesize sufficient vitamin B$_{12}$ in the digestive tract. The large intestine of the horse contains microorganisms that synthesize B$_{12}$, and the concentration of B$_{12}$ increases as digesta moves down the intestinal tract. Cobalt is the limiting factor for vitamin B$_{12}$ synthesis by ruminal microflora. This is probably true for the large intestinal microflora in the horse as well.

Vitamin B$_{12}$ is necessary for the metabolism of propionic acid, an important product of large intestinal fermentation in the horse. Experimental attempts to produce vitamin B$_{12}$ deficiency in the horse have not been successful. Excretion of large

TABLE 3. SUMMARY OF VITAMIN FUNCTIONS, DEFICIENCY SIGNS, AND FEED SOURCES

Vitamin	Some Functions	Some Deficiency Signs	Good Feed Sources	Poor Feed Sources
Vitamin A	Stability of lysosomal and other cell membranes; growth and development of epithelial cells; growth, development, and remodeling of bone; vision; dark adaptation; maintenance of visual purple	Night blindness; corneal cloudiness, keratinization; impaired growth; reproductive problems; inability to conceive; abortion; loss of libido in the male; testicular degeneration; convulsions; elevated cerebrospinal fluid pressure; decreased tissue and serum vitamin A concentration	Provitamin A is abundant in all green feeds; good quality, well-cured hay, especially alfalfa	All grains; poorly cured hays and those subjected to long storage in poor conditions
Vitamin D	Synthesis of intestinal calcium binding protein (CaBP); absorption of dietary calcium and phosphorus; resorption of calcium from bone; control of urinary calcium excretion	Skeletal disease; defective mineralization of newly formed bone, bone deformities; impaired growth; hypocalcemia; hypophosphatemia; elevated serum alkaline phosphatase	Sun-cured hay; vitamin D_3 formed in the skin of animals exposed to sunlight; fish oils; fish meal; irradiated yeast	Grains and grain byproducts
Vitamin E	Antioxidant in tissues: prevents peroxidation of lipids of cell membranes; cofactor in synthesis of ascorbic acid	Decreased serum tocopherol concentration; increased red blood cell fragility; elevated serum glutamic-oxaloacetic transaminase (SGOT) levels; muscular dystrophy	Grains; grain byproducts; green forages; hay	Solvent-extracted oil, meals
Vitamin K	Synthesis of blood clotting factors	Hemorrhagic disease in species that require the vitamin	All green feeds	
Thiamine	Serves as the coenzyme cocarboxylase for the enzymatic decarboxylation of α-ketoacids in energy metabolism	Accumulation of pyruvic and lactic acids in tissues; loss of appetite; weight loss; impaired growth; bradycardia; peripheral and central nervous system disturbances; incoordination, weakness in hindquarters, muscular weakness and twitching; hypoglycemia; elevated blood pyruvate; increased thiamine pyrophosphate effect; elevated sorbitol dehydrogenase and creatine in serum	Most horse feeds, especially grains and grain byproducts; brewers' yeast	Poorly cured hay
Riboflavin	Serves as a coenzyme (flavin mononucleotide—FMN—and flavin adenine dinucleotide—FAD) in many enzyme systems	Impaired growth and feed efficiency; photophobia; corneal vascularization; conjunctivitis; lacrimation	Leafy feeds, especially alfalfa, yeast	Cereal grains and byproducts
B_{12}	Coenzyme in several enzyme systems; involved in metabolism of propionic acid in ruminants	Deficiency signs have not been described in horses.	The vitamin is probably synthesized in adequate amounts in the tissues of the horse.	
Ascorbic acid	Important in collagen synthesis in the hydroxylation of proline and lysine to hydroxyproline and hydroxylysine	Deficiency of vitamin C has not been described in the horse.	The vitamin is synthesized in the tissues of the horse.	

amounts of B_{12} in feces and urine has suggested that the horse does not have a dietary requirement for the vitamin under normal circumstances. Excretion of B_{12} in feces has been found to be 0.5 mg per day and in urine to be 0.007 mg per day. This is several thousand times greater than the urinary excretion in humans and the fecal excretion of the vitamin in cattle. Serum vitamin B_{12} values have been found to be 6 to 7 µg per ml in the horse.

OTHER B VITAMINS

Other B vitamins and related compounds are known to be dietary essentials for one or more species. Among these are niacin, pantothenic acid, pyridoxine, biotin, choline, folic acid, and inositol. It is assumed that these substances are required by the horse as metabolic essentials, but it is not known if they are required in the diet of the horse. Feeds that are commonly fed to horses tend to be good sources of these compounds, and many of these and other B vitamins are synthesized in the lower bowel of the horse. Nevertheless, these and other substances are frequently added to vitamin premixes and to vitamin supplements for horses. The value of such supplements is not known.

Supplemental Readings

Cunha, T. J.: Horse Feeding and Nutrition. New York, Academic Press, 1980.

Maynard, L. A., Loosli, J. K., Hintz, H. F., and Warner, R. G.: Animal Nutrition, 7th ed. New York, McGraw-Hill Book Co., 1979.

National Academy of Sciences: Nutrient Requirement of Horses, 4th ed. Washington, DC, National Academy of Sciences–National Research Council, 1978.

Swenson, M. J. (ed.): Dukes' Physiology of Domestic Animals, 9th ed. Ithaca, NY, Comstock Publishing Associates of Cornell University Press, 1977.

Underwood, E. J.: Trace Elements in Human and Animal Nutrition, 4th ed. New York, Academic Press, 1977.

Feeding Programs

Harold F. Hintz, ITHACA, NEW YORK

The following section outlines feeding programs for the mature horse at maintenance, the working horse, the brood mare, the stallion, and growing horses. Sample rations are presented here and in the next section, but many different combinations of feedstuffs can be fed satisfactorily to horses, and of course there are differences of opinion as to the best methods of providing the nutrients. The sample rations were selected to reflect regional differences in relative availability of feedstuffs and to reflect differences in opinions of various authorities.

HOW MUCH HAY?

Most feeding programs are based on hay or pasture. How much hay *must* a horse be fed? The answer of course, is none. Hay is not essential. Fiber is essential, but many feedstuffs, for example, beet pulp, peanut hulls, or citrus pulp, can provide fiber. Nevertheless, when horses do not have access to pasture, the feeding of good-quality hay greatly simplifies ration formulation and is usually one of the easiest methods of providing needed nutrients. Hay intake is usually equivalent to 1 to 2 per cent of body weight.

MATURE HORSES

The feeding program for maintenance of the average mature horse can be very simple. Good quality hay consumed at a rate of 1½ to 1⅔ kg of hay per 100 kg of body weight, water, and trace mineralized salt fed free choice should supply all the needed nutrients. Additional mineral supplements may be needed if the hay was grown on soil lacking in minerals such as selenium, copper, or phosphorus. If the climate is harsh, energy requirements should be increased, and some grain will be needed. The preceding recommendation also assumes reasonable parasite control and no dental problems. Some highly nervous horses may require additional energy.

Merits of legume and grass hays were discussed on page 389. Average grass hay will provide the 8 per cent protein, 0.30 per cent calcium, and 0.20 per cent phosphorus needed by the mature horse. Legume hay will provide much more protein and calcium than needed. The excess is not likely to be harmful but could be expensive.

WORKING HORSES

One of the primary concerns in the development of working horse rations is energy intake, and of course energy need depends on the amount and type of energy expenditure. Horses used in equitation classes may be ridden several hours per day yet may not require a great deal of energy because the work is not intensive. Equitation horses at Cornell working two to three hours per day maintained weight when fed 8 kg of hay and 3 kg of oats. On the other hand, racehorses at the track work fewer hours but may require 7 to 10 kg of hay and 8 to 10 kg of grain daily.

Thus, it is difficult to provide simple guidelines on the energy intake of working horses. The values in Table 1 provide some information that can be used as starting points in the feeding of working horses, but the body condition of the horse is the best guide, and energy should be regulated accordingly (p. 387).

The protein requirement of the horse is not greatly increased by work. The nitrogen lost in sweat is easily compensated for by the increased intake of the total ration. High levels of protein (24 per cent) were neither beneficial nor harmful to horses ridden 50 miles per day at a rate of 9 miles per hour. However, the excess protein may increase the water requirement and thus may be detrimental if water availability is limited. Excess protein is also expensive. The effect of excess protein feeding on the performance of working horses requires further study. Some reports have suggested that the excess protein can increase heat production and decrease performance but no effects were found in other studies. There is no doubt that levels of protein greatly above the requirement will increase the water requirement because water is needed to excrete the additional nitrogen. Energy efficiency will be decreased because protein is not utilized as efficiently as carbohydrate for energy.

Although amino acids are often ingredients of supplements or injections given to performance horses, we are not aware of any controlled studies on their benefits, assuming the horse is fed a balanced diet.

Working increases the mineral requirements because of the losses in sweat, but, as with protein, if the diet contains a percentage of minerals adequate for maintenance, the horse will in most cases obtain additional minerals when eating to meet energy needs. There are exceptions, however. Electrolyte losses may be of particular concern in horses that sweat profusely, such as endurance horses or three-day event horses. Synchronous diaphragmatic flut-

ter (thumps) has been related to low serum Ca and K levels in endurance horses. Lewis suggested that electrolytes lost by endurance horses could be replaced by giving the horse 2 oz (57 gm) of three parts "lite" salt plus 1 part limestone just before an endurance race, at each watering during the race (which, preferably, will not be more than every two hours), after the race, and twice on the day following.

"Lite" salt is one-half sodium chloride, and one-half potassium chloride. Lewis suggested the electrolyte mixture could be added to a few ounces of water or molasses and squirted into the back of the horse's mouth, or it may be added to the feed. According to Lewis two ounces of the mixture in one gallon (15 gm/L) of water provides 50 mM of sodium and potassium, 100 mM of chloride, and 20 to 25 mM of calcium, and has an osmolality of 200 to 250 mOsm/L. He said that electrolytes should not be added to the drinking water, as doing so can decrease water consumption.

As energy intake increases, the requirement for B vitamins increases because the vitamins are co-factors necessary for energy utilization. Reports have suggested that some racehorses have a marginal intake of thiamine, a sign of which is anorexia.

BROOD MARES

Brood mares can be divided into three categories: open mares, pregnant mares, and lactating mares. Energy intake is often suggested to influence breeding performance. Underfeeding of the filly could delay the onset of first heat. Several studies have suggested that the mares gaining weight (flushed) during breeding season have increased chances of conception, but body condition at breeding time may be more important than flushing. Studies at Texas A & M indicated that Quarterhorse mares that were thin at foaling and then fed to reduce weight during the first 90 days after foaling were unlikely to conceive again. Thin mares fed to gain or maintain weight had a higher conception rate. But mares kept in good to fat condition also had high conception rates and did not respond to flushing.

Obesity can cause problems, but as Roberts pointed out, it is difficult to determine if some mares are barren because they are fat or fat because they are barren. If they do not have foals, their energy requirements are greatly reduced, and they are much more likely to gain weight.

The nutrient requirements of mares are summarized in Table 2. In the following text, the requirements of the 450 kg mare (open, pregnant, or lactating) will be used to illustrate the effect of physiologic condition on nutrient requirements.

TABLE 1. EXAMPLES OF FEED INTAKE OF HORSES AT WORK

Description of Work	Hay (Kg/Day)	Grain (Kg/Day)
Equitation classes	8–10	2–3
Standardbreds at the track	9–10	7–9
Thoroughbreds at the track	7–9	6–8
Polo ponies (indoor)	8–10	3–6
Draft horses—light work	7–8	2–3
(600 kg) —medium work	6–7	5–6
—heavy work	6–7	7–9

TABLE 2. NUTRIENT CONCENTRATION IN DIETS FOR MARES (EXPRESSED ON 90% DRY MATTER BASIS)

Mare	Digestible Energy (Mcal/kg diet)	Crude Protein (%)	Ca (%)	P (%)
Open	2.0	7.7	0.30	0.20
Pregnant (last 90 days)	2.3	10.0	0.45	0.30
Lactating (early)	2.6	12.5	0.45	0.30
Lactating (late)	2.3	11.0	0.40	0.25

An open mare weighing 450 kg needs 15 Mcal digestible energy. If the hay contains 2.15 Mcal per kg, the mare would need to eat 7 kg of hay daily or approximately 1.5 kg of hay per 100 kg of body weight. Of course, more than 7 kg of hay would need to be fed because some hay is usually wasted.

The National Research Council recommends that the ration of the open mare contain at least 7.7 per cent protein. Most hays and grains of average or greater quality contain at least 8 per cent protein. Thus, protein supplements are not usually needed by the open mare.

The ration of the open mare should contain at least 0.3 per cent calcium and 0.2 per cent phosphorus. As discussed earlier (p. 396), the mineral content of hay varies according to many factors, such as species, soil type, and age of the plant at harvest. Good-quality grass hay could be expected to contain at least 0.35 per cent calcium and 0.2 per cent phosphorus; legumes such as alfalfa may contain 1 to 1.5 per cent calcium and 0.2 to 0.25 per cent phosphorus. Thus, calcium and phosphorus problems would not be expected when the open mare is fed hay of reasonable quality.

Crops grown in many parts of the United States, such as the Northeast, eastern coast, and Northwest, contain low levels of selenium. It has been suggested that feeding rations with low levels of selenium may cause decreased fertility. The requirement for selenium has been estimated to be 0.1 ppm (p. 402).

One study suggested that high levels of vitamins A and E may improve reproductive performance of mares, but in another study no benefit of vitamin supplementation was found. The role of carotene was discussed earlier (p. 406). Of course, the basic ration must contain concentrations of protein, minerals, and vitamins that are adequate for maintenance.

The pregnant mare early in the gestation period does not have nutrient requirements greatly different from those of the open mare. During the last 90 days of gestation, the fetus is developing rapidly, and the mare's needs are increased. The National Research Council suggests that the energy requirement of the mare during the period of rapid fetal growth is about 12 per cent greater than for maintenance.

During the last 90 days of gestation, about 17 Mcal of digestible energy would be needed by the 450 kg mare. That amount of energy could be supplied by 5.5 kg of hay and 1.5 kg of grain daily.

The pregnant mare's need of protein, as for energy, is increased significantly over that of maintenance only during the last 90 days of gestation. The National Research Council estimates that at least 10 per cent protein is needed then. Even though the increase is 20 per cent above maintenance, the actual amount needed is not really high. Mares fed legume hays such as alfalfa or clover (usually 11 to 15 per cent protein) and grain such as oats (12 per cent protein) or corn (9 per cent protein) would not need a protein supplement. When a grass hay such as late-cut timothy hay is fed, a protein supplement may be needed. For example, if grass hay contains only 8 per cent protein and 5.5 kg of the hay and 1.5 kg of grain are fed, the grain mixture should contain about 16 per cent protein. Grain mixtures calculated to contain 16 per cent protein are shown in Table 3.

The calcium and phosphorus requirements, when expressed as a percentage of the diet, are similar for pregnant and lactating mares. Of course, total intake is much greater for the lactating mare because she eats more feed.

The pregnant or lactating mare needs 0.45 per cent calcium and 0.30 per cent phosphorus in the ration. Thus, the pregnant or lactating mare fed grass hay and grain would need a mineral supplement. When grass hay is fed, the grain mixture should contain at least 0.55 per cent calcium. The addition of 1 per cent dicalcium phosphate and 1 per cent limestone to the grain mixture usually supplies adequate levels of calcium and phosphorus. When legume hay is fed, a calcium supplement is usually not needed.

TABLE 3. EXAMPLES OF GRAIN MIXTURES (A, B, AND C) CALCULATED TO CONTAIN 12 OR 16% PROTEIN*

Ingredient	12% A	12% B	12% C	16% A	16% B	16% C
Corn	28	46	—	26	39	—
Oats	60	40	45	50	35	39
Barley	—	—	45	—	—	39
Soybean meal	6	8	4	18	20	16
Molasses	6	6	6	6	6	6

*Based on National Research Council (1978) reports of feed analysis

The energy needs of the lactating mare are a function of the level of milk production. The amount of milk produced varies greatly among mares, but the National Research Council states that some mares will produce amounts of milk equivalent to 2 to 3 per cent of their body weight during early lactation (1 to 12 weeks) and late lactation (13 to 24 weeks), respectively. A 450 kg mare milking at these levels would require about 70 per cent more energy during early lactation than for maintenance and about 48 per cent more energy during late lactation than for maintenance. A 450 kg mare producing 13.5 kg of milk would need almost 26 Mcal of digestible energy (about 6 kg of hay and 4.5 kg of grain daily). A mare producing 9 kg of milk would need about 22 Mcal of digestible energy (4.5 kg of hay and 3.5 kg of grain).

The lactating mare needs about 12.5 per cent protein in her ration. If 6 kg of alfalfa hay containing 14 per cent protein was fed, the 4.5 kg of grain mixture would need to contain about 11 per cent protein. When feeding oats containing 12 per cent protein and alfalfa hay, no protein supplement is needed, but if corn containing 9 per cent protein is fed, a protein supplement may be necessary. A grain ration containing 12 per cent protein would be reasonable to ensure adequate protein intake. Grain mixtures containing 12 per cent protein are shown in Table 3.

If the lactating mare is fed a hay containing 9 per cent protein, the grain mixture should contain 16 per cent protein (see Table 3).

Note that soybean meal is used as the protein in all the mixtures shown in Table 3. Soybean meal is recommended because it is of higher protein quality (better array of essential amino acids) than other vegetable proteins such as cottonseed meal.

Many horse owners give brood mares a supplement containing milk products or milk substitutes. Such products are usually excellent sources of amino acids and often of vitamins and minerals. Little benefit should be expected from the addition of such products to the mare's ration when the ration is adequately balanced.

The calcium and phosphorus requirements were discussed with those of the pregnant mare.

Estimates of hay and grain needed for various classes of mares are summarized in Table 4. Remember that many factors influence the energy requirement. Cold environment, parasites, or dental problems are examples of factors that can increase the energy needs. The total digestible nutrient (TDN) content of feeds varies. For example, the TDN content of some hays is different from that of others, but the estimates in Table 4 can be used as starting points. If the mare is too fat, the amount of feed, particularly that of grain, should be decreased.

TABLE 4. ESTIMATES OF DAILY FEED REQUIREMENTS OF MARES*

Mare	Feed†	Weight of Mare (Kg)				
		400	*450*	*500*	*550*	*600*
Open	Hay (kg)	6.4	6.9	7.4	8.0	8.6
Pregnant	Hay (kg)	5.0	5.4	5.9	6.3	6.6
	Grain (kg)	1.6	1.7	1.8	1.9	2.0
Lactating	Hay (kg)	4.5	5.0	5.4	5.8	6.1
(early)	Grain (kg)	4.0	4.5	5.0	5.5	5.9
Lactating	Hay (kg)	4.0	4.5	5.0	5.5	5.9
(late)	Grain (kg)	3.4	3.6	4.0	4.6	4.9

*Based on National Research Council (1978) report
†Values for hay and grain are based on representative analyses. Actual intake that is needed will depend on several factors such as quality of feed, environment, and individual status of the mare.

STALLIONS

Little research has been conducted on the effect of nutrition on stallion performance. Some stallion managers claim excess protein is detrimental to the proper production of sperm. However, there is no evidence to support such a theory, nor is there any evidence to suggest that the protein requirement of the stallion is significantly greater than for maintenance.

Ration formulation for the stallion is simple. Feed the same grain the mare receives plus good-quality hay, water, and trace mineralized salt free choice. A problem on many farms may be the amount of feed given. Stallions that are slightly to moderately overweight probably do not have impaired function, but it would seem prudent to attempt to keep stallions in good, trim condition—not too lean or too fat. Excessive fat has been shown to impair reproduction in other species. Furthermore, stallions that receive limited exercise and are chronically overfed are prime candidates for founder. In fact, several outstanding stallions have had their careers shortened because of founder.

GROWING ANIMALS

NEWBORN FOALS

Mare colostrum contains about five times the protein concentration and twice the energy concentration of mare milk. Furthermore, colostrum is an excellent source of vitamin A. Recent studies have demonstrated that foals deprived of colostrum have lower vitamin A stores. For example, when antibodies were provided by serum, the vitamin A intake was lower than when foals received colostrum. Therefore, it is recommended that supplemental vitamin A be given to foals deprived of colostrum. The requirement for foals is estimated to be about 4000 IU of vitamin A daily.

Foals that are much smaller at birth than normal foals may require additional care and may have difficulty nursing. Mares fed rations lacking in energy or protein or obese mares may have smaller foals than mares in good nutritional state. Although the heritability of birth weight is only 0.15 to 0.25, the size of the mare can greatly influence birth weight, presumably because of the environment and nutrition afforded to the fetus by the mare. That is, a large mare bred to a small stallion will probably have a larger foal than a small mare bred to a large stallion.

Dams younger than 8 years of age or older than 12 years of age are likely to have lighter, shorter foals than mares 8 to 12 years of age. The average colt is bigger than the average filly at birth. Foals born in May, June, or July are bigger at birth than foals born in January, February, or March.

ORPHAN FOALS

Orphans can be reared on nurse mares or even nurse goats. Cow's milk contains more fat and less sugar than mare's milk and should be modified if fed to foals. Many old-time recipes are available. For example, Morrison suggested one fourth pint of limewater and one teaspoonful of sugar be added to one pint of cow's milk and that the foal be fed about one half pint of the mixture every two hours for the first few days after birth. Fortunately, several commercial products such as Borden's Foal-Lac are now available, and they have been used successfully.

CREEP FEEDING

Creep feeding is often recommended because some mares do not produce adequate amounts of milk and because it is more efficient to feed the foal directly than feeding the mare to produce milk. It is also suggested that creep feeding allows the foals to grow faster and helps prevent setbacks at weaning. On the other hand, some authorities suggest that creep feeding may induce such rapid growth that the foals are predisposed to skeletal problems such as epiphysitis. Although there has been much speculation about the advantages and disadvantages of creep feeding and discussion of the pros and cons of rapid growth, few controlled studies have been conducted. In particular, much more research is needed to determine the effects of rate of growth on performance of the horse as a two-year-old and as a mature animal. Growth rate will be discussed in more detail in the section on the feeding of weanling foals.

The National Research Council recommends that creep rations contain 16 per cent protein, 0.8 per cent calcium, and 0.55 per cent phosphorus. The grain should be cracked, crimped, or rolled.

WEANLINGS

The weanling is much more susceptible than older horses to nutritional problems. The protein requirement, expressed as a percentage of the diet, is almost twice that of the mature horse at maintenance. The National Research Council estimates of the energy, protein, calcium, phosphorus, and vitamin A requirements of growing horses are shown in Table 5.

Of course, the requirements are dependent upon the desired rate of growth. The expected rate of growth (weight gain) is higher now than during the 1950s and before. For example, a 1978 NRC bulletin suggests that a six-month-old foal with an expected mature weight of 500 kg should gain about 0.8 kg per day. The 1949 bulletin suggests 0.6 kg per day. The 1978 bulletin indicates that a light horse should reach about 46 per cent of its mature weight at six months of age and 75 per cent of its mature weight at 12 months of age. The comparable values in the 1949 bulletin were 40 per cent and 56 per cent at six and 12 months, respectively.

The increased rate of gain requires careful nutritional considerations. For example, in 1951 Morrison suggested that good legume hay and oats would be satisfactory for weanlings. Such a diet might be expected to contain 13 per cent protein or less, which would not support the rate of gain expected by some owners. When protein is added to produce more rapid growth, the requirements for other nutrients are increased. When rapid growth is obtained but essential minerals are lacking, skeletal problems are likely to develop.

Problems Associated with Improper Nutrition of Growing Horses

The optimal growth rate of young horses varies with the type and use of the animal and the objectives of the owner. Several studies with other species have clearly demonstrated that longevity can be increased by feeding a balanced diet but at a level lower than that required for maximal growth rate. Studies with dogs and pigs indicate that young

TABLE 5. SUMMARY OF NUTRIENT CONCENTRATION NEEDED IN RATIONS OF GROWING HORSES*

	Digestible Energy (Mcal/kg diet)	Crude Protein (%)	Ca (%)	P (%)
Weanling (3 mos)	2.9	16	0.8	0.55
Weanling (6 mos)	2.8	14.5	0.6	0.45
Yearling (12 mos)	2.6	12	0.5	0.35
Long yearling (18 mos)	2.3	10	0.4	0.30

*90% dry matter basis

animals fed a highly palatable diet at high levels of intake may grow rapidly but develop a higher incidence of skeletal diseases such as osteochondrosis dissecans, hypertrophic osteodystrophy, enostosis, elbow dysplasia, and hip dysplasia. The conditions developed even though the diets were balanced according to present knowledge.

Overfeeding has long been claimed to cause problems in horses. Henry wrote that "liberal feeding must be counterbalanced by an abundance of outdoor exercise. In no other way can colts be ruined so surely and so permanently as by liberal feeding and close confinement." Henry recommended that colts 6 to 12 months of age be fed 1 to 1.4 kg of grain daily, which is considerably below most feeding standards of today. In 1968, Miller, a prominent breeder, trainer, and driver of Standardbreds, wrote: "Horsemen have preached for years that stock farms should market ready-to-race yearlings that are not 'hot-housed' and not stuffed with feed during the last few months before the sale. But it is also a fact that more owners and trainers, despite what their natural inclination might be, seem to prefer slick, stout yearlings that actually have been overfed. Apparently this is an occupational hazard of the yearling selection business and it is doubtful that it will ever change."

Stromberg reported an increasing incidence of osteochondrosis in young fast-growing horses. He postulated that a genetic predisposition is associated with rapid growth and excessively high energy feeding. Overfeeding also appears to be involved in the etiology of certain types of wobbles. Kronfeld suggested that overfeeding of genetically predisposed animals but not overfeeding per se might be responsible for skeletal disorders.

Epiphysitis. Epiphysitis has been claimed to be induced by overfeeding. This problem, characterized by abnormalities in the epiphyses of the long bones (particularly the distal epiphysis of the radius, metacarpus, tibia, and metatarsus) consists of enlargement and lipping of the physes, premature closure, and, frequently, metaphyseal osteosclerosis or osteomalacia.

Epiphysitis is perhaps most often seen when young animals are fed rations high in protein and energy and low in calcium, such as heavy concentrate feeding with grass hay as the main forage. However, even when calcium supplements are provided in these circumstances, the problem may still occur. Further studies are needed to define the relationship of diet to epiphysitis, but decreasing grain intake frequently seems to be of therapeutic value.

Contracted Tendons. The condition of "contracted tendons," generally affecting foals 4 to 12 months old, involving the superficial and/or the deep flexor tendons, can also be associated with overfeeding. However, further studies are needed to substantiate the role of nutrition in the development of contracted tendons. Evidence to support the hypothesis that the condition may be associated with undernutrition followed by overnutrition has been reported by Hintz et al. In this study, four of six foals weaned at four months of age and subsequently fed limited amounts of high-energy feed for four months developed a condition similar to "contracted tendons" within one to three months of being fed the diet free choice. None of the six control foals fed the same diet free choice from weaning developed the condition. Weight gains during the first four months for restricted and control foals were 0.23 kg per day and 0.85 kg per day, respectively, and during the second period 0.81 kg per day and 0.56 kg per day, respectively. Foals with restricted growth rates in their early months may require special consideration when growth-inhibiting factors are removed. If flexure abnormalities appear, measures to restrict growth rate may be helpful.

Enterotoxemia. Enterotoxemia may be caused by acute overfeeding, and although Diekie et al. claimed that "enterotoxemia in the foal occurs infrequently," Swerczek reported that the condition is one of the most important causes of mortality of young horses, accounting for the death of 28 of 935 foals necropsied at University of Kentucky from 1973 to 1975. The largest and most aggressive foals in group feeding situations are the most affected. The foals appeared healthy at feeding but were found dead shortly thereafter, often with no clinical signs, although flatulent colic and acute dyspnea were sometimes observed. Posterior ventral subcutaneous edema and emphysema were found at necropsy, and the gastrointestinal tract was filled with grain and was dilated from gas formation. The cortex of the kidneys was degenerative. It was concluded that the enterotoxemia was due to *Clostridium perfringens* Type D. As mentioned earlier, careful management is necessary to prevent acute overeating.

In summary, the optimal growth rate for young horses is not known, but the average light horse might be expected to obtain about 47 per cent, 67 per cent, and 80 per cent of mature weight by 6, 12, and 18 months, respectively. The average light horse obtains about 83 per cent, 91 per cent, and 95 per cent of mature height at the withers by 6, 12, and 18 months, respectively. Estimates of body weight at various ages for horses of various mature body weights are shown in Table 6.

EARLY WEANING

The average foal is now weaned at a younger age than in the past. Traditionally, many farm managers

TABLE 6. ESTIMATES OF BODY WEIGHT AT VARIOUS AGES FOR HORSES OF VARIOUS MATURE BODY WEIGHTS

Age (Months)	Mature Weight (Kg)					
	200	400	500	600	800	1000
2	60	105	130	155	150	210
4	85	150	180	220	250	315
6	110	185	230	275	340	420
8	125	220	275	320	400	500
10	140	245	310	360	450	565
12	150	270	335	400	500	630
14	160	290	360	435	540	670
16	165	305	380	460	580	730
18	170	320	400	480	620	780

weaned at six months of age or later. Weaning at four months or even two months is now common. Earlier weaning allows the mare to be returned to use sooner, makes more efficient use of feed, appears to cause less setback at weaning time, and may increase the growth rate of the foal. However, earlier weaning requires greater attention to the diet of the foal. A four-month-old foal given only oats and grass hay cannot be expected to grow and develop properly. The requirements for foals are shown in Table 5. Complete feeds, either pelleted or a mixture of chopped hay and grain, are useful for growing foals. Once the foals are adjusted to the

ration, the feed can be in front of the foals at all times without danger of overfeeding. The ratio of hay to grain in the mixture can be increased as the foal matures, thus preventing the animal from getting too much energy or becoming overweight. The complete feed makes the balancing of rations easier because the foals cannot sort the feed, and all foals in a group are eating the same percentage of hay. The complete feed may also save labor costs and works well with three-sided run-in shed arrangements. However, some long hay should be fed with complete feeds. Foals fed complete rations free choice may be expected to eat amounts equivalent to 3 per cent of their body weight. Some foals will consume even greater amounts. Estimates of daily feed requirements are shown in Table 7.

TABLE 7. ESTIMATES OF DAILY FEED REQUIREMENTS OF GROWING HORSES

Age of Foal (Mos)	Type of Feed	Expected Mature Weight (kg)		
		400	500	600
		Weight of feed (kg)*		
4	Hay	1.4	1.5	1.8
	Grain	3.0	3.5	4.2
6	Hay	1.6	1.8	1.9
	Grain	3.2	3.8	4.3
8	Hay	1.9	2.2	2.5
	Grain	3.4	4.1	4.7
12	Hay	2.7	3.2	3.7
	Grain	2.8	3.4	3.9
14	Hay	3.2	3.7	4.3
	Grain	2.7	3.3	3.7
18	Hay	3.7	4.3	4.9
	Grain	2.4	2.9	3.3

*Values may be used as initial guidelines. Amount of feed will vary according to desired rate of gain, quality of feed, individual status of the foal, and environmental conditions.

Supplemental Readings

Diekie, C. W., Klinkerman, D. L., and Petrie, R. J.: Enterotoxemia in two foals. J. Am. Vet. Med. Assoc., *173*:858, 1978.

Henry, W. A.: Feeds and Feeding. Madison, WI, published by author, 1901.

Hintz, H. F., Schryver, H. F., and Lowe, J. E.: Delayed growth response and limb conformation in young horses. Proc. Cornell Nutr. Conf., 94, 1976.

Hintz, H. F., Hintz, R. L., and Van Vleck, L. D.: Growth rate of Thoroughbreds. Effects of age of dam, year and month of birth and sex of foal. J. Anim. Sci., *48*:480, 1979.

Kronfeld, D.: Feeding practices on horse breeding farms. Proc. 24th Annu. Conv. Am. Assoc. Eq. Pract., 461, 1978.

Lewis, L.: Feeding and Care of the Horse. Philadelphia, Lea and Febiger, 1982.

Mayhew, I.: Spinal cord disease in the horse. Cornell Vet., *68*, Suppl. *6*:205, 1978.

Miller, D.: Feeding. *In* Harrison, J. C. (ed.): Care and Training of the Trotter and Pacer. Columbus, OH, United States Trotting Association, 1968.

Morrison, F. B.: Feeds and Feeding. Ithaca, NY, Morrison Pub. Co., 1951.

National Research Council. Nutrient Requirement of Horses. Washington, DC, National Academy of Sciences–National Research Council, 1978.

Owen, J. M.: Abnormal flexion of the corono-pedal joint or "contracted tendons" in unweaned foals. Equine Vet. J., *7*:40, 1975.

Roberts, S. J.: Veterinary Obstetrics and Genital Disease. Ithaca, NY, published by author, 1971.

Stromberg, B.: A review of the salient features of osteochondrosis in horses. Equine Vet. J., *11*:211, 1979.

Swerczek, T. W.: The etiology, pathology and pathogenesis of diseases of foals and weanlings. Proc. Soc. Theriogenol., 19, 1976.

Swerczek, T. W.: Experimentally induced toxicoinfectious botulism in horses and foals. Am. J. Vet. Res., *41*:348, 1980.

Swerczek, T. W., and Crowe, C. W.: Enterotoxemia in young horses due to *Clostridium perfringens* Type D. Chicago, Proc. 54th Conf. Res. Workers Anim. Dis., 1978.

Sample Rations and Commercial Feeds

Harold F. Hintz, ITHACA, NEW YORK

SAMPLE RATIONS

As stated earlier, many different combinations of feedstuffs can be fed satisfactorily to horses, and of course there are differences of opinion as to the best methods of providing the nutrients. Furthermore, local conditions such as availability and price of feedstuffs should influence formulation. Many companies also manufacture feeds specifically designed for various classes of horses.

It must be stressed, however, that the success of any feeding program depends on good management. Horses should be observed closely and frequently. Routine weighing (or estimating weight with tapes placed around the heart girth) is an excellent management aid, as even experienced horsemen can sometimes be fooled as to the extent of weight changes.

On many farms, a considerable amount of feed is wasted because of inadequate or poorly designed feeding equipment or because of carelessness. Also, many injuries to horses result because of feeding equipment that is not used properly or designed properly.

The results of surveys of feeding practices at four racetracks are shown in Table 1. In addition to hay and grains, almost all the trainers fed or injected vitamin and mineral supplements.

Rations for breeding animals are shown in Table 2. The rations vary from simple to complex. Unfortunately, the rations have not been compared with each other to determine which is best.

Rations for growing animals are shown in Tables 3 and 4. Amounts of feed were discussed in the article on feeding programs.

TABLE 2. EXAMPLES OF RATIONS SUGGESTED BY VARIOUS AUTHORITIES

Mares*	Gestation Per Cent by Weight	Lactation Per Cent by Weight
Oats	30	15
Corn or milo	10	10
Barley	12¼	26
Wheat bran	10	7
Soybean meal	11	13
Linseed meal	4	4
Alfalfa meal	10	7
Molasses	7	7
Dicalcium phosphate	2	1¼
Limestone	¾	¾
Salt	1	1
Vitamins	2	1

Lactating Mares (550 kg)†

1. Alfalfa hay (7.3 kg) and corn (2.7 kg)
2. Red clover hay (7.3 kg) and barley (1.3 kg), corn (1.3 kg)
3. Timothy hay (7.3 kg) and oats (1.3 kg), wheat bran (1.3 kg), soybean meal (0.45 kg) plus mineral supplement

Pregnant Mares‡

1. Grass-legume hay plus grain mixture containing 80 per cent oats and 20 per cent wheat bran; mineral mixture fed free choice
2. Grass-legume hay plus grain mixture containing 45 per cent barley, 45 per cent oats, and 10 per cent wheat bran; mineral mixture fed free choice

Pregnant or Lactating Mares§	Fed with Legume Hay (Per Cent)	Fed with Grass Hay (Per Cent)
Corn	43.0	38.0
Oats	40.5	35.5
Soybean meal	5.0	14.0
Molasses	6.0	6.0
Wheat bran	5.0	5.0
Dicalcium phosphate	0.5	0.5
Limestone	—	1.0

Fed with good-quality hay

*Cunha, T. J.: Horse Feeding and Nutrition. New York, Academic Press, 1980.

†Morrison, F. B.: Feeds and Feeding. Ithaca, NY, Morrison Pub. Co., 1951.

‡Ensminger, E.: Horses and Horsemanship, 5th ed. Davisville, IL, Interstate Pub. Co., 1977.

§Hintz, H. F.: Cornell University, unpublished information.

TABLE 1. SURVEY OF FEEDING PRACTICES AT FOUR RACE TRACKS

Track	Type	Average Weight of Horse (kg)	Hay* (kg)	Oats (kg)	Corn (kg)	Sweetfeed (kg)	Wheat Bran† (kg)
Roosevelt‡	Standardbred	475	8.8	4.4	0.5	1.8	0.2
Vernon Downs	Standardbred	452	8.3	4.5	0.5	1.6	0.2
Finger Lakes	Thoroughbred	489	6.6	6.2	—	1.0	0.5
Belmont	Thoroughbred	486	7.3	5.8	—	1.3	0.5

*Most trainers fed grass or grass-legume mixed hay. Ten percent fed alfalfa or clover hay or alfalfa cubes.

†Average of those trainers feeding wheat bran. Approximately 50 per cent of the trainers used wheat bran.

‡At least 10 trainers were surveyed at each track.

TABLE 3. EXAMPLES OF CREEP RATIONS

I*	Fed with Alfalfa Hay (Per Cent by Weight)	II†	Fed with Mixed Hay (Per Cent by Weight)
Cracked corn	38	Cracked corn	53
Crushed oats	38	Soybean meal	33
Molasses	6	Molasses	10
Soybean meal	17	Trace mineral salt	1
Dicalcium phosphate	1	Limestone	1
		Dicalcium phosphate	1
		Brewers' yeast	0.5
		Vitamin supplement	0.5

*Cornell University
†William Tyznik, Ohio State University

COMMERCIAL FEEDS

The sales of commercial horse feeds have increased greatly since the 1960s. It has been suggested that most modern horse owners have little experience in formulating rations and are not interested in mixing their own feed. Many suburban horse owners are much more comfortable buying a complete feed for their horses, just as they would buy one for their cats or dogs. Consequently, the sales of complete pelleted feeds have greatly increased.

Pellets have several advantages: decreased feed waste, economy of space in storage and transportation, more attractive horses because of loss of hay belly, more opportunities for mechanization of feeding, less labor, prevention of sorting of feed by the horse, and reduced dust. Complete pelleted diets also permit the use of properly supplemented byproducts, feeds, or ingredients that might not normally be accepted by horses.

The disadvantages of pellets include the cost of pelleting and increased incidence of vices such as wood chewing, tail chewing, and cribbing. The vices are probably due to boredom or perhaps simply a desire to chew. If complete pelleted rations are fed, some hay should be provided as a source of roughage. Some veterinarians have also reported that the feeding of pellets increases the incidence of choke. We have not observed this problem in our horses and ponies fed complete rations.

Many companies manufacture horse feeds, and most companies have different formulations for various classes of horses to give the horse owner a wide variety from which to select. Factors to consider when selecting feed include cost, nutrient content, quality control, reliability of the manufacturer, and services provided by the manufacturer. The feed tag should list the minimal amount of crude protein and crude fat and the maximal amount of fiber. Some companies also list the Ca and P content. Even if not listed, the latter information

TABLE 4. EXAMPLES OF RATIONS FOR WEANLINGS

I*	Fed with Alfalfa Hay (Per Cent by Weight)	Fed with Grass Hay (Per Cent by Weight)	II†	Per Cent
Corn	45	39	Oats	25.0
Oats	36	27	Corn or barley	30.8
Soybean meal	12	25	Milo or corn	15.0
Molasses	6	6	Soybean meal	15.0
Limestone	—	2	Dehydrated alfalfa meal	5.0
Dicalcium phosphate	1	1	Molasses	5.0
			Vitamin supplement	0.7
			Dicalcium phosphate	2.0
			Limestone	0.5
			Salt	1.0

Barley can replace corn and oats; steamed bone meal or a similar Ca-P supplement can replace dicalcium phosphate. Trace mineralized salt is given free choice. If hay is of poor quality, a vitamin supplement should also be fed.
*Hintz, H. F.: Cornell University, unpublished information.
†Cunha, T. J.: Horse Feeding and Nutrition. New York, Academic Press, 1980.

TABLE 5. ESTIMATES OF MINIMUM NUTRIENT CONTENT NEEDED IN COMMERCIAL FEEDS IN ORDER TO MEET NUTRIENT REQUIREMENTS FOR VARIOUS CLASSES OF HORSES

Class of Horse	Nutrient (Per Cent by Weight)	Type of Forage Feed			
		Legume Hay	Mixed Hay	Grass Hay	None*
Weanlings	Crude protein†	14.5	16	18	14.5
	Calcium	0.4‡	0.6	0.9	0.70
	Phosphorus	0.6	0.6	0.6	0.45
Yearlings	Crude protein	10	12	14	12
Mares	Calcium	0.1‡	0.3‡	0.7	0.50
Late gestation and lactation	Phosphorus	0.5	0.5	0.5	0.35
Mature horses	Crude protein	8	8	10	10
	Calcium	—§	—§	0.2‡	0.30
	Phosphorus	0.3	0.3	0.3	0.25

*Feeding small amounts of hay even when using complete feeds will help alleviate such vices as wood chewing.

†The protein should be of good quality; that is, it should supply the essential amino acids. Soybean meal, milk proteins, and meat meal are examples of reasonable protein sources.

‡Many mixtures will contain calcium levels greater than 0.4 per cent, but the extra calcium is not harmful when an adequate level of phosphorus is provided.

§The forage will normally provide all the calcium needed.

should be available from the dealer. Estimates of the amount of nutrients required in commercial feeds for various situations are shown in Table 5. The feed tag may also list ingredients, but most tags now list ingredients according to groups of feeds and not individual feeds. The tag may say cereal grain instead of corn or plant protein instead of soybean meal. The wording is more general so that companies can take advantage of low-cost formulas and thereby minimize feed cost. Sometimes the basic ingredients in any given brand of feed may vary greatly among shipments. Drastic changes in ingredient quality may influence the feed intake of horses.

Supplemental Readings

Cunha, T. J.: Horse Feeding and Nutrition. New York, Academic Press, 1980.

Ensminger, E.: Horses and Horsemanship, 5th ed. Davisville, IL, Interstate Pub. Co., 1977.

Morrison, F. B.: Feeds and Feeding. Ithaca, NY, Morrison Pub. Co., 1951.

Nutrition of the Sick Horse

Jonathan M. Naylor, SASKATOON, SASKATCHEWAN, CANADA

David E. Freeman, KENNETT SQUARE, PENNSYLVANIA

Recent work in horses and extrapolation from studies in other species have improved the ability to provide effective enteral and parenteral nutritional support to the malnourished sick horse. It has also been recognized that certain types of equine illness impose requirements for feeds with unusual physical properties, and this knowledge can be exploited therapeutically.

ASSESSMENT OF NUTRITIONAL STATUS

Evaluation of food intake and body condition should be part of the routine physical examination, improvement in voluntary food intake being one of the best indicators of recovery from illness. It is particularly important to establish whether cachexia is due to poor feed intake before proceeding with more specialized tests of digestive or metabolic function. Prolonged starvation can lead to intestinal epithelial hypoplasia and malabsorption.

The quality of the feed has to be evaluated before the adequacy of a given level of feed intake can be judged (see p. 387). Nutritional requirements may be elevated in sick horses because of fever, wound healing, and other factors. In some horses digestive derangements interfere with the efficiency of nutrient absorption (p. 102).

Body condition gives an assessment of long-term nutritional adequacy. In mature horses negative energy balance results in loss of fat and muscle but not skeletal structures. Thus, flesh "falls away" from the bones. "Body scoring" is better than weighing in assessing fat stores because it is less affected by differences in body frame. The most reliable site for body scoring is the rump. Flesh cover over the shoulder also has a reasonable correlation with total body fat. Contrary to popular opinion the amount of flesh over the ribs is poorly correlated with body condition. In general, fat horses have a well-rounded rump, an invaginated crease along the backbone and plenty of flesh over the shoulders. The inner thighs are thick with fat and there is bulging fat around the tailhead. Pads of fat may be apparent over the ribs, neck, and shoulders.

Very thin horses have little flesh over the rump, and the tuber coxae and tuber ischiae are prominent. There is loss of thigh musculature and the semimembranosus and semitendinosus are prominent on the plantar aspect of the limb. Flesh cover is poor over the spine and the tips of the spinous and transverse processes of the lumbar vertebrae are visible. The scapula and ribs are also prominent. Growing animals show similar patterns of weight loss. Stunting as a result of severe nutritional restriction results in horses that are tall and thin with a shallow thorax because bone growth is not matched by soft tissue growth. Moderate nutritional restriction, however, results in slow growth, but body proportions are similar to those seen in normal animals of the same weight. Nutritional status in growing horses is best assessed using expected weight for age growth curves (see Table 6, p. 418).

Blood chemistry offers some guidance to a horse's nutritional status. The best indices of food deprivation are plasma free fatty-acid and glycerol concentrations, but techniques for measuring these are not routinely available. Some laboratories measure serum triglycerides and give a normal range of 60 to 780 mg per L; mild elevations in the 1000 to 5000 mg per L range are usually consistent with a period of poor food intake. Normal serum triglycerides do not rule out poor food intake, since there is much variation in the triglyceride response to food deprivation. Also, a lag of more than 40 hours between the removal of food and an elevation in serum triglycerides is common. Studies in cattle indicate that changes in blood chemistry are most likely to be seen when very little food is eaten rather than when a prolonged but low-grade undernutrition is present. Low serum albumin values usually reflect protein-losing enteropathy or renal or liver disease rather than long-term protein deprivation.

EFFECTS OF UNDERNUTRITION

Anorexia, a common response to infections, may initially enhance the ability to overcome acute bacterial infections. However, prolonged undernutrition adversely affects immune function. Host defenses are compromised by three to five days of complete food deprivation. Wound healing is poor and there is greater susceptibility to postoperative problems.

In some chronic illnesses, cachexia is the cause of death. Losses of 20 to 30 per cent of normal body weight are incompatible with life. Cachexia can also limit the return of the horse to normal work. The equine gastrointestinal tract seems peculiarly sensitive to periods of starvation. Complete food deprivation for three to five days predisposes horses to diarrhea, which can be fatal. Cachectic adult horses can reagain normal body condition, but growth restriction in young foals can have permanent consequences, particularly if the restriction is severe and occurs early in development. Pony foals that were not allowed to gain weight between 6 and 12 months of age had delayed epiphyseal closure and exhibited compensatory growth when subsequently fed an adequate diet. They grew best if they were allowed to eat as much as they wanted of a balanced diet high in energy and protein during the rehabilitation period. However, at 18 months of age they were still 20 to 40 kg lighter than their normally fed compatriots, which weighed around 300 kg.

DIETS FOR SICK HORSES

The following sections discuss dietary regimens that can be used in treating horses. When making dietary changes it is important not to disturb gastrointestinal function with rapid changes of feed. Because sudden introduction of alfalfa hay can cause diarrhea, alfalfa should be gradually introduced over a five-day period. Rapid increments in grain feeding can result in founder; grain levels should not be increased faster than 0.5 kg a day for a 500-kg horse. Lush grass can also cause problems. Access should be gradually increased over a period of a week or more.

Trauma, Infection, and Surgery. In general, horses destined for surgery or recovering from infections or trauma require a diet that is palatable, digestible, and rich in nutrients. Nutrients such as protein and B vitamins that are stored in the body are of special concern. Gut synthesis of vitamins usually satisfies B vitamin needs; however, supplementation may be required if food intake is poor or intestinal function compromised. Protein balance is of major importance because in patients with infections or trauma, muscle protein is mobilized to supply amino acids needed for energy production, wound healing, and vital functions.

Useful feeds for these types of horses are alfalfa hay, which contains more high quality protein than other forages; young grass, which is palatable and high in protein; and soybean meal. Brewer's yeast is used as a protein-vitamin supplement. Commercial preparations can vary greatly in their protein content. Protein supplements are often mixed with grain and molasses, making the combination palatable and giving it a high energy density. Iron supplementation should be reserved for horses with iron deficiency demonstrated by anemia and deficient iron stores in the bone marrow.

Chronic Pulmonary Disease. Horses with chronic pulmonary disease usually do best at pasture. However, if kept indoors, they often improve if they are taken off hay, fed pelleted feeds, and placed in a well-ventilated stall. When hay has to be fed, it should be thoroughly soaked with water either with a hose or preferably placed in a net and completely immersed in a tub of water for at least five minutes. Soaked feed should be replaced frequently because it can easily mold. There will be less dust if hay cubes are fed in place of loose hay, but these should also be soaked.

Diarrhea. Some horses with diarrhea, particularly those fed high levels of grain and in good physical condition, will respond to decreasing the grain content of the ration and feeding more grass hay. In contrast, horses that have primarily large intestinal disease (such as chronic salmonellosis), which impairs fiber digestion, may maintain condition better on grain diets. In the latter case, the improvement in bodily condition is presumably due to increased absorption of nutrients in the small intestine even though fecal quality is not improved.

Colonic Impaction. Dietary management is useful in preventing recurrence of impaction colic. Fresh water should be freely available and the horse given regular exercise. Straw or excessively fibrous hays should be replaced with good-quality grass or legume hays. Some horses seem particularly prone to impactions and require a mildly laxative diet. Restricting hay intake and feeding a complete pelleted feed containing ground alfalfa softens the stool and decreases filling of the large intestine. The small particle size also reduces the resistance to flow through the gut. Young grass is another diet that often produces a soft stool. If it proves difficult to obtain soft feces by dietary manipulation, magnesium sulfate can be added to the diet at the rate of 100 gm a day for a 500-kg horse.

Intestinal Resection. Removal of more than 50 per cent of the horse's small intestine can produce a malabsorption-maldigestion syndrome. Although this problem has been well documented, there are no studies on the best methods of feeding horses with a short bowel. We recommend that these horses be fed frequently on energy-rich and protein-rich diets. They may also benefit from feeding good-quality alfalfa hay so that volatile fatty acids derived from fiber digestion in the cecum and colon can provide a source of energy. As these horses may develop preference for a certain type of food, they should be offered a variety of different food until they demonstrate a clear preference for one type over others. Ponies that have undergone extensive resection of the small intestine show a preference for roughage in the diet.

Choke. Horses that have been treated for esophageal obstruction should be fed a soft mush for several days. Horses prone to obstruction should not be fed pellets. If the horse is a greedy eater, large round stones placed in the grain will slow down the rate of eating and decrease the probability of further episodes of choke.

ANOREXIA

Although sick horses often become anorectic, the time at which the clinician should begin supplemental feeding has not been established. Improving voluntary feed intake is usually tried early in the disease, while tube feeding is reserved for horses that are physically unable to ingest feed. Intravenous nutrition allows precise control of nutrient intake.

IMPROVING VOLUNTARY FEED INTAKE

Palatable feeds are usually the first line of attack in improving voluntary feed intake. Young leafy grass is palatable and digestible and may be preferred by horses that refuse other foods. Alfalfa hay is more palatable than bran. "Sweet feeds"— usually mixtures of molasses and rolled grains—can often increase palatability when added to grain feeds. However, some sick horses will reject a good alfalfa hay and grain and will eat poor hay or their bedding. For this reason, it is important to offer the sick horse its choice of a variety of foods. There may be an initial preference for a novel food such as apples or carrots, but this can soon diminish, and the person who feeds the horse should be constantly searching for foods it prefers. The site at which food is offered can be important, as some horses prefer to eat from the ground rather than a manger or hay rack.

Bran mashes are a popular food for sick horses. Palatability can be improved by mixing a quart of oats with a quart of bran. The mixture is steeped with boiling water and served warm but not hot. Molasses (up to 250 ml) and up to 20 gm of salt can be added for flavoring. Steamed oats, barley, and well-boiled linseed meal may be particularly palatable to some horses and can be substituted for part of the oats in the mash.

Fever and pain depress feed intake and interleukin 1 (endogenous pyrogen) also stimulates catabolism of muscle protein. Nonsteroidal anti-inflammatory drugs can improve feed intake by blocking fever and reducing pain; they may also reduce degradation of muscle tissue. Anti-inflammatory drugs are not useful in improving feed intake in severely toxemic horses.

Feed stimulants such as diazepam directly stimulate feeding centers in the hypothalamus. Our experience in sick horses suggests that the tranquilizing and ataxia-producing effects of diazepam often predominate and we do not recommend its use. However, in some European countries, new derivatives are available that stimulate feed intake with minimal tranquilizing side effects. Anabolic steroids increase feed intake, but because the effect may take up to 10 days they are unlikely to be of use in the immediate treatment of the sick horse. However, they can be useful in the convalescent period.

Vitamin supplementation may be beneficial to some horses. Normally the diet and synthesis of vitamins by the gut flora provide plenty of B vitamins, and the average horse has adequate stores of vitamins for short-term food deprivation. Horses that have been off feed for a number of days and horses that have disturbed gut function because of diarrhea or oral antibiotic therapy may benefit from vitamin B complex administration.

FORCE FEEDING

There are two approaches to nutritional supplementation in sick horses unable or unwilling to eat. The first approach is to supplement part of the horse's requirements; the other is to provide all nutrients.

Partial supplementation, dosing with a high-protein food, is used in patients that are in fairly good bodily condition and still have some voluntary food intake. High-protein supplements improve the balance between protein requirements and protein intake and minimize catabolism of muscle protein. The horse is still in negative energy balance, and depot lipid is broken down to meet the energy deficit. One type of therapy involves the use of casein as a protein supplement. A dose syringe can be used to feed 50 gm of casein as a slurry three times a day. This provides less than a third of maintenance protein requirements but may convert a patient with marginal protein intake into positive protein balance. Casein is used as a supplement because it is 90 per cent digestible, its amino acid spectrum is particularly good, and the protein is likely to have a high biological value to the horse. Casein can either be used directly or, alternatively, some forms of dehydrated cottage cheese contain minimal lactose and fat and are rich in casein. We do not recommend the use of lactose-rich milk products because adult horses cannot digest lactose.

When horses cannot be fed orally because of derangements in gastrointestinal function, adding 5 per cent dextrose to the intravenous fluids will provide a small amount of calories and may reduce catabolism of protein.

COMPLETE NUTRITIONAL SUPPORT

Complete nutritional support is indicated in patients that are either severely cachectic or unable to eat for more than five days. Complete nutritional support may also be given early in the therapeutic regimen if it is thought that any further loss of body condition is undesirable—for example, in a horse that is recumbent and is losing body weight so that it cannot regain sufficient strength to stand. We tend to reserve complete nutritional support for horses wanting to eat but unable to ingest food because of painful, neurologic, or esophageal obstructive diseases.

Complete nutritional support can be given orally or intravenously. Intravenous therapy is both costly and time-consuming. Solutions and infusion sets must be sterile. Contamination of solutions occurs readily when additions are made to the intravenous fluid bottles, and bacterial contaminants multiply in the medium of the intravenous solutions. This is a special problem with intravenous feeding, since the bottle of nutrient solution can hang for long periods before being exhausted. Particular care must also be taken with catheter placement. Solutions are hypertonic, and the catheter should be in a large vessel to minimize the risk of thrombosis. The tubing and catheter should be changed regularly to decrease the risk of contamination (see p. 174).

Another problem with intravenous nutrition is that large loads of glucose are given by a route that bypasses many of the normal homeostatic mechanisms. Hyperglycemia may develop, particularly in septic patients, and can result in urinary loss of glucose and osmotic diuresis. Very high blood glucose concentrations may induce convulsions. Fat would be particularly useful as an alternative energy

TABLE 1. FORMULATION OF INTRAVENOUS FEEDING SOLUTION

Item*	Amount
5% amino acid solution	1000 ml
50% dextrose	500 ml
Potassium chloride	30 mEq
Sodium bicarbonate	30 mEq
Injectable multivitamins	

*These items are mixed aseptically to yield a solution with a final volume of 1500 ml. The solution is hypertonic and is administered at the rate of 3 L/day to a 45-kg foal.

Reproduced with permission, Compendium on Continuing Education, 6:S93, 1984.

TABLE 3. MAINTENANCE ORAL ELECTROLYTE MIXTURE*

Substance	Amount (gm)
Sodium chloride (NaCl)	10
Sodium bicarbonate (NaHCO$_3$)	15
Potassium chloride (KCl)	75
Potassium phosphate (dibasic anhydrous) (K$_2$HPO$_4$)	60
Calcium chloride (CaCl$_2$•2H$_2$O)	45
Magnesium oxide (MgO)	25

*One day's requirement for a 450-kg horse.

Reproduced with permission, Compendium on Continuing Education, 6:S93, 1984.

source, and a commercial preparation* used successfully in Europe is now available for this purpose in the United States.

Intravenous feeding can be useful in the feeding of foals. Their small size reduces the costs of feeding and the intravenous route circumvents problems due to disturbances in gastrointestinal function. A formulation based on recommendations for calves can be used (Table 1). One way to prepare the solution is to use an empty 1-liter sterile bottle and add half the ingredients to this. The partially emptied amino acid container can then be used for the other half of the ration. Mixing should be conducted in a clean environment, preferably under a laminar flow of filtered air. A syringe and needle should be used for the transfer. The solution should be mixed freshly each day and the bottles kept refrigerated until needed. With intravenous feeding, the flow of nutrients should be kept as even as possible. Nutrient intake should slowly be built up from half maintenance to maintenance over the course of two days. Additions to the fluid bottles should be restricted to the absolute minimum. Other medications are best given through a separate line.

Oral alimentation is the alternative to intravenous feeding and is used more frequently because it is

*Intralipid, Cutter Laboratories, Inc., Emeryville, CA

inexpensive and sterile solutions are not needed. Foals can be fed a commercial foal milk replacer,* and this can be given through a nasogastric tube if necessary (see p. 205).

Adult horses can be fed slurries of alfalfa meal or complete pelleted feeds. Alternating a liquid diet of electrolytes, dextrose, dehydrated cottage cheese, and dehydrated alfalfa meal can be used (Table 2). The electrolyte mixture is shown in Table 3. The mixture is low in sodium and rich in potassium, like many natural horse feeds. These proportions of electrolytes are suitable for maintenance purposes but not for replacement purposes. Horses with fluid losses as a result of diarrhea or sweating require additional sodium-rich replacement electrolyte solutions (p. 89). Horses have been successfully maintained on this electrolyte mixture for up to four weeks. Occasionally a mild hyponatremia may develop, and in these cases, 15 gm of sodium chloride can be added daily to the electrolyte mixture. Routine supplementation of additional sodium salts is not recommended. The diet is introduced gradually and slowly is increased to maintenance amounts (Table 2). The diet is rich in highly digestible protein and should induce positive balance. Figures for digestible energy contents in Table 2

*Foal-Lac, Borden International, New York, NY

TABLE 2. RECOMMENDED TUBE FEEDING SCHEDULE FOR A 450-KG HORSE*

Parameter	Day 1	2	3	4	5	6	7
Electrolyte mixture (gm)†	230	230	230	230	230	230	230
Water (L)	21	21	21	21	21	21	21
Dextrose (gm)	300	400	500	600	800	800	900
Dehydrated cottage cheese (gm)‡	300	450	600	750	900	900	900
Dehydrated alfalfa meal (gm)	2000	2000	2000	2000	2000	2000	2000
Energy (mcal)§	7.4	8.4	9.4	10.4	11.8	11.8	12.2

*These allowances should be divided and administered in three feedings daily. Maintenance requirements for a 450-kg horse are 13 mcal of digestible energy and 580 gm of crude protein.

†Mixture is listed in Table 3.

‡Dehydrated cottage cheese—82% crude protein with less than 2% lactose (American Nutritional Laboratory) or Casein (Sigma Chemical).

§Megacalories of digestible energy.

Reproduced with permission, Compendium on Continuing Education, 6:S93, 1984.

are estimates, but the diet gives close to the maintenance energy requirement of the normal horse. Water intake is more than sufficient for maintenance purposes, and the urine is often dilute. Sometimes an improvement in hydration is noted following the use of this regimen even though the horse had previously been receiving intravenous fluids.

This diet can be difficult to pass through a stomach tube because it is viscous. The limiting factor is the amount of dehydrated alfalfa meal added. Alfalfa swells on contact with water and should be added immediately before the mix is poured into the stomach tube. A large-diameter stomach tube facilitates passage of the mix, and if persistent difficulties occur, the alfalfa meal can be cut back to 600 gm per feeding.

Two problems in horses that are tube-fed this diet are diarrhea and laminitis. The risk of laminitis can be minimized by avoiding the diet in horses that are foundering, that have chronic laminitis, or that have rotation of the pedal bones. Diarrhea associated with tube feeding is not accompanied by fever or changes in the hemogram and responds to withdrawal of tube feeding and use of intravenous electrolyte solutions to maintain hydration. The incidence of diarrhea can be greatly reduced by making sure that alfalfa meal is not left out of the oral alimentation mix.

ESOPHAGOSTOMY

Oral alimentation diets are frequently fed through a nasogastric tube. Occasionally an indwelling esophagostomy tube may be preferred for protracted feeding regimens to avoid problems with nasal irritation and aversion to passage of a stomach tube. An indwelling esophagostomy may also be used following surgery to the upper esophagus, pharynx, or nares to spare abrasion to the healing surfaces. The esophagostomy should be placed at the junction of the middle and lower thirds of the neck. The esophagus is readily accessible and has little contact with major structures at this site. The horse is sedated and the site infiltrated with local anesthetic before surgery is begun. It is important to use a ventral midline approach to facilitate drainage. Passage of a medium-size nasogastric tube greatly facilitates identification of the esophagus. This tube is removed as the esophagostomy tube is inserted.

Cellulitis and edema are common postoperative complications of this surgery. Antibiotic therapy will often help control these problems. Delaying feeding for 12 to 24 hours after surgery allows a fibrin seal to form.

Premature removal of the esophagostomy tube can be a major problem. If the tube is inadvertently replaced in the periesophageal tissues and pushed into the mediastinum, the horse can die. The chances of premature removal can be minimized by placing the tip of the tube into the stomach and firmly suturing the tube in place. A neck rack should be used if the horse rubs the esophagostoma. Blocked tubes are best treated by back flushing rather than removing them for cleaning. A syringe can be attached to a small polyethylene tube. This is passed into the esophagostomy tube and the obstruction flushed away. When the tube is no longer needed, it can be removed and the site allowed to heal. However, tube removal should not occur until a fistula has formed 5 to 10 days after surgery. Premature removal of the tube results in peristomal inflammation and delayed healing.

Horses should be carefully selected for an esophagostomy. As well as the complications already discussed, damage to the left recurrent laryngeal nerve is also a possibility. Complications are also more likely to occur when the technique is used for the first time or when untested modifications are tried. The risk of complications should be carefully weighed and surgery reserved for those animals in which failure to perform the surgery will jeopardize life or seriously compromise well being.

Supplemental Readings

Baracos, V., Rodemann, P., Dinarello, C. A., and Goldberg, A. L.: Stimulation of muscle protein degeneration and prostaglandin E_2 release by leukocytic pyrogen (interleukin-1). N. Engl. J. Med., *308*:553, 1983.

Della Fera, M. A., Naylor, J. M., and Baille, C. A.: Benzodiazepines stimulate feeding in clinically debilitated animals. Fed. Proc., *37*:401, 1978.

Ellis, R. N. W., and Lawrence, T. L. J.: Energy under-nutrition in the weanling filly foal. 1. Effects on subsequent live-weight gains and onset of oestrus. Br. Vet. J., *134*:205, 1978.

Freeman, D. E., and Naylor, J. M.: Cervical esophagostomy to permit extraoral feeding of the horse. J. Am. Vet. Med. Assoc., *172*:314, 1978.

Hoffsis, G. F., Gingerich, D. A., Sherman, D. M., and Bruner, R. R.: Total intravenous feeding of calves. J. Am. Vet. Med. Assoc., *171*:67, 1977.

Kluger, M. J., and Rothenburg, B. A.: Fever and reduced iron: Their interaction as a host defense response. Science, *203*:374, 1979.

Naylor, J. M., and Kenyon, S. J.: Effect of total caloric deprivation on host defense in the horse. Res. Vet. Sci., *31*:369, 1981.

OCULAR DISEASES

Edited by M. B. Glaze

Examination of the Eye

Mary B. Glaze, BATON ROUGE, LOUISIANA

Even though ocular disease can disable a horse as surely as any lameness, it is seldom given equal diagnostic consideration. Hampered by poor examination facilities or an uncooperative patient, the busy practitioner may forego a thorough examination and rely on obvious signs of redness or cloudiness as the basis for therapy. The most obvious lesion may not be the most important, however, and the ocular problem may persist, resulting in chronic disease and blindness.

The risk to the animal's vision and performance is minimized by early diagnosis and appropriate therapy. The veterinarian should base that diagnosis on two sources of information: the owner's account of the ocular problem and a systematic examination of the eyes and surrounding structures.

HISTORY

A good ophthalmic history is an essential part of every patient's evaluation. Historical data focuses the clinician's attention during the ophthalmic examination and suggests subsequent laboratory work and therapy. In a large percentage of cases, the informed practitioner can arrive at a plausible diagnosis on the basis of history alone.

The process of history taking should be as orderly as the ocular examination itself. Owners may be given a simple form to complete (Table 1), but it is the veterinarian's task to refine that information. A standard format includes (1) signalment, (2) chief complaint, (3) history of present illness, (4) past history, and (5) family history.

Signalment refers to the breed, age, and sex of the horse. This information is useful in identifying the animal as well as in predicting the ocular lesion. Although sex-linked ocular abnormalities have not been identified in the horse, some conditions are more likely to occur in a specific breed or at a certain age. Equine night blindness, for example, would be suspected in a young Appaloosa with repeated injuries suffered at night. General information that may also be helpful in ophthalmic diagnosis includes the horse's primary use, housing, environment, vaccination status, diet, and contact with other animals.

The chief complaint is the first clue to the horse's problem. It should be stated in the owner's words since premature definition of the problem by the veterinarian may compromise objectivity during the examination. A "red eye" may suggest conjunctivitis, for example, but does not exclude subconjunctival hemorrhage, corneal vascularization, neoplasia, hyphema, or even protrusion of the nictitating membrane. Even when more significant problems are identified, the veterinarian must explain the meaning of the chief complaint and its proper management. It was, after all, the primary cause of the owner's concern.

The history of the present illness should describe the signs and the course of the disorder in detail. Most owners have difficulty providing precise descriptions, so the veterinarian should question the client until the problem is clearly understood. The time sequence should specify when, how fast, and in what order events occurred. Previous medication therapy should be identified by name, dosage, and

TABLE 1. OPHTHALMIC HISTORY FORM

1. What made you aware of your horse's eye problem?

   Rubbing at eye _____ Discharge from eye _____ Cloudiness of eye _____ Redness of eye _____ Eye held closed _____
   Loss of vision _____ Veterinarian noted problem _____ Other _____

2. How long has the problem been present? _____

3. Which eye is affected? Right _____ Left _____ Both _____ Unsure _____

4. Since you first noted the problem, has the eye changed?

   Yes, it is better _____ How? _____
   Yes, it is worse _____ How? _____
   No change _____

5. Has any medication been used for the eye(s)? Yes _____ No _____
   If so, what medication? _____

   How long? _____
   How often per day? _____
   Time last administered? _____
   Do you feel the medication is helping? Yes _____ No _____

6. Your horse's eyesight seems to be:

   Excellent _____ Poor _____ Blind in both eyes _____ Blind in one eye _____
   Poor in bright light _____ Poor in dim light _____ Do not know _____

7. Has your horse had any other eye problems? Yes _____ No _____

8. Has any surgery been performed on your horse's eye(s)? Yes _____ No _____

9. Have your horse's sire, dam, or siblings ever had any eye problems?

   Yes _____ What kind? _____
   No _____ Do not know _____

10. Is your animal receiving any other medication? Yes _____ No _____
    If so, what other drugs? _____

effect so any unsuccessful regimen is not repeated. Certain medications may also mask clinical signs.

The most relevant part of the past history asks if similar or related problems have occurred previously. Repeated episodes of a red, watery eye may indicate recurrent uveitis, for example. Past medical history should also be determined, since systemic diseases can have profound effects on the eye.

Heritability has been established in equine night blindness and in aniridia and is suspected in congenital cataracts. A patient's ophthalmic history should therefore consider past generations, i.e., family history.

RESTRAINT

Examination of the equine eye is more easily described than performed, for the horse with painful or blinding ocular disease can be ill-tempered and uncooperative. Adequate restraint is therefore critical for thorough evaluation, as well as for the safety of the examiner and the patient. A variety of techniques are available and can be tailored to the individual.

In some horses, a twitch may be sufficient to complete the examination, but animals that are in pain or are apprehensive due to vision loss may need chemical restraint. Intravenous xylazine* is commonly used for sedation at a dosage of 0.5 to 1.0 mg per kg and is effective for one to two hours. Analgesic effects last only 15 to 30 minutes, but minor surgical procedures can be performed following xylazine administration.

Parenteral agents for sedation have virtually replaced regional nerve blocks in ophthalmic practice. The horse's powerful orbicularis oculi muscle, innervated by the palpebral nerve, can nevertheless be a factor in the sedated animal with ocular pain. A field block around the orbital rim will produce akinesia with eyelid analgesia by affecting the terminal branches of the palpebral nerve as well as branches of the ophthalmic division of the trigeminal nerve. A successful motor block produces a narrowed palpebral fissure and a drooping upper eyelid.

Infiltration of the auriculopalpebral nerve at a site distant from the eye may be safer and will produce comparable akinesia. Anesthesia is *not* achieved by this technique. Five to 7 ml of 2 per cent lidocaine without epinephrine are injected near

_____
*Rompun, Haver-Lockhart, Shawnee, KS

the base of the ear using a 22- or 25-gauge needle inserted to a depth of one half inch. The landmark for needle placement is a depression located where a line paralleling the caudal aspect of the mandibular ramus intersects a line parallel to the dorsal rim of the zygomatic arch (specifically, the zygomatic process of the temporal bone).

An alternative method blocks the palpebral nerve as it crosses the dorsal border of the zygomatic arch just anterior to its highest point. The nerve is easily palpated in this area. One to 2 ml of local anesthetic are injected subcutaneously using a 25-gauge, five eighth-inch needle. Akinesia is not as profound as that following the auriculopalpebral block, but it is adequate for diagnostic purposes.

Blocks of the eyelids' four sensory nerves can augment motor paresis and are also indicated for surgical procedures when general anesthesia is not desirable. The frontal nerve emerges from the supraorbital foramen to innervate the middle two thirds of the superior lid. The nerve is found by grasping the supraorbital process between the thumb and middle finger. As the process widens medially, the supraorbital foramen can be felt with the index finger. A 25-gauge, five eighth-inch needle is inserted its full length into the foramen and 1 to 2 ml of anesthetic are injected. As the needle is withdrawn, another 2 to 3 ml are injected subcutaneously. This block may be sufficient to permit a thorough examination, since some palpebral branches are also located at this site.

The lateral canthus and lateral aspect of the upper eyelid are anesthetized by a block of the lacrimal nerve. Two to 3 ml of anesthetic are injected with a 25-gauge, five eighth-inch needle just under the dorsolateral orbital rim. Medial canthal anesthesia requires an infratrochlear nerve block. A notch at the dorsomedial orbital rim marks the site for needle placement. Two to 3 ml of anesthetic are injected along the medial orbital periosteum with a 25-gauge, five eighth-inch needle.

The zygomatic nerve innervates the middle two thirds of the lower lid. It is found by placing the index finger on the ventrolateral orbital rim, as it begins to rise. A 25-gauge needle is inserted medial to the finger and 2 to 3 ml of anesthetic are injected subcutaneously along the orbital rim. Figure 1 illustrates the sites for these local nerve blocks.

OPHTHALMIC EXAMINATION

The ideal facility for ocular examination is quiet and dimly lit. Noise can easily excite a visually compromised horse, while bright light produces reflections that obscure intraocular detail. If the horse must be examined in sunlight, a thick blanket can be used as a canopy to reduce glare. A good source of focal illumination is required. A Finoff transilluminator* on a fully charged direct ophthalmoscope handle is ideal. A dim or diffuse light source, such as an old disposable penlight, does not penetrate well through opaque ocular media. Magnifying loupes† (1.5 × to 4 ×) should also be considered in the ocular examination.

A list of tentative diagnoses evolves along with the horse's history. As examination of the eye begins, the clinician should keep in mind the physical and laboratory findings that will confirm or exclude each differential. A much more detailed examination of the involved area will be performed if a given problem is suspected.

The examination of the eye and periocular structures must be completed in a systematic manner, beginning superficially and progressing intraocularly, as summarized in Table 2. Obvious lesions are less likely to distract the practitioner who follows an orderly examination sequence. Remember, the most obvious abnormality may not be the most

---

*Welch Allyn, Inc., Skaneateles Falls, NY
†Optivisor, Donegan Optical Co., Kansas City, MO

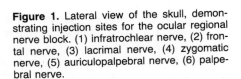

Figure 1. Lateral view of the skull, demonstrating injection sites for the ocular regional nerve block. (1) infratrochlear nerve, (2) frontal nerve, (3) lacrimal nerve, (4) zygomatic nerve, (5) auriculopalpebral nerve, (6) palpebral nerve.

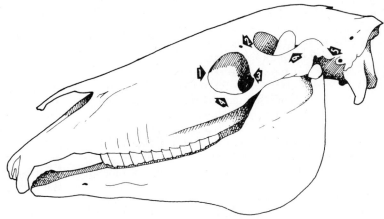

TABLE 2. STEPS IN EQUINE OPHTHALMIC EXAMINATION

Evaluate Globe-Orbit Relationship
Note size/position of globe
Note position of nictitans
Assess palpebral fissure

If Painful:
Regional nerve blocks, sedation

Adnexal Examination	**Anterior Segment Examination**	**Lens and Posterior Segment Examination**
1. Characterize Discharge	1. Determine Clarity	1. Dilate Pupil
If excessive:	Use tapetal reflection	1% tropicamide
Continue ocular exam		
Nasolacrimal flush	2. Evaluate Cornea	2. Evaluate Lens
If thick/purulent:	If curvature abnormal:	Clarity
Conjunctival culture	Culture margin of defect	Position
Consider Schirmer tear test	Fluorescein dye test	
Conjunctival cytology	Topical proparacaine	3. Evaluate Fundus
	Cytology of defect margin	Use ophthalmoscope
2. Evaluate Lids	Examination of posterior	Clarity of vitreous
Note margins/cilia	surface of nictitans	Size/color of disc
Examine inner surface	If surface dull/vascularized:	Character of vessels
(cilia/foreign bodies)	Consider Schirmer tear test	Tapetal reflectivity
	Fluorescein dye test	Nontapetal pigment
3. Evaluate Conjunctiva	Examine cul-de-sacs for foreign	
Note edema/irregularities	body/irregularities	
Characterize hyperemia;		
Pattern of redness	3. Evaluate Anterior Chamber	**If Abnormal**
(Localized/generalized)	Assess depth	Re-evaluate cornea
Vessels affected	Identify abnormal contents	Tonometry
(Conjunctival/ciliary)		Proceed to posterior
	4. Evaluate Iris	segment examination
4. Evaluate Nictitating Membrane	Assess pupillary light reflex	
Note position/size	Note pupil size	
Assess surface character	Evaluate pupil margin	

significant. Corneal edema secondary to an anterior lens luxation may be dramatic, but the abnormal lens position is much more important prognostically and therapeutically.

Ancillary diagnostic procedures are often incorporated into the basic ophthalmic examination. The practitioner should consider the effect of topical agents on corneal and conjunctival culture, Schirmer tear test, pupillary light response, and corneal sensation when planning these supplemental tests. Corneal and conjunctival cultures must be performed without topical anesthesia, since the anesthetic agent contains a bacteriostatic preservative. The Schirmer tear test, although seldom indicated in the horse, should be performed before topical anesthetics that alter reflex tearing and before manipulations that may increase tear formation. Pupillary light responses following mydriatic application are unreliable. Topical anesthetics reduce corneal sensation as well as the veterinarian's ability to assess trigeminal nerve integrity.

Great care must be taken when examining an injured eye. Pressure over the eye should be avoided when separation of the lids is attempted. If penetration of the eye is ascertained at any time, the examination should be stopped immediately to avoid further damage.

Vision. A horse's sight can be evaluated by several methods, although most are crude estimates of vision. Each eye should be assessed independently by blindfolding the opposite globe. The animal's age, temperament, and vision influence the response to a menacing gesture. Menace reflex is poor in very young foals. Normal adult horses vary in their response; some show little reaction to bold movements while others respond violently to slight motion. Noiseless materials, such as cotton balls or gauze pads, can be tossed into the horse's field of view to gauge the response to moving objects. Visually handicapped horses may be frightened or injured when put into an obstacle course of hay bales or plastic barrels. The horse should therefore be kept on a loose lead for reassurance as it makes its way through the maze.

Orbit. Before sedation, a general assessment of orbital symmetry, eyelid position, and the position of the eye within its bony socket should be made. The eyelashes are normally perpendicular to the corneal surface but may become more parallel if the upper lid droops abnormally. Globe-orbit relationship may be altered by tumor, inflammation, trauma, or developmental defects. Abnormal orbital tissue is suspected when firm pressure on the eye through closed lids cannot push the globe into the orbit.

Cranial Nerves. Examination of cranial nerves II through VII is more reliable if performed prior to sedation. Pupillary light responses are used to assess cranial nerves II and III. The reflex is evaluated in a darkened area with a bright focal light. Although direct pupillary response in the horse is normally brisk, response of the opposite pupil (consensual reaction) is usually limited. Frightened animals exhibit dilated, poorly responsive pupils due to endogenous epinephrine release. A normal pupillary response is not synonymous with vision.

Ocular position and ability to follow movement are used to assess cranial nerves III, IV, and VI, which innervate the extraocular muscles. Contraction of the retractor bulbi muscle, which is innervated by cranial nerve VI, causes retraction of the globe and passive prolapse of the nictitating membrane. Sensory innervation of the eyelids and cornea is derived through branches of cranial nerve V. Corneal sensitivity is evaluated by a small wisp of cotton touched to the cornea. Motor innervation to the eyelids is by the auriculopalpebral branch of cranial nerve VII.

Eyelids. Lid examination should ascertain how well the eyes are protected, because potentially serious damage may result from exposure when the lids do not close properly. Injuries to the equine eyelid are common and may result in altered function due to scar formation or tissue loss. The lid margins and direction of the eyelashes should be assessed. Masses within the lid may be felt by sliding the examining finger across the closed lid surface.

Lacrimal Apparatus. The nasolacrimal puncta are located in the medial upper and lower eyelids near the mucocutaneous junction. The distal orifice is located at the mucocutaneous junction on the floor of the nares. Obstructive lesions of the nasolacrimal drainage apparatus result in tearing. Inflammatory disorders are characterized by mucopurulent discharge.

Patency of the nasolacrimal apparatus is evaluated by fluorescein passage through the system and by nasolacrimal flush. These tests can alter the results of other diagnostic procedures and should be postponed until the conjunctiva and cornea are evaluated. Fluorescein passage is performed first. An ample volume of fluorescein dye is instilled into the conjunctival cul-de-sac. The dye can usually be detected at the distal nasolacrimal opening within five minutes. The system is flushed by cannulating the distal opening with a smooth, flexible polyethylene catheter and injecting 10 to 15 ml of sterile saline through the system. A twitch or sedation or

both are usually necessary. Mucopurulent material flushed from the puncta should be cultured. Nasolacrimal patency may also be evaluated by catheterization of the system and by dacryocystorhinography.

Conjunctiva. The conjunctiva lining the lids (palpebral) and the globe (bulbar) should be thoroughly examined. The bulbar conjunctiva is normally quite transparent, and the white color of the eye is due to the underlying sclera. Many small conjunctival vessels are normally visible. The bulbar conjunctiva is often pigmented temporally. The palpebral conjunctiva overlies fleshy tissue and therefore appears much redder than the bulbar conjunctiva. Although lymphoid tissue is present, lymphoid follicles are scant in the normal eye.

Conjunctival vessels must be differentiated from deeper ciliary vessels and the serious ocular diseases they represent. Conjunctival vessels move with the conjunctiva and branch profusely, whereas ciliary vessels remain stationary and have little branching. Conjunctival vessels will also blanch following application of 10 per cent phenylephrine; ciliary vessels are not affected.

Ocular discharge, ranging from serous to purulent, is common in conjunctival disease. Microbiological culture and antibacterial sensitivity should be considered in horses with purulent discharge or with severe conjunctivitis. The lower eyelid is everted to prevent contamination by the lid margin. A sterile cotton swab,* premoistened with sterile saline or transport medium, is gently twisted in the ventral cul-de-sac and then replaced in transport medium.

A tenacious mucopurulent discharge may indicate keratoconjunctivitis sicca or dry eye, a rare occurrence in the horse. Tear production is quantitated by the Schirmer tear test; commercial test strips are saturated in less than 30 seconds. Strips of Whatman 42 filter paper (80 mm × 7.5 mm), folded 10 mm from the end, have also been used. The folded portion is inserted into the lower conjunctival cul-de-sac for a minute. The distance that the tears diffuse along the strip is then measured. The mean reported value in the normal horse is 13 mm per minute. Values less than 5 mm per minute confirm inadequate tear production.

Conjunctival cytology may be used to demonstrate the intensity of inflammation and the presence of infection. Topical 0.5 per cent proparacaine† is applied, the lower lid is everted, and a stainless steel spatula is gently scraped across the conjunctival surface. Specimens are placed on glass slides and processed using Gram, Wright's, new methylene blue, or Wright-Giemsa–like‡ stains.

Nictitating Membrane. Examination of the nic-

---

*Culturette, Marion Scientific Corp., Rockford, IL
†Ophthaine, E. R. Squibb, Princeton, NJ
‡Diff Quik, American Scientific Products, McGaw Park, IL

titans requires topical anesthesia, for evaluation of the anterior and posterior surfaces is necessary if foreign bodies and masses are to be identified. The anterior surface is smooth with few, if any, lymphoid follicles; the leading edge is usually pigmented. A small fleshy nodule, or caruncle, is located at the base of the nictitating membrane, adjacent to the medial canthus. Thumb forceps are used to expose the posterior surface of the nictitating membrane. A few lymphoid follicles are normally present.

Cornea. Oblique illumination with a focused light source is particularly effective in demonstrating corneal abnormalities. The most common lesions of the cornea are ulcers and opacities. Severe and medically nonresponsive corneal ulcers should be cultured for bacteria and fungi. Topical anesthetics cannot be used prior to culture, even though the horse will resent corneal contact. Culture of the ulcer margin is preferred. The examiner must be prepared to quickly remove the swab to prevent contamination by the lids and nictitating membrane. Conjunctival culture is not a substitute for corneal culture.

Defects in the corneal epithelium are identified with the fluorescein dye test. Since dropper bottles of fluorescein are readily contaminated, fluorescein strips* should be used. The end of the strip is moistened with a drop of sterile saline and the dye is instilled at the medial canthus or along the everted lower lid. The dry strip can also be inserted into the lower cul-de-sac, allowing the tears to dissolve the fluorescein. If the strip contacts the cornea, excessive dye may be deposited, mimicking a corneal defect. Ulcers will stain a brilliant green if excess dye is washed out with saline.

Corneal cytology is indicated in cases of rapidly progressive or nonresponsive ulceration. The cytologic findings can be helpful in the initial choice of antibacterials or antifungals. Topical anesthesia is necessary for scrapings of the ulcer margin. A platinum spatula is preferred, although a cotton swab is potentially less traumatic in the uncooperative animal. Again, conjunctival cytology is not a reliable measure of corneal disease.

A Schirmer tear test should be performed when a mucopurulent discharge and a dull, vascularized cornea are noted.

Anterior Chamber. The depth of the anterior chamber is best evaluated from the side. Focal narrowing of the chamber may result from anterior synechiae or neoplasia. A generally shallow chamber is seen with inflammation and congestion of the iris. The anterior chamber should be examined for transparency of the aqueous humor. Intraocular inflammation causes an increase in aqueous protein and turbidity, known as *aqueous flare*. This can be

demonstrated by an intense focal beam of light traversing the anterior chamber, much like headlights on a foggy night. Abnormal components, such as blood, cysts, parasites, inflammatory debris, and neoplastic cells, should be noted.

Iris. Iridal color in most horses is a medium to dark brown. The pupil is rod-shaped and elongated horizontally. Multiple pigmented nodules, known as corpora nigra or granula iridica, are conspicuous along the dorsal pupillary margin and are also found at the ventral edge of the pupil. These masses should not be confused with iris cysts or melanomas.

The size and shape of the pupil are important considerations. Enlargement of the pupil (mydriasis) may be due to ocular injury, glaucoma, or parasympatholytic agents. Constriction of the pupil (miosis) is seen in iris inflammation, following application of parasympathomimetics such as pilocarpine, and physiologically in sleep. Irregularity of pupil contour is invariably abnormal, as in iritis, trauma, or developmental defects.

Intraocular Pressure. A crude estimate of intraocular pressure can be made by indentation of the eye with the fingers, but the technique can only detect gross pressure alterations. Greater accuracy requires a tonometer. The Schiotz tonometer is of no value in the standing horse since the cornea must be oriented horizontally for accurate pressure determinations. Applanation tonometers, such as the MacKay-Marg* and the Pneumotonograph,† are better suited to the horse, but their use is limited by their expense.

Lens. Evaluation of the lens and fundus requires dilation of the pupil. Dilating agents (mydriatics) should not be instilled until pupillary light responses are evaluated. Mydriatics are also contraindicated in elevated intraocular pressure. Several drops of 1 per cent tropicamide‡ are instilled into the ventral conjunctival cul-de-sac. Contamination of the multidose container can be avoided by drawing the solution into a syringe before instillation. A second dose is given after five minutes. Maximum dilation occurs in 15 to 20 minutes and lasts four to six hours. Atropine is unacceptable for routine diagnostic use, since one application may produce mydriasis lasting several days.

As light enters the posterior segment, the colorful tapetum reflects through the pupil. Small opacities in the lens or vitreous will obscure the reflected light and will appear as black defects against the bright background. Dense, diffuse cataracts will completely obscure tapetal reflection.

A shift in lens position is important prognostically and therapeutically, for the change may alter fluid dynamics within the eye. Variations in anterior

---

*Fluor-I-Strip, Ayerst Laboratories, Inc., New York, NY

*Biotronics, Redding, CA
†Alcon Laboratories, Inc., Fort Worth, TX
‡Mydriacyl, Alcon Laboratories, Inc., Forth Worth, TX

chamber depth and a fluttering motion by the iris are associated with changes in lens position.

Fundus. Direct ophthalmoscopy is the most common technique used for fundic examination, although indirect ophthalmoscopy using a focal light source and an aspheric lens provides a wider field of view. Disadvantages of the direct ophthalmoscope are its short working distance, which forces the examiner to stand only a few inches from the horse's head, and its limited ability to penetrate cloudy media.

The direct ophthalmoscope should be firmly braced against the practitioner's brow. The right eye should be used to examine the horse's right eye, and the left should be used to examine the horse's left. Although this stipulation is not as critical in evaluation of the equine eye, the technique should be reinforced for companion animal use. The ophthalmoscope lens is set at zero, and the examiner views the tapetal reflection from a distance of two feet, noting opacities that obscure the reflection. The examiner then moves within 3 to 5 cm from the eye, using a lens diopter setting of -3 to -5. The closer the instrument is to the eye, the larger the fundic area visualized.

A definite routine, beginning with the optic disc, should be followed in examination of the fundus. (1) The optic disc is the most conspicuous feature of the equine fundus and its size, shape, color, and margins should be evaluated. The horse's disc is characteristically oval, salmon-colored, and located in the nontapetal region. (2) The appearance of the retinal vessels can be affected by ocular and systemic diseases. Differentiation of arterioles and venules is impossible in the horse, whose 30 to 60 small vessels emerge at the optic disc margin and extend only a few disc diameters into the surrounding retina. (3) Reflectivity of the tapetum may be altered if retinal thinning is present. The normal tapetum is yellow to blue-green. Small dots distributed throughout the tapetum represent end-on choroidal capillaries and are referred to as "stars of Winslow." (4) The nontapetal fundus should be evaluated for depigmentation, especially in the area adjacent to the optic disc. The nontapetal fundus in most horses is dark brown to black, but may lose pigment following retinal and choroidal disease.

After completion of the fundus examination, the more anterior structures of the eye may be reevaluated by turning the lens wheel clockwise to the more positive lenses.

CONCLUSIONS

Equine ocular disease presents a diagnostic challenge to the veterinary practitioner. Often faced with an uncooperative patient, the veterinarian may base therapy on signs of redness, cloudiness, discharge, and/or diminished vision. Unfortunately, these findings are shared by diseases of diverse etiologies—and symptomatic treatment may be unable to prevent irreversible ocular damage. A horse's worth and productivity may well depend upon the equine practitioner's ability to perform a thorough examination of the eye and surrounding tissues. It is only through such systematic evaluation that accurate diagnosis and definitive therapy can be realized.

Supplemental Readings

Bistner, S. I.: Fundus examination of the horse. Vet. Clin. North Am. (Large Anim. Pract.), 6:541, 1984.

Gelatt, K. N.: Ophthalmic examination and diagnostic techniques. *In* Gelatt, K. N. (ed.): Veterinary Ophthalmology. Philadelphia, Lea & Febiger, 1981.

Merideth, R. E.: Ophthalmic examination and therapeutic techniques in the horse. Compend. Contin. Ed., 3:S426, 1981.

Algorithms for Ophthalmic Problems

Gretchen M. Schmidt, RIVERWOODS, ILLINOIS

An algorithm is a step-by-step method of solving a problem. Algorithms do not replace the complete ophthalmic examination but rather provide the framework for facilitating thought processes used in clinical problem solving.

The purpose of this chapter is to guide the equine practitioner in a logical approach to common ophthalmic problems. The algorithms are to be supplemented by the other chapters in this section as well as by other references and by consultation with veterinary ophthalmologists.

Algorithms are given for the problems of loss of vision, cloudy eye, red eye, protrusion of the third eyelid, and ocular discharge.

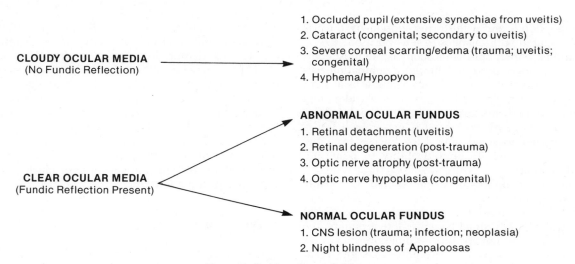

CLOUDY OCULAR MEDIA
(No Fundic Reflection)

1. Occluded pupil (extensive synechiae from uveitis)
2. Cataract (congenital; secondary to uveitis)
3. Severe corneal scarring/edema (trauma; uveitis; congenital)
4. Hyphema/Hypopyon

CLEAR OCULAR MEDIA
(Fundic Reflection Present)

ABNORMAL OCULAR FUNDUS

1. Retinal detachment (uveitis)
2. Retinal degeneration (post-trauma)
3. Optic nerve atrophy (post-trauma)
4. Optic nerve hypoplasia (congenital)

NORMAL OCULAR FUNDUS

1. CNS lesion (trauma; infection; neoplasia)
2. Night blindness of Appaloosas

Figure 1. Problem: Loss of vision.

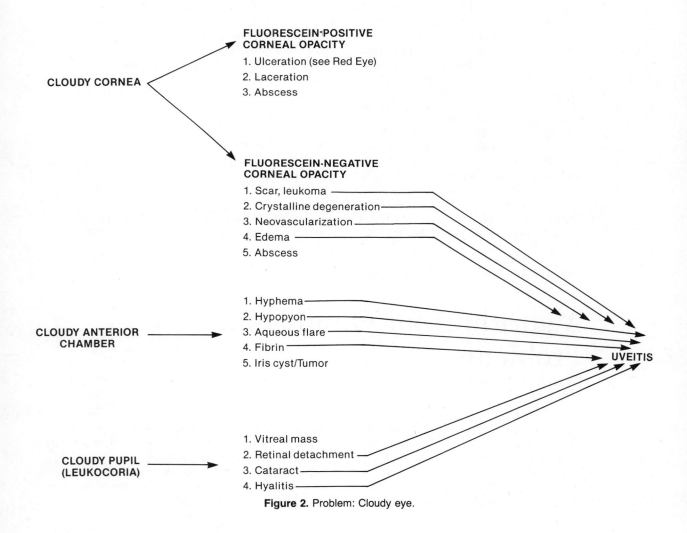

CLOUDY CORNEA

FLUORESCEIN-POSITIVE CORNEAL OPACITY

1. Ulceration (see Red Eye)
2. Laceration
3. Abscess

FLUORESCEIN-NEGATIVE CORNEAL OPACITY

1. Scar, leukoma
2. Crystalline degeneration
3. Neovascularization
4. Edema
5. Abscess

CLOUDY ANTERIOR CHAMBER

1. Hyphema
2. Hypopyon
3. Aqueous flare
4. Fibrin
5. Iris cyst/Tumor

UVEITIS

CLOUDY PUPIL (LEUKOCORIA)

1. Vitreal mass
2. Retinal detachment
3. Cataract
4. Hyalitis

Figure 2. Problem: Cloudy eye.

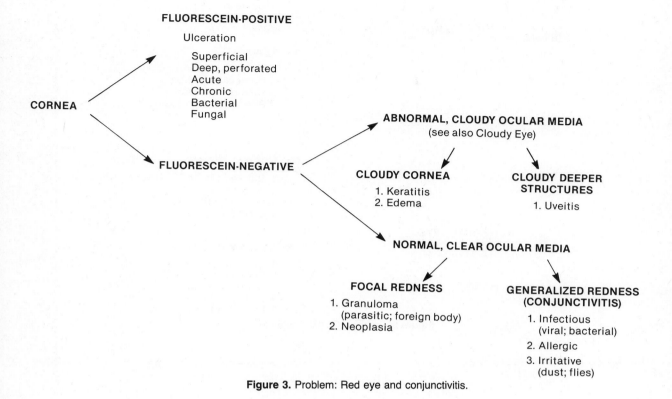

FLUORESCEIN-POSITIVE

Ulceration

Superficial
Deep, perforated
Acute
Chronic
Bacterial
Fungal

CORNEA

FLUORESCEIN-NEGATIVE

ABNORMAL, CLOUDY OCULAR MEDIA
(see also Cloudy Eye)

CLOUDY CORNEA

1. Keratitis
2. Edema

CLOUDY DEEPER STRUCTURES

1. Uveitis

NORMAL, CLEAR OCULAR MEDIA

FOCAL REDNESS

1. Granuloma
(parasitic; foreign body)
2. Neoplasia

GENERALIZED REDNESS (CONJUNCTIVITIS)

1. Infectious
(viral; bacterial)
2. Allergic
3. Irritative
(dust; flies)

Figure 3. Problem: Red eye and conjunctivitis.

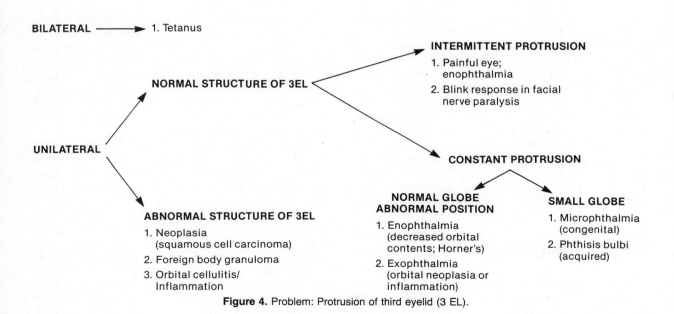

BILATERAL ⟶ 1. Tetanus

NORMAL STRUCTURE OF 3EL

INTERMITTENT PROTRUSION

1. Painful eye;
enophthalmia
2. Blink response in facial
nerve paralysis

UNILATERAL

CONSTANT PROTRUSION

ABNORMAL STRUCTURE OF 3EL

1. Neoplasia
(squamous cell carcinoma)
2. Foreign body granuloma
3. Orbital cellulitis/
Inflammation

NORMAL GLOBE ABNORMAL POSITION

1. Enophthalmia
(decreased orbital
contents; Horner's)
2. Exophthalmia
(orbital neoplasia or
inflammation)

SMALL GLOBE

1. Microphthalmia
(congenital)
2. Phthisis bulbi
(acquired)

Figure 4. Problem: Protrusion of third eyelid (3 EL).

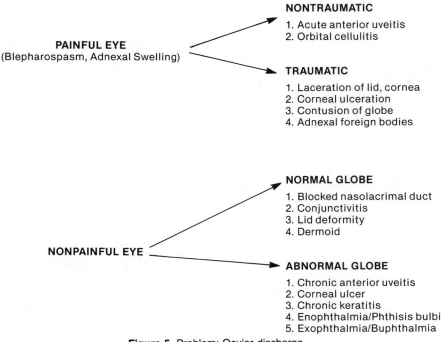

Figure 5. Problem: Ocular discharge.

Ocular Therapeutic Techniques

Mary B. Glaze, BATON ROUGE, LOUISIANA

A treatment plan must specify not only the therapeutic agent but also its route of administration. Succeeding chapters review the indications and dosages for specific ophthalmic drugs. The topic of delivery of medication to the equine eye is sufficiently challenging to warrant a chapter of its own.

The route of administration is dictated by the disease process and the horse's behavior. Ocular therapy may be delivered by topical, subconjunctival, retrobulbar, intraocular, or systemic routes. Multiple routes are combined to maintain effective drug levels in severe ocular disorders. Special therapeutic techniques are indicated in temperamental animals to ensure drug delivery to the eye.

TOPICAL ADMINISTRATION

Topical administration refers to the application of ointments or solutions around the eyelids and into the conjunctival cul-de-sacs. The topical route is effective in diseases of the eyelids, the nasolacrimal system, conjunctiva, cornea, and anterior uvea. Drug concentrations in the posterior ocular tissues are negligible following topical administration.

The efficacy of topical therapy is proportional to the frequency of drug administration. The nature of the horse and the owner must therefore be considered when choosing the topical route. The animal must tolerate repeated manipulation of the eye, and the owner should be both willing and able to treat the horse several times daily.

Topical administration of drugs can cause corneal damage in the uncooperative animal if the drug container inadvertently contacts the eye. An alternate therapeutic route may be chosen for the more fractious animal.

The increased contact time of oily or petrolatum-based ointments reduces the frequency of medication required, giving them an advantage over ophthalmic solutions and suspensions. Ointments are especially useful in blepharitis and conjunctivitis, although they do cause retention of exudate in the conjunctival cul-de-sacs. They should be avoided in perforated corneas, since the ointment base will produce inflammation upon entering the anterior chamber.

Ointments can be applied to the lids with a clean or gloved finger or with a cotton applicator. When administration of drug into the cul-de-sac is indicated, the lower lid is everted and a one fourth-inch ribbon of ointment is applied to the conjunctival surface. The practitioner should take care to avoid contaminating the tube tip. If the horse will not allow eversion of the lid, a small amount of ointment can be placed on a gloved or clean finger and pressed into the medial canthus. As the ointment warms to body temperature and liquefies, it will move across the conjunctiva and cornea.

Solutions and suspensions require more frequent application, since contact time is reduced by their liquid vehicle. Although drops can be applied directly from the container, contamination of the vial is avoided by drawing the solution into a tuberculin syringe. The liquid is placed in the inferior cul-de-sac by everting the lower lid. If the horse objects to such manipulation, the liquid can be squirted directly onto the conjunctiva or cornea when the lids are open. The horse will shy as the medication strikes the eye.

Less conventional forms of topical therapy are also available for use in the horse. Soft contact lenses* can be soaked in antibiotic solutions prior to insertion, functioning as a slow-release reservoir of drug. Medicated conjunctival inserts† are another means of sustained-release medication. These insol-

*Veterinary Hydrophilics, Edgewood, MD
†Alza Pharmaceuticals, Palo Alto, CA

uble devices are impregnated with drugs and are placed or sutured into the lower conjunctival cul-de-sac, anterior to the nictitating membrane. The device must be removed or replaced or both after depletion of the drug.

TOPICAL DELIVERY SYSTEMS

Although direct application of medication into the conjunctival cul-de-sac would seem a simple task, topical treatment is quite difficult in the horse with painful ocular disease and in the animal requiring frequent or prolonged therapy. One of three events may occur as the animal resists medication: contamination of the drug, iatrogenic damage to the cornea, or injury to the handler or horse or both. Topical application can be facilitated by a subpalpebral (Fig. 1) or nasolacrimal (Fig. 2) delivery apparatus, which reduces direct manipulation of the eye and allows medication administration from a site distant to the globe.

The subpalpebral system can be placed in the sedated horse. A local anesthetic injection is recommended in the area of needle insertion. Topical anesthesia with 0.5 per cent proparacaine* is achieved by conjunctival application every 15 seconds for two minutes. The hub of a 14-gauge needle is removed to reduce the risk of corneal damage and to allow the needle to traverse the eyelid.

*Ophthaine, E. R. Squibb, Princeton, NJ

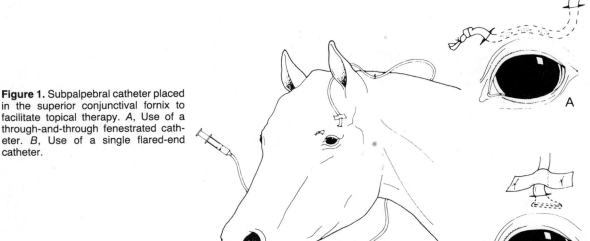

Figure 1. Subpalpebral catheter placed in the superior conjunctival fornix to facilitate topical therapy. *A*, Use of a through-and-through fenestrated catheter. *B*, Use of a single flared-end catheter.

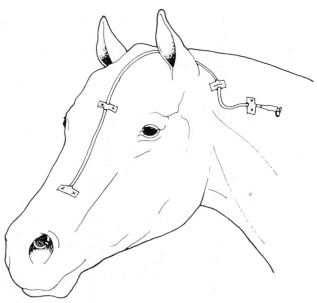

Figure 2. Nasolacrimal medication apparatus, with catheter seated in nasolacrimal duct to facilitate topical therapy.

The needle is introduced into the dorsolateral conjunctival fornix, with care taken to protect the cornea from the point as the needle is positioned. The needle, directed away from the eye, is inserted through the lid until it pierces the skin. Polyethylene tubing (PE 190) or a No. 5 French premature infant feeding tube* is inserted *toward* the eye through the needle lumen, and the needle is retracted along its original path. This positions the tubing laterally. The needle is then repositioned in the dorsomedial fornix and, with the point directed away from the eye, is pushed through the lid. The proximal end of the tubing is now directed *away* from the eye through the needle lumen. The needle is pulled completely through the lid, leaving the tube in place medially as well as laterally. A knot is tied in the end of the tubing where it exits medially to prevent its slipping out of position.

The portion of the tubing that lies in the superior fornix is fenestrated in two or three sites (Fig. 1A). Before the remainder of the tubing is secured, sterile saline should be flushed through the system to determine the adequacy of the fenestrations and the position of the fenestrations in the superior fornix. The tubing must be repositioned if swelling occurs during the infusion.

The external tubing is sutured in place with 2-0 nylon using adhesive tape tabs. The distal tubing extends from the eye posteriorly between the ears and is taped to the halter or sutured along the neck on the side opposite the affected eye. Such placement may alleviate the horse's apprehension during treatment. A 20- or 21-gauge needle with the point removed may be placed in the distal end, or an intravenous catheter and injection cap may be inserted.

An alternate subpalpebral system uses a single flared tube rather than the through-and-through tubing (Fig. 1B). The PE 190 tubing is flared by heating the end above a match flame. The flared end can be exaggerated by pressing it downward on a flat surface while still warm. The tubing is positioned laterally by placing the 14-gauge hubless needle in the superior fornix, penetrating the lid, and passing the nonflared portion of the tubing through the needle. The needle is pulled through the skin and removed. This positions the tip of the tube in the dorsolateral conjunctival fornix. The major disadvantage of the flared tube is its tendency to dislodge from the fornix and damage the cornea.

The subpalpebral system is generally well tolerated by most equine patients. Various drugs can be infused separately or in combination. Medication can be drawn into a tuberculin syringe for introduction into the tubing. Injection of 0.1 to 0.2 ml of solution is followed by a bolus of air to force the medication into the eye.

The nasolacrimal medication system utilizes the horse's nasolacrimal duct for catheter placement. The technique can be performed in the sedated animal, although local anesthetic injections may be indicated in the skin of the false nostril and adjacent to the nasolacrimal orifice. A small stab incision is made through the skin of the false nostril into the nasal vestibule using a 12-gauge hubless needle or a scalpel blade. The fenestrated end of a No. 8 French feeding tube is passed through the needle

*Bard-Parker, Rutherford, NJ

and both the needle and tubing are pulled into the vestibule. The needle is removed and the tubing is inserted 8 to 10 inches into the nasolacrimal duct. The tubing is sutured at the nasolacrimal orifice and at the false nostril using 2-0 nylon and adhesive tape tabs. The remaining tubing may be sutured at intervals along its length or taped to the halter. Whereas iatrogenic damage may occur with the subpalpebral technique, placement of the nasolacrimal catheter is done at a site distant from the eye. The system is therefore safer to establish. Both the subpalpebral and nasolacrimal systems can be used for several weeks without adverse effects.

SITES OF INJECTION

Subconjunctival. Subconjunctival injections are indicated in ocular disease requiring intensive therapy and cases in which client compliance or patient cooperation is lacking. Subconjunctival medication lavages the corneal surface by leaking slowly from the injection site. Drug penetration may also occur by diffusion across the sclera or following absorption by the limbal vasculature. The dorsal bulbar conjunctiva is the site of choice. Injection into the palpebral conjunctiva is less effective owing to the rapid absorption of the drug by the systemic circulation (i.e., the palpebral vessels). Sedation, an auriculopalpebral nerve block, and topical anesthesia will facilitate the injection, but some horses may only require a twitch and topical proparacaine.

A 25- or 27-gauge needle is inserted in the loose bulbar conjunctiva 3 to 4 mm from the limbus. The index finger should be positioned in readiness on the syringe plunger so the injection can be completed quickly. No more than 1 ml of solution should be injected. Subconjunctival injections can be repeated frequently, but some drug vehicles will produce plaques at the injection site.

Retrobulbar. The retrobulbar route is used primarily for regional anesthesia because of the serious complications that may occur following its use. A method to block the ophthalmic nerve and nerves innervating the extraocular muscles at the orbital foramen has been described for the horse. An 18-gauge, 4-inch needle is inserted at a 40-degree angle immediately caudal to the zygomatic process of the frontal bone, at the level of the supraorbital foramen. The needle is advanced ventromedially and caudal to the orbital foramen. Complications of retrobulbar injections include penetration of the globe, retrobulbar hemorrhage, and damage to the optic nerve.

Intraocular. Intracameral (injection into the anterior chamber) and intravitreal injections must be carefully considered because of the sensitivity of the intraocular tissues to most drugs. Intraocular injection may be used in the management of advanced intraocular infections, but only if there is immediate danger of losing the eye or if other conventional therapy has been ineffective. The globe must be immobilized for intraocular injections. General anesthesia is recommended for intracameral injection and required for intravitreal penetration. The volume of drug placed in the anterior chamber or vitreous should equal the amount of material removed.

Injection into the anterior chamber can be made with a 25- or 26-gauge needle inserted through clear cornea immediately adjacent to the lateral limbus. A 25-gauge needle can also be inserted through bulbar conjunctiva 3 to 4 mm from the limbus and advanced subconjunctivally to the limbus, where the needle is inserted into the chamber. For intravitreal injection, a 22-gauge needle is inserted 10 mm from the limbus through the sclera and lateral pars plana of the ciliary body. This will minimize intraocular hemorrhage and the possibility of further retinal damage.

SYSTEMIC ADMINISTRATION

Systemic therapy is often combined with the topical or subconjunctival route to ensure effective drug levels in severe ocular disease. Parenteral administration may be utilized to treat diseases of the anterior and posterior segments, orbit, sclera, and eyelids.

Supplemental Readings

Bistner, S. I.: Ocular therapeutics. *In* Kirk R. W. (ed.): Current Veterinary Therapy VII. Philadelphia, W. B. Saunders Company, 1980.

Gelatt, K. N.: Veterinary Ophthalmic Pharmacology and Therapeutics, 2nd ed. Bonner Springs, KS, VM Publishing, Inc., 1979.

Lavach, J. D., Roberts, S. M., and Severin, G. A.: Current concepts in equine ocular therapeutics. Vet. Clin. North Am. (Large Anim. Pract.), 6:435, 1984.

Diseases of the Adnexa and Conjunctiva

Claire Anne Latimer, COLUMBUS, OHIO

The eyelids, nictitating membrane, lacrimal apparatus, and conjunctiva are structures protecting the globe—particularly the cornea, which must remain clear and moist to maintain vision. Thus diseases of these protective structures not only may produce local irritation, inflammation, and infection, but may threaten the integrity of the globe through their secondary effects on the cornea.

THE EYELIDS AND NICTITANS

The eyelids are delicate, pliable folds of integument lined with palpebral conjunctiva. From their margins exit the cilia and the meibomian glands, contributors of the outermost oily layer of the precorneal tear film. The orbicularis oculi muscle, which encircles the palpebral fissure, is well developed in the horse, often necessitating akinesia (auriculopalpebral nerve block) to facilitate examination.

The nictitating membrane moves passively across the eye when the globe is retracted. In addition to this protective function, the nictitans contributes significantly to the serous portion of the precorneal tearfilm.

Blepharoedema. Blepharoedema is most commonly seen as the result of blunt trauma or as a sequela to the severe blepharospasm that may accompany corneal disease (e.g., ulcer, laceration) or anterior uveitis. If blepharoedema is traumatic in origin, the globe must be thoroughly examined to identify and address any concomitant lesions. In the absence of other abnormalities, nonsteroidal anti-inflammatory agents (flunixin meglumine,* phenylbutazone†) may hasten resolution of the swelling. Lid edema secondary to blepharospasm will resolve with alleviation of the ocular pain.

Other less common causes of palpebral edema are equine viral arteritis, babesiosis, allergy, and infestation of the conjunctival sacs with Thelazia spp.

Blepharitis. Blepharitis manifested as alopecia, excoriation, depigmentation, and crusted discharge is most often associated with fly bites and irritation in the summer months. These lesions are usually most prominent at the canthi, where the lids may be moist with tears and mucus. In addition to causing blepharitis, flies act as intermediate hosts for Thelazia spp. (see under conjunctiva) and Habronema spp. Control of the fly population is the necessary treatment. Ulcerative blepharitis due to the aberrant larval migration of the nematodes *Habronema muscae, H. microstoma,* and *Draschia megastoma* is discussed under Habronemiasis (see below).

Abnormal Cilia. Trichiasis, or deviation of the cilia toward the cornea, is seen secondary to traumatic eyelid lacerations that are not repaired or are inadequately repaired. Cilia that contact the corneal surface are a source of constant irritation and may cause lacrimation, blepharospasm, and corneal ulceration. Eversion of the eyelid margin with a modified Celsus surgical procedure relieves topical irritation while maintaining cosmesis and function.

Ectopic cilia exit through the palpebral conjunctival surface of the lid and cause corneal irritation and ulceration. I have seen an ectopic cilium cause chronic superficial corneal ulceration in a mature Thoroughbred. Epilation with a cilia forceps was curative.

Entropion. Entropion is a turning of the eyelid margin toward the globe with resultant irritation of the cornea and conjunctiva. The irritation causes lacrimation, blepharospasm, and corneal ulceration, which further exacerbates the entropion. In some patients, ocular irritation and blepharospasm may initiate the entropion. This cycle of irritation, pain, blepharospasm, and entropion must be broken to allow corneal healing and a return of the eyelid to a normal position. In most instances, temporary eyelid-everting sutures (e.g., two or three interrupted Lambert sutures of 4-0 nonabsorbable material placed perpendicular to the lid margin) are effective, and further surgical intervention is unnecessary. The temporary sutures are left in place for 10 days, during which time any secondary corneal lesions such as corneal ulcer are treated appropriately (see p. 451). Blepharoplasty is indicated to surgically reposition the eyelid when the lesion is severe.

Habronemiasis. The infective L_3 larvae of *Habronema muscae, H. microstoma,* and *Draschia megastoma* may escape from the mouthparts of adult stable flies or houseflies as they feed around wounds or moist areas on the body, including the medial canthus. These larvae then migrate aberrantly in the ocular adnexa, initiating severe granulomatous reactions in the periocular skin or conjunctiva.

Skin lesions are often slightly raised, ulcerated,

---

*Banamine, Schering Corp., Kenilworth, NJ
†Butazolidin, Coopers Animal Health Inc., Kansas City, MO

well-demarcated, and yellowish red in color with yellow, gritty, caseated or calcified particles interspersed in the granulation tissue. Nonulcerated intradermal nodules may also occur, and these may be distributed along the course of the nasolacrimal duct. Similar yellow, gritty nodules in the bulbar and palpebral conjunctiva are associated with conjunctivitis and secondary keratitis or corneal ulceration. Habronemic blepharoconjunctivitis must be distinguished from neoplasia, foreign body granuloma, phycomycosis, and cutaneous mastocytosis. Diagnosis is based on clinical appearance, cytology, and/or biopsy. Microscopic findings consist of inflammatory and necrotic reactions to the larvae. Larval fragments, eosinophils, and lesser numbers of plasma cells, histiocytes, and mast cells may be seen within a collagenous stroma.

Treatment of adnexal habronemiasis should be both larvicidal and anti-inflammatory. The efficacy of ivermectin* against Habronema spp. and *Draschia megastoma* makes this orally administered broad-spectrum antiparasitic agent a convenient larvicidal drug for adnexal lesions. Clinical improvement should be noted seven days after administration. A topical antibiotic-corticosteroid suspension or ointment such as neomycin, polymyxin-B, or dexamethasone† applied two or three times daily should speed resolution of the adnexal inflammatory response. An alternative treatment for conjunctival lesions is topical application of an ophthalmic organophosphate solution such as 0.03 per cent echothiophate‡ twice daily used in combination with a topical antibiotic-corticosteroid suspension or ointment. Excision of gritty raised lesions may be indicated to minimize secondary corneal and conjunctival lesions.

For skin lesions, an ointment mixture containing 9 gm, trichlorfon§ wettable powder, 224 gm water soluble nitrofurazone base,‖ 20 ml (40 mg) of dexamethasone solution¶ and 56 gm 90 per cent dimethyl sulphoxide** massaged into the affected tissue twice daily is an effective alternative to ivermectin.

Horner's Syndrome. Clinical signs of Horner's syndrome vary somewhat with the location of the lesion, but experimental preganglionic or postganglionic surgical sympathectomy produces similar signs. Ptosis of the upper eyelid, slight protrusion of the nictitans, slight enophthalmos, slight miosis with normal pupillary light reflexes, sweating and increased skin temperature at the base of the ear, on the side of the face, and down the neck to the level of the axis, and mild dilation of the nasal and conjunctival mucous membrane vasculature all occur. Signs will vary with the individual and the time from insult.

Horner's syndrome may be temporary or permanent depending on the cause. Neoplasia, injury, or focal abscesses may impinge upon the sympathetic fibers in the brain or spinal cord. Cranial thoracic lesions such as neoplasia, trauma (e.g., stake injury), or mediastinal lymphadenopathy may result in Horner's syndrome. Intramuscular injections, jugular venipuncture or perivascular injections, guttural pouch mycosis or guttural pouch surgery may affect preganglionic or postganglionic sympathetic fibers. When identified, the underlying cause may require specific treatment. Treatment of Horner's syndrome per se is not indicated and the pharmacologic tests used in other species to localize the lesion have not been evaluated in the horse. Topical application of 10 per cent phenylephrine ophthalmic solution* should resolve the ptosis, miosis, and protrusion of the nictitans, thus confirming the diagnosis of sympathetic denervation. Horner's syndrome is easily differentiated from facial nerve paralysis in which there is ptosis, lagophthalmos, and drooping of the ear ipsilateral to the lesion and deviation of the muzzle toward the contralateral side.

Neoplasia. A wide variety of neoplasms have been reported to affect the eyelids and nictitans including squamous cell carcinoma, sarcoid, melanoma, mastocytoma, basal cell carcinoma, adenoma, hemangiosarcoma, lymphosarcoma, schwannoma, fibrosarcoma, fibroma, and plasma cell tumors. Squamous cell carcinoma is the most common of these, occurring most frequently in horses with a mean age of 9 to 10 years. Solar radiation may induce squamous cell carcinoma, thus predisposing to this condition individuals that lack periocular pigment. Although periocular squamous cell carcinoma is locally invasive, metastasis to regional lymph nodes, salivary glands, and the thorax can occur. Squamous cell carcinoma most frequently presents as a proliferative and/or ulcerated mass affecting the nictitans, perilimbal conjunctiva, and cornea, or the skin. It may be confused with or complicated by granulation tissue, Habronema lesions, or local infection and should be considered in the differential diagnosis of all nonhealing ulcerative skin lesions.

Sarcoid is the second most frequent periocular neoplasm in the horse. This locally invasive fibro-

---

*Eqvalan, MSD-AGVET, Rahway, NJ

†Maxitrol Suspension or Maxitrol Ointment, Alcon Laboratories, Inc., Fort Worth, TX

‡Phospholine Iodide 0.03%, Ayerst Laboratories, New York, NY

§Dyrex, Fort Dodge Laboratories, Fort Worth, TX

‖Furacin Dressing, Norwich-Eaton Pharmaceuticals, Norwich, NY

¶Azium, Schering Corp., Kenilworth, NJ

**DOMOSO, Diamond Laboratories, Inc., Des Moines, IA

---

*Ak-dilate, Akorn, Inc., Metairie, LA

blastic neoplasm does not metastasize but frequently recurs locally following surgical excision or other treatment modalities. Sarcoid is not always clearly differentiated histologically from fibroma, fibrosarcoma, neurofibroma, schwannoma, and neurofibrosarcoma. However, these neoplasms that have been classified as fibrous connective tissue sarcomas have similar biologic behavior and require the same therapeutic considerations. They present as nonregressive smooth nodular, crusted nodular, ulcerated, or pedunculated lesions of the eyelids.

The only self-limiting periocular tumor is viral papilloma, which more commonly affects the muzzle. Viral papillomas are usually multiple, affecting yearlings and two-year-olds, and most regress spontaneously over a one- to three-month period.

Treatment of periocular neoplasms varies with the location, extent, and biologic behavior of the tumor, and the value and function of the patient. Excisional biopsy with histologic examination of the removed tissue is the ideal treatment. However, the extent or location of the lesion may necessitate use of other modalities either alone or in combination with surgical debulking.

Cryosurgery is used successfully for in situ periocular tumor destruction. Squamous cell carcinoma and sarcoid are responsive to this treatment modality. Basic principles of cryobiology must be followed including the use of a double cycle of rapid freeze to $-25°$ C and slow thaw. Adequate freezing and protection of surrounding normal tisses are ensured with the use of thermocouples placed 0.5 cm from the tumor base and margin. Care must be taken to protect the globe and perilesional tissues from accidental exposure to the cryogen. In addition to direct necrosis, cryosurgery may enhance the immune response of the host to neoplastic tissue, thus contributing to its effectiveness. Following separation of the resultant eschar from the underlying granulation bed, healing continues by epithelialization from the periphery with minimal cicatrization. Although poliosis and vitiligo are common sequelae to cryosurgery, pigmentation often returns over several months.

Radiotherapy is also used successfully for the treatment of periocular equine sarcoid and squamous cell carcinoma. Radon seed implantation following surgical reduction of the mass allows for a large local dose of radiation without the necessity for retrieval required when many types of radioactive implants are used. Radon has a half-life of 3.83 days and loses essentially all effective radioactivity by 30 days. However, its use is limited by the necessity for licensure to handle radioactive material, and the need to minimize human health hazard by provision of adequate isolation of the patient.

Radiofrequency hyperthermia is used successfully for management of squamous cell carcinoma of less than 5 cm diameter without deep invasion. Localized current field radiofrequency heating at 50° C for 30 seconds is controlled by a thermistor within one electrode. Cancer cells are sensitive to the thermal energy dissipation that occurs in the tissue just below and outside the electrodes. This treatment modality is thus limited to very shallow lesions.

Immunotherapy is used successfully for the treatment of equine sarcoid. Bacillus Calmette-Guerin (BCG),* an attenuated strain of *Mycobacterium bovis,* is a nonspecific biologic potentiator of the cellular immune system. Tumor regression is linked to the host's ability to develop a delayed hypersensitivity reaction to mycobacterial antigens. BCG is injected intralesionally every two to three weeks until tumor regression is noted. Four to six treatments are often required. Localized swelling, purulent discharge, and ulceration often occur after the first few injections. The use of BCG is not approved in horses, and adverse reactions have occurred with both killed cell wall and live vaccine products. Fatal anaphylaxis has occurred after the second injection of live BCG preparations, and transient malaise, anorexia, and nonfatal anaphylaxis have been observed with cell wall preparations. Pretreatment with flunixin meglumine (1 mg per kg intravenously) and prednisolone (1.0 mg per kg intramuscularly) or flunixin meglumine alone seems to prevent the anaphylactic response that has occurred on the second or subsequent injections.

Protrusion of the Nictitans. The nictitans is passively prolapsed across the surface of the cornea whenever action of the retractor oculi muscle causes the globe to become enophthalmic. Similarly, patients with enophthalmos caused by loss of orbital content or those with a small globe (microphthalmia or phthisis bulbi) will often have a prominent nictitating membrane.

In the normal horse, retraction of the globe occurs in response to superficial (e.g., corneal, conjunctival) pain. Thus, any horse with protrusion of the nictitans should be carefully evaluated for the presence of a foreign body, corneal ulcer, corneal laceration or other source of superficial pain. Bilateral prolapse of the nictitans should arouse suspicions of tetanus, which may occur as a complication of elective surgery or accidental wounds. Stiff gait and bilateral protrusion of the nictitans may be the most prominent clinical signs.

THE LACRIMAL APPARATUS

The lacrimal system is composed of the secretory glands, the precorneal tear film, and the nasolacri-

---

*BCG Vaccine U.S.P., Glaxo, Inc., Research Triangle Park, NC mal drainage apparatus. Diseases of this system fall into two basic categories: (1) those causing decreased or increased tear production, (2) those causing decreased drainage of tears. The main producers of the aqueous portion of the precorneal tear film are the lacrimal gland and the nictitans gland. These glands secrete in response to local stimulation of the fifth cranial nerve, a response called reflex tearing. Impaired function of the fifth cranial nerve, or interruption of the efferent arm of this reflex (the parasympathic fiber traveling with the facial nerve), will cause decreased tear production and result in keratoconjunctivitis sicca.

Keratoconjunctivitis Sicca. Keratoconjunctivitis sicca (KCS) is rarely diagnosed in the horse. Decreased tear production has been observed with locoweed poisoning, secondary to facial nerve damage associated with mandibular fracture, and as an idiopathic lesion. Patients with idiopathic KCS have been presented with ulcerative keratitis and conjunctivitis. Sulfonamide therapy has been incriminated as one cause of KCS in the dog, and its widespread use in the horse may prove a similar association in this species. Therapy for KCS regardless of cause must be directed toward tear replacement and control of the secondary keratoconjunctivitis. A topical parasympathomimetic such as pilocarpine may be used to stimulate tear production. A mixture containing 12 ml of a tear replacement solution such as Adapt,* 6 ml of 2 per cent pilocarpine,† and 2 ml (100 mg) of gentamicin sulfate‡ for injection administered topically is often effective in small animals with KCS. Frequency of application is determined by the severity of the KCS and the response to treatment. An animal that responds to six times per day administration with increased tearing and decreased keratoconjunctivitis might be placed on a four times a day schedule. If no response to this mixture occurs, a tear replacement ointment such as Duratears§ should be substituted because it will have a more prolonged wetting effect than the liquid medication. An antibiotic-corticosteroid ophthalmic ointment may augment the control of keratoconjunctivitis in the absence of corneal ulceration.

Excessive Lacrimation. Horses with excessive lacrimation should be evaluated for the many causes of ocular pain or irritation. Corneal ulceration, foreign body irritation, and uveitis are the most common causes of lacrimation, and they should be managed appropriately. Slaframine (derived from *Rhizoctonia leguminicola,* a soil fungus that infects certain legumes under particular climactic conditions) intoxication produces signs of parasympathetic stimulation including lacrimation.

Epiphora. Epiphora occurs when the nasolacrimal drainage apparatus is obstructed or impatent. Acquired obstructions may result from dacryocystitis, foreign bodies, or traumatic swelling and inflammation affecting the nasal mucosa or concha. Obstruction may also be secondary to fibrous osteodystrophy, chronic sinusitis and rhinitis, neoplasia, periodontitis, or osteomyelitis.

Nasolacrimal Duct Obstruction. Although congenital impatency of the nasolacrimal duct can occur anywhere along its length, atresia of the nasolacrimal meatus is most common. Epiphora is the earliest sign of obstruction; however, the discharge may not be noticed until it becomes copious and mucopurulent due to secondary dacryocystitis. The nature and amount of ocular discharge are inconsistent with the mild degree of conjunctivitis. Inspection of the nasal cavity reveals absence of the nasolacrimal meatus. The dilated duct can often be palpated as a soft tubular mass proximal to the expected location of the meatus. Incision over the tip of a No. 5 male urinary catheter or size 160 polyethylene tubing passed distally from the superior or inferior punctum lacrimale restores nasolacrimal duct patency in uncomplicated cases. After irrigating the duct until the effluent is clear, the tubing is advanced through the new orifice and brought back caudally through a 14-gauge hollow-point needle positioned in the false nostril. The tube is then sutured to the facial skin at both ends and left in place for 7 to 10 days. While the tube is in place, a topical antibiotic-corticosteroid ophthalmic solution is administered four times a day. Dacryocystorhinography is indicated to define the site of obstruction before attemped surgical correction when the distal duct is not readily identified by palpation.

THE CONJUNCTIVA

The conjunctiva is a mucous membrane that provides specific and nonspecific immunologic defense of the ocular surface through normal anatomic features and specific acquired and adaptive immunity. The conjunctival-associated lymphoid tissue is particularly important in the mobilization of a specific reaction against foreign molecules. The conjunctiva is capable of a variety of pathologic processes, the most common of which is inflammation (see Conjunctivitis).

Dermoid. A dermoid is a choristoma or focal skinlike differentiation of bulbar limbic conjunctiva or, less commonly, cornea or nictitans. Histologically, dermoids mimic skin; their cutaneous appendages (such as hair, keratinized epithelium, and

---

*Adapt, Alcon Laboratories, Inc., Fort Worth, TX
†Isopto Carpine, Alcon Laboratories, Inc., Fort Worth, TX
‡Gentocin, Schering Corp., Kenilworth, NJ
§Alcon Laboratories, Inc., Fort Worth, TX

fibrous tissue) often cause local irritation. Although complete excision is curative, the surgeon must be aware that corneal dermoids in the horse may extend into the deep stroma. Following excision and reapposition of the conjunctival margins, a topical antibiotic solution is recommended until corneal healing is complete.

Chemosis. Chemosis, or edema of the conjunctiva, occurs to some extent with any conjunctivitis. Following orbital fractures, allergic reactions, and acute orbital inflammation, extreme chemosis can prevent lid closure and corneal examination. The redundant conjunctiva is then subject to exposure, and desiccation will occur rapidly without provision of additional moisture. Treatment should be aimed at determination and correction of the underlying cause. Meanwhile, liberal frequent application of a topical antibiotic or antibiotic-corticosteroid ointment to prevent desiccation is indicated. In cases in which chemosis is secondary to orbital trauma, flunixin meglumine (1.0 mg per kg once a day orally) may speed resolution of the local swelling. When recovery is prolonged, a temporary tarsorrhaphy may be indicated to prevent exposure.

Hemorrhage. Subconjunctival hemorrhage may be seen in newborn foals and is presumed to result from compressive trauma during birth. The foal should be carefully examined to exclude the presence of other mucosal or cutaneous hemorrhage that might indicate a coagulopathy. Uncomplicated subconjunctival hemorrhage should resolve over 7 to 10 days without treatment. Conjunctival or subconjunctival hemorrhage in the mature horse must be carefully evaluated. Post-traumatic hemorrhage may be accompanied by other ocular lesions that may require treatment such as corneal injury, iridocyclitis, and lens luxation. Hemorrhages may occur with vasculitis, anemia, thrombocytopenia, or other coagulopathies. Petechial conjunctival hemorrhages have been described with equine viral arteritis and equine infectious anemia. Treatment, determined by the primary etiology, may be monitored by the change in conjunctival hemorrhage.

Conjunctivitis. Inflammation of the conjunctiva may be primary or secondary to other ocular or systemic disease. Clinical signs vary but may include hyperemia, chemosis, lymphoid follicles, and ocular discharge. Diagnosis is based on ocular and general physical examination along with evaluation of the environment and morbidity of the disease. Culture and exfoliative cytology are helpful in refractory lesions.

Mechanical irritants such as dust, flies, and fly spray cause conjunctivitis in animals of any age. Affected individuals are most often affected bilaterally, and the ocular discharge tends to be serous in the early stages. With chronicity, secondary bacterial infection may occur and the discharge may become mucopurulent. Treatment is based on identification and removal of the ocular irritant and topical antibiotic or antibiotic-corticosteroid ointments used three times a day to control secondary inflammation and infection,

Allergic conjunctivitis probably occurs in horses, although the diagnosis is often presumptive. Affected horses may have an acute onset of chemosis, blepharoedema, and serous ocular discharge. Signs abate with removal of the offending allergen, which may be identified by an observant owner. Treatment with flunixin meglumine or phenylbutazone and a topical antibiotic-corticosteroid ointment will hasten resolution of clinical signs. Occasionally, allergic conjunctivitis may be associated with a topical medication. Clinical signs are exacerbated with continued application and abate when the medication is discontinued.

The infectious agents involved in primary bacterial or viral conjunctivitis in the horse have rarely been identified. It is not uncommon to see groups of foals or yearlings affected with a mild to moderate self-limiting conjunctivitis without signs of systemic illness. Recovery is generally uneventful without any form of treatment. However, the group should be closely observed for signs of systemic disease, and conjunctival culture and cytology may be indicated if spontaneous recovery does not occur within 7 to 10 days. Several parasites have been incriminated as causative agents in equine conjunctivitis. *Thelazia lacrimalis* is a white nematode 10 to 25 mm long that may cause lacrimation, conjunctivitis, and blepharoedema. Manual removal of the parasite is facilitated by a topical organophosphate miotic and a topical anesthetic. A topical antibiotic-corticosteroid ointment may then be used to hasten resolution of the conjunctivitis. *Onchocerca* spp. have been identified in horses with bilateral interstitial keratitis and temporal perilimbal bulbar conjunctival vitiligo. However, conjunctival depigmentation is not an absolute indicator of microfilariasis and as an isolated clinical finding requires no treatment.

Conjunctival habronemiasis is manifested as conjunctivitis with congestion, mild chemosis, serous discharge, and raised, gritty yellow-white caseated particles 1 to 2 mm in diameter in the bulbar or palpebral conjunctiva. This form of habronemiasis may be treated with topical ophthalmic organophosphates (e.g., 0.03 per cent echothiophate) twice a day or oral ivermectin as the larvicidal agent and a topical antibiotic-corticosteroid ophthalmic solution or ointment to control the inflammatory reaction to the aberrant larvae. Surgical removal of irritating gritty plaques may be indicated if they cause corneal abrasion and discomfort.

Conjunctivitis may be seen secondary to a wide variety of systemic diseases, particularly those causing respiratory infections, such as rhinopneumonitis, influenza, *Streptococcus equi, Rhodococcus equi, Actinobacillus equuli,* and adenovirus. A careful ocular examination should be performed to rule out the presence of anterior uveitis that may accompany these systemic diseases. Treatment should be directed toward the systemic disease.

In general, horses with apparent conjunctivitis should be examined to determine whether the conjunctivitis is primary or secondary. In particular, the presence of attendant corneal or uveal disease should be ruled out. In many instances, conjunctivitis is probably self-limiting in horses. However, careful examination will reveal clinical signs that may indicate an etiologic agent requiring specific therapy, such as habronema or thelazia. Animals with a clear serous discharge are less likely to have bacterial involvement than those with a mucopurulent discharge, and treatment should be decided accordingly.

Neoplasia. A variety of neoplasms may affect the conjunctiva of the horse, and squamous cell carcinoma is the most frequently diagnosed. Any proliferative conjunctival mass that causes secondary ocular irritation and/or enlarges in size should be excised and submitted for histopathology. Although other treatment modalities such as cryotherapy, radiofrequency hyperthermia, and radiotherapy may be used instead of or in addition to excisional biopsy, tissue should always be submitted for histopathologic examination.

Supplemental Readings

Herd, R. P., and Donham, J. D.: Efficacy of ivermectin against cutaneous *Draschia* and *Habronema* infection (summer sores) in horses. Am. J. Vet. Res., 42:1953, 1981.

Mayhew, I. G.: Horner's syndrome and lesions involving the sympathetic nervous system. Equine Pract., 2:44, 1980.

Munger, R. J.: Equine onchocercal keratoconjunctivitis. Equine Vet. J., Suppl 2, p. 65, 1983.

Raphel, C. F.: Diseases of the equine eyelid. Comp. Cont. Ed., 4:S14, 1982.

Schmidt, G. M., Krehbiel, J. D., Coley, S. C., and Leid, R. W.: Equine ocular onchocerciasis: histopathologic study. Am. J. Vet. Res., 43:1371, 1982.

Intraocular Inflammation

Thomas J. Kern, ITHACA, NEW YORK

Inflammation of the iris, ciliary body, and/or choroid is a frequent cause of painful unilateral or bilateral ocular disease in horses. The sequelae of anterior uveitis (iris and ciliary body inflammation) and posterior uveitis (choroiditis) may well comprise the leading causes of equine blindness worldwide. These sequelae include secondary degeneration or dysfunction of the cornea, lens, vitreous, retina, and optic nerve.

Competent therapy of uveitis requires accurate diagnosis by recognition of the characteristic clinical signs. Prognosis for vision and for uveitis recurrence depends on the underlying cause and the response to therapy.

CLINICAL SIGNS AND OCULAR EXAMINATION

Owners' observations of horses with intraocular inflammation prompting veterinary consultation include the appearance of "red," "painful," "cloudy," and "blind" eyes. The accuracy of these observations depends, in part, upon the condition's duration and severity. Chronic inflammation may result in marked intraocular pathologic changes, but their gradual onset may go unnoticed. Conversely, acute uveitis may be so painful that intense blepharospasm prevents casual inspection of the eye.

Complete examination—external and intraocular—of both eyes must be carefully performed, even if the presenting ocular complaint is unilateral. When blepharospasm is moderate to intense, examination can be facilitated by auriculopalpebral nerve block to relax the orbicularis oculi muscle. Most significant lesions of the external eye and adnexa, as well as intraocular lesions anterior to the vitreous, can be identified and characterized by inspection with a bright light source (e.g., penlight, ophthalmoscope with or without a Finhoff transilluminator tip) and the observer's trained eye. Fundus examination, when not impaired by the clinical signs of uveitis themselves, may be performed with a penlight and indirect condensing lens or a direct ophthalmoscope. Mydriasis should be achieved when possible with topically applied 1 per cent tropicamide.* Pupillary dilatation allows more complete evaluation of lens, vitreous, and fundus—a major advantage when subtle lesions are present, as in the apparently "normal" opposite eye of horses afflicted with uveitis.

---

*Mydriacyl, Alcon Laboratories, Inc., Fort Worth, TX

The clinical signs observed during ocular examination vary with both the intensity and duration of uveitis. Horses with acute initial or recurrent episodes of uveitis may show clinical signs similar to those of horses with other painful external eye and adnexal disorders, such as corneal ulceration and blepharitis. Epiphora, blepharospasm, photophobia, conjunctival hyperemia, corneal opacity, hypopyon, and miosis all occur to at least some degree in acute uveitis.

Epiphora is a nonspecific sign due to either excessive lacrimation or nasolacrimal duct obstruction. Horses with uveitis are stimulated to tear profusely from the pain of ciliary muscle spasm and the accompanying photophobia. Moist facial dermatitis may occur if epiphora persists. Blepharospasm is, likewise, a nonspecific finding. Its intensity is generally proportional to the severity of uveitis. Spastic entropion causing secondary corneal ulceration may ensue if squinting becomes intense and persistent. Photophobia is manifested as squinting in moderate to bright light and is often relieved when surroundings are darkened. Photophobia is very suggestive of intraocular inflammation, as it is mediated in part through reflex ciliary muscle spasm. Conjunctival hyperemia is present in active uveitis. Its prominence seems proportional to the inflammation's severity. Circumciliary vascular injection—prominence of deeper blood vessels at the corneoscleral junction—is pathognomonic for uveitis. Both of these findings are present in active uveitis, although the latter requires close inspection, often aided by low magnification.

Corneal opacity occurs with uveitis caused by (1) stromal edema, (2) neovascularization, and (3) primary or secondary corneal ulceration. Stromal edema, which gives the affected cornea a "ground glass" appearance, is caused by endothelial dysfunction, usually promoted by the presence of protein and cells in the aqueous humor. If corneal endothelium is severely damaged, permanent corneal opacity results. While corneal edema often develops very quickly, corneal neovascularization does not become visible for several days. Circumciliary neovascularization of the peripheral cornea for its entire circumference—appearing like a "paintbrush" pattern—is pathognomonic for uveitis. It is most prominent in eyes with severe subacute to chronic uveitis.

Alterations in appearance of the anterior chamber, often confused with corneal changes, result from increased protein (aqueous flare), large accumulations of inflammatory cells (hypopyon), and clotted or unclotted blood (hyphema). Impairment of the normal blood-aqueous barrier in the iris and ciliary body vasculature owing to inflammation is the underlying cause of the clinical signs. When this impairment is severe, aqueous humor alterations are dramatically evident.

Iris changes nearly always accompany intraocular inflammation. These are most obvious when the inflammation seems centered in the iris and ciliary body, but even when active choroiditis is the most apparent problem, anterior uveal changes are usually attendant. Edema and cellular infiltration alter normal iris color. Spasm of the iris constrictor muscle results in miosis, a hallmark of active inflammation. Chronic or recurrent uveitis results in posterior and anterior synechiae, iris depigmentation, and atrophy. Extensive posterior synechia formation may cause iris bombé and secondary glaucoma.

In both acute and chronic uveitis, pathologic changes in the lens, vitreous, and retina are less apparent to horse owners and veterinarians. Except for acute changes such as posterior synechia formation most lens changes occur weeks or months after uveitis begins. Pigment flecks on the anterior lens capsule, even in quiet (nonpainful) eyes, suggest prior uveitis. Cataract development may occur focally at sites of synechiae or may involve large areas of lens cortex and nucleus. Lens luxation or subluxation may occur following chronic uveitis associated with zonular and vitreal degeneration.

Vitreal alterations include acute cellular exudation and chronic degeneration with liquefaction and collagen condensation ("floaters"). Retinal detachment may result from vitreal liquefaction or traction resulting from linear bands of fibrotic tissue.

Retinal changes accompanying or following uveitis include active chorioretinitis, atrophic chorioretinal scars, and retinal detachment. Active chorioretinitis with exudation or cellular infiltration causes dullness and loss of apparent detail in the affected areas of the fundus; the nontapetal area is more commonly involved than the tapetal area. Both active and inactive lesions are commonly reported adjacent to the optic disc nasally and temporally following the retinal vascular distribution. Inactive peripapillary lesions consisting of multifocal hyperpigmented and depigmented foci constitute a so-called "butterfly" lesion adjacent to the disc. Retinal detachment is promoted by choroidal exudation, vitreal liquefaction, and vitreal traction. If retinal degeneration is extensive, optic disc atrophy, characterized by disc pallor and retinal vessel paucity or absence, ensues.

Intraocular pressure (IOP) is usually decreased in acute uveitis owing to decreased aqueous production and possibly altered aqueous outflow. Documentation of IOP in horses is difficult. Conventional Schiotz tonometry cannot be readily performed on horses; applanation tonometry may be used but instruments are prohibitively expensive. Digital palpation of the affected eye often suggests whether IOP is extremely low or high but is *not a reliable indication of normal IOP*. Chronic glaucoma, resulting in buphthalmos, is an occasional sequela to chronic uveitis.

The severity of vision loss in an individual horse is determined by the combination of acute and chronic ocular lesions which afflict its eyes.

ETIOLOGY

Identification of the causative factor(s) in acute or chronic equine uveitis is usually difficult. Uveitis in the horse, as in other species, can be a manifestation of other systemic diseases or a component of a primary ocular disorder. A summary of known and suspected causes is presented in Table 1.

THERAPY

Therapy for equine uveitis is almost exclusively targeted toward eyes with active inflammation. Quiet (nonpainful) eyes blinded by uveitis sequelae in general neither require nor benefit from treatment. The objectives of therapy are (1) reduction of uveal inflammation, (2) preservation of pupil size and motility, (3) pain relief, (4) prevention of blinding sequelae, and (5) resolution of associated exogenous or endogenous causes, if possible. The first four objectives are best served through the combined use of steroidal and nonsteroidal anti-inflammatory agents and mydriatic and cycloplegic drugs. Specific pharmacotherapy for purported individual causative agents should accompany the former, essentially symptomatic treatment.

TABLE 1. CAUSATIVE FACTORS IN EQUINE UVEITIS

Exogenous Factors
Corneal ulceration: infectious, sterile
Trauma
    Blunt: direct, contrecoup
    Penetrating: ± infection, ± lens injury
    Foreign body: extraocular, intraocular
    Postsurgical

Endogenous Factors
Infectious diseases ↔ Immune-mediated disorders
  Leptospirosis   Cell-mediated immunity?
  Onchocerciasis   Humoral immunity?
  Streptococcus equi
  Viral arteritis
  (Brucellosis?)
  (Toxoplasmosis?)
  Bacterial septicemia
  Others?
  Idiopathic

An algorithm for initial therapy of acute uveitis is presented in Table 2.

CORTICOSTEROIDS

Corticosteroids can be administered topically, subconjunctivally, or systemically, or by a combination of these. Suppression of uveitis and pain relief are determined by both administration frequency and the routes used. For treatment of mild clinical signs, relatively infrequent (e.g., three to four times a day) topical administration may be

TABLE 2. TREATMENT PLANS FOR ACUTE UVEITIS OF UNKNOWN CAUSE

Initial Treatment
Rule out corneal ulceration
Maxitrol— every 2 to 4 hrs
Atropine—every 2 to 4 hrs
Flunixin IV BID

Re-evaluate after 24 hours

If Improved
Repeat flunixin or phenylbutazone IV
Continue topical drug regimen every 4 hrs
Assess gastrointestinal motility
Re-evaluate in 2–3 days

If Improved
Reduce atropine frequency (SID-TID)—continue to effect
Maxitrol every 2 to 4 hrs—continue to effect
Discontinue flunixin or phenylbutazone

If Not Improved
Rule out corneal ulceration
Continue topical drug regimen every 2 to 4 hrs
Flunixin or phenylbutazone PO or IV BID
Assess gastrointestinal motility
If mydriasis incomplete, add 10% phenylephrine topically every 2 to 4 hours
Consider subconjunctival corticosteroids
Re-evaluate daily

If Not Improved
Consider consultation/referral

effective and sufficient. For moderately severe clinical signs, frequent (every four to six hours) topical administration combined with subconjunctival injection of a repository preparation may be optimal. For fulminant uveitis, intensive (every two hours) topical treatment, combined with subconjunctival injection and oral or parenteral administration, may be necessary to quell the inflammation. In all of these instances, the use of nonsteroidal anti-inflammatory agents and mydriatic and cycloplegic drugs is indicated.

Topical corticosteroid preparations' efficacy is limited by the frequency with which they are used and their relatively short contact time with the eye. Both ophthalmic solutions and ointments are acceptable formulations for use in horses; in fact, their combined use is often the optimal way to ensure adequate treatment response. Many specific products may be used successfully. Prednisolone acetate,* distinguished by its excellent intraocular penetration, is an ophthalmic solution of choice. Potent dexamethasone preparations† are available as both solutions and ointments and can be used together to tailor effective treatment regimens. Topical administration of drug solutions in many horses that are fractious or in pain can be facilitated by use of subpalpebral or nasolacrimal lavage systems (see p. 436). These are especially useful when protracted topical therapy is prescribed or anticipated.

An adjunct or alternative administration route to frequent topical treatment is subconjunctival injection of repository corticosteroids. Ten to 40 mg of methylprednisolone acetate‡ in a 0.5 to 1 ml volume injected beneath the bulbar (*not* palpebral) conjunctiva may prove beneficial for one to four weeks. Prednisolone acetate§ (10 to 25 mg in 0.5 to 1 ml volume) administered similarly gives rapid but short-lived (24 to 48 hours) benefit. Triamcinolone‖ (3 to 6 mg in a 0.5 to 1 ml volume) injected subconjunctivally yields an intermediate effect, over three to seven days, but has been reported to cause laminitis. Clinical judgment and follow-up examination findings should determine whether repeated injection is indicated.

Systemic corticosteroid administration is warranted for severe uveitis when either topical or subconjunctival corticosteroids or both fail to effect improvement. Because of the notable potential side effects of systemic corticosteroids, the relatively safer nonsteroidal anti-inflammatory agents should probably be prescribed *first*. If they prove ineffec-

tive or insufficient, dexamethasone* (20 mg intramuscularly twice a day) may be given daily for up to five days. Longer term systemic administration is discouraged.

While drugs of this class are beneficial as the mainstay of uveitis therapy, nonetheless they may promote undesirable, even catastrophic, side effects.

1. They suppress corneal epithelial and stromal healing and potentiate endogenous corneal collagenolytic enzyme activation; therefore, their use in the presence of corneal ulceration is almost always *contraindicated*. If ulceration is present, systemic nonsteroidal anti-inflammatory drugs and topical mydriatic and cycloplegic agents should be used *first*.

2. Immunologic defense of the ocular surface is compromised and alteration of normal external ocular microflora may result. Corticosteroids potentiate both bacterial and mycotic keratitis. Chronic corticosteroid usage may be the *single greatest risk factor for equine keratomycosis*.

The best ocular corticosteroid therapy is that administered in the lowest dose by the safest route with the least frequency to be effective.

NONSTEROIDAL ANTI-INFLAMMATORY AGENTS

The initiation, promotion, and maintenance of ocular inflammation are associated with complex prostaglandin metabolism within the uveal tract. The drugs of this class useful in equine uveitis management have antiprostaglandin activity. Adjunct use of low-dose antiprostaglandins is indicated in most equine uveitis cases. Their benefit is often striking, minimizing the role that corticosteroid therapy plays in uveitis management. Three antiprostaglandins are currently in widespread use in equine practice. Phenylbutazone,† given orally or intravenously at a dosage of 3 to 5 mg per kg twice a day, has good ocular anti-inflammatory and analgesic effects. It may be most effective for mild and moderate uveitis as well as for chronic low-dose oral prophylaxis for horses with intractably recurrent uveitis. Flunixin meglumine‡ has remarkably potent anti-inflammatory, analgesic, antispasmodic, and antipyretic activities. This drug is the antiprostaglandin of choice in treatment of moderate to severe uveitis, administered orally, intravenously, or intramuscularly once to twice a day at 1.0 mg per kg. Although clinically less potent than phenylbutazone or flunixin, aspirin (15 mg per kg twice a day orally) has been used successfully as prophylaxis against chronic recurrent uveitis after acute uveitis has been managed with other drugs.

---

*Pred-Forte, Allergen Pharmaceuticals, Irvine, CA
†Maxitrol, Maxidex, Alcon Laboratories, Inc., Forth Worth, TX
‡Depo-Medrol, Upjohn Company, Kalamazoo, MI
§Prednisolone Acetate, Carter-Glogan Laboratories, Inc., Glendale, AZ
‖Vetalog, E. R. Squibb, Princeton, NJ

*Azium, Schering Corp., Kenilworth, NJ
†Butazolidin, Coopers Animal Health, Inc., Kansas City, MO
‡Banamine, Schering Corp., Kenilworth, NJ

Potential side effects of antiprostaglandins include gastric ulceration and possibly renal dysfunction. Flunixin may be the most commonly implicated agent.

MYDRIATIC AND CYCLOPLEGIC DRUGS

Every horse with uveitis must be treated with a parasympatholytic mydriatic and cycloplegic agent. Pupillary dilatation decreases lens-to-iris contact, minimizing risk of pupil seclusion by posterior synechiae, and may reduce aqueous flare by promoting iris vasoconstriction. Mydriasis also may allow useful vision throughout an episode of uveitis.

Topical application of 1 to 4 per cent atropine solution or ointment is indicated every one to two hours until the pupil dilates. Once it dilates, mydriasis may be maintained by less frequent administration, e.g., every 6 to 12 hours. The inflamed uveal tract is markedly resistant to atropine's effects. If mydriasis is slow or incomplete, 10 per cent phenylephrine hydrochloride* may be administered in conjunction with atropine, or methylscopolamine-phenylephrine† may be substituted for both. *Caution:* Frequently applied topical phenylephrine may cause corneal ulceration.

Horses receiving mydriatic and cycloplegic drugs should be monitored for signs of colic, although this development is uncommon. Pupillary dilatation may persist for up to four weeks following cessation of treatment; owners should be informed accordingly.

ANTIBIOTICS

Indications for topical antibiotic therapy of uveitis are the presence of corneal ulceration, and the inability to rule out an exogenous or endogenous infectious cause. In actual practice, topical corticosteroid therapy is usually accompanied by use of broad-spectrum antibiotics such as bacitracin-neomycin-polymixin B combinations, gentamicin, and chloramphenicol. In most adult horses without corneal ulceration, nonseptic immune-mediated inflammation is the cause of uveitis; therefore, topical or systemic antibiotic therapy is not expected to be effective. Topical antibiotics may temporarily discourage overgrowth of pathogenic bacteria during intensive corticosteroid treatment.

Indications for systemic antibiotic therapy are septicemic uveitis (most frequent in foals) and documented or strongly suspected leptospiral infection. For septicemic uveitis, broad-spectrum parenteral antibiotics, such as aminoglycosides, are indicated for life-saving therapy. The occasional horse with documented serially increasing leptospiral titers should be suspected of harboring viable organisms and treated with appropriate systemic antibiotics, such as penicillin-streptomycin.

OTHER DRUGS

The role of *Onchocera cervicalis* infection in acute and recurrent uveitis is unclear and has recently been disputed. Until the existence of a relationship is conclusively verified or disproved larvicidal therapy may be considered for horses with uveitis in which dermal and conjunctival biopsies show microfilaria. This is discouraged during active uveitis episodes because microfilarial death may exacerbate inflammation.

Treatment should be delayed until uveitis is quiescent, and even then horses should be prophylactically treated with corticosteroids and antiprostaglandins. Two microfilaricidal compounds are available. Diethylcarbamazine citrate may be administered orally at a dosage of 4 mg per kg body weight once daily for 21 days. Ivermectin* may be administered as a single treatment at a dosage of 200 μg per kg body weight orally. The increasingly widespread use of this drug by veterinarians and horse owners has not as yet been associated with the initiation or exacerbation of uveitis in large numbers of horses. The clinician should be wary, however, of this potential complication if classic concepts of the onchocercal pathogenesis of uveitis are correct.

OTHER MODES OF THERAPY

Vaccination. *Only* in bands of horses in which leptospiral infection has been reasonably well documented in association with uveitis should periodic leptospiral vaccination be considered. Credible documentation should include (1) affliction of several horses with acute or recurrent uveitis in one location, (2) serial positive leptospiral serology from affected and/or (as yet) unaffected horses, and (3) exposure to infected cattle. *Caution:* Exacerbation of leptospiral uveitis might occur following leptospiral vaccination. Therefore, indiscriminate vaccination is probably unwise.

Surgery. Chronic, intractable, or recurrent uveitis frequently causes chronic pain, secondary glaucoma, and phthisis bulbi. Options for surgical management are enucleation and evisceration of the globe with silicone prosthesis† implantation.

Therapy for Nonpainful Eyes. No treatment is warranted for nonpainful eyes with lesions from chronic uveitis. Some horses require chronic, lowest-effective-dose treatment with aspirin, phenyl-

---

*Neo-Synephrine, Winthrop-Breon Laboratories, New York, NY

†Murocoll No. 2, Muro Pharmacal Laboratories, Inc., Tewksbury, MA

---

*Eqvalan Paste 1.87%, MSD-AGVET, Rahway, NJ
†Jardon Plastics, Southfield, MI

butazone, or flunixin meglumine for maintenance of ocular comfort and function.

PROGNOSIS

The outlook for retention of useful vision is related to the frequency and severity of uveitis recurrences as well as to the success of their treatment. No data are available to objectively predict the likelihood of uveitis recurrence. Thus, the long-term prognosis for vision in horses with unilateral or bilateral uveitis is guarded.

Supplemental Readings

Cook, C. S., Peiffer, R. L., and Harling, D. E.: Equine recurrent uveitis. Equine Vet. J., 2:48, 1983.

Glaze, M. B.: Red, painful eyes (uveitis). In Robinson, N. E. (ed.): Current Therapy in Equine Medicine, 1st ed. Philadelphia, W. B. Saunders Company, 1983, pp. 382–385.

Matthews, A. G., and Handscombe, M. C.: Uveitis in the horse: A review of the aetiological and immunopathological aspects of the disease. Equine Vet. J., 2:61, 1983.

Rebhun, W. C.: Diagnosis and treatment of equine uveitis. J. Am. Vet. Med. Assoc., 175:803, 1979.

Trogdon-Hines, M.: Immunologically mediated ocular disease in the horse. Vet. Clin. North Am. (Large Anim. Pract.), 6:501–512, 1984.

Diseases of the Cornea

Cecil P. Moore, MADISON, WISCONSIN

The avascular, transparent cornea is composed of the epithelium with its basement membrane, the corneal stroma, the endothelial basement membrane (Descemet's membrane), and a monolayer of endothelial cells. The epithelium, which is five to seven cell layers thick, provides an effective superficial barrier to microbes, excessive fluid entry, and particulate matter. The stroma accounts for over 90 per cent of the total corneal thickness and consists of an orderly arrangement of stromal cells (keratocytes) and collagen lamellae. The optical function of the corneal stroma depends on its compactness and state of dehydration. The endothelium and Descemet's membrane serve as an inner barrier for the cornea. The corneal endothelium maintains the stroma in a dehydrated state. Since the cornea is avascular it is nourished by the tears externally and by the aqueous humor internally. Nutrients may also diffuse into the peripheral cornea from the limbal capillaries.

The horse eye is prominent and the cornea is visible as a slightly oval dome that is broader nasally. The axial cornea is thicker than the perilimbal cornea. In many horses, a white crescent is noted at the corneoscleral junction nasally and temporally. In some animals the entire limbus may be involved. These normal structures represent areas of insertion of the pectinate fibers of the iridocorneal angle from the base of the iris to the inner surface of the cornea. The scleral shelf is frequently more prominent dorsally and ventrally, resulting in reduced visualization of the iridocorneal angle in these areas.

Equine corneal diseases may be categorized as congenital or acquired. Congenital corneal diseases are frequently inherited.

CONGENITAL KERATOPATHIES

DERMOIDS

A choristoma is a congenital mislocation of normal tissue. Dermoids, a type of choristoma, are the most common congenital abnormalities of the equine cornea. Dermoids are skinlike masses with hair follicles, sebaceous glands, and other dermal structures. Equine corneal dermoids commonly involve the lateral aspect of the cornea, although any area of the cornea or the entire cornea may be involved.

Depending upon the size, location, and the presence of bristly hairs, dermoids may cause localized frictional irritation and visual disturbance. The clinical characteristics of the dermoid and the presence or absence of other ocular anomalies will dictate whether surgical excision is feasible. Two types of dermoids may be observed in the foal. One form is a thick localized tissue mass with a distinct tuft of hair. This well-differentiated dermoid is usually superficial and may be locally excised by superficial keratectomy. Following surgical removal of the dermoid, the eye is treated for the postsurgical ulceration. Some degree of postoperative corneal scarring is usual.

A less common dermoid may be associated with multiple ocular anomalies such as microcornea, persistent pupillary membranes, and anterior segment cleavage anomalies. It tends to be flattened, poorly differentiated, and intensely pigmented with multiple depigmented (pink or white) foci representing hair follicles with or without visible cilia. In general, surgical excision of this type of dermoid cannot be recommended.

CORNEAL OPACITIES ASSOCIATED WITH PERSISTENT PUPILLARY MEMBRANES

Persistent pupillary membranes are strands of mesodermal tissue that arise from the anterior iris surface and may attach to the endothelial surface of the cornea, resulting in focal corneal opacities (leukomas). Treatment is not indicated unless iris movement causes tension on the corneal endothelium with progressive corneal edema. In such instances surgical transection of the membranes might be considered.

CORNEAL MELANOSIS

An anterior corneal melanosis involving the epithelium and superficial stroma of the central cornea has been described in the foal. Corneal neovascularization may be a component of this congenital opacity. Congenital corneal melanosis may also be observed with corneal dermoids or persistent pupillary membranes. When corneal melanosis presents a cosmetic or functional problem and in the absence of intraocular anomalies, superficial keratectomy might be considered.

OTHER CONGENITAL CORNEAL LESIONS

Microcornea usually accompanies microphthalmia with multiple ocular anomalies. Nonprogressive, noninflammatory congenital corneal opacities of Thoroughbred foals have been recently reported. Among affected foals some had superficial irregular punctate opacities that occurred as a transient condition. Deep corneal, linear, and band opacities with histologically abnormal Descemet's membrane appear to be associated with congenital thinning of this layer. Although lines of edema may be associated with the defective membrane, this condition is nonprogressive. No treatment is either available or indicated for the condition.

ACQUIRED KERATOPATHIES

TRAUMATIC KERATOPATHIES

Trauma may result in a wide range of corneal lesions varying from focal superficial corneal abrasions through blunt nonulcerative injury to perforation and rupture of the eye. Causes of trauma include scratches and penetrations from plant material, injury from tack or stable hardware, injuries related to training, racing, or loading, and injury inflicted by handlers while attempting to restrain or discipline an animal. Nonulcerative injury of the cornea is discussed here. The management of ulcerative keratitis following trauma will be considered in the following section. The management of corneal lacerations is discussed under the heading of Ocular Emergencies (see p. 460).

Blunt nonulcerative injury of the equine cornea may result in endothelial contusion and corneal edema. Contusion may indent the cornea sufficiently to allow contact between the endothelium and the anterior lens capsule. This may result in anterior capsular lens opacities associated with corresponding areas of corneal edema. Mild to moderate corneal edema may be observed with blunt injury to the epithelium and anterior stroma. Severe corneal edema, characterized by an intense blue appearance of a markedly thickened cornea, is typical of extensive endothelial damage. Bullous keratopathy may result from edema following severe endothelial injury or from blunt trauma with sufficient force to separate the corneal layers. Occasionally, nonpenetrating trauma causes separation of stromal lamella creating intrastromal spaces that fill with fluid while the overlying epithelium remains intact.

Conservative therapy consists of topical 5 per cent sodium chloride ointment applied four times daily to reduce corneal edema during the initial post-traumatic period. Topical broad-spectrum antibiotics are indicated should the epithelium or superficial stroma subsequently slough. Topical corticosteroids may be useful in treating concurrent traumatic uveitis. Corticosteroids should be discontinued immediately if ulceration occurs. Fibrovascular infiltration may occur before resolution of post-traumatic nonulcerative keratopathy, particularly if anterior stromal lamellae have been separated or severe edema is present. When this occurs, superficial or stromal neovascularization should not be discouraged, because it is usually necessary for corneal healing. Following neovascularization, there will be some degree of corneal scarring.

Whenever surface ocular injury has occurred, the clinician must assess the deeper ocular structures for damage. Traumatic uveitis, ruptured or dislocated lens, intraocular hemorrhage, and retinal or optic nerve contusion are possible sequelae of acute ocular trauma. Ocular ultrasonography can be used to assess deep intraocular structures when the anterior ocular media are opaque. The assessment and management of intraocular trauma are discussed further under the heading of Ocular Emergencies (see p. 460).

ULCERATIVE KERATITIS

Corneal ulcers are usually due to trauma. With superficial ulceration only the epithelium is lost. Squinting, photophobia, and lacrimation are observed clinically. Upon closer examination the corneal surface usually appears slightly irregular and mildly edematous. Application of fluorescein solution to the eye delineates the ulcerated area. Healing of epithelial defects normally occurs rapidly by migration and mitosis of epithelial cells. Depending upon the total area involved, an epithelial defect may heal in two to eight days without scar formation.

Regrettably, corneal ulcerations frequently involve the stroma, which is slower to heal than the epithelium. Stromal defects present more readily visible changes in corneal contour, variable degrees of opacification, and moderate to severe ocular pain with reflex pupillary constriction. Healing usually occurs after inflammatory cell infiltration, dissolution of damaged stroma by degradative enzymes, neovascularization, and reformation of collagen. Focal or diffuse ulcerations in which the entire corneal stroma has been lost, leaving only Descemet's membrane and the endothelium to prevent aqueous loss, are termed *descemetoceles*. Repair of Descemet's membrane requires regeneration by endothelium. The corneal endothelium has limited potential for healing and repair occurs primarily by sliding of cells rather than by mitosis.

An accurate and carefully acquired history provides useful information to formulate the initial therapeutic plan. Frequently after the initial corneal trauma, opportunistic microorganisms, enzymatic degradation of the corneal stroma, mechanical irritants, corneal desiccation and inappropriate therapy can delay and complicate healing. Corneal penetration by plant foreign material suggests the inoculation of fungi into the corneal stroma. Topical corticosteroids account for a high incidence of mycotic keratitis, while resistant bacterial organisms commonly follow unsuccessful treatment with topical antibiotics. A rapidly progressive keratopathy with degradation of the corneal stroma indicates excessive enzymatic activity. Pseudomonas organisms and certain genera of fungi such as Aspergillus may produce collagenase. When combined with enzymes from degranulating inflammatory cells and proliferating fibrocytes, collagenase results in rapid destruction of corneal tissue.

Therapy

Diagnostic and therapeutic measures for ulcerative keratitis depend upon the history and the extent of the ulcer. Acute, focal, superficial ulcers may be treated empirically with topical broad-spectrum antibiotics such as gentamicin, chloromycetin, or triple antibiotics (neomycin, bacitracin, and polymixin B). Ointments are preferred when treating uncomplicated ulcers because of their prolonged contact time. Antibiotic ointment applied three or four times daily and topical 1 per cent atropine ointment applied to effect pupillary dilation will usually allow rapid healing of an uncomplicated traumatic ulcer.

Complicated corneal ulcers are generally subacute, infected, and progressive with varying degrees of keratomalacia and neovascularization. Aggressive diagnostic and therapeutic measures are necessary. Corneal cultures and scrapings are essential to determine the presence of opportunistic microorganisms. Following tranquilization and eyelid anesthesia, a sterile cotton or Dacron swab moistened with transport medium is applied to the margin of the ulcer and submitted to the laboratory for aerobic bacterial culture. Topical anesthetic is applied to desensitize the cornea and a scraping of the ulcer margin is obtained for cytology and fungus culture. For a corneal scraping, some affected corneal stroma dislodged for cytologic analysis is most reliable for locating and identifying fungi. Corneal scrapings are placed on glass slides for Wright's and Gram stains. A small specimen of tissue is placed on Sabouraud's medium for fungus culture.

Initial therapy of complicated ulcers requires aggressive antimicrobial therapy on the basis of history, clinical findings, and results of cytology (see Table 1). Results of bacterial culture and susceptibility tests may indicate that therapy should be modified at 48 to 72 hours. If gram-negative rods are identified cytologically, gentamicin (20 mg) or carbenicillin (100 mg) is injected subconjunctivally. When gram-positive organisms are observed, cefazolin (50 mg), chloromycetin (40 mg), methicillin (5 mg), or ampicillin (50 mg) may be injected subconjunctivally. The relatively rare identification of gram-negative cocci requires penicillin G subcon-

TABLE 1. INITIAL LOCAL ANTIBIOTIC THERAPY OF CORNEAL ULCERS

Organism(s)	Local Antibiotic	
	Subconjunctival *(may be repeated in 24 hrs)*	Topical *(every 1 to 4 hrs)*
Gram-positive cocci	methicillin* (50 mg) or cefazolin‡ (50 mg)	triple antibiotic† or chloromycetin§
Gram-negative rod	gentamicin‖ (20–25 mg)	gentamicin** or tobramycin††
Gram-negative cocci	penicillin‡‡ (250,000 IU)	triple antibiotic or tetracycline§§
Mixed bacteria	gentamicin‖ (20–25 mg) and methicillin* (50 mg)	triple antibiotic† or gentamicin‖
Fungi	miconazole‖‖ (10 mg)	miconazole‖‖ or natamycin***

Based on Gram staining characteristics of bacteria observed on cytologic examination.
*Staphcillin, Bristol Laboratories, Syracuse, NY
†Neosporin, Burroughs Wellcome Co., Research Triangle, NC
‡Kefzol, Eli Lilly & Co., Indianapolis, IN
§Chloroptic, Allergan Pharmaceuticals, Irvine, CA
‖Gentocin (Injectable), Schering Corp., Kenilworth, NJ
**Gentocin Ophthalmic, Schering Corp., Kenilworth, NJ
††Tobrex, Alcon Laboratories Inc., Fort Worth, TX
‡‡Penicillin G potassium, E. R. Squibb, Princeton, NJ
§§Achromycin, Lederle Laboratories, Wayne, NJ
‖‖Monistat IV, Janssen Pharmaceutica Inc., New Brunswick, NJ
***Natacyn, Alcon Laboratories, Forth Worth, TX

junctivally (250,000 units). When two or more bacteria are present, methicillin and gentamicin may be used simultaneously subconjunctivally if injected at different sites. When fungal elements are present or suspected, miconazole (10 mg) is administered subconjunctivally.

Following initial subconjunctival injections, topical antimicrobial solutions should be applied a minimum of every two hours or ointments every four hours. Hourly application of solutions may be necessary in rapidly progressive cases of Pseudomonas or Aspergillus keratitis or in cases of very deep ulcers of unknown cause. Antibacterial solutions available commercially for topical administration include gentamicin, chloromycetin, triple antibiotic solution, and tobramycin. Other solutions may be formulated using sterile injectable preparations with artificial tear diluents. Antibiotic ointments commercially available include gentamicin, chloromycetin, triple antibiotic, erythromycin, tobramycin, and tetracycline. Commercially prepared antifungals are limited to natamycin, which is available as a 5 per cent suspension. Although not approved for use in the eye, miconazole 1 per cent solution may be used topically and appears to be safe and effective in treating fungal keratitis. Topical dermatologic creams containing miconazole have also been used in the eye for two to three weeks without complications.

In addition to eliminating infectious agents, other goals of therapy are removing mechanical irritants, preventing further enzymatic destruction of the cornea, relieving pain and concurrent uveitis, ensuring adequate moisture to the eye, and providing surgical support of the cornea in cases of deep ulcerations.

Therapy for rapidly progressive infected ulcers with extensive keratomalacia consists of the topical application of an antibiotic, an antifungal, a cycloplegic and an anticollagenase preparation. Therapy must be initially intensive and often prolonged. Miconazole (10 mg per ml), gentamicin solution (3 mg per ml) and 1 per cent ophthalmic atropine and 5 per cent acetylcysteine have been successfully applied sequentially every one to two hours. Alternate therapy might include tobramycin substituted for gentamicin and natamycin suspension in place of miconazole solution. Tobramycin and natamycin are generally effective but expensive.

A subpalpebral or nasolacrimal infusion tube may greatly enhance the administration of liquid drugs. After 48 to 72 hours, therapy may be modified according to the results of bacterial culture and sensitivity tests. Common opportunistic bacterial isolates include Streptococci, Staphylococci, Pseudomonas, and coliform organisms. As the ulcer begins to heal, frequency of topical solutions may be reduced to every three to four hours. If destruc-

tion of the cornea is controlled and healing is indicated by re-epithelialization and neovascularization, gentamicin and atropine ophthalmic ointments and miconazole dermatologic cream may be substituted for solutions. Ointments are applied four times daily for an additional two weeks and the acetylcysteine solution may be discontinued.

Superficial and deep corneal neovascularization occurs in many cases of infectious keratitis. This normal healing response should not be inhibited by corticosteroids until the affected area has completely vascularized and epithelialized as evidenced by a lack of retention of fluorescein stain. Frequently this requires three to four weeks. Following complete healing, topical corticosteroid antibiotic combinations will hasten the regression of the fibrovascular infiltrates. The degree of scarring is directly related to the degree of initial corneal involvement and may vary from transient focal superficial scarring to diffuse deep stromal scarring that may be permanent or, at best, remodel slowly with some clearing over several years.

In cases of severe keratomalacia or descemetocele formation surgical intervention may be indicated. A temporary tarsorrhaphy or a third eyelid flap may be used as a short-term emergency measure to keep the eye moist and to support and protect it until more definitive surgical repair can be attempted. A temporary tarsorrhaphy is recommended before transporting an animal with a deep corneal ulceration or corneal staphyloma. Two horizontal mattress sutures of 0 Supramid or silk are usually adequate.

Third eyelid flaps are difficult to perform successfully in the horse. Three to four horizontal mattress sutures are generally necessary. These are placed through the upper eyelid with deep bites into connective tissue on the anterior side of the third eyelid. The use of upper eyelid stints will prevent the suture from cutting into the eyelid. The most common complication is the suture pulling through the third eyelid conjunctiva. Third eyelid flaps have been used to support healing in cases of granulating staphylomas with protrusion of tissue beyond the normal corneal curvature.

Focal perforated ulcers may be sutured with 6-0 to 7-0 Dexon, Vicryl, or silk if the ulcer margins are healthy enough to support the suture. Principles of surgical repair of the cornea are discussed on p. 461. Deep, nonvascularizing ulcers or descemetoceles may be treated with conjunctival flaps. Whether a simple advancement flap, a pedicle flap, a bridge flap, or a 360-degree flap, the conjunctiva is meticulously dissected free from the underlying bulbar connective tissue. A properly dissected conjunctival flap should be quite thin and nearly transparent. Opaque thick flaps result when epibulbar connective tissue (Tenon's layer) is dissected with the conjunctiva. Conjunctival flaps provide support for the weakened cornea and serve as a source of nutrition and fibrocytes to the healing cornea. Large corneal defects may be repaired by performing a corneal-limbal-conjunctival transposition or full-thickness corneal graft. Detailed discussion of these surgical procedures is beyond the scope of this chapter.

Soft, hydrophilic contact lenses have been used in equine ulcerative keratitis to support and protect the cornea and to reduce the pain associated with an ulceration. When presoaked in antimicrobial solutions, lenses may provide a constant perfusion of medications to infected corneal tissue. Although therapeutic soft contact lenses for horses have become more readily available in recent years, cost of the lenses and variations in surface curvature of equine corneas have limited their widespread use.

Providing additional moisture to the ulcerated eye is usually not necessary because profuse lacrimation characterizes most cases. If facial nerve paralysis accompanies ocular trauma, atony of the orbicularis oculi muscles and inability to blink may cause neuroparalytic keratitis. Characteristically the inferior central cornea dries and ulcerates diffusely, necessitating tear supplementation, application of lubricant ointments, or a temporary tarsorrhaphy. Motor innervation of the palpebral muscles often returns in such cases within four to six weeks.

Inapparent, persistent, mechanical irritants may cause recurrent corneal ulceration. Frictional irritants include masses, foreign bodies of the bulbar surface of the third eyelid, distichiasis, ectopic cilia, chalazia. Masses or foreign bodies may involve the eyelid margin or palpebral conjunctiva. Irregularities of the eyelid margin, such as notching or scarring of the eyelid, and misdirected eyelid hairs from previous injury must not be overlooked as possible causes of corneal irritation. A thorough systematic external ocular examination, performed with a bright focal light and magnifying source in a darkened area, is essential in every case of ulcerative keratitis.

SUPERFICIAL KERATITIS

Uniocular superficial keratitis, presumably viral, has been described in horses in Great Britain. Presumptive diagnosis was based on clinical improvement following antiviral therapy with 0.5 per cent idoxuridine ophthalmic ointment topically administered 5 times daily for 5 to 14 days. One form of disease is a superficial lacelike opacity with or without punctate staining; another form is a corneal ulcer with peripheral punctate staining and lacelike opacity; a third form is diffuse superficial corneal opacity with no staining. Whether these clinical entities represent phases of the same disease or different diseases is unknown.

Equine herpesvirus I has been isolated from the surface epithelium of horses with multiple punctate, whitish epithelial lesions. The significance of this finding is not clear. Punctate keratitis may also occur with ocular onchocerciasis.

INDOLENT ULCERS

Chronic nonhealing ulcers characterized by epithelial undermining or lack of neovascularization are not common but present a therapeutic challenge. Differential diagnoses for indolent ulcers include viral keratitis, resistant bacterial keratitis, mycotic keratitis, drug-induced keratopathy (as from phenylephrine), low-grade frictional irritant, and tear film deficiency. One type of indolent ulcer is a static superficial stromal ulcer, which over a period of several weeks or months does not vascularize or epithelialize. A second type is a superficial epithelial ulcer with undermining around its rim. Therapy may include debridement of undermined epithelium with a dry cotton swab or superficial keratectomy if a static stromal ulceration is present. Cautery with 7 per cent tincture of iodine may remove devitalized tissue and stimulate neovascularization. Empirically, hypertonic solutions or ointments may be used to allow local dehydration of the epithelium and encourage attachment to its underlying basement membrane. Hydrophilic soft contact lenses used as a physiologic bandage allow contact and encourage adherence of the epithelium while protecting the cornea. Lubricant antibacterial ointments may be helpful to sterilize the ulcer and reduce frictional rubbing from the third eyelid or eyelid margins. More extensive surgical procedures such as conjunctival flaps might be considered, particularly with an indolent stromal ulcer. The use of topical corticosteroids in treating indolent ulcers in horses is controversial at this time and is not recommended.

NONULCERATIVE KERATOPATHIES

Corneal fibrosis (scarring), stromal abscessation, interstitial keratitis associated with anterior uveitis (keratouveitis), corneal degeneration, and striate keratopathy are nonulcerative lesions that may opacify the cornea.

Inflammation of the cornea frequently results in fibrovascular infiltrates into the corneal stroma. While these infiltrates are essential to the repair of the cornea, they leave scars. Opacities associated with corneal scars result from deposition of irregular fibrocytic collagen in contrast to the regular (transparent) arrangement of collagen normally produced by stromal keratocytes. The deeper and more diffuse the initial corneal lesion, the more extensive and the more opaque the scar. In heavily pigmented eyes, melanocytic migration will frequently accompany the final stages of granulation resulting in a pigmented scar.

Heavily pigmented scars tend to lose pigmentation and become more white after several months. A pigmented scar is often more acceptable to the owner than an intense white area. As the corneal stroma remodels, the appearance of scars may change. Focal or superficial corneal scars may become faint and regress in a period of 6 to 18 months. Extensive deep stromal scars are usually accompanied by persistent vascular infiltrates. These may be visible with a focal light source or may be seen as "ghost" vessels with a slit lamp biomicroscope. Dense scars with active or latent vascularization undergo only minimal changes with time. Corneal tattooing or colored contact lens application are cosmetic procedures that may improve the appearance of a scarred cornea.

Nonulcerative corneal abscesses may occur as single or multifocal areas of yellow-white stromal infiltrates. These are most commonly caused by introduction of pyogenic microorganisms, such as Pseudomonas, Streptococci, Staphylococci, and E. coli, or opportunistic fungi into focal puncture wounds. Corneal scrapings, cytology, and bacterial and fungal cultures are indicated. Occasionally cases of nonseptic corneal stromal abscessation are encountered.

Nonulcerative corneal stroma abscesses frequently ulcerate spontaneously or from diagnostic scraping and superficial debridement. Therapy is the same as for complicated corneal ulcerations. Broad-spectrum antibiotics (gentamicin or methicillin) may be administered subconjunctivally. Antibiotics (gentamicin, chloromycetin, or triple antibiotic combination) and a mydriatic (1 per cent atropine) should be administered topically. Fungal elements on stained scrapings, a history of plant puncture, or topical corticosteroid application merit initiation of topical antifungal agents such as 1 per cent miconazole. Culture and susceptibility testing will determine maintenance antimicrobial therapy. Progressive keratomalacia may dictate the application of anticollagenase preparations to the cornea. When rapid progression and extensive ulceration occur, surgical intervention may be necessary. Endophthalmitis secondary to corneal abscessation is an indication for systemic antibiotics such as ampicillin or tribrissen.

Intraocular inflammatory diseases commonly cause corneal opacities. Intraocular exudates may adhere to the endothelium, resulting in an endothelialitis observed as focal or geographic plaquelike lesions. Clumping of anterior chamber exudates (keratic precipitates) onto the corneal endothelium may result in chronic inflammatory changes characterized by deep corneal fibrovascular infiltrates. Varying degrees of corneal edema may accompany acute and chronic uveitis. The amount of edema depends on the extent of endothelial damage.

Deep corneal vascularization (interstitial keratitis) is frequently seen following recurrent uveitis. In the subacute form fibrovascular infiltrates may appear as pink focal or diffuse pre-Descemet's lesions. Fibrosis of these granulomatous-appearing lesions occurs as the condition becomes chronic, leaving areas of deep corneal scarring. Chronic uveitis may result in lens luxation or, in a small percentage of cases, secondary glaucoma. Diffuse corneal edema is not uncommon in such cases and is usually accompanied by chronic fibrovascular infiltrates from previous episodes of uveitis. Glaucoma may also result in buphthalmos and striate opacities from breaks in Descemet's membrane.

Onchocerca larvae migrating through the cornea may result in linear stromal opacities. These opacities usually occur in the mid to deep corneal stroma. Punctate epithelial lesions and focal subepithelial opacities are also associated with ocular onchocerciasis. Parasitic migration tracks in the cornea may occur as isolated lesions or as part of a generalized keratouveitis.

Opacities that contain lipid or mineral deposits (usually calcium) occur secondary to previous inflammatory processes or the treatment of a prior corneal disease. Corneal lipidosis and calcium deposition are usually associated with corneal vascularization. Predisposing causes include ulcerative keratitis, neovascularization, recurrent uveitis, and local administration of corticosteroids. The clinician must realize that these degenerations are secondary to previous inflammatory disease. Treatment is not indicated unless the lesion impairs vision and is superficial so that a lamellar keratectomy might be considered. Since surgical invasion of the cornea incites additional inflammation, the risk of recurrence of the degeneration must be recognized.

A noninflammatory keratopathy may occur following radiation treatment of ocular neoplasms. Corneal epithelial bullae, progressive corneal edema, and nonhealing erosions characterize this apparently uncommon entity. Since the capacity of the cornea to heal is reduced by radiation therapy, even minor insults may result in ulceraton. Treatment is empirical to prevent secondary problems such as drying and infection.

Corneal dystrophies are noninflammatory, spontaneously occurring corneal opacities involving primarily one layer of the cornea. They are frequently bilateral, often symmetrical, and generally familial. Adult-onset corneal dystrophy has not been observed in the horse. A transient superficial corneal dystrophy has been seen in Thoroughbred foals (see Congenital lesions). Post-inflammatory corneal degeneration should not be confused with corneal dystrophy, which implies a genetic cause.

Primary tumors of the cornea are extremely rare. Squamous cell carcinomas arise at the limbus and extend to the adjacent cornea. Mast cell tumors, hemangiomas, hemangiosarcomas, adenomas, adenocarcinomas, and lymphomas originate from the anterior uvea, sclera, conjunctiva, or third eyelid, and corneal involvement is quite uncommon. Older animals that lack perilimbal pigmentation have a higher incidence of limbal squamous cell carcinoma probably due to chronic exposure of nonpigmented tissues to actinic radiation. Limbal squamous cell carcinomas may be treated successfully if diagnosed early by biopsy and histopathology. In the majority of cases the characteristic rough, elevated, nonpigmented mass remains superficial, and a lamellar keratectomy and conjunctivectomy effectively remove the neoplasm. Strontium 90 (Sr^{90}) beta radiation is used as an adjunct to superficial keratectomy. A calculated absorbed dose of 10,000 rads is safe and effective. Higher doses may be used safely, but latent adverse side effects have been reported.

Postoperatively the eye is treated for the iatrogenic ulceration by application of a broad-spectrum antibiotic ophthalmic ointment every 8 hours and 1 per cent atropine ophthalmic ointment as needed to maintain moderate mydriasis. Corticosteroids are applied topically if fibrovascular infiltration occurs at the surgical site and only after reepithelialization is complete. Alternative modes of therapy include hyperthermia and cryosurgery.

Suggested Readings

Barnett, K. C., Rossdale, P. D., and Wade, J. F. (eds.): Equine Ophthalmology Supplement, Equine Vet. J., Suppl 2, November, 1983.

Moore, C. P. (ed.): Large Animal Ophthalmology. Vet. Clin. North Am. (Large Anim. Pract.), 6, No. 3, November 1984.

Riis, R. C.: Equine Ophthalmology. In Gelatt, K. N. (ed.): Veterinary Ophthalmology. Philadelphia, Lea and Febiger, 1981.

Cataracts

R. David Whitley, GAINESVILLE, FLORIDA

Cataracts are opacities of the ocular lens or its capsule. Such opacities must be differentiated from other causes of leukokoria in the horse: vitreous opacity, retinal detachment, intraocular tumor, hypopyon, and fibrin. Cataracts may occur as congenital or acquired defects. Congenital cataracts are present at birth or within the first three months after birth and are an important cause of blindness in horses. In one report of congenital ocular defects in horses, the most frequent was cataracts. Affected foals may be presented with complaints of visual deficits, clumsiness, or repeated lacerations of the face, forelimbs, neck, or chest.

Although the precise cause of most congenital cataracts in horses is unknown, heritable, traumatic (prenatal and foaling), nutritional, and post-inflammatory (in utero infection) etiologies have been proposed. Heredity can rarely be documented, but dominant inheritance has been reported in the Thoroughbred and in Belgian horses with aniridia. Anterior subcapsular cortical cataracts have been observed in a Welsh Thoroughbred filly with aniridia. Nonprogressive nuclear cataracts that have no appreciable effect on vision have been described in the Morgan horse. Congenital cataracts may be associated with other ocular defects such as microphthalmia, aniridia, and persistent pupillary membranes.

Acquired cataracts in horses are frequently secondary to equine recurrent uveitis or to trauma.

Juvenile-onset cataracts, as seen in many breeds of dogs, are uncommon in the horse. Senile cataracts that interfere with vision are also uncommon. Nuclear lenticular sclerosis is often seen in old horses; however, their vision is clinically normal.

Regardless of cause, cataracts may involve the lens diffusely or focally. Diffuse (total) cataracts produce severe visual impairment or blindness. Focal cataracts may involve any area of the lens. Suture line and nuclear cataracts may not progress or cause visual deficits. Anterior and posterior cortical cataracts are more prone to progression and resulting visual impairment. Focal central (axial) cataracts may interfere with vision in bright light when the pupil is constricted; topical mydriatics will allow vision around axial cataracts. Peripheral opacities of the lens rarely affect vision; however, they may progress to complete cataracts.

TREATMENT

Several medical regimens have been proposed for cataract resolution in humans and animals. These have included administration of acetazolamide, calcium, cysteine, iodine, orgotein, selenium-tocopherol injections, sulfonamides, sulfadiazine, and injection of cytolyzed culture of *Actinomyces bovis* followed by horse serum extract. Medical treatment of cataracts is currently a highly questionable mode of therapy owing to lack of controlled studies.

Although some rapidly progressing cataracts in foals may show spontaneous resorption without surgery, surgical removal of cataracts is usually recommended if the owner desires therapy. Four surgical techniques have been described to remove cataracts from the equine eye: aspiration, phacofragmentation with aspiration, extracapsular extraction, and intracapsular extraction.

Currently the most common technique used for removal of congenital cataracts is a two-needle discission-aspiration technique, by which lens material is removed from the eye through a large-gauge needle. Phacofragmentation is also an excellent technique for removing congenital cataracts in foals and for some traumatic cataracts in adult horses. The procedure involves the use of ultrasonic fragmentation of the lens followed by aspiration. Although extracapsular and intracapsular techniques have been used to remove acquired cataracts in horses, phacofragmentation is suggested when cataract removal is indicated in the adult animal. Details of surgical procedures are beyond the scope of this book.

Selection of surgical candidates is important. By temperament, the horse must be amenable to handling and the frequent giving of medication. Halterbroken animals are preferred. The presence of other ocular or systemic abnormalities is justification for postponing or canceling surgery.

Cataract surgery is more successful when performed before six months of age; therefore, a thorough physical and ophthalmic examination is recommended in foals during the first month of life. Medical history should include ophthalmic status of the sire, dam, and siblings; pedigree analysis; health and diet of the dam during gestation; and exposure of the dam to drugs, chemicals, radiation, or infectious diseases. In adult horses, recurrent ocular disease or previous trauma should be documented.

The animal's eyesight should be carefully assessed. Weak, disoriented foals may have other neurologic abnormalities without lesions of the visual system. Pupillary response to light is not a dependable measure of vision, since the reflex is retained in blindness of central origin as well as in early stages of retinal disease. The menace reflex is also unreliable in very young foals. Adult horses may be led through an obstacle course, but foals seldom cooperate in maze testing.

The eyes should be evaluated for other developmental anomalies or concurrent ocular disease. Foals with microphthalmia and aniridia or horses with cataracts secondary to uveitis are unsuitable surgical candidates. Blepharitis, conjunctivitis, ulcerative keratitis, and uveitis must be controlled before cataract surgery. The pupils should be dilated with 1 per cent tropicamide to allow complete evaluation of the lens. Lenses with anterior capsular opacities may also have posterior capsular densities that will compromise vision postoperatively. A preoperative electroretinogram should be considered in the Appaloosa, a breed with heritable nyctalopia (night blindness).

PROGNOSIS

Location of the cataract may be useful in predicting its progression. Table 1 summarizes the likelihood of further opacification on the basis of position of the cataract. The success rate for cataract extraction in foals less than six months of age is 75 to 80 per cent. The percentage decreases in older foals, which are more difficult to medicate postoperatively and which have a higher incidence of hypermature cataracts and lens-induced uveitis.

Complications of cataract surgery in the horse are often related to synechiae and iridocyclitis. Intense postoperative uveitis with fibrin and inflammatory cells aggregating on the corneal endothelium may result in moderate to severe corneal edema. Persistent corneal edema may also result from extensive endothelial cell loss associated with overzealous irrigation or touching the endothelium with instruments during surgery. Fibropupillary membranes, secondary cataracts, recurrent uveitis, and phthisis bulbi are other potential complications of cataract surgery in the horse.

Following lens aspiration, secondary cataracts may develop from opacification of remnants of the anterior lens capsule, retained cortical material, or posterior capsular opacities. Vision reduction depends on the location and extent of opacification. Some owners and trainers have reported visual impairment at night or in dim light in animals with apparently normal day vision following cataract surgery. This may be related to secondary cataract formation. Other complications include self-trauma, periorbital edema, corneal ulceration, mycotic keratitis, superficial and deep corneal fibrovascular infiltrates, chronic corneal edema, recurrent uveitis,

TABLE 1. PROGNOSIS FOR CATARACTS ON THE BASIS OF ANATOMIC LOCATION

Position of Opacity	Prognosis
Anterior capsule	Usually nonprogressive
Anterior cortex	Progressive
Perinuclear	Usually nonprogressive
Nuclear	Usually nonprogressive
Posterior cortex	Progressive
Posterior capsule	Unpredictable
"Y" suture	Usually nonprogressive

and retinal detachments. Systemic illness following cataract surgery is often related to the stress of anesthesia or hospitalization.

Soundness following cataract surgery is of concern to the surgeon and the owner. Many foals may have adequate vision for training and riding after cataract surgery. Evaluation of vision should be performed postoperatively with an obstacle course in bright and dim illumination. The horse's temperament, whether it is affected unilaterally or bilaterally, the experience of the rider, and the complexity of the maneuvers required of the animal are additional factors that determine the animal's suitability to be ridden following cataract surgery. Although the genetics are poorly defined at this time, breeding of animals affected with congenital cataracts is not recommended.

Supplemental Readings

Bistner, S. I., Aguirre, G., and Batik, G.: Surgery of the lens. *In* Bistner, S. I., Aguirre, G., and Batik, G. (eds.): Atlas of Veterinary Ophthalmic Surgery. Philadelphia, W. B. Saunders Company, 1977.
Gelatt, K. N., Myers, V. S., and McClure, J. R.: Aspiration of congenital and soft cataracts in foals and young horses. J. Am. Vet. Med. Assoc., *165*:611, 1974.
Riis, R. C.: Equine ophthalmology. *In* Gelatt, K. N. (ed.): Veterinary Ophthalmology. Philadelphia, Lea & Febiger, 1981.
Whitley, R. D., Moore, C. P., and Slone, D. E.: Cataract surgery in the horse: A review. Equine Vet. J., *15*(Suppl. 2):127, 1983.

Diseases of the Retina and Optic Nerve

William C. Rebhun, ITHACA, NEW YORK

Diseases of the retina and optic nerve may occur in horses without obvious anterior segment inflammatory diseases. In these cases, the owner may observe reluctance to perform, shying, nervous behavior, or fear of strange environments in the affected horse. Many horses with retinal and optic nerve lesions, however, show no clinical signs and continue to perform well. These animals that have adjusted to their visual handicaps are diagnosed only during soundness examinations; therefore, medicolegal problems may occur with these cases.

CLINICAL SIGNS

In unilateral retinal or optic nerve lesions, direct pupillary light response in the affected eye may be absent or depressed. Consensual light responses are variable depending on whether total or partial retinal or optic nerve damage is present. Clinical signs are usually more obvious if both eyes are affected. In bilateral cases, both pupils may respond poorly or not at all to direct light stimulation and the eyelids tend to be held widely open since the horse is "light hungry" and apprehensive. Owners' observations of decreased vision are more emphatic in horses that are affected bilaterally. These observations include balking, shying, apprehensive behavior, or reluctance to carry out previously normal performance. In unilateral lesions, owners may observe that the horse is apprehensive only on one side, tilts its head to look at objects, shies, or fails to take certain leads. They may observe that the horse works better in specific lighting circumstances. Some patients are presented for recurrent or frequent corneal abrasions due to poor vision of which the owner is unaware. It must be emphasized, however, that some horses with partial or complete unilateral blindness are asymptomatic because they have adjusted to their handicap.

In addition to direct and consensual pupillary light responses, funduscopic examination with an ophthalmoscope is imperative to document retinal or optic nerve lesions. The examiner must be familiar with the paurangiotic equine fundus, the normal color variants encountered, and the differences between the tapetal and nontapetal fundus. Most horses, except those with partial albinism, have a tapetal layer within the choroid. This tapetum is not part of the retina but is responsible for light reflection from the tapetal choroid back through the retina. This process allows the retina two opportunities to absorb light messages. The tapetal color is usually blue or green in black or bay horses and may vary toward yellow in palomino horses. Paints, pintos, and ponies can have partially albinotic fundi with choroidal vessels being apparent as large orange-red linear vessels showing through the retina in areas where the tapetum is partially missing or absent. The optic disc lies below the tapetal and nontapetal border within the nontapetum. It is located ventral and slightly temporal to the visual axis.

Almost all equine fundic lesions appear in the nontapetum or are located in the peripapillary area. Therefore, the examiner must concentrate on examining the ventral fundic areas when looking for lesions. The optic disc should be pinkish white with 50 to 75 small vessels radiating from the peripheral border of the disc into the adjacent retina in a circumferential manner for a distance of approximately one disc diameter. Extreme pallor of the optic disc with absence of retinal vessels indicates optic atrophy. Hemorrhages or exudates on the optic disc are definitely abnormal and indicative of traumatic or inflammatory optic neuritis. Active lesions of optic neuritis-retinitis may also show perivascular cuffing that appears as radiating white bands extending along the retinal vessels. Areas of active retinitis in the nontapetal area appear as white or gray raised focal areas. Areas of active retinitis in the tapetal area are gray and make the tapetum appear dull or grayish. It is much more common to observe healed or inactive retinal or chorioretinal lesions that are actually scars from previous inflammation, infarction, or trauma. These healed areas appear as depigmented circular, vermiform, or streaklike lesions in the nontapetum; they tend to have central areas of pigmentation from retinal pigment epithelial hypertrophy. In the tapetal zone, they appear as hyperreflective areas because the retina overlying the reflective tapetum has been destroyed. Ventral to the optic disc, these scars, although multifocal, may assume a linear pattern. Experience with such lesions as well as the historic data and pupillary light responses all must be considered in assessing the visual significance of lesions.

Ancillary procedures to document visual handicaps should be used at this point of the examination. Alternate blindfolding of both eyes is useful when interpreting the relative visual loss in each eye. Silent objects such as white gauze or cotton balls may be thrown into the visual fields of each eye to assess response of the horse to moving objects. Tacking or harnessing the animal and making it perform are also useful means to document the owner's observations of visual or performance problems. Menacing is a helpful but very crude means of assessing visual loss unless the loss is complete in the eye being tested.

SPECIFIC CONDITIONS

Orbital or Skull Trauma. The most common sequelae to this problem are optic nerve trauma, hemorrhage, and avulsion. Vision is absent in the affected eye and there is minimal or no pupillary response to direct light in the affected eye. The optic nerve may appear normal or may show hemorrhage or edema. Treatment consists of steroidal and nonsteroidal anti-inflammatory agents in normal dosages. If other neurologic signs are present, intravenous dimethylsulfoxide (DMSO) may be administered at 1 gm per kg body weight intravenously diluted with an equal volume of 5 per cent dextrose. In acute cases, response should be noted within several days if the optic nerve has not been permanently damaged. If the nerve is permanently damaged, the eye will remain blind and unresponsive to direct light, and the optic nerve will develop the typical appearance of optic atrophy over the ensuing weeks or months.

Another serious fundic lesion has been attributed to severe skull trauma or blood loss in horses. These animals have a diffuse retinopathy with multifocal streaks and vermiform lesions in the fundus as well as optic atrophy. The pathophysiology is unknown but may be either an infarctive or anoxic lesion. No treatment is possible in these cases.

Retinopathies Secondary to or Associated with Respiratory or Septicemic Diseases. Although specific etiologies are vague, multifocal small circular areas in the nontapetum have been observed in foals and horses with concurrent septicemia or severe respiratory infections. I have observed these in foals with influenza and they have been reported following *Streptococcus equi* infections. These lesions are white or gray lesions when active and appear as "bullethole" lesions with depigmented periphery and pigmented center when healed. Therapy in acute cases should include specific therapy for any primary systemic disease, nonsteroidal anti-inflammatory agents at standard dosages, and topical corticosteroids that penetrate the eye well.* If the lesions are no longer active, therapy is not likely to be helpful.

Retinopathies Secondary to Vascular Occlusion, Thrombosis, or Thromboembolism. Many of the retinopathies in horses have unknown causes. However, in those multifocal retinopathies that are arranged in a horizontal band extending ventral to the optic disc, vascular infarction has been suggested as a cause. Lesions in the nontapetal zone that are arranged in a perfectly horizontal fashion suggest infarction of a major choroidal vessel or short ciliary artery branch. In addition, in some of these cases, concurrent neurologic disease has been shown to be caused by infarctive lesions in the brain. These findings suggest further investigation into vascular infarction as a cause of equine retinopathies.

Peripapillary Inflammation. Nearly all cases of peripapillary inflammation in horses are associated

---

*Pred Forte, Allergan Pharmaceuticals, Irvine, CA

with uveitis and therefore are discussed under intraocular inflammation (p. 445). Onchocerciasis and leptospirosis have both been proven causes of peripapillary inflammation. When active, these lesions appear as grayish white, fluffy areas adjacent to the optic disc or grayish streaks and exudates extending from the optic disc along the retinal vessels. When inactive, they appear as depigmented scars containing spots of pigmentation adjacent to the optic disc. These lesions have been described as "butterfly lesions" when they involve both the nasal and temporal borders of the optic disc in an alar form. They are important to identify from the standpoint of their possible relationship to equine uveitis.

Retinal Detachments. Most retinal detachments in horses are secondary to vitreoretinal adhesions caused by equine uveitis. Those detachments may occur at the time of active inflammation in the affected eyes but, more commonly, occur long after the initial inflammation owing to slow fibrosis and contracture of the vitreoretinal adhesions. Therefore, a horse can become slowly or acutely blind with a noninflamed eye because of retinal detachment that has been developing since the time of the prior uveitis.

Detachments may be complete and appear as gray veils attached only at the optic disc and floating in the ventral vitreous. They may also appear as a "sunburst" detachment with multiple radiating bands of detachment extending from the optic disc into the vitreous. These detachments secondary to uveitis are not amenable to any therapy.

Rarely, retinal detachments occur secondary to severe skull trauma in the horse. If complete detachment has occurred, no treatment is possible. Theoretically, if a partial serous detachment occurs, diuretics and anti-inflammatory agents systemically would be indicated for therapy.

CLIENT EDUCATION FOR THE VISUALLY HANDICAPPED HORSE

Each horse with less than normal vision must be treated as an individual case when counseling owners concerning its usage. It must be realized that racing animals often must attempt to continue to perform to realize economic gains for the owners unless they have breeding potential. Many Standardbred horses and, to a lesser extent, Thoroughbred horses can actually race with rather severe visual handicaps. These owners have to be aware of the animal's limitations; if the visual handicap results in balking, shying, breaking, or other abnormal behavior, racing will not be possible.

For the pleasure and performance horse, the question of visual soundness is extremely important. The higher the level of performance expected from the horse, the less visual handicap that can be tolerated. In addition, the age and experience of the rider are of the utmost importance since the visually imperfect horse may, *at any time,* show abnormal behavior or "spook," and the rider must be prepared to control a frightened, unpredictable animal. Therefore, a small child would not be a suitable rider for the average horse with limited vision. Many tractable horses that have adjusted to their visual handicap continue to be able to perform as trail horses or at other tasks not requiring total vision when guided by experienced riders.

Supplemental Readings

Gelatt, K. N.: Ophthalmoscopic studies in the normal and diseased ocular fundi of horses. J. Am. Hosp. Assoc., 7:158, 1971.
Rebhun, W. C.: Equine and retinal lesions and retinal detachments. Equine Vet. J., Suppl 2, p. 86, 1983.
Rubin, L. F.: Atlas of Veterinary Ophthalmoscopy, Philadelphia, Lea & Febiger, 1974.

Ocular Emergencies

John D. Lavach, FORT COLLINS, COLORADO

ADNEXAL INJURIES

Injuries to the ocular adnexa are caused by various activities, including struggling during anesthesia recovery or induction, restraint, training, and working. Often the mere size of a horse combined with impact with fixed objects results in the transmission of a tremendous amount of energy resulting in tissue damage. In addition, kinetic energy is transmitted through the adnexa to the eye and may produce severe intraocular or retrobulbar damage.

The veterinarian must perform a complete ophthalmic examination to ascertain which tissues are damaged and prescribe appropriate treatment. A tetanus immunization is recommended with all ocular or periocular injuries.

Bruising. Concussive trauma to the eyelids will cause bruising. The eyelids are extremely vascular and extravasation of blood into the tissues may be extensive. Usually the injury is not serious; however, function of the eyelids may be compromised. The examiner must determine if eyelid function is adequate to protect the cornea. Local nerve damage may cause a partial or complete facial paralysis or a transient or permanent decrease in tear production. If tear production or eyelid function is compromised, a temporary tarsorrhaphy should be performed. Care of the bruised eyelids and periocular tissues is symptomatic. Often systemic anti-inflammatory treatment such as flunixin meglumine for five days will decrease local pain and inflammation. Topical dimethyl sulfoxide (90 per cent solution) seems to reduce tissue swelling. If possible, the owner may apply compresses to the bruised area. Alternating warm and cool compresses for five to 10 minutes two or three times each day is beneficial but not always possible or practical.

The horse should be sedated and the rim of the orbit palpated for fractures. Radiographs are indicated if there is any doubt about the integrity of bony tissue. Fractures with displacement should be surgically repaired to prevent malformation of the orbit and displacement of the eye.

Abrasions. Abrasions to the eyelids and periocular skin are slightly more severe than bruising. All of the previously mentioned treatments are applicable. The abraded tissue should be gently cleansed. Warm saline will help wash away particulate debris. A nitrofurazone ointment "sweat bandage" may be applied to help soften dried exudate and necrotic tissues. The ointment is liberally applied to the abrasion and is covered with gauze sponges, plastic kitchen wrap, or a plastic wastebasket liner. The entire area is bandaged with gauze and tape. After 4 to 24 hours the bandages are removed and the wounded tissue evaluated. Usually, gentle washing with saline will reveal a clean wound. A saline-diluted 1:50 povidone-iodine solution can be used to irrigate the wound to reduce the possibility of bacterial infection. Treatment is minimal and symptomatic. During fly season the tissue should be protected. A fly fringe, goggles, or simply an insecticide cattle eartag may be attached to the halter to prevent fly strike.

Lacerations. Eyelid lacerations in horses are treated by primary wound repair as described for other species. Minimal debridement with care to preserve the eyelid and its mucocutaneous junction is extremely important. Even lacerations with a large flap of eyelid tissue and a small attaching bridge should not be excised. Contaminated or infected wounds should be treated with a nitrofurazone bandage before surgery. This will also help the surgeon differentiate necrotic and viable tissue. Systemic antibiotics are recommended for five days.

The upper and lower puncta should be identified and catheterized during surgery if they are near the wound. Punctal or canalicular lacerations are complications to consider during wound repair. A polyethylene tube or male canine urinary catheter may

be left in the nasolacrimal system for three to four weeks if a canalicular laceration is present. Usually the canaliculus will heal and remain functional if this extra treatment is provided. Failure to recognize and treat this injury will result in chronic epiphora.

Lacerations of the third eyelid are infrequent but are easily sutured with absorbable suture material. Suture knots should be placed on the tarsal surface of the third eyelid to prevent rubbing on the cornea. If suturing is not permitted or possible, any loose flaps may be trimmed to prevent corneal irritation. Exposed cartilage should be covered by suturing adjacent conjunctiva over the cartilage. Necrosis and chronic irritation may result from leaving the cartilage exposed.

Conjunctival lacerations may be associated with other ocular or eyelid injuries. Wounds in the tarsal conjuctiva do not require surgical repair. Full-thickness lacerations of the bulbar conjunctiva should be sutured with absorbable material to prevent herniation of orbital fat. The fatty tissue may not be herniating initially but with movements of the globe will gradually migrate forward and may even be misdiagnosed as a neoplasm in the future.

CORNEAL INJURIES

All horses sustaining ocular or periocular injury should have the cornea examined before and after the application of fluorescein. Superficial injuries may not be seen without fluorescein, and deeper wounds are more easily evaluated after staining. Superficial corneal abrasions and injuries causing a loss of a full thickness of corneal epithelium are treated as ulcers (see p. 451). A blunt injury to the eye may cause a flap of corneal epithelium to separate from the stroma or an anterior stromal split to occur. The flap is often rolled up and attached to the edge of the wound. Amputation of the flap and topical treatment for a superficial ulcer is more rewarding than attempting to suture the flap back to the cornea.

Lacerations into the stroma may be left to heal by epithelialization and fibrosis. However, they are better managed by surgery. Primary wound closure using 6–0 to 8–0 size absorbable suture will decrease the inflammatory reaction and reduce healing time. The major benefit will be a smaller area of scarring and less interference with vision. Sutures should be placed to the bottom of the defect to prevent wound gaping. Postoperative care includes routine treatment for corneal ulcers. Systemic treatment including anti-inflammatory therapy for the uveitis is important. Any keratitis in the horse is likely to have a concurrent iritis or iridocyclitis; it is better to treat this condition unnecessarily rather than to fail to treat it.

Perforating corneal and scleral lacerations represent a serious group of ocular injuries warranting a guarded to poor prognosis in most cases. Since considerable time and expense are incurred with primary wound repair and postsurgical nursing care, a thorough presurgical evaluation is mandatory so the owner can be accurately informed.

The horse should be placed in a room that can be darkened. Sedation is necessary to prevent sudden movements that might further injure the eye during the examination. Pupillary light reflexes should be evaluated. In a dark room a focal light source should be directed by oblique angles to help the examiner determine the condition of the intraocular tissues. The examiner should try to identify the pupil and iris. The presence or absence of any formed anterior chamber is important. The iris may be pushed against the cornea, closing the iridocorneal filtration angle and producing glaucoma. After topical anesthesia the cornea should be touched gently with the finger to assess intraocular tension. A traumatized eye may be exceptionally soft or hard.

Favorable findings include an eye with a small perforation caused by a sharp object. A formed anterior chamber with a fibrin clot and uveal tissue closing the wound with minimal intraocular damage is favorable. Hyphema occupying less than half of the anterior chamber and a miotic pupil are also encouraging.

Large wounds with major distortion of the intraocular structures such as lens luxation, lens rupture, and vitreous movement into the anterior chamber warrant a poor prognosis. Wounds caused by blunt trauma are usually associated with severe intraocular damage. A globe that has collapsed without reformation of the anterior chamber represents a poor chance for restoring vision. Hyphema occupying more than half of the anterior chamber or continuous bleeding from the corneal wound indicates a major uveal tract injury and a poor prognosis.

A detailed discussion of the surgical treatment is beyond the scope of this chapter. It is important not to overlook the uveitis associated with any wound of the eye. Systemic anti-inflammatory agents must be used and will not compromise corneal wound healing. Failure to use high enough levels or for a long enough time period will result in secondary uveal complications including synechia formation, cataract formation, and phthisis bulbi.

FOREIGN BODIES

Foreign bodies are associated with a wide variety of ocular diseases. Every ophthalmic examination initiated by trauma, ulcers, or pain should include a systematic examination to establish an etiology. Foreign objects may be concealed by edematous bulbs of conjunctiva, perforate the conjunctiva, become trapped behind the third eyelid, or penetrate into the eye or nasolacrimal system.

Foreign bodies on the conjunctiva or cornea can often be irrigated from the surface. A gentle prodding from a lacrimal needle may be necessary in some instances because they tend to melt into the epithelium, and a rim of epithelial tissue usually attempts to overgrow the edges. The foreign material should be removed from the conjunctival sac. Failure to remove the object may result in the foreign body regaining its original position after a few blinks from the eyelids. Treatment for a superficial ulcer is usually all that is necessary; however, caution should be exercised to ensure prompt healing. Secondary infection by bacteria or fungal organisms is possible.

Subconjunctival plant material may form a nodule or granulomatous mass that must be distinguished from a neoplasm. A biopsy may reveal foreign material such as plant awns or porcupine quills, or histopathology may be necessary to confirm the diagnosis.

Foreign objects are occasionally seen embedded in the cornea. If the object can be secured with a forceps it may be easily removed. If this occurs the wound should be irrigated with a dilute povidone-iodine solution. Thorough examination with magnification is necessary to ascertain complete removal of all material. When the object cannot be removed through the original entry wound, a 25-gauge needle on a tuberculin syringe may be used to enlarge the wound and remove the foreign debris from the cornea. Routine treatment for a corneal ulcer with follow-up to ensure uncomplicated healing is important.

Horses with objects that perforate the cornea, enter into the anterior chamber, and cannot be retrieved from the original wound should be prepared for intraocular surgery. A limbal approach should be used rather than enlarging the corneal perforating wound. This will minimize the scar at the site of the perforation. The limbal wound will heal more rapidly and will have scarring away from the center of the visual axis.

Lead shot in the eye is usually better left alone since it will not incite a metallic reaction. Other metals such as iron and copper compounds will oxidize and cause chronic inflammation and an attempt should be made to remove them as soon as possible. Cataracts caused by a foreign body injury are permanent and irreversible.

HYPHEMA

Hyphema (blood in the eye) may be caused by trauma, iridocyclitis, and systemic diseases such as lymphoma and thrombocytopenia. A bilateral hyphema is more suggestive of a systemic disorder and deserves a complete investigation. Acute hemorrhage into the anterior chamber that does not clot will clear within two to three days. Clotted blood disappears more slowly, often requiring two to three weeks depending on the volume of blood and the cause.

In general, smaller hyphemas or those occupying less than half of the anterior chamber warrant a better prognosis than larger hyphemas. Also, chronic hyphemas or those that have recurring episodes have a poorer prognosis. If the anterior chamber is filled with blood for several days and takes on the characteristic deep purple to black color of the "eight ball" hemorrhage, the prognosis is poor. Chronic iridocyclitis eyes will often have a layering of blood described as marbling. The inferior layer is darker in color than the more recent superficial layers that are lighter. Eyes that continue to hemorrhage or hemorrhage intermittently probably are blind (or will be soon) and often become painful. Enucleation may be necessary to stop the pain.

An acute hyphema of any cause may be treated with topical 1 per cent epinephrine or 10 per cent phenylephrine. Systemic treatment for iridocyclitis is important. Topical treatment with atropine is of questionable value but may help re-establish endothelial integrity and reduce pain associated with iris and ciliary body muscle spasm. Additional supportive care such as forced rest as provided in a darkened box stall and tranquilization may help stop the bleeding. The clot should not be surgically removed unless the veterinarian is absolutely sure intraocular pressure is rising. The act of decompression may stimulate more hemorrage. The presumed etiology of hyphema in chronic hemorrhaging eyes is from neovascularization of the uveal tract and has a poor prognosis.

ACUTE BLINDNESS

Acute vision loss may be unilateral but is often not recognized by the owner unless both eyes are affected. Retinal detachments, iridocyclitis, and optic neuritis affecting one or both eyes occur in horses (see other sections for therapy). Acute bilateral blindness in horses has been diagnosed in association with chronic epistaxis or severe blood loss from other sites. The mechanism is not understood but a bilateral exudative optic neuritis is present. Unfortunately, the process has not responded to intensive treatments and the horses have remained blind.

Supplemental Readings

Brooks, D. E., and Wolf, E. D.: Ocular trauma in the horse. Equine Vet. J., Suppl 2, p. 141, 1983.
Lavach, J. D., Severin, G. A., and Roberts, S. M.: Lacerations of the equine eye: A review of 48 cases. J. Am. Vet. Med. Assoc., *184*:1243, 1984.
Munger, R. J.: Equine ophthalmic emergencies. Vet. Clin. North Am. (Large Anim. Pract.), 6:467, 1984.
Riis, R. C.: Equine ophthalmology. *In* Gelatt, K. N. (ed.): Veterinary Ophthalmology. Philadelphia, Lea & Febiger, 1981.

PROBLEMS OF THE PERFORMANCE AND ENDURANCE HORSE

Edited by R. J. Rose

Physiological Responses to Exercise; Effects of Training

Jennifer R. Allen, PULLMAN, WASHINGTON

Equine exercise physiology is a rapidly expanding field of study. The goals of modern sports medicine include assessment of potential performance, estimation of fitness, critical evaluation of existing training methods, and development of new training techniques to improve performance and minimize risk of injuries. An understanding of the physiology of exercise and training is imperative if these goals are to be attained.

Aerobic and Anaerobic Exercise

All exercise involves the conversion of stored chemical energy to mechanical energy manifest as locomotion. Discussion of the energy sources and pathways in exercising horses is beyond the scope of this section. However, it is necessary to define two categories of energy production. Fuel sources (glucose, fatty acids) may be metabolized by oxidative phosphorylation (aerobic), or by glycolysis (anaerobic) to yield energy via the intermediary of adenosine triphosphate (ATP).

Traditionally, aerobic exercise has been regarded as exercise of submaximal intensity in which all energy demands can be met by metabolism occurring in the presence of oxygen. Anaerobic exercise has been defined as short-duration, high-intensity effort that necessitates the use of anaerobic glycolytic pathways to meet energy needs. The concept of the "anaerobic threshold" has been widely used to describe the transition point between the two forms of energy production. However, the two systems are not mutually exclusive. Some lactate production occurs in all muscles at all levels of exercise intensity. Conversely, oxygen consumption, and hence aerobic metabolism, continues to increase at exercise intensities well above those producing initial increases in blood lactate. The relative contributions of anaerobic glycolysis and oxidative phosphorylation during exercise are influenced by a number of factors including the intensity of the exercise, level of conditioning, diet, and warm-up received before exercise.

Oxygen Uptake

The rate of oxygen consumption ($\dot{V}O_2$) during exercise indicates the level of aerobic metabolism occurring. Maximum oxygen uptake ($\dot{V}O_2$ max) reflects the maximum aerobic capacity of an individual, that is, the workload that can be sustained before the onset of rapid increases in anaerobic energy production. Maximum oxygen uptake in the horse is approximately 120 to 160 ml per kg per minute, compared with 40 to 80 ml per kg per minute in man. $\dot{V}O_2$ depends on both rate of oxygen delivery to and rate of oxygen extraction and utilization by the working muscle. It is thus the product of heart rate (HR), stroke volume (SV), and arteriovenous oxygen difference $C(a-v)O_2$.

$$\dot{V}O_2 = HR \times SV \times C(a-v)O_2.$$

From this equation it is apparent that oxygen consumption is influenced by a number of factors, summarized in Table 1. $\dot{V}O_2$ max can be increased by training in human athletes, but no studies have examined this response in the horse.

EFFECTS OF EXERCISE

CARDIOVASCULAR SYSTEM

During strenuous exercise the horse is capable of a 35-fold increase in oxygen uptake, compared with the 10-fold to 12-fold increase seen in man. This remarkable adaptation is brought about primarily through changes in cardiovascular function.

Heart Rate. The resting heart rate of the horse ranges from 30 to 40 beats per minute, with maximal heart rates varying from 215 to 240 beats per minute during exercise. A close linear correlation between heart rate and workload exists for heart rates up to approximately 210 beats per minute. At very low exercise intensities, psychogenic influences exert proportionally greater effects on heart rate. As exercise approaches maximal intensity, the incremental heart rate response to increasing speed levels off. However, between these extremes the heart rate under standardized exercise conditions is a reliable indicator of workload. This has application both during training workouts for quantification of work intensity and in standardized exercise tests used for predictive, comparative, or monitoring purposes.

Stroke Volume and Cardiac Output. Cardiac output (volume flow of blood, $\dot{Q}$) is the product of heart rate and stroke volume. The cardiac output of a 500-kg horse at rest is approximately 30 to 40 L per min. Increases of more than eight times resting

values have been recorded during exercise. The majority of this elevation is achieved through increased heart rate. Stroke volume at rest is approximately 900 mL in a 500-kg horse; this changes little with exercise. Increases of 15 to 40 per cent have been measured during submaximal exercise. It is likely that at very high heart rates reduced diastolic filling time becomes a limiting factor to stroke volume.

Distribution of Blood Flow. Redistribution of blood flow during exercise constitutes an important adaptation, which has two effects. First, constriction of venous capacitance vessels increases venous pressure and promotes ventricular filling. Second, skeletal muscle vasodilation combined with vasoconstriction in regions of lower metabolic activity causes a marked increase in blood flow to active muscles. It is estimated that skeletal muscles receive 15 per cent of cardiac output at rest compared with more than 70 per cent during strenuous exercise.

Hemoglobin Concentration. Sympathetically mediated splenic contraction begins before exercise as part of the anticipatory response. During exercise, the degree of erythrocyte mobilization depends on workload intensity. Red cell concentration increases by more than 60 per cent during maximal exercise, resulting in a marked increase in oxygen-carrying capacity of the blood. It has been suggested that at very high red cell concentrations this benefit may be partially offset by alterations in blood flow dynamics due to increased blood viscosity.

SKELETAL MUSCLE

Irrespective of exercise type, activation of skeletal muscle is a common denominator of athletic activity. A commonly raised question concerns the extent to which skeletal muscle capacity limits performance. The application of the percutaneous needle biopsy technique has facilitated studies of the type, size, and biochemical characteristics of muscle fibers and their adaptive responses to training.

Muscle Fiber Types. Some of the characteristics of different muscle fiber types are presented in Table 2. Numerous fiber classification systems exist, based on either contractile or metabolic properties or both.

The *contractile speed* of a fiber is related to the structure of its myosin molecule. Slow-twitch (ST) and fast-twitch (FT) fibers can be differentiated according to their histochemical staining patterns after treatment with acid or alkali. In general, three types of fiber have been recognized by this method (types ST, FTa, and FTb). More recently up to five fiber types have been detected according to the time course of their acid lability. *Metabolic classification* involves histochemical staining to demonstrate oxidative or, less commonly, glycolytic capacity. In general, ST fibers stain intensely for oxidative

TABLE 1. FACTORS AFFECTING OXYGEN CONSUMPTION

1. Cardiac output
   Heart rate
   Stroke volume
2. Arterial oxygenation
   Pulmonary ventilation
   Hemoglobin concentration and saturation
3. Rate of oxygen utilization
   Regional distribution of blood flow
   Capacity of the oxidative enzyme systems of skeletal muscle

TABLE 2. GENERAL CHARACTERISTICS OF MUSCLE FIBER TYPES

| | Slow Twitch | Fast Twitch | |
	Type I	Type IIA (FTa)	Type IIB (FTb)
ATPase staining after pretreatment at pH			
4.3	Dark	Light	Light
4.6	Dark	Light	Intermediate
10.3	Light	Dark	Dark
Contractile speed	Slow	Fast	Fast
Metabolic Classifications	**ST**	**FTH (FOG)***	**FT (FG)†**
Oxidative capacity	High	Intermediate-high	Low
Glycolytic capacity	Low	Intermediate-high	High
Lipid content	High	Intermediate	Low
Glycogen content	Intermediate	High	High
Capillary density	High	Intermediate	Low
Fatigability	Low	Intermediate	High

*Fast twitch high oxidative (fast twitch oxidative-glycolytic)
†Fast twitch (fast twitch glycolytic)

enzymes while certain FT fibers are low in oxidative capacity and others are intermediate or high. However, a spectrum of oxidative potentials exists, especially among the type II fibers, and this may be greatly affected by training.

Muscle Fiber Recruitment. During exercise, controlled development of appropriate muscle tension is achieved through selective fiber recruitment. With very low intensity exercise only the relatively fatigue-resistant ST and some type FTa fibers may be utilized. As exercise intensity increases there is progressive recruitment of more FTa and finally FTb fibers. Fiber recruitment is determined by both speed and duration of exercise. Thus recruitment of Type FTb fibers occurs both in short-duration, high-speed (maximal) exercise such as galloping and in extremely prolonged submaximal (endurance) exercise.

EFFECTS OF TRAINING

Training refers to performance of repeated sessions of physical exercise with the aim of increasing physical fitness or performance. In the horse as in humans, two broad categories of training are recognized. The term endurance training is applied to conditioning programs involving submaximal exercise, usually at an intensity of around 70 to 75 per cent of $\dot{V}O_2$ max. Sprint training refers to short bouts of high-intensity (supramaximal) exercise. The training response is affected by both intensity and duration of the exercise sessions. However, interaction between these two variables results in a spectrum of possible training regimes. This concept is of importance in the training of horses, in which musculoskeletal injuries associated with conventional strenuous training programs result in substantial losses.

CARDIOVASCULAR SYSTEM

Few controlled studies on the cardiovascular effects of training have been performed in the horse. At this time, data are available only from examination of submaximal exercise programs. This is currently an active area of study of several research groups.

Heart Rate, Stroke Volume, and Cardiac Output. The resting bradycardia known to occur in well-conditioned human athletes is generally not seen in horses. This is possibly due to the high degree of vagal tone that exists in all resting horses. However, heart rates at given (submaximal) workloads are lower in trained than in untrained horses. Recovery heart rates are also lower in the fit horse, with a more rapid return toward the resting value. Limited studies to date have not found significant changes in stroke volume with training. Hence cardiac output tends to be slightly decreased at the same submaximal workload following training.

Oxygen Uptake. Longitudinal studies using inclined treadmill exercise have found no difference in oxygen uptake at submaximal workloads following training. This is consistent with observations in humans. Performance of a given submaximal workload requires a given amount of energy. The $\dot{V}O_2$ required is therefore the same irrespective of training. Constant $\dot{V}O_2$ in the presence of decreased cardiac output results from increased $C(a–v)O_2$, that is, improvement in arterial oxygenation or peripheral oxygen extraction or both.

Blood Volume and Red Cell Count. Significant increases in blood volume and total red cell mass occur with training. Good correlations have been demonstrated between aerobic working capacity and both total blood volume and total body hemoglobin in the horse.

SKELETAL MUSCLE

Fiber Types, Fiber Area, and Capillary Density. Fast- and slow-twitch fiber interconversion has not been demonstrated with normal training. Alterations in the type FTa to FTb ratio have been reported both in humans and the horse following prolonged training. However, interpretation of changes in fiber type percentages is hindered by the considerable variation encountered with repeated sampling.

In general, endurance training produces a decrease in muscle fiber areas, whereas sprint training results in few changes in fiber area. An increase in the number of intermyofibrillar capillaries associated with each fiber type occurs with training in humans. Interestingly, in the horse, increased capillarity following various types of training has been found associated with FTb but not with ST or FTa fibers. It is suggested that these fiber types exhibit a higher capillary density in untrained horses than in sedentary humans.

Biochemical Characteristics. A fundamental effect of training is the increase in oxidative capacity induced in skeletal muscle. This change parallels increases in total mitochondrial volume. It is quantified biochemically by measurement of concentrations of key enzymes in the aerobic pathways. Enzymes commonly used include succinate dehydrogenase (SDH) and citrate synthase (CS), from the tricarboxylic acid (Krebs) cycle, and beta-hydroxyacylCoA dehydrogenase (HAD), from the beta (fatty acid) oxidation pathway. A number of longitudinal studies have demonstrated 1.5 to two-fold increases in concentrations of SDH or CS and HAD in horses following endurance, submaximal treadmill, and conventional race training, with the greatest increases following endurance training.

With increasing oxidative capacity there is a shift in emphasis from carbohydrate to fat metabolism during submaximal exercise. This results in sparing of intramuscular glycogen stores. Since intramuscular glycogen depletion is correlated with the onset of fatigue, the trained horse performing submaximal exercise is able to sustain greater workloads for longer periods. It should be remembered that aerobic capacity is also of importance in maximal exercise (racing) since high lactate levels are associated with fatigue. Increased oxidative capacity allows performance of a workload of greater intensity before the onset of rapid increases in blood lactate concentration.

In contrast to studies of aerobic exercise, the biochemical responses of muscle to anaerobic training regimes have received scant attention. However, the vast majority of published reports have shown no increase in concentration of glycolytic enzymes during conventional race training in either Thoroughbreds or Standardbreds. It is postulated that the horse has a very high innate glycolytic capacity and that glycolytic enzyme concentrations are not a limiting factor in maximal exercise. Suggested mechanisms contributing to the beneficial effects of sprint training include increased muscle glycogen stores, increased metabolism of lactate or tolerance to it, and increased capacity of intramuscular buffering systems.

INFLUENCE OF TYPE OF TRAINING

No controlled studies have been attempted to examine the effects within a group of horses of varying the nature of the training workload. However, a recent detailed study using rats provided information of interest to trainers of both human and equine athletes. The study concluded the following:

(1) the training response of skeletal muscle depends on both the intensity and duration of daily exercise.

(2) There is an interaction between intensity and duration, with similar increases in oxidative capacity achieved after either a high intensity–short daily duration or a lower intensity–prolonged daily duration exercise program.

(3) the extent of the training response varies between fiber types, according to their recruitment threshold. In other words, for any improvement in oxidative potential to occur in a given fiber type, that fiber type must be recruited by the training exercise, while for maximal training response, 100 per cent recruitment of the fiber type is desired. In rats, 100 per cent recruitment (maximal training response) was found in fast-twitch high oxidative fibers at 80 per cent of $\dot{V}O_2$ max. No training response occurred in fast-twitch glycolytic fibers at low exercise intensities. Maximal response (100 per cent recruitment) in these fibers was not achieved at the highest intensity used (116 per cent of $\dot{V}O_2$ max).

(4) Lower exercise intensities result in slower rates of response, i.e., longer training time to achieve the same response.

Detailed studies of specific responses of equine muscle are lacking. However, glycogen depletion studies during various forms of exercise indicate that muscle fiber recruitment occurs at similar relative exercise intensities to those shown in humans and the rat. Thus this work has potential implications in formulation of training programs for horses.

TRAINING REGIMENS

The specificity of the training response is such that training exercise must employ energy pathways and muscle fiber types that will be utilized in competition. The relative contributions of each energy source can be assessed from the duration of the competition exercise. Thus, in "explosive" exercise such as Quarterhorse racing, the creatine phosphate (CP) system provides important energy for several seconds and the remainder is supplied almost exclusively anaerobically. Racing lasting one to two minutes also has an important requirement for the CP pathway and is predominantly anaerobic. In longer "staying" races, aerobic energy production is a significant contribution to total energy used. Events requiring a combination of speed and "endurance," such as three-day eventing or polo, utilize all energy sources available, while most endurance competitions involve purely aerobic work. Maximal conditioning of racing horses cannot be achieved without a component of "sprint" work, recruiting the FTb fibers and utilizing anaerobic energy pathways. However, aerobic capacity is also critical to these horses. Furthermore, risks are imposed on the musculoskeletal system by fast work, particularly in the immature horse. The slow rate at which the osseous and tendinous structures are strengthened during chronic exercise is well known. A lengthy aerobic conditioning phase before introduction to fast work is advantageous although seldom emphasized in conventional training regimes.

Workload intensity is readily quantified using the exercise heart rate. It has been estimated that a work intensity producing a heart rate of 60 to 70 per cent of $\dot{V}O_2$ max (approximately 140 to 160 bpm) is necessary to elicit aerobic training responses. A workload of around 85 per cent of $\dot{V}O_2$ max (approximately 200 bpm) corresponds to the so-called aerobic–anaerobic transition in the horse, since small increases in blood lactate (up to 4 mmol per L) occur. This has been suggested as the optimal work intensity at which a training stimulus to both aerobic and anaerobic energy systems is provided.

A downward trend in human track times following the introduction of "interval training" has generated interest in this method for conditioning horses. The technique utilizes repeated sessions of high-intensity exercise with interspersed rest periods. This allows imposition of more intense training stress than would be possible with a constant workload. Aerobic ATP replenishment occurs in the rest periods, resulting in less lactate accumulation and less fatigue. The work intensity, "rest intensity," and work:rest ratio vary according to the desired training effect. Limited controlled data using the technique in horses are available. A recent study could demonstrate no difference in heart rate, cardiac output, and blood lactate levels between Standardbreds trained by conventional or interval techniques. However, the interval technique was thought to reduce the risk of fatigue-associated injuries.

Supplemental Readings

Dudley, G. A., Abraham, W. M., and Terjung, R. L.: Influence of exercise intensity and duration on biochemical adaptations in skeletal muscle. J. Appl. Physiol., 53:844, 1982.

Persson, S. G. B.: Evaluation of exercise tolerance and fitness in the performance horse. In Snow, D. H., Persson, S. G. B., and Rose, R. J. (eds.): Equine Exercise Physiology. Cambridge, Granta Editions, 1983, pp. 441–457.

Saltin, B., Nazar, K., Costill, D. L., Stein, E., Jansson, E., Essen, B., and Gollnick, P. D.: The nature of the training response: Peripheral and central adaptations to one-legged exercise. Acta Physiol. Scand., 96:289, 1976.

Snow, D. H.: Skeletal muscle adaptations: A review. In: Snow, D. H., Persson, S. G. B., and Rose, R. J. (eds.): Equine Exercise Physiology. Cambridge, Granta Editions, 1983, pp. 160–183.

Thomas, D. P., Fregin, G. F., Gerber, N. H., and Ailes, N. B.: Effects of training on cardiorespiratory function in the horse. Am. J. Physiol., 245:R160, 1983.

Poor Performance Syndrome: Investigation and Diagnostic Techniques

Reuben J. Rose, SYDNEY, AUSTRALIA

Reduced or inadequate performance is a common reason for horses to be presented to the veterinarian. While many of these horses are suffering from a basic lack of ability, the majority have had a previous history of good performance with a sudden unexplained reduction. This type of animal can be found among racehorses, endurance horses, three-day event horses, and others in such events. Some horses have subclinical lameness or problems such as chronic obstructive pulmonary disease. These can generally be diagnosed by a complete physical examination together with special techniques such as radiology and blood gas analysis. More problematic are the horses that are completely normal on clinical examination and require more specialized diagnostic techniques to help in elucidating the problem.

HISTORY

It is important to take a careful history. The performance history usually falls into one of two categories: the horse performs badly throughout the event or the horse begins well but has no stamina to put in a final finishing effort. Sometimes a horse will pull up very distressed, but often no signs of abnormality will be noted. In these animals, the problems are often difficult to elucidate and a full range of diagnostic tests may be necessary. In other cases of poor racing performance, the history may give a much better guide to the problem. This happens in those horses with respiratory viral infections, which will have histories of nasal discharge and coughing. Such infections can leave the horse chronically debilitated, and racing performance can be impaired for as long as 6 to 12 months. However, in the past a "virus" has been blamed for poor racing performance when a more precise diagnosis could not be reached.

APPROACH TO INVESTIGATION

.Because the respiratory, cardiovascular, musculoskeletal, and hematopoietic systems are all interrelated in competitive performance, it is of little use to isolate one of these systems and focus all attention on its investigation. A detailed clinical examination should be carried out, concentrating particularly on the cardiovascular, respiratory, and musculoskeletal systems. If no abnormalities are found, the next step is the use of various diagnostic aids. Hematology and plasma biochemistry should be undertaken to establish any abnormal values. This is usually of most help if previous samples have been collected to establish the individual horse's "normal" values. The next test is the electrocardiogram (ECG); a high percentage of horses with poor performance will have abnormalities of the T wave. Endoscopy, which may be combined with bronchoalveolar lavage, is also useful for ensuring that no abnormalities exist in either the upper or lower respiratory tracts. In some cases muscle biopsy may also be indicated. Finally, standardized exercise tests may be useful to quantify more accurately the performance problem.

DIAGNOSTIC AIDS

Depending on the degree of sophistication of the practice facilities, some or all of the tests to be discussed may be performed. No one test will invariably show the reason for the horse's performance problem, but judicious use of the techniques may identify reasons for suboptimal performance.

HEMATOLOGY AND PLASMA BIOCHEMISTRY

The use of hematology and plasma biochemistry has long formed the basis for evaluating fitness and performance problems in horses. This is probably because these tests are relatively easy to carry out in practice. However, in many cases, small deviations from normal are incorrectly interpreted as being the cause for the horse's problem. Normal values for the various hematologic measurements will not be considered in this section and can be found in the section on hematopoietic diseases and in the Appendices.

Hematology. The popularity of hematologic measurements in the evaluation of equine performance problems appears to be based on the relationship between hemoglobin and oxygen carriage. A correlation between hemoglobin levels and performance has been demonstrated in Standardbred horses, but this correlation was with total hemoglobin rather than resting hemoglobin levels. No correlation was found between the resting level of hemoglobin and the total body hemoglobin or circulating red cell mass. For this reason, the value of resting hematology for the asssessment of fitness or performance problems is quite limited, despite the increase in total body hemoglobin in response to training. Most horses that are normal on physical examination will have hematology values that lie within normal ranges. To measure the total hemoglobin or total red cell mass requires collecting a blood sample after strenuous exercise (to mobilize the splenic red cell reserve) and determining plasma volume using a technique such as Evan's Blue dye dilution. This may be undertaken in a practical way by collecting a blood sample in the first five minutes after exercise. If the horse has exercised at speeds in excess of 500 meters per minute, the splenic red cell pool will be mobilized and the total circulating red cell mass can be estimated, ignoring the variations between horses in plasma volume. Many veterinarians regard resting hematocrits of less than 35 per cent as being abnormal and likely to cause suboptimal racing performance, but values as low as 30 per cent have been found in normal Thoroughbred racehorses. Endurance and eventing horses will usually have mean resting hematocrit values that are lower than racehorses.

The resting leukocyte count is also relied upon to indicate overtraining in a performance horse. Decreases in the neutrophil:lymphocyte (N:L) ratio are often reported as indicating that the horse is "training off." However, the N:L ratio is variable in the individual horse depending on when the blood sample is collected after exercise. In racehorses, the N:L ratio decreases quite markedly immediately after exercise due to lymphocyte release from splenic reserves. After several hours, however, the ratio increases in response to elevated plasma cortisol values. On the other hand, endurance horses have a marked elevation of the N:L ratio immediately following exercise, and in severely stressed or exhausted horses there is usually a significant left shift in the neutrophil population. For these reasons, N:L ratios should be interpreted carefully, and the time of day in relation to any exercise performed must be taken into account. If conditions for collection are standardized, the N:L ratio may have some relevance. In Standardbred horses suffering overtraining, resting plasma cortisol values are depressed, the response to an ACTH stimulus is diminished, and the N:L ratio is deviated.

Plasma Biochemistry. With the advent of autoanalyzers, plasma biochemistry "profiles" have become commonly used for evaluating horses with performance problems. While these profiles are useful, it must be remembered that when a large number of measurements are performed, a high statistical probability exists that one or two values could be outside the normal ranges. This is because the normal range is usually defined as including 95 per cent of the population and so some apparent abnormalities may not be of clinical relevance. However, plasma biochemical profiles are of value in detecting subclinical myositis (rhabdomyolysis) and disturbances of liver function.

The measurements usually included in a plasma biochemistry profile to examine performance problems are aspartate aminotransferase (AST), creatine kinase (CK), alkaline phosphatase (AP), gamma glutamyl transferase (GGT), creatinine, urea, sodium, potassium, chloride, and bicarbonate. Other biochemical measurements are usually performed as part of the screen, but most of these are of little clinical relevance. Although plasma biochemistry measurements have been used to assess fitness, longitudinal studies of horses during training have not shown any changes relating to increasing fitness in samples collected either at rest or during exercise. A possible relationship between plasma or serum electrolyte disturbances and poor racing performance has been reported, and at the University of Sydney we have confirmed that such abnormalities can be significant. However, the normal range of electrolytes is quite wide and it must be remembered that plasma electrolyte values are affected by diurnal variation, feeding, and exercise.

Electrocardiography. An electrocardiogram often provides useful information in evaluation of these horses. The recording technique used at the University of Sydney utilizes four limb leads and a chest electrode placed approximately 5 cm behind the elbow point on the left side of the chest. The horse is usually stood on a rubber mat and positioned so that its left front leg is slightly in front of its right front leg. The leads recorded are 1, 2, 3, aVR, aVL, aVF, the unipolar chest lead CV, and the bipolar chest leads CR, CF, and CL. It is most important to ensure that the horse is quiet during the recording, with a heart rate less than 42 beats per minute. In this way consistent recordings are possible, including the T waves in the various leads. The T wave of the equine ECG is notable for its lability, particularly at elevated heart rates. The details of electrocardiography in the horse and interpretation of various abnormalties have been covered in the section on cardiovascular diseases. However, in the performance horse that is clinically normal, it is unusual to find major conduction abnormalities, which is probably the reason that few veterinarians have an ECG machine.

At the University of Sydney we examined the relationship of some ECG abnormalities to poor racing performance. In almost 50 per cent of horses with a history of reduced racing performance, there were abnormal T wave changes in the ECG chest leads. These abnormalities consisted of positive and peaked T waves in contrast with normal horses, which had diphasic T waves in the chest leads. The pathologic significance of these changes is somewhat debatable, although histologic evidence of myocarditis was found in a series of autopsied horses. Certainly the correlation of poor performance with the finding of abnormal T waves in the resting ECG is very clear. Our studies have shown a significantly higher incidence of horses with T wave abnormalities in a poorly performing group than in a group presented with musculoskeletal abnormalities or for heart score determination. When horses with these abnormal T wave findings are rested for periods of 6 to 12 months, many will return to normal. However, after the horses were returned to training the majority of their ECGs showed abnormal T waves once again. The condition appears to be training-related, because in 50 Thoroughbred yearlings that had ECGs recorded before training, none had abnormalities of the T waves. When these horses were followed up after eight weeks in training the incidence of abnormal T waves was up to 25 per cent, with some horses from certain training stables having a high incidence. While all the factors involved in these T wave abnormalities are imprecisely understood, a relationship exists between the finding of abnormal T waves on the ECG and poor racing performance.

The other major use of the resting ECG has been for assessment of performance potential by heart score measurement. The heart score concept was first proposed by Steel, who found that the mean QRS duration in leads 1, 2, and 3 expressed in milliseconds (the "heart score") was strongly correlated with heart weight and significantly correlated with prize money won by racehorses. On this basis, veterinarians in Australia and New Zealand are often asked to perform ECGs on yearlings to assess their future potential. While the heart score has been shown to be a useful measurement in the clinical situation, great care has to be taken when attempting to use any one measurement to assess potential, as performance requires the integration of a number of different body systems.

The heart score concept has also been widely criticized as being unphysiologic and there is no doubt that recording and measurement of the QRS complexes requires expertise. Artifact-free QRS complexes are necessary for evaluation and a 8–10 × magnifier is essential for accurate measurement. In spite of the problems in the measurement of heart score and criticisms of the basis of its use, it has been found to be a useful practical measurement to give a guide to cardiac capacity.

Muscle Biopsy. Muscle biopsy is a simple procedure to carry out with a minimum of equipment, although the laboratory facilities needed for the biochemical and histochemical analyses are quite complex. While a large number of muscles have been studied, the most consistently used muscle has been the middle gluteal. This muscle appears to be active at all intensities of exercise and is probably representative of locomotor muscles in general.

A number of different muscle biopsy needles are now available, consisting of three parts. The *outer needle* varies in diameter from 3 to 7 mm and has a side window into which the muscle is pushed during the biopsy; an *inner cutting sleeve* cuts the piece of muscle that is forced into the window; and a *stylet* fits down the inside of the sleeve and pushes the muscle sample out. Taking the muscle biopsy involves shaving a small area of skin, approximately 12 to 15 cm caudodorsal to the tuber coxae. Following skin disinfection, 1 ml of a nonirritant local anesthetic such as 2 per cent prilocaine or 2 per cent mepivacaine is injected subcutaneously and an incision made through the skin and fascia with a No. 10 scalpel blade. The biopsy needle is then inserted, with the cutting cylinder depressed, to a depth of 8 to 10 cm. The cutting cylinder is withdrawn to allow exposure of the window in the biopsy needle, and the tip of the needle is pushed slightly up into the muscle. The cutting cylinder is then depressed to cut off the piece of muscle pushed into the window. This procedure can be repeated three or four times so that a total of 200 to 300 mg of muscle is obtained for analysis. When the needle is withdrawn there is occasionally some slight bleeding from the wound, but this is easily controlled by digital pressure with gauze swabs for a minute or two. The skin wound is left unsutured and the horse is given tetanus prophylaxis.

If biochemical measurements are to be performed, the muscle is placed directly into liquid nitrogen. However, if histochemistry is to be undertaken for the determination of muscle fiber types, the muscle must be oriented so that the fibers run longitudinally. In this way tranverse sections of muscle can be obtained when the sections are cut on a cryostat. The oriented muscle is mounted on a small piece of cork using a small drop of a methylcellulose solution and the muscle either coated with talc before freezing in liquid nitrogen or placed in a solution of isopentane chilled to $-80°$ C. These techniques prevent the formation of ice crystals in the muscle fibers during freezing. Storage of the muscle should be at or below a temperature of $-80°$ C.

The information that can be derived from a muscle biopsy specimen depends on the range of analyses performed. Histochemical staining for the presence of myosin ATPase will allow determination of the percentage of slow- and fast-twitch muscle fibers in the muscle. If acid preincubation at a pH of 4.6 is used, the fast-twitch fibers may be further subdivided into FTa(IIa) and FTb(IIb). FTa fibers are on the whole more oxidative than FTb fibers, which have a greater glycolytic capacity. In general, horses suited for short-distance fast exercise have a greater percentage of fast-twitch fibers in the middle gluteal muscles than horses suited for longer distance events, which have a higher percentage of slow-twitch fibers. This finding has led to interest in the predictive value of muscle biopsy for the assessment of performance potential. While a relationship to performance may be found, muscle fiber type distribution is only one of the factors involved in equine performance. Therefore it is important not to make extravagant interpretations of the results of muscle fiber distributions. Nonetheless, we have found that a reasonable correlation exists between muscle fiber type and performance in endurance horses. Horses with less than 20 per cent slow-twitch fibers are seldom successful in endurance events. In racehorses (trotters and gallopers) it appears advantageous to have a high FTa:FTb ratio (except for those competing over distances less than 1200 meters).

The other measurements that may be made from resting muscle biopsy specimens, previously frozen in liquid nitrogen, are key enzyme concentrations in homogenized muscle. The enzymes usually measured are citrate synthase (CS) or succinic dehydrogenase (SDH), which are citric acid cycle enzymes; 3-hydroxyacyl coenzyme A dehydrogenase (HAD), which is a marker of fat metabolism, and one or several of the glycolytic enzymes such as lactate dehydrogenase (LDH), phosphorylase, and phosphofructokinase (PFK). Concentrations of these enzymes in skeletal muscle can provide some information on the fitness of the horse, as CS, SDH, and HAD all tend to increase in response to training and give a good guide to aerobic fitness. However, the glycolytic enzymes do not show such a training response, even with high-intensity training programs, and so the anaerobic capacity of the horse cannot be assessed in this way. Some recent work in humans has indicated that the buffering capacity of muscle may improve in response to high-intensity training, but this has not yet been evaluated in the horse.

Exercise Testing. When attempting to elucidate the causes of poor performance in competitive horses, most of the tests undertaken at rest provide only limited information. In many cases, clinical examination followed up with hematology, plasma biochemistry, and ECG examination may reveal no abnormalities. In these cases clinical exercise testing, which involves measurement of various values during and after exercise, can give precise information concerning a horse's reduced performance. Exercise testing can be complex or relatively simple, depending on the equipment and facilities available. However, it involves use of a standardized exercise test over a known distance at a set speed, to give an indication of exercise capacity.

The simplest form of exercise test involves the measurement of heart rate during exercise using a cardiotachometer, of which there are several available commercially.* Because of the linear relationship between heart rate and exercise intensity, in the heart rate range 150 to 210 beats per minute (BPM), the fitness or work tolerance of an individual horse can be assessed. It has been established that the horse's speed at a heart rate of 200 BPM (V200) is a good predictor of the horse's aerobic capacity. The V200 changes with the degree of fitness and will be altered in disease states such as chronic obstructive pulmonary disease and cardiac insufficiency. With increasing fitness the V200 will increase. Therefore, if a repeatable exercise test can be devised, the response of a horse to training can be monitored. Conversely, in a horse presented for reduced exercise tolerance, a low V200 will establish that its aerobic capacity is reduced and so the various systems in the oxygen transport chain can be investigated. Such testing at the racetrack is difficult because of variations in track surface. Thus it is not easy to completely standardize the test.

Measurement of the blood lactate response to exercise is another approach to assessing exercise tolerance. This can be included with measurement of exercising heart rates to give additional information as to the horse's fitness. At low to moderate exercise intensities (less than 450 m per min) there is little lactate accumulation in most horses. However, at speeds above this, a point is reached when lactate begins to accumulate in the blood, the *onset of blood lactate accumulation* (OBLA). The speed at which OBLA is reached varies with the individual horse's fitness and exercise capacity. The point of OBLA can be determined for an individual horse by exercising it over a set distance at increasing speeds. Usually four steps are used, with a rest period of three to five minutes between each step. This allows the blood, for lactate determination, to be collected as the blood lactate continues to rise for up to five minutes after exercise because of efflux of lactate from muscle. The speeds usually chosen give heart rates of 170 to 180 BPM (step 1), 190 to 200 BPM (step 2), 210 to 220 BPM (step 3), and greater than 220 BPM (step 4). This will produce an exponential increase in blood lactate after step 2 so that the point of OBLA, which is usually defined as a lactate value of 4 mmol per liter, can be calculated using regression analysis. If this is related to the speed of the horse the V4 (speed at a blood lactate value of 4 mmol per liter) and the HR4 (heart rate at a lactate value of 4 mmol per liter) can be calculated. The value of expressions such as V200, V4, and HR 4 is that they provide standards against which individual improvements in fitness can be assessed and objective comparisons made between horses.

It is obvious that exercise testing is not a simple procedure, but it can be much more rewarding in information gained than performing resting hematology or other simple tests. Exercise tests can be conducted at racetracks, but the recent availability of relatively inexpensive high-speed treadmills,* has simplified exercise testing considerably. With these machines, horses can be exercised at speeds up to a full gallop under completely standardized conditions. In the future these machines will become increasingly used by veterinarians who specialize in performance horse medicine.

CONCLUSIONS

The investigation of poor racing performance must be detailed and thorough, as more than one body system may be involved. The use of diagnostic aids such as hematology and plasma biochemistry, endoscopy, ECG, and muscle biopsy will help to reach a diagnosis in many cases. However, care must be taken not to overinterpret small deviations from normal. Ultimately, the use of high-speed treadmills for exercise testing will help to define more specifically problems that lead to reduction in racing performance.

The therapy used in horses with poor performance problems is still an area of art more than

---

*EKEG, Vancouver; EQB, Pennsylvania; Hospimedi, Belgium; Ingenieurburo Isler Bioengineering, Switzerland.

*Sato, Sweden; Beltalong, Australia

science. Many drugs, vitamins, and electrolytes are commonly used by veterinarians on an entirely empiric basis. A more scientific approach to performance medicine in the future could enable evaluation of efficacy of these treatments.

Supplemental Readings

Mumford, J. A., and Rossdale, P. D.: Virus and its relationship to the "poor performance" syndrome. Equine Vet J., *12*:3, 1980.

Persson, S. G. B.: Evaluation of exercise intolerance and fitness in the performance horse. *In* Snow, D. H., Persson, S. G. B., and Rose, R. J. (eds.): Equine Exercise Physiology. Cambridge, Granta Editions, 1983, pp. 441–457.

Snow, D. H.: Skeletal muscle adaptations: A review. *In* Snow D. H., Persson, S. G. B., and Rose, R. J. (eds.): Equine Exercise Physiology. Cambridge, Granta Editions, 1983, pp. 160–183.

Steel, J. D.: Studies on the Electrocardiogram of the Racehorse. Sydney, Australasian Medical Publishing Co., 1963.

Stewart, J. H., Rose, R. J., Davis, P. E., and Hoffman, K.: A comparison of electrocardiographic findings in racehorses presented either for routine examination or poor racing performance. *In* Snow, D. H., Persson, S. G. B. and Rose, R. J. (eds.): Equine Exercise Physiology. Cambridge, Granta Editions, 1983, pp. 135–143.

Wilson, R. G., Isler, R. B., and Thornton, J. R.: Heart rate, lactic acid production and speed during a standardized exercise test in standardbred horses. *In* Snow, D. H., Persson, S. G. B., and Rose, R. J. (eds.): Equine Exercise Physiology. Cambridge, Granta Editions, 1983, pp. 487–496.

Causes of Fatigue

David R. Hodgson, PULLMAN, WASHINGTON

Muscular fatigue can be defined as the inability to maintain a given exercise intensity. The process of fatigue appears to be task specific and its causes multifactorial. In humans, both central (within the central nervous system) and peripheral (within the muscles themselves) causes of fatigue have been described. Although central fatigue is likely to occur in the horse, assessment and description of the particular factors involved is not possible. In contrast, many factors causing peripheral fatigue have been described. These include impairment of excitation-contraction coupling, impairment of energy production, and limitations in fuel supply. The particular processes that result in the production of fatigue are related to the type or intensity of work the horse is required to perform. Therefore, given the large number of tasks equine athletes are asked to undertake, it is most useful to characterize the causes of fatigue in relation to the imposed workload.

FATIGUE DURING HIGH-INTENSITY EXERCISE

A number of mechanisms have been postulated to explain fatigue during extremely heavy exercise in which muscular force can only be maintained for a maximum of several minutes. One view ascribes fatigue to a reduction in the efficiency of muscular excitation at the neuromuscular junction. An alternative hypothesis suggests that the fatigue results from events at or beyond the muscle t-tubular system. Although fatigue at the level of the neuromuscular junction has not been demonstrated in the horse, several of the changes occurring within the muscle cell itself, known to be associated with the production of fatigue, have been described.

Of these intracellular events, depletion of the phosphagen pool, which is composed of adenosine triphosphate (ATP) and creatine phosphate (CP), and the accumulation of lactate appear to be important processes contributing to fatigue. Although cellular homeostatic mechanisms are designed to maintain the levels of ATP within working muscle, short-term exhaustive exercise produces initial depletion of CP stores, with subsequent reduction in intramuscular ATP levels. There is a resultant diminution of the force-producing potential of the working muscle. Accumulation of lactate within working muscle reduces intracellular pH to 6.3 or lower, from a resting value of 7.0 to 7.1. Such changes in pH probably exert their effects in several ways. Protons may displace calcium ions from troponin, interfering with the actomyosin contractile machinery. Additionally, as intracellular pH falls, several of the key enzymes within the major metabolic pathways are progressively inhibited. The net result of these processes is a reduced availability or production of ATP for muscular contraction, with a subsequent decrease in the ability to perform muscular work. Progressive lactate accumulation in the working muscle of horses usually occurs at or above speeds of approximately 600 meters per minute. Decreases in the concentration of intramuscular ATP per se have only been reported following short-term exhaustive exercise (speeds greater than 800 meters per minute). Therefore it is important to realize that the accumulation of lactate, even at somewhat slower speeds, ultimately undermines the force-producing capacity of muscle.

FATIGUE DURING PROLONGED SUBMAXIMAL EXERCISE

Many factors—including disturbances in thermoregulation, hydration, and ionic balance, and depletion of muscle glycogen stores—have been implicated, both singularly and collectively, as causes of fatigue during prolonged submaximal exercise.

The energy that allows continued muscular contraction is provided by the enzymic degradation of substrates within the muscles themselves. One of the consequences of these metabolic processes is the liberation of large amounts of heat. To dissipate this heat and avoid hyperthermia, horses are endowed with a finely controlled thermoregulatory system, based primarily on the evaporation of sweat. However, as ambient temperature increases, the efficiency of this mechanism is reduced, potentially resulting in hyperthermia and a decreased capacity to perform endurance exercise. Increases in heart rate and cardiac output are necessary to increase peripheral blood flow for heat dissipation. It is likely that a similar sequence of events occurs in the horse in response to "heat stress." As sweating is the most important mechanism for heat dissipation in the horse during prolonged submaximal exercise, large volumes of fluid may be lost via this route. In humans, dehydration equivalent to approximately 5 per cent body weight is associated with a marked reduction in the capacity to perform endurance exercise. As the state of dehydration increases, this diminution in exercise capacity becomes more pronounced. This relationship between alterations in fluid balance and fatigue would also appear to be critical for the horse.

Horse sweat is hypertonic, and the potential exists for dramatic electrolyte losses during prolonged exercise. Sodium and chloride are the major ionic constituents of sweat, and sodium loss appears to have the most pronounced effects on body function. Due to the central role of sodium in fluid homeostasis, the major signs resulting from the loss of sodium and associated fluid are those of decreased circulatory function and poor organ perfusion. Such alterations in homeostatic mechanisms could be intimately related to reductions in athletic performance.

During exercise, potassium is liberated from working muscle. This potassium enters the circulation with some being liberated in sweat. However, most of the potassium is taken up by nonworking muscle. Studies in humans have demonstrated that if exercise of moderate to high intensity is continued to exhaustion, decreases in the intracellular potassium concentration of working muscle, from resting values of approximately 160 mEq/L to as low as 130

mEq/L, are possible. Such alterations in potassium concentration have been related to decreases in the force-producing potential of the muscle and would therefore contribute to fatigue. This effect is relatively transient, as on cessation of exercise there is rapid repletion of the potassium deficits within the working muscle.

Calcium ions (Ca^{2+}) have been reported to increase in the mitochondria of working muscle during prolonged submaximal exercise. These ions are liberated from the sarcoplasmic reticulum during excitation–contraction coupling and some may be sequestered by the mitochondria. This process requires the consumption of oxygen and therefore may reduce the potential of mitochondria to phosphorylate adenosine diphosphate (ADP) to ATP, which in turn may result in fatigue.

Regardless of the causes of fatigue just described, there does appear to be one common element associated with fatigue during prolonged exercise of moderate to high intensity. This is closely related to a depletion of the intramuscular glycogen store. It occurs in a selective manner in given muscle fibers (fiber types) as a function of the intensity or duration or both of the exercise. Depletion of glycogen from within muscle fibers is associated with a decreased force-producing capacity of the fibers. Although muscle fibers are selectively recruited during submaximal exercise, with new ones being added as others become exhausted, eventually many fibers are depleted of their glycogen stores and the overall force-producing capacity of the muscle is reduced. The depletion of glycogen, despite the fact that fats are the major substrate for muscular work during this type of exercise, indicates that glycogen is vital if exercise is to continue. When horses undergo endurance training, one of the major metabolic adaptations is to further increase the ability of working muscle to utilize fats during submaximal exercise. This has the effect of reducing the rate of glycogen utilization and therefore delays the onset of fatigue.

In summary, the inability to maintain a given exercise intensity depends on several factors, including the nature of the exercise, the physiologic or training status of the horse, the environmental conditions, and other (poorly defined) psychologic considerations. At times, the inability to continue exercise at a given intensity depends on the availability of a key metabolite within a particular tissue. Under other conditions abnormal or inadequate interaction of several individual systems may result in the onset of fatigue. However, as physiologic systems are often matched in their capacities, it may be extremely difficult to identify precisely the factor or factors that result in a decrease in exercise capacity.

Supplemental Readings

Karlsson, J.: Localized muscular fatigue: Role of muscle metabolism and substrate depletion. Exercise Sport Sci. Rev., 7:1, 1979.

Sahlin, K.: Intracellular pH and energy metabolism in skeletal muscle of man. (With special reference to exercise.) Acta Physiol. Scand., Suppl. 455, 1978.

Sjogaard, G., Adams, R. P., and Saltin, B.: Water and ion shifts in skeletal muscle of humans with intense dynamic knee extension. Am. J. Physiol., 24:R190, 1985.

Snow, D. H., Harris, R. C., and Gash, S. P.: Metabolic response of equine muscle to intermittent maximal exercise. J. Appl. Physiol., 58:1689, 1985.

Clinical Assessment of Performance Horses

David R. Hodgson, PULLMAN, WASHINGTON

Endurance rides and the cross-country phase of event competition constitute two of the most demanding forms of equine exercise. The aims of participants in both these forms of equestrian endeavor are to complete the competition at the highest level of performance, yet still have the horse in sufficiently good condition to be able to continue if asked to do so. Successful participation requires optimal use of an adequately conditioned horse, with the speed of exercise being adjusted appropriately to prevent injury or excessive fatigue. Although many decisions regarding a horse's condition are ultimately made by the rider, astute judgments by the supervising veterinarian may often reduce the incidence of injuries and unnecessary stress on the horse. Therefore, the attending veterinarian's primary goal should be to prevent such occurrences. Because this is not possible under all circumstances, early recognition of medical problems and rapid institution of the appropriate therapy are extremely important. An organized and careful clinical examination is fundamental in achieving these aims.

Official veterinarians are often required to make a clinical judgment of an individual horse's ability to continue in the competition. Without access to sophisticated laboratory equipment, accurate assessment of any underlying biochemical disturbances is impossible. As a result, judgments are frequently made on the basis of physical examination, which should include determination of heart and respiratory rates, body temperature, and an assessment of hydration. It is preferable to record baseline values of these parameters with the horses at rest before the competition. By comparing these values with those obtained following cessation of the exercise, a better overall impression of the horse's condition is often obtained. If any doubt exists as to a horse's condition these measurements should be repeated on several occasions. Determination of the horse's general appearance, gait, attitude, desire or lack of desire to drink, sweating rate, appetite, intestinal motility, and anal tone may also provide useful information when attempting to make assessments regarding a horse's response to the exercise. In addition, particular examination should be made for the presence of lameness, obvious stiffness, exertional myopathies, lacerations, ocular injuries, saddle sores, and girth galls.

HEART RATE

Although assessment of horses during strenuous athletic events requires complete clinical assessment, repeated measurement of the heart rate provides valuable objective assessment of the degree of fatigue. In a study involving endurance horses in Australia, elevated heart rates 30 minutes after cessation of exercise and delayed heart rate recoveries following competition correlated closely with the degree of stress and biochemical derangement, particularly in endurance horses. Horses with heart rates greater than 60 to 65 beats per minute 30 minutes following cessation of exercise were more dehydrated, had greater disturbances in renal, muscle, and liver function, and had greater depletion of intramuscular energy reserves than those with heart rates less than 60 beats per minute. The horse's heart rate immediately after exercise only reflects the average speed of the ride and does not correlate with the existence of metabolic derangements.

RESPIRATORY RATE

Few useful correlations exist between respiratory rate and the various biochemical indicators of exhaustion. A persistently elevated respiratory rate following exercise may be associated with hyperthermia, dehydration, and fatigue, but there is no consistent correlation between the degree of metabolic derangement and respiratory rate. This is not to say that the measurement or respiratory rate is not useful. For example, horses suffering from the so-called "exhausted horse syndrome" may have elevations in respiratory rate for variable periods of time following cessation of the exercise, possibly the result of metabolic abnormalities and attempts by the horse to dissipate body heat via the respiratory tract.

RECTAL TEMPERATURE

Continued muscular contraction requires a constant supply of energy. This energy is provided by the enzymic degradation of substrates accompanied by the liberation of large amounts of heat. As a result, a horse's body temperature rises in response to physical activity. Rectal temperatures in the range of 39° to 40° C are not uncommon following prolonged strenuous exercise, particularly when ambient temperatures are high. Normally, rectal temperatures begin to return to normal within 20 to 30 minutes following cessation of exercise. Horses with rectal temperatures in excess of 40.5° C to 41° C should be regarded as abnormal. Such horses are usually encountered when the ambient temperature and humidity are high and when the animals have derangements in fluid and electrolyte balance. These animals should be observed closely and their riders should be strongly discouraged from allowing the horse to continue further exercise. Persistent elevations in rectal temperature (above 40.5° C) may also be associated with elevations in the horse's core temperature, which may be manifested clinically as altered central nervous system function.

HYDRATION

Sweating provides the most important mechanism for heat loss in the horse during prolonged submaximal exercise. As a result, up to 25 to 50 liters of fluid may be lost during endurance rides. Assessment of hydration therefore plays a pivotal role in the evaluation of horses performing prolonged exercise. Heart rate or heart rate recovery provides a useful guide to the degree of dehydration. Other parameters that may be useful for the assessment of hydration include changes in skin turgor or elasticity, capillary refill time, jugular distensibility, and pulse pressure. Dehydration produces hypovolemia and a decrease in peripheral perfusion, which in turn is often reflected by a decrease in skin elasticity, an increase in capillary refill time (often in association with dry mucous membranes), a decrease in the rate of jugular filling, and a decrease in peripheral pulse pressure. If the dehydration is severe enough, some horses may fail to sweat, even in the presence of elevated rectal temperatures (see p. 187).

Supplemental Readings

Carlson, G. P.: Thermoregulation and fluid balance in the exercising horse. *In* Snow, D. H., Persson, S. G. B., and Rose, R. J. (eds.): Equine Exercise Physiology. Cambridge, Granta Editions, 1983, pp. 291–309.

Rose, R. J.: An evaluation of heart rate and respiratory rate recovery for assessment of fitness during endurance rides. *In* Snow, D. H., Persson, S. G. B., and Rose, R. J. (eds.): Equine Exercise Physiology. Cambridge, Granta Editions, 1983, pp. 505–509.

Thermoregulatory Problems

Gary P. Carlson, DAVIS, CALIFORNIA

Exercise requires a massive increase in the metabolic rate of working muscle. However, only a portion of the available energy can be effectively utilized for this work and the remaining energy accumulates as heat. This heat must be removed by the vascular system, which serves to transport heat from core areas to the skin where heat exchange with the environment can occur. One of the major problems facing the equine athlete is the dissipation of this excess body heat. When exercise is performed in a hot or humid environment, competing demands for heat dissipation and maximal exertion limit performance and may result in serious heat-associated illness. For these reasons thermoregulatory processes are of particular relevance to the practitioner working with performance horses.

Core temperature is critical and is normally maintained within relatively narrow limits. The processes by which this is accomplished are controlled by the thermoregulatory center located in the midbrain. This center integrates input from the central as well as the peripheral nervous systems and is responsive to local concentration changes of specific electrolytes, hormones, and certain chemical mediators. The center establishes a set point or threshold temperature at which increased heat production (e.g., shivering) or increased heat dissipation (e.g., peripheral vasodilatation, vascular redistribution, and sweating) are brought into play. Alteration of this set point is one of the important adaptive responses to physical training in humans. Thermal balance represents careful regulation of factors responsible for metabolic heat production and heat loss or gain from the environment. Failure to maintain this balance may lead to progressive elevation of core temperature, altered CNS function, collapse, and death.

Heat is lost from the body by four basic processes: radiation, conduction, convection, and evaporation. The effectiveness of the first three processes as means of heat dissipation are all dependent upon a favorable temperature gradient between the subject and the environment. For this reason exercise in cool climates is rarely associated with thermoregulatory problems. As environmental temperature increases and approaches that of body temperature the first three of these processes become ineffective. Evaporative processes, particularly sweating, are the most important means of heat dissipation for the exercising horse. Race horses may lose up to 10 L of sweat in an attempt to disperse the excess body heat generated in a one-mile race that can be run in less than two minutes. Exercise performed by endurance horses is at a much slower pace but must be maintained for hours. On hot days rectal temperatures of these horses often exceed 40° C, and sweat losses may exceed 10 to 15 L per hour. Clinically normal endurance horses may accumulate transient fluid deficits of 20 to 40 L (4 to 10 per cent of body weight), and significant electrolyte deficits are associated with sweat losses of this magnitude. The combined effects of fluid and electrolyte losses in sweat may have profound physiologic effects as detailed in the subsequent section on the exhausted horse syndrome. Dehydration and hypovolemia have adverse effects on heat transfer and the rate of sweating, thus impairing the ability of the horse to dissipate excess body heat. Human athletic performance is compromised by net fluid deficits of 2 to 5 per cent of body weight.

The effectiveness of evaporative thermoregulatory processes is a function of the rate of heat production, environmental temperature, relative humidity, and wind velocity. High relative humidity interferes with sweat evaporation and thus impairs the principal means of heat dissipation. A variety of heat stress indexes have been developed to assess these factors in human subjects, including effective temperature index, equivalences en sejour, and the wet bulb globe temperature index. There have been no comparable indexes developed for the horse. An arbitrary system using a combination of temperature in degrees Fahrenheit and relative humidity in percent has been proposed for use in the horse. In this system the sum of the relative humidity and temperature in degrees Fahrenheit is made. If the value is less than 120, there are no problems; if the value is greater than 150 care should be exercised. Values over 180 will severely compromise thermoregulation.

HEAT STROKE

Heat stroke occurs when the normal thermoregulatory processes fail. It may occur when an unacclimatized horse is suddenly exposed to a hot humid climate. Most often heat stroke occurs during transport in overheated, poorly ventilated trailers or with vigorous and protracted exercise in a hot and humid environment. Dehydration associated with sweat losses compromises thermoregulatory response and is considered to be a major contributing factor in the development of heat stroke. Obesity, long hair coat, heavy blanketing, extensive skin damage as the result of dermatitis or burns, and anhidrosis impede sweating or effective sweat evaporation and may also be contributing factors in the onset of clinical signs.

Horses with heat stroke may proceed from a state of restlessness and anxiety to depression, stupor, disorientation, collapse, and death. Sweating may be profuse in some cases but is generally less than anticipated for a given circumstance and the skin is hot to the touch. Heart rate and respiratory rate are elevated and pulse pressure may be weak. Rectal temperature is 40° C or greater and may actually increase. These horses are in critical condition and emergency therapy is indicated.

Therapy. The first and foremost therapeutic objective is control of body temperature. This can be accomplished by rigorous sponging or spraying of cold water or alcohol over the large vessels of the distal extremities, head, and neck. The horse should be placed in a shady area with good ventilation. Air movement is critical; advantage should be taken of any available wind or electric fans. Cold water enemas may be of benefit in extreme situations. Intravenous fluids are an important component of successful therapy. Sodium-containing polyionic fluids such as lactated Ringer's solution are suitable, although saline fortified with potassium at 10 to 15 mEq per L may more closely match likely deficits. Fluids should be given rapidly to effect and 10 to 20 L or more may be required. Antipyretics such as dipyrone, phenylbutazone, and flunixin meglumine are generally given but care should be taken to restore hydration if these agents are to be used.

ANHIDROSIS

Anhidrosis (failure to sweat under appropriate stimulus) is a condition that occurs exclusively in horses maintained in the tropics, where there is persistently high temperature and humidity. Anhidrosis has been reported as a special exercise-associated problem in individual performance horses moved from a temperate to a tropical climate. Recent epidemiologic studies indicate that the problem may also occur in stabled sedentary horses and horses native to tropical areas. There is no breed or sex predisposition, but the condition is definitely exacerbated by exercise. Further details are provided on pg. 187.

Supplemental Readings

Nadel, E. R., Wenger, C. B., Roberts, M. F., Stolwijk, J. A., and Cafarelli, E.: Physiological defenses against hyperthermia of exercise. Ann. N.Y. Acad. Sci., *301*:98, 1977.

Wyndham, C. H.: The physiology of exercise under heat stress. Ann. Rev. Physiol., *35*:193, 1973.

Wyndham, C. H.: Heat stroke and hyperthermia in marathon runners. Ann. N.Y. Acad. Sci., *301*:128, 1977.

Fluid, Electrolyte and Acid-Base Disturbances Associated with Exercise

Reuben J. Rose, SYDNEY, AUSTRALIA

Exercise in the horse produces a variety of changes in fluid, electrolyte, and acid-base values. Some of these changes, for example the severe acidosis of high-speed exercise, may limit the actual performance of the horse, while other changes may have a more severe effect after the exercise session. As noted in the chapter on thermoregulation, evaporative cooling is the principal means of heat loss in the horse; therefore, extensive losses of both fluid and electrolytes can occur during long-distance exercise. Understanding the nature and extent of these losses can provide a basis for the rational treatment of horses with exercise-induced fluid, electrolyte, and acid-base disturbances.

INTERPRETATION OF PLASMA ELECTROLYTE VALUES

The measurement of plasma electrolyte values provides the key to assessment of disturbances of electrolyte balance. However, changes in the major plasma electrolytes do not always indicate net gains or losses. When plasma values are interpreted, taking into account changes in body weight and the distributions in the body, it is possible to obtain a relatively accurate guide to total body electrolyte balance. While calcium and magnesium are important electrolytes, major disturbances associated with exercise are rare. This chapter will therefore be restricted to consideration of sodium, potassium, chloride, and bicarbonate.

Sodium. Plasma sodium values provide no guide to body sodium balance. Sodium is the most important of the extracellular fluid solutes in determining osmotic activity. Because of this, plasma sodium values provide a guide to total body osmotic equilibrium, because the intra- and extracellular fluids are in osmotic equilibrium. Thus the plasma sodium provides a guide to body fluid tonicity and is more an indicator of relative water balance than of sodium balance. The plasma sodium is affected by the changes in the exchangeable sodium (Na exch), the exchangeable potassium (K exch), and total body water. This is expressed by the equation:

$$\text{Plasma Na (mmol/l. H}_2\text{O)} = \frac{\text{Na exch} + \text{K exch}}{\text{total body water}}$$

As approximately 60 per cent of the body weight consists of water, it can be seen that by measuring changes in body weight together with plasma sodium concentrations an estimate of the sodium and potassium deficit can be obtained. If the electrolyte composition of the source of the fluid and electrolyte losses can be obtained—for example, in sweat loss, the sodium:potassium ratio is about 3:1—then the separate sodium and potassium losses can be estimated.

Potassium. One of the major problems in assessment of body potassium status is that the plasma values provide little guide to total body potassium. Only 400 mmol of potassium, or approximately 1.4 per cent of the total body potassium store, is contained in the extracellular fluid. Because of the intracellular location of potassium, it is intimately bound up in the relationship between cell structure and function. Disturbances of potassium balance can result in signs such as muscle weakness and cardiac arrhythmias, and may be involved in the pathogenesis of some exercise-related muscle disorders. For the interpretation of plasma potassium, low values generally indicate total body potassium depletion. However, quite severe potassium deficits can also exist without the plasma potassium values being outside the normal range. The best estimates of potassium loss are made from the equation given. Thus it is possible to calculate the total body potassium status quite accurately, once the body weight loss, plasma sodium values, and relative distributions of sodium and potassium losses are known.

Chloride. Chloride is the major anion in the extracellular fluid. While it tends to behave passively in the body and inversely reflects changes in bicarbonate values, exercise-induced alterations are common due to high concentrations of this electrolyte in the sweat. Because the bulk of the chloride in the body is contained in the extracellular fluid, the plasma values tend to reflect net gains or losses.

Bicarbonate. Bicarbonate concentrations accurately reflect the nonrespiratory component of acid-base disturbances. Acid-base disturbances of respiratory origin are seldom encountered, apart from transient changes during exercise. Lower than normal bicarbonate values indicate an acidosis, which is usually due to lactic acid production during high-intensity exercise. Increased bicarbonate concentrations indicate an alkalosis, which is sometimes found in endurance horses after competing in hot conditions.

ALTERATIONS IN ELECTROLYTE BALANCE

Sodium. During endurance exercise, there are extensive losses of sodium, and total body sodium deficits in excess of 4000 mmol can occur as a result of 160-km endurance rides in hot weather. Although such losses are common, it is unusual to find plasma sodium values greatly outside the normal range. This would seem to indicate that sweat electrolyte losses are largely isotonic or otherwise hypo- or hypernatremia would be found. If a horse with a normal plasma sodium value following an endurance ride consumes 20 L of water, the plasma sodium may decrease quite substantially. This indicates that electrolyte replacement must be undertaken in addition to fluid replacement.

In most forms of short-distance, high-intensity exercise, there is an increase in plasma sodium values. This occurs not from a net sodium gain but from fluid movement out of the extracellular fluid. In the majority of horses, the plasma sodium values have returned to normal by 30 to 60 minutes after exercise. However, some horses that sweat heavily while being transported to the races or when excited can lose substantial amounts of sodium.

Potassium. Losses of potassium during endurance exercise can be in the order of 1000 to 2000 mmol. This results in some reduction in the plasma concentrations after endurance exercise. Additionally, there is movement of potassium into cells after exercise, so that if plasma potassium is measured 30 minutes after an endurance ride, the values are much lower than immediately following exercise.

Increases in plasma potassium values are found immediately after high-intensity exercise. This appears to be the result of both hemoconcentration and the extracellular movement of potassium. Plasma values remain elevated for only a short time after maximal exercise and are usually within the normal range by 30 to 60 minutes afterward. As with endurance exercise, there is a post-exercise movement of potassium into cells so that plasma potassium values 30 to 60 minutes after exercise are usually lower than normal. It is important to be aware of these effects when interpreting plasma electrolyte concentrations.

Chloride. Major changes in plasma chloride values are usually only found associated with endurance exercise. This is because prolonged sweating is necessary to produce sufficient chloride loss to result in hypochloremia. Hemoconcentration may result in a transient increase in plasma chloride values.

In tropical climates, where more extensive losses of sweat can be found in racehorses in training, horses may develop hypochloremia if they are not given a dietary electrolyte supplement.

Bicarbonate. Abnormalities of plasma bicarbonate are quite unusual in blood samples collected from horses at rest. The low bicarbonate values following high-speed exercise and the elevated values sometimes found after endurance exercise are only transient. Therefore, therapy directed at acid-base disturbances is seldom necessary in the average performance horse.

ALTERATIONS IN FLUID AND ACID-BASE BALANCE

Fluid Balance. During all types of exercise there are fluid shifts between the extracellular and intracellular fluid compartments. Even with intense short-distance exercise fluid shifts out of the vascular system, there being elevations of plasma protein values. These fluid shifts are transient, and in most cases pre-exercise values are regained by 30 to 60 minutes after exercise. The most common route of fluid loss during exercise is sweat, although minor losses can occur from the urinary, gastrointestinal, and respiratory systems. During high-intensity exercise, fluid losses in the range of 5 to 10 liters can occur. However, more extensive losses may arise from the transport of horses and the extensive sweating that sometimes takes place before racing. During endurance exercise, evaporative sweat loss provides the main mechanism for thermoregulation. Under hot conditions, the fluid losses in sweat may be as much as 10 to 15 liters per hour. Several reports have indicated that the mean fluid losses following endurance riding are between 20 and 40 liters. Interestingly, although these losses sometimes represent up to 10 per cent of the horse's body weight, clinical signs of hypovolemia seldom occur. This is probably because the majority of the losses are quickly replaced when the horse has access to water and electrolytes.

Acid-Base Balance. Although major disturbances in acid-base balance take place during exercise, in most cases these changes are short-lived. With all forms of exercise, there is an increase in the production of lactate in skeletal muscle. The diffusion of lactate into the circulation results in an increase in blood lactate, which at values of 4 mmol per L or greater will produce a systemic metabolic acidosis, with a decrease in blood pH. After endurance exercise, the increase in blood lactate is usually in the range 1 to 2 mmol per L and therefore insufficient to produce a change in acid-base status. At higher intensities of exercise such as those performed by Thoroughbred and Standardbred racehorses, large increases in blood lactate are found, with post-exercise values in excess of 30 mmol per L. This degree of increase in blood lactate will lead to a profound metabolic acidosis with blood pH values in the vicinity of 6.8. The acidosis following high-intensity exercise is most profound in the first five minutes after the exercise ceases. Although the rate of lactate metabolism varies between individual horses, most horses have returned to normal acid-base status by one hour after exercise. Because of this rapid metabolism of lactate by the body, a continuing metabolic acidosis is not found in performance horses. Therefore, commercial feed supplements that are purported to treat acidosis in racehorses are of no value. Recent studies in human athletes have shown that increasing the alkali reserve by administration of oral bicarbonate before sprint exercise can lead to an improvement in performance times. Whether such an effect exists in the horse is unknown at this time.

In horses performing in endurance or trail rides in hot weather, metabolic alkalosis may occur. This is thought to be caused by the high chloride content of equine sweat, resulting in hypochloremia. In an attempt at maintaining electroneutrality, bicarbonate is retained by the kidney, resulting in an increase in blood bicarbonate and an increase in pH. For this reason, bicarbonate therapy is inappropriate when treating most fluid and electrolyte disturbances in endurance horses.

THERAPY

In the case of horses performing endurance exercise, the most common therapeutic requirement is fluid and electrolytes, to replace losses in sweat. While most horses will be able to replace these losses by the provision of water and salts, some exhausted horses will not drink. The therapeutic regimens for these horses are discussed in the chapter on the exhausted horse syndrome.

Fluid may be administered by stomach tube or intravenously. If administered by stomach tube, isotonic or hypotonic solutions should be given and not more than 9 liters administered at any one time. Intravenous fluids are necessary only when there are signs of hypovolemia or a lack of response to the oral fluids. Because of the possibility of metabolic alkalosis, bicarbonate solutions should not be given. In general, a polyionic fluid that contains electrolytes in the normal ranges for equine plasma is the fluid of choice. Should intravenous fluid therapy be indicated, a minimum of 15 to 20 liters of fluid needs to be administered at a rate of 6 to 8 liters per hour.

With horses performing maximal exercise, the disturbances in fluid, acid-base, and electrolyte balance seldom require intensive therapy. However, as a result of fluid and electrolyte losses in the sweat and deficiency of green feed in most racehorses' diets, it is possible to find abnormalities of both electrolyte and fluid balance in horses in training. The most common abnormalities are hypokalemia and hypochloremia with or without dehydration. These can be treated with dietary addition of an electrolyte supplement. The common use in racetrack practice of the saline drench may be of some benefit if the horse will not eat the electrolytes in its feed. However, the practice of the administration of 1 to 2 liters of intravenous fluids the day before racing is of no therapeutic value.

Supplemental Readings

Carlson, G. P.: Thermoregulation and fluid balance in the exercising horse. *In* Snow, D. H., Persson, S. G. B., and Rose, R. J. (eds.): Equine Exercise Physiology. Cambridge, Granta Editions, 1983, pp. 291–309.

Edelman, I. S., Leibman, J., O'Meara, M. P., and Birkenfeld, L. W.: Interrelationships between serum sodium concentrations, serum osmolality, and total exchangeable sodium, total exchangeable potassium and total body water. J. Clin. Invest., 37:1236, 1958.

Rose, R. J.: A physiological approach to fluid and electrolyte therapy in the horse. Equine Vet. J., *13*:7, 1982.

Snow, D. H., Kerr, M. G., Nimmo, M. A., and Abbott, E. M.: Alterations in blood, sweat, urine and muscle composition during prolonged exercise in the horse. Vet. Rec., *110*:377, 1982.

Snow, D. H., Mason, D. K., Ricketts, S. W., and Douglas, T. A.: Post-race blood biochemistry in Thoroughbreds. *In* Snow, D. H., Persson, S. G. B., and Rose, R. J. (eds.): Equine Exercise Physiology. Cambridge, Granta Editions, 1983, pp. 389–407.

The Exhausted Horse Syndrome

Gary P. Carlson, DAVIS, CALIFORNIA

Fatigue or exhaustion is a physiologic result of relatively brief maximal exercise or protracted submaximal exercise. With maximal exertion in racehorses, there is rapid depletion of readily available muscle energy stores (creatine phosphate, ATP). Exhaustion is closely correlated with the development of a severe metabolic lactic acidosis. With protracted submaximal or endurance exercise, energy is supplied by aerobic metabolism of both fatty acids and carbohydrates with minimal changes in acid-base status or lactic acid concentration. Fatigue after endurance exercise is less well-understood but may be associated with depletion of energy substrates, muscle glycogen, as well as fluid and electrolyte imbalances and their attendant pathophysiologic effects. Most endurance rides are conducted in the summer months when high environmental temperature imposes an additional stress to which these horses must respond. Both the incidence and severity of exercise-associated medical problems are greater during such periods of high environmental temperatures or humidity or both. Although a variety of factors contribute, fluid and electrolyte losses via sweating play a central role in the genesis of the exhausted horse syndrome.

Before proceeding, it may be advantageous to consider some of the factors that contribute to fluid and electrolyte imbalance in these horses. During 50- to 100-mile rides, particularly those held on very hot humid days, most horses drink copious amounts of water. It is generally recommended that horses exercising under these conditions be allowed to drink at every opportunity. Despite frequent access to water, many endurance horses, even those performing normally, develop clinical signs of slight to moderate dehydration during the course of a ride. Dehydration, as assessed by both clinical and laboratory evaluation, appears to be maximal in most horses at or near the midpoint of these rides. Medical problems also tend to occur most frequently in association with maximal dehydration or after rides on particularly stressful terrain and not necessarily at the end of a ride. Horses that successfully complete these rides and continue to eat and drink appear to replenish a substantial portion of their fluid losses by the end of the ride or early in the recovery period after the race.

Protracted exercise at the pace of endurance rides requires an energy expenditure 10 to greater than 20 times that of the basal metabolic rate. This rate of energy expenditure results in a massive metabolically generated heat load, which must be dissipated to maintain thermal balance. Since horses normally do not pant, sweating is the primary means of thermoregulation for horses exercising under these conditions. Measured weight change as an index of net change in water balance indicates that many horses will have fluid deficits of 20 to 40 L or more. There are no accurate quantitative data on total body sweat electrolyte losses in exercising horses. There are data, however, on the relative electrolyte losses in equine sweat. As a rough approximation, for each 100 mEq of sodium, 30 mEq of potassium and 130 mEq of chloride are lost in equine sweat. Significant amounts of calcium and magnesium are also lost in sweat. When sweat losses are maximal, there are normally compensating reductions of fluid and electrolyte losses by other routes.

Serum electrolyte concentrations tend to change in a predictable fashion with protracted exercise in hot environments while relatively few changes are observed in moderate to cooler climates. Sodium and potassium concentrations tend to decrease during the course of an endurance ride but generally remain within the broadest range of normal values. Decreased sodium concentration reflects a combination of water and electrolyte loss followed by partial replacement of the water deficit by drinking. There are no clear-cut differences between normal and exhausted endurance horses in regard to the concentration of these two cations, although a number of the latter group of horses develop significant hypokalemia. Hypochloremia is a consistent feature in all profusely sweating horses. Plasma chloride concentrations of 90 mEq per L or less are common and may be less than 80 mEq per L in some dehydrated, exhausted horses. The hypochloremia reflects the relatively high concentration of chloride lost in equine sweat. Calcium and magnesium concentrations tend to decline with endurance exercise while phosphate concentration increases. The most consistent acid-base alteration associated with endurance exercise in hot environments is a mild metabolic alkalosis. The metabolic alkalosis appears to be associated with the developing hypochloremia and hypokalemia that result from heavy sweating and may not be seen with exercise in cooler environments.

The combination of dehydration and sodium depletion results in decreased plasma volume evidenced by increased packed cell volume (PCV) and plasma protein concentration (TPP), increased blood viscosity, inadequate tissue perfusion, and inefficient oxygen and substrate transport. This may contribute to impaired renal function and lead to partial renal shutdown as part of the overall cardiovascular effects. Chloride depletion may contribute to the development and persistence of metabolic alkalosis. This acid-base disturbance associated with depletion of potassium, calcium, and magnesium may alter membrane potential and neuromuscular transmission, and contribute to gastrointestinal stasis and cardiac arrhythmias, as well as muscle cramps and spasms including synchronous diaphragmatic flutter (SDF). When severe, the combined depletion of both water and electrolytes may result in diminished sweat production. Impairment of the normal means of heat dissipation may result in persistently elevated body temperature with attendant heat-induced injury to a variety of tissues, including the central nervous system. Fluid and electrolyte alterations affect the cardiovascular, neuromuscular, digestive, and urinary systems, in which they either evoke a response or impair normal function.

RECOGNITION OF EXHAUSTION

There are variations in the severity of signs of exhaustion in individual horses. Most problems are recognized at veterinary checkpoints or at mandatory rest stops. All affected horses will have elevated rectal temperatures and pulse and respiratory rates, and variable dehydration on arrival at these stops. The most reliable quantitative guides to impending exhaustion are pulse and respiratory recovery rates. At mandatory rest stops pulse and respiratory rates taken 30 minutes after arrival must return to acceptable levels, usually 60 to 70 per minute and 40 per minute, respectively. At the veterinary checkpoints where horses are held for shorter periods, slightly higher values may be used. No horse should be allowed to proceed until pulse and respiratory rates have recovered sufficiently. Riders are informed of specific ride criteria to be used and should be encouraged to monitor their horse's pulse and respiratory rates to pace their ride and thus avoid problems.

Severely exhausted horses are readily recognized. They are usually severely depressed with little interest in food or water despite apparent dehydration. Most will continue to sweat although at apparently reduced rates. Pulse and respiratory rates generally remain elevated despite the period of rest. Pulse pressure and jugular distensibility are often markedly decreased, capillary refill time prolonged, and cardiac irregularities may be noted.

Muscle cramps and spasms are often evident. There is usually a marked diminution or absence of intestinal sounds and a lack of anal tone. Exhausted horses require prompt and vigorous therapy with careful monitoring to ensure that they respond fully to therapy. Some horses will also develop SDF. This contraction of the diaphragm is recognized as a tick or spasm in the muscles of the flank, which is synchronous with the heart beat and will be discussed further on page 485.

TREATMENT OF EXHAUSTION

Horses manifesting depression and persistently elevated pulse and respiratory rates as their only problems may respond to rest, cooling out, and access to salt, clean feed, and water. A return of appetite and water consumption are exceedingly important factors in the recovery process. Horses should be closely watched and, if there is no improvement in 30 minutes, they should receive fluids orally or intravenously or by both routes.

Rectal temperatures in most normal horses begin to return toward normal in 15 to 30 minutes. It may be possible to hasten this process by external application of water. On hot humid days most experienced riders will make rigorous efforts to assist in the cooling-out process. Cool water is applied by a hose, sprayer, sponge, or towels over the large vessels of the distal extremities, head and neck, and over the jugular veins. This is most effectively done in an open area with free circulation of air, in a breeze or in front of a fan. It is a general practice to avoid pouring very cold water over the large muscle masses as there is concern of inducing muscle spasms. Cold alcohol leg wraps are used by some individuals and are said to reduce filling of tendon sheaths. In hot climates riders are well advised to carry sponges so that water can be applied to the horse whenever available. External means of removing excess body heat becomes a critical factor when a combination of high humidity and dehydration render the normal thermoregulatory mechanisms ineffective. Rapid cooling of horses with marked or peristently elevated rectal temperatures (in excess of 40.5° C) and signs of altered central nervous system function is essential. Cold water enemas may benefit these horses in addition to the rigorous cooling procedures described. Intravenous fluid therapy should be employed as well.

The most important aspect of treatment of severe exhaustion is prompt and vigorous fluid therapy. The aims of fluid therapy are restoration of the effective circulating blood volume, correction of electrolyte deficits, and provision of readily metabolizable energy as glucose. Since the principal problems in these horses are dehydration and sodium and chloride depletion, rapid restoration of the plasma and extracellular fluid (ECF) volume with sodium-containing replacement fluids is essential. Polyionic replacement solutions such as Ringer's solution are commonly utilized and effective. Saline contains sodium and chloride in proportions that approximate deficits likely to occur with heavy sweat loss. Potassium should be added to these solutions so as to provide at least 10 mEq per L. Glucose as an energy source can be supplied as 5 per cent dextrose or 50 per cent dextrose may be added to the polyionic fluids to deliver between 50 and 100 gm per hour. This readily metabolizable energy source is extremely beneficial in horses with marked hypoglycemia. Horses with SDF almost invariably have intestinal atony, which may contribute to inappetence and thus a failure to replace deficits by voluntary consumption. These horses generally respond promptly to calcium solutions (100 to 300 ml of 20 per cent calcium borogluconate) given intravenously. Administration of calcium solutions should be at a relatively slow rate, given to effect, and should be discontinued if cardiac irregularities develop.

Intravenous fluids can be supplemented or, in many cases, supplanted by fluids administered by a stomach tube. Fluids administered by this route appear to be well-tolerated and fairly rapidly absorbed. This route of fluid administration offers the advantages of low cost, speed, and convenience but should not be used in horses that are recumbent or manifesting signs of colic. Volumes of 5 to 8 L are given at one time and may be repeated every 30 minutes to an hour as required. It is thus possible to deliver 15 to 24 L in an hour. Fluid administration via this route should be discontinued if there is evidence of discomfort or gastric reflux. Fluids administered via nasogastric tube should be isotonic or hypotonic. Markedly hypertonic salt solutions should not be administered since the osmotic gra-

dient created may draw water into the bowel from the already compromised ECF. The composition of commonly used intravenous fluids and oral electrolyte supplements is given in Table 1. A simple inexpensive and useful isotonic fluid can be prepared by the addition of one level tablespoon of common table salt (NaCl) and one of Lite Salt* (NaCl + KCl) per gallon of water. Twenty-four liters (just over 6 gallons) of this fluid will provide 2570 mEq of sodium, 670 mEq of potassium, and 3200 mEq of chloride. This is similar to the theoretic estimates of electrolyte deficits in moderately dehydrated endurance horses. This preparation or minor variants has been used by experienced veterinarians working with endurance animals with a good response. The addition of a soluble carbohydrate such as dextrose is reported to enhance gastrointestinal absorption of electrolyte solutions in calves. Whether this is true for the adult horse is not known. Many of the electrolyte and energy replacement combinations contain dextrose and may be of benefit. Care should be taken that the product does not contain large amounts of bicarbonate or bicarbonate precursors. If these products are used the actual electrolyte content should be determined because label recommendations for additions to drinking water may result in very dilute solutions.

The volume, rate, and route of fluid administration should vary with the severity of the presenting problems. Since under field conditions absolute losses are unknown, quantitative estimates provide a guide to fluid and electrolyte requirements. Volume requirements may range from 20 to 40 L or more. In severely affected horses, sodium-containing fluids should be administered intravenously at a rate of 10 to 20 L per hour in addition to the fluids given by nasogastric tube. Potassium-supplemented saline, lactated Ringer's solution, or one of

*Morton Thiokol, Inc., Chicago, IL

TABLE 1. COMPOSITION OF COMMON INTRAVENOUS FLUIDS AND ORAL ELECTROLYTE SUPPLEMENTS

Fluid		Na	K	Cl	HCO$_3$	Calories (Kcal/L)
				(mEq/L)		
Saline		154	—	154	—	—
Lactated Ringer's		130	4	109	28	9
5% dextrose		—	—	—	—	170
5% NaHCO$_3$		600	—	—	600	—
Oral Supplements				(mEq)		(Kcal)
NaCl	1 tbs (16.6 gm)	284	—	284	—	—
KCl	1 tbs (16.2 gm)	—	217	217	—	—
Lite Salt	1 tbs (16.9 gm)	144	113	256	—	—
Eltrad*	8 oz packet	570	39	415	—	724

A. The theoretical optimal ratio of electrolyte replacement for massive sweat loss is: Na 100 mEq, K 30 mEq, Cl 130 mEq.

B. One level tablespoon each of common salt (NaCl) and Lite Salt (NaCl + KCl) in 4 L of water (just over 1 gallon) provides a solution with the following composition: Na 107 mEq/L, K 28 mEq/L, Cl 135 mEq/L.

*Eltrad 4000, Haver-Lockhart, Shawnee, KS

the other polyionic sodium-containing replacement fluids should be used. Responses to therapy include improvement in capillary refill time, pulse pressure, and jugular distensibility. The PCV and TPP concentrations will decline toward normal values, whereas sodium concentration is usually unaltered. There should be a marked improvement in attitude and appetite. Establishment of normal urine flow is also a good indicator of the adequacy of volume replacement. Once the horse begins to eat substantial quantities of good-quality hay, potassium deficits are readily replaced from this potassium-rich source. The principal objective of fluid therapy in these horses is the partial restoration of homeostasis so that the horse recovers sufficiently to replenish the remaining accumulated deficits by voluntary consumption.

PRECAUTIONS

Nonsteroidal anti-inflammatory agents are often used in exhausted horses for their analgesic, anti-inflammatory, and antipyretic effects. While these drugs do have beneficial actions, they also have the potential to produce toxicity when administered at high dosages to dehydrated, volume-depleted patients. Extra precaution should thus be taken to restore and maintain hydration if these drugs are to be used. The use of potent glucocorticoids in ex-

hausted horses is the subject of some controversy. The anti-inflammatory and metabolic effects should aid in the prevention of hypovolemic shock. However, an acute and severe laminitis may develop as a sequela to exhaustion and some veterinarians believe that exogenously administered corticosteroids play a causal role. Hypotensive drugs such as the phenothiazine-derived tranquilizers should not be given to volume-depleted patients as they may cause collapse and even death. If these drugs are to be considered in the therapeutic plan they should be employed only after rigorous fluid therapy has corrected the volume depletion.

Supplemental Readings

Carlson, G. P.: Thermoregulation and fluid balance in the exercising horse. *In* Snow, D. H., Persson, S. G. B., and Rose, R. J. (eds.): Equine Exercise Physiology. Cambridge, Granta Editions, 1983, p. 291.

Carlson, G. P.: Medical management of the exhausted horse. *In* Robinson, N. E. (ed.): Current Therapy in Equine Medicine. Philadelphia, W. B. Saunders Company, 1983, p. 318.

Fowler, M. E.: Veterinary problems during endurance trail rides. J. South Afr. Vet. Assoc., *51*:87, 1980.

Rose, R. J., Atkins, J. E., and Martin, I. C. A.: Blood gas, acid-base, and haematological values in horses during an endurance ride. Equine Vet. J., *11*:56, 1979,

Snow, D. H., Kerr, M. G., Nimmo, M. A., and Abbott, E. M.: Alterations in blood, sweat, urine and muscle composition during prolonged exercise in the horse. Vet. Rec., *110*:377, 1982.

Synchronous Diaphragmatic Flutter

Gary P. Carlson, DAVIS, CALIFORNIA

Synchronous diaphragmatic flutter (SDF) is a condition seen most frequently in endurance horses performing in hot climates. It has also been reported in horses with transit tetany and lactation tetany, and in association with electrolyte imbalances due to digestive disturbances. Some horses may develop SDF after a race following administration of furosemide as a prerace medication for exercise-induced pulmonary hemorrhage. Synchronous diaphragmatic flutter has been iatrogenically and experimentally produced by massive administration of oral sodium bicarbonate to volume-depleted and chloride-depleted horses. Trauma is also reported to cause SDF. It is possible that some horses with chronic recurring SDF may have an anatomic alteration of the phrenic nerve or its myelin sheath that predisposes them to recurring problems.

CLINICAL SIGNS

Synchronous diaphragmatic flutter is the result of a contraction of the diaphragm that is synchronous with the heartbeat. It is apparent as a twitch or contraction in the flank, which may be right-sided, left-sided, or bilateral. The twitch is not related to normal respiratory movements and may become sufficiently violent to produce an audible thumping sound, hence the descriptive word "thumps." Placement of one hand over the flank while auscultating the heart with a stethoscope will demonstrate that contraction is indeed synchronous with the heartbeat. In the horse, SDF is associated with atrial depolarization, while in humans and dogs the diaphragmatic contraction is synchronous with ventricular depolarization. It is thought that acid-base and electrolyte imbalances may alter the membrane potential of the phrenic nerve, allowing it to discharge in response to the electrical impulse generated during myocardial depolarization. Synchronous diaphragmatic flutter is often placed in the same category as the exhaustive disease syndrome. Indeed, many exhausted endurance horses will have SDF along with signs of dehydration and volume depletion. Other horses develop SDF with little other indication of exhaustion. Synchronous diaphragmatic flutter by itself is probably not dangerous. In most cases, however, it is an index of significant electrolyte imbalance and as such is generally considered grounds for removal of the horse from endurance competition. Some horses that repeatedly develop SDF without exhaustion are reported to complete rides without developing complications if allowed to continue. At present there are no data that would allow veterinarians to separate these few horses from others in which SDF may be an early sign of impending disaster.

THERAPY

The most characteristic pattern of electrolyte alteration associated with SDF is a hypochloremic metabolic alkalosis with hypocalcemia, hypokalemia, and hypomagnesemia. The condition is generally transient provided that the underlying electrolyte and acid-base alterations are resolved. Unless the signs are severe or persistent, specific therapy may not be required if the horse begins to eat and drink normally. Intravenous calcium results in a prompt cessation of clinical signs. Calcium should be administered slowly to effect with careful monitoring of heart rate and rhythm. Ordinarily 100 to 300 ml of 20 per cent calcium borogluconate is required. The products that contain calcium, magnesium, phosphate, and glucose used to treat milk fever and grass tetany are also widely utilized. If these preparations are diluted 1:4 with saline or dextrose the fluid can be administered more rapidly with reduced chances of inducing cardiac arrest. Response is evident by relaxation and increased alertness of the patient as well as return of gastrointestinal motility and cessation of the SDF.

PREVENTION

Electrolyte supplementation during endurance rides may help some horses with recurrent SDF. Of particular importance is the provision of chloride and potassium along with sodium. These salts will help to prevent volume depletion and the metabolic alkalosis associated with SDF. Some horses may benefit from supplemental calcium and magnesium given during the ride. It is believed by some endurance riders and veterinarians that horses fed diets high in calcium, such as alfalfa hay, are more frequently affected by SDF. This theory is similar to one involving cows with milk fever in which diets high in calcium lead to dependence on the rapid absorption of dietary sources for maintenance of serum calcium concentration. When increased demand is placed on the system (by lactation in cows or sweat loss in horses), stress-associated release of adrenal hormones suppresses calcium mobilization from bone stores and, additionally, diminished intake or inappetence contribute to the development of hypocalcemia. These theories have led to the recommendation that horses with recurrent SDF be fed a diet relatively low in calcium just before a major endurance event. The objective of this dietary maneuver is to stimulate the normal homeostatic mechanisms to initiate mobilization of calcium reserves. It is to be hoped that these horses will be less dependent on immediate dietary sources for maintenance of serum calcium concentrations. A combination of electrolyte and acid-base alterations is associated with this disorder. The developing metabolic alkalosis may alter the ratio of free and protein-bound calcium. Since only the free form is biologically active, the acid-base alteration may be of major importance in the development of SDF.

Supplemental Readings

Baird, J. D.: Lactation tetany (eclampsia) in a Shetland pony mare. Aust. Vet. J., 47:402, 1971.

Hinton, M., Yeats, J. J., Hastie, P. S., McGuiness, A., and Constance, L.: Synchronous diaphragmatic flutter in horses. Vet. Rec., 99:402, 1976.

Hutyra, F., Marek, J.: Special Pathology and Therapeutics of the Diseases of Domestic Animals. Chicago, Alexander Eger, 864, 1920.

Mansmann, R. A., Carlson, G. P., White, N. A., and Milne, D. W.: Synchronous diaphragmatic flutter in horses. J. Am. Vet. Med. Assoc., 165:265, 1974.

White, N. A., and Rhode, E. A.: Correlation of electrocardiographic findings to clinical disease in the horse. J. Am. Vet. Assoc., 164:46, 1974.

Exertional Rhabdomyolysis

David R. Hodgson, PULLMAN, WASHINGTON

Exertional rhabdomyolysis, also known as azoturia, "Monday morning disease," "tying up," paralytic myoglobinuria, and myositis, occurs as the result of a number of predisposing factors that may act individually or in combinations. Some of these are:

Diet/Exercise. Classically the disease is observed in horses undergoing training that are rested for one or more days while being maintained on full rations. When returned to exercise, these animals frequently suffer the myopathy.

Training Status. Sudden elevations in the duration and/or intensity or both of the training stimulus may be accompanied by rhabdomyolysis. In addition, exertional myopathies are commonly observed in animals, particularly endurance horses, that are inadequately trained for competition.

Endocrine Factors. Fillies and mares, especially those that are nervous or "high strung," are reported to be more commonly affected than colts, possibly suggesting some endocrine influence in the disease. Decreased thyroid function has also been implicated as a predisposing factor.

Genetic Factors. When compared with the equine population as a whole, certain breed lines or families of horses are reputed to suffer from a higher incidence of the disease. Given the large number of potential predisposing factors, strictly controlled longitudinal studies are required to further investigate these claims.

Previous History. Once affected, it is not uncommon for horses to suffer repeated episodes of the myopathy.

Other Factors. This group includes factors that alter the blood supply of working muscle, derangements in fluid and electrolyte balance, and a number of other unidentified or poorly understood factors.

CLINICAL SIGNS

The clinical signs vary considerably, a factor that may make diagnosis difficult. By definition exertional rhabdomyolysis involves muscular degeneration. Many of the signs associated with this disease are a direct reflection of the degree of muscle pathology occurring in the animal. A mild condition frequently observed in endurance horses, particularly when the ambient temperature is high and the animals are dehydrated, produces transient mild to moderate gait abnormalities and may be associated with little if any detectable muscle pathology. The most commonly observed clinical manifestations of the disease include stiff or stilted gait. Hindlimb and back muscles are most commonly affected, and severely affected animals may suffer marked muscle dysfunction and cramping resulting in reluctance or inability to move. In extreme cases, animals may become recumbent and incapable of rising.

Affected horses are often anxious; they sweat and have elevated heart and respiratory rates and increased body temperature. Pain may be associated with deep palpation of the back and hindlimb muscles. Attempts to move affected animals may result in extreme pain, obvious anxiety, and possible exacerbation of the condition.

Differential diagnosis of exertional rhabdomyolysis should include colic, laminitis (p. 277), lactation tetany (p. 189), pleuritis (p. 592), tetanus (p. 370), aortic-iliac thrombosis (p. 175), and other primary musculoskeletal disorders. Exertional myopathy may occur concurrently with other disease processes in some horses—for example, in the poorly understood post-exhaustion myopathy laminitis syndrome.

LABORATORY FINDINGS

Laboratory data provide a useful guide to the extent of the metabolic disturbances and muscular damage in affected animals. When muscle tissue is damaged, there is leakage of cellular constituents into the surrounding tissues and subsequently into the circulation. By measuring the levels of specific enzymes within the serum, assessments of the degree of myodegeneration are possible. Creatine kinase (CK) is the most sensitive and specific indicator of muscle pathology in the horse, rising rapidly to a peak within six hours at levels from 1000 to greater than 400,000 IU per L and declining within two to three days. Aspartate aminotransferase (AST) rises more slowly, peaking within 24 hours, at levels greater than 1000 IU per L, and declines within 7 to 14 days. Aspartate aminotransferase may also be elevated in response to hepatocellular or red blood cell damage. Lactate dehydrogenase (LDH) is found in many tissues and must be electrophoretically separated into its isoenzyme fractions before definitive evidence of myodegeneration can be obtained. In cardiac muscle LDH_1 and LDH_2 predominate, whereas high levels of LDH_4 and LDH_5 are found in skeletal muscle. Lactate dehydrogenase tends to peak within 12 hours of cellular breakdown and to remain elevated for up to 7 to 10 days.

Horses suffering from exertional rhabdomyolysis often experience concurrent alterations in fluid and electrolyte balance. Dehydration, hypochloremia, and hypocalcemia have all been reported. Estimations of the degree of hemoconcentration and dehydration are possible by the determination of packed cell volume (PCV) and total plasma protein. However, it must be remembered that alterations in the whole body status of certain electrolytes, specifically potassium, are poorly reflected by measurement of their plasma concentrations.

Pigmenturia resulting from renal myoglobin excretion is a common finding in horses with exertional rhabdomyolysis. Although specific identification of myoglobin in urine is a complex procedure, urinalysis test strips* designed to detect the presence of hemoglobin will also yield a positive reaction to myoglobin. From a practical point of view, a positive urine strip test for heme pigments, an elevated plasma CK level, and appropriate clinical signs are sufficient to diagnose exertional rhabdomyolysis.

The results of muscle biopsies may produce useful information. Collection of samples is relatively uncomplicated and many histopathology laboratories are able to process the fixed tissues. Biopsy samples should be obtained from affected muscles and, if possible, from another muscle showing no evidence of disease. Muscle samples may be collected using either surgical (open) or needle (percutaneous) biopsy techniques. After collection the samples should be fixed in 10 per cent formalin prior to routine histopathologic examination. In the first 24 hours after the onset of signs, demonstrable pathologic changes may include diffuse interstitial edema, fiber degeneration with altered fibers often displaying segmental derangement, and the accumulation of mononuclear cells in the endomysium.

PATHOPHYSIOLOGY

The pathophysiology of this disease remains relatively obscure. It is most likely that a variety of factors produce the muscle dysfunction associated with exertional rhabdomyolysis. Originally the condition was thought to be the result of increased muscle lactate production as the disease occurred following exercise in draft horses fed large amounts of molasses. However, this hypothesis is not supported by more recent studies involving Standardbred horses. Elevated muscle lactate levels were found in only 4 to 12 horses suffering acute exacerbations of the disease. In addition, most horses afflicted with exertional myopathies do not have metabolic acidosis, and if an alteration in acid-

base balance exists, it is most commonly a mild metabolic alkalosis. There does appear to be a correlation between intake of grain, breaks in the exercise routine, and the incidence of exertional rhabdomyolysis. Horses fed diets containing large amounts of grain, and given one or more days rest while being maintained on full rations, have an increased incidence of this myopathy when subsequently returned to normal training.

Alterations in the blood supply to the muscles of locomotion may be important in the pathogenesis of this disease. Light microscopic studies indicate that fast-twitch muscle fibers undergo the most severe pathologic changes, with the slow-twitch fibers often being spared. Fast-twitch muscle fibers are usually much larger and have fewer capillaries surrounding them than slow-twitch fibers. This has led to the suggestion that a local hypoxia occurs in the fast-twitch fibers during exercise, resulting in the pathologic changes observed within these fibers.

Although associations have not been clearly demonstrated in the horse, it is likely that alterations in fluid and electrolyte balance as a result of exercise, training, diet, climate, or other management factors may influence local blood supply, which could result in exertional rhabdomyolysis. This may also explain why fast-twitch fibers are predominantly affected in this disease as they would possibly be more susceptible to ischemic damage if reductions in local blood flow were to occur.

Horses undergoing the stress of training and racing can be subjected to periods of suppressed thyroid function. Some of these animals experience exercise-related episodes of muscular pain and stiffness, which produce only moderate elevations in the plasma concentrations of muscle enzymes, leading to the suggestion that the myopathy is related to hypothyroidism. Despite this, considerable debate still exists as to whether hypothyroidism is a legitimate concern when considering the pathogenesis of exertional myopathies in horses.

Other factors implicated in the etiology of exertional rhabdomyolysis include selenium and/or vitamin E deficiency, excitement, influenza virus, endocrine factors, and a number of other poorly defined disease complexes. Clearly, no single cause for exertional rhabdomyolysis can be identified, and a combination of causes should be considered.

TREATMENT

The aims of treatment are to limit further muscle damage, restore fluid and electrolyte balance in order to decrease the chances of renal impairment, and reduce pain. Following the onset of exertional rhabdomyolysis, further exercise is contraindicated, although not all investigators agree with this dictum.

---

*Multistix, Ames Company, Elkhart, IN

In some horses further movement, even walking, can markedly exacerbate the muscle damage. Such animals should be kept quiet and given access to water until specific treatment is available. Horses suffering from relatively uncomplicated muscle spasms and cramps, and in which little if any muscle damage has occurred, often demonstrate marked improvement in response to light exercise such as walking. Obviously, astute clinical judgment is necessary to differentiate between the relatively benign and transient condition of muscle spasm and cramping and the potentially devastating syndrome of exertional rhabdomyolysis. If any doubt exists, cessation of exercise should be encouraged.

Nonsteroidal anti-inflammatory agents are indicated and give good symptomatic relief. Phenylbutazone,* flunixin meglumine,† and meclofenamic acid,‡ given at relatively high-dose rates, all yield good results. Severely affected, recumbent animals may require more potent analgesics such as meperidine hydrochloride,§ butorphanol ‖ or the other narcotic derivatives to aid in the relief of pain and anxiety. Unfortunately, these agents have only a relatively short duration of action. Tranquilizers such as acetylpromazine¶ and the other phenothiazine derivatives have been recommended to aid in the relief of anxiety and may improve peripheral blood flow by creating alpha-adrenergic blockade. If these agents are to be employed, it is *imperative* that the animal's circulatory status be adequate, as the peripheral redistribution of blood flow may have catastrophic effects in an animal already suffering from circulatory compromise. Small doses of xylazine** or diazepam†† may be more desirable in such cases.

Corticosteroids may be indicated in cases of exertional rhabdomyolysis as these agents are reported to produce relaxation of capillary sphincters and should theoretically improve tissue perfusion. In addition, they may aid in reducing continued muscle damage by stabilizing cellular membranes. If steroids are to be used, they are probably only beneficial during the first few hours of illness.

Dantrolene sodium,‡‡ at a dose rate of 2 mg per kg, diluted in normal saline and given via stomach tube, is recommended for the treatment and prophylaxis of this disease. This agent has been successfully employed in the prevention of stress-related myopathies in humans and pigs and may prevent progression of muscle damage in acute cases of exertional rhabdomyolysis.

Recently, the muscle relaxant methocarbamol,* 15 to 25 mg per kg by slow intravenous injection, has been used in cases of exertional rhabdomyolysis. This agent has central nervous system activity and is believed to reduce pain by relieving muscle spasm. If necessary, the dose can be repeated up to four times per day. Following administration some horses may become ataxic and depressed. In my experience methocarbamol has limited efficacy.

If laboratory facilities are available, assessment of fluid and electrolyte imbalances can be made and plans for replacement therapy initiated. In the absence of such facilities, when horses are showing obvious clinical evidence of exertional rhabdomyolysis, hemoconcentration, and/or myoglobinuria, the first priority is to re-establish fluid balance and induction of diuresis. Affected animals are usually alkalotic, making bicarbonate therapy inappropriate. Therefore, balanced electrolyte solutions† or the balanced electrolyte concentrates,‡ diluted with sterile water, are most desirable, although in many cases Ringer's§ or lactated Ringer's solution‖ may be suitable. In addition, fluids may be administered orally, as this provides a convenient and physiologic route for the rehydration of the animal. Because myoglobin is nephrotoxic in the dehydrated animal, fluid therapy should be maintained until urine is clear.

If laboratory facilities are available, reassessment of the PCV, total plasma protein, and serum electrolytes after the initial period of therapy should provide a guide as to the effectiveness of the therapeutic regimen. In severely affected animals, regular monitoring of BUN or serum creatinine or both is advised to assess the extent of renal damage. Although diuretics have been suggested as useful in the treatment of this condition, they are *contraindicated*. If diuresis is required, the safest method of induction is by fluid therapy.

Severely affected recumbent animals require good bedding, warmth, and adequate nursing care. Forcing these animals to stand may only exacerbate the myopathy. However, if the animals are given adequate fluids, food, pain relief, and judicious assistance in standing, results may be favorable when they are sufficiently strong.

PROPHYLAXIS

Dietary management is vitally important in the prevention of exertional rhabdomyolysis. It is desir-

---

*Butazolidin, Coopers Animal Health Inc., Kansas City, MO
†Banamine, Schering Corp., Kenilworth, NJ
‡Arquel, Parke-Davis, Morris Plains, NJ
§Demerol, Winthrop-Breon Laboratories, New York, NY
‖Stadol, Bristol Laboratories, Syracuse, NY
¶Acepromazine, Ayerst Laboratories, New York, NY
**Rompun, Haver-Lockhart, Shawnee, KS
††Valium, Roche Laboratories, Nutley, NJ
‡‡Dantrium, Norwich-Eaton, Pharmaceuticals, Norwich, NY

---

*Robaxin, A. H. Robins Co., Richmond, VA
†Normosol R, Abbott Laboratories, North Chicago, IL
‡Eltrad 4000, Haver-Lockhart, Shawnee, KS
§Ringer's Injection, Travenol Laboratories Inc., Deerfield, IL
‖Lactated Ringer's Injection, Travenol Laboratories Inc., Deerfield, IL

able to establish a well-balanced feeding program that meets, but does not exceed, the horse's nutritional requirements. Obviously if the horse's daily exercise routine varies, its dietary intake should also vary. Unfortunately, what may be suitable in the prevention of exertional rhabdomyolysis in one horse may not prove successful in another. However, attempts to maintain adequate dietary control and regular exercise programs should always be encouraged.

Dantrolene sodium has been evaluated for the prophylaxis and treatment of exertional rhabdomyolysis. Recommended dose rates are 2 mg per kg per os once a day for three to five days, followed by 2 mg per kg every third day for a month. Although some practitioners have maintained horses on this treatment regimen for several months with no apparent untoward effects, the drug may be hepatototoxic and its use is questionable.

Vitamin E and selenium* have long been used in attempts to prevent exertional rhabdomyolysis. Although no scientific evidence exists to support the efficacy of this treatment, there are some reports suggesting that therapy helps to prevent recurrence. The diets of susceptible horses should be supplemented at up to five times the currently recommended 0.1 ppm of selenium.

In hot, humid climates, in which horses may be prone to excessive sweating, supplementation of feed with 30 to 60 grams per day of potassium chloride is reportedly beneficial. If hypothyroidism is suspected, thyroid function tests and supplementation are indicated (see p. 185). Horses with hypothyroidism often have improved exercise tolerance when given levo-thyroxine sodium† at a dose of 0.01 mg per kg per os once a day or iodinated casein* 6 to 14 mg per kg per os once a day.

In anxious performance horses prone to repeated episodes of exertional myopathy, small doses of phenothiazine tranquilizers such as acetylpromazine at a dose rate of approximately 0.01 mg per kg, administered about 30 minutes before exercise, have been suggested to decrease the incidence of the condition. These small doses are reputed to afford a protective effect against the myopathy without associated decrements in performance. Phenothiazine derivatives are prohibited by most racing authorities.

Recently, anecdotal reports have suggested that dimethylglycine (DMG)† at a dose rate of 1 mg per kg in the diet reduces the incidence of rhabdomyolysis. This agent is present in many foods and is reputed to increase oxygen utilization and decrease blood lactate levels during high-intensity exercise. If DMG does reduce the incidence in exertional myopathies, the mechanism by which it creates this effect is unclear.

*Protomome, Agri Tech, Kansas City, MO
†Vetri-cine, Sports and Stress Nutrition, Inc., Spearman, TX

*E-S, Burns-Biotech, Omaha, NB
†Thyro-Tabs, Vet-A-Mix Inc., Shenandoah, IA

Supplemental Readings

Lindholm, A., Johnasson, H., and Kjaersgaard, P.: Acute rhabdomyolysis ("tying up") in Standardbred horses. Acta Vet. Scand., *14*:325, 1974.
Koterba, A., and Carlson, G. P.: Acid-base and electrolyte alterations in horses with exertional rhabdomyolysis. J. Am. Vet. Med. Assoc., *180*:303, 1983.
Sjogaard, G., Adams, R. P., and Saltin, B.: Water and ion shifts in skeletal muscle of humans with intense dynamic knee extension. Am. J. Physiol., *248*:R190, 1985.
Waldron-Mease, E.: Hypothyroidism and myopathy in racing Thoroughbreds and Standardbreds. J. Equine Med. Surg., *3*:124, 1979.

Photoperiod and Artificial Lighting

Dan C. Sharp, GAINESVILLE, FLORIDA

Environmental photoperiod is the main driving force for seasonal estrous activity in mares. No other environmental factor (temperature, humidity, rainfall) is as consistent or predictable from one season, or year, to the next. The two objectives of an annual breeding season are to control the timing of parturition and to aid neonatal survival rather than mating. Therefore, mechanisms for seasonal control must be capable of predicting environmental conditions at least a gestation length into the future. Annual changes in photoperiod provide that predictive reliability.

After winter anestrus, mares enter the breeding season with remarkable precision. Despite marked yearly differences in temperature, rainfall, and forage growth, there is relatively little variation in the date of first ovulation (diagnosed by serial ovarian palpation, per rectum) in mares. In a seven-year study, the mean date of first ovulation in Thoroughbred and Quarterhorse mares was April 1st (day 91 ± 16) and in pony mares was May 6th (day 127 ± 21).

The fact that the onset of the breeding season can be manipulated by altering the photoperiod or the way the brain interprets it suggests that photoperiod is the primary regulatory factor. Burkhardt first exposed anestrous mares to artificially length-ened days beginning on January 1st and significantly advanced the onset of the breeding season. He increased day length at twice the natural rate, so that by March 22nd (spring equinox) day length was equivalent to the longest day (June 21st). Mares started estrous cycling in March as opposed to April for control mares. Since these first experiments, many different artificial lighting regimens have been used with apparent success.

LIGHT INTENSITY AND WAVELENGTH

Light intensity and wavelength are not critical as long as certain minimal criteria are met. As the eye is the primary photoreceptor, the light source must satisfy the principles of visual physiology. Rhodopsin, the main photoactive chemical of the retinal rods, is activated optimally by light with a wavelength of 550 nm (yellow-green); fortunately this range extends to between 450 and 650 nm (blue-green and orange-yellow) so that most commercially available lightbulbs produce satisfactory wavelengths. Fluorescent bulbs emit light energy from blue to orange, with varying maxima, and incandescent bulbs emit light energy from blue-green to infrared. The light intensity threshold is as yet

491

unknown, but satisfactory results have been obtained with as little as 10 to 12 foot-candles. Thus, in practical terms, one 200-watt incandescent bulb per 12 by 12-foot stable is recommended.

A simple method of testing the intensity of light in a stable is to use a 35-mm camera with a through-the-lens light meter. With the film speed setting at ASA 400 and the shutter speed setting at 0.25 seconds, a clean, plain white Styrofoam cup is placed over the lens. This simple device acts as a diffuser and averages the light from all the point sources in the stable. The meter is turned on and the aperture setting is viewed through the viewfinder, with the camera held level at about the height of a horse's eye. Readings should be taken at different areas in the stable. Aperture readings of greater than f4 indicate a light intensity of more than 10 to 12 foot-candles, which is an adequate level of artificial lighting to induce early estrous cyclical activity.

The timing of artificial lighting regimens is important, particularly the time they are begun. The true (ovulatory) season is preceded by a prolonged transitional phase, on the average lasting approximately 40 days in horse mares and approximately 60 days in pony mares. This produces a considerable lag period before cyclic estrus; for mares to ovulate in February, lighting adjustments should begin in mid-November to early December.

DURATION OF LIGHTING

The duration of lighting through the day is also important. Horses, as most other animals do, have a "biological clock." Exposure to 14 to 16 hours of daylight "sets" the clock to long-day or summertime activity. For unknown reasons, there appear to be times of light sensitivity and insensitivity during the day, however. Anestrus mares can be stimulated to cycle earlier by adding 2.5 hours of artificial light after sunset but not before sunrise. A single one-hour pulse of artificial light given 9 to 10 hours after natural sunset has been shown to produce early cyclical estrus in mares. Caution must be used in the interpretation of night interruption studies, as mares are then exposed to two periods of light and two of darkness within 24 hours and it becomes impossible to say which light period is interpreted as sunrise.

Nevertheless, both extension of the day at sunset

and interruption of the night appear to produce effects that have practical applications. Extension of the day is particularly suited to paddock lighting. Mares are put into the paddock at the end of the working day and lights-on can be controlled by a photo-cell or an electric timer. After two and a half hours, the lights can be automatically turned off and the gates automatically opened to allow the mares to return to pasture.

Although the precise mechanisms controlling light-stimulated early sexual recrudescence are not fully understood, it is now clear that the pineal gland is a mediator. Pinealectomy abolishes the stimulatory effects of additional artificial light. Melatonin, a pineal hormone secreted during darkness, may transmit information about the photoperiod to the brain. Melatonin secretion begins at sunset; therefore, two and a half hours of artificial light, administered at that time, delays the timing of melatonin secretion. The exogenous administration of melatonin during artificial light administration abolishes the light's stimulatory effect; this suggests that light stimulates by delaying melatonin secretion. This interesting concept deserves further research.

There is still much to be learned about the seasonal breeding cycle of mares. However, artificial light regimens are being used to stimulate early sexual recrudescence with a high degree of success and practical advantage.

Supplemental Readings

Burkhardt, J.: Transition from anestrus in the mare and the effects of artificial lighting. J. Agric. Sci. (Camb.), 37:64, 1947.

Cooper, W. L., and Wert, N. E.: Wintertime breeding of mares using artificial light and insemination: Six years experience. Proc. 21st Annu. Conv. Am. Assoc. Eq. Pract., 1973, pp. 245–253.

Kooistra, L. H., and Ginther, O. J.: Effects of photoperiod on reproductive activity and hair in mares. Am. J. Vet. Res., 36:1413, 1975.

Loy, R. G.: Effects of artificial lighting regimens on reproductive patterns in mares. Proc. 14th Annu. Conv. Am. Assoc. Eq. Pract., 1968, pp. 159–167.

Palmer, E., and Driancourt, M. A.: Photoperiodic stimulation of the winter anestrus mare: What is a long day? Photoperiodism and Reproduction. International Colloquium, Nouzilly, France, 1981.

Sharp, D. C., and Ginther, O. J.: Stimulation of follicular activity and estrous behaviour in anestrus mares with light and temperature. J. Anim. Sci., 41:1368, 1975.

Sharp, D. C.: Environmental influences on reproduction in horses. Vet. Clin. North Am. (Large Anim. Pract.), 2:207, 1980.

Exogenous Control of the Breeding Season

Peter D. Rossdale, NEWMARKET, ENGLAND

The horse is a seasonally polyestrous species. Evolution has produced an endocrine system with an inherent rhythm and a fertile breeding season during the late spring and summer. Typically, following winter anestrus, mares undergo a transitional period of erratic or subdued cyclical activity before the fertile, regularly cyclic true breeding season starts. This transitional period is highly variable between individuals in character and length. It is a period that happens to coincide with the start of the arbitrarily imposed breeding season, and is thus the source of frustration among mare owners who wish their mares to become pregnant at an early stage for commercial advantage. Veterinarians are encouraged therefore to attempt exogenous control of the mare's reproductive functions to stimulate fertile estrus during February, March, and early April in the northern hemisphere and August and September in the southern hemisphere.

Over recent years, people have selected mares to suit the pattern of their own requirements. Thus, within a population of any breed, individuals may have changed their inherent reproductive pattern and undergone fertile estrous cycles early in the year, even throughout the winter. These mares need no exogenous help unless their cyclical activity becomes suppressed during the arbitrary or natural breeding season.

BASIC CONSIDERATIONS

The control of the breeding season is fraught with the difficulties inherent in the control of biological mechanisms in general. All forms of veterinary treatment should be given on the basis of specific diagnoses; however, with current techniques we cannot accurately assess the exact physiologic status of an individual.

The most commonly used but frequently imprecise aids in determining whether a mare is in estrus are teasing, vaginal examination, palpation of ovaries, and measurement of hormone levels. Teasing assesses the mare's behavioral receptivity to a male horse. In some individuals, especially in an unfamiliar environment, atypical teasing behavior or the unfamiliarity of personnel responsible may result in an inaccurate interpretation of reproductive status. Unfamiliar environments and new personnel are frequently encountered by Thoroughbred mares, which are usually bred at a different stud farm each year. Vaginal examinations are used to assess the state of relaxation, moisture, and color of the cervix. During the transitional phase, appearances are frequently misleading. Rectal palpation of ovaries is used to assess ovarian size and follicular activity. Serial examinations are required to give a functional assessment, which is often retrospective. The use of ultrasound echography has demonstrated the potential inaccuracy of this traditional technique.

Plasma progestogen assays detect the presence or absence of a functional corpus luteum. The measurements do not reflect the activity of the hormone at its target site, the rate of synthesis by the endocrine gland, or the relationship with other hormones. The practical application of gonadotropin and estrogen assays has yet to become apparent.

By repeating the aforementioned examinations over a period of days or weeks a more reliable assessment of the reproductive status of an individual mare may be achieved. This is not always practical, however, because owners are anxious for immediate positive action. Veterinarians are therefore often pressed, against their better judgment, to embark upon the premature use of hormone therapy, which may fail or even be counterproductive.

TREATMENTS

The following methods are currently used to encourage the early onset of fertile estrous cycles.

Artificial Daylight. It has been recognized, since the pioneering days of John Burkhardt, that increasing daylight by artificial means causes transition from acyclic anestrus to cyclic estrus (see p. 491). If this method is used in December and January (in the southern hemisphere, July and August), some mares may be induced to cycle early in the arbitrary breeding season. Sixteen hours of daylight (100- to 200-watt bulbs, suspended within about four meters of the mare) to eight hours of darkness are recommended, starting six to eight weeks before the effect is required. Some management systems claim high success rates following the use of artificial lights, but more fundamental knowledge is required to explain those cases in which the system fails.

Gonadotropin-Releasing Hormone (GnRH). Gonadotropin-releasing hormone (0.04 mg. Buserelin*) has been used to stimulate cyclic estrus; however, the results have been poor as compared with those for artificial light programs. This may not be a reflection of the products available but may be a function of dosage and frequency of administration. Bolus doses are unphysiologic and may even cause suppression of gonadotropin release. Pulsatile doses or continuous infusions or both may be necessary. Pulsatile-release (e.g., timed doses as used in other species) or slow-release implants may give better results in the future.

Progestogens. Progesterone, or more recently progestogen (27.5 mg allyl trenbolone,† orally, daily for 10 consecutive days) prevents gonadotropin release. On removal of the block, the accumulated gonadotropins are released to initiate estrus cyclical activity (usually three to four days after cessation of treatment). Mares in the transitional phase rather than in deep anestrus, and those showing prolonged, nonprogressive "spring" estrus, are suitable for treatment. The use of estrogens and/or testosterone therapy with progestogens has been reported for the synchronization of fertile estrus (see p. 495).

Prostaglandins. Natural (e.g., 5 mg dinoprost‡) and synthetic (e.g., 250 to 500 μg cloprostenol§) prostaglandin $F_{2\alpha}$ is highly successful in inducing cyclical activity in mares that are acyclic because of persistent corpora lutea. Those mares with plasma progestogen levels greater than 1 ng per ml (most reliably greater than 4 ng per ml) and mature corpora lutea (greater than five days old) respond well to treatment.

Persistence of the corpus luteum reflects a cyclic variant rather than a true acyclic state. By maintaining high progesterone levels, this produces a somewhat similar effect to that of feeding allyl trenbolone. As the block has usually been in place for more than 10 days, the hypothalamic-pituitary-ovarian pathway is better primed and the response to removing the block by luteolysis is better.

MANAGEMENT REQUIREMENTS

Achievement of early cyclical activity should start with management. Mares showing estrus early in the breeding season should be given a good plane of nutrition. Light and warmth should be provided with controlled environments, with housing in well-insulated buildings and sheltered paddocks. Artificial light must be given well before the desired effect is required and continued until natural daylight reaches 16 hours.

---

*Receptal, American Hoechst Corp., Somerville, NJ
†Regumate, American Hoechst Corp., Somerville, NJ
‡Lutalyse, Upjohn Co., Kalamazoo, MI
§Estrumate, ICI Pharmaceuticals, Mississauga, Ontario

CONCLUSIONS

For induction of cyclic activity early in the breeding season, drug therapy should only be used as a last resort. At present, the following approach to exogenous control is recommended:

1. Start an artificial light program in December (July in southern hemisphere).
2. Tease all nonpregnant mares regularly from February 1st (August 1st in southern hemisphere).
3. Examine all mares that show no signs of receptivity for more than three weeks by vaginoscope, rectal palpation of ovaries, and plasma progestogen assay.
4. Treat those with signs of persistent corpora lutea (active ovaries, tight, pale, dry cervix, and plasma progestogen greater than 1.0 ng per ml) with prostaglandins.
5. Treat those in transitional phase (active ovaries, relaxed, pale, dry cervix, and plasma progestogen less than 1.0 ng per ml) and those in prolonged estrus with oral allyl trenbolone.
6. Treat those in deep winter anestrus (inactive ovaries, relaxed, pale, dry cervix, and plasma progestogen less than 1.0 ng per ml) with patience and, if satisfactory treatment protocols become available, GnRH.

The truth remains that the best solution to this problem would be to change the arbitrary breeding season to coincide with the natural breeding season, for those breeds in which asynchrony occurs. In the Thoroughbred this would be a reversion to the situation that applied before 1833, when the Jockey Club moved the registration date to January 1st for the convenience of the racing calendar. Before that date there was lack of uniformity, but May 1st was commonly used as the official birthdate.

Supplemental Readings

Allen, W. R., and Rossdale, P. D.: Preliminary studies upon the use of prostaglandins for inducing and synchronizing oestrus in Thoroughbred mares. Equine Vet. J., 5:137, 1973.

Allen, W. R., Urwin, V., Simpson, D. J., et al.: Preliminary studies on the use of oral progestagen to induce oestrus and ovulation in seasonally anoestrous Thoroughbred mares. Equine Vet. J. 12:141, 1980.

Evans, M. J., and Irvine, C. H. G.: Induction of follicular development and ovulation in seasonally acyclic mares using gonadotropin releasing hormones and progesterone. J. Reprod. Fert., Suppl. 27:113, 1979.

Irvine, C. H. G.: Pituitary hormones—basic aspects. J. Equine Vet. Sci., 3:203, 1979.

Palmer, E., Driancourt, M. A., and Ortavant, R.: Photoperiodic stimulation of the mare during winter anoestrus. J. Reprod. Fert., Suppl. 32:275, 1982.

Sharp, D. C., Grubaugh, W., Berglund, L. A., McDowell, K. J., Killmer, D. M., and Peck, L. S.: Effects of pinealectomy in pony mares. J. Reprod. Fert., Suppl. 32:297, 1982.

Webel, S. K., and Squires, E. L.: Control of the oestrus cycle in mares with altrenogest. J. Reprod. Fert., Suppl. 32:193, 1982.

Synchronization of Estrus

F. Bristol, SASKATOON, SASKATCHEWAN, CANADA

The objective of synchronization of estrus in mares is to reduce and concentrate the time spent on estrus detection and reduce the number of matings per mare. Detection of estrus in horses is time-consuming because of its variable length and the variable response of mares to the presence of the stallion. A great deal of time is spent teasing unreceptive mares that are in the diestrus phase, most stallions being reluctant to tease mares not showing obvious signs of estrus. While acceptable methods for estrous synchronization have been developed, synchronization of ovulation to allow a single breeding at a predetermined time has not been notably successful (see p. 499). Recently a combination of progesterone and estradiol-17β has been used to synchronize both estrus and ovulation in recipient and donor mares undergoing embryo transfer.

It is extremely important to thoroughly evaluate all stallions before they are used in a synchronization program to ascertain their capability to produce sufficient normal and progressively motile spermatozoa to repeatedly inseminate the allocated number of synchronized mares (see p. 557). A minimum of 100 million progressively motile sperm per insemination is required for normal fertility. Most stallions will produce an adequate number of spermatozoa for 15 to 20 mares when semen is collected every second day. Although the foaling period is not as concentrated as the breeding period because of the variation in gestation length, adequate personnel and facilities should be available for foaling.

Although artificial insemination has been used in most estrous synchronization programs, pasture breeding can also be successful. For the latter method, it is extremely important to use experienced stallions that not only have excellent semen quality but also good libido. Provided these criteria are met, pregnancy rates of 70 to 95 per cent have been reported when a stallion:mare ratio of 1:20–25 was used.

METHODS OF SYNCHRONIZATION

There are three methods for synchronizing estrus in normally cycling mares.

1. Use of two injections of prostaglandin.
2. Use of short-term progestogen treatment together with a single injection of prostaglandin at the end of progestogen therapy.
3. Use of short-term progesterone and estradiol-17β treatment, with or without prostaglandin.

Prostaglandin. Prostaglandin $F_{2\alpha}$ (5 mg dinoprost tromethamine)* and its analogues (3 mg alfaprostol,† 0.250 μg fluprostenol,‡ 2 mg prostalene§) are luteolytic in mares except during the five days immediately following ovulation. The synchronization of estrus in a large group of mares that may be at all stages of the estrous cycle will necessitate the use of two intramuscular injections given 14 to 18 days apart. The onset of estrus is then relatively well synchronized. Approximately 60 per cent of mares will begin estrus four days after the second injection and by six days about 90 per cent will have shown estrous behavior. On the other hand, ovulation is not well synchronized and can occur from 2 to 12 days after the second prostaglandin treatment. Mares can be artificially inseminated every second day during estrus or inseminated at predetermined times without estrus detection. With the latter method it is best to inseminate four times on alternate days beginning four days after the second prostaglandin injection.

Conception rates are normal when mares are bred during a synchronized estrus. When timed inseminations have been used, conception rates are somewhat lower if mares are not inseminated at least four times.

An intramuscular injection of between 1500 and 3300 IU human chorionic gonadotropin (hCG) can be used to hasten ovulation in normally cycling mares when administered on the first or second day of estrus. The prostaglandin regimen can be combined with hCG to try and decrease the variation in the interval from the second prostaglandin treatment to ovulation. A single injection of hCG can be given following the second prostaglandin treatment or it can be given after both the prostaglandin treatments. An example of such a treatment regimen is shown schematically in Figure 1. I have found that when hCG is used in a synchronization program during the middle of the natural breeding season (June), it has little effect on ovulation and the duration of estrus. However, it may be of more benefit when mares are synchronized early in the breeding season.

The use of two prostaglandin injections has the advantage that the mares must be handled only twice for treatment; however, adequate handling

---

*Lutalyse, Tuco Products Co., Orangeville, Ontario
†Alfavet, Hoffmann-La Roche Inc., Nutley, NJ
‡Equimate, ICI Pharmaceuticals, Mississauga, Ontario
§Synchrocept, Diamond Laboratories Inc., Des Moines, IA

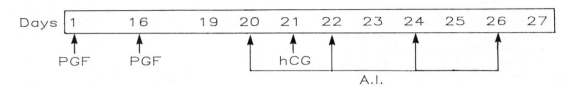

Figure 1. Procedure for synchronization of estrus in mares using PGF and hCG (PGF = Prostaglandin $F_{2\alpha}$ or an analogue; hCG = human chorionic gonadotropin).

facilities are required. All mares must have ovulated at least five days before the second prostaglandin treatment. Therefore, this method is best suited for use during the natural breeding season. Postpartum mares should have foaled at least 18 days before the second prostaglandin injection.

Progestagen and Prostaglandin. The progestagen altrenogest (allyl trenbolone)* can be used successfully to synchronize estrus in mares. It is administered orally at a rate of 0.044 mg per kg for 8 to 12 days using a dose syringe, or it can be incorporated into the grain ration. Experimentally it has been administered by means of vaginal sponges impregnated with 0.5 gm of altrenogest. This may provide a useful alternative to breeders who may have difficulty with oral administration. Because mares may develop follicles, ovulate, and form new corpora lutea during progesterone or progestagen treatment, it is necessary to give an injection of prostaglandin on the last day of altrenogest treatment to cause luteolysis of any corpora lutea that may be present (Fig. 2).

---

*Regumate, American Hoechst Corp., Somerville, NJ

Most mares will begin to show estrus two to five days after the last day of treatment. The distribution of ovulations is similar to that observed for prostaglandin synchronization, with the majority of mares ovulating between 8 and 15 days after withdrawal. Synchronization of ovulation can be improved by giving 2500 IU hCG intramuscularly to mares on the first or second day of estrus or at a fixed time five to seven days after altrenogest withdrawal. Fertility following this regimen is similar to that after the use of prostaglandin. A pregnancy rate of 71 per cent has been reported when mares are inseminated every second day during estrus; however, when they are inseminated at a predetermined time, the rate is lower.

Altrenogest is the drug of choice for synchronization of estrus in mares during the transitional phase or early part of the breeding season because it is particularly effective in those mares cycling irregularly, especially those having prolonged estrus. It can be easily administered by the owner but must be given daily for at least eight days. If the drug is mixed with the feed, each mare must receive the appropriate dose. Therefore, individual feeding facilities are required and each mare must consume

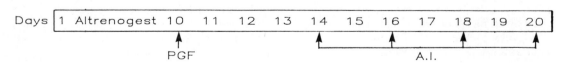

Figure 2. Procedure for synchronization of estrus in mares using altrenogest, prostaglandin $F_{2\alpha}$ (PGF), and human chorionic gonadotropin (hCG).

all of the medicated feed. If the drug is administered by dose syringe, adequate restraint, personnel, and facilities are required. The use of altrenogest-impregnated intravaginal sponges, if successful, will alleviate the problem of daily administration. Altrenogest has been used in combination with photoperiodic stimulation for estrous sychronization during the nonbreeding season or early part of the imposed breeding season (see p. 493). Mares require at least 60 days of photoperiodic stimulation (see p. 491) before progestagen therapy is begun to ensure that most will begin some cyclic activity. Again, this has the advantage of reducing the incidence of abnormally long estrus periods.

Progesterone and Estradiol-17β. A regimen consisting of 10 daily intramuscular injections of 150 mg progresterone and 10 mg estradiol-17β, combined with prostaglandin $F_{2\alpha}$ on the last day of treatment, is effective for synchronization of both estrus and ovulation in normally cycling mares. The prostaglandin treatment is necessary because some mares may ovulate shortly after the beginning of treatment and develop a corpus luteum without showing signs of estrus.

When this regimen is used during the natural breeding season, most mares show estrus five and seven days after withdrawal and ovulate between 10 and 12 days after the last day of treatment. At the present time this method appears to result in the best synchronization of ovulation. If used during the transitional phase of the breeding season there is greater variation from the end of treatment to the onset of estrus and ovulation.

POSTPARTUM MARES

Prostaglandins are not effective for synchronization of estrus in mares before 18 days postpartum because, although some mares ovulate as early as six days after parturition, the proportion of mares in a large group that will have a mature corpus luteum is not high enough to ensure good estrous synchronization. However, postpartum estrus can be delayed and then synchronized with a combination of steroids.

The method to be discussed is primarily used to synchronize estrus in a group of mares foaling in a relatively short span of time. Mares are given a varying number of daily injections of progesterone and estradiol-17β beginning on the day of parturition. It is important to give the first injection as soon after parturition as possible because some mares may develop follicles, ovulate, and form a corpus luteum during the course of treatment, which will delay the onset of estrus following withdrawal. Although the day on which treatment begins varies because the mares foal on different days, treatment for all mares is withdrawn on the same day and mares are given an injection of prostaglandin $F_{2\alpha}$ or its analogue (Fig. 3). Most mares will show estrus five to seven days and ovulate 9 to 14 days after the end of treatment. Fertility is similar to, or higher than, that of mares bred at first postpartum estrus.

Although the progesterone and estradiol-17β combination appears to be the best method of synchronizing both estrus and ovulation, daily injections are time-consuming. This method has the greatest potential for synchronization of estrus in recipient and donor mares for embryo transfer. At present several potential recipient mares must be prepared in order to ensure good synchronization of ovulation between donor and recipient. The method may also be useful for delaying and scheduling estrus in some mares when stallions have a particularly busy breeding schedule.

CONCLUSIONS

Synchronization of estrus in mares is not as successful when used early during the imposed breeding season as when used during the natural breeding season when most mares are showing normal estrous cycles. Because many mares are mated during the early months of the year, the use of estrous synchronization will be limited. It will primarily be restricted to those breeds allowing artificial insemination. Although it has been used successfully with

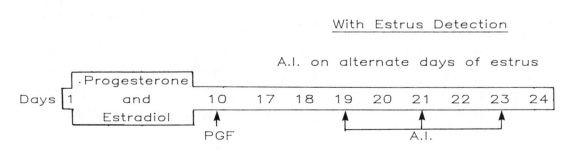

Figure 3. Procedure for synchronization of estrus in mares using progesterone, estradiol-17β, and prostaglandin $F_{2\alpha}$ (PGF).

natural breeding at pasture, it is doubtful that it could be usefully applied in situations in which hand breeding is used.

Although all methods are satisfactory for synchronizing estrus in mares, only the progesterone and estradiol-17β combination, when used during the natural breeding season, will result in adequate synchronization of ovulation.

Supplemental Readings

Bristol, F.: Studies on estrus synchronization in mares. Proc. Ann. Mtg. Soc. Therio., 1981, pp. 258–264.

Bristol, F., Jacobs, K. A., and Pawlyshyn, V.: Synchronization of estrus in postpartum mares with progesterone and estradiol 17B. Theriogenology, 19:779, 1983.

Hyland, J. H., and Bristol, F.: Synchronization of estrus and timed insemination of mares. J. Reprod. Fert., Suppl. 27:251, 1979.

Loy, R. G., Pemstein, R., O'Canna, D., and Douglas, R. H.: Control of ovulation in cycling mares with ovarian steroids and prostaglandin. Theriogenology, 15:191, 1981.

Palmer, E.: Different techniques for synchronization of ovulation in the mare. Proc. 8th Int. Congr. Anim. Reprod. & A. I., Krakow, 1976, pp. 495–498.

Palmer, E.: Reproductive management of mares without detection of estrus. J. Reprod. Fert., Suppl. 27:263, 1979.

Palmer, E., and Jousset, B.: Synchronization of estrus in mares with a prostaglandin analogue and hCG. J. Reprod. Fert., Suppl. 23:269, 1975.

Squires, E. L., Shideler, R. K., Voss, J. L., and Webel, S. K.: Clinical applications of progestins in mares. Comp. Cont. Ed., 5:S16, 1983.

Sullivan, J. J., Parker, W. G., and Larson, L. L.: Duration of estrus and ovulation time in nonlactating mares given human chorionic gonadotropin during three successive estrous periods. J. Am. Vet. Med. Assoc., 162:895, 1973.

Ovulation Management

Steven M. Hopkins, AMES, IOWA

Induction or synchronizaton of ovulation by the use of a variety of hormonal treatments is attempted in modern stud farm medicine. Induction, or "hastening," of ovulation reduces the number of matings or inseminations per estrus per mare, and helps to conserve a busy stallion's libido, semen quality, and energy. Ovulation induction may also be indicated in mares in which ovulation is persistently and unphysiologically delayed. Accurate synchronization of ovulation is essential in embryo transfer programs.

HORMONES USED

Hormone treatments involve either single injections or combinations of gonadotropins, ovarian steroids, or prostaglandins. The commercially available gonadotropins include purified luteinizing hormone (LH), human chorionic gonadotropin (hCG), and gonadotropin-releasing hormone (GnRH).

Because of price differential, GnRH (synthetic analogue buserelin*) is used more widely in Europe than in the United States. Experience suggests that

*Receptal, American Hoechst Corp., Somerville, NJ

GnRH is as effective as hCG in inducing ovulation in normally cycling mares and may not induce antibody production as readily. Gonadotropin-releasing hormone may induce ovulation more successfully in mares with larger and thicker-walled follicles.

Luteinizing hormone (extracted from pituitary glands of domestic animals) gives less consistent results than hCG (obtained from the urine of pregnant women). The latter is widely used and induces ovulation in the majority of normally cycling mares. Naturally occurring prostaglandin ($PGF_{2\alpha}$) and various analogs stimulate myometrial activity and luteolysis (if given when the corpus luteum is more than four days old). This effect is used, in combination with hCG, for estrus and ovulation synchronization. When ovarian steroids (progesterone and estradiol-17β) are used to suppress estrus and follicular development, hCG is then used for estrus and ovulation synchronization.

ROUTINE STUD FARM MEDICINE

Commercial stud farms aim to provide maximum fertility with the minimum number of matings or inseminations. This avoids stallion overuse, particularly in the early breeding season, and minimizes uterine contamination by penile and other environmental microorganisms, particularly in subfertile mares. For these reasons, ovulation induction is routine on some farms. The most consistent indications for ovulation induction are (1) when the mare repeatedly fails to ovulate within 48 hours of mating, and (2) when repeated follicular regression or excessive enlargement occurs. In general, follicles that are destined to regress do not respond to hCG, and there is clinical evidence to suggest that GnRH may more successfully induce ovulation in such follicles, and also in large, thick-walled follicles. GnRH (buserelin) is given at a dose rate of 0.04 mg intramuscularly six hours before mating. Human chorionic gonadotropin seems to induce ovulation more successfully during the ovulatory phase rather than during the transitional phase of the breeding season.

Human chorionic gonadotropin should be given during early estrus when there is one large dominant, palpable ovarian follicle having a diameter equal to, or greater than, 35 mm. This may be at the first mating, at the second (repeat breeding or "cross" cover), or alternatively hCG can be given routinely on the second day of estrus. Mares responding to hCG usually ovulate within 48 hours of treatment and there is no demonstrable difference in conception rates between those mares receiving hCG and those that do not. It may be preferable to treat mares less than six hours before mating. However, some stud farm managers are reluctant to allow this in case there is some unavoidable and unexpected delay and the mare is unwilling to accept the stallion.

Research evidence suggests that the optimal hCG dosage is 2000 to 3000 IU given intravenously, while dosages greater than 4500 IU may depress conception rates. If multidose vials are used, unused quantities must be refrigerated and used within 30 days to maintain potency.

Antibody production to the human globulin component of hCG has been demonstrated in mares following single or multiple treatments, and titers may persist for several months. There is no cross-reaction with endogenous LH. No evidence exists to suggest that the production of antibodies blocks or delays ovulation.

Although gonadotropin-releasing hormone is often used in an attempt to induce ovulation in transitional phase persistent follicles, the results are often unsuccessful because of insufficient quantities of stored endogenous LH. Human chorionic gonadotropin hormone may thus be more beneficial at this time. Some follicles appear unresponsive to hCG during the ovulatory season, perhaps because of an individual deficiency or immaturity of LH receptors. Repeated treatments are not indicated.

OVULATION SYNCHRONIZATION

A greater degree of accuracy can be achieved with estrous synchronization than with ovulation synchronization (see p. 495). Synchronization techniques are essential for embryo transfer and may be helpful for artificial insemination. Synchronized mares may have lower conception rates than non-synchronized mares.

The aim of synchronization is to induce ovulation in the recipient mare within 24 hours of the donor mare's ovulation. Two treatment regimens (Table 1) have been recommended for randomly cycling mares.

The two injections of hCG in Schedule B encourage more mares to ovulate by days 8 and 9. This increases the number of mares that have responsive corpora lutea at the time of the second prostaglandin injection.

A third treatment (Schedule C, Table 1), although more costly, has been recommended to more accurately induce ovulation in diestrous mares. Treatment begins between days 4 to 12 after ovulation.

The estradiol-17β causes regression of large follicles that could ovulate prematurely after the withdrawal of progesterone. The prostaglandin causes luteolysis of any persistent corpora lutea remaining from a previous estrus.

MULTIPLE OVULATIONS

Induction of ovulation may lead to an increased incidence of multiple ovulations. Nevertheless, evidence from ultrasound echography suggests that multiple ovulations are far more common than has been suspected by palpation alone. Also, a uterine mechanism exists that encourages the elimination of multiple conceptuses; therefore, this worry may be of little practical consequence. Evidence now clearly shows that avoidance of mating in the presence of palpable multiple ovarian follicles reduces

TABLE 1. TREATMENT REGIMENS FOR RANDOMLY CYCLING MARES

Schedule A	Schedule B
PGF$_{2\alpha}$ on day 0	PGF$_{2\alpha}$ on day 0
PGF$_{2\alpha}$ on day 15	hCG on day 6
hCG on day 20	PGF$_{2\alpha}$ on day 14
62% ovulate by day 22	hCG on day 20
	79% ovulate by day 24

Schedule C

150 mg progesterone + 10 mg estradiol-17β, daily for 10 days
PGF$_{2\alpha}$ on the 1st and 10th day
hCG 48-72 hours after the last progesterone + estradiol-17β treatment
   95% ovulate within 24 hours

the number of potential single pregnancies. If mares with multiple follicles are bred, facilities for the early detection of twin pregnancy by ultrasound echography should be available.

CONCLUSIONS

The success of ovulation induction depends less upon the hormone treatments used than upon other factors such as nutrition and housing, alterations in photoperiod (see p. 491), and the skill and experience of those responsible for detection of estrus and ovarian palpation. Suboptimal housing and nutrition may result in delays in transition from anestrus to cyclic estrus; it is in the latter situation that hormone treatments are most successful. Skill and experience with estrus detection and ovarian palpation become more important as the management system deviates from "normality," e.g. with estrus and ovulation synchronization for embryo transfer or artificial insemination. It must also be said that, under conditions of commercial stud farm medicine, it is difficult to prove that ovulations are being induced by hormone treatments, as it is impossible to prove that

follicles would not have spontaneously ovulated at a similar stage. Thus, the opinions of experienced clinicians still vary on the use of these techniques in normally cycling mares.

Supplemental Readings

Ginther, O. J., and Douglas, R. H.: The outcome of twin pregnancies in mares. Theriogenology, *18*:237, 1982.

Hyland,, J. H., and Bristol, F.: Synchronization of oestrus and timed insemination of mares. J. Reprod. Fert., Suppl. *27*:251, 1979.

Loy, R. G., and Hughes, J. P.: The effects of human chorionic gonadotropin on ovulation, length of estrus, and fertility in the mare. Cornell Vet., *56*:41, 1966.

Neely, D. P.: Hormone therapy in mares. *In* Neely, D. P., Liu, I. K. M., and Hillman, R. B. (eds.): Equine Reproduction, Veterinary Learning Systems Co. Inc., 1983.

Palmer, E., and Jousset, B.: Synchronization of oestrus in mares with a prostaglandin analogue and hCG. J. Reprod. Fert., Suppl. *23*:269, 1975.

Roser, J. F., Kiefer, B. L., Evans, J. W., Neely, D. P., and Pacheco, D. A.: The development of antibodies to human chorionic gonadotropin following its repeated injection in the cyclic mare. J. Reprod. Fert., Suppl. *27*:173, 1979.

Sanderson, M., and Allen, W. R.: Fertility statistics in mares. Equine Vet. J. (in press).

Ovarian Abnormalities

Irwin K. M. Liu, DAVIS, CALIFORNIA

Abnormalities of the ovary are relatively uncommon and may be classified as pathologic or functional abnormalities.

PATHOLOGIC ABNORMALITIES

NEOPLASIA

The most common neoplasms are the granulosa–theca cell tumor and the teratoma. Melanomas, epitheliomas, cystadenomas, dysgerminomas, hemangiomas, adenocarcinomas, arrhenoblastomas and hemoblastomas have also been reported. There is no obvious age or breed predilection and metastasis is rare. A presumptive diagnosis is based on palpation of a persistently large (6 to 40 cm in diameter), firm unilateral ovarian mass and ultrasound echograph (Fig. 1). In most tumors other than granulosa–theca cell tumors, the contralateral ovary remains functional and of normal size. A definitive diagnosis is made by gross and microscopic examinations following surgical removal of the ovary.

Arrhenoblastoma. In one case reported, testosterone levels were elevated, the mare showed stallionlike behavior, and the contralateral ovary was small, firm, and inactive.

Teratoma (Germ cell tumors). Teratomas contain misplaced embryonic structures such as bone, skin, teeth, cartilage, nerves, blood vessels, and hair.

Granulosa–Theca Cell Tumors (Stromal Tumors). Granulosa–theca cell tumors are composed predominantly of neoplastic granulosa cells, frequently with theca cell involvement. Clinical signs include nymphomaniac, anestrus, and stallionlike behavior. Abdominal discomfort, physical change with development of a heavy, crested neck and increased foreleg and chest musculature have been reported. Mares with stallionlike behavior may exhibit Flehmen reaction and may tease and mount estrous mares. This behavior may also occur in fillies that have received excessive doses of anabolic steroids, in those with testicular feminization (Tfm), and occasionally in mares during apparently normal pregnancy. In these cases, there is no palpably enlarged ovary. Stallionlike behavior during preg-

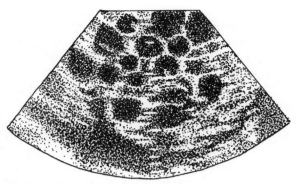

Figure 1. Granulosa theca cell–ovarian tumor. Diagram of the characteristic honeycomb appearance on ultrasound echography.

nancy usually occurs between approximately 40 and 120 days of gestation but may persist to term. In these mares, testosterone levels may rise significantly (more than 50 pg per ml) at 40 to 45 days and these levels may persist throughout pregnancy.

Rectal palpation of a granulosa–theca cell tumor reveals a large, multicystic mass involving one ovary. This mass may increase in size over a period of several months, whereas the contralateral ovary remains small, firm, and inactive. Ultrasound echography (Fig. 1) reveals a multilocular "honeycomb" appearance. Testosterone levels are usually elevated (more than 50 pg per ml) regardless of behavior, but this is not a specific diagnostic aid. Definitive diagnosis is made by histologic examination of the abnormal ovary, following surgical removal.

Granulosa–theca cell tumors may be first diagnosed during pregnancy but it is believed that conception occurs before development of the neoplasm and subsequent endocrine abnormality. After the neoplasm develops, ovarian steroid production may exert a negative feedback suppression of pituitary gonadotropins, which prevents follicular development in the contralateral ovary and renders the mare infertile until the affected ovary is removed.

Surgical removal is the treatment of choice for all forms of ovarian neoplasia. Vaginal, flank, and abdominal approaches have been used depending on the size, age, and temperament of the mare. In the majority of mares with granulosa–theca cell tumors, the remaining ovary returns to normal cyclic activity, and cyclic estrous behavior is restored by the following breeding season. In occasional cases the remaining ovary may remain inactive for up to one and half years. After ovarian function is restored, normal fertility returns.

GONADAL DYSGENESIS

Gonadal dysgenesis is occasionally seen in infertile phenotypic females with evidence of chromo-

some abnormality. The most common abnormality is the XO genotype (63, XO; that is, one X chromosome missing from the normal sex pair). The mare presents as a "barren maiden;" rectal palpation reveals extremely small, firm, and inactive ovaries. If examined histologically, these may contain little if any recognizable ovarian tissue. The cervix is pale and dilated (as in anestrus) and the uterus is small and flaccid. The mare may be physically small for her breed and may show erratic estrous behavior. These mares are sterile.

The 64,XY genotype ("testicular feminization") has been recorded. The mare presents as a barren maiden with stallionlike behavior. Some mares are large for their breed and have the appearance of stallions or geldings that have been castrated later in life. Rectal palpation reveals small, firm, and inactive ovaries. The cervix is usually pale and dilated and the uterus small. These mares show erratic estrous behavior and are sterile. I have seen one 64,XY mare with no uterus or cervix but with rudimentary testes in the ovarian position.

Sex chromosome mosaics have also been reported; for example, 63,XO/64,XX; ,63,XY/64,XX; 63,XO/64,XY; 65,XYY/64,XX; 65,XXX;65,XXY;64,XX and 64,XX? del 2q. These mares present with infertility and small, minimally active ovaries. Mares with gonadal dysgenesis show marked endometrial hypoplasia. Endometrial biopsy is a useful diagnostic aid, especially when the clinician does not have ready access to chromosome analyses. In one random sample of 60 fillies, one showed a sex chromosome mosaic (XO/XX). A much larger study is required to investigate the incidence and natural variability of sex chromosome abnormalities in mares and stallions before their significance in relation to fertility can be fully understood.

FUNCTIONAL ABNORMALITIES

HEMATOMAS

Hematomas are relatively common and can vary in size from 50 mm to 50 cm. Hemorrhage occurs normally during ovulation, but if this persists abnormally, a variable sized ovarian distention is formed. There is no obvious effect on the released ovum, which may be fertilized, as is normal.

Hematomas may persist for two weeks to six months depending on the original size. They may be differentiated from ovarian neoplasia by their sudden formation following estrus, ultrasound echography (Fig. 2), progressive reduction in size over a period of two weeks, and continuing normal cyclic activity of the mare. Ovarian hematomas resolve without treatment.

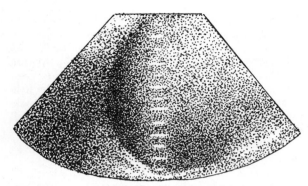

Figure 2. Ovarian hematoma. Diagram of the appearance seen with ultrasound echography. Note the diffuse echogenic mottling within the ovarian perimeter.

PERSISTENT (PROLONGED) CORPUS LUTEUM

Persistent diestrus (less than three months with a mean of two months) occurs in the non-pregnant mare, associated with a failure of normal luteolysis, presumably caused by a deficiency of prostaglandin release. Follicular activity may continue, with occasional diestrus ovulations, but most follicles formed during prolonged luteal function do not ovulate. Clinical examination reveals typical diestrous characteristics—that is, tight pale cervix, moderate to good uterine tone, and active ovaries. An accurate differentiation from early pregnancy may now be made using ultrasound echography.

Treatment is by the injection of a luteolytic dose (10 mg per 450 kg intramuscularly) of prostaglandin $F_{2\alpha}$* or its synthetic analogues. The interval between treatment and ovulation varies considerably depending upon the size of ovarian follicles at the time of treatment. One study demonstrated that of 34 mares with ovarian follicles larger than 40 mm during prolonged diestrus, 21 ovulated 5.1 ± 0.3 days after treatment. The remaining 13 mares underwent follicular regression followed by development of another follicle, which ovulated 9.0 ± 0.7 days after treatment. Of 62 mares studied, 61 (98.4 per cent) ovulated at an average of 6.8 days after treatment and pregnancy rate following mating was 58 per cent.

FOLLICULAR ATRESIA

Follicular atresia with ovulation failure may occur at any stage during the breeding season. The precise pathogenesis remains obscure, but it has been postulated that the 3-cm diameter stage is a critical maturation point because at this stage threefold increases in estrogens and androgens occur. Palpably, the follicle becomes firmer and smaller on serial examination rather than softer and larger as would be expected for a maturing follicle.

At the stage that a diagnosis can be made, treatment is probably inappropriate. When serial palpation suggests that a previously maturing follicle has become "arrested" in its development, treatment with gonadotropin-releasing hormone (GnRH)* may be indicated.

"CYSTIC OVARIES"

The typical condition that is seen in cows, in which a deficiency of luteinizing hormone is thought to result in large follicular and luteal cysts, does not occur in mares. A misdiagnosis by clinicians more experienced in bovine practice is frequently made in mares with large or multiple follicular development, hematomas, and/or prolonged estrus.

Mares may occasionally exhibit prolonged estrus (six to eight days) due to the development of multiple follicles, which may ovulate synchronously or asynchronously. Two adjacent ovarian follicles may be palpably indistinguishable from an abnormally large single follicle. When twin follicles occur, the first follicle often develops to maturity but then fails to ovulate until the second follicle has matured, producing a double ovulation.

Ovulation fossa "cysts" have been described in mares of all ages but most commonly in aged mares with ovaries that are hard, multifollicular (like a bunch of grapes) and that do not palpably change during the estrous cycle. Estrous behavior may be erratic and difficult to monitor accurately by serial palpation. Small (1 to 2 mm), fibrous capsuled subepithelial cysts, which contain clear serous fluid, occur at the ovulation fossa and may cause mechanical obstruction. These cysts are thought to originate from fimbrial tissue and fulfil the histologic criteria for classification as germinal inclusion cysts. Surgical wedge resection is attempted in some species. In some mares with persistent multifollicular ovaries and erratic or quiescent estrous behavior, repeated high doses of human chorionic gonadotropin (hCG)† (9000 IU on 2 consecutive days) followed seven days later by one dose (500 μg) fluprostenol‡ has been reported to reduce ovarian size markedly and to be followed by normal estrous cycles.

Paraovarian cysts occur quite frequently in the tissues surrounding the ovary but are of no clinical significance.

OVARIAN "SENILITY"

In some multiparous mares 20 years old or more, ovarian activity appears to decline to complete inactivity. Endometrial biopsy reveals persistent endometrial atrophy, even when some follicular activity is present. Before complete inactivity, there

---

*Prostin, Upjohn Co., Kalamazoo, MI

---

*Receptal, American Hoechst Corp., Somerville, NJ
†Pregnyl, Organon Pharmaceuticals, West Orange, NJ
‡Equimate, ICI Pharmaceuticals, Mississauga, Ontario

is a transitional phase in which follicles fail to mature and ovulate and during which time estrous behavior may be passive or erratic.

This condition requires further study and adequate documentation but appears to parallel that of premenopause, menopause, and premature menopause as seen in women. Daily oral progesterone (150 mg) and estrogen (10 mg) supplementation of cases in the early transitional phase may maintain cyclic activity.

Supplemental Readings

Hughes, J. P., Kennedy, P. C., and Stabenfeldt, G. H.: Pathology of the ovary and ovarian disorders in the mare. Proc. 9th Intnl. Congr. Anim. Reprod. Artif. Insem., *1*:203, 1980.

Kenney, R. M., Condon, W. A., Ganjam, J. K., and Channing, C.: Morphological and biochemical correlates of equine ovarian follicles as a function of their state of viability or atresia. J. Reprod. Fert., Suppl. 27:163, 1979.

Loy, R. G., Buell, J. R., Stevenson, W., and Hamm, D.: Sources of variation in response intervals after prostaglandin treatment in mares with functional corpora lutea. J. Reprod. Fert., Suppl. 27:227, 1979.

Meagher, D. M., Wheat, J. D., Hughes, J. P., Stabenfeldt, G. H., and Harris, B. A.: Granulosa cell tumors in mares—a review of 78 cases. Proc. Ann. Conv. Am. Assoc. Eq. Pract., 1977, pp. 133–143.

Prickett, M. E.: Pathology of the equine ovary. Proc. 12th Ann. Conv. Am. Assoc. Equine Pract., 1966, pp. 145–154.

Rossdale, P. D., and Ricketts, S. W.: Equine Studfarm Medicine, 2nd ed. London, Bailliere Tindall, 1980.

Stabenfeldt, G. H., Hughes, J. P., Kennedy, P. C., Meagher, D. M., and Neely, D. P.: Clinical findings, pathologic changes, and endocrinological secretory patterns in mares with ovarian tumors. J. Reprod. Fert., Suppl. 27:277, 1979.

Trommershausen-Smith, A., Hughes, J. P., and Neely, D. P.: Cytogenetic and clinical findings in mares with gonadal dysgenesis. J. Reprod. Fert., Suppl. 27:271, 1979.

Uterine Abnormalities

Sidney W. Ricketts, NEWMARKET, ENGLAND

The uterus is of fundamental importance for sperm transport, receipt of the fertilized ovum, and maintenance of pregnancy. Myometrial activity is necessary during parturition, which is followed by rapid uterine involution before the first postpartum estrous period (foal heat). The stallion ejaculates semen through the mare's open estrous cervix into the uterus, challenging the endometrium with microorganisms and other foreign proteins. This challenge results in recurrent endometritis. In contrast to endometritis, neoplasia and endocrine-induced endometrial pathology are not commonly diagnosed in mares.

The horse breeding industry aims for maximum efficiency; owners would like mares to produce single foals annually throughout their lives. However, the repeated challenge of coitus, endometritis, pregnancy, and parturition followed by involution is associated with a comparatively high incidence of uterine disease. Progressive endometrial pathology is a major factor in producing the linear fall in Thoroughbred fertility with age. A knowledge of the pathogenesis of progressive endometrial disease, its treatment, and the application of managerial and veterinary preventive measures is in part responsible for the comparatively high degree of efficiency now seen in the more intensive areas of the horse breeding industry.

The diagnosis of equine uterine abnormality may require a study of the gynecologic history, examination of the external genitalia, vaginoscopic examinations, palpation of the internal genitalia per rectum, bacterial, cytologic and histologic examination of endometrial swab, smear and biopsy samples, ultrasound echography, hysteroscopy, laparoscopy, endocrinologic analysis, and leukocyte karyotyping. In unusual cases, a definitive diagnosis is made only after laparotomy or necropsy.

DEVELOPMENTAL AND FUNCTIONAL ABNORMALITIES

These are unusual in the mare. Cases of persistent hymen are easily corrected by digital or surgical rupture. Before this is attempted, however, care should be taken to exclude the possibility of vaginal or uterine discontinuity. This is rare but these mares are clearly unsuitable for reproductive purposes.

Endometrial Hypoplasia. Underdevelopment or delayed development of the endometrium may be observed in some "barren maiden" mares. This condition, which is usually suspected following palpation of the uterus, may be confirmed by endometrial biopsy. These cases may be associated with ovarian abnormalities (see p. 500) gonadal dysgenesis, ovarian neoplasia, or immaturity.

GONADAL DYSGENESIS. Chromosome abnormalities, most commonly 63X0 and XX/XXY mosaics, result in extreme endometrial epithelial and glandular hypoplasia. Typical cases involve persistently very small (usually less than 1.0 cm) or absent ovaries (see p. 501), a palpably small, flaccid uterus, persistent anestrus, or irregular periods of behavioral estrus. Some mares may appear small in stature. The precise genetic abnormality may be defined following leukocyte karyotyping; confirmed cases are unsuitable for reproductive purposes.

OVARIAN NEOPLASIA. Granulosa cell tumor may occur in mares of any age including immature mares (two- and three-year-olds) (see p. 500). Mares usually show persistent anestrus and have endometrial epithelial, and glandular hypoplasia, which may be confirmed by biopsy. The ovarian abnormality is diagnosed by palpation and ultrasound echography. Following surgical removal of the affected ovary, the other ovary, which is typically small and inactive, usually develops and functions normally and the endometrial hypoplasia resolves.

IMMATURITY. Immaturity may result in degrees of endometrial epithelial and glandular hypoplasia. Mares less than seven years old may have relatively small (less than 3.0 cm) ovaries with little evidence of follicular activity, a small uterus, persistent anestrus, and subestrus. The latter is characterized by prolonged estrous periods or weak behavioral estrus, more typical of the transitional phase. Mating is unproductive and is followed by a relatively high incidence of persistent acute endometritis associated with penile and perineal contaminant microorganisms. Patience is recommended as most cases not associated with gonadal dysgenesis or ovarian neoplasia show improvement in time. Secondary acute endometritis should be treated as described below.

Endometrial Hyperplasia. Endometrial glandular hyperplasia, with gross thickening of the uterus, may be suspected following palpation per rectum and may be confirmed by biopsy. It can be caused by or accompany delayed uterine involution, or persistent acute endometritis.

DELAYED UTERINE INVOLUTION. Endometrial hyperplasia most commonly accompanies delayed endometrial involution following parturition or gestational failure. There is often a concurrent acute endometritis. A relatively high proportion of "first foal" mares suffer from this problem and often end their second breeding season barren. Provided there are no other gynecologic abnormalities, the prognosis for the next breeding season is good. Apparently "arrested" involution has been observed up to six weeks following parturition and up to three months after gestational failure.

If there is delayed postpartum uterine involution, mares should not be mated at the "foal heat" period; treatment with intravenous oxytocin (60 IU in 500 ml saline) is recommended. Acute endometritis should be treated by intrauterine antibiotic irrigation as described on p. 505. In diestrous mares not immediately postpartum, estrus may be induced with exogenous prostaglandin treatment before use of oxytocin. Antibiotic irrigation usually produces luteolysis after two to three days, and oxytocin treatment may be delayed until this occurs.

The response to treatment should be monitored by repeat palpation and by endometrial swab, smear, and biopsy examinations. Mating should then be conducted, when appropriate, using suitable minimal contamination techniques.

PERSISTENT ACUTE ENDOMETRITIS. Endometrial glandular hyperplasia accompanies some cases of long-standing, persistent acute endometritis. These mares often show shortened diestrous periods and may have pyometra. A diagnosis is based on the results of rectal palpation and on endometrial swab, smear, and biopsy examinations. Successful treatment of the endometritis usually results in resolution of the endometrial hyperplasia without specific treatment. If medical treatment is unsuccessful, endometrial curettage (see p. 506) followed by further medical treatment gives useful results. The treatment of pyometra is more difficult.

Cystic Glandular Hyperplasia. This is unusual in mares but has occasionally been seen in association with pyometra or mucometra. The diagnosis is based on gross examination of the uterine contents, rectal palpation, ultrasound echography, and endometrial biopsy. The glands are diffusely and uniformly distended with an amorphous, eosinophilic, PAS-positive glandular secretion. The cause of this condition is unknown but excessive glandular secretory activity is postulated. Treatment is as for pyometra (see p. 507) and the prognosis for breeding is poor.

ENDOMETRITIS

Acute Endometritis. Polymorphonuclear leukocytic (PMN) infiltrations of the endometrial epithelia and stroma are common in mares in response to challenge by microorganisms or foreign proteins or both. During estrus, the normal mare exhibits a low-grade stromal PMN infiltration but this is insufficient to constitute a "leukocytic tide" as seen in some other species and is insufficient to produce cytologic evidence of acute endometritis. Acute endometritis follows coitus, artificial insemination, parturition, and veterinary invasion of the uterine lumen. In the genitally healthy mare, this acute endometritis is transient. In older mares with either an apparent local defense mechanism deficit (see p. 508), or perineal, vaginal, or cervical abnormality (see pp. 516 and 518), the acute endometritis persists, causing subfertility or infertility.

Diagnosis of acute endometritis is made by the observation of a mucopurulent vulval discharge, vaginoscopic examination, and the results of endometrial swab, smear, and, if necessary, biopsy examinations.

INFECTIOUS ACUTE ENDOMETRITIS. This occurs following contamination of the uterus with microorganisms, which invade via the cervical canal. Microorganisms can be aspirated during estrus in cases of pneumovagina (see p. 518), or following parturition, or occasionally during pregnancy, if the cervix relaxes and pneumovagina occurs. During pregnancy, infection may result in placentitis and fetal death. The uterine lumen is also contaminated by penile, perineal, and vaginal microorganisms during coitus, and environmental microorganisms may be introduced during artificial insemination and veterinary invasion.

Veterinarians have concentrated on aerobic bacteria as causal agents for acute endometritis. *Streptococcus zooepidemicus*, *Escherichia coli*, and *Staphylococcus aureus* are the most commonly isolated potential pathogens, whereas *Streptococcus faecalis*, α-hemolytic and nonhemolytic streptococci, *Staphylococcus albus*, Corynebacterium spp., and Anthracoides spp. are more commonly isolated as nonpathogenic contaminants. *Klebsiella pneumoniae* and *Pseudomonas aeruginosa* are occasionally isolated in cases of acute endometritis, and some strains such as *K. pneumoniae* capsule types 1, 2, and 5 appear to be capable of causing true epidemic venereal disease (see p. 513). In the case of these latter organisms, a carrier mare may contaminate a stallion's penile skin, which then transmits the organisms during coitus. This produces endometritis in mares with previously healthy uteri as well as those with deficient local defense mechanisms. Since 1977, the microaerophilic gram-negative coccobacillus *Taylorella equigenitalis* (*Haemophilus equigenitalis*, also known as contagious equine metritis organism [CEMO]) has been recognized as a potential cause of acute endometritis and of epidemic venereal disease. A number of other anaerobic bacteria, such as *Bacteroides fragilis*, Peptostreptococcus spp., and Peptococcus spp. may be isolated from endometrial swab samples, sometimes associated with acute endometritis, usually together with aerobic bacteria, or as apparently nonpathogenic contaminants. Fungi and yeasts are present in the perineal environment and are sometimes associated with acute endometritis (see p. 511). It is probable that other microorganisms as yet unrecognized, such as viruses, mycoplasmas, and Chlamydia spp., may also be capable of causing endometritis.

The diagnosis of acute endometritis should be primarily based on the presence of a discharge containing PMNs and/or tissue infiltration by PMNs, rather than the isolation of a particular microorganism. Many veterinarians now routinely use concurrent cytologic and bacteriologic examinations for mares during early estrus, with major improvements in diagnostic accuracy.

With the diagnosis confirmed and a pathogen isolated, treatment is based on removal of the pathogen by appropriate antimicrobial therapy and the identification and removal of any predisposing factors, such as poor vulval conformation (see p. 518), cervical damage (see p. 516), and deficiencies in local defense mechanisms (see p. 508).

Systemic antibiotic treatment alone is seldom effective against acute endometritis. Similarly, the induction of estrus by exogenous prostaglandins is not as effective in mares as it is in some other species. In fact, many mares with acute endometritis have repeated short diestrous periods rather than prolonged diestrus. The most effective treatment remains daily or twice-daily uterine irrigation with antibiotic solutions to which the pathogen has been shown to be sensitive by in vitro tests. Irrigation may be performed via a sterile insemination pipette, Nielsen catheter, or indwelling uterine infuser.* The latter avoids daily internal interference and is usually retained in place provided that the mare does not come into estrus soon after placement. The catheter is anchored to the skin at the vulval-buttock junction by loosely tied stay sutures.

Nonirritant, water-soluble, low-residue antibiotic preparations should be selected for uterine use or a persistent noninfectious acute endometritis may be induced. For this reason, pessary preparations and some ampicillin and tetracycline preparations are contraindicated. Unless isolated pathogens are not sensitive, a water-based intramammary mixture of neomycin sulphate (1 gm), furaltadone (600 mg), and polymixin B sulphate† (40,000 units) is dissolved in 100 ml sterile water. Five million units sodium benzylpenicillin‡ is added when appropriate. This mixture is therapeutically effective without producing overgrowth of *P. aeruginosa*, *K. pneumoniae*, fungus, or yeast. The response to treatment is monitored by repeat endometrial swab, smear and, if necessary, biopsy examinations.

Intractable cases, often involving deficient local uterine defense mechanisms, have been treated with intrauterine homologous plasma or colostrum (see p. 508). Weak solutions of hydrogen peroxide have been recommended as a treatment for acute endometritis and certainly appear helpful when there is debris such as pus in the uterine lumen. When there is advanced chronic stromal fibrosis, dimethyl sulphoxide (DMSO) (1 ml per dl infusion mixture) may be added to aid antibiotic penetration. Anaerobic bacterial infections are treated with intrauterine infusion of 0.5 per cent metronidazole§ solution. In cases refractory to all forms of medical treatment, endometrial curettage followed by further medical treatment is useful.

---

*Arnolds Ltd, England
†Univet 2 Ltd, Bicester, England
‡Crystapen, Glaxo, England
§Flagyl, Searle Pharmaceuticals Inc., Chicago, IL

NONINFECTIOUS ACUTE ENDOMETRITIS. This may occur following the intrauterine introduction of irritant chemicals such as chlorhexidine, or irritant or persistent vehicles and residues. If it is only transient, this response may not be unwelcome, being a form of "chemical curettage," but these effects are uncontrollable and best avoided. An endometrial biopsy often reveals large numbers of eosinophils in addition to PMNs.

Noninfectious endometritis may also follow local endometrial responses to sperm and seminal proteins when the normal luminal epithelial "barrier" is breached, allowing antigenic access to the tissues. This is most likely to occur during the postpartum period when morphologic and functional repair may be incomplete. In some mares, even when gynecologic, cytologic, and bacteriologic examinations suggest that satisfactory uterine involution has occurred, a persistent acute endometritis, which may be refractory to treatment for a prolonged period, follows coitus. An endometrial biopsy reveals a PMN infiltration, often with large numbers of eosinophils. Occasionally, a similar response may occur to milk and other "foreign" proteins in seminal extenders used during the postpartum period.

Treatment by intrauterine saline irrigation is performed to remove remaining antigenic material. Suitable antibacterial preparations are added to prevent the introduction of secondary infection. Rest from mating activity is recommended.

Chronic Endometritis. Mononuclear cell infiltrations, glandular degeneration, and the formation of fibrous tissue in the stroma are all features commonly seen in the endometrium of multiparous mares. They appear to be unavoidable consequences of the cycle of endometrial challenge that occurs in the brood mare. Diagnosis is made by histologic examination of endometrial biopsy specimens. Acute endometritis or parturient trauma may accelerate development of these changes to a degree considered excessive for the age of the mare.

CHRONIC INFILTRATIVE ENDOMETRITIS. Histiocytes, lymphocytes, and plasma cells are seen in the endometria of mares following antigenic challenge and are a normal manifestation of local immune mechanisms. There are no indications for specific treatment unless other pathologic features are present. Infiltrations may be marked in degree following persistent acute endometritis and when luminal epithelial cell damage has allowed "access" of microorganisms to the tissues. Some bacteria, notably *T. equigenitalis, K. pneumoniae,* and *Ps. aeruginosa,* elicit a marked plasma cell response. Concurrent acute endometritis should be treated as described earlier.

CHRONIC DEGENERATIVE ENDOMETRITIS. Glandular degenerative changes, such as cystic distentions or "nesting" in thick sheaths of encircling fibrous tissue, with flattened or sometimes atrophic epithelia and periglandular or diffuse stromal fibrosis, are part of the progressive pathology seen in the endometria of multiparous mares. It is thought that these degenerative changes play an important part in reducing fertility with age. As with mononuclear cell infiltrations, some mares develop lesions that are excessive in relation to their age. If this is confirmed with a uterine biopsy, attempts may be made by curettage to reduce the degree of chronic degenerative endometritis.

There is no analogy between human and equine endometrial curettage. The human uterus is smooth-surfaced and pear-shaped, and it is menstrual. Total curettage strips the endometrium and new tissue regenerates during the following cycle. The equine uterus is tubular, its surface is highly folded, and it is nonmenstrual. Mechanical curettage merely produces a controllable and quite minimal degree of physical stimulation, but experience suggests that this may be beneficial.

With the mare bridled, restrained, and prepared as for a routine gynecologic examination, the rectum is evacuated and the uterus palpated. The perineum is then washed and the curette* introduced with a gloved arm into the vagina and through the cervix into the uterus. Maintaining the curette in place, the arm is then withdrawn from the vagina and placed in the rectum, where the curette may be palpated in the uterus. The curette is positioned in one of the uterine horns, which is manually stretched cranially, and the endometrium is scraped using multiple longitudinal strokes all around the diameter of the uterine tube. This process is repeated in the other uterine horn and in the body of the uterus prior to careful withdrawal of the instrument through the cervix and vagina. An indwelling uterine infuser is then fitted and irrigations with saline and antibiotics, as described for acute endometritis, are performed for five to seven days. This provides antibacterial coverage after uterine invasion and avoids the theoretic possibility of transluminal adhesion formation. The latter has not been recognized as a complication with use of this technique.

TRANSLUMINAL ADHESIONS. These may follow the use of chemical irritants such as Lugol's iodine and may be diagnosed by manual palpation or hysteroscopy, often in association with acute endometritis. If extensive, no treatment is likely to be satisfactory and the best advice is to retire the mare. If the adhesions are focal and easily broken down by manual manipulation, a course of intrauterine saline and antibiotic irrigations (as described earlier) should be given in addition to the daily topical application of corticosteroid ointment to deter reformation. The prognosis for all cases of transluminal uterine adhesions should be very guarded.

---

*Rockel of London Ltd, London, England

PYOMETRA. When functional or structural abnormalities such as cervical or caudal uterine adhesions prevent drainage of uterine contents, purulent exudate and endometrial glandular secretions accumulate. Sometimes the uterus distends and resembles a balloon. Echographically it contains fluid with "scintillating" particles, throughout both horns and body. When the cervical seal is broken or the adhesions are parted, a viscid, brownish-cream fluid may be collected. This fluid contains many degenerate leukocytes and sometimes bacteria.

Mares with pyometra seldom show systemic illness. The condition appears more common in hot, dry, and thus probably dusty geographic areas such as South Africa, India, North Africa, and the southwestern United States, where the incidence of *P. aeruginosa* is higher. In these cases, extensive endometrial damage results in severe fibrosis and glandular atrophy. This may in turn cause persistent diestrus, presumably associated with inadequate endogenous prostaglandin production and failure of luteolysis. Pyometra appears to be less common in more northern, colder, wetter, and less dusty environments. In these locations, the mares usually have less extensive endometrial damage, they may have endometrial glandular hyperplasia, and the recurrent inflammatory stimulus appears to result in premature prostaglandin release, luteolysis, and "short cycling." *Streptococcus zooepidemicus* or *E. coli* or both are sometimes cultured from the accumulated purulent material.

If the uterine fluid is a viscid, grayish color, bacteriologically sterile, amorphous, and eosinophilic, and if it contains few leukocytes and appears to be accumulated glandular secretion, the condition is called *mucometra*.

Treatment of pyometra requires drainage and flushing out of the accumulated material by frequent, large-volume saline, antibiotic, and hydrogen peroxide flushes. These may be administered through a stomach tube placed in a uterine horn and drained out of another stomach tube, placed just inside the cervix. A variety of antiseptics and irritants have also been used. Intrauterine homologous plasma may be used to provide opsonins (see p. 510). When cervical or endometrial adhesions are present, these are broken and treated with local corticosteroid preparations. Unfortunately, treatment often results in only temporary resolution of the problem; reversion usually occurs spontaneously or after mating, even when minimal contamination methods are used. The most practical advice to give an owner of a mare with pyometra is usually to retire the mare from breeding.

LYMPHATIC CYSTS AND LACUNAE. Stromal fluid accumulations and thin-walled fluid filled cysts that project into the uterine lumen are seen in most multiparous mares over the age of 14 years. They contain lymphatic fluid and sometimes large numbers of lymphocytes and may result from the stenosis of lymphatic ducts. These lesions vary in size, some being as large as 6 to 10 cm in diameter, but most are less than 2 cm. Cysts may be multiple or solitary and may be diagnosed by ultrasound echography (in which case differentiation from a three-week pregnancy can sometimes be difficult), manual palpation, or hysteroscopy.

These lesions represent chronic uterine degenerative changes. However, unless they are large, multiple, and extensive enough to cause gestational failure through poor placental perfusion, specific treatment is not indicated. Large lymphatic cysts may be ruptured by mechanical curettage (see earlier discussion). Cysts usually re-form at the same or different sites and thus curettage may be repeated, as indicated, during a barren year.

ATROPHY

Ventral Dilatation and Mucosal Atrophy. Areas of endometrial and myometrial degeneration occur in the implantation site area in some older mares. A saccular, poorly tonic area of "pendulous" uterine horn may be palpated and hysteroscopy may reveal an area devoid of endometrial folds. There are no specific data in relation to fertility. However, this abnormality is usually seen in association with more widespread chronic degenerative endometritis or atrophy, and the breeding prognosis is usually poor. Although treatment with warm hypertonic saline uterine irrigations has been recommended, it seldom appears successful.

Endometrial Atrophy. Diffuse glandular atrophy may be diagnosed by endometrial biopsy, and is a normal physiologic feature during periods of prolonged ovarian inactivity, such as winter anestrus. It is important to recognize this when interpreting endometrial biopsy specimens during the winter period, and thus it is preferable to complete routine examinations of barren mares in the autumn, while mares are still showing cyclic estrus. In aged mares over 17 years, diffuse glandular atrophy may be seen in association with endometrial and sometimes ovarian senility. The luminal epithelium often remains cuboidal in spite of behavioral estrous activity and, sometimes, ovarian follicular activity. In my experience, the breeding prognosis for these mares is hopeless; no effective treatment has been found.

ENDOMETRIAL NEOPLASIA

Endometrial tumors are rare in mares. Leiomyomas or fibroleiomyomas are the most common, usually in older mares, and are usually small, 2.5 to 5 cm diameter, sometimes multiple, firm, and often occur in the posterior uterine body, sometimes involving the cervix. In this form, unless they interfere with cervical function, they appear to have no effect on fertility and behave benignly. Occasionally, they may occur more anteriorly in the uterine body or horn, may become large (5 to 10 cm in diameter), pedunculated, and secondarily infected, and may result in persistent vulval hemorrhage. Such large lesions may be diagnosed by palpation or hysteroscopy and are best removed surgically.

There have been isolated reports of endometrial fibromas, fibroadenomas, adenosarcomas, and a malignant adenocarcinoma with pulmonary metastases.

Supplemental Readings

Greenhof, G. R., and Kenney, R. M.: Evaluation of reproductive status of non-pregnant mares. J. Am. Vet. Med. Assoc., *167*:449, 1975.

Hughes, J. P., Stabenfeldt, G. H., Kindahl, H., Kennedy, P. C., Edqvist, L. E., Neely, D. P., and Schalm, O. W.: Pyometra in the mare. J. Reprod. Fert., Suppl. *27*:321, 1979.

Jeffcott, L. B., Rossdale, P. D., Freestone, J., Frank, C. J., and Towers Clark, P. F.: An assessment of wastage in Thoroughbred racing from conception to four years of age. Equine Vet. J., *14*:185, 1982.

Kenney, R. R.: Cyclic and pathologic changes of the mare endometrium as detected by biopsy with a note on early embryonic death. J. Am. Vet. Med. Assoc., *172*:241, 1978.

Kenney, R. M., and Ganjam V. K.: Selected pathological changes of the mare uterus and ovary. J. Reprod. Fert., Suppl. *23*:335, 1975.

Knudsen, O.: Partial dilatation of the uterus as a cause of sterility in the mare. Cornell Vet., *54*:423, 1964.

Ricketts, S. W.: The technique and clinical application of endometrial biopsy in the mare. Equine Vet. J., 7:102, 1975.

Ricketts, S. W.: Histological and histopathological studies on the endometrium of the mare. Fellowship Thesis, Royal College of Veterinary Surgeons, London, 1978.

Ricketts, S. W.: Endometrial curettage in the mare. Equine Vet. J., 17:324, 1985.

Rossdale, P. D., and Ricketts, S. W.: Equine Studfarm Medicine, 2nd ed. London, Bailliere Tindall, 1980.

Wingfield Digby, N. J., and Ricketts, S. W.: Results of concurrent bacteriological and cytological examinations of the endometrium of mares in routine studfarm practice 1978–1981. J. Reprod. Fert., Suppl. *32*:181, 1982.

Failure of Uterine Defense Mechanisms

Atwood C. Asbury, GAINESVILLE, FLORIDA

Reproductive efficiency in mares is directly correlated with the ability of the uterus to maintain an environment that is compatible with embryo development, fetal growth, and normal parturition. Repeated contamination of the uterus with environmental microorganisms followed by endometritis occurs throughout the mare's reproductive career—at mating, at parturition, during veterinary examinations, and continually or intermittently in mares with perineal conformational defects. Natural defense mechanisms are required to remove these contaminant organisms, preventing persistence of the endometritis. Failure or incompetence of these natural defense mechanisms is a major cause of equine infertility.

The equine embryo descends from the oviduct into the uterus between five and six days after ovulation. Postcoital endometritis must have been resolved by this time or embryonic death and premature lysis of the corpus luteum may occur. For successful resolution, pathogenic microorganisms, cellular debris, and inflammatory byproducts must have been rapidly cleared. The large number of mares that foal each year and are then successfully mated again, often within 10 days, demonstrates how efficient these natural defense mechanisms are in the majority of mares. However, the clinician involved in stud farm practice must identify incompetence in individual mares and must compensate for it by treatment and prophylactic regimens. Until recently, these techniques were based on the use of intrauterine antibiotic treatments, before or after mating or both (see p. 505). However, increased research interest in this area has led to the use of more specific techniques.

UTERINE DEFENSE MECHANISMS

Although uterine immunologic mechanisms remain poorly understood, it appears that the primary defenses are local and nonspecific, the most important being the phagocytosis of bacteria by polymorphonuclear leukocytes. IgA binding of organisms at the luminal epithelial cell surface (providing surface protection) and direct, nonspecific bacterial inhibition by microbicidal factors in uterine secretions have now been demonstrated and are undoubtedly also important. Specific humoral or cell-mediated immunologic responses have not been demonstrated and would probably not be activated quickly enough to provide the rapid clearance necessary. Physical responses involving uterine myometrial and cervical activity are important in the mare.

Contamination of the uterine lumen with micro-organisms initiates a chain response. Chemotactic signals attract very large numbers of neutrophils from the uterine circulation, where, during early estrus, they normally marginate in the small superficial endometrial vessels. Serum proteins, containing complement and antibody, migrate into the uterine lumen. These opsonins bind organisms together into large complexes and to the neutrophil cell membrane, where they can then be phagocytosed in large numbers rather than individually. Phagocytosis involves engulfing the clumps of organisms and then destroying them by complex biochemical reactions using oxidative cell metabolism and the production of byproducts such as peroxide, and enzymatic reactions involving cell granules. Although phagocytic efficiency varies with bacterial species, common equine uterine contaminants are readily destroyed by these processes.

The phagocytosed organisms are then removed from the uterine lumen, primarily by mechanical evacuation. The normal uterus responds to inflammation by contracting and pushing luminal contents through the open cervical, vestibular, and vulval "valves," which are normally "one-way." Ciliary action at the luminal epithelial surface is also important.

FAILURE OF NATURAL DEFENSE MECHANISMS

When these natural defense mechanisms fail, uterine contamination is followed by persistent endometritis, which leads to infertility. Individual mares, which thus become susceptible to uterine infection, require special management. This may include reduced exposure to contamination (see p. 505), antibiotic treatments (see p. 505), and/or anatomic corrections (see pp. 516 and 518). Eventually, such procedures are no longer effective and the mare becomes infertile, often with low-grade persistent endometritis. Definition of the cause of such immune failure is thus required before specific treatment can result in improved fertility.

Studies in uterine phagocytosis have suggested a reduced chemotactic response in uterine neutrophils in mares with degenerate endometria. Other in vitro studies have suggested reduced opsonization in susceptible mares possibly associated with uterine complement abnormality. The latter theory is supported by clinical trials using complement (in the form of intrauterine plasma infusions) to treat and to prevent the recurrence of persistent endometritis. These studies form the basis for treatment programs suggested later.

Anatomic defects may cause or contribute to failure of natural uterine defense mechanisms in individual mares. Old mares with pendulous, atonic uteri may not be able to evacuate luminal contents. Cervical integrity must allow evacuation but prevent further contamination. Perineal conformation must not predispose to pneumovagina, urovagina, or fecal contamination of the vestibule. All these features must be assessed and corrected, if possible, before specific immune defects are suggested.

DIAGNOSIS OF REDUCED UTERINE IMMUNE COMPETENCE

At the present state of our knowledge, the diagnosis of susceptibility to uterine infection is made retrospectively—i.e., after the mare has demonstrated repeated postcoital persistent endometritis following normal precoital examinations. A detailed history including the results of gynecologic examinations should be obtained. The presence of acute endometritis may be determined by visual signs of vaginitis and cervicitis with purulent exudate in severe cases. In less severe cases, the diagnosis is made on the basis of cervical cytologic examinations and, in some cases, by histologic examination of endometrial biopsy specimens. The presence of neutrophils in the uterine lumen suggests active antigenic stimulation and inadequate evacuation and is probably the most reliable diagnostic criterion.

TREATMENT

Correction of Anatomic Defects. Abnormalities such as cervical lacerations, urovagina, thinning of the perineal body, and vulval incompetence must be identified and corrected (see p. 518).

Uterine Flush. Large-volume saline irrigation mechanically removes uterine exudate and reduces bacterial numbers. The technique dilates the uterine wall and mildly irritates the endometrium, which may also be beneficial, stimulating young neutrophils to migrate into the lumen accompanied by serum proteins including opsonins. Hot saline (50° C) appears to be additionally beneficial, and in mares with a thick-walled or pendulous uterus its effect can be palpated before and after irrigation.

Uterine irrigation is best performed using a No. 24 or 30 French Foley catheter with a 75-ml inflatable retaining balloon.* An 80-cm autoclavable catheter designed for this purpose is now available.† Saline is infused by gravity in 1-liter quantities and is then recovered into a large vessel. This allows

---

*C. R. Bard, Inc., supplied by Wise Surgical Supply, Gainesville, FL

†Equine Uterine Flush Catheter, EUF-80 Bivona Inc., Gary, IN

inspection for degree of cloudiness, which correlates well with the amount of exudate present. The volume infused and then recovered should be measured, as this may be helpful in assessing dilution. To achieve complete recovery, uterine manipulation per rectum may be required.

Plasma Infusion. Homologous plasma (which is technically more convenient than serum, both of which are sources of complement), has been used as an intrauterine infusion on the basis of studies that have suggested a defect in opsonization. The use of heterologous plasma would be convenient; however, at present the possibility of sensitization of the uterus to foreign protein cannot be ruled out.

The technique is to collect blood, aseptically, into sterile containers, using either heparin (5 to 10 units per ml blood) or standard dilutions of citrate anticoagulant. Complement is unstable at ambient temperatures and thus the plasma should be separated aseptically as soon as possible and infused immediately or frozen for subsequent use. Cold centrifugation is the ideal separation technique; when sedimentation by gravity is used, this should be performed in a refrigerator. Opsonins in plasma have been shown to be stable at domestic freezer temperatures for longer than 100 days. Repeated thawing and refreezing may denature proteins and therefore should be avoided. It is convenient to freeze the separated plasma in 50 to 100 ml aliquots, and 6 oz sterile, disposable plastic bags* have been used successfully. Plasma should be thawed slowly in lukewarm water just before infusion. One hundred milliliter quantities are infused using aseptic technique.

Combined Antibiotic and Plasma Treatment. Some antibiotics are more compatible with the phagocytic process than are others. In vitro studies have shown that in concentrations commonly used for intrauterine infusion, amikacin sulfate† and gentamicin sulfate‡ inhibit neutrophil phagocytosis, whereas potassium penicillin G§ and disodium ticarcillin‖ do not. Following these studies, a number of mares were treated with plasma infusions to which saline dilutions of penicillin or ticarcillin had been added, just before use. Results of this treatment were good.

Hydrogen Peroxide Infusion. During neutrophil phagocytosis, bacteria are destroyed at least in part by the products of oxidative metabolism, which include hydrogen peroxide. With this in mind, mares have been treated with 60 to 250 ml of a solution of one part 3 per cent hydrogen peroxide to four parts normal saline, by intrauterine infusion

daily for three days late in diestrus. The mares are then mated at the next estrous period and the results have been encouraging, particularly when *Pseudomonas aeruginosa* and *Klebsiella pneumoniae* infections are involved.

Streptococcal Filtrate Infusion. This technique has recently been suggested for the treatment of low-grade recurrent endometritis and has now been used with some apparent success. A bacteria-free filtrate of *Streptococcus zooepidemicus* is prepared by inoculating brain-heart infusion broth with the bacteria, incubating the broth, and then passing it through a small-bore filter; 50 to 80 ml filtrate is infused into the uterus, eliciting a severe acute endometritis. Large numbers of neutrophils and probably serum proteins migrate into the uterine lumen without the presence of bacteria.

TREATMENT STRATEGIES

The various treatments just described may be used for mares with active or low-grade recurrent acute endometritis. In mares with deficient uterine defense mechanisms they may be temporarily successful, but additional prophylactic techniques must be employed at the time of mating to prevent the re-establishment of persistent endometritis. Treatment strategies have thus been designed to suit the individual mare.

Active Acute Endometritis. In over 60 cases that were refractory to conventional antibiotic treatment, mares were given a 3-liter (at least) uterine flush, on the first day of treatment, during estrus. When the uterus had been evacuated as much as possible, plasma was infused. Plasma infusions were repeated daily for a minimum of five days and uterine flushes were repeated on alternate days until the recovered saline was visibly clear. It was sometimes necessary to repeat the treatments at successive estrous periods before the endometritis was resolved and then the mare was mated using a postmating treatment, as described later. Approximately 50 per cent of the mares treated conceived and carried a normal foal to term.

Infusions of plasma with added antibiotics have recently been used when bacteriologic examinations revealed a specific pathogen. Although the selection of antibiotic was guided by in vitro sensitivity tests, early impressions suggest that 3 to 6 gm ticarcillin disodium is particularly suitable.

Peroxide infusions and streptococcal filtrates have been used for cases of active endometritis, with some apparent success.

Recurrent Acute Endometritis. After a period of time, a persistent endometritis may subside in intensity and may be demonstrable only by endometrial cytologic or histologic examinations. Mating during this condition will usually result in severe

*Whirl-Pak Bags, Nasco, Fort Atkinson, WI
†Amiglyde-V, Bristol Laboratories, Syracuse, NY
‡Gentocin, Schering Corp., Kenilworth, NJ
§Squibb, Princeton, NJ
‖Ticar, Beecham Laboratories, Bristol, TN

acute endometritis. Therefore, treatments as just described have been used at the estrus before mating or for a few days during early estrus before mating. When saline flushes are used, the appearance of the recovered saline may be used as a prognostic guide. When the recovered saline appears clear, the mare may be mated and postmating treatment used.

The use of streptococcal filtrates to convert long-standing, low-grade recurrent endometritis into severe acute endometritis, with recruitment of young neutrophils and opsonins, appears theoretically sound and deserves clinical evaluation.

Postmating Treatment. Spermatozoa reach the oviducts within minutes of natural mating or artificial insemination and the embryo is retained there for at least five days after ovulation. The uterotubal junction prevents fluids infused by gravity into the uterus from entering the oviducts. The corpus luteum is refractory to prostaglandins until about five days after ovulation. For these reasons, uterine infusions of saline, antibiotics, and/or plasma may be administered as early as one hour after mating and may be repeated daily until the third or fourth day after ovulation without harm to the embryo.

A regimen that has been apparently successful in many cases of impaired natural uterine defense mechanisms is as follows:

1. At 24 hours after mating, repeated large-volume saline flushes are given until the recovered saline is visually clear.

2. This is followed immediately with an infusion of homologous plasma with or without added antibiotics, as appropriate.

3. Saline flushing followed by plasma infusion is repeated daily until all the recovered saline is clear or the third day after ovulation is reached.

4. Plasma infusion alone is administered on the day following the last saline flush if the third day after ovulation has not been passed.

Accurate timing of ovulation is imperative for this regimen, and thus daily ovarian palpation during this period is necessary.

MANAGEMENT CONSIDERATIONS

In addition to uterine treatments, management techniques designed to reduce uterine contamination at mating should be used. These include limiting the number of matings, ideally to one per estrus, by serial ovarian palpation and the administration of 2000 to 3000 IU chorionic gonadotropin* intravenously, 12 to 18 hours before mating. Artificial insemination, ideally with washed and antibiotic-treated semen, is recommended in areas where registration authorities allow this technique. If this is not appropriate, antibiotic-containing semen extenders can be infused into the uterus just before mating. Good hygienic examination, treatment, and mating techniques are essential.

---

*Chorisol, Burns-Biotec, Omaha, NE

Supplemental Readings

Asbury, A. C.: Uterine defense mechanisms in the mare: The use of intrauterine plasma in the management of endometritis. Theriogenology, 21:387, 1984.

Asbury, A. C., Gorman, N. T., and Foster, G. W.: Uterine defense mechanisms in the mare: serum opsonins affecting phagocytosis of *Streptococcus zooepidemicus* by equine neutrophils. Theriogenology, 21:375, 1984.

Couto, M. A., and Hughes, J. P.: Intrauterine inoculation of a bacteria-free filtrate of *Streptococcus zooepidemicus* in clinically normal and infected mares. J. Equine Vet. Sci., 5:81, 1985.

Liu, I. K. M., Cheung, A. T. W., Walsh, E. M., Miller, M. E., and Lindenberg, P. M.: Comparison of peripheral blood and uterine derived polymorphonuclear leukocytes from mares resistant and susceptible to chronic endometritis: Chemotactic and cell elastimetry analysis. Am. J. Vet. Res., 46:917, 1985.

Fungal Endometritis

Murray G. Blue, STRATFORD, NEW ZEALAND

Mycotic infections of the nonpregnant equine uterus occur most frequently under intensive reproductive management systems with the widespread use of antibiotics. However, fungi and yeasts are common environmental contaminants and may be isolated in genital swab cultures in the absence of uterine disease. The most commonly reported organisms are Candida spp., particularly *C. albicans*, and *Aspergillus fumigatus*.

CLINICAL SIGNS

Clinical signs vary in severity from none, in cases in which there is no tissue invasion, to severe purulent endometritis with chronic infertility. Seldom are there signs of systemic illness.

PATHOGENESIS

Fungi, bacteria, and other environmental microorganisms invade the uterus via the cervix, during estrus, in cases of pneumovagina, at coitus, following parturition, and during gynecologic examinations and/or manipulations. The ensuing endometritis produces a purulent fluid in which the fungi may grow. When normal uterine defense mechanisms prevail, the purulent material containing the fungi is spontaneously eliminated within three to four weeks, without tissue invasion having taken place. When uterine defense mechanisms are compromised, often for unknown reasons, or when inappropriate or excessive antibiotic treatment encourages growth of fungi and sometimes the more resistant bacteria such as Pseudomonas spp. and Klebsiella spp., the organisms are not eliminated and tissue invasion occurs. In pregnant mares, fungi can produce abortion in late gestation, but recovery is usually spontaneous and subsequent fertility is not affected.

DIAGNOSIS

The commonly isolated fungi and yeasts grow in ordinary blood agar, in aerobic culture, and thus may be identified in routine swab examinations, often in association with bacteria. Fungi and yeasts are not normal inhabitants of the uterus, but because of technical difficulties in obtaining truly representative uterine swab samples, false-positive and false-negative results may be obtained. It is thus important to clarify the significance of isolates by use of multiple sampling and further diagnostic techniques and by consideration of the case history and clinical signs.

The cytologic examination of cervical or endometrial smear samples or both is a helpful diagnostic aid. In cases of fungal endometritis, even when a purulent discharge is not evident, neutrophils are almost invariably present in cervical smears. Fungal or yeast elements may be identified using most routine cytologic stains or, if necessary, special stains.

The histologic examination of endometrial biopsy samples can define whether tissue invasion has occurred and the degree and character of the endometritis. Fungal elements may be identified in the endometrial tissues or uterine lumen, or both by using special stains such as periodic acid-Schiff (PAS), Gomori's methenamine silver, and Grocott's or Gridley's methods. Although it is often suspected

that the fungus has invaded endometrial tissues, this can be extremely difficult to prove.

TREATMENT

In mares with normal uterine defense mechanisms, fungal infections usually resolve spontaneously with time. During the breeding season, time is at a premium and treatment is usually undertaken. When tissue invasion has occurred, or there are concurrent bacterial infections and genital abnormalities such as defective perineal conformation, treatment of all these is important. Unfortunately, clinical trial data for the efficacy and dosage of specific antifungal treatments are not available for the horse. Extrapolation has been made from human and tissue culture data.

Prior to the use of specific antifungal treatment, it may be beneficial to irrigate the uterine lumen repeatedly with a minimum of 250 ml sterile saline to remove accumulated inflammatory fluids. Dilute iodine solutions, although not specific for fungal infections, have been commonly used. Three to five daily intrauterine infusions of 250 ml 10 per cent povidone-iodine* (1 per cent available iodine) in saline solution is recommended.

Most fungi, including Candida spp. and A. *fumigatus*, are inhibited by amphotericin B† in vitro, at a dosage rate of 0.03 to 1.00 μg per ml. Cytotoxicity and adverse reactions are reported in human medicine. Yeasts and probably some fungi are inhibited by nystatin in vitro, at a dose rate of 100 units per ml. The suspension is not cytotoxic at this dosage and is not absorbed through intact mucous membranes. If indicated, nystatin and amphotericin B are used at concentrations known to be effective in vitro, as intrauterine infusions (250 ml), daily for three to five days.

Human antifungal vaginal suppositories, e.g., nystatin tablets.‡ (100,000 units) and clotrimazole tablets§ (100 mg), have been used for intrauterine treatment in mares, at extrapolated dosage rates.

The response to treatment should be monitored by repeated endometrial swab, smear, and biopsy tests. Spontaneous recovery in mares with normal uterine defense mechanisms complicates the evaluation of treatments.

PROGNOSIS

In mares with normal uterine defense mechanisms, uncomplicated cases of fungal endometritis

---

*Betadine, Purdue Frederick Co., Norwalk, CT
†Fungizone Intravenous, Squibb, Princeton, NJ
‡Mycostatin, Squibb, Princeton, NJ
§Gyne-Lotrimin, Schering Corp., Kenilworth, NJ

usually resolve satisfactorily with or without treatment. When tissue invasion has occurred and when there is concurrent infection with Pseudomonas spp. or Klebsiella spp., intensive and sometimes repeated courses of specific antifungal and antibacterial treatments may be needed before sustained

recovery occurs. In mares with abnormal uterine defense mechanisms, with multifactorial endometrial disease including persistent fungal infection, the response to treatment and subsequent fertility is poor.

Venereal Diseases of Mares

D. J. Simpson, NEWMARKET, ENGLAND

There are five important venereal diseases that affect mares: three bacterial infections—contagious equine metritis (CEM), *Klebsiella pneumoniae* and *Pseudomonas aeruginosa*—and two viral infections—coital exanthema (CE) and equine viral arteritis (EVA). Combinations of these infections rarely occur. Recent emphasis to control bacterial infections, stimulated by CEM outbreaks, has reduced their incidence, particularly in countries where there is veterinary supervision of horse breeding.

CLINICAL SIGNS OF BACTERIAL INFECTIONS

Venereal infections should be suspected when genital inflammation and vaginal discharge occur in several mares mated by an individual stallion. Previously healthy mares may return to estrus unexpectedly, often with shortened diestrus. The systemic spread of these infections is rare. Carriers of both sexes showing no clinical signs allow persistence of the infection within a horse population. Control of infection is by detection and treatment before mating. Routine screening of mares and detection of infected horses during an outbreak of bacterial venereal disease are achieved by collecting appropriate swab samples for bacterial culture. Laboratories must be experienced in the isolation and identification of the specific organisms incriminated in venereal disease.

All CEM organisms isolated from Thoroughbreds have proven potentially pathogenic, but some appear to be carried by European non-Thoroughbred populations without ill effect. In the case of *K. pneumoniae* and *P. aeruginosa*, it is important to differentiate between strains that form part of the normal flora and those that are venereal pathogens. Capsule types 1 and 5 are now the common *K. pneumoniae* pathogens in England. *Pseudomonas aeruginosa* strains are more difficult to categorize and thus the safest approach would be to regard all

isolates as potentially pathogenic and withhold mating until the affected mare has been successfully treated.

TREATMENT

Before either a diseased or a carrier mare is treated, the extent of the infection must be determined by collecting swabs from all the possible sites of infection—that is, endometrium and/or cervix, vestibule, and clitoral fossa and sinuses. Culture results from cervical and endometrial swabs are more reliable when samples are collected during estrus. Uterine treatment is of primary importance in acute infections. Carrier mares are often free of uterine infection but may have a well-established clitoral colonization. Treatment regimens are selected according to the site of infection.

Systemic. Systemic treatment is more useful in acute or chronic metritis and in the occasional ascending urinary tract infection. Systemic treatment alone is less effective than intrauterine treatment and a combination of both may be helpful in persistent uterine infections. Systemic treatment is usually parenteral, and a five-day course of therapy is minimal.

Intrauterine. Solutions or suspensions are preferred for intrauterine treatment even though some drugs are available in pessary or paste form. Infusion of volumes of liquid in excess of 200 ml provokes straining by the mare, resulting in a fluid loss from the uterus. Although volumes as low as 20 ml disperse through the uterus effectively, 50 to 100 ml is the optimal volume. A large syringe and bovine-type uterine catheter provide the easiest method to administer intrauterine medications. The catheter is passed by dilating the cervix with a gloved finger and guiding the catheter tip into the lumen of the uterus. Infusate flows most freely when the catheter tip is in the uterus. Indwelling catheters are convenient if frequent treatment is required, or when it is necessary for an inexperienced person to perform this therapy. Treatment should be given at 12- to 24-hour intervals for at least five days.

Topical. Topical treatment is used for clitoral or vestibular infections. It requires cleansing followed by the application of a cream or ointment, which should persist to give adequate drug levels for a reasonable period of time.

The following technique is recommended for clitoral treatment:

1. The clitoral fossa is opened and flushed with warm water from a syringe or pressure spray. The clitoral sinuses should also be flushed after their contents have been expressed.

2. When cleansing solution is used, approximately 4 ml is infused into the clitoral sinuses and fossa through the nozzle of a disposable syringe. A smaller cannula may be required for infusions if the lateral sinuses are deep. Following infusion of the cleansing solution, the fossa is closed over the clitoris by gripping the two sides between thumb and forefinger, allowing the fluid to be massaged into the folds and crevices.

3. Excess fluid and loosened smegma are wiped away and the area is partly dried. Three to four milliliters of antibacterial ointment or cream are put into the sinuses and fossa and distributed as described.

Clitoral treatment must be repeated at 12- or 24-hour intervals for at least five days. When uterine and clitoral infections are treated concurrently, external dressings should begin one or two days before intrauterine therapy to reduce the risk of contaminating the uterine catheter during its introduction into the vagina.

If clitoral sinus infection survives protracted and vigorous treatment, clitoral sinusectomy may be necessary. Sinusectomy is a simple procedure that need not cause disfigurement and is often effective when allied with postoperative topical dressing. After topical treatment of the clitoris and clitoral sinuses, introduction of a broth culture of normal clitoral flora may prevent reinfection, especially by *P. aeruginosa* and *K. aerogenes*. This therapy has proved valuable in the treatment of penile bacterial infections (p. 570).

Selection of Antibiotics and Other Drugs. Drugs used for treatment of bacterial venereal infections must be effective against the causative organism. The choice of agent is determined by both in vitro sensitivity testing and clinical experience. It is often necessary to consider a wider range of antibiotics than those included in the standard veterinary range. Some clinicians add dimethylsulfoxide (DMSO) or estrogens to intrauterine infusion mixtures to improve penetration and absorption of antibiotics. To reduce the development of antibiotic resistance, antibacterial agents other than antibiotics should be considered. The drug should be convenient to administer and free from side effects such as local irritation and systemic toxicity.

Antibiotic Dosage Rate. Systemic antibiotics are administered at the recommended therapeutic level. If higher dose rates for longer periods are necessary for persistent infections, possible toxicity must be considered, particularly with aminoglycoside antibiotics. The dosage of antibiotics recommended for parenteral administration can be used as a guide for intrauterine treatment. Tissue levels can be raised by increased dosage or more frequent treatments. Because drugs infused into the uterus may be absorbed through the inflamed endometrium, intrauterine infusion of large doses of some drugs may result in systemic toxicity.

When selecting external treatments, the clinician should remember that topical preparations can cause local irritation. Finding a suitable preparation is often more of a problem than dosage.

CONTAGIOUS EQUINE METRITIS

The contagious equine metritis organism is sensitive to a wide range of antibacterial agents, but the most commonly isolated strain is streptomycin-resistant. Acute endometritis is best treated with intrauterine infusions of penicillin, ampicillin, or amoxicillin. Solutions and suspensions of these antibiotics are readily available. Solutions may be prepared in normal saline or sterile water, and suspensions can be obtained from multidose vials prepared for intramuscular injection, e.g., procaine penicillin. Ampicillin and amoxicillin may be available in pessary form. Although many acute endometritis cases resolve without treatment, the risk of chronic endometritis or persistent clitoral contamination is greater if treatment is withheld.

For treatment of chronic endometritis, possibly complicated by salpingitis, simultaneous systemic and local treatment is recommended. Ampicillin or amoxicillin is injected and penicillin is infused into the uterus or vice versa. A 7- to 10-day treatment period is recommended, during which time the animal should be observed for diarrhea, indicating a disturbance of intestinal flora.

Although penicillins may be used for topical clitoral treatment, a combination of chlorhexidine and nitrofurazone is the most successful treatment. After local cleansing with chlorhexidine surgical scrub (4 per cent weight for volume), the clitoral fossa is packed with 0.2 per cent nitrofurazone soluble ointment daily for five days. If longer courses of therapy result in local irritation caused by the chlorhexidine, nitrofurazone should be used alone.

In the small proportion of cases of CEM that do not respond to medical treatment, sinusectomy may be necessary to eliminate infection.

KLEBSIELLA PNEUMONIAE INFECTION

Outbreaks of Klebsiella infection are usually less acute than outbreaks of CEM, and a smaller proportion of exposed mares becomes infected. Treatment is mostly required for well-established infections, in which prolonged systemic and local treatment are required. The therapeutic approaches to Klebsiella infection and CEM are similar, but selection of antibacterial agents for Klebsiella infection is more difficult. The organism capsule type and sensitivity to a wide range of antibiotics must both be determined.

The aminoglycoside antibiotics are the most effective against *K. pneumoniae*, in vivo, but toxicity and untoward local reactions may limit their clinical use. Although gentamicin gives the best result, it is expensive; neomycin is therefore often used as a first line of therapy. Framycetin, kanamycin, and amikacin may also be used. *K. pneumoniae* is sometimes sensitive in vitro to polymixin B, chloramphenicol, and the tetracyclines, but the results obtained in vivo are often disappointing.

Mild liquid soap or detergent may be used as a clitoral cleansing agent before application of 0.3 per cent gentamicin cream. Clitoral infections usually respond satisfactorily to treatment.

PSEUDOMONAS AERUGINOSA INFECTION

Pseudomonas aeruginosa is the most difficult of the bacterial pathogens to eliminate from the reproductive tract, sometimes reappearing several weeks after apparently successful treatment. *P. aeurginosa* can become endemic on breeding farms, causing recurrent low-grade infection rather than acute outbreaks of venereal disease. Fertility is depressed, especially in "newly introduced" and aging mares. Because elimination of infection can be extremely difficult, suppression of infection by prophylactic treatment may be all that can be accomplished.

It is essential to select therapy on the basis of a wide range of antibiotic sensitivity tests and to provide a therapeutic dosage for an adequate period. The aminoglycosides are the most useful antibiotics, gentamicin and amikacin giving the best results. Other useful antibiotics include streptomycin, framycetin, neomycin, polymixin B, and carbenicillin. Combined and prolonged systemic and intrauterine treatment may be indicated for persistent endometritis.

Clitoral treatment is enhanced by flushing with 0.5 to 1 per cent silver nitrate solution before applying 0.3 per cent gentamicin cream. The silver nitrate acts as a desiccant but may cause irritation after two to three days. One per cent silver sulphadiazine cream has been used topically but appears less effective than silver nitrate solution. Some clinicians claim that povidone-iodine surgical scrub is a useful cleanser in *P. aeruginosa* infections. Clitoral sinusectomy or clitoridectomy may have value in cases of clitoral infection that persistently fail to respond to medical treatment.

A single clitoral treatment with silver nitrate and gentamicin cream, on the day before mating, may reduce venereal transmission when *P. aeruginosa* has become endemic.

POST-TREATMENT ASSESSMENT

The accepted standard for the assessment of success following treatment is three negative sets of clitoral and endometrial swabs, taken at weekly intervals, commencing more than seven days after the end of treatment. While this is a practical compromise, it may not be a complete safeguard. Organisms such as *K. pneumoniae* and *P. aeruginosa* may reappear later. A small percentage of mares remain unresponsive to all forms of treatment and are thus permanently unsuitable for mating.

VIRAL INFECTIONS

Coital Exanthema. Equine herpesvirus III can remain dormant until conditions favor the spread and development of clinical disease. Some mares, as well as stallions, appear particularly susceptible to recurrent outbreaks of clinical disease.

Small vulval vesicles appear, surrounded by inflamed mucosa. Usually, lesions are close to the mucosal margin of the vulva toward the lower commisure, sometimes involving the clitoral body and fossa. A brief period of local irritation ends when the vesicles rupture, leaving small punctate ulcers. In severe cases, there is spread to adjacent perineal skin and ulcers become confluent. The appearance is characteristic and has produced the colloquial name "spots." Nonspecific secondary bacterial infection may occur, occasionally involving *P. aeruginosa*.

Venereal spread follows a short incubation period, conception rate is not depressed, and healing is rapid (7 to 10 days). Permanent loss of pigmentation may occur at the site of the healed lesions.

Mares are suitable for mating at the next estrus and treatment is usually unnecessary. Symptomatic treatment with soothing antiseptic creams or powders or both may prevent or treat secondary bacterial infection. A careful watch should be kept for spontaneous development of clinical signs following minor vulval abrasions, stretching, or episiotomy. In such cases mating should be postponed until healing is complete.

Equine Viral Arteritis. The recent outbreak of equine viral arteritis in Kentucky has demonstrated the potential for venereal transmission of this disease. The virus persists in the semen of infected stallions for long periods after clinical signs have resolved. During mating, the virus is readily transmitted to susceptible mares, which may show typical signs of the acute febrile disease 7 to 10 days later. A proportion of mares become chronic carriers of the infection, with virus excretion in the urine completing the cycle of venereal transmission. When the disease has become endemic and a population contains carriers of both sexes, vaccination appears to be the most promising control method.

Supplemental Readings

Animal Health Trust: Proceedings of the International Symposium on Equine Venereal Diseases, Lanwades Park, Kennett, Newmarket, England, 1979.

Asbury, A. C.: Infectious causes of infertility. *In* Equine Medicine and Surgery, 3rd ed., Mansmann, R. A., McAllister, E. S., and Pratt, P. W. (eds.), Vol. 2, Chap. 23, Santa Barbara American Veterinary Publications, 1982.

Powell, D. G., David, J. S. E., and Frank, C. J.: Contagious equine metritis. The present situation reviewed and a revised code of practice for control. Vet. Rec., *101*:20, 1978.

Simpson, D. J., and Eaton-Evans, W. E.: Laboratories for contagious equine metritis. Vet. Rec., *102*:48, 1978.

Wingfield-Digby, N. J., and Ricketts, S. W.: A method for clitoral sinusectomy in mares. In Practice, *4*:154, 1982.

Cervical Abnormalities

Harry C. Frauenfelder, HAHNDORF, SOUTH AUSTRALIA

The cervix constitutes the third line of defense of the uterus against external contamination, after the vulval lips and the constrictor muscles of the vaginal vestibule. Although abnormalities of the vulval and caudal vagina are commonly recognized and treated (see p. 518), the cervix is often overlooked as a source of reproductive problems in mares.

The sphincter action of the equine cervix is provided by the longitudinal and circular layers of smooth muscle, which are continuations of the myometrium. The equine cervix lacks the rigid and nondistensible annular rings characteristic of the cow, goat, sheep, and pig. Thus its shape and structure are dependent on hormonal balance during the estrous cycle. During estrus, when circulating progesterone levels are low, the cervix relaxes, is difficult to palpate per rectum, and its external os lies flat on the vaginal floor. This state allows accurate apposition of cervix and glans penis during coitus, allowing normal ejaculation of semen into the uterine lumen. Material from the cranial vagina (e.g., feces or urine) can also enter the uterus, but contamination is reduced by the outward movement of uterine secretions and exudate. During diestrus and pregnancy, when circulating progesterone levels are high, tone increases in the cervical circular muscles. The cervix can be readily palpated per rectum (approximately 5 to 7 cm long and 4 cm wide). The external os closes, and the continuity between the uterus and vagina is eliminated. When cervical abnormality leads to failure of closure, infertility commonly follows.

DIAGNOSIS

Cervical abnormalities are usually traumatic in origin (congenital abnormalities are rare) and may be suspected in the following circumstances:

1. There has been a spontaneous or assisted traumatic parturition.

2. An old or small mare has produced a markedly oversized foal.

3. The uterus has been irrigated with irritant solutions (e.g., tincture of iodine).

4. A mare has suffered repeated pregnancy failures and has no demonstrable endometrial or perineal abnormality.

5. An abnormally shaped cervix is observed during vaginoscopic examination or palpated during cervical manipulations per vagina, as during endometrial biopsy or cervical culture.

Examination of the Cervix. Rectal palpation of the shape, size, and consistency of the cervix may provide information regarding pregnancy or stage of the estrous cycle. However, direct observation (via a vaginoscope) and digital palpation per vagina are essential for accurate detection and definition of cervical abnormalities. Examination during estrus facilitates the detection of cervical canal lesions, whereas cervical tone and competence are best assessed during diestrus or pregnancy. Palpation during pregnancy should be performed carefully and infrequently, as stimulation of endogenous prostaglandin release may jeopardize the pregnancy. The most common cervical abnormalities recognized are mucosal defects, adhesions, lacerations, and incompetence.

TREATMENT

The aim is to restore normal cervical function—that is, tight closure during diestrus and throughout pregnancy—with adequate relaxation during estrus and parturition. As the majority of abnormalities are structural, surgical treatment is usually appropriate. In the absence of obvious structural damage, treatment with progesterone supplementation has been used.

Mucosal Defects. Many acute mucosal lesions go undetected and heal spontaneously by epithelialization, without adhesion formation. Nevertheless, in all cases of prolonged spontaneous or assisted parturition, detailed vaginoscopic examination and digital palpation is advisable wtihin three to five days, to detect mucosal defects in the cervix or vagina.

Early detection can prevent fibrous adhesion formation, either within the lumen of the cervical canal or between the external os and the vaginal wall. Areas of roughened mucosa or exposed submucosa should be cleansed with a dilute solution of aqueous povidone-iodine before antibiotic ointment is applied liberally. In most cases, lesions will have epithelialized by the first postpartum estrus ("foal heat"). When large areas of ulceration are present, treatment should be repeated every three to four days for up to two weeks. Intermittent massage with ointment has given better results than administration via a self-retaining catheter.

Adhesions. Fibrous adhesions are formed when mucosal defects allow exposed submucosal tissues to lie in apposition. As organization and contraction occur in this scar tissue, the cervical canal may be distorted or obliterated, which may lead to cervical incompetence (inability to close the external os) and pregnancy failure.

Immature adhesions should be manually debrided and antibiotic ointment applied every three days for 7 to 10 days to encourage epithelialization of the small areas of exposed submucosa. Mature adhesions are best treated by surgical resection and debridement. If this produces areas of exposed submucosa greater than 1 cm across, the mucosal edges should be undermined and reapposed with polyglycolic acid sutures in a continuous horizontal mattress pattern, aiming for first-intention healing to avoid excessive fibroblastic activity.

Lacerations. Excessive cervical stretching during parturition can cause total disruption of the muscularis and of the vaginal and cervical mucosal layers. A wedge-shaped defect can be palpated in the body of the cervix, with its base at the external os. Before surgical correction is attempted, it is wise to examine the complete genital tract (including endometrial biopsy examination) to establish that the mare has a reasonable breeding prognosis.

Surgical repair is best performed with the mare restrained in a standing position, using epidural anesthesia. The layers of the cervix are more easily delineated during diestrus. A course of antibiotics, such as systemic procaine penicillin, is begun preoperatively, and tetanus prophylaxis is advisable. The rectum is evacuated to maximize vaginal diameter and to prevent defecation during surgery. The base of the tail and a large area of the perineum and buttocks should be clipped, washed, and surgically scrubbed, as the surgical field is very difficult to drape. The tail is bandaged and tied forward.

Two heavy-gauge coated multifilament sutures are placed through each caudal edge of the defect and are then gently retracted to bring the cervix as close to the vulval lips as possible, thus improving surgical access. These retention sutures may then be held by assistants or may be attached to Balfour retractors. The retractors are used to dilate the caudal vagina and may be placed over the base of the tail, obviating the need for manual retraction. Access to the cervix is improved, compared to that obtained by use of the Caslick's speculum. With the cervix retracted, long-handled instruments are used to debride the edges of the wedge-shaped defect, exposing the two mucosal layers and the muscularis.

For dorsal cervical defects, a continuous horizontal mattress suture pattern is placed in the cervical canal submucosa. Suturing is begun cranially, at the apex of the defect, and continued caudally (toward the surgeon). The sutures are placed in the submucosa and evert the mucosa into the lumen of the cervical canal. For ventral or ventrolateral defects, the suture line is placed in the vaginal submucosa, and the mucosa is everted into the lumen of the vagina, away from the cervical canal. For both types of defect, the muscularis layer is then closed with a simple continuous pattern, the sutures being placed close together and well back from the edge of the defect. The remaining mucosal layer is apposed using a continuous horizontal mattress pattern in the submucosa.

The course of systemic antibiotics should be maintained for three days. In order to minimize adhesion formation between the suture line and the vaginal wall, gentle manipulation and application of nitrofurazone ointment may be performed on days 4, 8, and 12 postoperatively. Alternatively, elevation of the cervix from the vaginal floor may be achieved by passing the tension sutures through a loop of multifilament suture in the vaginal roof, and then attaching them to the vestibule. Mating should not be allowed for at least 30 days following surgery.

A guarded long-term breeding prognosis must be given following the repair of a cervical laceration, although at least one successful pregnancy can usually be expected. The cervix may be lacerated again at subsequent foalings, but the defect is usually not so extensive and the cervix may remain competent. The appearance of the cervix following surgery is usually far from normal. However, examination during diestrus will give an indication of the success of the surgery in re-establishing the competence of the uterovaginal sphincter.

Incompetence. This defect results from tearing of the circular cervical muscularis without any associated mucosal damage. It can also result from poor healing following surgical closure of a cervical laceration if submucosal tissue becomes trapped between the edges of the muscularis. Surgical repair essentially consists of converting the defect to a cervical laceration by resection of the redundant mucosal layers. Special care must be taken during debridement to ensure total exposure of the edges of the muscularis so that they can be accurately apposed during closure.

A retention suture of nonabsorbable Mersilene has been used as an additional support for the incompetent cervix. The suture is placed submucosally during the first two days after breeding and ovulation. However, the suture must be removed before foaling, or the resultant cervical damage may be irreparable. Cervical injury is always a serious threat to a brood mare's career, but careful treatment with particular attention to detail may produce useful results and is thus worth attempting.

Supplemental Readings

Evans, L. H., Tate, L. P., Cooper, W. L., and Robertson, J. T.: Surgical repair of cervical lacerations and the incompetent cervix. Proc. 21st. Annu. Conv. Am. Assoc. Eq. Pract., 1980, pp. 483–486.

Roberts, S. J.: Infertility in the mare. *In* Roberts, S. J.: Veterinary obstetrics and genital diseases. Published by the author, Ann Arbor, 1971.

Sisson, S.: Urogenital System. *In* Getty, R. (ed.): Sisson and Grossman's the anatomy of domestic animals. Philadelphia, W. B. Saunders Company, 1975.

Walker, D. F., and Vaughan, J. T.: Surgery of the cervix and uterus. *In* Walker, D. F., Vaughan, J. T.: Bovine and Equine Urogenital Surgery. Philadelphia, Lea & Febiger, 1980.

Perineal Conformation Abnormalities

Sidney W. Ricketts, NEWMARKET, ENGLAND

In 1937, Caslick first described deteriorations in perineal conformation that caused pneumovagina, cervicitis, endometritis, and subfertility in Thoroughbred mares. The "normal" mare has three functional genital seals forming a barrier between the external environment and the uterine lumen: the vulva, the vestibule, and the cervix. During estrus the vulva and cervix relax, leaving the vestibule as the sole seal. When the vulva is high in relation to the pelvic brim, the vestibular seal is compromised and pneumovagina occurs. When the vulva slopes cranially toward a "sunken" anus, pneumovagina is complicated by fecal material falling into the vestibule. When the vestibule and urethral opening are displaced cranially, urovagina may occur.

SURGICAL REPAIR METHODS

CASLICK OPERATION

The Caslick operation is an important procedure in equine stud farm medicine. Under local anesthesia a thin strip of the mucocutaneous junction is removed from either side of the vulva from the upper commisure to the level of the pelvic brim. The exposed submucosal tissues on either side of the vulva are sutured together to close it. This reduces the vulval aperture and usually prevents pneumovagina and fecal contamination of the vestibule.

Once the vulva has been sutured, an episiotomy must be performed before foaling or major damage may occur. An episiotomy must also be performed on "tightly stitched" mares before natural coitus, or injury to the stallion's penis or mare's vulva may occur. The episiotomy wound must be repaired after foaling or coitus to prevent pneumovagina. Repeated episiotomy followed by closure leads to loss of vulval tissue, poor healing, and, on occasion, major veterinary and management problems. In mares with a concave, sloping vulva, the results of Caslick's operation are often poor even though the vulval lips have been sutured to the level of the clitoris. The procedure has no effect on urovagina.

POURET'S PROCEDURE

In an attempt to overcome unwelcome sequelae of the Caslick operation, Pouret described an alternative operation that does not reduce the size of the vulval aperture, and corrects pneumovagina and urovagina. Pouret suggests that as mares become older, abdominal muscles slacken and the intestinal tract displaces cranioventrally. This results in a cranial displacement of the rectum and anus, which, because of their intimate muscular and ligamentous connections with the caudal vagina (Fig. 1), results in cranial displacement of the upper commisure of the vulva. Surgical sectioning of these muscular and ligamentous connections allows the rectum and anus to displace cranially and the vagina and vulva to return caudally to their normal position, producing a vertical vulva (Fig. 2). The vestibule, including the urethral opening, moves caudally, allowing improved voiding of urine.

Ideally, the mare is restrained, bridled, in stocks. Tranquilization is recommended. I have found that detomidine hydrochloride* at a dose rate of 8 μg per kg intravenously, is particularly useful because, in addition to its analgesic effects, it helps to immobilize the patient. Tetanus vaccination status is supplemented as necessary. Antibacterial treatment is started before surgery, and trimethoprim sulphonamides by intravenous injection are recommended. Using standard methods, epidural anesthesia is performed. To avoid residual sensitivity

---

*Domosedan, Farmos Group, Turku, Finland

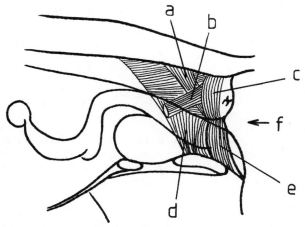

Figure 1. Diagram of lateral view of the pelvic organs of a mare with a sloping vulva. Anatomical relationships of the perineal muscles and ligaments are shown.

a, Vulval suspensory ligament; b, anal retractor muscle; c, anal sphincter muscle; d, vulval constrictor muscle; e, caudal vulval constrictor muscle; and f, plane of surgical dissection. (Adapted from Pouret, E. J. M.: Surgical technique for the correction of pneumo- and urovagina. Equine Vet. J. *14*:249, 1982.)

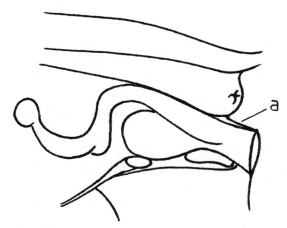

Figure 2. Diagram of lateral view of the pelvic organs of a mare following surgery, showing the horizontal anovulval shelf (a) that has been created.

from incomplete epidural block, local infiltration anesthesia is recommended. Approximately 20 ml of local anesthetic is infiltrated into the rectovaginal shelf and under the vulvoanal skin. Adrenalin in the local anesthetic may perform a useful hemostatic function. Feces are removed from the rectum, and the perineum is thoroughly cleansed and scrubbed. The bandaged tail is held or tied out of the surgical site.

A 4 to 5 cm horizontal skin incision is made halfway between the anus and vulva. The subcutaneous tissues are separated with scissors and the upper skin margin is elevated, by an assistant, with Aliss' tissue forceps. Straight Mayo scissors are used and the points are kept slightly down to avoid accidental rectal penetration; sharp and blunt dissection is made cranially and laterally to split the rectovaginal shelf. For a right-handed surgeon, it is helpful to place the left hand into the vagina to aid orientation. At approximately 10 cm cranial to the perineum, muscular tissue disappears at the level of the peritoneal reflection. It is then important to section any residual muscular tissue laterally along the line of dissection. During the dissection, the cranial displacement of the anus and the caudal return of the vulva become progressively apparent and a horizontal perineal shelf forms. No attempts are made to close the subcutaneous "dead space." However, the skin must be sealed carefully to obtain primary intention healing. I recommend a 00-gauge monofilament nylon suture and a T-shaped closure (Fig. 3) to make maximal use of the horizontal perineal shelf.

Postsurgical swelling is minimized with 1 gm phenylbutazone given intravenously at the end of surgery. Antibacterial cover is maintained with trimethoprim sulphonamides given orally or by injection. The wound is cleansed and antibacterial pow-

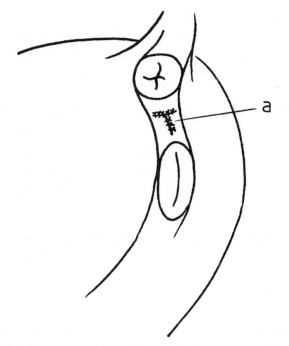

Figure 3. Diagram of rear view of the perineum of a mare following surgery, showing the T-shaped skin closure (*a*), which helps to maximize and maintain the horizontal shelf.

der applied daily until sutures are removed at 10 days. Walking exercise is given from day 1 and natural coitus is avoided for three weeks.

Pouret reported 19 surgical cases and, to date, I have operated on 20 mares. No serious untoward sequelae have been encountered during or after this operation, or later during coitus or parturition. Wound breakdown has occurred in five cases, four of which were associated with seroma formation and one an acute inflammatory response, but all eventually healed satisfactorily. All procedures have resulted in improvements in perineal conformation. Less satisfactory results, in terms of conformation improvement, were obtained in two mares in which lateral dissection was incomplete.

The Pouret perineal reconstruction operation is recommended for mares with poor perineal conformation. Many of the mares operated on so far have been older mares, with poor breeding histories, multiple genital abnormalities, and previously sutured vulvas. Postsurgical fertility can thus not be used as a measure of success. It is hoped that as the technique becomes more widely used, increased confidence will lead to its use as a "first-choice" operation. A reduction in the incidence and degree of vulval suturing in the brood mare population would provide an important management advantage.

Supplemental Readings

Caslick, E. A.: The vulva and vulvo-vaginal orifice and its relation to genital health of the Thoroughbred mare. Cornell Vet., 27:178, 1937.

Pouret, E. J. M.: Surgical technique for the correction of pneumo- and urovagina. Equine Vet. J., *14*:249, 1982.

Abortion

John Hyland, MELBOURNE, AUSTRALIA
Leo B. Jeffcott, MELBOURNE, AUSTRALIA

Abortion is the expulsion of a nonviable fetus before day 300 of gestation. This chapter is intended to give the reader a practical overview of abortion; we shall refer to abortion as meaning loss of a nonviable fetus from day 40 to term. Early embryonic mortality (see p. 525), placental defects (see p. 528), and the effects of twinning (see p. 532) are dealt with elsewhere in this section.

Estimates of the incidence of abortion in mares vary from 2 to 14 per cent. The wide range arises because many abortions are not observed, recording methods vary, and many different systems of stud management are involved. As a rule, abortions occur sporadically with the exception of those due to equine herpesvirus (EHV-1) infection, which can be responsible for abortion "storms." Mares rarely abort in consecutive years with the exception of mares that repeatedly conceive twins.

CLINICAL SIGNS

Frequently there are no observed premonitory signs of abortion. The mare may simply be empty at the end of gestation, the autolyzing fetus may be found in the paddock or stable, or the fetal membranes may be seen hanging from the vulval lips. When abortion is a sudden event, there may be a short first stage of labor followed by delivery of the fetus by the mare in lateral recumbency. More often, however, the abortus is simply expelled by the standing mare. The fetal membranes are usually delivered with the fetus.

A mucopurulent vaginal discharge is usually an indication of chronic fungal or bacterial placentitis. However, a vulval discharge will also be present if the fetus becomes autolyzed in utero or remains in the vaginal vestibule for periods of 24 hours or more. Mummification of equine fetuses is rare except in the cases of twin and triplet pregnancies. Fetal resorption is common in mares in which early embryonic mortality occurs.

In the more protracted abortions involving some degree of placental separation there is often premature mammary development. Lactation (running of milk) can occur in some instances for weeks before the abortion. Signs of impending parturition are frequent, and the mare may separate from the others a short time before aborting. Dystocia is uncommon with singleton pregnancies because of the relatively small size of the fetus, which can often be delivered despite abnormal position or presentation. However, twin fetuses occasionally present at the pelvic inlet together, resulting in dystocia. Complications of abortion are infrequent, although uterine infection and laminitis may occur in association with retained fetal membranes. Less frequently, uterine prolapse and rupture of the utero-ovarian artery may occur.

PATHOGENESIS

The causes of equine abortion can be conveniently grouped under the headings of *noninfectious* and *infectious* (Table 1). Twinning is the most important cause of abortion, and infectious abortions are usually much less common than noninfectious ones.

Abortion presumably results from the release of prostaglandins, which cause cervical dilatation and uterine contractions. Fetal death may be caused by hematogenous spread of bacteria or viruses through the placenta, killing the fetus directly or indirectly because of placental damage. Torsion of the umbilical cord and other physical disturbances may cause fetal death by asphyxiation and cardiac arrest. Fetal death is not always the cause of abortion; occasionally, the fetus is born with a beating heart and respiratory movements. In these cases placental pathology or maternal endocrinologic disturbances are responsible for expulsion of the fetus, which is unable to survive outside the uterus.

NONINFECTIOUS CAUSES OF ABORTION

Placental Defects. A mild degree of twisting of the umbilical cord often occurs in normal pregnancies and may be accompanied by small urachal dilatations. Pathologic twisting of the cord is much more dramatic, with swelling, congestion, large urachal dilatations, and impairment of blood supply. The result is fetal anoxia and death followed by an abortion usually between six and nine months' gestation. The underlying cause is not certain, but the cord is often abnormally long, greater than 90 cm. Strangulation of the cord around the fetal neck or trunk is rare.

The normal site of implantation in the mare is at the junction of the uterine body and uterine horns. Occasionally, attachment may occur only in the body (i.e., body pregnancy). This leads to placental insufficiency and generally results in abortion at around eight months of gestation. Bicornual pregnancy has also been recorded, but this condition usually results in dystocia rather than abortion.

Other placental problems involve a degree of separation of the placenta before term or just before second-stage labor. The pathogenesis of this condition is not known, but it is assumed to be associated with a hormonal imbalance.

Maternal Stress. Stress due to psychologic influences or systemic illness may precipitate an abortion, although the role of stress is difficult to prove. Abortion from physical causes is uncommon, although there have been cases in which several mares aborted soon after being disturbed by low-flying aircraft. Most owners will not transport mares long distances in the latter stages of gestation. Colics and other types of debilitating disease sometimes result in abortion.

Immunologic Incompatibility. This is occasionally stated as a possible cause of abortion. The epitheliochorial placenta of the mare is impermeable to large molecules from the fetal circulation so that the maternal immune system should not be stimulated to reject the fetus during pregnancy. Furthermore, the fetus contains paternal antigens, and the

TABLE 1. MAJOR CAUSES OF ABORTION IN THE MARE

Noninfectious Causes	Infectious Causes
Placental Defects	Bacterial
Umbilical cord defects	*Streptococcus zooepidemicus*
Abnormal implantation	*Escherichia coli*
Premature placental	*Staphylococcus aureus*
separation	*Pseudomonas aeruginosa*
Twinning	*Salmonella abortus equi*
Maternal Stress	*Klebsiella aerogenes*
Immunologic Incompatibility	*Brucella abortus*
Chromosomal Defects	Leptospira spp.
Iatrogenic	Viral
Nutritional and Toxic	Equine herpesvirus (EHV-1)
	Equine viral arteritis (EVA)
	Fungal
	Aspergillus spp.
	Mucor spp.
	Allescheria boydii

fact that the vast majority of mares carry foals successfully suggests that this immunologic difference between mother and fetus is unrecognized. In rare cases in which fetal red blood cells escape into the maternal circulation through the placenta, autoimmune hemolytic disease occurs in the foal (see p. 244).

Chromosomal Defects. There are no documented accounts of chromosomal defects being responsible for abortion in mares. The major problem in studying the chromosomal composition of aborted fetuses is the technical difficulty of culturing explants of the fetus after death. There is a high incidence of chromosomal anomalies in spontaneous abortions from women and it is likely that chromosomal defects contribute to the overall reproductive wastage in mares. Chromosomal defects may be reflected as an increase in embryonic mortality rather than abortion.

Iatrogenic Abortion. The main indication for induction of abortion in the mare is twin pregnancy. Abortion is usually performed as early in gestation as possible so that the mare can be bred again the same season. Multiple injections of prostaglandin or prostaglandin analogs have been used with varying degrees of success; 20 to 100 IU oxytocin given intramuscularly has achieved a high success rate as an abortifacient in mares 280 to 327 days pregnant. Infusion of 1 to 3 liters of hypertonic saline (1700 to 2350 mOsm) via the cervix into the amniotic sac has also been effective in inducing abortion in mares at 99 to 153 days of gestation.

It has been suggested that veterinary drugs given to mares during susceptible periods of fetal growth may result in teratogenicity and abortion.

Nutritional and Toxic Causes of Abortion. Poor nutrition may play a role in equine abortion, although this has yet to be definitely proven. Van Niekerk recorded embryonic resorption in mares grazing poor-quality pasture, although two of five mares in the same study that received supplementary feeding also suffered embryonic loss. On well-managed stud farms in developed countries, lack of energy intake is unlikely to be a cause of abortion.

Various plant species have been incriminated in abortions occurring during late gestation in mares. Fescue grass has been suspected of predisposing to abortion and agalactia. The cause may be a selenium deficiency. Selenium supplementation in combination with vitamin E* can be given intramuscularly (11 mg selenium and 100 mg vitamin E per 100 kg body weight every 2 weeks). Sorghum and Sudan grasses have also been associated with abortions in mares, but a direct cause-effect relationship has not been established. On sorghum and Sudan grass

*E-Se Injection, Burns-Biotec, Omaha, NB

pastures, iodine deficiency may occur, resulting in abortion of goitrous foals with long hair and muscle wasting. Iodine supplementation via salt licks may be indicated in mares grazing these types of pastures.

Certain types of pastures in Kentucky have also been incriminated in abortions occurring between two and four months of gestation. Most abortions occur in May and June, suggesting that the stage of pasture growth is important. These mares had conceived early in the breeding season and physiologic signs of estrus during pregnancy may have predisposed these mares to ascending genital infection.

Some anthelmintics, such as carbon tetrachloride, phenothiazine, and the organophosphates, have been associated with equine abortions. It is recommended that these compounds not be used in pregnant mares.

INFECTIOUS CAUSES OF ABORTION

Bacterial. Bacterial abortions constitute up to 13 per cent of all equine abortions. The most commonly isolated types are beta-hemolytic streptococci, *Escherichia coli*, pseudomonas spp., *Staphylococcus aureus*, and Enterobacter spp. Contagious abortion caused by *Salmonella abortus equi* was common 50 years ago, but it has disappeared from most parts of the world. There are three possible routes of infection that result in abortion: (1) hematogenous spread to the fetus via intercurrent infection of the mare, (2) local spread from foci of deep-seated endometritis, and (3) ascending infection via the cervix of the mare, causing placentitis.

Ascending infection is the most common means by which bacteria cause abortion in mares. The placentitis can be recognized as a thickened edematous area in the chorioallantois, commencing from the cervical star. The affected chorion may be covered with a thick brown exudate, consisting of sloughed microvilli and blood. There is usually a definite demarcation line separating the diseased placenta from the normal chorioallantois. The fetus may become infected by direct spread through the allantoic and amniotic cavities into the fetal stomach and lungs, or via the allantoic veins. Pregnancy continues until the remaining area of functional placenta is insufficient to maintain pregnancy, causing fetal distress or death or both, which precipitates parturition. Alternatively, septicemia may occur first, resulting in fetal death and abortion. The fetus may be stunted and emaciated because of the progressive placental insufficiency. This type of ascending placentitis has been caused by *S. zooepidemicus*, *E. coli*, *P. aeruginosa*, *S. aureus*, *K. aerogenes*, and *Enterobacter agglomerans*. Presumably, these organisms enter the cervix as a result of faulty vulval conformation and associated pneumovagina. Mares in which abortions are suspected to be caused by ascending infection of the placenta should undergo Caslick's operation as soon after service as is practicable. The use of minimal contamination breeding techniques or artificial insemination should also be considered.

Mycotic. Fungi are responsible for up to 10 per cent of all abortions in mares. The most common fungi involved are Mucor spp., Aspergillus spp., and *Allescheria boydii.* A mare may run milk for days or even weeks before abortion, and occasionally a thick brown, sticky vulval exudate may be seen. Mycotic abortions occur in the latter part of gestation (8 to 11 months). The fetus is usually small and emaciated and is sometimes born alive but almost invariably succumbs soon after birth.

The fungi are opportunist agents and enter the uterus via the cervix, causing ascending placentitis. There is thickening and necrosis of the maternal chorionic surface and, presumably, lesions on the endometrial surface of the uterus. In 10 per cent of cases the amniotic membrane contains a series of irregular necrotic plaques. Rarely, there are lesions within the fetus and these consist of grayish-white nodules in the lungs. In these cases, the amnion is invariably involved, the amniotic fluid becomes infected, and the fetus takes the fungal hyphae into its lungs during respiratory movements. The placental lesions cause a reduction of nutrients available to the fetus, resulting in the abortion of emaciated foals.

After abortion, there may be a purulent vulval discharge for some days that resolves spontaneously; intrauterine treatment is not usually necessary (see p. 505). However, mares should not be mated until recovery is confirmed by endometrial culture and cytologic examinations. Because veterinary gynecologic examinations before service may introduce fungi into the reproductive tract of the mare, such examinations should be performed in a hygienic manner.

Viral

EQUINE HERPESVIRUS TYPE 1. The most frequent cause of infectious equine abortion is equine herpesvirus type 1 (EHV-1). The virus is transmitted via the respiratory tract, by ingestion of contaminated feedstuffs, or by fomites. Immunity to abortion is of short duration, persisting for only four to six months, and so repeated abortions may occur in successive years. Pregnant mares exposed to infection may abort within three weeks to four months. They do so without premonitory signs and the fetus is usually enclosed in its membranes. Although the virus survives for 14 days outside the body, occasionally survival may be extended to 40 days if the virus is dried on horse hairs.

The incidence of viral abortion is variable (1 to 5 per cent), and abortion "storms" are occasionally recorded. Abortion occurs from five months of gestation onward but more commonly between nine months of gestation and term. Sometimes the foal is born alive, but death frequently ensues in a few hours to a few days.

Characteristic lesions are seen at postmortem examination in most aborted fetuses. The most consistent gross lesion is severe edema of the lungs, these organs being heavy and rubbery with a pitting response to pressure and edema of the interlobular septa. Other findings include excessive clear fluid in the pleural cavity, edema of the pharyngeal tissues and subcutis, and slight jaundice of the mucous membranes. Hepatic lesions consist of small, grayish-white foci of necrosis from pinpoint size to 5 mm diameter, seen under the capsule. Pericardial effusion occurs occasionally, with numerous petechiae on the epicardium. The placenta is sometimes edematous but exhibits no other lesions typical of EHV-1 infection.

Histologically, the lesions in the liver, lung, and spleen are necrotic without cellular infiltration. Although intranuclear inclusion bodies may be found in several tissues, they occur most frequently in the liver and lungs. Numerous small necrotic foci occur in the liver with evidence of nuclear damage. The surrounding parenchymal cells contain specific quadrilateral intranuclear, acidophilic inclusions, typical of the herpesviruses (Cowdray; type A). Bronchiolitis, with small amounts of catarrhal exudate in the affected bronchioles, can usually be found in the lungs. Inclusions can sometimes be seen in the nuclei of the bronchial and alveolar epithelial cells. In the spleen there is enlargement of the malpighian corpuscles, necrosis of lymphocytes and hemorrhages in the splenic pulp. No microscopic changes have been described in the placenta in field cases of abortion.

There are currently two EHV-1 vaccines commercially available, one an attenuated live-virus formulation and the other a killed preparation of the virus. Only the killed vaccine is recommended for protection of mares from abortion caused by EHV-1. A series of inoculations must be given to mares at five, seven, and nine months of gestation. It has also been suggested that mares should be vaccinated at two to three months of pregnancy to eliminate early abortions that may be caused by the virus. Use of the EHV-1 vaccines coincided with a reduction in diagnosed EHV-1 abortion from 25 to 10 per cent in Kentucky between 1950 and 1980.

Mares that have aborted and that are suspected to be infected with EHV-1 should be isolated until the diagnosis is confirmed. Any bedding used by the mare should be burned. Staff attending the mare should wear plastic gloves and rubber boots, which must be thoroughly disinfected before other mares are attended. The mare's reproductive tract should be irrigated with an antiseptic solution such as cetrimide and the tail and perineal region must be thoroughly cleansed. Bridles and other equipment used for these mares must not be applied to other horses before they are thoroughly cleaned and disinfected. If the abortion has occurred in a paddock it should be cleared of all horses for a period of four weeks. A mare is considered noninfectious four weeks after the abortion has taken place. The aborted fetus and the placenta should be placed in a plastic bag and taken directly to a diagnostic laboratory for pathologic examination.

EQUINE VIRAL ARTERITIS. Equine viral arteritis (EVA) virus has caused abortion in mares between 5 and 10 months of gestation. In the 1950s the virus occurred frequently on farms in the United States and was responsible for many abortions.

The virus is transmitted between horses as an aerosol and the disease has an incubation period of 7 to 10 days. Unlike EHV-1 abortions, in which the mare is unaffected, EVA causes moderate to severe depression, high temperature, leukopenia, keratitis, palpebral edema, photophobia, and edematous swellings of the extremities and ventral abdomen. Fetal death is followed by abortion 7 to 10 days after first signs of illness in the mother. The fetus is often autolyzed; however when it is fresh there may be no lesions observed on gross autopsy. Occasionally, pleural effusion and petechial hemorrhages on the pleura may be seen. Immunofluorescent tests on fetal tissue and serum neutralization tests on the sera of infected mares are used for definitive diagnosis of EVA abortion.

In 1984 the Kentucky breeding season was disrupted by an outbreak of EVA in a number of stallions and mares on different stud farms. The disease was apparently transmitted venereally, with the EVA virus detected in the semen of nine of the stallions. A blood testing program revealed that 55 of 630 (8.7 per cent) stallions showed a positive reaction, indicating exposure to EVA. Of the 55 reactors, 37 had been vaccinated. No field abortions were recorded in affected mares. However, research with the EVA virus at the University of Kentucky produced abortions in 5 of 14 experimental mares, with the earliest abortion occurring at 100 days of gestation. Subsequently, one of these mares developed a carrier state, shedding the virus in urine while remaining clinically healthy. Vaccination is effective and it has been recommended that all Thoroughbreds over the age of four months be vaccinated.

Although other viruses such as equine infectious anemia (EIA) virus and coronavirus have been found to be associated with abortion, their involvement is circumstantial.

GENERAL CONSIDERATIONS

TREATMENT

In cases of noncontagious abortion, the main consideration is to return the mare to a satisfactory condition for mating. If the abortion has been diagnosed as due to an infectious agent, the mare should be treated for endometritis. Intrauterine infusion of the appropriate antibiotic or antiseptic solution for several days is indicated (see p. 505). Abstinence from mating for the ensuing breeding season may be necessary. Uterine involution may be aided by administration of oxytocin. An endometrial bacteriologic culture and cytologic examination should be carried out at the next estrus. If this indicates no evidence of endometritis, the mare may be mated at that estrus. If abortion occurs early in gestation, the mare may not commence estrous cycles for several months. In these cases, initial treatment should be given and endometrial examination performed when the mare begins cycling in the breeding season. Noninfectious abortions usually do not require antibacterial treatment unless secondary infection occurs.

PREVENTION

It is doubtful that abortion can be successfully prevented using current knowledge and technology. Prediction of which mares are likely to undergo abortion is impossible, whether it be of infectious, hormonal, or genetic origin. If genetic abnormalities are present in a fetus the sooner the mare aborts the better.

The most common prophylactic measure is to treat mares with exogenous progesterone, either by oral or parenteral administration. Doses of depot progesterone in the order of 1 gm intramuscularly twice per week need to be given to maintain adequate blood levels for early pregnancy in ovariectomized mares. Once the placenta has taken over progesterone production from the ovaries (around day 70 of gestation) exogenous supplementation is unlikely to be necessary.

Endometrial incompetence may be a cause of nonepidemic abortion in older mares. In this case, treatment is unlikely to be successful because of fibrotic changes occurring in the endometrium. An attempt to improve the condition of the endometrium may be made by curettage (see p. 506) or intrauterine plasma infusion (see p. 510).

CONCLUSIONS

Much has been learned in recent years about the nature of equine pregnancy and abortion. However, there is still a great deal unknown, particularly about noninfectious causes of abortion. The overall incidence of abortion in the Thoroughbred, with the possible recent exception of that caused by twin pregnancy, has not been significantly reduced in the last 30 years in spite of modern methods of husbandry, diagnosis, and control. In order to minimize the risks of abortion, the following recommendations are made:

1. Clinical examination of the mare before mating.
2. Endometrial bacteriologic and cytologic examination before mating if necessary, but certainly after an abortion. It is important that known infectious mares *not* be mated without veterinary advice.
3. Hygienic measures at mating and parturition to minimize the entry of microorganisms into the uterus. Vaccination of mares against viral abortion if this is indicated.
4. Attention to the health and husbandry of brood mares throughout gestation.
5. Isolation and sanitary precautions for mares and stables after an abortion has occurred.
6. Pathologic examination of all aborted fetuses *and* the fetal membranes to determine the infective nature of an abortion and prevent its spread.

Supplemental Readings

Bosu, W. T. K., and McKinnon, A. O.: Induction of abortion during midgestation in mares. Can. Vet. J., 23:358, 1982.
Neely, D. P., and Hawkins, D. L.: A two-year study of the clinical and serologic responses of horses to a modified live-virus equine rhinopneumonitis vaccine. J. Equine Med. Surg., 2:532, 1978.
Neely, D. P.: Causes and prevention of abortion. *In* Robinson, N. E. (ed.) Current Therapy in Equine Medicine, 1st ed. Philadelphia, W. B. Saunders Company, 1983.
Rossdale, P. D., and Ricketts, S. W.: Equine Studfarm Medicine, 2nd ed. London, Bailliere Tindall, 1980, pp. 195–206.
van Niekerk, C. H.: Early embryonic resorption in mares (a preliminary report). J. S. Afr. Vet. Med. Assoc., 36:61, 1965.
Whitwell, K. E.: Investigations into fetal and neonatal losses in the horse. Vet. Clin. North Am. (Large Anim. Pract.), 2:313, 1980.

Early Fetal Death

Kerstin Darenius, UPPSALA, SWEDEN

Early fetal death (EFD) is defined as death of the conceptus before 150 days of gestation. It can be divided into embryonic and fetal death with the dividing line at day 40 of gestation, when organogenesis is complete.

The incidence of EFD reported in the literature ranges from 5 to 45 per cent, which reflects both diagnostic difficulties and differences between horse populations. Use of ultrasound echography has increased the accuracy of routine early pregnancy diagnosis. The incidence of EFD under conditions of modern stud farm management is usually 10 to 15 per cent.

No category of mares—lactating, maiden, or barren—has been proved to be especially susceptible to pregnancy loss. Lactating mares have a relatively high incidence of EFD when mated during postpartum estrus but not when mated during later estrous periods.

PATHOGENESIS

Few cases of EFD have been studied in detail and their causes established. Experimentally, maternal malnutrition has been shown to cause EFD between 25 and 31 days of gestation. Bacterial endometritis is one of the most important causes of EFD. In the acute form, at the time of mating, this often results in conception failure. However, low-grade persistent endometritis after mating may result in EFD. Embryonic or fetal death may occur following direct infection or following infection of the placental membranes. Recurrent acute endometritis can also result in diffuse endometrial fibrosis, which may cause abnormal placental function and fetal loss.

Genetic factors are known to be major causes of EFD in other species and are thus also suspected in the horse. The genetic factors involved are not necessarily inherited by the parents; indeed, the majority probably arise anew in each parent generation and some are likely to arise in the definitive gametes, as a result of aging. Chromosome defects that may arise during early embryonic cell division may adversely affect organogenesis and may result in death at a later stage. The diagnosis is difficult to make since the products of EFD in mares are rarely available for examination and chromosome studies require fresh tissues.

Inbreeding, a common feature in most modern horse populations, has been thought to reduce fertility. Although not a proven cause of EFD, the resulting increased homozygosity and increased genetic similarity between dam and embryo may not be conducive to normal pregnancy.

Early fetal death is relatively common in mares with twin pregnancies. Double ovulations increase the likelihood of conception but also the risk of EFD to one or both conceptuses.

Maternal stress during pregnancy can cause EFD. Severe pain, infectious diseases, emotional disturbance, and exogenous corticosteroid administration have been shown to depress plasma progestagen levels in pregnant mares. Many mares are subjected to long, tiring journeys that might be unduly stressful. The period of pregnancy most susceptible to stress has not been identified. However, it would be wise to avoid the 20- to 45-day stage when critical events such as transition from yolk sac to chorioallantoic placentation, development of endometrial cups, attachment, and organogenesis are occurring.

DIAGNOSIS

Repeated gynecologic examinations are often required to make an accurate diagnosis of EFD. Ultrasound echography has made confirmation possible at 14 to 40 days. A relatively high incidence of EFD is suspected during the first 14 days of gestation. This is seldom diagnosed because luteolysis and return to estrus occurs at the same time as for nonpregnant mares. If EFD occurs after day 15, the primary corpus luteum may persist for 30 to 90 days, resulting in persistent diestrus or "pseudopregnancy." The cervix remains tightly closed, the ovaries have multiple follicular development, and the uterus is tense and tubular. The diagnosis of nonpregnancy is made by the absence of a fetal bulge and conceptus (confirmed by ultrasound echography). If EFD occurs after endometrial cup formation—that is, after 36 days—the mare may not return to fertile estrus until 90 to 150 days after conception. Even if luteolysis is induced with exogenous prostaglandins during this period, circulating equine chorionic gonadotropin (eCG), produced by the endometrial cups, appears to inhibit normal estrus. Sometimes erratic estrus occurs, with multiple ovarian follicular development without subsequent ovulation. Plasma progesterone concentrations then gradually increase and the follicles become palpably firmer. The conception rate for mares mated during these abnormal estrous periods is poor.

RECTAL PALPATION

Between 17 and 21 days of gestation, rectal palpation reveals an increase in uterine tone, often before a conceptual swelling is accurately detectable. This feature has been used as an indication of early pregnancy. However, variations in tone within pregnant mares, nonpregnant mares, and mares with EFD make an accurate diagnosis at this stage difficult. At 40 to 45 days the fetal sac can normally be palpated as a distinct enlargement of the uterine horn, 4 to 10 cm in diameter. Palpation findings in EFD depend on the interval between embryonic or fetal death and collapse of the fetal sac. During the embryonic stage of pregnancy these events usually coincide, causing the uterine contents to become diffuse and giving the uterus a somewhat enlarged and doughy consistency. This state can persist for many weeks, making subsequent differentiation between normal pregnancy and EFD difficult. When EFD occurs during the fetal stage, the sac may remain intact for some time. In one mare serially studied with ultrasound echography, EFD occurred at day 50 but the sac remained intact until day 110, when it collapsed and abortion occurred. This situation demonstrates the limitations of pregnancy diagnosis by rectal palpation alone.

ULTRASOUND ECHOGRAPHY

Real-time ultrasound echography has provided major improvements in the accuracy of pregnancy diagnosis and early confirmation of EFD. The condition should be suspected in the following situations:

1. The circular dark-colored fluid image is "small for dates." A 16- to 20-day conceptus should be at least 20 mm in diameter, but serial examinations are essential to differentiate EFD from a small but viable conceptus possibly undergoing embryonic "rest" or diapause. Although an endometrial cyst (see p. 507) may also be confused with a small conceptus, the former often has a strongly echogenic cyst wall.

2. The fluid image is irregular in outline and has a speckled or granular appearance. It must be remembered that the conceptus normally becomes less circular in outline between 20 and 30 days, due to increased uterine tone.

3. No fetus is detectable after 30 days of gestation.

4. No fetal heart beat is detectable after 30 days of gestation. Between 30 to 50 days the fetal heart should be demonstrable, but later the increased size of the fetus sometimes makes this more difficult. Fetal limb and body movements may then be more easily seen.

LABORATORY TESTS

High blood levels of estrone sulphate detected by radioimmunoassay after 85 days of gestation will help to confirm that the fetus is alive. A positive eCG test does not prove fetal viability or that a fetus was present at the time of sampling, but it does prove that a conceptus was present at 35 to 40 days and that endometrial cups were formed. Once the cups have formed, eCG continues to be produced after fetal death and even abortion.

Blood and milk progesterone tests are a measure of luteal function but do not aid in the diagnosis of pregnancy or viability of the fetus.

TREATMENT

Once EFD has been accurately diagnosed, treatment is directed toward returning the mare to estrus as soon as possible and making sure that her uterus is in optimal condition for mating.

Before 36 days, prostaglandin treatment usually results in luteolysis followed by estrus with relaxation of the cervix and, in most cases, ejection of the dead fetus and placental membranes. After 36 days, circulating eCG appears to completely or partially block the effect of exogenous prostaglandins, and repeated daily or twice daily injections may be required to produce estrus. Estrous periods induced at this stage have lowered fertility. Occasionally, irrigation of the uterus with saline solution is required to complete evacuation of the uterus. The endometrium is in a relatively susceptible state to succumb to infection; thus it is always prudent to include suitable antibiotics in the irrigation mixture (see p. 505). When uterine conditions are considered satisfactory for re-mating, it is recommended that minimal contamination techniques be used.

PROPHYLAXIS

As uterine infection is an important cause of EFD, measures should be taken to avoid mating mares with acute endometritis. Routine endometrial swab samples should be collected for bacteriologic and cytologic examination before each mating period. When signs of acute endometritis are found, mating should be delayed until treatment has been undertaken. To reduce the risk of reinfection, matings should be restricted to one per estrous period, when possible, and minimal contamination techniques should be used.

In mares with a history of repeated EFD, endometrial biopsy may be useful. The histopathologic features may provide a prognosis and a basis for rational treatment (see p. 503).

Because aging gametes are known to predispose to EFD in other species, it is wise to time matings as close as possible to ovulation.

Serial pregnancy diagnoses, using rectal palpation and ultrasound echography, will help to make an early diagnosis of EFD. Ideally, it is recommended that examinations be made at: (1) 16 to 20 days after ovulation, (2) 28 to 30 days when twin pregnancy is suspected, (3) 40 to 45 days of gestation; and (4) 60 to 90 days of gestation.

An early decision regarding the management of twin pregnancy should be made, although the fact that approximately 50 per cent reduce to singletons before 25 to 30 days of gestation makes the correct decision difficult. The success rate for manual rupture of one twin conceptus decreases with advancing gestational age (see p. 532).

Undue maternal stress such as long exhausting journeys should be avoided between days 20 and 45 of pregnancy. Adequate nutrition should be provided to maintain the early pregnant mare in positive energy balance. Lactating mares often require supplementary feeding.

Despite the absence of experimental evidence that progesterone deficiency is a significant cause of equine pregnancy failure, mares throughout the world are commonly given natural progesterone or synthetic progestagens at arbitrary and highly variable dose rates and intervals during gestation. The fall in plasma progesterone concentration following experimental stress (see above) has not been proved to be the cause of EFD in such cases, but this possibility still remains. Administration of progesterone to mares with histories of repeated EFD should be considered only as a last resort after the exclusion of all other possible causative factors. If progesterone supplementation is used, intramuscular doses of at least 200 mg progesterone in oil daily or 1 gm repositol progesterone every three or four days have been recommended. To avoid the common problem of injection site reactions, 22 mg allyl trenbolone may be given daily by mouth.

Many questions regarding progesterone treatment remain unanswered. If exogenous progesterone is given to a pregnant mare, the question remains as to when it is safe to discontinue treatment without causing abortion via a withdrawal effect. Exogenous administration may result in a suppression of endogenous production by a negative feedback effect; therefore, it is probably wise to continue supplementation at least until after 150 days of gestation when the placenta has taken over progesterone production from the ovaries.

Supplemental Readings

Allen, W. R.: Is your progesterone therapy really necessary? Equine Vet. J., *16*:496, 1984.
Bergin, W. C.: A survey of embryonic and perinatal losses in the horse. Proc. 15th Annu. Conv. Am. Assoc. Eq. Pract., 149, 1969.

Bishop, M. W. H.: Paternal contribution to embryonic death. J. Reprod. Fert., 7:383, 1964.

Chevalier, F. and Palmer E.: Ultrasonic echography in the mare. J. Reprod. Fert., Suppl. 32:423, 1982.

Ginther, O. J.: Reproduction in mares. Ann Arbor, McNaughton & Gunn, Inc., 1979.

Kenney, R. M.: Cyclic and pathologic changes of the mare endometrium as detected by biopsy, with a note on early embryonic death. J. Am. Vet. Med. Assoc., 172:241, 1978.

Kindahl, H., Knudsen, O., Madej, A., and Edquist, L-E.: Progesterone, prostaglandin $F_{2\alpha}$, PMSG, and estrone sulphate during early pregnancy in the mare. J. Reprod. Fert., Suppl. 32:353, 1982.

van Niekerk, C. H.: Early embryonic resorption in mares. J. S. Afr. Vet. Med. Assoc., 36:61, 1965.

van Niekerk, C. H. and Morgenthal, J. C.: Fetal loss and the effect of stress on plasma progestagen levels in pregnant Thoroughbred mares. J. Reprod. Fert., Suppl. 32:453, 1982.

Fetal Membrane Abnormalities

Katherine E. Whitwell, NEWMARKET, ENGLAND

A high proportion of equine fetal and neonatal foal deaths are accompanied by pathologic changes in the fetal membranes—that is, in the allantochorion (chorion), allantoamnion (amnion), or the umbilical cord, or in all three. In normal membranes, the outer surface of the chorion is covered by vast numbers of tiny villous tufts that interdigitate with the maternal microcotyledons. At the fetomaternal epithelial junction is a microvillous border. Fetal well-being depends on the integrity of the junction and the ability of the maternal and fetal placental components to expand and mature together. Abnormalities can lead to fetal growth defects, death, or expulsion, or all three. Following fetal death or parturition, blood flow ceases in the chorionic vessels. However, when the fetomaternal junction remains intact, there may be a sufficient oxygen-nutrient gradient to preserve the villous epithelium and even the core of the villus, such as at the tip of the nonpregnant horn in a retained placenta.

The mare has a diffuse epitheliochorial placenta. Hence, following dehiscence, the outer surface of the chorion presents a mirror image of the luminal topography of the endometrium: many lesions in the former are reflections of lesions in the latter. Deeper placental pathology may also reflect or cause fetal abnormalities. The nature of parturition and placental dehiscence may influence the appearance of the membranes. These should be examined carefully, as information gathered may prove to be diagnostically relevant or of value in the subsequent management of the mare and her foal.

METHOD OF PLACENTAL EXAMINATION

Placental examination is most conveniently performed by spreading the membranes on an approximately 1.5-meter square washable board. Notes and measurements are recorded on a placental "map." A swab should be taken routinely from the surface of the cervical star and additional swabs where indicated by the gross appearance. Any surface exudate should be examined microscopically for fungal hyphae. Both surfaces of the chorion, the amnion, the fetal fluids, the umbilical cord, and the yolk sac remnant are all examined. Note should be made of tears, missing parts, abnormalities of size, weight, shape or color, shreds of adherent endometrial tissue, and the length, attachment site, and degree of twisting of the umbilical cord. Spatial orientation of the chorion, as it would have been in utero, can be achieved by observing the manner in which the horns hang down when their tips are elevated. Routine histologic assessment of the cervical star and any areas of special interest can greatly assist in interpreting placental changes.

INFECTIVE CONDITIONS

EQUINE HERPESVIRUS 1 (EHV-1, RHINOPNEUMONITIS VIRUS)

No specific lesions have been noted in the placental membranes. However, nonspecific gross changes are often seen—more than one third of placentas from mares with EHV-1 infections have edematous, overweight chorions (greater than 4 kg); 30 per cent have no rupture of the cervical star. In over half of cases of virus abortion the fetus is found still attached to its membranes. They are expelled without warning. In a proportion of cases premature placental separation occurs, causing the intact chorion to bulge through the vulval lips. The fetus is either born inside intact membranes or the chorion ruptures transversely across its body, followed by rapid dehiscence, with the chorion villous side outermost.

Premature placental separation is not specific for EHV-1 infection and can cause stillbirth in otherwise healthy foals. Occasionally it has been seen in elective induction of parturition. The foal dies from anoxia because placental detachment occurs before it can breathe air. It may survive if the membranes are manually ruptured and birth is assisted. When a premature placental separation occurs, EHV-1 investigations should be made if the foal is stillborn or weak.

BACTERIA AND FUNGI

Bacterial and fungal infections are generally recognized from five months of gestation onward and are responsible for approximately 13 per cent of abortions and stillbirths. Most commonly, incompetent cervical defenses allow vaginal or cervical organisms to cause an ascending chorionitis at the cervical pole of the chorion. Well-established necrotizing chorionitis makes the chorion appear thickened and discolored, with villous loss or overlying exudate or both. Exceptionally, the entire uterine body may be affected, but it is more common for a smaller area (approximately 5 to 25 per cent of the chorionic surface area) to be involved. This reduction in functional chorionic surface area may be responsible for the growth retardation often noted in the fetus.

A wide variety of organisms have been associated with chorionitis, with beta-hemolytic streptococci and *Aspergillus fumigatus* being the most common bacteria and fungi isolated. In many cases, infection is restricted to the chorion, but fetal infection may occur centripetally via the allantois and amnion or be blood-borne via the umbilical vein. With the latter route, the fetus may have focal inflammatory liver lesions. With amniotic spread there may be pulmonary lesions, and organisms may be isolated from the lungs and stomach contents. Occasionally, fungal granulomatous lesions spread to the fetal organs, particularly with *Absidia ramosa* infection. Bacterial placentitis results in abortions at any stage in gestation, whereas fungal placentitis is usually chronic and causes abortions from 10 months onward.

Foals born alive, if not already septicemic, are predisposed to postnatal infection because they pass through an infected birth canal. They are often premature or weak or both, the dam's colostrum may be absent or of low immunoglobulin content (often because of premature lactation), and in some foals the lymphoreticular system may be atrophic at birth. Donor colostrum and a course of prophylactic antibiotics is therefore recommended.

Pregnant mares with premature lactation or vulval discharge or both should be examined by vaginoscopy and the discharge examined for microorganisms and inflammatory cells. The vaginitis or cervicitis or both should be treated with appropriate antimicrobial therapy and vulval surgery performed, if it is suspected that poor vulval conformation is causing pneumovagina (p. 518). If the condition is treated early, pregnancy may continue to term. Vaginitis can occur without penetration of infection through the cervix or development of placentitis. Early acute chorionitis, occurring immediately before or during parturition, may be difficult or impossible to recognize macroscopically and may only be diagnosed histologically. Rarely, mares with chorionitis have died from septicemia, following abortion. Infrequently, uteroplacental infection originates from the maternal circulation, sometimes after a period of pyrexia. The foci of chorionitis are then unassociated with the cervical star.

It has been postulated that a single persistent focus of uterine infection present before the pregnancy may result in the development of a focal chorionitis, as in one uterine horn, but proof is lacking. Infection overlying a fallopian tube ostium could lead to ascending salpingitis. A possible case was seen in a pregnant mare with repeated unexplained colic. After she aborted, a focal chorionitis was found at the tip of the left horn and a firm swelling was palpated adjacent to the left ovary. The colic ceased after a course of antibiotics.

To hasten recovery following chorionitis, the concurrent endometritis should be treated by appropriate antimicrobial therapy. It may also be necessary to enhance uterine involution with oxytocin therapy (see p. 548). These measures aim to reduce the risk of early fetal loss in subsequent pregnancies. Mapping of the chorionic lesions may help in the assessment of these mares, using endometrial biopsy. Mares may suffer chorionitis from different microorganisms during consecutive pregnancies suggesting a "new" infection on each occasion. In mares that are considered "susceptible" to infection, measures designed to avoid genital infections, such as vulval surgery and minimal contamination techniques at mating, are recommended.

NONINFECTIVE CONDITIONS

TWINS

The endometrial surface available for placental attachment is finite and is shared by the individual placentae of twin and triplet pregnancies. As there is a close correlation between chorionic surface area and fetal weight, twins invariably show growth retardation. Anatomic insufficiency of the placenta may be an important contributory factor in causing abortion in twin pregnancy.

When a single aborted fetus is found, the placenta must be examined for evidence of twin pregnancy. Characteristically there is a totally avillous area on each chorion at the site where they abut. The chorions may be easily separated or may be adhesed by tissue bridges and sometimes pseudoanastomoses. When membranes are badly torn, areas of very differing states of preservation suggest multiple pregnancy.

Udder development and premature lactation appear to be associated with the chorionic separation that accompanies death of one twin fetus. When early death of a twin fetus does not provoke abortion, fetal and placental dehydration and eventual mummification ensue. The dead tissues are gradually invaginated into the live twin's chorion. The latter may then expand into the vacated part of the uterus; the surviving fetus may develop to term and become a viable foal. When one twin fetus survives, existing interchorionic anastamoses may permit survival of small areas of well-vascularized viable tissue on the necrotic chorion of the dead twin, at or beyond the avillous in-contact area. When the viable tissue includes villi, this constitutes a small auxillary placenta for the surviving twin.

UMBILICAL CORD ABNORMALITIES

Factors governing the ultimate cord length are unknown. A few mares have been known to produce foals or fetuses with abnormally long cords in successive pregnancies, with associated defects. Cord abnormalities are discussed in succeeding paragraphs.

Obstruction to Blood Flow. Cords that are longer than normal (more than 80 cm) have a tendency to excessive twisting or looping around fetal appendages, with compression of the umbilical veins and fetal death. In these cases there are antemortem changes indicative of excessive twisting and vascular compromise, such as local edema, tearing, hemorrhage, and constriction. There may be calcification in the chorionic vessels and stroma.

Obstruction to Urachal Urinary Flow. This often accompanies signs of vascular obstruction, but alone does not usually cause fetal death. Some degrees of urachal dilatation are frequently seen in normal foals. Severe proximal obstructions have been associated with bladder and sometimes abdominal distention, which may be of sufficient degree to cause dystocia at parturition. More uncommonly hydroureter, hydronephrosis, or rectal prolapse may also be present. Prenatal urinary retention may also predispose to pervious urachus, or to "ruptured bladder" in foals.

Premature Cord Rupture During Parturition. This occurs rarely when the cord is abnormally short (less than 40 cm). Foals may die from intrapartum anoxia, and there is excessive umbilical bleeding.

Anomalies. Discrepancy in the size of the umbilical arteries is common in twins and in the occasional normal foal with certain types of asymmetric chorionic vascular pattern. Extreme hypoplasia (thread-like) or absence of one artery may be accompanied by serious developmental vascular and organ system defects. Such foals should be examined carefully for cardiac and other vascular abnormalities. Anoma-lous allantochorionic cord attachment sites are seen in 2.5 per cent of normal foals but are more common in aborted or defective foals. Their exact significance is uncertain. Herniation of intestines into the proximal cord may be accompanied by intestinal stenosis or atresia with resultant proximal intestinal dilatation. The presence of such defects should be ascertained during attempts at surgical correction. Vestigial yolk sac remnants, usually less than 2 cm in diameter, occur in all normal cords and frequently contain bony plaques. Larger anomalous ones of more than 10 cm are fairly common, but very large ones (over 20 cm diameter) are rare. Occasionally the larger ones become pedunculated and may loop around and strangulate an otherwise normal cord. These remnants should not be described as an anomalous twin (amorphus globosus).

Ischemic Necrosis of the Chorion. Clearly defined, full-thickness necrosis at the cervical pole may cause abortion. The precise mechanism is uncertain but in most cases the cord is abnormally long, and sometimes intimal "cushions" are seen obstructing main arteries. Occasionally, a second necrotic area, supplied by the same umbilical artery, is present at the tip of one horn. The thin, necrotic chorion may leak fetal fluids, causing a vulval discharge. Abortion may be delayed and fetuses are usually growth retarded or have skeletal deformities or both.

Posterior Birth Presentation. In these cases, umbilical cords are usually longer than normal.

NONINFECTIVE LESIONS OF THE VILLOUS SURFACE OF THE CHORION

Histologic examination is necessary to define the true nature of pallid or discolored areas of the villous surface.

Villus Atrophy. Focal placental separation may cause degeneration and atrophy of previously normal villi with accumulation of endometrial secretions. This is a consistent finding in normal placentas at the edematous tip of the pregnant horn at term and at the cervical star, but only affects fetal health when it is extensive. It is seen in cases in which excessive twisting of the cord causes poor vascular perfusion of villi.

Villus Hypoplasia. The villi are short and simple rather than branched and there may be areas of total villous aplasia. A reciprocal hypoplasia of the maternal microcotyledons is present, and the condition is probably associated with uterine stretching or endometrial disease. By mapping of the affected areas, the corresponding areas of endometrium may be investigated at a later date. Circular areas of villus hypoplasia, with coincident chorionic diverticula, indicate space-occupying endometrial lesions, most commonly luminal cysts. Their position can be confirmed by ultrasound echography. In one growth-retarded fetus, approximately one third of the chorionic body showed villus hypoplasia. At necropsy of the mare, a corresponding area of chronic endometrial atrophy with fibrosis was found in the uterine body.

Raised Linear Folds. These are sometimes seen along the chorionic horns in mares with a history of infective endometritis. They may reflect endometrial scarring and are often associated with fetal growth retardation.

Neoplasia. Placental neoplasms are very rare. I have seen single chorionic papillomas (3 to 4 cm diameter) on the outer surface of the chorions of two 12-year-old mares, originating from the edge of an endometrial cup site. Neither lesion was considered to be of clinical significance.

Abnormal Chorionic Dimensions

Absolute deviations from normal placental dimensions can be objectively assessed by reference to published values of linear measurements. Changes in the relative shapes of horns and body can only be evaluated subjectively.

Hydroallantosis. Some fetal losses are associated with an excessively large chorionic body, such as 55 to 65 cm wide in Thoroughbreds, and surface area. The horns are of normal size and the umbilical cord is usually long. In these cases the mare has an abnormally distended abdomen. It is not clear whether fetal loss is primarily caused by hydroallantois or that this merely reflects other lethal influences.

Body Pregnancy. Mares with this rare condition abort usually at eight or nine months of gestation. The chorionic horns are attenuated (22 to 55 cm long), often with partial obliteration of their lumens, and the fetus is in the body only. The uterine body and the mare's abdomen are wider than normal. Fetal growth retardation occurs and there are often congenital deformities and abnormalities of internal organs. The umbilical cord is frequently either abnormally short (27 cm) or long (80 to 134 cm). There may be allantoitis and cervical necrosis with no significant bacterial isolations seen on aerobic and microaerophilic culture. Leptospira (subtype Australis) was isolated from one case. However, the conditions giving rise to body pregnancy remain unknown.

Unicornual Allantochorion. This has been associated with fetal growth retardation and is an indication for a thorough investigation of the mare's uterus for congenital abnormalities and transluminal adhesions.

Foal Skeletal Deformities or Positional Abnormalities. Mechanical molding pressure on the developing fetus is generated by the uterine wall, the size and shape of which is reflected by the size and shape of the chorion. The chorions are found to be of abnormal shape in foals born with certain congenital deformities or positional abnormalities (such as parallel curvature of the limbs, mutual deformity of adjacent skeletal structures, and deviation of the ears). The chorions are also of abnormal dimensions in bicornual pregnancy.

Amniotic Lesions

Multiple foci of calcification (associated with hippomane material), adherence of innocuous fetal debris, focal edema, and parturient hemorrhage occur on the amnion of normal foals. Extensive green staining of the amnion is caused by fetal diarrhea. Although this may occur terminally in EHV-1 infection, it is also seen in the "chronic fetal diarrhea syndrome," which is of unknown etiology. Foals born alive may have meconium inhalation, pneumonia, and diarrhea from birth and may require intensive care. The mare and foal should be isolated pending examinations for EHV-1.

Perforation of the amnion may occur during pregnancy, associated with traumatic or ischemic lesions or with conditions leading to urine accumulation within the amniotic cavity. When allantoic and amniotic fluids mix, there is a diffuse allantoitis, shrinkage, fibrosis, and sometimes eversion of the amnion and occasionally intra-amniotic adhesions. One fetus was found to have ensnared two limbs beneath such an adhesion, causing ischemic amputation of one foot and asymmetrical growth of the other limb. Prolonged contact with allantoic fluid may be toxic to the fetus.

Supplemental Readings

Ginther, O. J.: Reproductive biology of the mare. Basic and applied aspects. O. J. Ginther, Cross Plaines, WI, 1979.

Jeffcott, L. B., and Whitwell, K. E. Twinning as a cause of fetal and neonatal loss in the Thoroughbred mare. J. Comp. Path., 83:91, 1973.

Mahaffey, L. W., and Adam, N. M.: Abortions associated with mycotic lesions of the placenta in mares. J. Am. Vet. Med. Assoc., 144:24, 1964.

Platt, H.: Infection of the horse fetus. J. Reprod. Fert., Suppl. 23:605–610, 1975.

Prickett, M. E.: The pathology of the equine placenta and its effects on the fetus. Proc. Ann. Conv. Am. Assoc. Eq. Pract., 1967, pp. 201–214.

Prickett, M. E.: Abortion and placental lesions in the mare. J. Am. Vet. Med. Assoc., 157:1465, 1970.

Vandeplassche, M.: The normal and abnormal presentation, position and posture of the foal-fetus during parturition and at presentation. Vlaams. Diergeneesk. Tijdsch., 26:4, 1957.

Whitwell, K. E.: Morphology and pathology of the equine umbilical cord. J. Reprod. Fert., Suppl. 23:599–603, 1975.

Whitwell, K. E.: Investigations into fetal and neonatal losses in the horse. Vet. Clin. North Am. (Large Anim. Pract.), 2:313, 1980.

Whitwell, K. E.: A critical assessment of the criteria for diagnosing virus abortion: A review of 100 cases. J. Reprod. Fert., Suppl. 32:632, 1982.

Whitwell, K. E.: Triplet pregnancy in two Thoroughbred mares. Equine Vet. J., 16:393, 1984.

Whitwell, K. E., and Jeffcott, L. B.: Morphological studies on the fetal membranes of the normal singleton foal at term. Res. Vet. Sci., 19:44, 1975.

Twin Pregnancy

Peter D. Rossdale, NEWMARKET, ENGLAND

Twin pregnancies often terminate in abortion during the last third of pregnancy. In Thoroughbred horses twins represent 20 to 30 per cent of all abortions, and the incidence of reported twin pregnancy is about 0.5 to 1.0 per cent of conceptions. Of these pregnancies, 65 per cent are aborted, in 21 per cent one twin is born alive, and in 14 per cent both are born alive. Twins are a naturally induced situation of dysmaturity because the competition between the two placentas causes damage to both (see p. 529).

Twin pregnancy has been a continuing source of financial loss to owners and of embarrassment to clinicians who practice pre-service examinations and early pregnancy diagnosis. Failure to deal effectively with the problem has, in many instances, cast doubt on the usefulness of these procedures.

As the majority of equine twins are thought to be dizygotic, emphasis has traditionally been placed on the avoidance of mating when more than one apparently mature ovarian follicle is palpated. Recent surveys have shown that multiple ovulation is far more common than is detected by rectal palpation, that twin pregnancy occurs more frequently following asynchronous rather than synchronous double ovulations, and that the correlation between palpation of twin ovulation and twin pregnancy is poor. Although a slightly higher incidence of twin pregnancy follows palpable multiple ovulation, early death of one fetus appears common. In many cases a normal singleton pregnancy evolves.

DIAGNOSIS OF TWIN PREGNANCY

The diagnosis of twin pregnancy in most mares, by rectal palpation alone has been inaccurate up to 30 days of gestation. Thus, the success of the deliberate elimination of one twin with the maintenance of the other to term has been poor. However, with the introduction of ultrasound echography into routine stud farm medicine, there is now a substantial possibility that the incidence of twins can be reduced significantly.

Ultrasonic examinations are most commonly performed with a real-time, B mode, linear array scanner, using a 3 or 5 mHz transducer inserted into the rectum following the removal of feces. The transducer is lubricated with coupling gel and is enclosed in a disposable plastic sleeve for hygienic reasons. Although sector scanners have been used for pregnancy diagnosis in mares, their advantages for use appear to accrue during late rather than early pregnancy.

The transducer is moved over the whole of the uterine horns and body, repeatedly, deliberately, and methodically. A thorough search must be made because embryonic sacs may migrate throughout the uterine lumen at least up to 16 days after ovulation. Once the conceptus is identified, the echogenic frame is "frozen" and measurements are made of its diameters and surface area. The features of the echogenic content of the sac are noted.

The fluid-filled yolk sac vesicle may first be identified as a circular dark area within the uterus at about 14 days after ovulation, but for practical reasons most early pregnancy examinations are made between 17 and 23 days. The shape of the echogenic image may change because of uterine contractions, pressure of viscera from outside the uterus, or peristaltic movements of the intestine against the uterine wall. An embryonic mass may be identified by about day 22 and a heartbeat may be detected in a live fetus after about day 25.

It is important that an early accurate diagnosis of twin pregnancy be made to facilitate an early decision regarding appropriate treatment. The unnecessary elimination of a singleton fetus is as unfortunate as is the failure to diagnose the presence of twins. A fetal sac must be distinguished from an endometrial cyst (see p. 507), with which it might be confused in the early stages of pregnancy. Diagnoses should be confirmed when necessary by serial scans with measurements.

Fetal sac size *per se* does not appear to indicate the presence of twins, nor does the presence of excess echogenic material. The presence of two embryos with two heartbeats is an obvious confirmatory sign when it is detected. Dividing lines and irregular or unusual shapes at any stage of pregnancy must be regarded with suspicion. At 25 to 40 days following ovulation, the junction between the yolk sac and the chorioallantoic placentas may be seen as a distinct echogenic line across the conceptus. This must not be mistaken for evidence of twin pregnancy.

Twin fetal sacs may occur either one in each uterine horn or two in one uterine horn. The latter may be close together or apart.

ELIMINATION OF ONE CONCEPTUS

Twins in separate horns may be successfully treated by manual rupture of one conceptus, if this is performed before day 30 and preferably before day 22. Each fetal sac is identified echographically and, if possible, by manual palpation. A decision is made as to which sac should be "squeezed" on the basis of size, shape, and clarity, suggesting potential viability. When the sacs are similar, this decision is arbitrary. Rupture is performed in three ways: by placing the base of the uterine horn between the thumb and finger, or pressing the uterine horn against the pelvic brim, or a combination of these two methods. Pressure is applied until the sac can be felt to rupture. If this is not felt, a repeat scan should provide evidence as to whether the procedure has been successful.

Twins in the same horn, positioned apart, may be successfully treated by manual rupture of one conceptus. However, this sometimes results in the loss of both. This more often occurs if the sacs are touching, and is thought to be stimulated by endogenous prostaglandin release. Treatment with exogenous prostaglandin synthetase inhibitors such as meclofenamic acid has been tried, either before or at the time of rupture, with somewhat equivocal results. When twins occur in the same uterine horn, the best approach may be to terminate both pregnancies with exogenous prostaglandin treatment.

The success rate for rupture of one fetal sac, between 17 and 30 days' gestation, is about 80 per cent. When twins occur in the same horn, the success rate is much lower. Of twin pregnancies diagnosed but not treated, about 70 per cent continue and terminate in the abortion or delivery of twins near to term. Therefore, about 30 per cent may progress to normal singleton full-term pregnancies. The final decision regarding the management of a diagnosed twin pregnancy must be a joint one, involving owner and veterinarian, made on the basis of stage of pregnancy and breeding season and statistical chances of success.

CONCLUSIONS

Experience to date suggests that the most reasonable approach to the twin pregnancy problem is as follows:

1. Mate all mares, when appropriate, irrespective of numbers of palpable mature ovarian follicles.

2. At 17 to 23 days following ovulation examine all mares by rectal palpation and ultrasound scan, looking carefully for signs of twin pregnancy.

3. Repeat these examinations as frequently as appears necessary, depending on individual considerations, to enable an early diagnosis and decision on treatment to be made.

4. As a general rule, treat twins in separate uterine horns by manual rupture, and those in the same horn by exogenous prostaglandin termination.

It is to be hoped that this approach will reduce the incidence of twin pregnancy. It would be naive, however, to suggest that one could expect 100 per cent accuracy. Mare owners must not be allowed to asssume that the problem of twin pregnancy can be eliminated entirely.

Supplemental Readings

Allen, W. E., and Goddard, P. J.: Serial investigations of early pregnancy in pony mares using real time ultrasound scanning. Equine Vet. J., *16*:509, 1984.

Ginther, O. J.: Twinning in mares: A review of recent studies, J. Equine Vet. Sci., 2:127, 1982.

Jeffcott, L. B., and Whitwell, K. E.: Twinning as a cause of foetal and neonatal loss in the Thoroughbred mare. J. Comp. Path., *83*:91, 1973.

Pipers, F. S., Zent, W., Holder, R., and Asbury, A.: Ultrasonography as an adjunct to pregnancy assessments in the mare, J. Am. Vet. Med. Assoc., *184*:328, 1984.

Rossdale, P. D., and Ricketts, S. W.: Equine Studfarm Medicine, 2nd. Edit., London, Bailliere Tindall, 1980.

Simpson, D. J., Greenwood, R. E. S., Ricketts, S. W., Rossdale, P. D., Sanderson, M., and Allen, W. R.: Use of ultrasound echography for early diagnosis of single and twin pregnancy in the mare, J. Reprod. Fert., Suppl. 32:431, 1982.

Torbeck, R. L., and Rantanen, N. W.: Early pregnancy detection in the mare with ultrasonography, J. Equine Vet. Sci., 3:204, 1982.

Whitwell, K. E.: Investigations into fetal and neonatal losses in the horse. Vet. Clin. North Am. (Large Anim. Pract.), 2:313, 1980.

Induction of Parturition

Robert B. Hillman, ITHACA, NEW YORK

Induction of parturition has become a routine procedure in many equine practices. Despite the success achieved by most practitioners, reports of complications persist primarily when induction is attempted before full term. The procedure is not without risks and it is essential to carefully evaluate each case before attempting induction. When proper guidelines are observed, this procedure ensures the presence of professional assistance at foaling and is of particular advantage when employed on mares that have experienced previous foaling difficulties. Once a successful induction has been performed, it is often difficult to curb the owners' enthusiasm for inductions at their convenience rather than waiting until the mare is ready. To succumb to this enthusiasm is to invite disaster. Induction of parturition is a critical procedure, and strict adherence to rigid guidelines is essential to ensure success. It is necessary to understand the limitations of this technique, to carefully select the cases in which it is to be employed, and, once started, to continually monitor the foaling through to its completion.

INDUCTION SITE

Mares should be placed in the area to be used for foaling at least a month before the estimated due date. This permits the mare to relax and become familiar with the environment and allows time for her to develop antibodies against any pathogens present so that the colostrum will provide specific protection for the newborn foal. The foaling area and pregnant mares should be isolated from persons transiently entering the stud farm. The pregnant mare should receive a tetanus toxoid booster upon arrival at the foaling area. Other vaccinations deemed necessary by past farm experience can also be administered at this time to ensure maximal colostral protection for the foal.

The foaling stable should be of ample size (12 ft × 12 ft), dry, warm, well-bedded, and provided with good ventilation but free of drafts. It should allow observation without disturbing the mare.

INDICATIONS

Induction of parturition in the mare has been recommended for many clinical conditions as well as for managerial, teaching, and research purposes. Mares in the following categories are candidates for induction of parturition.

1. Mares that reach term and appear ready to foal, with colostrum in the udder and with relaxed vulva, sacrosciatic ligaments, and cervix, but that do not go into labor because of uterine atony.

2. Mares previously producing dead or severely hypoxic foals owing to premature placental separation associated with delayed parturition.

3. Mares that have suffered injuries or tears at previous foalings and that require professional assistance at foaling.

4. Mares in which gestation is prolonged beyond 365 days and is associated with a very large fetus. Such mares require careful supervision at foaling. However, mares that carry beyond 365 days may produce a foal of normal or even small size. These mares usually do not require veterinary assistance.

5. Mares in which there is impending rupture of the prepubic tendon due to prolonged excessive ventral edema or hydrops of the amnion.

6. Mares that have produced icteric foals (foals with neonatal isoerythrolysis). Induction of parturition at term allows prevention of ingestion of colostrum before it can be tested for compatibility with the newborn foal's blood.

7. Nurse mares for a valuable orphan foal, a foal whose dam fails to lactate, or a foal rejected by its dam.

Prefoaling loss of colostrum, which has been listed as a reason for inducing parturition, is better handled by milking the mare and freezing the colostrum.

MANAGERIAL INDICATIONS

When a mare has a history of foaling problems and veterinary assistance will probably be necessary, it is desirable to schedule the foaling at a time convenient for the veterinarian and the stud farm management. Most mares foal at night. Therefore, scheduling an induced foaling during the day, in addition to being more convenient, eliminates the expense of emergency night calls and false alarms. It also reduces the need and expense of prolonged night watches. Also, scheduling an induced foaling enables observation of the entire birth process and postpartum care for teaching purposes.

INDUCTION CRITERIA

The criteria used to select the proper time for induction are (1) length of gestation, (2) udder enlargement with the presence of milk, (3) relaxation of the sacrosciatic ligaments, and (4) cervical softening.

Length of Gestation. It is essential that induction take place when the fetus is mature enough to adapt to the extrauterine environment. Normal gestation in the mare ranges from 320 to 360 days or more. A minimum of 330 days' gestation ensures adequate fetal maturity at the time of induction if all other criteria are fulfilled. In the absence of the other criteria, foals induced after a 330-day gestation may show signs of prematurity.

Udder Enlargement with Presence of Milk. Mammary development begins approximately four weeks before parturition and is maximal at the time of foaling. The teats distend just a few hours prior to foaling. The udder secretion at first is scant, thick, sticky, and of amber color. As foaling becomes imminent, the quantity of secretion increases, its viscosity decreases, and its color changes to gray or yellow-white. Induction can begin when the udder is enlarged and the teats are distended with an ample supply of smokey gray to yellow-white colostrum. A sufficient supply of colostrum in the udder is the most important indicator of fetal maturity.

Relaxation of the Sacrosciatic Ligaments. Sufficient relaxation of the sacrosciatic ligaments is indicated by a softening of either side of the tailhead. Maximum relaxation at foaling is accompanied by relaxation and lengthening of the vulva just before foaling.

Cervical Relaxation. After the previously listed criteria have been carefully evaluated, the degree of cervical relaxation is determined by gentle vaginal examination or by careful rectal palpation. The vaginal examination is performed after wrapping the tail and thoroughly cleaning the vulva with a disinfectant soap. A well-lubricated, gloved hand is inserted into the vagina to locate the cervix and determine the degree of relaxation. A mare that is eligible for induction must have a soft easily compressed cervix or a cervix that is starting to dilate. It is not necessary to penetrate the cervix to determine the extent of relaxation. Gentle palpation through the vaginal wall will enable the clinician to determine the position of the fetus. Cervical softness and compressibility can also be determined by careful rectal palpation, which eliminates the need for preparing the mare for a vaginal examination and avoids unnecessary vaginal exploration.

Studies of prepartum mammary secretions by biochemical methods have demonstrated a significant rise in calcium and magnesium as parturition approaches. Recently water hardness test strips* have been successfully used as a quick and simple test to detect these electrolyte changes. The colostrum must be diluted 1:6 with distilled water. The test strip is dipped quickly into the solution and a color change from green to red-violet is observed after a minute if magnesium and calcium levels are elevated. There are four test zones on each strip and if none change, parturition is at least four days away. When four zones change for the first time, 21 per cent of mares foal within 24 hours and a further 21 per cent foal within 48 hours.

METHOD OF INDUCTION

Oxytocin. Oxytocin was the agent first used to induce parturition in mares and is still used by many practitioners. When oxytocin is used on properly evaluated mares, induction is rapid and safe to both the mare and the foal. A dosage of 20 IU given intramuscularly causes a slow, quiet foaling, whereas doses of greater than 100 IU result in the rapid completion of a more active foaling. Forty to 60 IU of oxytocin given intramuscularly provide a quiet, safe foaling that will be completed in less than one hour.

---

*Merchoquant Water Hardness Test Strip No. 10 025; E. Merck, Post Fach 4119, 6100 Darmstadt, West Germany

Intravenous doses of 2.5 to 10 IU of oxytocin given as a bolus are also effective for initiating parturition. Some clinicians use 120 IU of oxytocin in 1 L normal saline administered intravenously at the rate of 1 L per hour until labor proceeds to the point at which delivery is assured. Smaller doses are probably more physiologic and reduce the chances of possible complications such as hyperstimulation of the myometrium, myometrial spasm, premature placental separation, and malpresentation. Whereas these complications—which are seen in women—have not been reported in mares, their potential argues for the use of low doses of oxytocin and mandates the careful monitoring of an induced parturition.

The clinical signs observed in induced parturition following the administration of oxytocin mimic natural foalings. Approximately 10 minutes after injection, there is frequent passage of small amounts of feces. Fifteen minutes after injection, sweat appears on the neck and gradually spreads over the shoulders. By 20 minutes the mare appears slightly anxious, swishes her tail, drips milk, and begins to quietly walk around the stable. At 20 to 25 minutes, the mare lies down and straining begins. If the fetal membranes are not observed at the vulva by 30 minutes, a vaginal examination is cleanly and carefully performed to confirm the proper position of the fetus. Correction of any malpresentation is easily accomplished at this time. Should the red, velvet-like chorioallantosis with the cervical star be presented at the vulva, it is opened within the vagina to allow passage of the amnion and foal. Failure to do this will allow premature placental separation and can result in a mildly to severely hypoxic foal. Retention of the fetal membranes beyond three hours after foaling has not been observed in most trials, and fertility following oxytocin inductions is not impaired.

Estrogens were formerly used to relax the cervix before induction with oxytocin. The dosage of diethylstilbestrol varied from 10 to 30 mg and was administered 8 to 12 hours before the oxytocin injection. Exogenous estrogen is not necessary, as natural relaxation of the cervix is a valuable guide to the proper time for induction.

Corticosteroids. While glucocorticoids induce parturition in the ewe, sow, cow, and rabbit when administered late in pregnancy, initial trials with horses were uniformly unsuccessful. Later trials using massive doses of dexamethasone (100 mg per day) starting at 321 days of pregnancy for a four-day treatment schedule induced foalings from six and a half to seven days after starting the injections. Resultant foals were small and weak but were healthy and grew at normal rate. The necessity of repeated dosing and the delay in completion of foaling have combined to deter acceptance of this technique.

Prostaglandins. Prostaglandins have been successfully used to induce foaling in mares between 325 and 367 days of gestation and before the development of signs of imminent parturition. Mares receive flumethasone (10 to 15 mg) and stilbestrol (30 mg) 24 hours before prostaglandin $F_{2\alpha}$ (10 mg). Several mares received an additional 5 mg flumethasone 12 hours after the initial treatment. Of five mares receiving the two doses of flumethasone, two foaled within three hours of the administration of prostaglandin, and the remaining three foaled within three hours of a second injection of prostaglandin (7.5 mg) given three hours after the first one. In all cases, foaling was uneventful, and placental expulsion occurred within an hour.

Fluprostenol, a synthetic prostaglandin analogue, has also been used to induce foaling in mares not showing signs of imminent foaling. Pony mares received 250 µg, while full-sized mares received 1000 µg intramuscularly. All the mares showed first-stage labor (uneasiness, sweating, and mild abdominal discomfort) within 30 minutes. The onset of second-stage labor varied from one half hour to three hours and lasted for five to 33 minutes. The fetal membranes were expelled within two hours. Of 17 foals from fluprostenol inductions, 13 were healthy during the adaptive period. Foal health might have been better if mares had met the established criteria for determining optimal time of induction. While it would be convenient to be able to induce parturition without waiting for all the criteria, further studies are required before routine applications of this technique can be recommended.

CARE OF THE MARE AND FOAL

Aftercare of the mare and foal is vital in ensuring the successful outcome of any foaling, but it takes on extra importance following induction, since any problems that develop are invariably attributed to this technique. With this in mind, the entire induction process should be accomplished in as quiet and unobtrusive a manner as possible. After the second stage of labor is completed and a check has been made to ensure that the foal is breathing normally with its head free of the amnion, the mare and foal are allowed to lie quietly with the umbilical vessels intact for several minutes. This minimizes loss of placental-fetal blood and results in strong, more vigorous foals. Once the mare stands and the umbilical cord has separated, the foal's navel is dipped in mild iodine solution, or an antibiotic powder is applied. A warm, gentle enema is administered to enhance passage of the meconium. Whenever foaling is induced, we milk 300 to 500 ml of colostrum from the mare and administer it to the foal using a well-lubricated soft rubber stallion catheter passed through the nose into the stomach. This ensures the presence of an ample supply of colostrum in the foal's digestive tract at the time of maximal immunoglobulin absorption. While some researchers have reported decreased passive transfer of immunoglobulin in foals from mares induced before maximum mammary development, foals induced after the previously stated criteria were met have attained acceptable levels of protection. My colleagues and I have not found it necessary to administer prophylactic antibiotics following most inductions but do not hesitate to do so if there is any indication of infection such as a weak, listless foal, evidence of fetal diarrhea, or passage of a heavy, inflamed placenta. Problems with weak, immature foals have been reported when parturition is induced before the preinduction criteria are met.

ELECTIVE ABORTION

The indications for elective abortion are (1) mismating, (2) pregnancy discovered in a supposedly nonpregnant performance mare that has been purchased, and (3) twin pregnancy.

TECHNIQUES

Intrauterine Infusions. Intrauterine infusions of saline, antibiotic solution, or a mild iodine solution have been used successfully for many years. The mare's perineum is cleaned, the vagina examined, and the cervix dilated by gentle digital pressure. A catheter is passed into the uterus, and 500 to 1000 ml of solution is infused. Abortion usually occurs within 48 hours. Before inducing abortion, it is best to wait at least one week after mating to ensure the presence of the embryo within the uterus. If the mare is to be mated again in the same season, it is equally important that the intrauterine flush be accomplished before 35 days of gestation to prevent the formation of the endometrial cups. Once these structures form, the mare usually does not return to estrus until the cups are rejected by the uterine tissue at about 120 days.

Prostaglandins. A single injection of prostaglandin or its analogue administered after the formation of a mature corpus luteum (five days after ovulation) and before the formation of endometrial cups (35 days), will cause lysis of the corpus luteum, loss of the pregnancy, and return of the mare to estrus. If prostaglandin is used after the formation of the endometrial cups, it must be administered at daily intervals for four days. Mares that are aborted after 35 days do not return to estrus until the endometrial cups cease functioning.

TWIN PREGNANCY

Mares carrying twins usually abort from mid to late pregnancy when remating is no longer feasible.

The few mares that carry twins to term usually produce small, weak foals that fail to grow or perform well and therefore cannot be marketed profitably. For these reasons, when twin pregnancies are diagnosed early, many owners elect to induce abortion in an effort to get the mare remated and pregnant with a single fetus. Either of the previously described techniques can be used to terminate the pregnancy. Another option practiced by veterinarians is to rupture one embryonic vesicle in the hope that the remaining vesicle will survive and produce a single healthy foal (see p. 532). The routine employment of ultrasound for early pregnancy diagnosis in the mare provides early detection of twins.

Elective abortion of mares after four months of gestation is usually contraindicated because of complications that may arise owing to the large size of the fetus. Once the placenta has taken over the role of supplying the hormones necessary to maintain pregnancy, prostaglandins are ineffective in precipitating abortion.

Supplemental Readings

Alm, C. C., Sullivan, J. J., and First, N. L.: Induction of premature parturition by parenteral administration of dexamethasone in mares. J. Am. Vet. Med. Assoc., *165*:721, 1974.

Douglas, R. H., Squires, E. L., and Ginther, O. J.: Induction of abortion in mares with prostaglandin $F_{2\alpha}$. J. Anim. Sci., *39*:404, 1974.

Hillman, R. B.: Induction of parturition in mares. J. Reprod. Fert., Suppl. 23:641, 1975.

Jeffcott, L. B., and Rossdale, P. D.: A critical review of current methods of induction of parturition in the mare. Equine Vet. J., 9:208, 1977.

Leadon, D. P., Rossdale, P. D., Jeffcott, L. B., and Allen, R. W.: A comparison of agents for inducing parturition in mares in the pre-viable and premature periods of gestation. J. Reprod. Fert., Suppl. 32:597, 1982.

Ousey, J. C., Dudan, F. E., and Rossdale, P. D.: Preliminary studies of mammary secretions in the mare to assess fetal readiness for birth. Equine Vet. J., *16*:259, 1984.

Pashen, R. L.: Low doses of oxytocin can induce foaling at term. Equine Vet. J., *12*:85, 1980.

Rossdale, P. D., Pashen, R. L. and Jeffcott, L. B.: The use of synthetic prostaglandin analogue (fluprostenol) to induce foaling. J. Reprod. Fert., Suppl. 27:521, 1979.

Rossdale, P. D., and Silver, M.: The concept of readiness for birth. J. Reprod. Fert., Suppl. *32*:507, 1982.

Prepartum Complications and Dystocia

M. Vandeplassche, GHENT, BELGIUM

PREPARTUM COMPLICATIONS

Prepartum pregnancy complications may seriously endanger the life of a mare and her fetus and an early diagnosis followed by appropriate treatment is essential. Clinical signs usually include colic of uterine origin. When this is seen late in pregnancy, the most common causes are premature parturition, uterine dorsoretroflexion, uterine torsion, and placental hydrops. Bicornual pregnancy and prolonged gestation are prepartum complications that may cause dystocia.

PREMATURE PARTURITION

Colic in a preterm mare may always be a sign of premature parturition or abortion. There may be no mammary development, the vulva is dry, the vagina is moist and slippery rather than sticky, and the cervical plug is absent. The allantochorion may bulge through the half-opened cervix and will eventually rupture under pressure during abdominal straining. If the mare is seen at an earlier stage, rectal palpation demonstrates that the fetus is entering the birth canal. When the aforementioned signs are present, the only appropriate treatment is to facilitate atraumatic delivery of the fetus by correcting any malposition or malpresentation.

UTERINE DORSORETROFLEXION

I have seen 30 referred cases of uterine dorsoretroflexion, between seven and a half and 11 months of gestation, over a period of 15 years. Clinical signs are acute colic, repeated lying down and then getting up, depressed appetite, difficulty in defecation, violent abdominal straining, and swelling of the vulva and perineum. There is little or no response to analgesic therapy.

Rectal palpation reveals a live fetus, sometimes with head and legs in the birth posture, enclosed in a hypertonic uterus inside the pelvic canal, sometimes close to the anus. When the fetus is pushed downward, the mare shows severe acute colic and the fetus quickly returns to its previous position in the pelvis. Examination of the vagina reveals it to be sticky, with the cervical plug intact. Characteristically the fetus may be palpated dorsal to the vagina. The pathogenesis of this condition is unclear. Observations suggest that an accumulation of fetal fluid occurs, resulting in abnormal uterine expansion forming a dorsal uterine body distention that projects toward the pelvic inlet. Uterine wall stretching and fetal stress probably provoke spasmodic uterine contractions, resulting in colic. In some cases, the fetus assumes the birth posture with stretched head, neck, and forelimbs pushing into the pelvic canal, which induces abdominal straining.

Treatment is by the administration of smooth muscle spasmolytic drugs such as 200 mg isoxsuprine lactate* intramuscularly or the longer-acting 200 μg clenbuterol hydrochloride† by slow intravenous or intramuscular injection. Signs of colic disappear within 15 minutes and the fetus can be repelled in an anteroventral direction, per rectum. In some cases, one injection is sufficient. In others, treatment must be repeated at three- to six-hour intervals over one to two days. Normal fetal posture is regained even when the birth posture was previously assumed. Restrictions of food intake and regular walking exercise encourage a return to normal within a few days and relapses are uncommon.

UTERINE TORSION

Approximately 50 per cent of cases of uterine torsion develop between 8 to 10.5 months of gestation. Clinical signs are varying degrees of colic with difficulty in defecation.

Sixty per cent of torsions occur in an anticlockwise (to the left) direction. At rectal examination it is often difficult to advance the arm, and the fetus usually cannot be reached. The uterine broad ligaments should be carefully examined, starting at the dorsal lumbar region and following them in a ventral direction until they join where they pass under the uterus. The more caudal ligament indicates the direction of the torsion. Starting ventrally, the caudal and tighter ligament rises in a vertical direction whereas the cranial and slacker ligament crosses horizontally over the uterus toward the opposite side of the abdomen. An examination in this manner confirms the diagnosis, direction, and severity of the torsion. Vaginal examinations are usually unproductive because torsions invariably occur cranial to the cervix.

In some cases of colic associated with large intestinal displacements, it may be difficult to differentiate stretched mesenteric bands from uterine ligaments, but there is no palpable fetus with the former condition. Once the diagnosis has been confirmed, the torsion should be corrected without delay. The operation is best performed with the mare standing restrained in stocks with hindquarters elevated. Fluid therapy should be given when indicated to correct shock and electrolyte imbalance. Tranquilization is recommended before epidural and then local infiltration analgesia of the upper flank on the side of the torsion (left flank for an anticlockwise torsion).

Two surgeons should be available for this operation. An incision is made in the abdominal wall of the flank, just large enough for one surgeon to insert the hand and arm without allowing intestinal prolapse. The arm is passed under the uterus and, with a lifting and rotating movement, the torsion can usually be corrected gradually and quite easily. Correction in this manner becomes more difficult toward term. In difficult cases, the aid of the second surgeon, via a flank incision on the opposite side of the mare, may be helpful. To check for adequate correction, both broad ligaments must be carefully palpated either via the peritoneal cavity, when two flank incisions have been made, or by rectal palpation by the second surgeon, when there is only one flank incision.

Following satisfactory correction of the torsion, the uterus should be palpated for signs of edema, congestion, and hematomas that might adversely affect fetal viability and postpartum uterine involution. When a live fetus is present, treatment with clenbuterol hydrochloride during the first 24 hours after surgery is recommended. When there is, without doubt, a dead fetus, parturition usually commences soon after surgery. Treatment should be directed toward aiding atraumatic delivery with a minimum of abdominal straining and damage to the abdominal suture line.

PLACENTAL HYDROPS

I have been involved in treating 15 cases of placental hydrops over a 20-year period. The mares were between 6 to 20 years old and none were primiparous. This condition is much more common than is realized. Depending on its degree, many mares may show little or no obvious clinical signs, even with placental fluid quantities of 100 liters or more.

The history is of an apparently normal pregnancy until seven and a half to 11 months of gestation, when a sudden excessive distention of the abdomen occurs associated with variable degrees of colic, and difficulty in defecation. This is followed by loss of appetite, difficulty in walking, and dyspnea during recumbency. Eight of the 15 mares began spontaneous parturition soon after arrival at the clinic, possibly induced by the stress of transport. The loss

---

*Duphaspasmin, Philips-Duphar, Netherlands. Vasodilan, Mead Johnson & Co., Evansville, IN
†Planipart, Boehringer-Ingelheim, Ingelheim, West Germany

of allantoic fluid clearly resulted in a marked improvement in their clinical condition.

In the remaining seven mares, parturition was induced because of marked dyspnea, cyanosis, and elevated pulse rate. Rectal temperature was normal. Rectal palpation revealed retained mucus-covered feces; passage of the arm was made difficult by the pressure of the distended uterus closing the rectal lumen. When the placental membranes had not ruptured, a diagnostic feature was that the fetus could not be palpated, externally or by rectal or vaginal examinations. When the chorioallantois had ruptured, the uterus felt flabby. In these cases, the fetus could be easily palpated. In cases in which spontaneous parturition had started, vaginal exploration revealed large quantities of allantoic fluid in which the amnion and fetus were not easily palpable. In such cases, the history and clinical signs allow a differentiation from twin gestation, ascites, and exudative peritonitis.

In the majority of cases, the condition is progressive and very few of such pregnancies reach term and produce a live foal. Induction of parturition is indicated when the mare's clinical condition is seriously affected. Oxytocin infusions are usually ineffective in these cases. Hot water irrigation of the cervix for 10 to 15 minutes causes sufficient cervical relaxation to allow manual rupture of the allantochorion, which is sometimes surprisingly flabby. Only small quantities of allantoic fluid escape spontaneously; therefore, it is necessary to siphon as much of the remaining fluid as possible from the uterus.

In the 15 cases seen, all fetuses were alive, eight were malformed and one (11 months' gestation) survived. Quantities of allantoic fluid measured ranged from 110 to 230 liters and amniotic fluid measured from 6 to 15 liters.

As soon as 50 to 60 liters have been siphoned off, 50 to 100 IU oxytocin should be administered by intravenous drip to induce uterine contractions and to prevent blood pooling in the splanchnic circulation. Fluid therapy and 100 mg dexamethasone, intravenously, help to control cardiovascular shock, which was the cause of death in two mares in the series reported. Retention of the placenta occurred in 11 cases. This was successfully treated by oxytocin therapy, which, in the case of two mares, required administration over three days. Eight of the 15 mares were subsequently mated; six became pregnant and produced normal healthy foals at term.

BICORNUAL PREGNANCY

In these cases, the fetus develops in both uterine horns instead of the normal one horn and uterine body position. The condition occurs in only one in 500 pregnancies but causes dystocia and is responsible for 50 per cent of the cesarean sections at this clinic. Bicornual pregnancy leads to marked abdominal distention, and fetal hypermotility can be observed in both flanks. The start of second-stage labor may go undetected because the allantochorion does not rupture; consequently, reflex abdominal straining is not initiated. The fetus remains in transverse presentation and can often be palpated only with the tips of the fingers. Prompt cesarian section usually delivers a viable fetus, as the placental attachments are seldom significantly disrupted. However, many of these fetuses are malformed with signs of torticollis and scoliosis.

PROLONGED GESTATION

Approximately 1 per cent of pregnancies continue for longer than 370 days. In spite of owner's fears, the majority of cases produce an apparently normal healthy foal following a normal parturition. I have seen 19 single pregnancies ranging from 372 to 395 days and five twin pregnancies ranging from 370 to 399 days of gestation. In some cases there was an apparent delayed conceptual development at approximately 20 to 40 days, which resulted in a negative blood PMSG test until 66 days of gestation. It is postulated that there was a three- to four-week period of embryonic "rest" at this time, characterized by and possibly associated with a drop in blood progesterone level. As long as there are no signs of ill health, prolonged gestation is not an indication for therapeutic induction of parturition.

DYSTOCIA

MANAGEMENT OF THE PREPARTUM MARE

Sudden changes in diet should be avoided and exercise is beneficial to both mare and fetus. In exceptional cases, excessive milk production may cause discomfort, necessitating milking and storing the colostrum to be fed to the foal postpartum. Foaling should be unobtrusively observed in a manner that will not disturb the mare but will allow the early diagnosis of abnormality so that assistance may be given when indicated. Indirect observation, using closed-circuit television or microelectronic teledetectors,* can be useful additional aids to supervision. The latter equipment, contained in a harness, detects increased neck skin electroconductivity as sweating occurs and transmits a signal to a remote receiver less than 500 meters away, setting off an alarm.

OBSTETRIC EXAMINATIONS AND TREATMENT

An accurate diagnosis of the condition of both mare and fetus is an essential prerequisite to the

---

*Rheintechnik, Bendorf, Koblenz, West Germany

treatment of dystocia. In addition to a general physical examination, detailed examinations of mammary development, swelling and relaxation of the vulva, vestibule, vagina and cervix, uterine wall tension, and placental adherence may be made. The fetal position, posture, viability, and size relative to the pelvic diameter should be established. In protracted cases, fetal viability may be assessed in anterior presentation by digital pressure on the base of the tongue and the throat to elicit a swallowing reflex, and in posterior presentation by palpation of the umbilical artery.

Treatment should aim to maximize the chances of survival of mare and fetus, but the choice will depend upon the diagnosis and the viability of the fetus.

Reposition

Uterine Torsion. This may present at term causing dystocia. When a hand can be passed through the cervix, the fetal head or preferably the trunk should be grasped. Epidural analgesia and elevation of the hindquarters will reduce straining and increase abdominal space for manipulation. A semicircular movement of the hand and arm, with fetal movements, may correct the torsion, allowing the fetus to be delivered. When the cervix cannot be penetrated, cesarian section is indicated.

Fetal Reposition. This is more difficult for presentation than for position and posture. Ropes, used as snares, and manual manipulation are preferred to the use of instruments. When there is no contracture, forelimbs are more easily repositioned than hindlimbs. Epidural analgesia and elevation of the hindlimbs reduce straining and increase the abdominal space, greatly facilitating manipulation. Adequate lubrication is essential and mineral oil or carboxyl-methylcellulose gel may be pumped deep into the uterus. Spasmolytic agents will cause uterine relaxation and will aid manipulation. Following reposition, uterine motility can be re-established with oxytocin.

When the head and neck are flexed, eye hooks, in the hands of an experienced obstetrician, may be helpful. When the fetus is dead and in cases of head scoliosis and torticollis, partial embryotomy may be indicated. With hip or hock flexion, transverse fetal presentation, and bicornual presentation, embryotomy or cesarian section is usually indicated.

Traction

This is indicated when uterine contractions and abdominal straining are inadequate, not to provide "forced extraction" but to supplement the natural parturient forces. The mare should be in lateral recumbency, the birth canal fully relaxed and copiously lubricated. Traction should be synchronized with natural contractions. With the fetus in anterior presentation, especially when dead, traction should be applied to the forelimbs and head, in line with the mare, deviating occasionally laterally to the right and left. No more than three men should be used—occasionally four are necessary with heavy breeds of mare.

If a dead foal becomes impacted at the pelvis ("hiplock"), transverse fetal section in the lumbar region, followed by longitudinal bisection of the hindquarters, will allow delivery by traction.

Uterine inertia is an important indication for traction and may occur in consecutive parturitions. Uterine involution and placental detachment may begin, endangering the life of the fetus. Manipulation and massage of the vagina and cervix followed by gentle traction will provoke abdominal straining and the release of oxytocin, allowing expulsion of the fetus.

Embryotomy (Fetotomy)

A high-quality tubular wire-saw embryotome (Thygesen) is recommended. This comprises (1) a long (90 cm) embryotome; (2) a flexible wire-saw (Liess) composed of $3 \times 3 \times 3$ or 27 steel wires and two hand grips; (3) a threader and wire saw introducer (one light "Schriever" type and one heavier type, capable of sinking downward); (4) a double hook (Krey). For mares, partial rather than total embryotomy is usually indicated—that is, one or two (exceptionally three) sections in order to reduce fetal diameter to allow reposition and expulsion.

Embryotomy is best performed with the mare standing, under the effects of epidural analgesia, a tranquilizer, and a spasmolytic such as isoxuprine lactate, which relaxes the uterus around the fetus. The operation should be performed hygienically, with frequent copious lubrication of the fetus and vagina. The surgeon should carefully plan the position, direction, and order of the sections before fixing the relevant part with a snare or double hook. For transverse and oblique sections, the head of the embryotome should be introduced, in the palm of the hand, over the dorsal half (preferably the dorsal limb) of the fetus and should reach its final position *before* any attempt is made to push the wire-saw ring forward. During the introduction of the embryotome, the operator's finger should remain in contact with the fetus. A final check of the position of the head of the embryotome and the wire-saw ring should be made before sawing is started. This should be performed using long rather than short strokes to spread the wear on the wire. Sawing should be periodically stopped to check the position of the embryotome and wire. When the section is complete, the embryotome should be removed first, guarded in the palm of the hand. Some specific indications for embryotomy follow.

ANTERIOR PRESENTATION

FLEXED HEAD AND NECK ("Wry-Neck"). This is the cause of approximately 50 per cent of cases of dystocia in mares. When the fetus is dead, the operator should pull on its neck, using a fixed double hook, to enable passage of an introducer with a wire-saw dorsally over and then around the neck, before the head and neck are removed. If it is not possible to pass the introducer around the neck, an oblique section through the axilla should be made to remove the easiest limb to reach (usually the most dorsal one opposite the neck deviation). This reduces the fetal diameter substantially so that traction on the other leg allows advancement to a position at which the head and neck can be removed followed by the remaining torso.

POSTERIOR PRESENTATION

This occurs in approximately 2 per cent of pregnancies and 12.5 per cent of cases of dystocia, indicating a predisposition to postural abnormalities such as hock and hip flexion.

FLEXED HOCK. Embryotomy is indicated and quite simple when the fetus is dead and when reposition might injure the mare. The introducer with wire-saw is passed around the tarsal joint and the head of the embryotome is fixed below the tarsus. A longitudinal section is made between the os calcis and the dorsal epiphysis of the metatarsus and the amputated portion is removed. The limb is then stretched posteriorly to prevent stump trauma to the uterine wall. If the other hindlimb is abnormally presented, it is similarly removed and stretched and the fetus expelled after adequate lubrication.

If the fetus is alive and reposition is impossible, cesarian section may be indicated. Other skeletal malformations of the head, neck, and forelimbs are common in these cases and it is seldom possible to save a fetus with hock flexion.

FLEXED HIP ("Breech Presentation"). With a small live foal, manual reposition may occasionally be successful, or cesarian section should be attempted. With a dead foal, embryotomy is indicated but is rather difficult. Isoxuprine lactate should be administered and the uterus pumped full of oil or lubricant. An epidural anesthetic should be administered followed by general anesthesia (such as 30 to 50 gm glyceryl guaiacolate with chloral hydrate), then positioning of the mare in lateral recumbency with elevated hindquarters. A heavy wire-saw introducer is passed dorsally between the trunk and the most accessible flexed hindleg before sectioning it through the hip. This leg is removed and then the second leg, by an identical technique. Copious lubrication then allows delivery of the fetus.

ABNORMAL PRESENTATION

BICORNUAL TRANSVERSE PRESENTATION. The fetus may be out of reach or too difficult to manipulate and in these cases cesarian section is indicated.

VENTROVERTICAL PRESENTATION ("Dog-Sitting Position"). The head and forelimbs protrude from the vulva while the hindlimbs lie on the pelvic brim. The latter have often not been detected until traction has been applied and the fetus is dead and firmly impacted. Isoxuprine lactate should be administered and the uterus pumped full of oil or lubricant. An epidural anesthetic is administered followed by general anesthesia, then positioning of the mare in lateral recumbency with elevated hindquarters. An oblique section is made to amputate the head and complete neck with, if possible, two withers vertebrae. The threaded embryotome is then passed over the dorsal half of the fetus to remove the withers. A forelimb may be removed if necessary. There will then be more space within the vagina. It is often possible to repel the hind feet anteriorly before removing the fetus.

VENTROTRANSVERSE PRESENTATION. After preparation as described for ventrovertical presentation, a forelimb is first amputated followed by the head and neck. It may then be possible to repulse the cranial part of the fetus, and by traction on the hindlimbs achieve the longitudinal posterior presentation. The fetus is then rotated into the dorsal position, from which it may be removed.

The experienced obstetrician should be able to correct over 90 per cent of cases of dystocia by reposition, traction, and embryotomy. Thus *cesarian section* (see p. 542) may be indicated as a primary obstetric treatment in 5 to 10 per cent of cases.

POSTOPERATIVE CARE

Obstetric manipulation traumatizes the genital tract of the mare. There is an increased incidence (greater than 20 per cent after embryotomy) of retained placenta and delayed uterine involution. Necropsy examinations have shown severe uterine wall hemorrhages, often complicated by intravascular thrombosis of veins and arteries. Mucosal damage to the vagina and cervix can result in adhesions. All these features, singly or in combination, can seriously jeopardize subsequent fertility.

It is therefore important to minimize trauma and infection and to promote postpartum involution. An intravenous drip infusion of 30 IU oxytocin given over 30 to 60 minutes is recommended, and this can be repeated over the next few days. Systemic and intrauterine antibacterial treatment is indicated. Uterine washings should be made using warm saline solution and not antiseptics, which inhibit leukocyte phagocytosis important to the recovery process.

In spite of all preventive measures and experienced treatment, the subsequent fertility of some mares will be depressed following dystocia.

Supplemental Readings

Freytag, K.: Zur Eihautwassersucht beim Pferd, Tierärztl. Umschau., 33:327, 1978.

Muylle, E., Vandeplassche, M., Nuytten, J., Oyaert, W., Vlaminck, K., and Bonte, P.: The parturient dorsoflexio uteri in the mare, VI. Diergeneesk. Tijdschr., 50:155, 1981.

Vandeplassche, M.: The normal and abnormal presentation, position and posture of the foal-fetus during gestation and at parturition. Mededel., 1:No.2, 1–68, VI. Diergeneesk. Tijdschr., Vol. 26, 1957.

Vandeplassche, M.: Obstetrician's view of the physiology of equine parturition and dystocia. Equine Vet. J., 12:45, 1980.

Vandeplassche, M.: Stimulation and inhibition of phagocytosis in domestic animals. Proc. 10th. Int. Congr. Anim. Reprod. A.I., Urbana, Champaign, Illinois, 3:475, 1984.

Vandeplassche, M., Bouters, R., Spincemaille, J., and Bonte, P.: Dropsy of the fetal sacs in mares. Vet. Rec., 99:67, 1976.

Vandeplassche, M., Simoens, P., Bouters, R., De Vos, N., and Verschooten, F.: Etiology and pathogenesis of congenital torticollis and head scoliosis in the equine fetus. Equine Vet. J., 16:419, 1984.

Cesarean Section

H. Pearson, BRISTOL, ENGLAND

Cesarean section in the mare is a relatively uncomplicated procedure that generally carries an excellent prognosis. The procedure should be performed as early as possible in the course of dystocia and not as a last resort after protracted and possibly traumatic attempts at vaginal delivery. The equine fetus cannot survive lengthly dystocia; clinicians will realize the necessity for prompt surgery if a live fetus is not to die before surgical delivery. If the fetus is already dead, general anesthesia of the mare may facilitate vaginal manipulation and successful delivery but at the risk of seriously traumatizing the soft tissues of the birth canal.

ANESTHESIA

The choice of anesthetic technique depends on the facilities available; however, hypotensive drugs and those having a marked depressant effect on the foal's respiration after birth should be avoided. Anesthesia can be induced with thiopentone sodium or brietal sodium, or with the combination of glyceryl guaiacolate followed by either of these short-acting barbiturates and maintained with halothane vaporized in oxygen delivered through an endotracheal tube. Adequate oxygenation throughout the operation is essential to maintain fetal viability. If available, positive pressure ventilation may be helpful. Intensive supportive fluid therapy is advisable to maintain maternal blood pressure and compensate for inevitable blood loss during the operation.

SURGICAL APPROACH

Of the alternative laparotomy sites, the linea alba has distinct advantages in allowing an incision of adequate length for optimal access to the uterus with minimal disruption of muscle tissues. For this approach, the mare is placed in dorsal recumbency but tilted slightly to one side to avoid compression of the caudal vena cava by the heavily gravid uterus. The incision is made in the midline extending through the umbilicus to a site immediately cranial to the udder. The relatively few bleeding points in subcutaneous tissues are ligated before the subperitoneal fat and peritoneum are perforated. If uterine torsion is present, an excessive quantity of blood-tinged peritoneal fluid may be evident at this stage.

Even after protracted dystocia and loss of uterine fluids, the uterus is seldom so tightly contracted that a fetal limb cannot be drawn into the abdominal wound. The hysterotomy is ideally sited on the greater curvature of the gravid horn away from the ovary. By grasping a limb, this segment of uterine wall is exposed and surrounded by protective towels to minimize contamination of the peritoneal cavity with uterine contents that are probably no longer bacteriologically sterile.

Incision of the uterus results in profuse endometrial bleeding. This can be controlled by inserting a continuous polygalactic or polyglycolic acid suture, using an atraumatic needle along the edges of the uterine incision after first separating the placenta. The exposed limb and its counterpart are then carefully drawn from the uterus, with maximum use made of joint flexibility so as not to tear the uterine incision. If the forelimbs are first extracted, the head and neck are then exposed. By gentle traction, the trunk is withdrawn and placed on the mare's abdomen with the umbilical cord still intact. If the foal is drawn head first, the hindlimbs may remain partly in the uterus until the umbilical cord is divided. If the foal is alive, pulsations will be felt in the umbilical cord that is left intact until respiration begins and cord pulsations subside.

Ligation of the cord predisposes to umbilical infection and it is better divided simply by traction, approximately 10 cm from the umbilicus. Persistent cord hemorrhage is stopped with swab pressure or temporary clamping. If the fetus is already dead, the placenta may have separated and is then easily removed from the uterus. Manual separation of the placenta is unwise because residual microvilli may lead to puerperal metritis.

The hysterotomy incision is repaired with two rows of continuous Lembert inversion sutures of polygalactic or polyglycolic acid on an atraumatic needle. Excessive tension is to be avoided because of the risk of tearing and bleeding along the suture line.

When torsion is present, the uterus is repositioned after hysterotomy, with care taken not to perforate the friable uterine wall. Careful repair of the midline laparotomy incision is essential because of the risk of incisional hernia or dehiscence, particularly as the abdominal wall at this stage of pregnancy is stretched and thin. Interrupted sutures of a nonabsorbable material such as steel or preferably monofilament nylon on a noncutting needle are placed not more than 2 cm apart, through both edges of the abdominal wall but not including the peritoneum and subperitoneal fat. The subcutaneous tissues and skin are then sutured separately, the latter with eversion sutures.

POSTOPERATIVE CARE AND COMPLICATIONS

After the operation, the mare is given 50 IU oxytocin, over 30 to 60 minutes in a saline infusion and tetanus antitoxin, if she is not adequately protected by vaccination. Parenteral antibiotic treatment may be initiated at this stage, but in latent carrier mares this may precipitate clinical and potentially fatal salmonellosis, with profuse acute diarrhea, secondary dehydration, and toxemia, usually starting on the second day following surgery. Thus, if a live foal is born, it may be prudent to withhold antibiotic treatment of the mare unless signs of infectious peritonitis develop.

Most mares recover without untoward complications except for a variable degree of ventral edema, which develops over the first five days or so and then slowly subsides. Most maternal deaths result from a combination of surgical and endotoxemic shock and occur within 24 hours of the operation, in spite of intensive fluid and, if necessary, blood replacement therapy. Uncommonly, a mare may regain consciousness but be unable to stand. After dorsal recumbency, myopathy of the gluteal muscle masses, resulting from hypoperfusion, may prevent normal hindlimb function and the mare may remain recumbent or may adopt a crouching stance when trying to stand. If the mare is bilaterally affected the prognosis is poor, but two to three days should elapse before it is considered hopeless.

Placental retention for more than 24 hours may occur despite oxytocin therapy. In these cases, repeated oxytocin treatment and antibiotics are indicated (see p. 548). If the placenta is still retained, most clinicians would remove it manually on the second postoperative day. In the heavier breeds of horse, placental retention may result in a serious septic metritis and laminitis syndrome with clinical signs of pyrexia, dyspnea due to pulmonary edema, lameness and reluctance to move, and vulval discharge of accumulated infected uterine fluids. If these mares are to survive, evacuation of all uterine contents and irrigation of the uterine lumen are immediately necessary, followed by symptomatic treatment for the other signs of illness.

Following inevitable delayed uterine contraction, manual manipulation of the uterus, per rectum, on the third to fourth postoperative day has been recommended to break down perimetrial adhesions. This procedure may be repeated at weekly intervals if significant adhesions are found.

In one published series, despite an 81 per cent maternal recovery rate, only 50 per cent of mares that were subsequently mated actually conceived and some aborted before term. The operation thus has an adverse effect on both fertility and the ability to maintain a normal pregnancy, probably due to uterine adhesions and fibrosis.

Supplemental Readings

Vandeplassche, M., Spincemaille, J., and Bouters, R.: Aetiology, pathogenesis, and treatment of retained placenta in the mare. Equine Vet. J., 3:144, 1971.

Vandeplassche, M.: Cesarian section in horses. *In* C. S. G., Grunsell, and F. W. H., Hill (eds.): The Veterinary Annual. Bristol, England, John Wright, 1973.

Vandeplassche, M., Bouters, R., Spincemaille, J., and Bonte, P.: Cesarian section in the mare. Proc. 23rd Annu. Conv. Am. Assoc. Eq. Pract., 1977, pp. 75–79.

Postpartum Complications

Walter W. Zent, LEXINGTON, KENTUCKY

A variety of injuries and disorders develop during foaling and the immediate postpartum period that can have serious consequences for the mare. The age and breed of the dam have some influence on the incidence of these complications, but many are purely accidents associated with the rapid and often violent birth process. Frequently, diagnosis is difficult because the clinical signs of many postpartum problems are nonspecific. Early recognition of postpartum disorders may improve the success rate of treatment.

PROLAPSED UTERUS

The mare uterus is composed of a body and two horns suspended cranially and laterally by the broad ligaments. The cranial attachment of the broad ligaments makes uterine prolapse less likely than in the cow. Uterine prolapse can occur after normal delivery, but is more common following dystocia or retention of placental membranes. It is my opinion that uterine prolapse is more common in Standardbreds than in Thoroughbreds.

Occasionally the tip of one uterine horn may partially prolapse after foaling, causing pain and straining, frequently resulting in a total eversion of the organ. Recurrences after subsequent foalings are more likely in mares having a history of previous uterine prolapse. Such mares should be observed closely during the early postpartum period. The principles in treating uterine prolapse are (1) controlling straining, (2) cleaning and replacing the uterus, and (3) preventing recurrence. Straining is best controlled by first sedating the mare with moderate doses of xylazine* and pentazocine,† followed by epidural anesthesia with 8 to 10 ml of 2 per cent lidocaine.‡

The uterus should be carefully and thoroughly washed with a dilute solution of mild disinfectant such as povidone-iodine solution.§ If the placenta can be easily removed, it is advantageous to do so before replacing the uterus. The uterus is examined for lacerations and carefully replaced, with an attempt to straighten out the horns as completely as possible. Antibiotic boluses are placed into the uterine lumen and the vulva sutured with a heavy material such as umbilical tape to prevent reprolapse.

Systemic antibiotics are indicated to control infection. Kanamycin* at 5 mg per kg given twice daily and procaine penicillin,† at 10 million units given twice daily, make a satisfactory broad-spectrum combination. If the mare's vital signs remain normal, no attempt should be made to medicate the uterus for several days. If there are signs of toxemia or an elevated temperature, the uterus should be examined and, if necessary, treatment for metritis should be instituted.

UTERINE RUPTURE

Uterine rupture may occur during dystocia or normal delivery. If the rupture is large, the mare will rapidly show signs of hemorrhagic shock and may die. If the serosa remains intact, there are signs of hemorrhage and colic, but the mare will usually survive. Smaller uterine ruptures such as those produced by perforation during dystocia may not be apparent until several hours after the initial injury. Signs of peritonitis gradually become evident after this time. Antibiotic therapy may control some of these infections, but the prognosis is grave. Intravenous gentamicin,‡ 2 mg per kg four times a day, and sodium penicillin,§ 10 million units twice a day, is one choice of antibiotic combination. The tear in the uterus may be difficult to find. However, if antibiotics fail to bring about improvement, surgical repair may be accomplished through a midline laparotomy.

UTERINE HEMORRHAGE

Hemorrhage from a uterine artery is common in older mares and is a significant cause of death in aged brood mares. Multiparous mares over 11 years of age are the prime candidates; however, a postpartum hemorrhage can occur rarely in younger horses. Peripartum hemorrhage can occur before, during, or after foaling. Dystocia does not seem to affect the incidence.

Uterine hemorrhages are not always fatal. If the broad ligament that surrounds the artery remains

---

*Rompun, Haver-Lockhart, Shawnee, KS

†Talwin, Winthrop-Breon Laboratories, New York, NY

‡Xylocaine, Astra Pharmaceutical Products, Inc., Westboro, MA

§Betadine, Purdue Frederick Co., Norwalk, NC

---

*Kantrim, Bristol Laboratories, Syracuse, NY

†Crysticillin, Squibb, Princeton, NJ

‡Gentocin, Schering Corp., Kenilworth, NJ

§Sodium Penicillin G, Squibb, Princeton, NJ

intact, the ligament may contain the hemorrhage and cause the blood to dissect between the myometrium and the serosa of the uterus, forming a hematoma. The resulting clot controls the arterial bleeding and the mare may survive depending on the quantity of blood lost. If the broad ligament ruptures with the artery or if the uterine serosa ruptures during hematoma formation, the blood quickly moves out into the peritoneal cavity and survival is less likely.

Clinical signs of postpartum hemorrhage include mild-to-severe colic, sweating, pale mucous membranes, and elevated pulse rate. Shock and death may be ultimate results. The most successful treatment is to keep the mare quiet using mild sedation if necessary. Blood transfusions, plasma expanders, and fluid therapy do not seem to alter the course of these cases and may even be contraindicated if the mare becomes excited by the treatment procedures. Naloxone* was used on an experimental basis during the 1984 breeding season on several mares with signs of postpartum hemorrhage. Eight milligrams of naloxone was given intravenously one time. The results were encouraging.

Some management practices are logical to minimize arterial rupture in older mares during the periparturient period. Because it is prudent to minimize handling of older mares, shipping, deworming, foot care, and minor surgery should be scheduled during a safer time period. Additionally, the routine Caslick's operation after foaling should be delayed a few days to minimize excitement and stress.

CERVICAL LACERATION

Laceration of the mare's cervix can occur during parturition and is commonly associated with dystocia. The injury may be produced by an oversized fetus, obstetric chains, or fetotomy wire. Although small cervical lacerations that do not interfere with closure of the os during diestrus are of no consequence, serious trauma can have a profound effect on future reproductive performance. I favor attempting to repair cervical lacerations during estrus when exposure and retraction are easier. When attempting repair of the injuries, it is important to free all of the adhesions between the cervix and the vaginal wall. The integrity of the lumen of the cervical canal must be maintained. For a more detailed discussion of the repair of the damaged cervix, see page 516.

Many cervical lacerations can be prevented. Sufficient time should be allowed for maximal dilation to occur before attempting to deliver a foal. Cutting

instruments that might predispose to cervical trauma should not be passed through the cervix. In difficult cases of dystocia, cesarean section should be considered if excessive manipulation or fetotomy is needed for vaginal delivery. The future reproductive potential of the mare following cesarean section is greater than following vaginal delivery with cervical damage.

VAGINAL RUPTURE

Vaginal rupture can occur by perforation of the foal's foot through the vaginal wall, or as a result of obstetric procedures. The dorsal vaginal wall is more susceptible when the feet of the foal are the cause. The vagina may rupture at any point from the cervix caudally. Cranial vaginal ruptures communicate directly with the peritoneal cavity. Concurrent damage to the colon or rectum need not occur. In mares in which a dorsal vaginal injury is not discovered at the time of foaling, the presenting signs are those of peritonitis, appearing as early as a few hours postpartum. There is seldom a prolapse of bowel through a laceration in this location.

Repair of dorsal vaginal rupture is most easily accomplished in the standing animal. The mare should be restrained in stocks and sedated. Epidural anesthesia with 10 ml of 2 per cent lidocaine is indicated. Intraperitoneal administration of an antibiotic solution such as 10 million units of sodium penicillin and 500 mg of gentamicin, buffered with sodium bicarbonate* (1 ml 7.5 per cent $NaHCO_3$ per 50 mg gentamicin), is easily accomplished through the tear in the vagina before repair. The volume of the infusion should be at least 500 ml. Stay sutures placed adjacent to the cervix may permit some retraction of the wound to a more accessible area, but the heavy postpartum uterus may make retraction difficult.

The edges of the laceration should be apposed with resorbable sutures. Completely sealing the wound is not necessary if the major portions of the edges are apposed. Following repair, a Caslick's operation will reduce the chances of air aspiration into the peritoneal cavity.

When laceration of the ventral wall of the vagina occurs, a frequent sequela is herniation of portions of the viscera, usually small intestine. If this prolapse occurs before delivery of the foal, it may complicate the dystocia. Vigorous attempts to deliver the foal vaginally can lead to serious trauma and contamination of the gut. Immediate cesarean section is therefore indicated. It is helpful to suture the labia completely before anesthesia induction to protect the herniating intestine.

---

*Narcan, DuPont Pharmaceuticals, Inc., Manati, Puerto Rico

*Sodium Bicarbonate Sterile Solution 7.5%, Med Tech, Inc., Elwood, KS

If the prolapsed gut has been badly damaged before the clinician's arrival, the only choice may be euthanasia of the mare to salvage the foal. The ideal approach to this problem is to shoot the mare and to immediately remove the foal through a slash incision. Chemical euthanasia greatly reduces foal survival.

RECTOVESTIBULAR INJURIES

Rectovestibular injuries occur during foaling when a foot fails to pass the vaginovestibular sphincter and the abdominal contractions of the mare force the foot dorsally and caudally. The resulting injury is a perforation of the vestibular roof and the rectum. If the situation is detected at this time and the foal is repelled and delivered vaginally, the more serious third-degree perineal laceration can be prevented.

In the case of either injury, repair should not be attempted for several weeks to allow resolution of edema and inflammation. Some rectovestibular fistulas will heal without surgery. Details on repair of these perineal and rectovestibular problems appear elsewhere (p. 550).

VULVAR LACERATION

Vulvar lacerations are common aftermaths of foaling. One of the frequent causes is failure to adequately open the previous year's Caslick's operation. If the laceration is severe, time must be allowed for resolution of inflammation before repair is attempted.

Extensive pressure on the labia during delivery can disrupt the circulation, resulting in vulvar necrosis. The resulting damage may reduce the amount of tissue remaining and may require a deeper closure than the simple Caslick's procedure. In the worst of these cases, it is often prudent to delay repair until after the mare is mated, thus allowing more healing time.

GASTROINTESTINAL COMPLICATIONS OF FOALING

A variety of intestinal complications can follow parturition in the mare, ranging from simple constipation to a ruptured viscus. The signs observed are often confusing and make the differential diagnosis challenging. Constipation is a frequent occurrence following delivery of the first foal. Bruising of the vagina and perineal area cause pain, which makes the mare reluctant to defecate. The resulting constipation is generally mild and will usually respond to mineral oil, 4 liters orally, and a little time.

A more serious intestinal problem follows bruising of the small colon when this organ is compressed between the uterus and pelvis during delivery. These mares will show signs of constipation soon after foaling. By the second day postpartum, signs of mild colic appear, and temperature may be elevated. At about 72 hours, signs of peritonitis are evident, such as fever, congested mucous membranes, elevated white blood cell count, and colic of increasing severity. Rectal examination at this time will usually reveal a large sausage-shaped mass involving the small colon. Immediate surgical intervention to resect the damaged bowel is indicated. Any delay will increase the possibility of further breakdown of the colon wall with resulting irreversible peritonitis.

The most serious intestinal problem related to parturition is rupture of the rectum, small colon, or cecum. Rectal and small colon rupture follows entrapment of the organs and compression during delivery. Cecal rupture, usually at the base of the cecum, occurs because of distention of the organ at the time of delivery. Abdominal compression is apparently forceful enough to cause the rupture. These mares develop peritonitis within a few hours with fatal results.

One management technique that may reduce the incidence of cecal rupture is the reduction of roughage intake by mares in the last few days prepartum. Most mares voluntarily eat less hay as parturition nears, but individual animals, especially in groups that compete for feed, may lose this natural instinct.

Rectal prolapse is occasionally an aftermath of foaling (p. 73). Immediate replacement of the prolapse may appear to be a satisfactory solution, but the short mesentery of the rectum may have been damaged in the process with compromise in the blood supply as a sequela. Cases in these mares follow the same pattern as cases involving bruised colon, with necrosis of the avascular portion of the rectal wall leading to leakage and peritonitis.

Surgical correction of rectal damage is difficult owing to the limited access to the area. One approach is to reprolapse the rectum and anastomose the healthy ends outside of the anus. It may help to have a second operator working through a ventral midline incision. This allows delineation of the damaged area of the rectum and can provide extra stretching of the mesentery to make it more accessible.

METRITIS-LAMINITIS-TOXEMIA SYNDROME

Postpartum metritis, while not common, is extremely serious because of the rapid development of laminitis, septicemia, and toxemia. Acute metritis may result from dystocia, retained placenta, or any massive contamination of the uterine lumen. The mare is usually depressed and anorectic 24 to 36 hours after foaling. The rectal temperature may range from 38.5° C to 41° C. The mucous membranes become congested, then muddy or purple. Depression progresses rapidly. There may be an increase in the digital pulse at any time, signifying the onset of laminitis.

The uterus usually contains several gallons of a chocolate-colored, fetid fluid, which distends the organ and pulls it over the pelvic brim. A small piece of placenta is frequently found in one horn. This membrane should be removed if it is readily lifted out without tearing. If the placenta is tightly adherent to the endometrium it is best left until complete separation has occurred.

Treatment should be directed at evacuation of the uterus to eliminate toxins. Large volumes of dilute povidone-iodine solution are pumped into the uterus using a stomach tube, pump, and a five-gallon bucket. The contents are then siphoned off. This washing procedure is repeated until the character of the fluid drained off is similar to that being pumped in. The entire procedure should be repeated at least twice a day.

After the uterus is emptied, antibiotic boluses should be introduced into the lumen. Systemic antibiotic therapy is imperative. Sodium penicillin (10 million units intravenously twice a day) with kanamycin (10 mg per kg twice a day) or gentamicin (2 mg per kg four times a day) offer broad-spectrum coverage. When acute metritis is treated vigorously from the onset, laminitis is an infrequent sequela. When laminitis does occur, however, it may develop very quickly and with dire consequences. Puerperal laminitis often results in sloughing of the hooves, necessitating euthanasia. The laminitis should be treated with anti-inflammatory drugs such as phenylbutazone* (4 gm daily) or dexamethasone† (20 mg daily).

If the mare can be kept on a three- to four-inch bedding of sand, uniform sole pressure is maintained, which reduces the chance of coffin bone rotation. Ice is helpful in reducing the inflammation of the feet, and forced exercise, when possible, will improve blood flow from the feet and help prevent rotation. It must be remembered that the laminitis in these cases is secondary to the metritis, so prompt and diligent treatment of the uterus is essential to correct the entire problem. Metritis-laminitis-toxemia syndrome is often fatal in mares that do not receive adequate care.

---

*Butazolidin, Jensen-Salsbery Labs, Kansas City, MO
†Azium, Schering Corp., Kenilworth, NJ

Supplemental Readings

Richter, J., And Gotze, R.: Tiergeburtshilfe, 3rd ed. Berlin, Verlag Paul Parey, 1980.
Roberts, S. J.: Veterinary Obstetrics and Genital Diseases, 2nd ed. Ithaca, published by author, 1971.
Vandeplassche, M.: Obstetrician's view of the physiology of equine parturition and dystocia. Equine Vet. J., 12:45, 1980.

Retained Placenta

J. Pierre Held, KNOXVILLE, TENNESSEE

A review of equine placentation is helpful in understanding the physiologic process involved in the normal expulsion of fetal membranes and in the etiology of retained placenta. Placentation in the mare is epitheliochorial, which means that the fetal membranes do not invade the uterine tissue, other than in the endometrial cup area where trophoblast cells infiltrate the uterine epithelium. The fully developed organ of nutrient exchange, the microcotyledon, is an interdigitation of chorionic and endometrial epithelium. After the microcotyledons are fully formed (approximately 150 days), the placental barrier is confined to the villi and crypts of the microplacentomes. Several areas of the chorion are devoid of villi. These are (1) the cervical star, located at the internal os of the cervix (during parturition the allantochorion breaks at this location); (2) the tip of both horns opposite the fallopian tube opening; (3) the endometrial cup site; and (4) invaginated placental folds, which usually occur over major allantoic vessels. At most of the avillous areas, glandular secretions accumulate between the chorion and endometrial epithelium.

Retained placenta has long been thought to be caused by placental edema preventing normal release of the membranes. This belief led to the rule of thumb that any placenta weighing more than 6.3 kg (14 lb) had some degree of pathology. In a study involving over 200 normal foalings, however, the normal weight for an equine Thoroughbred placenta varied between 4 and 8 kg (8.8 and 17.6 lb). It has also been shown that placentae are most frequently retained in the nonpregnant horn even though the incidence of edema is higher in the pregnant horn. Clinical experience indicates that delayed separation of the allantochorion seems to be a fairly localized phenomenon. If manual separation is attempted, areas of loose placenta alternate with areas in which the fetal membranes remain firmly attached.

Factors predisposing to retained placenta include induction of parturition before all signs of impending foaling are present (see p. 534), cesarean section, delayed uterine involution, and any obstetric manipulation, including fetotomy. The thickness of the allantochorion, its degree of folding, the length of the villi, as well as the degree of attachment are greater in the nongravid than the gravid horn. These factors may explain the greater frequency of retained placental membranes in the nonpregnant rather than the pregnant uterine horn.

MANAGEMENT OF RETAINED PLACENTA

Removal of the Placenta

Several different approaches are advocated for the removal of the placental membranes. The advantages and disadvantages of these methods are listed in Table 1.

Oxytocin Bolus. An intramuscular injection of oxytocin gives satisfactory results in some cases of retained placenta. Early postpartum doses greater than 60 IU can cause spasmodic contraction of the whole myometrium and are therefore of little value. When bolus injections are used, a dose of 30 to 40 IU should be given intramuscularly at intervals of 60 to 90 minutes. If parturition has occurred over 24 hours before oxytocin is injected, the dosage can be safely increased to 80 to 100 IU intramuscularly. Another approach for such cases is to inject repeated boluses intravenously (30 to 60 IU) until an adequate

response is detected by rectal palpation of the uterus.

Oxytocin Infusion. Intravenous oxytocin infusion is in my opinion the method of choice for placental removal. Eighty to 100 IU of oxytocin is prepared in 500 ml saline. The speed of infusion is adjusted according to the mare's reactions, the flow rate being slowed if excessive abdominal pain occurs. With this method, the retained membranes are generally expelled within 30 minutes. Gentle traction on the placenta will speed up expulsion. In cases treated several days after parturition, rapid infusion of up to 300 IU of oxytocin may be necessary before an adequate increase in uterine motility occurs.

Uterine Infusion. Infusion of a large volume of a povidone-iodine solution is another way to stimulate uterine contraction. Povidone-iodine solution* diluted 1:10 (10 to 12 liters) is infused into the allantochorionic space using a stomach tube. At the end of the infusion, the stomach tube is withdrawn and the opening in the fetal membranes tied with umbilical tape. At this point, the membranes may be squeezed to force the fluid into the uterus. The pressure of the fluid expanding the uterus, vagina, and cervix will stimulate endogenous oxytocin release. Membranes are usually expelled within 30 minutes. The main advantage of this method is that the uterus is not invaded; therefore, the risk of contamination is reduced. Such treatment should, however, be used only in early cases of retained placenta. If the mare starts straining excessively, the procedure should be discontinued to prevent occurrence of vaginal or uterine prolapse. In protracted cases, the allantochorion may rupture under the pressure of the fluids.

Manual Removal. Manual separation of the allantochorion is still used by some clinicians. The risk of damage to the uterus as well as the increased chance of infection is high with this traumatic

---

*Betadine, Purdue Frederick Co., Norwalk, CT

TABLE 1. ADVANTAGES AND DISADVANTAGES OF VARIOUS METHODS
FOR REMOVAL OF RETAINED PLACENTA

Method	Advantage	Disadvantage
Oxytocin; repeated bolus injections	Easy to apply; no special equipment needed; might be given by owner	Possibility of uterine cramps; may cause excessive discomfort to mare
Oxytocin; as a drip	Can be given to effect; method giving the most reliable results	Time involved to place catheter and set up infusion equipment
Povidone-iodine solution into allantoic space	Most physiologic method, as it stimulates endogenous oxytocin release	Time involvement; possibility of membrane rupture before expulsion; difficult to perform clean and leakless application, especially on restless mares
Manual separation	None	Danger of excessive bleeding; several attempts might be needed; increased uterine contamination. Microcotyledonary villi may remain in crypts

method. Limited manual separation at the time of a cesarean section is, however, useful to prevent postsurgical retention caused by inadvertent suturing of the membranes to the uterine incision.

Following removal, the placenta should be carefully examined to ensure that all the membranes have been expelled (see p. 528). In some instances, especially if the membranes have been manually extracted, the placenta may tear near the tip of the horn. The preferred treatment for this partial retention is either oxytocin injection or manual removal if the membranes are not too firmly attached. Antimicrobial therapy (see below) might also be instituted. Repeated oxytocin injection, 12 to 24 hours apart, is indicated in any case in which delayed uterine involution is diagnosed. Rectal examination is, therefore, an important clinical tool to monitor the status of the uterus.

CHEMOTHERAPY

In addition to the removal of all placental membranes from the uterus, antibiotics and anti-inflammatory drugs are often indicated in the treatment of retained placenta, especially in protracted cases or in cases in which severe uterine contamination is suspected (Table 2). During the first six to eight hours after foaling, bacterial growth remains minimal. If the placenta is retained for more than eight hours, bacteria multiply rapidly, and antimicrobial therapy should be instituted immediately.

Antimicrobial Treatment. A characteristic of uterine infections postpartum is the presence of a mixed bacterial population, which may include beta-hemolytic streptococci as well as coliforms. When these organisms are found, a broad-spectrum antibiotic effective against both gram-negative and gram-positive bacteria must be chosen. Some of the available antimicrobial agents that are particularly useful against mixed bacterial infections are listed in Table 3. When the route of administration is selected, it is important to remember that damaged uterine tissue may absorb intrauterine antibiotics poorly and consequently endometrial tissue levels may not exceed the minimal inhibitory concentration (MIC) of the infecting organism. In protracted cases of retained placenta, treatment should include both systemic and intrauterine infusion of antibiotics.

Anti-inflammatory Medication. Flunixin meglumine* or phenylbutazone† at the manufacturers recommended dosage may be helpful in preventing the metritis-laminitis-toxemia syndrome (see p. 546) following placental retention. The analgesic properties of these antiprostaglandin agents may also eliminate excessive abdominal pain caused by rapid uterine involution.

REFRACTORY CASES OF RETAINED PLACENTA

On occasion, routine therapeutic procedures fail to achieve delivery of the retained placenta, and a tightly adhered area of allantochorion may be palpable. The danger of forcibly stripping these membranes away from the endometrium should be recognized. Permanent endometrial damage may occur, resulting in a compromise of the mare's reproductive future.

In these protracted cases, chemotherapy combining local and systemic antibiotics and oxytocin infusions as well as phenylbutazone should be instituted. Each time the uterus is treated, the site of

---

*Banamine, Schering Corp., Kenilworth, NJ
†Butazolidin, Jensen-Salsbery Laboratories, Kansas City, MO

TABLE 2. SUPPORTIVE THERAPY FOLLOWING REMOVAL OF RETAINED PLACENTA

	Intrauterine Antibiotic Treatment	Parenteral Antimicrobial Therapy	Flunixin Meglumine or Phenylbutazone	Oxytocin
Placenta removed in less than 5 hrs postpartum without invading uterus	None	None	None	None
Placenta removed in less than 5 hrs after obstetrical manipulation minimal contamination	One treatment after placenta has been removed	None	None	One IV infusion after delivery of the foal
Placenta removed in less than 5 hrs after obstetrical manipulation marked contamination	One treatment after placenta has been removed	3–4 days	None	Two IV infusions or IM boluses 12 hrs apart
Membranes removed after more than 5 hrs	One treatment or as needed if delayed uterine involution with fluid pooling is present	3–4 days or as needed	2–3 days or as needed	Daily IV infusion for 2–3 days or as needed

TABLE 3. ANTIBIOTICS USED IN TREATMENT OF PROTRACTED RETAINED PLACENTA

Antibiotic	Intrauterine	Dosage Intramuscular	Intravenous
Procaine penicillin	1–5 Million IU	20,000 IU/Kg BID	—
Ampicillin	3 gm	10 mg/kg TID	10 mg/kg TID
Ticarcillin	1–3 gm	40–80 mg/kg BID	40–80 mg/kg BID or TID
Gentamicin	2–3 gm	2–4 mg/kg TID	—
Amikacin	2 gm	—	—
Kanamycin	2–3 gm	5–10 mg/kg TID	—
Polymyxin B	10,000–500,000 IU		

placental attachment may be explored for signs of release. Usually no more than three or four days of treatment are needed even in the most stubborn cases. If prolonged intrauterine antibiotic treatment is necessary and sensitivity tests are unavailabe, the use of amikacin will decrease the risk of bacterial resistance over most other antibiotics. If systemic and local treatment is necessary the combined use of intrauterine amikacin and intramuscular or intravenous ticarcillin would be a therapeutically compatible combination.

CONCLUSIONS

The key to successful treatment of retained placenta is the promotion of rapid uterine involution combined with antimicrobial therapy when indicated. The importance of limiting intrauterine ma-nipulation cannot be stressed enough. Even with strict aseptic conditions, the introduction of contaminants will increase the danger of subsequent metritis-laminitis-toxemia syndrome.

Supplemental Readings

Ayliffe, R. R., and Noakes, D. E.: Some preliminary studies on the uptake of sodium benzylpencillin by the endometrium of the cow. Vet. Rec., 102:215, 1978.

Burns, S. J., Judge, N. G., Martin, F. E., and Adams, L. G.: Management of retained placenta in mares. Proc. 23rd Annu. Conv. Am. Assoc. Eq. Pract., pp. 381–390, 1977.

Samuel, C. A., Allen, W. R., and Steven, D. H.: Studies on the equine Placenta. II. Ultrastructure of the placental barrier. J. Reprod. Fertil., 48:257, 1976.

Vandeplassche, M., Spincemaille, J., and Bouters, R.: Etiology, pathogenesis and treatment of retained placenta in the mare. Equine Vet. J., 3:144, 1971.

Whitwell, K. E., and Jeffcott, L. B.: Morphological studies on the fetal membranes of the normal singleton foal at term. Res. Vet. Sci., 19:44, 1975.

Parturient Perineal and Rectovestibular Injuries

Rolf M. Embertson, LEXINGTON, KENTUCKY
James T. Robertson, COLUMBUS, OHIO

Several types of injuries may be associated with parturition in the mare. These include vaginal and cervical contusions and lacerations, uterine rupture or prolapse, urinary bladder eversion or prolapse, and perineal lacerations, including rectovestibular fistulas. Perineal lacerations are probably the most common type of injury that require surgical repair.

The majority of perineal lacerations occur in the ceiling of the vestibule beginning at or just caudal to the vaginovestibular junction. This is located at the cranial aspect of the transverse fold that covers the external urethral orifice. This fold continues dorsally as the hymen in young healthy mares. Vaginal lacerations occur infrequently cranial to the vaginovestibular junction and only occasionally enter the peritoneal cavity.

Perineal lacerations are classified by the extent and severity of tissue damage:

1. First-degree lacerations involve the mucosa of the vestibule and skin of the dorsal commissure of the vulva.

2. Second-degree lacerations involve the vestibular mucosa and submucosa, skin of the dorsal commissure of the vulva, and perineal body musculature, including the constrictor vulvae.

3. Third-degree lacerations involve the ceiling of the vestibule, floor of the rectum, perineal septum and musculature, and anal sphincter.

4. Rectovestibular fistulas involve the ceiling of the vestibule, floor of the rectum, and a variable amount of the perineal septum and musculature.

Perineal lacerations usually result from delivery of a malpositioned or oversized fetus and occasionally from overzealous assistance during foaling. Third-degree lacerations and rectovestibular fistulas are more commonly seen in the primiparous mare; the forefoot of the fetus may catch on the dorsal transverse fold of the vaginovestibular junction. Continued expulsion drives the foot up through the dorsum of the vestibule and into the rectum. If this situation is corrected by manual assistance or spontaneously, the result is a rectovestibular fistula. With no correction, the expulsive efforts of delivery result in a third-degree laceration.

TREATMENT

FIRST-DEGREE LACERATIONS

These can be repaired using Caslick's operation. This will return the tissue at the dorsal aspect of the vulva to its previous appearance. This injury can be repaired in the acute state or after the inflammation subsides. Dietary management is unnecessary.

SECOND-DEGREE LACERATIONS

These require reconstruction to repair the damaged perineal body and vestibular sphincter. A simple Caslick's operation usually leaves a sunken perineum, which predisposes to pneumovagina and its associated problems. Dietary management is unnecessary as the rectum is not involved. Repair may be performed under epidural or local analgesia with the mare standing in stocks.

A triangular section of mucous membrane is removed from the ceiling and dorsal walls of the vestibule. The base of this triangle is the mucocutaneous junction of the vulva with the apex located in the vestibule. The incised edges of vestibular mucosa are sutured together, as are the exposed submucosal surfaces and the edges of cutaneous perineum. Natural breeding is delayed for four to six weeks to allow adequate time for healing.

THIRD-DEGREE LACERATIONS

Preoperative Considerations

Surgical repair during the acute state is seldom successful. The response to perineal trauma, bacterial contamination, tissue inflammation, edema, and some devitalization create a poor environment for successful surgery. If immediate repair is attempted, it should be performed within the first few hours after injury with adequate debridement of devitalized tissue and strict adherence to the principles of repair.

Following the acute injury, daily cleansing of the wound during the first week is beneficial and ensures examination for potential complications. Antibiotics and nonsteroidal anti-inflammatory therapy is appropriate for three to five days and current tetanus prophylaxis is mandatory. A minimum of three to four weeks delay in repair is necessary to allow for resolution of the inflammation, wound margin epithelialization, and wound contracture. The dimensions of the wound will decrease significantly during this period.

Extensive lacerations that penetrate the vaginal wall and peritoneal reflection are rare. These require immediate attention with closure of the vaginal perforation to prevent evisceration and peritonitis.

If there is a live foal, it is usually advisable to delay repair until weaning. Confinement to a hospital environment restricts the foal's exercise and exposes it to hospital infections and other hazards. In addition, management of the mare's diet may adversely affect lactation.

Soft feces that are reduced in volume are important to the success of the repair. Several different feeding and laxative regimens have been used including lush green grass, pelleted rations, wet bran mashes, magnesium sulfate, mineral oil, and dioctyl sodium sulfosuccinate (DSS),* all with reported success. Abrupt changes in feeding should be avoided by making adjustments over a four- to five-day period. Prolonged fasting to empty the intestinal tract has been recommended, but this is unnecessary and may predispose to enteritis.

Treatments necessary to produce and maintain soft feces will vary between mares. Lush green grass pasture with mineral oil is sufficient for some. If this is not available, the following regimen may be used on healthy mares with normal hydration:

1. Gradually discontinue feeding hay and change to a pelleted ration.

2. Provide a wet bran mash with sweet feed and mineral oil twice daily.

3. Administer magnesium sulfate (0.5 to 1.0 gm per kg) dissolved in two gallons of water once daily via a nasogastric tube.

---

*Dioctynate, The Butler Co., Columbus, OH

4. On alternate days, DSS (0.02 to 0.04 gm per day) is added until the feces are soft, at which time the surgery is performed.

Fasting the mare 24 hours before surgery is desirable to reduce the amount of feces in the operative and immediate postoperative period.

Phenylbutazone (4 mg per kg intravenously) and procaine penicillin G (20,000 IU per kg intramuscularly) are administered three to four hours preoperatively, ensuring effective blood levels during surgery. Phenylbutazone may help in the immediate postoperative period to decrease inflammation and swelling and lessen the mare's tendency to strain. Although no definite advantage for antibiotic use has been shown, the inevitable contamination of the surgery site and the large anaerobic bacterial population in the feces justifies the use of penicillin.

Preparation

The mare is placed in stocks and tranquilized. Acepromazine HCl* (0.05 mg per kg intravenously) and xylazine† (0.4 mg per kg intravenously) can be used together or individually. The diuretic effect of xylazine may cause intraoperative micturition. During lengthy procedures the mare may become uncooperative, requiring a trustworthy handler at her head to lessen the anxiety level of both the mare and the surgeon. Additional doses of xylazine (0.8 mg per kg intramuscularly) and occasionally butorphanol tartrate‡ (0.02 mg per kg intravenously) may be indicated.

The tail is bandaged and the tail head is clipped and prepared for epidural analgesia. Six to 9 ml of 2 per cent lidocaine or mepivacaine HCL§ should provide adequate regional analgesia for a 450-kg mare for about two hours. More than 9 to 10 ml may cause posterior ataxia or even recumbency. General anesthesia is indicated in those mares that become recumbent and uncontrollably frightened. Although positioning becomes a problem, the procedure can be completed in dorsal or ventral recumbency under general anesthesia or postponed. Recumbent mares that are quiet should be kept comfortable until they can stand.

The tail is tied securely to the top cross bar of the stocks to remove it from the surgical field and provide posterior support if the mare becomes ataxic. The rectum is manually evacuated. The rectum, vestibule, and perineum are thoroughly cleansed with a mild soap, then sprayed with povidone-iodine solution.||

---

*Acepromazine, Ayerst Laboratories, New York, NY
†Rompun, Haver-Lockhart, Shawnee, KS
‡Stadol, Bristol Laboratories, Syracuse, NY
§Carbocaine, Winthrop-Breon Laboratories, New York, NY
||Prepodyne Solution, West Chemical Products Inc., Princeton, NJ

Balfour retractors or stay sutures placed through the labia and perineal tissue can be used to aid exposure. Either can be sutured to the skin or held by an assistant. A surgical light or a head lamp worn by the surgeon provide illumination of the surgical site.

Principles of Repair

Successful repair depends on careful observation of basic surgical principles, preparation of the patient, and postoperative care. The suture material used must be of sufficient strength and should cause minimal tissue reaction. Hand ties and surgeon's knots are necessary to snugly place sutures no more than 1.0 to 1.5 cm apart, thus producing firm tissue apposition. This is aided by adequate dissection to create generous flaps of the rectal and vestibular walls. Loosely placed sutures lead to poor tissue apposition, fistulation, and possible repair dehiscence. Excessive hemorrhage is unusual but should be controlled, as hematomas in the repair are undesirable.

Operative Techniques

The variety of surgical techniques currently employed involve two phases of repair: (1) dissection and reconstruction of the rectovestibular septum and (2) dissection and reconstruction of the perineal body.

The surgery can be performed in one stage, wherein both phases of the repair are completed in one procedure or in two stages, wherein the second phase is done about two weeks after the first. The two-stage repair allows the mare to defecate more easily during the early healing of the rectovestibular septum because of the larger anal orifice. This may reduce the incidence of postoperative rectal impactions. The advantage of a single stage repair is less need for preoperative and postoperative care, less time for hospitalization, and one surgical procedure (unless the repair breaks down).

Two surgical techniques will be described: (1) the six-bite vertical suture pattern (modified Goetze pattern) and (2) the rectal pull-back technique.

Both procedures are performed in one stage. The dissection is similar for both techniques, except the rectal pull-back technique requires a more generous cranial dissection. The intact portion of the rectovestibular shelf is incised cranially 2 to 8 cm, determined by the surgical technique planned, in a horizontal plane. Dissection is then directed caudally on each side along the junction of the rectal and vestibular mucosa and continued to the cutaneous perineum. The tissue flaps created should be thicker on the rectal side than the vestibular side if the six-bite vertical suture pattern is used. Flaps of equal thickness are appropriate for the rectal pull-back technique.

The six-bite vertical suture pattern repair (Fig. 1) uses nonabsorbable, noncapillary, synthetic suture material and a large half-circle cutting edge needle. Each suture is knotted in the vestibule leaving long (10 cm) ends for easy removal in 14 days. The first bite starts in the vestibule and is placed deep through the left vestibular flap emerging in the plane of dissection. The second bite is placed through the left rectal flap emerging just below the rectal mucosa. The third bite is placed in the right rectal flap emerging in the plane of dissection. The fourth bite goes deep through the right vestibular flap emerging in the vestibule. The fifth bite is placed up through the right vestibular flap near its edge and the sixth bite is placed down through the left vestibular flap near its edge and emerging in the vestibule. The suture is tied by hand under tension, which will abut the rectal flaps and invert the vestibular flaps into the vestibule. This pattern is started in the cranial pocket created in the rectovestibular septum by dissection and continued caudally to a point 4 to 6 cm from the cutaneous perineum. Sutures must not penetrate the rectal mucosa. The perineal body is then reconstructed as previously described.

The rectal pull-back technique (Fig. 2) starts by placing four long Allis tissue forceps in the rectal submucosa along the caudal margin of the dissected rectal shelf. The dissection should be adequate to allow the rectal floor to be pulled caudally to the level of the anal sphincter. The rectovestibular septum is reconstructed by placing No. 3 chromic

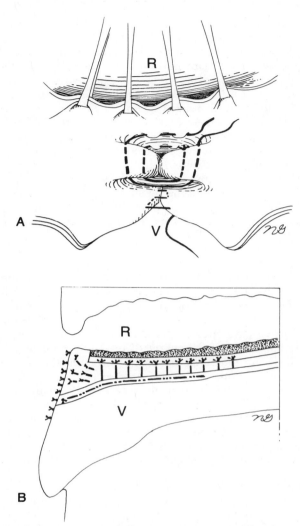

Figure 2. *A,* The rectal pull-back technique used in repair of third-degree perineal lacerations. Shown are suture placement and Allis tissue forceps grasping the rectal floor. R, rectum; V, vestibule. *B,* The rectal pull-back technique, depicting a sagittal view of the finished surgery. R, Rectum; V, vestibule.

gut or No. 2 polygalactin 910* sutures in an interrupted purse string pattern, starting at the most cranial aspect of the dissection and continuing caudally. The tissue incorporated in each suture includes (in order): right perivestibular tissue, right vestibular submucosa, left vestibular submucosa, left perivestibular tissue, left rectal submucosa, and right rectal submucosa. With each suture, the rectal floor is retracted caudally before the rectal submucosal bites are placed. The suture does not penetrate the rectal or vestibular mucosa. The purse string pattern is continued caudally about one third of the length of the laceration. A continuous horizontal

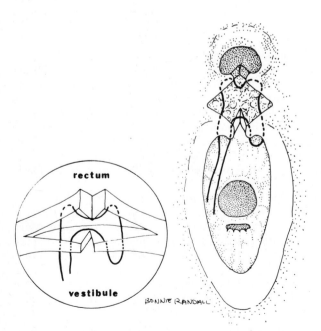

Figure 1. The six-bite vertical suture pattern used in repair of third-degree perineal lacerations. Suture placement is shown.

---

*Vicryl, Ethicon Inc., Somerville, NJ

mattress pattern is then placed in the edges of the vestibular flaps using No. 0 chromic gut or No. 0 polygalactin 910. This pattern inverts the edges of the vestibular flaps into the vestibule and is continued to the point at which the purse string pattern ended. It is then tied, and the remainder left in the vestibule until needed again. In this manner, the two-suture patterns are alternated to the point at which the perineal body reconstruction (phase 2) is started. Occasionally, the intact rectal floor cannot be pulled caudally to the anal sphincter. If this happens, the purse string pattern is continued past the caudal edge of the intact rectal floor, creating a floor or apposing the submucosa of the remaining left and right rectal flaps. The perineal body is then reconstructed.

Postoperative Management

The mare should remain on the same diet and receive laxatives as needed to keep the feces soft for two weeks postoperatively. Phenylbutazone and penicillin therapy are continued for another three to five days after surgery. Excessive postoperative examination of the surgical site should be avoided. Only in the case of an impacted rectum should the rectum be manually evacuated or enemas administered. The nonabsorbable sutures used in the six-bite technique are removed 12 to 14 days after surgery. The reproductive tract should be examined in four to six weeks. If it appears healthy, artificial insemination is possible in six to eight weeks, but natural breeding should wait at least three months.

RECTOVESTIBULAR FISTULAS

The surgical preparation, analgesia, principles of repair, and postoperative management for rectovestibular fistulas are the same as discussed for third-degree perineal lacerations. Immediate repair in the acute state is rarely successful. The recommended delay leads to a dramatic decrease in the size of the fistula, with spontaneous closure in rare cases.

As with third-degree lacerations, different repair techniques have been used with successful results. The different techniques include a horizontal perineal approach, the creation and repair of a third-degree laceration, a vestibular approach, and a rectal approach. The horizontal perineal approach produces the most consistent results. Creation and repair of a third-degree laceration is generally not recommended unless there is just a narrow strip of perineal tissue separating the anus and vulva. Although this wound is a rectovestibular fistula by strict definition, it is essentially a third-degree laceration and should be repaired as such.

The horizontal perineal approach (Fig. 3) requires a horizontal perineal incision midway between the anus and vulva. Dissection through the rectovestib-

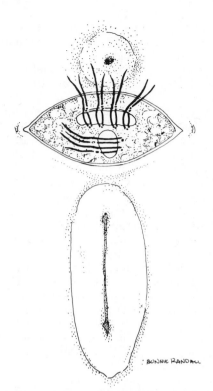

Figure 3. The horizontal perineal approach to repair of a rectovestibular fistula. Suture placement is shown.

ular septum is performed carefully so that no perforations are made into the rectum or vestibule. The dissection is continued 3 to 4 cm cranial to the fistula, incising its edges along the rectal and vestibular mucosal junction.

The principal lines of stress in the rectal wall occur at right angles to its longitudinal axis. Fistulas closed along these lines of stress (transversely) are subjected to less distracting forces than when closed against these lines of stress (longitudinally). Sutures of sufficient strength are preplaced longitudinally in the rectal submucosa using an interrupted Lembert pattern. These sutures are tied to convert the fistula to a transverse closure and to invert the rectal mucosa into the rectum. Sutures must not perforate the rectal mucosa.

The vestibular side of the fistula is closed in a similar manner (inverting the vestibular mucosa into the vestibule) except the sutures are placed transversely, creating a longitudinal closure. The space created by dissection is then closed in an interrupted purse string suture pattern and the cutaneous perineum is closed with simple interrupted sutures. Alternatively, this space can be packed with gauze, which is gradually removed over four to five days, allowing the wound to fill with granulation tissue.

PROGNOSIS

The breeding prognosis for mares with repaired perineal lacerations and rectovestibular fistulas is good. Concurrent vaginitis or endometritis usually resolves during the first postoperative estrus, following appropriate treatment as necessary. With attendance and proper care at subsequent foalings, additional severe perineal injuries are unusual.

Supplemental Readings

Asbury, A. C.: The reproductive system. *In* Mansmann, R. A., McAllister, E. S., and Pratt, P. W. (eds.): Equine Medicine and Surgery, 3rd ed. Santa Barbara, CA, American Veterinary Publications, 1982, pp. 1305–1367.

Colahan, P. T.: Female urogenital surgery. *In* Mansmann, R. A., McAllister, E. S., and Pratt, P. W. (eds.): Equine Medicine and Surgery, 3rd ed. Santa Barbara, CA, American Veterinary Publications, 1982, pp. 1367–1384.

Turner, A. S., and McIlwraith, C. W.: Techniques in Large Animal Surgery. Philadelphia, Lea & Febiger, 1982, pp. 177–182.

Vaughan, J. T.: Equine urogenital system. *In* Jennings, P. B. (ed.): The Practice of Large Animal Surgery. Philadelphia, W. B. Saunders Company, 1984, pp. 1122–1150.

Walker, D. F., and Vaughan, J. T.: Surgery of the perineum, vagina, and rectum. *In* Bovine and Equine Urogenital Surgery. Philadelphia, Lea & Febiger, 1980, pp. 197–213.

Evaluation of Stallion Fertility

John P. Hurtgen, NEW FREEDOM, PENNSYLVANIA

A fertility evaluation should assess libido, mating ability, and the quality of the semen ejaculated. This evaluation may be indicated before or after the purchase of a proved or unproved stallion, in a stallion with suspected subfertility or infertility, or as a management aid to maximize efficiency in a breeding program.

The best measurement of a stallion's fertility is the foaling rate of a large group of mares mated by him under optimal conditions of management. Nevertheless, a fertility evaluation is recommended for stallions before their first breeding season. No single physical characteristic or test of semen quality will accurately predict stallion fertility. Therefore, a series of observations, involving libido, mating behavior, external and internal genitalia, and semen quality, are used.

HISTORY AND PHYSICAL EXAMINATION

A complete history should be obtained, including age, previous management, use, and, if appropriate, frequency of ejaculation, present level of fertility, and previous fertility evaluation findings. Information should be obtained on factors that could influence libido and semen quality: severity and duration of illness or injury; medication history with particular reference to anabolic steroids, corticosteroids, and gonadotropins; and vaccination history.

General health and bodily condition may reflect disease or management conditions. Conditions seen in the stallion or his offspring that may have a heritable basis (umbilical hernia, cryptorchidism, parrot mouth, wobbler syndrome, and combined immunodeficiency disease) should be particularly noted.

OBSERVATION OF LIBIDO AND MATING BEHAVIOR AND SEMEN COLLECTION

An estrous mare is usually the most satisfactory mount for semen collection. Some stallions have been trained to or are willing to mount a phantom or "dummy" mare. The mount mare's tail is wrapped with gauze or placed in a plastic sleeve, fastened at the base of the tail with adhesive tape. The mare's buttocks and perineum are cleansed in a routine manner and the mare is restrained with a twitch.

Semen is collected using an artificial vagina. The inner liner jacket of the device is filled with warm water so that its internal temperature is 44 to 48° C at the time of semen collection. The liner should be lubricated with nonspermicidal lubricant. Collection should take place in a spacious area for the safety of all concerned. The semen should be protected from drafts, sunlight, and contamination with dust and water. A condom or "breeder's bag" may also be used for semen collection, but contamination and loss of the sample limit the use of this method. Dismount semen samples are unsuitable for evaluating stallion fertility.

The stallion is introduced to the estrous mare in a chute or at a teasing rail or board until erection occurs. The penile urethra, fossa glandis, and prepuce may be swabbed, using suitable transport media, for bacteriologic examinations. The stallion, when prepared, is allowed to mount the mare in a controlled manner. The penis is directed into the artificial vagina, which is held firmly against the mare's thigh during thrusting until ejaculation occurs, when urethral pulsations (three to nine) can be palpated at the ventral surface of the penis.

Immediately after dismount the penis can be maintained in a semierect state by an encircling grip around its base. A postejaculatory swab for bacteriologic examination can then be taken while the urethra is dilated. The artificial vagina is taken to the laboratory where the collection vessel is removed. Any gel is removed by filtration or aspiration with a syringe, the volume of the sample is measured, and its color is noted.

SEMEN EVALUATION

All laboratory equipment used to handle the semen should be prepared warm and free of chemical contamination. A small drop of raw semen is placed on a microscope slide, under a coverslip, and viewed at 40, 100, or 400 × magnification, for an estimation of the total percentages of motile and progressively motile sperm. The presence and relative numbers of erythrocytes, leukocytes, and spermatocytes are also noted as these cell types may not be easily visible in stained smears. Additional estimates of sperm motility can be made with semen diluted in a suitable extender.

The longevity of motility in raw and extended semen samples is a useful test, particularly in some infertile stallions. Aliquots of semen are placed in plastic tubes, capped and free of air, then incubated at 22° C in a dark, draft-free area. Motility is estimated at one- to two-hour intervals until the progressive motility falls to less than 10 per cent. Seminal extenders may enhance or adversly affect sperm motility. Some individuals' semen may respond differently to seemingly "acceptable" extenders. The pH should be measured with a pH meter immediately after collection and should register between 7.35 and 7.7. Measurements using pH paper are too inaccurate to be of value.

It is recommended that two or three smears should be made from each ejaculate for immediate staining with eosin-nigrosin.* Cells are examined for morphologic characteristics at 1000 × magnification using an oil immersion objective. As leukocytes and spermatocytes cannot be identified using this background stain, an additional one or two smears should be made for subsequent staining with hematoxylin and eosin.

Artifactual damage to sperm morphology may be caused by using slides at less than 35° C, by delays in smear preparation, and by the staining itself. Acrosome and midpiece damage, including loss of acrosome, are the most commonly induced artifacts. In order to obtain more repeatable, artifact-free morphology estimations, four to six drops of raw semen are fixed in 2 ml buffered formol saline or buffered glutaraldehyde before examination as a wet mount using phase contrast microscopy.

Sperm concentration can be determined using a spectrophotometer, after a standard curve has been developed, or with a hemocytometer. For the spectrophotometer, the percentage transmittance of semen diluted 1:10 or 1:20 in formol saline is measured at 525 µ. The hemocytometer should be used for low sperm density samples or for those with a high proportion of nonsperm cells or debris. Raw semen or formol saline–diluted semen is examined at dilutions ranging from 1:20 to 1:100. The erythrocyte dilution pipette is commonly used. Commercially available diluting systems* designed for peripheral blood samples are also useful for the dilution of semen samples. The total number of spermatozoa in the ejaculate is determined by multiplying the volume of gel-free semen by the sperm concentration.

EXAMINATION OF THE GENITALIA

The penis, prepuce, urethral process, and fossa glandis are carefully examined before semen collection. The testes and epididymes are palpated after semen collection for their presence, location, size, consistency, and shape. The length, width, and height of each testicle is measured using calipers. The testes are held in the ventral aspect of the scrotal sac and the total width of the scrotum and testes is measured. The head, body, and tail of each epididymis are carefully palpated.

The internal genitalia are palpated per rectum, provided that adequate facilities for restraint are available. Using the pelvic urethra as a landmark, the vesicular glands and ampullae are located and their presence, size, and consistency are noted. The bulbourethral glands cannot be identified per rectum. The vasa deferentia are often difficult to examine in their entirety, from the ampullae to the internal inguinal rings. The degree of patency of the internal inguinal rings is noted.

INTERPRETATION OF FINDINGS

Although lower foaling rates are accepted in the horse breeding industry, highly fertile stallions repeatedly achieve foaling rates of greater than 80 per cent when mated with reproductively healthy mares under good management conditions. As foaling rates are determined by the percentage of mares that

---

*Morphology stain, Society for Theriogenology, Association Bldg., 8th and Minnesota Sts., Hastings, NB 68901

*Unopette Test 5851 or 5855, Becton-Dickinson, Rutherford, NJ

deliver foals following mating throughout an entire breeding season, stallion fertility may be influenced by managerial factors such as the number of estrous cycles in which the mares are mated. Stallions with a large "book" of mares may be limited to mating each mare too infrequently to achieve maximal potential fertility. Management factors must therefore be considered in any stallion fertility assessment. Libido, behavior toward handlers and mares, mounting ability, and efficiency of ejaculation are particularly important for assessment. In some cases, these factors may be difficult to assess on the basis of one examination; for these cases repeated examinations, over a period of time in a variety of circumstances, may be indicated. Behavioral or mating problems can often be overcome in time to avoid delays if evaluations are made sufficiently in advance of the breeding season.

Factors such as stallion age, medication, frequency of ejaculation, staining methods, interval from semen collection to evaluation, type of extender used, method of semen collection, and experience of the examiner can all influence semen quality results. Factors such as the intended frequency of ejaculation, method of mating, interval between evaluation and the breeding season, breeding hygiene, and reproductive health of the mares to be mated can influence the relationship between results of semen quality and fertility achievable. Fertility evaluations must therefore be performed in a systematic and thorough manner.

Daily sperm output averages 4×10^9 in normal young stallions and 6×10^9 in normal mature stallions. There is a direct correlation between testicular size and daily sperm output. The dimensions of normal testes are approximately 9 to 10 cm in length, 5 to 6 cm in width, and 5 to 6.5 cm in height. Total scrotal width should be greater than 10 cm in mature stallions. To estimate daily sperm output, it is necessary to collect one ejaculate per day for seven days. This is impractical under most circumstances.

Stallions in regular use (3 to 7 ejaculates per week) that ejaculate less than 3×10^9 sperm per day should be viewed with suspicion and the reason for the low sperm output sought. Common causes are small testes, testicular degeneration, overuse, incomplete ejaculation, and administration of some drugs such as exogenous hormones. If low sperm output is noted outside the physiologic breeding season, the evaluation should be repeated during the season.

The effects on semen quality of racing or performance and the associated stresses of transportation, housing, and training are unknown. Similarly, the effects on semen quality and subsequent fertility of many drugs commonly administered to stallions is unknown. Exogenous testosterone, estrogen, and certain anabolic steroids, if administered in sufficient dosage frequently enough, will decrease sperm output and testicular size. Similar abnormalities of semen quality occur in testicular hypoplasia and chronic degenerative atrophy. Therefore, a careful interpretation of such abnormalties is required when they are detected in colts in training, destined for a stud career.

Sperm motility recordings are estimates and are frequently lower during periods of mating inactivity than during regular use. Progressive motility estimates are lower in those stallions whose sperm tend to agglutinate, for as yet unknown reasons. The significance of this phenomenon in terms of fertility is unknown. Temperature shock and increased incidence of tail and midpiece abnormalities decrease sperm motility. There is a wide variation in motility estimates between examiners and by the same examiner; however, the second ejaculate should be as motile or more so than the first ejaculate.

Highly fertile stallions ejaculate semen with 50 per cent or more progressively motile sperm. At least 10 per cent of sperm from such stallions in regular use should remain progressively motile for six or more hours after collection when stored in a dark draft-free environment at room temperature. Stallions which produce semen with less than 30 per cent immediate progressive motility in raw semen or have less than 10 per cent progressive motility two hours after collection should be suspected of having reduced conception rates per estrous cycle. The pH of normal semen ranges from 7.35 to 7.7 and is usually the same or slightly higher in the second ejaculate as compared with the first. A high pH may occur with ejaculatory failure, incomplete ejaculation, urospermia, or inflammatory conditions of the internal genitalia. The pH of preejaculatory fluid is usually 7.8 to 8.2. Sperm with morphologic abnormalities are found in the semen of all stallions. Normal sperm have abaxial attachment of the midpiece to the head, no proximal or distal midpiece cytoplasmic droplets, and a straight midpiece and tail.

Morphologic sperm abnormalities may arise in the testes or epididymes following impaired spermatogenesis or maturation or may be induced by semen handling or storage. Loss of acrosome, fraying or thickening of the midpiece, slight bending of the tail, and detachment of the sperm heads can result from temperature shock, storage of raw semen, and staining. Immediate fixation of the sample after collection in buffered formol saline or glutaraldehyde and examination of a wet mount under a phase contrast microscope can avoid induced abnormalities. Although the causes of many sperm abnormalities remain unknown, it is reasonable to assume that, above certain levels, fertility will be depressed by high proportions of abnormal sperm.

The effects of morphologic abnormalities on sperm viability and fertilizing ability has not been determined in detail.

Acrosome and head shape abnormalities, proximal cytoplasmic droplets, tightly coiled tails, detached heads, and midpiece abnormalities are most commonly associated with impaired spermatogenesis and infertility. Although the significance of distal cytoplasmic droplets on fertility is unknown, they appear to be of little importance. Their incidence decreases as ejaculation frequency increases. Increased proportions of distal cytoplasmic droplets, bent tails, and detached heads may be seen in stallions during periods of mating inactivity.

Although wide variations in the proportions of sperm abnormalities may be acceptable for normal stallions, most highly fertile stallions in regular use have less than 10 to 15 per cent of any single morphologic defect and have more than 60 per cent morphologically normal sperm. There are usually less than 5 per cent acrosome or midpiece abnormalities.

It is commonly recommended that mares be inseminated with 100 to 500 $\times$ 10^6 progressively motile, morphologically normal sperm. The number of spermatozoa needed to achieve acceptable fertility under conditions of natural mating is unknown.

The fertility of an individual stallion can be significantly influenced by factors such as the frequency of use, breeding potential of mated mares, timing and method of mating, and stallion behavior. Under certain management conditions, subfertile stallions may achieve acceptable foaling rates or normally fertile stallions may perform poorly. Information gained during a fertility evaluation may provide management assistance in optimizing fertility for an otherwise subfertile stallion.

Supplemental Readings

Society for Theriogenology: Manual for Clinical Fertility Evaluation of the Stallion. Published by the Society for Theriogenology, Hastings, NB, 1983.

Stallion Genital Abnormalities

John P. Hurtgen, NEW FREEDOM, PENNSYLVANIA

Stallion infertility may be associated with seminal abnormality (see p. 564), behavioral and mating disorders (see p. 555), venereal diseases (see p. 567), and abnormalities of the genitalia. The latter category includes traumatic injury, abnormalities of the penis or urethral process, contamination of the semen with urine or blood, and infection of the internal genitalia.

TRAUMATIC INJURIES

PENIS AND PREPUCE

Traumatic injuries to the penis and prepuce may be caused by a kick from a mare during mating, or may be the result of improperly fitted stallion "rings" and trauma from vulval "breeding stitches." Adequate restraint of the mare during mating is essential. A twitch should be applied to the upper lip and if the mare starts to kick, the stallion handler should pull the mare's head toward the stallion so that the mare's buttocks move away from the stallion. Padded felt boots can be fitted to the hind feet of mares to ameliorate the effects of a kick, should one occur. Individual mares may require tranquilization.

When artificial insemination is used, penile injuries may be caused by improperly fitted, cracked, or wrinkled phantom covers. When artificial vagina liners are secured by rubber bands, these may occasionally slip onto the penis during thrusting. If they are quickly stripped off the penis, a seroma may result. The penis should be gripped proximal to the band, which is then cut and removed. Stallion paddocks should be separated from mare paddocks by double fencing, at least 10 feet apart, or the stallion may attempt to mate across the fence, resulting in trauma to the external genitalia.

Extreme care must be exercised when catheterizing the stallion's urethra because of the risk of causing urethral irritation and bacterial contamination. The fossa glandis is a common source of both potentially pathogenic and nonpathogenic bacteria. The end of the penis and urethra should be thoroughly cleansed before catheterization is attempted, using sterile gloves and a sterile catheter. Repeated catheterization of the same stallion should be kept to a minimum.

Trauma to the penis and prepuce may result in edema or hemorrhage. Preputial edema is usually generalized whereas penile edema may be localized. The penis may prolapse from the preputial sheath, often bowing in a caudal direction. The edematous penis or prepuce should be elevated and supported to aid fluid return from the damaged tissues. This can be achieved using a stallion "supporter" or an encircling abdominal bandage that can include the penis and prepuce. If only the penis is damaged, this can be supported in the prepuce with temporary retention sutures, which close the preputial orifice. The penis must be periodically withdrawn for cleansing; ointments are used to prevent the penile skin from drying and cracking. Pressure bandaging may prevent further penile swelling and may reduce existing edema. When paraphimosis occurs, exercise should be limited to avoid further damage to the injured penis. Cold water hydrotherapy and massage (30 minutes per treatment, two to four times daily) may prevent further fluid accumulation. After the threat of further edema or hemorrhage has passed, warm water hydrotherapy may help to disperse fluid from the affected tissues.

Antibiotic ointments should be applied if there are penile or preputial lacerations or abrasions. Systemic antibiotic treatment is recommended for deeper lacerations. Phenylbutazone, aspirin, and flunixin meglumine are helpful as anti-inflammatory agents and analgesics. Treatment may be necessary for as short a period as two to three days or as long as two to three months.

Tranquilizers are contraindicated in cases of paraphimosis or penile injury as they cause further penile prolapse and edema. Sexual arousal should be avoided as attempts at erection will increase penile blood pressure, which may cause further hemorrhage or edema.

Paraphimosis may also occur as a secondary phenomenon in equine infectious anemia, purpura hemorrhagica, rhinopneumonitis, exhaustion, starvation, and penile paralysis. The prolapsed penis should be supported and moistened with ointments to prevent traumatic injury.

PENILE PARALYSIS (PRIAPISM)

Penile paralysis may follow local neurologic damage, rabies infection, and the use of phenothiazine tranquilizers. With the latter (proprioromazine and acepromazine but not xylazine) there appears to be a partial erection of the penis with a uniformly filled corpus cavernosum but no edema. The penis is painful on deep palpation for about two weeks after the onset of paralysis. Although the condition is usually seen in stallions, it also occurs in geldings receiving exogenous testosterone therapy. In most cases, amputation of the penis is necessary and this is best performed after the acute inflammation of the corpus cavernosum has subsided. If abrasions, lacerations, or hematoma have not occurred and avoidance of amputation is desired, a penile retraction operation (e.g., the Bolz technique) may be performed. Some breeding stallions with penile paralysis may be trained to ejaculate into an artificial vagina with increased water temperature. Retraining is likely to require substantial time and effort. Alternatively, recanalization of the organized corpus cavernosum hematoma, which may take four months or more, may be encouraged by sexual stimulation three times daily for 15 to 30 minutes per session.

URETHRAL TRAUMA

Urethral inflammation or stricture formation may be caused by direct penile trauma, urethral calculi, repeated catheterization, injudicious urethral endoscopy, tight stallion rings, and irritant chemicals. Minor lacerations of the urethral process may be cauterized with silver nitrate; care must be taken that none gains acess to the urethra.

TESTICULAR AND EPIDIDYMAL TRAUMA

This may be caused by a kick during mating and usually results in scrotal edema, elevated scrotal temperature, pain, hematocele, and, uncommonly, enlargement of the testis. Acute orchitis usually results in temporary or permanent testicular atrophy, the testis becoming small and fibrotic. Treatment is by support of the scrotum and testes, cold water hydrotherapy, systemic analgesics, anti-inflammatory drugs, and prophylactic antibiotics. Success depends on the early initiation of treatment. Unilateral castration may be indicated to prevent inflammatory and degenerative changes from ocurring in the other testis.

True epididymal obstruction or aplasia is very rare. Trauma to the scrotal contents may result in an epididymal duct blockage, resulting in the ejaculation of sperm-free seminal fluid. This may also occur in a syndrome thought to be caused by a unilateral or bilateral stasis of sperm in the ampullae. Stallions with epididymal duct blockage ejaculate sperm-free seminal fluid in their first ejaculates. Vigorous massage of the enlarged, turgid ampullae or vasa deferentia and prolonged sexual excitement (repeated attempts to collect semen) result in the ejaculation of dense clumps of dead, tail-less sperm. Subsequent ejaculations usually contain normal motile sperm and are fertile. The condition may recur in the same individual. For these, regular semen collection or natural mating throughout the year are logical prophylactic measures.

GENITAL NEOPLASMS AND TUMORLIKE LESIONS

PENILE NEOPLASMS

Tumors of the penis may interfere with intromission and frequently cause hemospermia. Squamous cell carcinomas are the most common penile tumors. The lesions tend to affect nonpigmented areas and are locally invasive and granulomatous in appearance. Metastasis to regional lymph nodes has been reported. Cryosurgical excision is recommended for small localized lesions. For larger and locally invasive lesions, radical surgical excision or penile amputation may be necessary.

Melanomas, sarcoids, hemangiomas, and fibropapillomas of the penis and prepuce have been reported. Stallions with fibropapillomas (viral warts) should not be used for natural mating during the period of infectivity. Although these lesions regress spontaneously, surgical excision is recommended to speed recovery. Autogenous vaccines have been used but their efficacy is questionable. Melanomas of the prepuce or scrotum are relatively common in gray horses. They do not affect fertility and only rarely require surgical excision.

HABRONEMIASIS

Advanced lesions on the skin of the penis or prepuce or urethral mucous membranes may be confused with neoplasia. *Habronema muscae* deposit their eggs on the moist surfaces of the urethral process or prepuce. The eggs hatch and the larvae invade the local tissues, facilitated by lacerations or breaks in the skin or mucous membranes. This results in edema, inflammation, and granuloma formation. Early acute localized edema of the urethral mucosa may result in sporadic hemospermia. Chronic cases involve ulceration and granulomatous lesions; if the lesions are on the urethral process, hemospermia is commonly seen. Blood is usually seen only at the end of ejaculation unless the lesions are extensive. Hematuria is uncommon.

Because the larvae in the lesions are usually dead, systemic treatment with organophosphorus anthelmintics seldom produces satisfactory resolution. It is reported that systemic treatment with ivermectin* is helpful in early cases. Topical and systemic treatment with anti-inflammatory drugs produces temporary inhibition of granuloma formation, but inflammation continues following cessation of treatment. Surgical amputation of the urethral process is frequently performed for distal pedunculated lesions. The incised mucocutaneous junction is sutured; however, areas frequently undergo dehiscence and may require cautery with silver nitrate. Sexual stimulation should be avoided for at least two weeks. The healed surgical site is susceptible to bleeding following the trauma of natural mating or semen collection because the healed mucosa is often slightly everted. Habronema lesions may regress during the cold months of the year. *Collitroga hominivorax* (screwworm fly) and Onchocerca spp.

larvae have also been incriminated in similar lesions of the penis and prepuce.

TESTICULAR NEOPLASMS

Testicular neoplasms include seminomas, lipomas, teratomas, and Sertoli cell and interstitial cell tumors. They are unusual but occur most commonly in older stallions, the seminoma being the most common. The tumors are usually unilateral and result in swelling that may be fluctuant and painful. These lesions are often not noticed by owners. They must be differentiated from abscesses or hematomas, which may also cause a localized, firm, space-occupying mass. Tumors cause testicular degeneration; therefore, the ejaculate contains low numbers of sperm and a high proportion of abnormal sperm and spermatocytes. Libido is not affected unless the lesion is painful. Unilateral castration is the treatment of choice. Metastasis is rare but palpation of the inguinal lymph nodes and histologic examination of the excised testis and spermatic cord are advised.

TESTICULAR TORSION

Acute 360-degree torsion of the stallion's testis, although rare, must be differentiated from tumors. In contrast to tumors, acute testicular torsion is usually seen in young stallions and causes signs of acute colic. A unilateral or bilateral 180-degree rotation is more commonly observed, sometimes during a routine examination. The tail of the epididymis is directed cranially on the affected testis. Libido and semen quality are not affected. This malposition is thought to occur during testicular descent.

SEMINAL CONTAMINATION

HEMOSPERMIA

Blood in the semen lowers fertility to a degree proportional to the amount of contamination. Hemospermia may be constant or intermittent, is always secondary to a penile, urethral, or internal genital lesion, and may be associated with pain on ejaculation. Treatment is directed at diagnosis and treatment of the underlying causal lesion.

The diagnosis is best made by a semen collection using an artificial vagina. The color of the ejaculate—pink or bright red—reflects the degree of contamination, which usually increases with the frequency of ejaculation. As erythrocytes agglutinate sperm, the proportion of progressively motile sperm decreases. Erythrocytes may be demonstrated using a Wright's or hematoxylin and eosin stain on an air-dried smear. Although simple occult blood tests may be used to monitor hemospermia, normal semen will give a slightly positive reaction. The source of the bleeding can often be readily

---

*Eqvalan, MSD/AGVET, Rahway, NJ

identified externally, e.g., traumatic wounds, viral papillomatosis of the penis, and cutaneous habronemiasis of the distal urethral process. These lesions must be differentiated from tumors. Bacterial urethritis, urethral ulceration, or rupture of urethral subepithelial vessels can also cause hemospermia. These conditions can be diagnosed by penile and pelvic urethral endoscopy using a small-diameter, flexible fiberoptic endoscope. This must be at least 100 cm long. A subischial urethrostomy is not necessary with this instrument. Inflammation of the internal genitalia may cause hemospermia.

In stallions used for natural mating, blood may be seen on the stallion's penis or the mare's vulva after mating. This bleeding may be unaccompanied by hemospermia and may result from rupture or stretching of the hymen, vaginal lacerations or bruising, rupture of the vagina, and vulval tears.

Cessation of mating and specific treatment for the causative lesion are indicated in hemospermia. Antibiotic ointments should be applied to superficial lacerations of the urethral process, glans, or shaft of the penis. Systemic anti-inflammatory agents and topical corticosteroids, if applied to early Habronema lesions, may allow mating to continue until the lesions regress or can be surgically removed. If the distal urethral process is amputated, adequate time for healing must be allowed before mating is resumed. In most of these cases, some form of focal cautery of the stump is required. This is best performed using silver nitrate, and great care must be taken to ensure that none gains access to the urethral lumen. Fibropapillomas usually regress spontaneously; however, if they do not, they should be removed surgically.

In stallions with early Habronema lesions or inflammation of the distal urethra, blood-free part ejaculates can sometimes be collected using a Polish type open-ended artificial vagina. This is useful when mares may be artificially inseminated.

In cases of bacterial urethritis or internal genital infection, the causative organism should be identified and the antibiotic sensitivity determined before systemic and local treatment are instituted. The response to treatment is often poor. When persistent genital infection occurs in the absence of hemospermia or pus in the semen, semen extenders can be used for artificial and natural mating programs to avoid transmission of organisms that cause endometritis.

UROSPERMIA

Ejaculates containing urine are usually light yellow to amber in color. They have an elevated pH, low sperm motility, and high osmotic pressure, may smell of urine, and contain sediment. The pH level depends on how much urine enters the collection vessel; therefore, some specimens remain within the normal range for stallion semen. The most useful tests for the presence of urine in semen appear to be urea and creatinine measurements. Semen creatinine levels above 2.0 mg per dl (177 μmol per L) or urea nitrogen levels above 30 mg per dl (5 mmol per L) indicate urospermia. Under conditions of natural mating, urospermia is seldom suspected and is often diagnosed only after investigations for lowered fertility.

Fertility of urospermic ejaculates is depressed by the effect on sperm quality and the effect on the mare's endometrium. The causes of urospermia are unknown and the condition may be intermittent. In the majority of cases, urination occurs near the end of ejaculation.

The effects of treatment are difficult to assess because of the intermittent and sometimes unpredictable nature of this condition. Under conditions of artificial insemination, each ejaculate may be examined for urine content and contaminated samples should be discarded. In known cases, mating or semen collection should be performed only after urination has occurred. Urination can be stimulated by exercise, exposure to heterologous feces, feeding, fresh stable bedding, and sometimes in response to whistling. Diuretic and ephedrine sulfate administration before ejaculation is not beneficial. Under conditions of artificial insemination, the collection of the early urine-free ejaculate jets using a Polish type open-ended artificial vagina may be helpful.

INFECTION OF THE INTERNAL GENITALIA

Contamination of semen with bacteria is unavoidable. Extreme caution must be used before genital infection is diagnosed, unless the organisms concerned are venereal disease producers, e.g., *Taylorella equigenitalis (Haemophilus equigenitalis)* contagious equine metritis organism (CEMO), *Klebsiella pneumoniae* (capsule types 1 and 5), and *Pseudomonas aeruginosa* (see p. 568), unless repeated semen samples contain pure cultures of the same potential pathogens, unless the semen contains abnormally high numbers of leukocytes (see p. 564) or unless mares mated are consistently returning to estrus with acute endometritis associated with the same bacterial species. The majority of young and genitally healthy mares are able to overcome the bacterial challenge to the endometrium that normally occurs at natural mating. Acute endometritis can be minimized in mares with apparently compromised natural defense mechanisms by use of minimal contamination mating techniques which include the use of semen extenders containing suitable antibiotics.

In stallions that persistently shed pathogenic bacteria in the semen, an attempt should be made to locate the source of the bacteria. Bacterial urethritis, frequently associated with cystitis, is probably the most commonly diagnosed inflammatory condition of the stallion's genital tract. Hemospermia and an increased number of mounts per ejaculate are frequently associated with urethritis. Systemic antibiotic treatment may be helpful in such cases; however, limited vascular supply to the urethra and failure of many drugs to be excreted via the urinary system limit the success of this route of therapy. Local irrigation with nonirritating antibacterials is also used. Rest from mating is indicated.

Seminal vesiculitis and ampullitis are rare. During the acute phase of inflammation, these organs are enlarged and painful on palpation. In chronic cases, although the organs are nonpainful, enlargement or induration may be palpable. Inflammation of the prostate and bulbourethral glands have not been reported.

Fiberoptic endoscopic examination of the penile and pelvic urethra should be performed in suspected cases of internal genital organ infection, particular attention being paid to the ducts and bladder opening. Fluids can be collected directly from the vesicular glands by passing a sterile flexible catheter into the pelvic urethra following sexual stimulation, which causes the vesicular glands to fill with fluid. With the catheter in position, fluid from each vesicular gland is manually expressed by compression of the glands per rectum. The fluid can be bacteriologically and biochemically analyzed.

The pre-ejaculatory fluid, which drips from the urethra during sexual stimulation, is thought to originate from the bulbourethral glands, and analysis of this fluid may allow evaluation of this organ. At present, palpation per rectum appears to be the only method of evaluating the ampullae.

Although bacterial epididymitis may occur, palpation is the only means of evaluation of the epididymes. Direct invasion of the epididymis is likely to result in the formation of adhesions and duct blockage. Orchitis may occur following trauma or bacterial infection with *Streptococcus equi* (strangles) or other systemic infections. Acutely, the testes are enlarged, warm, and painful on palpation. The scrotum may be edematous, and epididymal injury is common. Treatment with systemic antibiotics and cold water hydrotherapy must be initiated promptly. Elevation of the enlarged and painful testes is indicated. Chronic orchitis or unsuccessful treatment of acute orchitis usually results in the affected testis becoming small, firm, and frequently nodular in consistency. Sperm production is low, with increased numbers of morphologically abnormal cells.

Supplemental Readings

Rasbech, N. O.: Ejaculatory disorders in the stallion. J. Reprod. Fert., Suppl. 23:123, 1975.

Society for Theriogenology: Manual for Clinical Fertility Evaluation of the Stallion. Published by the Society of Theriogenology, Hastings, NB, 1983.

Walker, D. F., and Vaughan, J. T.: Bovine and Equine Urogenital Surgery. Philadelphia, Lea & Febiger, 1980, pp. 125–169.

Ejaculatory Failure

Erich Klug, HANNOVER, WEST GERMANY

Although accurate data are not available, it is probable that the incidence of ejaculatory failure among stallions is higher than is suspected. When it occurs and is recognized, this abnormality provides a challenging problem to breeding farm management.

CLINICAL SIGNS

The characteristic signs of ejaculatory failure, which results in aspermia, may be seen in stallions of all ages. These stallions have normal or often excessive libido and normal penile erection; they achieve normal intromission. The greater than 10 pelvic thrusts appear normal and full erection of the glans penis occurs. Ejaculation, however, does not occur, or does so only occasionally. Signs suggesting ejaculation, e.g., tail flagging and urethral pulsations, are sometimes detected, but no semen is produced. Repeated unproductive attempts by the stallion lead to behavioral signs suggesting frustration, sometimes aggression. If not interrupted, the stallion eventually becomes physically exhausted.

DIAGNOSIS

Ejaculatory failure should be considered when a change in stallion mating behavior is reported and when dismount seminal fluid ejection is consistently not seen. When tail flagging and urethral pulsations occur, a sudden decrease in conception rate may be the first indication recognized.

The stallion should be given a detailed physical examination, including examinations of the locomotor system, rectal palpation of the pelvic viscera, and detailed observations of repeated mating attempts performed under ideal conditions in familiar surroundings. Particular attention should be given to counting pelvic thrusts and noting full erection of the glans penis at dismount. Between mating attempts the stallion should be allowed to relax, with withdrawn penis, and then encouraged to remount at will. After four to five unsuccessful mounts, the urinary bladder should be catheterized and the contents collected, or if necessary, aspirated after the infusion of 500 ml 0.9 per cent saline solution, and examined for the presence of sperm.

It is theroretically possible for retrograde ejaculation of semen to occur into the urinary bladder. Although I have not been able to conclusively prove this, it must be considered a possibility, especially in those stallions that exhibit tail flagging and urethral pulsations. Evidence of urospermia was found in one physically weak stallion, suspected of being able to ejaculate in both a retrograde and antigrade direction and also showing an apparently normal refractory behavior after each ejaculation. In this context, retrograde ejaculation must be considered a variant of ejaculatory failure.

Horses with ejaculatory failure must be differentiated from horses that require repeated mounting before normal ejaculation occurs and from horses whose mating is interrupted shortly after intromission without full erection of the glans penis. This behavior is frequently associated with management problems, especially involving handling during mating, and is thus relatively easy to remedy.

PATHOGENESIS

Neurologic abnormality results in failure of contraction or asynchronous contraction of the urethral smooth muscle. Primary causes are often not known. However, in some stallions abnormalities of local blood flow may be involved, as similar but permanent ejaculatory failure is sometimes seen when pelvic arterial thrombosis is present.

Ejaculation is the result of a reflex chain of physiologic events. Transduction (also termed emission) of the contents of the cauda epididymides, ductus deferentia, ampullae, prostate gland, and seminal vesicles into the pelvic urethra occurs simultaneously with the closure of the neck of the urinary bladder, followed by ejection of the formed semen through the penile urethra. Transduction is controlled by the sympathetic nervous system and ejection by sympathetic stimulus, with parasympathetic involvement. Ejaculatory failure results when transduction does not occur. Nerve impulses come from the ejaculatory center through the caudal thoracic and cranial lumbar cord medulla. They are transmitted in postganglionic sympathetic fibers through alpha receptors, which predominantly induce contraction, and through beta receptors, which predominantly cause muscle relaxation. Catecholamines are the chemical mediators in these receptors.

TREATMENT

Treatment is directed toward correction of the abnormal neural transmission affecting the ejaculatory process and is based upon the use of synthetic sympathetic receptor agonists and antagonists. Successful treatment was achieved in 17 of 24 stallions by enhancing sympathetic-induced smooth muscle contraction with alpha-adrenergic agonists and by inhibiting sympathetic-induced smooth muscle relaxation with beta-adrenergic blockers.

L-norepinephrine,* an alpha-agonist, should be injected 0.01 mg per kg intramuscularly 15 minutes before mating, and carazolol,† a beta-adrenergic blocker, should be injected (0.015 mg per kg) 10 minutes before mating. It is important that the dose rates should be exactly adhered to, because beta blockers have, in addition to their sympatholytic effect, an intrinsic sympathomimetic action.

Beta blockers reduce the maximum heart rate achievable during ejaculation. The treatment is contraindicated in stallions with chronic obstructive pulmonary disease (COPD) because the sympatholytic effects aggravate this disease. Alternatively, it is possible but not proved that bronchodilators used for the treatment of COPD may have an untoward effect on urethral smooth muscle, and thus could adversely affect ejaculation.

---

*Levophed, Winthrop-Breon Laboratories, New York, NY
†Suacron, Praemix, Mannheim, West Germany

Supplemental Readings

Hurtgen, J. P.: Disorders affecting stallion fertility. *In* Robinson, N. E., (ed.): Current Therapy in Equine Medicine, 1st ed., Philadelphia, W. B. Saunders Company, 1983.

Klug, E., Markt, H. M., von Lepel, J. D., and Blobel, K.: Urospermie bei einem Hengst mit Hinterhandparese. Tiefgefrierkonservierung von befruchtungsfahigem Samen. Tierarztl. Umschau., 33:324, 1978.

Klug, E., Deegen, E., Lazaraz, R., Rojem, I., and Merkt, H. M.: Effect of adrenergic neurotransmitters upon the ejaculatory process in the stallion. J. Reprod. Fert., Suppl. 32:21, 1982.

Merkt, H. M.: Veranderungen von Sameneigenschaften und Herz-Kreislaufparametern beim Pferd nach Verabreichung von Bunitrolol, Clenbuterol und Arterenol bei der Samenentnahme. Vet. Med. Diss., Hannover, 1981.

Rasbech, N. D.: Ejaculatory disorders of the stallion. J. Reprod. Fert., Suppl. 23:123, 1975.

Seminal Abnormalities

K. F. Dowsett, BRISBANE, AUSTRALIA

Seminal testing is only part of the complete examination of a stallion for breeding soundness. Breeding soundness examination should include identification of the stallion, physical examination, and assessment for use as a sire, with any heritable conditions noted. Recent history, such as retirement from racing, exposure to infectious diseases, vaccinations, stresses of environment and transportation, and reproductive management have important implications when results are interpreted. Seminal abnormalities can be manifested in several ways. They may be caused by a variety of physiologic, pathologic, and managerial problems. Factors such as age and breed, season of the year, heat stress, service frequency, and treatment with anabolic steroids influence the semen and spermatozoa of stallions. Spermatogenesis takes approximately six weeks. This should be considered when a diagnosis is made of the likely cause of a problem and when possible treatments are weighed.

Careful palpation and measurement of the testes, palpation of the spermatic cord and head and body (not always readily palpable) and tail of the epididymides, and examination of the erect penis are essential. The seminal vesicles, ampullae, and vasa deferentia should be palpated per rectum, although the latter may be difficult to locate. The stallion must be adequately restrained for rectal examination.

SEMEN AND SPERMATOZOAL EXAMINATION

Bacteriology. Swabs should be taken from the urethra, urethral diverticulum (fossa glandis), prepuce and semen, placed into a suitable transport medium (Stuart's or Amies), and sent to a laboratory for culture and sensitivity tests. Obtaining swabs can be hazardous with stallions not used to having the penis handled before mating. In these cases it is preferable to take swabs immediately following collection of semen, just as the stallion is dismounting.

The external genitalia and semen have their own "normal" flora, which generally have no deleterious effects on stallion fertility. Organisms that may be associated with reduced fertility include (*Taylorella equigenitalis* (*Haemophilus equigenitalis*), beta-hemolytic streptococci, *Escherichia coli*, *Pseudomonas aeruginosa*, and *Klebsiella pneumoniae* (Table 1). The presence of these organisms on the external genitalia and even in the semen, without the presence of inflammatory cells, may not affect fertility. However, urethritis, cystitis, epididymitis, orchitis, or seminal vesiculitis, which may have deleterious effects on fertility, can be associated with the presence of such organisms. Differences in host susceptibility to or pathogenicity of organisms influence the severity of the infection and its effect on both stallion and mare fertility. Capsule types 1, 2, and 5 of *K. pneumoniae* are associated with outbreaks of sexually transmitted endometritis in mares, whereas capsule type 7 (frequently isolated from stallion genital swabs) is not.

Treatment of infections, particularly *Pseudomonas*, is expensive and often ineffectual. Gentamicin or tobramycin is likely to be effective against *Pseudomonas;* however, these agents are nephrotoxic when used in high doses. Other infections may be treated systemically with a suitable antibiotic or locally with nonirritant antiseptic washes or ointments. Because washing of the stallion's penis, even with soap, before or after service can

TABLE 1. RESULTS OF BACTERIAL CULTURES FROM THE SEMEN, URETHRA, URETHRAL DIVERTICULUM, AND PREPUCE OF 40 STALLIONS WITH REDUCED FERTILITY

Type of Bacteria	Semen	Urethra	Diverticulum	Prepuce
Mixed growth	0	1	1	1
Bacillus spp.	2	5	12	12
Corynebacterium spp.	7	16	22	20
Enterobacter spp.	3	3	1	7
Escherichia coli	6	4	7	3
Klebsiella spp.	1	0	1	1
Micrococcus spp.	5	7	2	2
Pasteurella spp.	0	1	1	1
Proteus spp.	1	1	4	1
Pseudomonas spp.	11	7	4	4
Staphylococcus spp.	9	9	9	8
α-hemolytic streptococcus spp.	2	1	5	0
β-hemolytic streptococcus spp.	4	1	2	0

alter the bacterial flora and favor the growth of more pathogenic organisms, sexual rest for a period of three to six months is often the most effective therapy for genital tract infections.

Semen Evaluation. Once a suitable semen sample has been collected, care must be taken to prevent cold stress to the spermatozoa. The characteristics listed in Table 2 should be evaluated at the collection site, in a position protected from sunlight, wind, and dust.

Density and Mass Activity. Immediately following collection, a drop of gel-free semen is placed on a prewarmed (37° C) microscope slide and viewed under low power (100 × magnification) to assess the density and mass activity of the sample. Density is an estimate of the spermatozoal concentration. Mass activity is an estimate of the overall activity of the population of spermatozoa and is a function of density and motility.

Spermatozoal Motility. Following assessment of density and mass activity, a prewarmed (37° C) glass coverslip is placed over the drop of gel-free semen. An estimate is then made of progressive motility (percentage of normally motile spermatozoa) at 400 × magnification. Oscillatory motility without progression is not considered normal.

Percentage Live Spermatozoa. One or more drops of gel-free semen are pipetted into a prewarmed (37° C) vial (0.35 ml, 8 drops) of nigrosin eosin stain, which is gently shaken and left for exactly three minutes. A drop of this mixture is smeared on a prewarmed microscope slide and allowed to air dry. At least 200 spermatozoa are examined, unmounted, under oil immersion (1000 × magnification) to determine the percentage of unstained (live) spermatozoa. This smear can also be used to observe morphologic abnormalities.

Volume of Ejaculate. On completion of the microscopic examination, the volumes of the gel-free and gelatinous fractions are measured.

Semen Color. The color of stallion semen varies according to the density from clear, watery gray, grayish-white, white, to milky white. The presence of blood, urine, or cellular debris alters the color of the semen, giving a yellowish, brownish, pinkish, or reddish discoloration. Any discoloration should be noted and considered indicative of a pathologic condition.

pH of Gel-Free Semen. A portable pH meter calibrated with buffer solutions and adjusted for ambient temperature is used to measure the pH of gel-free semen.

Concentration of Spermatozoa. A sample (0.1 ml) of the gel-free semen is pipetted into a McCartney bottle containing 4.9 ml of buffered formol saline and used to estimate the concentration of spermatozoa on a hemocytometer or spectrophotometer.

Total Number of Spermatozoa. This is estimated by multiplying the sperm concentration by the volume of gel-free semen.

Morphologic Examination. Semen samples for the morphologic examination of spermatozoa should be prepared and either sent to a laboratory or examined by the veterinarian.

Head and Midpiece Morphology. A drop of gel-free semen is placed on a prewarmed (37° C) microscope slide; a thin smear is made and allowed to air dry. This is stained with a modified Williams' stain or other suitable stain and used for the classification and counting of sperm heads and midpieces under oil immersion (× 1000 magnification).

Tail and Midpiece Morphology and Protoplasmic Droplets. One or more drops of gel-free semen are pipetted into a prewarmed vial (0.5 ml) of buffered formol saline. This sample is used for the classification and counting of abnormal tails and midpieces and to determine the presence of retained protoplasmic droplets under oil immersion (× 1000 magnification) and phase contrast illumination.

Giemsa Stain. If inflammatory cells are observed in the gel-free semen, an air dried smear is stained with Giemsa and examined for leukocytes under oil immersion (× 1000 magnification).

Morphologic Classification. Traditionally spermatozoal abnormalities are classified as primary, secondary, or tertiary. Primary abnormalities, associated with spermatogenesis, involve the head and midpiece of the sperm cell but can include some tail abnormalities. Secondary abnormalities associated with passage through the excurrent ducts usually affect the midpiece and tail of the cell but can involve the acrosome. Tertiary abnormalities are associated with poor handling technique after collection. These can be prevented by competent semen-handling techniques. This classification system, which has been criticized, has generally been superceded by a more detailed classification of spermatozoal abnormalities (Table 3).

Head Abnormalities. Abnormal heads may be

TABLE 2. SEMEN CHARACTERISTICS TO BE EVALUATED AT THE SITE OF COLLECTION*

Characteristic	Mean	Standard Deviation
Total volume (ml)	44.53	2.33
Gel-free volume (ml)	33.70	2.13
Gelatinous volume (ml)	2.88	5.09
Density score (0–3)	2.03	0.69
Mass activity score (0–3)	2.07	0.79
Percentage motile spermatozoa	76.44	1.75
Percentage live spermatozoa	82.56	1.93
Sperm concentration (× 10^6/ml)	164.13	39.35
Total number of sperm (× 10^6)	6342.40	1934.29
pH of gel-free semen	7.61	0.31

*Overall means and standard deviations for 536 ejaculates collected from 168 stallions.

TABLE 3. SPERMATOZOAL ABNORMALITIES*

Characteristic	Mean	Standard Deviation
Abnormal heads (%)	5.40	1.91
Proximal droplets (%)	6.66	2.55
Distal droplets (%)	4.79	2.69
Abnormal midpieces (%)	0.35	2.31
Abaxial midpieces (%)	12.92	2.31
Abnormal tails (%)	7.54	2.20
Loose heads (%)	1.51	2.93

*Overall means and standard deviations of 531 ejaculates collected from 168 stallions.

classified as follows: narrow, narrow at base, pear-shaped, large, small, broad, round, and undeveloped. Other abnormalities include spermatids; swollen, dislodged, or damaged acrosomes; and multiple heads. Loose or tail-less heads are recorded as a separate abnormality.

Midpiece Abnormalities. Midpieces are classified into normal, abaxial attachment, and abnormal, which can be further divided into the following descriptive groups: thin, kinked, coiled, thick, double, split, knob, bent or broken, defective attachment, vestigeal or "off-shoot defect," and pseudo-droplets. The presence of retained proximal or distal protoplasmic droplets on the midpiece is noted.

Tail Abnormalities. Abnormal tails are classified as single bend, double bend, or coiled.

CAUSES OF REDUCED FERTILITY

Semen and Spermatozoal Abnormalities. Stallions that produce ejaculates containing no spermatozoa (azoospermia) or totally dead spermatozoa are probably the only ones that can be definitely classified as infertile. No definite relationships have been shown between morphologically abnormal stallion spermatozoa and fertility. The only characteristics of stallion semen found to have any meaningful relationship with fertility and their threshold levels are (1) total volume, 35 ml, (2) gel-free volume, 25 ml, (3) sperm concentration, 20×10^6 per ml, (4) total number of sperm in the ejaculate, 1300×10^6, and (5) total number of live sperm, 1100×10^6. However, the presence and type of sperm abnormalities and inflammatory cells in the ejaculate may help to determine whether an infertility problem is associated with such conditions as aberrant spermatogenesis, testicular degeneration, orchitis, seminal vesiculitis, and epididymitis.

The use of testosterone or anabolic steroid "therapy" for poor libido or semen abnormalities is contraindicated. These hormones reduce ejaculate volume, spermatozoal concentration and motility, total number of spermatozoa in the ejaculate, and testicular size. Reduction in testicular size is due to degeneration of the seminiferous tubules and may or may not be permanent. Some evidence exists that the use of human chorionic gonadotro-

pin* (1500 to 2000 IU three times weekly for three weeks), pregnant mare serum gonadotropin (1000 IU three times weekly for three weeks), follicle-stimulating hormone† (10 to 50 mg three times weekly for three weeks), or gonadotropin-releasing hormone (200 μg twice daily for 21 days) may have beneficial effects in stallions with small testes or an undescended testis or in stallions suffering from mild and early testicular degeneration.

Overuse. This is probably the most common cause of reduced fertility in the stallion, particularly early in the breeding season when mares are in "spring estrus" and daily sperm production and daily sperm output is not maximal. Overuse can also be a problem at the end of the breeding season, when libido tends to be low and daily sperm output may not be sufficient to meet the demand to service all the mares still not pregnant. Some stallions are capable of consistently mating only twice daily if they are to remain capable of producing sufficient numbers of spermatozoa for optimal fertility (between 1100×10^6 and 4000×10^6 per ejaculate). Spacing of matings by at least six hours and preferably 12 hours will help to maintain the total number of spermatozoa per ejaculate above the limit required for acceptable fertility.

Age of Stallion. The use of "stallions" that are less than three years old is not recommended, as their spermatozoal concentration, total number of spermatozoa per ejaculate, and percentage of live spermatozoa are generally below what is required for acceptable fertility. If they are to be used, they should be expected to service only up to 12 mares and should be limited to one service per day.

There is a tendency for stallion fertility to decline with age after 10 years. Therefore, stallions 11 years and older should be managed carefully. Their semen should be monitored for any decline in sperm numbers and an increase in spermatozoal abnormalities that may indicate testicular degeneration or epididymal pathology. However, stallions up to the age of 26 years have been examined and found to have normal semen.

*Chorionic gonadotropin, Med-Tech Inc., Elwood, KS
†F.S.H.-P., Burns-Biotec, Omaha, NE

Supplemental Readings

Dowsett, K. F., and Pattie, W. A.: Collection of semen from stallions at stud. Aust. Vet. J., 56:373, 1980.

Dowsett, K. F., and Pattie, W. A.: Stallion semen characteristics and fertility. J. Reprod. Fert., Suppl. 32:1, 1982.

Dowsett, K. F., Osborne, H. G., and Pattie, W. A.: Morphological characteristics of stallion spermatozoa. Theriogenology, 22:463, 1984.

Gebauer, M. R., Pickett, B. W., and Swierstra, E. E.: Reproductive physiology of the stallion. II. Daily production and output of sperm. J. Anim. Sci., 39:732, 1974.

Pickett, B. W., Sullivan, J. J., and Seidel, Jr., G. E.: Reproductive physiology of the stallion. V. Effects of ejaculation frequency on seminal characteristics and spermatozoal output. J. Anim. Sci., 40:917, 1975.

Venereal Diseases of Stallions

J. M. *Bowen*, COLLEGE STATION, TEXAS

The recognized venereal diseases that affect stallions are caused by protozoa, viruses, and bacteria.

PROTOZOAL VENEREAL DISEASES

DOURINE (MAL DE COIT)

This protozoan infection now occurs in Central and South America, North and South Africa, the Middle East, and Asiatic Russia, having been eradicated from Europe and North America. The causal agent *Trypanosoma equiperdum* produces low morbidity but high mortality. The disease onset is slow, with an incubation period of one to two weeks. The first signs are mucoid urethral discharge and low-grade recurrent pyrexia followed by nonpainful, cold swellings of the prepuce, scrotum, and penis. Raised skin plaques, 2 to 10 cm in diameter, then appear on the lower parts of the body. These are considered pathognomonic and usually appear and disappear within hours; however, if they persist, they leave depigmented areas. Later the penis shows signs of paralysis and while the stallion retains libido, penetration of the mare is impossible. Emaciation and lameness followed by posterior incoordination, paralysis, and death usually occur.

The protozoan can sometimes be demonstrated in urethral fluid, in the plaques, and occasionally in blood samples. Confirmation is by complement-fixation (CF) test; however, cross reactions can occur in geographic areas where *T. evansi* and *T. brucei* coexist. The disease may be symptomless in some stallions, which then become lifelong carriers.

Treatment is attempted with quinapyramine sulfate.* The dosage (3 mg per kg subcutaneously) should be split to avoid toxicity. It is not known whether treated and recovered stallions are safe for breeding purposes. This and the very specific method of transmission make the disease more appropriately treated by eradication than by medication.

Control is best achieved by slaughter of infected animals and strict quarantine of contacts. The latter should be screened by the CF test and cleared after passing three consecutive monthly tests. If breeding is to be continued, an artificial insemination program should be implemented within the controlled area, with only uninfected stallions being used.

VIRAL VENEREAL DISEASES

Several virus diseases affect horses, and while true venereal spread is recognized in only two viruses, the presence of virus in semen as in all body fluids during the viremic phase must not be overlooked.

EQUINE HERPESVIRUS I (EHV-I, RHINOPNEUMONITIS)

There is no documented evidence of venereal transmission; however, the nature of herpesviruses and evidence of vaginal and nasopharyngeal transmission in other species suggest that this may occur.

EQUINE HERPESVIRUS II (EHV-II, CYTOMEGALOVIRUS)

Little is known of the pathogenicity of this infection, other than it can be identified in respiratory disease. It has been isolated from equine mammary and vaginal secretions and could be venereally transmitted.

EQUINE HERPESVIRUS III (EHV-III, COITAL EXANTHEMA)

This is a relatively common venereal disease that produces small vesicles on the shaft of the penis. The stallion may be temporarily depressed, pyrexic, and unwilling to mate. The vesicles burst and evolve into small (3 to 10 mm) ulcers that granulate and heal in 10 to 21 days, often leaving small depigmented areas. These must be differentiated from early signs of squamous cell carcinoma.

Serious secondary bacterial infection is unusual and treatment consists of three weeks' rest from mating activity with the use of demulcent ointments such as Furacin, lanolin, and petroleum jelly to prevent preputial adhesion formation. The use of antiviral drugs such as 5 per cent Acyclovir ointment (used for *H. simplex* and *H. zoster* infections in humans) for EHV-III infections in stallions has not been reported, and because of the benign nature of the disease, is probably not indicated.

Viral recrudescence may occur, either spontaneously or following a period of stress.

EQUINE VIRAL ARTERITIS (EVA)

This togavirus infection causes influenzalike respiratory signs in susceptible horses, with a characteristically marked conjunctivitis. In its mildest form, the infection causes no clinical signs. Serologic evidence in some horse populations suggests a 25 to 50 per cent exposure rate. Mild signs are similar to influenza but there is less coughing, and secondary bacterial infection is unusual. More virulent forms can cause diarrhea, ventral edema involving the abdomen, legs, scrotum, and prepuce, and urticaria. Abortion commonly occurs in mares at any stage of pregnancy, associated with marked pyrexia and usually within 14 days of exposure.

*Antrycide sulfate, ICI America, Wilmington, DE

Confirmation is by viral isolation and virus neutralization (VN) blood tests. A more rapid but possibly less specific enzyme-linked immunoabsorbent assay (ELISA) is available and may have an important diagnostic role to play.

The outbreak of EVA in Kentucky in 1984 has clearly shown that venereal spread of the virus in the semen of viremic and recovered stallions can be most important in a breeding population. Recovered stallions are now known to be capable of excreting virus for more than 7 months; expert opinion suggests that this may persist lifelong.

Treatment is confined to the control of secondary bacterial infection, if this occurs. Otherwise, rest, an elevated plane of nutrition, and isolation are sufficient.

In view of the proven venereal component of this disease, it is now clear that the first course of action to take in the face of an EVA outbreak in a breeding population is to suspend mating, identify infected animals, and isolate them. An experimental vaccine was used in the Kentucky outbreak but failed to fully protect horses from the virulent virus. A commercially prepared vaccine is planned for the American market for early 1985.* It must be remembered, however, that vaccination usually produces lifelong VN titers and this may render valuable bloodstock unexportable to many countries, under current export reglations. As of this writing, mare owners must remember that VN-positive stallions may remain a potential source of venereal infection.

EQUINE INFECTIOUS ANEMIA (EIA, SWAMP FEVER)

This retrovirus infection persists lifelong and causes periodic pyrexia, anemia, and sometimes emaciation. There is ventral edema and splenomegaly. Confirmation is by agar gel immunodiffusion (AGID or Coggins) blood test.

Infected horses become lifelong carriers and are intermittently or permanently viremic. The virus is spread by an intermediate host, the biting Tabanid fly, and also in blood transfusions and by veterinary instruments. The virus has been isolated from equine semen samples and there is somewhat equivocal evidence for intrauterine transfer. No appropriate treatments exist other than symptomatic ones and control is by the identification of infected horses and their slaughter or permanent isolation in fly-proof stables. The use of disposable syringes and needles has been a major factor in reducing the incidence of disease in endemic areas such as Texas. AGID-positive horses should not be used as blood donors.

VESICULAR STOMATITIS (VSV)

This rhabdovirus infection causes mucosal lesions in horses, cattle, and pigs. Venereal transmission

has not been proved. However, as transmission is linked to the presence of abrasions and injuries, it is conceivable that the infection could be transmitted by this route.

BACTERIAL VENEREAL DISEASES

Many bacteria may be isolated from the external genitalia of stallions (see p. 564). A differentiation must be made between those that are potential venereal disease inducers and those that are not. Most are harmless skin commensals relating to the local environment, the horse's feces, and stable bedding and are affected by housing and management procedures. They grow in penile and preputial smegma, which, with its normal microflora, tends to discourage the growth of pathogenic bacteria. Some pathogenic bacteria are capable of producing true venereal disease in mares while others cause only individual cases of acute endometritis in susceptible mares (see p. 513).

While *Streptococcus zooepidemicus* and *Escherichia coli* are commonly found in penile smegma and in individual acute endometritis cases, they seldom if ever produce outbreaks of true venereal disease in groups of mares mated to the same stallion. However, some strains of *Klebsiella pneumoniae* (especially capsule types 1 and 5), some strains of *Pseudomonas aeruginosa* (not as yet definable in vitro) and the contagious equine metritis organism (CEMO, *Taylorella equigenitalis*) have demonstrated their ability to cause outbreaks of contagious acute endometritis (see p. 513).

Neither *K. pneumoniae, Ps. aeruginosa,* nor CEMO cause lesions or systemic disease in stallions (with the exception of *K. pneumoniae* urethral lesions that may occasionally cause hemospermia), but may live in and be mechanically transmitted by penile smegma. Ascending infection may sometimes occur with *K. pneumoniae,* causing symptomless urinary tract contamination. Their persistence in carrier stallions and the difficulty in treating mares infected with *K. pneumoniae* and *Ps. aeruginosa* make these organisms a particular challenge to stud farm management, demonstrating the need for careful screening and control policies.

In the United Kingdom, Eire, and France, a common code of practice for the control of equine venereal diseases recommends that all Thoroughbred stallions be swabbed from the urethra, urethral fossa, preputial smegma, and preejaculatory fluid on two occasions more than seven days apart, before the start of each breeding season. The swabs are taken into suitable transport media and are cultured under aerobic and microaerophilic conditions by experienced, quality-controlled, and designated laboratories for the presence of CEMO, *K. pneumoniae,* and *Ps. aeruginosa.* Stallions that pass these tests receive certification for visiting mare owners

---

*Arvac: Fort Dodge Laboratories, Fort Dodge, IA

to see. Animals with positive results are considered unsuitable for breeding purposes until treatment followed by a series of three sets of similar swabs, taken at intervals longer than seven days demonstrates freedom from contamination. There is no doubt that this program (and its counterpart in mares [see p. 513]) has been highly successful in eradicating the disease in those countries in which it has been consistently and conscientiously used.

Washing the Penis. An important management factor is the custom of penile washing. At one time, only mild soaps and water were used to clean stallions before mating. However, in recent years, especially after the emergence of CEM, it has become fashionable to vigorously scrub the penis with more potent antiseptic cleansers such as povidone-iodine or chlorhexidine. Although this technique has been used in an attempt to reduce the spread of bacterial venereal infection, it has had the opposite effect. The incidence of *K. pneumoniae* and *Ps. aeruginosa* penile contamination has increased. Antiseptic washing removes the normal penile skin commensal flora, allowing these resistant organisms to multiply without ecologic competition and eventually colonize the penis in virtually pure culture. Thus, at mating, a pure culture of large numbers of *K. pneumoniae* or *Ps. aeruginosa* are deposited in the mare's uterus. The chances for the establishment of a persistent acute endometritis are increased, even in young, previously healthy mares.

An experiment was done to measure the effects of washing equine penises with different cleansing agents (water only, Ivory soap and water, and povidone-iodine surgical scrub and water, with a two-week rest period between each washing period). It showed that water had little effect except when a pathogen was present at the outset. In this situation the maintenance of this pathogen was encouraged. Ivory soap encouraged colonization with coliform bacteria, and povidone-iodine encouraged the establishment of *Ps. aeruginosa* colonization on the penis of all the stallions washed in this way. The alteration of the flora was most marked during the recovery period following the end of the washing period. The increase in number of pathogens cultured from penises with increasing bactericidal efficiency of cleansing agent is seen in Figure 1. In a report it is claimed that washing merely reduces the total numbers of bacteria on the penis. This does not alter the fact that washing produces a detrimental change in the demographic structure of the bacterial population rather than the numbers of colony-forming bacteria found on culture.

Treatment. Treatment of bacterial venereal infections in stallions is governed by five factors.

1. The lack of a systemic or even tissue-invasive response to infection, making parenteral treatment usually inappropriate. If this is used it is difficult to produce bactericidal antibiotic concentrations at the skin level.

2. The difficulty of removing smegma that contains pathogenic bacteria from all the crevices of the prepuce and penile skin.

3. The resistance of *K. pneumoniae* and *Ps. aeruginosa* to most antiseptics and antibiotics. In vitro sensitivity tests should be performed for each isolate. The aminoglycoside antibiotics gentamicin, amikacin, kanamycin, and carbenicillin have been found to be most useful.

4. The sensivity of the penile area to drug irritation. Ointments are preferred to creams as they persist longer, they are miscible with the oily smegma, and they are less likely to cause chapping of the delicate penile skin.

5. Untoward sequelae resulting from alterations of the normal penile microflora following treatment.

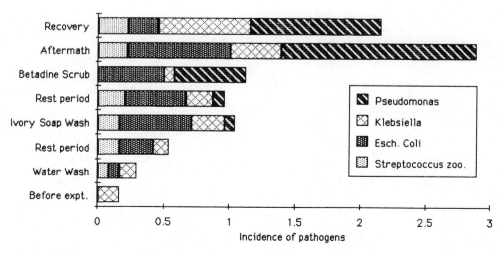

Figure 1. The effects of various washing agents on the bacterial flora of the stallion penis.

Penile contamination by CEMO may resolve without treatment provided that penile washing is not performed, but its capacity to persist in the urethral fossa makes specific treatment usually indicated. Contagious equine metritis organism is sensitive to most antibiotics and antiseptics, except streptomycin. Topical treatment with chlorhexidine surgical scrub and nitrofurazone ointment has been widely used. However, there is no doubt that chlorhexidine has major disadvantages in its irritant nature and its capacity to encourage the growth of *K. pneumoniae* and *Ps. aeruginosa*. Therefore, washing with mild soapy liquid, followed by the application of penicillin ointment to the shaft of the penis, the prepuce, and the fossa glandis daily for 12 days is recommended.

K. pneumoniae and *Ps. aeruginosa* penile contamination seldom if ever resolves without extensive treatment. Aminoglycoside antibiotic ointments are recommended, but these may cause irritation in individual stallions. Following treatment, recolonization of the "sterilized" penile skin with similar pathogens may occur and applications of normal commensal microflora is recommended. This may be achieved by taking smegma from a normal unwashed stallion or gelding, mixing it with petroleum jelly, and smearing the mixture over the erect penis. It may also be achieved by using repeated applications of a laboratory-prepared broth culture of penile and clitoral commensal bacteria. These applications are followed by a period of rest from mating activity, and efficacy is monitored by repeated post-treatment swabbing.

For *Ps. aeruginosa* contamination, a prolonged course (greater than 30 days) of treatment with 1 per cent silver nitrate solution (a desiccant) has been used with some apparently useful results. Silver nitrate can be sprayed over the erect penis using a household plant sprayer and has not been found to cause irritation. In urethral infections the solution may be deposited inside the urethral lumen, using a syringe and flexible polythene tube, without producing signs of irritation. Silver sulfadiazine cream (used for Pseudomonas skin infections in humans) appears to be of little value for stallions.

Prevention. For bacterial venereal diseases, prevention is far more satisfactory than control and treatment. The following points should be emphasized.

1. A strict screening program should be routine policy at all stud farms.

2. The custom of washing the penis of stallions should be discontinued. The removal of innocuous and protective bacteria is both pointless and detrimental. When it is necessary to remove excessive accumulations of irritant smegma, washing with water and mild soapy liquid is recommended. The penis should be blotted dry and lightly coated with petroleum jelly in order to replace lost skin oils.

3. When venereal disease is diagnosed, the first and immediate control measure is to cease mating. Delays result in unnecessary spread of infection.

4. All infected individuals should be identified and treated. The success of treatment should be monitored by repeated post-treatment bacteriologic examinations, and stallions should not resume mating until results are satisfactory.

5. Artificial insemination remains an obvious means of eliminating the spread of bacterial venereal diseases within the horse population. The use of small seminal volumes alone reduces the bacterial numbers deposited in the mare's uterus, lowering the challenge to her local immune system and making self-cure more likely. When indicated, antibiotic-containing seminal extenders are useful. All horse registration authorities should be prepared to authorize the sensible, controlled use of artificial insemination for specific veterinary indications such as venereal disease control.

OTHER PATHOGENS

Candida albicans and *Candida rugosa* have been isolated from stallions with cases of urethritis; thus these yeasts could conceivably be spread venereally. The role of anaerobic bacteria such as *Bacteroides fragilis* and Peptostreptococcus spp. that have been isolated from the genitalia of mares and stallions has yet to be defined. They may have a symbiotic role and aid the persistence of other genital aerobic bacteria. Chlamydia spp. and ureaplasmata occur in horses but have not yet been implicated in venereal disease.

Supplemental Readings

Bowen, J. M., Tobin, N., Simpson, R. B., Ley, W. B., and Ansari, M. M.: Effects of washing on the bacterial flora of the stallion's penis. J. Reprod. Fert., Suppl. 32:41, 1982.

Burns, S. J.: Equine viral arteritis. Proc. Eq. Conf. Texas A & M, 1984, pp 1–18.

Carter, G. R.: Diagnostic Procedures in Veterinary Bacteriology and Microbiology, 4th ed. Springfield, Charles C Thomas 1984.

Coggins, L.: Equine viral arteritis. *In* Robinson, N. E., (ed.): Current Therapy in Equine Medicine, 1st ed. W. B. Saunders Company, 1983

Liu, I. K. M.: Equine herpesviruses. *In* Robinson, N. E. (ed.): Current Therapy in Equine Medicine, 1st ed. W. B. Saunders Company, 1983.

Robertson, A. R. (ed.): Handbook of animal diseases in the Tropics, 3rd ed. London, British Veterinary Association, pp. 196–209, 1976.

Tillman, H., Meinecke, B., and Weiss, R.: Genitalinfektionen beim Pferd. In Tieratztl. Prax. 10, Munchen, Hans Marseille Verlag GmbH., 1982.

Cryptorchidism

John E. Cox, LEAHURST, ENGLAND

A cryptorchid horse is one with one or two testes retained somewhere along the normal pathway of descent. The condition is classified by type according to the area of retention: type 1, temporary inguinal; type 2, permanent inguinal; type 3, complete abdominal; and type 4, incomplete abdominal.

Temporary Inguinal Retention. This occurs predominantly in ponies and is characterized by small testes, which are usually readily palpable in the anesthetized horse in dorsal recumbency. If these testes are not removed, they grow and descend into the scrotum usually before the animal becomes a three-year-old.

Permanent Inguinal Retention. This occurs in all types of horse. It is characterized by testes that generally weigh more than 40 gm and may be misshapen.

Complete Abdominal Retention. Both testis and epididymis are completely retained within the abdomen. Figure 1 shows a dissection of an animal with such a testis. The animal's body wall has been opened and most of the intestines removed to expose the dorsal area of the abdomen. The bladder has been placed over the pelvic brim to show the rectum, the cut end of which can be seen. Exposed on the dorsal surface of the bladder are the vasa deferentia, which meet here to discharge into the urethra. On the animal's left, the vas can be seen passing towards the epididymal tail. A fold of peritoneum (the mesorchium) suspends the testicular

vessels, the testis, the epididymal tail, and the ligament of the tail of the epididymis (distal part of the true gubernaculum) from the dorsal body wall. At its caudal end this fold enters a small vaginal process that has developed as an outpouching of the peritoneal cavity through the deep inguinal ring. The opening to this diverticulum is known as the vaginal ring. In such a case it should be possible to find, on the inguinal side of the deep inguinal ring, the vaginal process and attached cremaster muscle and a few fibrous strands running distally from its tip toward the scrotum.

Incomplete Abdominal Retention. The vaginal process is well developed; it has an attached cremaster muscle and contains the epididymal tail. The deferent duct and the body of the epididymis pass proximally from the epididymal tail through the vaginal ring (Fig. 2).

PALPATION IN THE FOAL

Palpation of the scrotum of the newborn foal can be extremely confusing. At this stage the gubernacular complex is large, and it and the epididymal tail may together be larger than the testis. If the epididymal tail has descended, therefore, the foal may be believed to be normal even though the testis is in the abdomen. Even when the testis and epididymis both remain within the abdomen, the gubernacular complex may be so large as to be mistaken for a small testis.

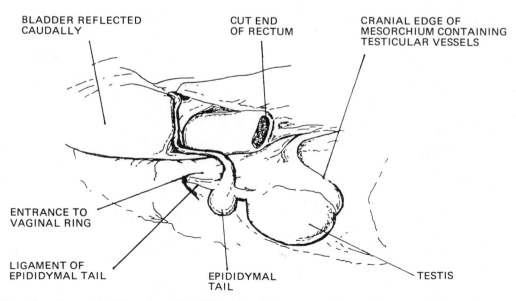

BLADDER REFLECTED CAUDALLY

CUT END OF RECTUM

CRANIAL EDGE OF MESORCHIUM CONTAINING TESTICULAR VESSELS

ENTRANCE TO VAGINAL RING

LIGAMENT OF EPIDIDYMAL TAIL

EPIDIDYMAL TAIL

TESTIS

Figure 1. Dissection of a cryptorchid to show the relationships of an abdominally retained testis. (Reproduced with permission, Department of Veterinary Clinical Medicine, University of Liverpool.)

FALSE RIGS

Not all animals that behave like stallions and that are without palpable testes are cryptorchids. Some are false rigs—geldings that, for a variety of reasons often associated with the social environment in which they live or work, develop the behavior patterns of complete males.

DIAGNOSIS

Any horse in which two testes are not visible and readily palpable in the scrotum must be suspected of being a cryptorchid. Careful examination in the standing horse, possibly after tranquilization, may allow a testis to be palpated that has been temporarily retracted under the influence of fear, cold weather, or cold hands, or that has been retained (type 1) just dorsal to the scrotum. Deep palpation of the inguinal region may allow an inguinal testis to be palpated. However, structures other than testes, such as remains of a spermatic sac or a spermatic sac containing an epididymal tail, may be present in this area and may be difficult to distinguish from a testis by palpation alone. Moreover, not all inguinally retained testes are palpable, especially those of type 2.

Rectal examination of the vaginal ring is said to allow inguinal cryptorchidism to be distinguished from abdominal cryptorchidism. However, it is rarely possible to palpate the testis; therefore, the evidence on which a diagnosis may be made is indirect. Only in type 3 will there be no palpable structure passing through the vaginal ring. In type 4 the efferent duct and the body of the epididymis pass through the ring. It is difficult to distinguish these from cases in which the testis, deferent duct, and testicular vessels have passed through the vaginal ring.

Blood Tests. In animals showing male behavior without palpable testes and with an unknown or uncertain history, surgery should not be undertaken without the supporting evidence of a blood test. Two blood tests for cryptorchidism exist, the age of the horse determining which one to apply. In horses of three years and older a single plasma or serum sample should be submitted to a laboratory for measurement of estrone sulfate concentrations. Cryptorchids have concentrations in excess of 400 pg per ml, false rigs less than 100 pg per ml. Donkeys of any age and horses less than three years old do not always produce significant quantities of estrone sulfate. In these cases diagnosis must be based on testosterone concentrations in a pair of samples, one taken before and the second 30 to 120 minutes after intravenous injection of 6000 IU of human chorionic gonadotropin (hCG). Cryptorchids have basal concentrations in excess of 100 pg per ml and should respond to hCG with a rise in concentration. False rigs have less than 40 pg per ml and do not respond to hCG.

TREATMENT

In my opinion, treatment of a cryptorchid in an attempt to give it the appearance of a normal stallion should not be undertaken. The condition is un-

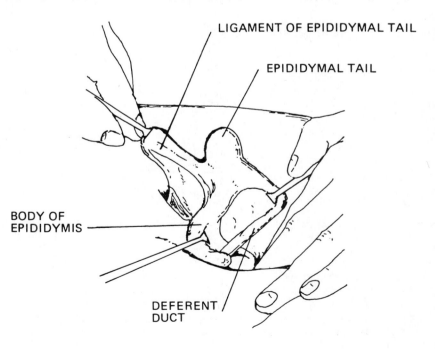

Figure 2. Surgical findings in a case of incomplete abdominal testicular retention. The vaginal tunic has been incised to expose the contents. (Reproduced with permission, Department of Veterinary Clinical Medicine, University of Liverpool.)

LIGAMENT OF EPIDIDYMAL TAIL

EPIDIDYMAL TAIL

BODY OF EPIDIDYMIS

DEFERENT DUCT

doubtedly inherited, although not in the simple way often quoted, and an animal exhibiting the trait should, therefore, be castrated. Surgical correction in humans is attempted partly for psychologic reasons and partly to reduce the risk of metastatic carcinoma developing later in life. The procedure must be attempted well before puberty and few male horses are recognized as cryptorchids at that age.

Medical therapy with repeated injection of hCG has no beneficial effect. If the testis is retained in the abdomen, it cannot descend through the inguinal canal beyond the first few weeks of life. If the inguinally retained testis is of type 2, it cannot be made to descend because its vaginal tunic is too short. If the retained testis is of type 1, it will descend in time. Moreover, hCG injections increase testicular size by edema rather than true growth and the testis is, therefore, not normal.

Surgical removal of an inguinally retained testis is a simple matter in an anesthetized horse placed in dorsal recumbency. The most important rule, in exploring the inguinal region for a testis, is never to cut deeper than the skin with a scalpel as there are numerous large tributaries of the external pudendal veins just under the skin. The inguinal region should always be explored surgically rather than relying solely on palpation.

Removal of an abdominal testis can be accomplished via the inguinal canal. The older procedure of pushing through the body wall close to or actually through the canal have now been replaced by the more sophisticated procedure of identifying the ligament of the epididymal tail in its vaginal tunic in the inguinal region and applying traction to this. The former techniques have a high rate of failure in inexperienced hands. Large testes can be re-moved only with unnecessary trauma and postoperative discomfort. I would recommend the technique of suprapubic paramedian laparotomy. This surgical approach is simple, and the testis itself is usually easily located and removed, whatever its size. Controlled repair of the incision is possible, postoperative complications are rare, and the dangers of postoperative prolapse of bowel, even in inexperienced hands, is almost entirely eliminated.

The approach is made through a 10 to 12 cm skin incision, level with the opening of the sheath, about 10 cm away from the midline and parallel to it. The incision is continued through the subcutaneous fascia and the yellow abdominal tunic with the adherent tendons of the oblique muscle. The exposed straight abdominal muscle is split along its fibers. The underlying transverse muscle tendon is split along its fibers at right angle to the straight muscle, thus creating a self-closing incision. The testis is usually found close to the deep inguinal ring. If not, it may be found by locating the ductus deferens on the bladder roof, and following this to the epididymal tail and thence to the testis.

Supplemental Readings

Adams, O. R.: An improved method of diagnosis and castration of cryptorchid horses. J. Am. Vet. Med. Assoc., *145*:439, 1964.

Cox, J. E.: Some observations of the behaviour of false rigs. Vet. Rev., 25:85, 1979.

Cox, J. E.: Surgery of the reproductive tract in large animals, 2nd ed. Liverpool University Press, 1981.

Cox, J. E.: Testosterone or oestrone sulphate assay for the diagnosis of cryptorchidism. J. Reprod. Fert., Suppl. *32*:625, 1982.

Cox, J. E., Edwards, G. B., and Neal, P. A.: Suprapubic paramedian laparotomy for abdominal cryptorchidism in the horse. Vet. Record, 97:428, 1975.

Embryo Transfer

Edward L. Squires, FORT COLLINS, COLORADO

The first successful equine embryo transfer was reported in 1972. Since that time, pregnancy rates resulting from embryo transfer have steadily improved. More widespread use is limited by the attitudes of breed registration authorities. Embyro transfer can be used to obtain more offspring from superior-performance mares. It can also get foals from old valuable mares with uterine degeneration, from two-year-old mares, from competing mares, and from mares foaling late in the season. The success of the technique has been limited by in-ability to superovulate mares, by poor results obtained with frozen semen, and by the failure of breed societies to register more than one foal per mare per year.

SELECTION AND MANAGEMENT OF DONOR AND RECIPIENT MARES

Before beginning an embryo transfer program, the regulations of the breed society should be checked. Some societies have minimal qualifying restrictions while others stipulate age and number of years a mare must have been barren before being used as a donor. For optimal chances of success, *donor* mares should be in good physical condition and should be cycling normally and located on the same premises as the stallion. The latter allows greater familiarity with cyclic behavior and the frequency of mating required for maximal reproductive efficiency.

Each donor should receive a thorough examination of the genitalia, including uterine culture and biopsy. If signs of infection are detected, the uterus should be flushed with 1 to 3 liters of sterile saline and the flushings examined for turbidity. Endometritis must be treated (see p. 505) so that the mare will be suitable for insemination before embryo recovery.

Donor and recipient mares should be teased daily and estrous mares examined daily by rectal palpation until ovulation is detected. Ideally, the donor mares should have a normal estrous cycle before insemination on day 2 or 3 of estrus and then daily or every other day until ovulation. Ovulation is day 0. The donor mare is flushed for embryo recovery on day 6 to 8, after which prostaglandin is administered to ensure return to estrus. If the recovered fluid is clear and debris-free, the donor mare may be inseminated again next estrus and the procedures repeated at subsequent cycles until the desired number of pregnancies is obtained.

The selection of known fertile, well-handled *recipient* mares is vital to the success of embryo transfer. Mares should be 3 to 10 years old, 450 to 600 kg, have no evidence of endometritis, and a "grade 1" biopsy result. One to two recipients should be available for each donor. Teasing and gynecologic examinations are as described for donor mares, and dates of ovulation are recorded. As with recipients, two to three previous normal cycles are preferable. Ideally, recipients should be assessed by embryo recovery after test insemination. In some cases, estrus synchronization is achieved by exogenous hormone therapy (see p. 495). Selected recipients should ovulate one day before (+1) or three days after (0, −1, −2, −3) the donor mare.

After surgical transfer, recipients receive 900,000 IU penicillin intramuscularly for five days. They are housed in individual stalls or pens and their rectal temperature and general health is monitored during this period. If there are no complications, the mares are returned to the herd on day 6 following surgery. Mares are returned to the herd immediately after nonsurgical transfer.

Pregnancy examinations are performed at day 15 after ovulation using ultrasound echography and repeated at days 20, 35, 50, and 60, after which they are allowed to return to their stud farm of origin. If the procedure has been unsuccessful, embryo transfer is repeated once only.

EMBRYO RECOVERY AND IDENTIFICATION

Commercial embryo recovery is attempted at days 7 to 8 after ovulation. Extended two-way, size 30 French Foley catheters,* individually packaged and sterilized with ethylene oxide, are air dried for at least 48 hours before use. A donor mare, in stocks, is prepared by wrapping the tail, surgically scrubbing the perineum and rinsing with a 5 per cent tamed-iodine solution.† A sterile surgeon's glove over a palpation sleeve is worn when the catheter is placed approximately 5 cm anterior to the internal os of the cervix. The cuff is inflated with 60 ml sterile saline or water and the catheter is pulled back to form a tight seal with the cervix (Fig. 1).

One liter of prewarmed (32 to 35°C) modified Dulbecco's phosphate-buffered saline (PBS) with 1 per cent heat-inactivated steer serum is infused into the uterus and allowed to return out by gravity flow through a 75-micron filter,‡ ensuring that at least 20 ml fluid remains in the filter cup. This infusion and recovery is repeated twice, making a fluid total of three liters. Recovery of fluid is assisted by uterine massage, per rectum. Approximately 96 per cent of the infused fluid should be recovered, clear and free from debris. The fluid from the filter cup is poured into a sterile search dish§ and 30 ml PBS is flushed through the filter via the outlet tube. An additional 30 ml PBS is used to rinse the cup and these washings are added to the search dish.

A stereo dissection microscope, with a 15× magnification, is used to search the fluid for an embryo. When it is located, it is moved into culture medium using a fire-polished glass pipette attached to a 1 or 3 ml glass syringe. The culture medium is prepared by aspirating 9 ml PBS into a 10 ml syringe, then adding 1 ml heat-inactivated steer serum before mixing. A sterile disposable 0.22 micron millipore filter is attached to the syringe and the culture medium is dispensed into three 35× 10 mm sterile culture dishes. The embryo is rinsed by being transferred from one dish to another and is then maintained at room temperature until transfer, within one to two hours after collection.

---

*Franklin Medical Ltd., High Wycombe, Bucks, England
†Betadine, Purdue Fredrick Co., Norwalk, CT
‡Immuno Systems, Kennebunk, ME
§V.W.R. Scientific, South Plainfield, NJ

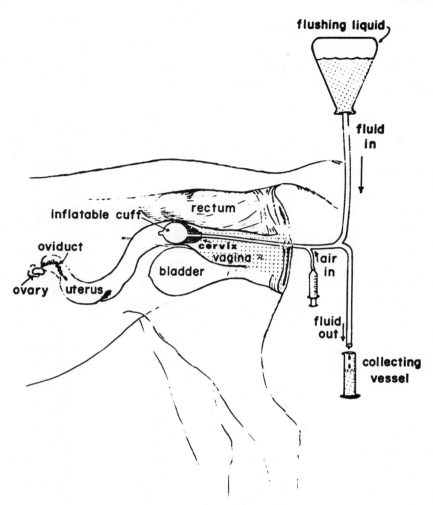

flushing liquid

fluid
in

inflatable cuff

rectum

oviduct

cervix
vagina

ovary   uterus

bladder

air
in

fluid
out

collecting
vessel

Figure 1. Technique for embryo collection. Catheter positioned within the reproductive tract and cuff inflated.

FACTORS AFFECTING EMBRYO RECOVERY

Table 1 shows the embryo recovery rate for experimental mares flushed between days 6 to 9 after ovulation. Days 7 to 8 are recommended because there is a 10 to 15 per cent better recovery rate than for day 6. Recovery at day 9 is not recommended because these larger, older embryos have poor viability.

Stallion fertility and seminal treatment methods affect embryo recovery and thus recovery rates may

be used to assess these experimentally. For example, recovery rates are higher for mares inseminated with raw semen or semen in skim milk extender than for those in which semen in EDTA-lactose extender is used.

The reproductive history of the donor mare has the greatest influence on embryo recovery. Between 1979 and 1980, 10 embryos were recovered from 36 attempts with infertile mares whereas 128 embryos were recovered from 160 attempts with normal fertile mares. Fluid recovery was not the problem, suggesting that fertilization failure or poor egg and/or sperm transport prevented embryos from reaching the uterus. Embryo recovery rates for infertile mares are 22 to 30 per cent, in contrast to 50.6 per cent in normal fertile mares.

EMBRYO SIZE AND MORPHOLOGY

Table 2 shows the average diameter of embryos collected between six and nine days after ovulation. The equine embryo, at this stage, doubles in size every 24 hours; therefore, ovulation must be accu-

TABLE 1. EFFECT OF
DAY ON EMBRYO RECOVERY RATES
FROM EXPERIMENTAL MARES

Day of Attempt	No. Attempts	No. Embryos Recovered	% Recovery
6	137	86	62.0
7	96	73	76.0
8	293	218	74.4
9	53	43	81.1

TABLE 2. EFFECT OF DAY OF COLLECTION
ON EMBRYO SIZE

Day	No.	Size (mm)
6	121	.208
7	144	.406
8	142	1.132
9	41	2.220

rately determined to avoid collecting large fragile embryos. Day 6 embryos are morulae with a thick zona pellucida or early blastocysts. Most of day 7 and all of day 8 and 9 embryos are expanded blastocysts. Their inner cell masses are easily distinguished from the trophoblast; however, the zona can be distinguished only at 20 to 30× magnification.

The equine embryo does not "hatch," as in the cow—instead, the zona becomes progressively thinner and forms a protein layer. Normally only fertilized ova reach the uterus. The unfertilized ones remain in the oviducts and degenerate, but occasionally an unfertilized ovum is recovered by flushing. Only 3 to 5 per cent of recovered embryos are considered unfit for transfer.

EMBRYO TRANSFER

The pregnancy rate using nonsurgical transfer is 45 to 66 per cent. Surgical transfer using midline or flank laparotomy results in pregnancy rates of 55 to 60 per cent and 65 to 72 per cent, respectively. The midline laparotomy has been largely replaced by the flank approach. The recipient mare is restrained in stocks and tranquilized with acepromazine maleate and xylazine hydrochloride. A 35 × 45 cm sublumbar fossa skin area is clipped, shaved, and prepared for surgery. Approximately 50 ml 2 per cent lidocaine hydrochloride is used to provide a vertical line block for the skin incision. The subcutaneous tissues and muscles are bluntly dissected, using a grid approach. The peritoneum is penetrated and the tip of the uterine horn is exteriorized and penetrated at its most avascular site using a cutting edged needle. The embryo is aspirated into a fire-polished pipette and transferred into the uterine lumen. The muscles, subcutaneous tissues, and skin are then closed using standard surgical techiques.

Improved results with fast, inexpensive, efficient, nonsurgical techiques may in the future make this the approach of choice. Three methods have been evaluated over six years.

Unguarded. The embryo is positioned in a sterile 55 cm insemination pipette, between two fluid columns and two air spaces. The embryo is deposited approximately 5 cm anterior to the cervix, in the uterine body.

Guarded. The embryo, inside the insemination pipette, is placed inside the sheath of a uterine culture instrument.* Once through the cervix, the cap of the instrument is pushed off and the embryo is deposited as in the unguarded method.

Cassou Nonsurgical Bovine Instrument. The embryo is loaded into a straw, between fluid and air columns, as described. Once inside the uterus, the straw is extended and the plunger depressed to expel the embryo.

Table 3 shows that pregnancy rates for nonsurgical methods were initially low but that they improved with the use of the guarded method. The best results (16 of 24 embryos transferred) were obtained in 1984. These results are similar to those obtained by surgical transfer.

FACTORS AFFECTING PREGNANCY RATES AFTER EMBRYO TRANSFER

Age and Size of Embryo. Higher pregnancy rates have been obtained with day 8 embryos (32 per cent) than with day 9 embryos (4 per cent), suggesting that the latter, with their larger ratio of fluid volume to surface, may be more easily damaged during collection and transfer. Table 4 shows pregnancy rates for days 6, 7, and 8 embryos transferred surgically and nonsurgically. The age effect is less at this stage but is more noticeable with nonsurgical techniques. Nevertheless, collecting and transferring embryos from mares on days 6, 7, or 8 after ovulation allows flexibility.

Synchrony of Recipients. Table 5 shows pregnancy rates following surgical embryo transfer into recipients that had ovulated more than two to less than three days relative to the donor (0 days = exact synchrony). There was no significant difference in these results, which suggests that the degree of synchrony is not as critical as was previously thought.

---

*Kalayjian Industries, Inc., Long Beach, CA

TABLE 3. PREGNANCY RATES AFTER
NONSURGICAL TRANSFER

Method of Transfer	No. Transfer	No. Pregnancy	% Pregnant 50 Days
Unguarded			
1979	15	4	27
1980	14	1	7
1981	26	6	23
Guarded			
1981	13	7	54
1982	40	18	45
Cassou Gun			
1984	24	16	67

TABLE 4. EFFECT OF AGE OF EMBRYO ON PREGNANCY RATE

| Age (days) | Method of Transfer | | | | | |
| | Nonsurgical* | | | Surgical (Flank) | | |
	No. Transfer	No. Pregnant	%	No. Transfer	No. Pregnant	%
6	10	7	70	5	5	100
7	20	10	50	159	113	71
8	44	21	48	33	24	73

*Includes only nonsurgical transfers performed with the guarded instrument or Cassou bovine instrument.

Method of Transfer and Technician. Pregnancy rates for nonsurgical transfer are improving progressively and now equal those for surgical techniques when performed by experienced technicians. When sufficient technical expertise is not available, the surgical approach is recommended.

Culture Medium and Embryo Storage. Storage of equine embryos for six hours or more, in vitro, results in poor pregnancy rates. Recent studies show that Ham's F10* is a better culture medium for embryo storage than PBS or MEM (minimal essential medium). Embryos stored in Ham's F10 for 12 hours and then transferred nonsurgically resulted in pregnancies at rates comparable to those transferred at less than an hour.

CRYOPRESERVATION

Six-day equine embryos appear relatively tolerant to freezing, with glycerol as a protectant. In one study, 32 embryos were collected nonsurgically at day 6 after ovulation and stored in 0.5 ml plastic straws or 1 ml glass ampules. A programmable, automatic freezer provided the following cooling rate: 4° C per minute from room temperature to −6° C, seeded at −6° C and held for 15 minutes, 0.3° C per minute to −30 or 35° C, and 0.1° C per minute to −33 or −38° C.

The embryos were then plunged into liquid nitrogen and stored for 1 to 60 days before thawing in a 37° C water bath. The glycerol was removed by a six-step dilution method and the embryos were cultured for 24 hours at 37° C in Ham's F10 plus 5 per cent fetal calf serum. The embryos frozen in straws and plunged at −33° C were found to be of

*Sigma Chemical Co., St. Louis, MO

TABLE 5. EFFECT OF SYNCHRONY ON PREGNANCY RATES AFTER SURGICAL TRANSFER (1982–84)

Synchrony	No. Transfers	No. Pregnant	% Pregnant at 50 Days
−3	17	11	64.7
−2	26	22	84.6
−1*	62	42	67.7
0	79	56	70.9
+1†	20	13	65.0
+2	2	2	100.0

*Denotes recipient ovulated 1 day after the donor.
†Denotes recipient ovulated 1 day prior to the donor.

better quality than those frozen in ampules and plunged at −38° C. Therefore, the former method was used for a surgical transfer study involving 23 day 6 embryos. On thawing, six embryos were found to be of poor quality and were discarded. Of the remaining 17 transferred embryos, nine resulted in pregnancies. These results are similar to those reported for the transfer of bovine frozen and thawed embryos.

SUPEROVULATION

The mare appears relatively refractory to attempts at superovulation. Crude pituitary extracts appear to give better results than FSH in cycling mares. There is a higher mortality rate for multiple embryos, which may negate the advantage achieved. However, this is less obvious in multiple embryos collected at six days after ovulation. Superovulation may thus be of some value if embryos are collected at day 6; however, the chances of a mare producing more than four to six embryos per year appears slim.

FUTURE CONSIDERATIONS

The technology and expertise for embryo transfer and semen and embryo freezing and storage is advancing more rapidly than its acceptance by the horse industry. Embryo micromanipulation can be used for splitting equine embryos, and identical twins have been born alive. In vitro fertilization techiques are badly needed for some infertile mares and these will undoubtedly be available in time. Progress is being made in the sexing of embryos by the detection of HY antigen, and this may prove to be of great interest to breeders in the near future.

Supplemental Readings

Douglas, R. H.: Some aspects of equine embryo transfer. J. Reprod. Fert., Suppl. 32:405, 1982.
Imel, K. J., Squires, E. L., Elsden, R. P., and Shideler, R. K.: Collection and transfer of equine embryos. J. Am. Vet. Med. Assoc., *179*:987, 1981.
Squires, E. L., Cook, V. M., and Voss, J. L.: Collection and transfer of equine embryos. Animal Reproduction Laboratory, Colorado State University, Bulletin No. 1, 1985.
Squires, E. L., Imel, K. J., Iuliano, M. F., and Shideler, R. K.: Factors affecting reproductive efficiency in an equine embryo transfer programme. J. Reprod. Fert., Suppl., 32:409, 1982.
Squires, E. L., Iuliano, M. F., and Shideler, R. K.: Factors affecting the success of surgical and nonsurgical equine embryo transfer. Theriogenology, *17*:35, 1982.

Evaluation of the Respiratory System: Diagnostic Techniques

Frederik J. Derksen, EAST LANSING, MICHIGAN

This chapter will briefly describe selected diagnostic techniques used in evaluation of horses with respiratory disease. Interpretation of test results will be discussed in subsequent chapters.

AUSCULTATION

In spite of its limitations, auscultation is one of the most sensitive, qualitative methods of evaluation available to the equine clinician. However, because of improperly used techniques, confused nomenclature, and overinterpretation of findings, auscultation has been de-emphasized. Auscultation should be carried out using a quality stethoscope that fits the operator's ears tightly and comfortably. Because the lung sounds audible at the horse's chest are of low intensity, auscultation should be carried out in a quiet area. Breath sounds may be accentuated by exercise before auscultation or by the use of a rebreathing bag.

Breath sounds are produced by turbulent air flow in the large airways and are conducted through the lung parenchyma and chest wall to the stethoscope. The intensity of breath sound production varies directly with air flow velocity. Therefore, breath sound production may be enhanced by increased ventilation and by ventilation through partially obstructed airways and decreased by complete obstruction of airways. Conduction of breath sounds is enhanced by lung consolidation or atelectasis and reduced by lung inflation or pleural fluid accumulation. The intensity of breath sounds heard at the chest wall in disease is a combination of changes in sound production and transmission.

In disease, abnormal lung sounds (adventitial sounds) may be superimposed on normal breath sounds. Adventitial sounds are classified as crackles or wheezes. Crackles are short, nonmusical, sharp, explosive sounds while wheezes are musical, high-pitched sounds of variable duration. The primary mechanism of crackles production is thought to be the equalization of pressure when a collapsed region of lung is reinflated. Crackles are uncommon in horses and are associated with restrictive lung disease including pulmonary edema, atelectasis, diffuse fibrosis, and interstitial pneumonia. Wheezes are produced by vibrations of airway walls and in the horse are associated with obstructive lung diseases, including bronchopneumonia and chronic obstructive pulmonary disease. Although auscultation may allow the clinician to establish the presence of respiratory disease, conclusions regarding etiology or pathology of the disease process should be drawn with caution.

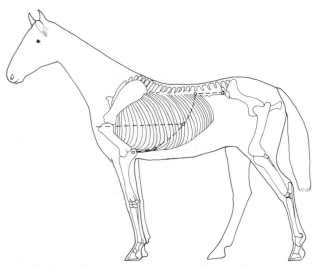

Figure 1. Percussion boundaries of the equine lung.

PERCUSSION

Percussion is accomplished using a rubber hammer (plexor) and a flat hard instrument (pleximeter) and helps delineate the boundaries of the lung. The cranial and dorsal percussion borders of the normal equine lung are the heavy shoulder and back musculature, respectively. The caudal-ventral border is marked by the 17th intercostal space at the level of the tuber coxae, the 11th intercostal space at the level of the point of the shoulder, and the point of the elbow (Fig. 1). Percussion allows identification of areas of lung consolidation, pleural fluid accumulation, and extension of the lung field.

TRANSTRACHEAL ASPIRATION

Transtracheal aspiration is indicated when a culture or cytologic evaluation of the lower respiratory system is required. A 5 cm square area is clipped on the ventral midline of the midcervical region where the trachea is easily palpable. The area is surgically prepared and analgesia is achieved by injecting 2 ml of local anesthetic solution subcutaneously. A stab incision is made through the skin and a trochar* is inserted between adjacent tracheal rings into the trachea. A catheter is inserted through the cannula and directed down the trachea. Fifty ml of physiologic saline solution is injected into the catheter and immediately aspirated. The aspirate is submitted for bacteriologic culture and cytologic evaluation. Cytologic evaluation is performed using Gram and Wright-Giemsa–stained preparations.

*Nested Trocar Set, Miltex Instruments Co., Lake Success, NY

THORACOCENTESIS

Thoracocentesis is a valuable diagnostic technique when evaluating horses with pleural disease. In the right hemithorax, thoracocentesis may be performed at the level of the point of the elbow in the seventh intercostal space. In the left hemithorax the procedure is performed 4 to 6 cm above the point of the elbow in the eighth or ninth intercostal space. A 5 cm square area is clipped and surgically prepared. Following desensitization of the skin and underlying musculature with approximately 5 ml of a local anesthetic solution, a stab incision is made through the skin. A 3-inch teat cannula or blunt catheter is attached to a 3-way stopcock. The catheter is inserted into the thoracic cavity along the cranial border of the rib, with care taken to avoid the lateral thoracic vein. A distinct release of tension is felt when the thoracic cavity is entered. In the normal horse, pleural pressure is negative relative to atmospheric pressure and air rushes into the pleural cavity when the stopcock is opened. Aspiration yields 1 to 2 ml of straw-colored fluid. In cases of pleural effusion, fluid will drain freely from the cannula. Pleural fluid is submitted for bacteriologic and cytologic evaluation. Following completion of the procedure the thoracocentesis site is covered with an antiseptic cream and bandaged. Thoracocentesis is a simple and safe technique; complications are uncommon.

BRONCHOALVEOLAR LAVAGE

Bronchoalveolar lavage has recently been adapted to the horse and allows for collection and quantitation of cells from the lung. Cell counts obtained by this method correspond well with results obtained through lung biopsy. Horses are tranquilized with xylazine (0.5 mg per kg intravenously) and a 180-cm long fiberoptic endoscope is passed via the nostrils into the trachea. Two ml of 0.5 per cent lidocaine solution is injected through the biopsy channel to desensitize the airways. The fiberoptic endoscope is gently wedged in a lower lobe bronchus and three 100-ml aliquots of body-temperature saline is infused through the biopsy channel and gently aspirated. Bronchoalveolar lavage fluid recovered is filtered through a single layer of gauze and the volume is measured. A differential cell count of 500 consecutive cells is performed using a Wright-Giemsa–stained preparation. Table 1 gives normal values used in our laboratory.

ARTERIAL BLOOD GAS ANALYSIS

Arterial blood gas analysis is one of the simplest and most practical quantitative tests of pulmonary

TABLE 1. CELL COUNTS PER µl ($\bar{X} \pm$ SEM) IN BRONCHOALVEOLAR LAVAGE FLUID OF NORMAL HORSES

Total cells	184 ± 59
Neutrophils	4 ± 1.5
Macrophages	64 ± 13
Lymphocytes	101 ± 49
Eosinophils	0.2 ± 0.2
Mast cells	11 ± 4
Epithelial cells	3 ± 1

function available to the practicing veterinarian. Arterial blood gas can be sampled from the carotid artery or the greater metatarsal artery, and in the newborn foal also from the femoral artery. Blood is collected in a heparinized syringe, air is expelled, and the syringe is sealed using a cap or rubber stopper. When transported on ice, samples remain stable for four to five hours. Arterial carbon dioxide tension is an indicator of alveolar ventilation while arterial oxygen tension reflects the gas exchange function of the lung.

LUNG BIOPSY

Percutaneous lung biopsy using a biopsy needle is an invasive technique that is easily performed but is associated with a variety of complications including hemoptysis, neurogenic shock, and death. The procedure should be performed only if a definitive diagnosis is essential for the management of the case and when other less invasive diagnostic methods have been tried. The preferred biopsy site is located at the level of the point of the shoulder in the eighth right intercostal space. Following aseptic preparation of the biopsy site, the skin and underlying musculature are desensitized using 5 ml of a local anesthetic solution. A stab incision is made through the skin and a 14-gauge biopsy needle* is advanced 2 cm into the lung parenchyma. The needle's obturator is pushed forward into the lung and stabilized. The cannula is advanced to procure the specimen. The biopsy site is covered with an aseptic ointment and bandaged.

---

*Trucut, Travenol Laboratories, Deerfield, IL

Supplemental Readings

Kotlikoff, M. I., and Gillespie, J. R.: Lung sounds in veterinary medicine, Part I. Terminology and mechanisms of sound production. Comp. Cont. Ed., 5:634, 1983.

Kotlikoff, M. I., and Gillespie, J. R.: Lung sounds in veterinary medicine, Part II. Deriving clinical information from lung sounds. Comp. Cont. Ed., 6:462, 1984.

Mansmann, R. A, and Knight, H. D.: Transtracheal aspiration in the horse. J. Am. Vet. Med. Assoc., 160:1527, 1972.

Raphel, C. F., and Gunson, D. E.: Percutaneous lung biopsy in the horse. Cornell Vet., 71:439, 1981.

Viral Respiratory Disease

David G. Powell, LEXINGTON, KENTUCKY

The "virus" is currently blamed for many equine respiratory ailments ranging from an individual horse suffering from acute respiratory disease to a stable of horses that have apparently lost their form but are showing little or no signs of illness. The range of respiratory illness attributable to viral infections is similar to that occurring in the human population, with various viral groups contributing to a complex etiologic and epidemiologic pattern. In addition to the recognized causes of viral respiratory disease such as influenza and equine herpesvirus, other groups of viruses including adenovirus, reovirus, rhinovirus, and other picornaviruses have been implicated either alone or more often in combination with other viruses and bacteria.

Factors that have contributed to an apparent rise in the incidence of viral respiratory disease include an increase in the horse population, especially of North America and Europe, with the associated tendency to house horses together in greater numbers. In addition, many horses are stabled under poor environmental conditions that are conducive to the spread of viral infection. The dramatic increase in the rapid international transportation of horses, usually by air, has also affected the spread of a variety of respiratory infections, notably equine influenza.

Alongside these changes in the management of horses have been improvements in diagnostic methods. They include better tissue culture techniques to isolate virus and greater use of the electron microscope to identify viruses. Use of more sophisticated serologic methods has also enhanced the clinician's ability to make a rapid and accurate diagnosis. No equivalent progress has been made in treatment of viral conditions of the horse; antiviral drugs have yet to be evaluated as a practical form of treatment in this species. Therapy still involves use of antibacterial drugs to control secondary infection. A number of antiviral drugs, including acyclovir, amantadine, and others, have been shown to be effective against equine herpesvirus and influenza, and their further evaluation may provide encouraging results. Some progress has been made in the control of a number of equine viral infections, notably influenza and equine herpesvirus type 1, with the development of inactivated vaccines. In both cases efficacy of the vaccines is limited by the short duration of immunity following vaccination.

ADENOVIRUS

Equine adenovirus type 1 was initially isolated from a foal with respiratory disease in 1969, and antigenically related viruses have been subsequently isolated from both healthy and sick foals as well as adult horses in many parts of the world. A second adenovirus, considered distinct from adenovirus type 1, has been isolated from the feces of a foal with diarrhea. The peculiar susceptibility of Arabian foals to fatal pneumonia associated with adenovirus infection has been linked to a combined immunodeficiency (CID) of genetic origin.

Pathogenesis

In the adult horse no clinical signs may be present but in the young foal characteristic signs of upper respiratory disease may be observed. Foals develop a nasal discharge, coughing, difficult breathing, conjunctivitis, fever, and occasionally diarrhea. This is associated with mild lymphopenia followed by leukocytosis. Arabian foals are more susceptible if they are immunodeficient, and mortality in this breed may reach 100 per cent. Other breeds of foals may develop only mild or inapparent signs. Pathologic changes include interstitial pneumonia, which may resolve spontaneously if the condition is uncomplicated. In the immunodeficient foal the lesions are more general and may include a suppurative bronchiolitis. Other changes include pancreatitis and enteritis with the presence of inclusions in the nuclei of urinary tract epithelial cells.

Diagnosis

Virus may be isolated in tissue culture from infected tissues or from nasopharyngeal and ocular swabs and identified by electron microscopy. Cell smears prepared from nasal or conjunctival epithelium can be examined by immunofluorescence to demonstrate either viral particles or inclusion bodies. Antibody measured by serum-neutralizing (SN), hemagglutination inhibition (HI), and precipitin techniques may be used to confirm infection.

Epizootiology

Adenovirus infection is common among the horse population throughout the world. The majority of infection occurs in early life and it is likely that foals acquire the virus from their dams during the suckling period. The virus persists in the upper respiratory tract of the adult horse so that individual animals act as carriers or reservoir hosts. The resistance of the virus to temperature and pH plus the shedding of virus in the urine, feces, and mucus of infected animals helps to disseminate the virus among the susceptible population. It seems unlikely that infection with adenovirus in the immunologically competent horse is of great consequence, but mixed infection with other viruses—especially equine herpesvirus type 1—and bacteria are of significance. No commercial vaccine is available, although an inactivated vaccine has been shown to elicit an antibody response in foals.

AFRICAN HORSE SICKNESS (AHS)

With the possible exception of Venezuelan equine encephalomyelitis, African horse sickness is the most important viral disease of equids causing widespread mortality during an epidemic. African horse sickness causes disease in horses, mules, and donkeys, with up to 95 per cent mortality among susceptible animals. Epizootics of AHS have been recorded in Africa over the centuries and evidence of endemic infection exists for most of Africa south of the Sahara. The disease does occur outside of Africa, most recently in southern Spain during 1965 and 1966 and the Middle East between 1959 and 1961. The virus is classified in the family Reoviridae, nine serotypes having been identified to date. The disease is arthropod-borne, the main vector being nocturnal biting insects Culicoides. Areas currently free of the disease are the Americas, Europe, Asia, and Australasia.

Pathogenesis

Horses appear to be the most susceptible, having high morbidity and mortality. Among mules the morbidity is high and mortality low, with donkeys being the least sensitive showing only a mild febrile response and no mortality. The clinical disease has been described under four distinct types: (1) the peracute or pulmonary form, (2) the subacute, edematous, or cardiac form, (3) the acute or mixed form, and (4) horse sickness fever.

The peracute form has a short incubation period for 3 to 5 days with obvious pyrexia and marked respiratory distress accompanied by spasmodic coughing and frothy fluid exuding from the nostrils. Death usually occurs within a few hours because of excess fluid in the lungs. This form affects susceptible animals exposed to a highly virulent strain of AHS. The subacute form has an incubation of 7 to 14 days. The major clinical sign is edema of the head, neck, trunk, and limbs. Death occurs from cardiac failure in approximately 50 per cent of affected animals. This form of AHS is usually associated with virus strains of lower virulence or occurs in animals with some degree of immunity. The acute form represents a combination of the peracute and subacute forms and is usually recognized at postmortem following an incubation period of 5 to 7 days. The mortality rate is about 80 per cent, death occurring three to six days after the onset of pyrexia. Horse sickness fever is the mildest form, with an incubation period of 5 to 14 days resulting in a febrile reaction lasting for several days. Other clinical signs may include respiratory distress, anorexia, depression, and reddening of the mucous membranes. This form of the disease is usually observed in animals with a degree of immunity or in resistant species such as donkeys and zebra.

Postmortem lesions are strongly influenced by the clinical form of the disease manifested before death. Edema of the lungs, hydrothorax, and fluid in the pericardium are consistent findings, with enlargement and edema of the lymph nodes of the thorax and abdominal cavities. Histopathologic examination of various organs does not reveal specific changes. It has been suggested that the variable clinical response is most strongly influenced by the degree of pneumotropism of the virus population. Those strains with pneumotropic properties give rise to the greatest degree of pulmonary involvement and hence to the peracute and acute form of the disease.

Diagnosis

African horse sickness virus may be isolated by taking a heparinized blood sample from the animal and inoculating into mice, embryonated eggs, and various cell cultures including monkey cell line. In addition, blood may be given intravenously into a known susceptible horse. Confirmation of virus isolation may be made by the complement-fixation (CF) or the neutralization test. Several serologic tests are available, including SN, CF, HI, fluorescent antibody (FA), and agar gel immunodiffusion (AGID).

Epizootiology

African horse sickness is restricted to warm, moist low-lying or coastal regions in valleys, swamps, and river basins. The disease occurs during the summer months and terminates with the onset of the colder weather. In view of its marked susceptibility and high mortality rate, the horse may be regarded as an accidental or indicator host. The horse is therefore not essential for the long-term survival of the disease. Whatever the true natural host, it is restricted to the tropical regions of Africa and is unlikely to manifest clinical signs of the disease. This would explain the failure of the disease to become established outside of tropical Africa despite the fact that epidemics have occurred. Zebra are susceptible but experience subclinical infection. A high percentage of elephants have been shown to possess circulating antibody to AHS. There is no evidence at present to suggest that once a horse has recovered from AHS it remains a carrier. The viremic phase is not known to exceed 21 days. AHS is not contagious even under conditions of very close contact. The virus is transmitted biologically by tiny midges (Culicoides) that are normally active from dusk until dawn. These insects are weak fliers but can travel long distances on air currents, which could contribute to the spread of the disease.

Prevention

Polyvalent and, to a limited extent, monovalent attenuated live vaccines have been successfully developed over the years to protect horses in geographic areas where the disease is enzootic. There is some cross-protection between certain serotypes. Traditionally, the virus was attenuated by serial intracerebral passage in adult mice. The disadvantage of this method was that it resulted in excessive neurotropism with an associated loss of immunogenicity. Administration of this vaccine even on an annual basis was not found to give polyvalent protection until after the third or fourth annual revaccination. More recently polyvalent cell culture vaccines have been developed that do not require annual revaccination.

In enzootic areas during the summer months it is wise to protect horses from insect bites by use of insect repellents and stabling in fly-proof accommodation. This is especially important from late afternoon to dawn.

EQUINE VIRAL ARTERITIS (EVA)

Equine viral arteritis was first distinguished from equine influenza and equine rhinopneumonitis in the United States during the 1950s following isolation of the virus during an outbreak of abortion and severe illness on a stud farm in Bucyrus, Ohio. Equine viral arteritis, which has the characteristics of the RNA togavirus, causes an acute infectious illness, the worldwide distribution of which is not precisely known.

Pathogenesis

The clinical signs of EVA include pyrexia, depression, edema of the limbs and less frequently of the head and trunk but including the external genitalia of the stallion, conjunctivitis, increased respiratory rate, and occasionally a skin rash. When an outbreak occurs the signs vary considerably from one horse to another. Some field strains of the virus appear to be relatively avirulent, causing only subclinical infection. Clinical disease is therefore rarely diagnosed but does occur in an epidemic form on racetracks and stud farms. A limited outbreak, the first reported among thoroughbred animals in the United States, occurred in central Kentucky during the summer of 1984. Although some strains of the virus are fatal when administered under experimental conditions, mortality under field conditions is invariably negligible. The incubation period ranges from 3 to 14 days with an average of 7 days. Abortion occurs during or shortly after the acute phase of febrile illness. EVA has a selective affinity for the media of small arteries throughout the body, causing necrosis of the muscle cells. This gives rise to edema and infiltration with leukocytes. The increased permeability of the small arteries produces generalized edema and hemorrhage with thrombosis formation in the vessels of the intestine and spleen. Abortion is the result of fetal death occurring in utero. It follows severe necrosis of the myometrium of the uterus leading to edema, which causes placental detachment.

Diagnosis

A clinical diagnosis in the individual animal may not be possible because of the range of clinical signs associated with EVA infection. Confirmation is obtained by isolation of the virus from the upper respiratory tract during the early acute phase of illness and demonstration of a rise in serum-neutralizing antibody between acute and convalescent sera. Virus may also be isolated from buffy coat, urine, and semen. EVA grows readily in rabbit kidney, equine fetal kidney, and equine dermal cells. Neutralizing antibody develops rapidly within a week or two after challenge and persists indefinitely. Reports suggest that following abortion from EVA, diagnosis is based on confirmation of disease in the mare because there are no characteristic lesions in the fetus.

Epizootiology

Although the majority of studies on EVA have been undertaken in the United States, the disease has been reported in Europe including Poland, Austria, and Switzerland. Seroepidemiologic studies suggest that the virus is especially prevalent among Standardbred and Saddlebred horses in the United States. The prevalence among the Thoroughbred population both in the United States and elsewhere is only about 2 per cent. Transmission of EVA occurs by the venereal and respiratory routes, and

isolation of the virus from the urine of mares several months after infection suggests that EVA may localize in the urinary system, giving rise to a carrier state. Accurate descriptions of a disease resembling EVA at the beginning of this century suggested that stallions infected mares over several seasons. The recent isolation of virus from the semen of stallions during the postrecovery period confirms this observation. Why EVA under experimental conditions causes more severe illness than is seen in natural outbreaks is not understood. The possibility exists that the variation in signs between field outbreaks of the disease may be attributable to variations in the virulence of the virus, but this has yet to be demonstrated.

Treatment and Prevention

The majority of infected animals, given sufficient rest for several weeks, recover spontaneously without resort to therapy. Antibiotic and sulfonamide therapy may reduce the possibility of secondary infection, especially in the young foal. A live modified EVA vaccine was developed during the 1960s at the University of Kentucky by successive passage of the Bucyrus strain of EVA in equine kidney, rabbit kidney,'and equine dermal cells. The vaccine appears to be safe and produces a demonstrable and persistent level of protection. Due to the lack of disease outbreaks the vaccine was not used until 1984 when it was administered intramuscularly to horses to control the outbreak on stud farms in central Kentucky. Subsequently the vaccine has been developed commercially and was licensed for general distribution within the United States during 1985. Other measures to control the spread of EVA include isolation of infected animals, restriction of movement, and closure of the breeding sheds. As the EVA virus is enclosed in a lipid envelope it is susceptible to the majority of disinfectants and detergents.

EQUINE HERPESVIRUS

Herpesvirus infections of the horse are very common indeed. Three antigenically distinct types of equine herpesvirus are recognized, equid herpesvirus type 1 (EHV-1, equine rhinopneumonitis), equid herpesvirus type 2 (EHV-2, cytomegalovirus, or slow-growing herpes), and equid herpesvirus type 3 (EHV-3, coital exanthema virus).

EQUID HERPESVIRUS TYPE 1

EHV-1 is a major cause of respiratory disease, abortion in the mare, sporadic outbreaks of paralysis, and perinatal mortality. Although these clinical signs have been attributed to one serotype, there is now increasing evidence that subtype 1 or fetal strain causes abortion and paralysis and a subtype 2 or respiratory strain is associated with rhinopneumonitis. This has led to the proposal that the virus be reclassified: the subtype 1 as EHV-1 and the subtype 2 as EHV-4. This reclassification is not yet universally accepted.

Pathogenesis

Horses acquire EHV-1 infection by inhalation of virus particles in aerosol droplets. The virus replicates in the epithelium of the nasal passages, pharynx, trachea, and bronchi, from which it is disseminated to the lymphoid follicles of the pharynx and respiratory tract. In foals, virus may invade the lower respiratory tract and cause viral bronchopneumonia.

Respiratory disease attributable to EHV-1 is prevalent among young horses under three years of age. The incubation period may be as short as two days or as long as ten. Acute disease is characterized by pyrexia, depression, and a serous nasal discharge that becomes mucopurulent because of secondary bacterial infection, usually streptococcal. Pathologic changes include extensive necrosis of the epithelial cells of the upper respiratory tract accompanied by an acute inflammatory response. Adult horses develop mild or subclinical signs as a result of repeated exposure to the virus, as it has long been recognized that immunity following natural infection is short-lived, two to three months. Mortality following respiratory infection is rare. However, if secondary bacterial infection occurs, bronchopneumonia may result and death can occur. Postmortem examination reveals severe bronchopneumonia, cellular infiltration around the bronchi and blood vessels, and serofibrinous exudate in the alveoli. Necrosis and intranuclear inclusions may be observed in the germinal centers of the bronchial lymph nodes.

In recent years perinatal infection with EHV-1 has been described in which weak foals die within 24 hours of birth. Foals that are apparently healthy at birth may also develop respiratory distress and die within one to three days. The principal postmortem lesion involves the respiratory tract. Lungs are firm on palpation and plum-purple in color; massive atelectasis is present. Microscopic lesions include profuse cellular infiltration around the bronchi, bronchioles, and blood vessels with serofibrinous exudate (hyaline membrane formation) in the alveoli. Intranuclear inclusions are also present in the lungs and bronchial lymph nodes.

Abortion in mares is considered a sequela to respiratory infection. Cell-associated viremia results in infection of the fetus and placenta. Loss of the fetus occurs between 14 and 120 days after exposure. Although abortions may occur as early as the fourth month of pregnancy, the majority occur during the last half of pregnancy, especially between 9 and 11 months. Mares do not show clinical signs, and abortion occurs suddenly. The fetus is usually dead at parturition; it dies of suffocation following separation of the placenta from the endometrium. There is usually very little autolysis of the fetus, suggesting that abortion occurs very quickly after death of the fetus. The majority of outbreaks of abortion involve only one or two pregnant mares; however, "abortion storms" in which 50 per cent of the potential foal crop is aborted have been recorded. Following an EHV-1 abortion the reproductive efficiency of the mare is not impaired. Postmortem findings in the fetus include jaundice, petechiation of mucous membranes, accumulation of pleural fluid, pulmonary edema, splenic enlargement with prominent lymphoid follicles, and white foci of hepatic necrosis. Characteristic microscopic lesions include bronchiolitis, severe necrosis of the splenic white pulp, and focal hepatic necrosis accompanied by a marked inflammatory response. Intranuclear inclusions are widely distributed in the tissues.

Disease of the nervous system associated with EHV-1 infection has been reported with increasing frequency over the last 15 years. Natural outbreaks have usually been associated with abortion and respiratory disease, but there are reports of ataxia occurring with no other concurrent problems. The early reports described the condition in pregnant and postpartum mares. More recently, however, reports have described the disease among foals, geldings, stallions, and fillies at stud farms, racetracks, and stables. Signs vary from mild ataxia to complete recumbency with forelimb and hindlimb paralysis. In severe cases there is also urinary and fecal incontinence. The incubation period is usually about seven days. Although no obvious macroscopic lesions of the nervous system are apparent, histologic lesions include vasculitis of the small arterioles of the brain and spinal cord. Paralysis may be caused as a result of ischemia and metabolic changes in the central nervous system. EHV-1 virus has been isolated only infrequently from the nervous tissues of affected horses. This may be a consequence of viral antibody complexes formed either in vivo or in vitro during the preparation of tissues for the inoculation into cell culture.

Diagnosis

Respiratory disease attributable to EHV-1 may be confirmed by viral isolation from nasopharyngeal swabs using a variety of cell cultures including RK13 and equine cell lines. A rise in serum antibody levels between acute and convalescent samples indicated by the serum neutralization, complement-fixation, or ELISA test is necessary to confirm a diagnosis of EHV-1 infection. Until recently, subtype identification of EHV-1 was a lengthy and highly specialized procedure. However, with the advent of subtype-specific monoclonal antibody reagents, differences between subtype 1 and 2 strains can be identified very quickly. When cases of abortion occur, EHV-1 is commonly isolated from lung, liver, and thymus of the fetus. Rapid diagnosis may be achieved by applying the immunofluorescence test to sections of frozen lung and liver. Histologic sections of lung and liver show the characteristic intranuclear inclusions. Diagnosis of the neurologic form is more difficult and is based on history, clinical signs, and histologic examination of central nervous tissue supported occasionally by virus isolation. Single cases of the paralytic form may be mistaken for other neurological disorders including the "wobbler" syndrome, protozoal myeloencephalopathy, arboviral encephalitides, and trauma to the brain or spinal cord. High levels of EHV-1 antibody in the blood and cerebrospinal fluid may be of value in the differential diagnosis.

Epizootiology

In recent years our understanding of the epizootiology of EHV-1 infection has undergone a radical change, primarily because of the introduction of more sophisticated techniques for isolation and typing of strains of EHV-1 virus. It now appears that EHV-1 is not a single virus but two genetically and antigenically distinct viruses causing different disease patterns. Historically, it was considered that EHV-1 isolated from aborted fetuses belonged to subtype 1, and those recovered from the respiratory tract were placed in subtype 2. Recently the technique of restriction endonuclease analysis of viral DNA, or "fingerprinting," has revealed the great genetic disparity between the two subgroups and has led to the suggested change in classification.

Studies in the United States and Australia using fingerprinting methods have demonstrated that subtype 2 strains are rarely the cause of abortion and have never been connected with multiple cases of abortion, perinatal foal mortality, and EHV-1 paralytic disease. Subtype 2 strains, however, are frequently isolated from outbreaks of respiratory disease in young horses. Thus the concept that outbreaks of respiratory disease in foals and yearlings attributable to EHV-1 posed a threat of abortion and neurologic disease in older horses is now without foundation.

Restriction endonuclease typing has made it possible to identify a number of strains within each subtype, including live vaccine strains. The vast majority of EHV-1 abortions occurring in central Kentucky between 1960 and 1982 were caused by two genotypes designated as 1B and 1P. The 1P genotype was responsible for 86 per cent of EHV-1 abortions between 1960 and 1980, but since 1980 the 1B type has emerged as the major cause of abortion. Such changes may have an influence on the choice of viral strains to be incorporated in a vaccine and emphasize the necessity for continued and detailed surveillance of outbreaks of EHV-1 infection. Within the subtype 2 group of EHV-1 viruses a much greater variety of DNA genotypes have been observed with no one type dominating the pattern of isolates.

Despite the fact that differences between subtype 1 and 2 have been demonstrated, it is still recognized that there is considerable antigenic cross-reactivity between the two subtypes using conventional polyclonal and the recently introduced monoclonal antibody reagents to a variety of serologic tests. As a consequence, repeated infection of young horses with respiratory subtype 2 viruses may result in the development of immunity to abortigenic subtype 1 viruses in later life.

In many instances the origin of an EHV-1 outbreak of abortion in a closed herd has remained a mystery. One of the hallmarks of herpesviruses is their capacity to persist in the tissues of the host in a latent state following primary infection. Months and years after primary infection, the latent virus may undergo recrudescence with the potential to cause disease and act as a focus of infection to incontact animals. Evidence of latent EHV-1 infection in the horse is currently circumstantial; those factors that might stimulate recrudescence of latent EHV-1 in the horse have not been accurately defined. However, there have been a number of reports of EHV-1 respiratory disease developing following vaccination against influenza and African horse sickness and after stress situations such as weaning, castration, and transportation. The location of the virus's hibernation during the latent period has not been conclusively demonstrated; however, it has been suggested that the leukocyte fraction of the buffy coat may harbor EHV-1.

Factors that influence the initiation of a respiratory outbreak of EHV-1 include a high contact rate and a population of susceptible animals. Such conditions are met at the time of weaning and the assembly of yearlings at the sales barns and at the racetracks. Factors influencing the initiation of the central nervous form of EHV-1 infection are not understood. It is obvious that great gaps still exist in our knowledge of the pathogenesis and epizootiology of EHV-1 infections. Now that sophisticated techniques of identification and typing are being applied to the equine herpesviruses it is imperative that disease outbreaks attributable to EHV-1 be investigated in detail. By correlation of clinical observations with the various EHV-1 genotypes and their changing patterns, a more rapid understanding of this complex disease syndrome may be achieved.

Treatment and Prevention

The possibilities of treating the various clinical manifestations of EHV-1 are evidently limited, although the development of certain antiviral drugs including acyclovir present the distinct possibility that perinatal and respiratory disease in foals can be treated. Currently, however, therapy is limited to controlling secondary bacterial infection in animals suffering the respiratory form of the disease. In these instances parenteral treatment with penicillin and oral therapy with sulfonamide drugs is recommended. Greater problems are faced by the veterinarian trying to cope with an outbreak of the paralytic form of the disease. Attempts to save severely affected recumbent animals by the use of slings have not been successful, although providing such animals with deep bedding and frequent rolling may enable them to survive the paralytic phase. Following this, some animals make an uneventful recovery.

The major efforts of preventing EHV-1 infections should be directed toward management and vaccination programs. Management practices should be designed to prevent the spread of EHV-1 and include the avoidance of stress that might lead to recrudescence of latent virus. It is important to prevent the possible introduction of EHV-1 virus from an outside source. The provision of proper isolation facilities for all incoming animals is therefore essential at stud farms and stables. Horses may be isolated for a period of 14 days to allow them to recover from the stress of a long journey. At the same time, animals should be checked for clinical signs of disease. The segregation of animals into small self-contained groups provides an effective barrier to the spread of infectious disease. Should an abortion occur on the stud farm, all members of the staff should be aware of a series of precautions that must be undertaken. These include submission of the fetus and placenta to an appropriate laboratory for postmortem examination, immediate isolation of the involved mare, prompt cleaning and disinfection of the stall, and destruction of bedding and other contact materials. When cases of paralysis attributable to EHV-1 occur, no animals should enter or leave the group until three weeks have elapsed from the time of recovery of the last clinical case. If possible, splitting of the in-contact animals into smaller isolated groups soon after the appearance of the initial case will limit the spread of the disease.

In support of the various management practices, there are two vaccines to control the spread of EHV-1 infection, one dead and one live. Vaccines are limited in their efficacy by the short duration of immunity they confer and the fact that both vaccines contain antigen or viral particles prepared from a single subtype 1 genotype.

To overcome the short duration of immunity, a program of repeated vaccinations is advocated. The killed inactivated vaccine* first became available in 1979 and is administered to pregnant mares during the fifth, seventh, and ninth month of each pregnancy. In young animals, two doses should be given at intervals of four to six weeks apart followed by booster vaccination at six-monthly intervals. When a large proportion of the pregnant mare population has received the killed vaccine, there is good evidence to suggest that it has reduced the level of abortion attributable to EHV-1.

The modified live vaccine† is primarily recommended to control the respiratory form of EHV-1 but may be given to pregnant mares. The vaccination schedule requires two doses at intervals of four to eight weeks followed by booster vaccination at intervals of six months. Field and experimental evidence indicates that neither vaccine is effective in preventing clinical respiratory disease caused by EHV-1. However, animals that have been on a regular vaccination program show reduced severity of clinical signs compared with nonvaccinated animals and excrete virus from the respiratory tract for a shorter period. Greater vaccine efficacy may result from the incorporation of more suitably immunogenic strains as well as ensuring that they are closely related to current strains circulating within the equine population. However, it must be remembered that complacency leading to overcrowding, increased movement of animals, and inadequate vaccination schedules has led to apparent breakdowns in the vaccination program.

EQUID HERPESVIRUS TYPE 2 (EHV-2)

EHV-2 is an extremely successful parasite; the majority of horses become infected and remain lifelong carriers and constant shedders of the virus. A multiplicity of antigenic types have been isolated from the respiratory and genital tract, conjunctiva, rectum, buffy coat and equine tissues prepared for cell culture. Because of the ubiquitous nature of EHV-2, assigning clinical significance to infection with it has been difficult. Some evidence exists that following experimental infection foals develop a chronic pharyngitis associated with lymphoid hyperplasia but no obvious clinical signs. The prevalence of antibody to EHV-2 is widespread among horse populations throughout the world.

EQUID HERPESVIRUS TYPE 3 (EHV-3)

EHV-3 is a venereal infection causing small pustular vesicles on the vulva of the mare and the penis of the stallion. The vesicles usually ulcerate and scabs develop that persist for two to three weeks.

---

*Pneumabort K, Fort Dodge Laboratories Inc., Fort Dodge, KS

†Rhinomune, Norden Laboratories, Lincoln, NE

The incubation period ranges from two to ten days. EHV-3 does not affect fertility in the stallion or mare; however; if the lesions are severe in the stallion, copulation and ejaculation may be inhibited. Respiratory disease following experimental intranasal infection has been reported and respiratory signs have been observed during natural outbreaks of the disease. Young horses up to three years of age infrequently possess antibody whereas antibody is present in a high proportion of older horses. Stallions with significant levels of neutralizing antibody but showing no clinical signs may act as carriers of EHV-3.

Tissue culture isolation of EHV-3 from lesions of the penis and vulva and the demonstration of a rise in serum neutralization antibody is evidence of infection.

Antibacterial ointment applied to affected areas of the penis and vulva will assist in preventing secondary bacterial infection. Rest from mating activity is essential as continued mating activity delays recovery and enhances transmission of EHV-3 to susceptible mares (see p. 567).

EQUINE INFLUENZA

Equine influenza has been recognized as a cause of epizootic respiratory disease for several centuries. It was only in the 1950s that the causal agent, an influenza type A virus, a member of the family Orthomyxoviridae, was isolated. Two antigenic subtypes are recognized: equine 1 (H_7N_7), first isolated from horses in Prague, Czechoslovakia in 1956, and equine 2 (H_3N_8), isolated from horses in Miami, Florida during 1963. The prefixes H and N refer to the surface antigens, hemagglutinin, and neuraminidase, which are subject to antigenic variability. A minor change in the hemagglutinin or neuraminidase is known as antigenic *drift*, whereas a major change as occurred with the appearance of equine 2 in 1963 is known as antigenic *shift*. Such antigenic changes have considerable significance with reference to the efficacy of vaccines. Inactivated vaccines containing equine 1 and 2 antigens have been used in North America and Europe since the 1960s.

Pathogenesis

The clinical signs of influenza in the horse are similar in many respects to the disease in humans. They include a dry hacking cough, pyrexia, nasal discharge, anorexia, muscular soreness, and secondary bacterial infections. Coughing is the most obvious sign. It develops during the first two or three days after onset. The cough is dry and hard and decreases rapidly after the first few days. If the horse is given complete rest the cough should disappear within one to three weeks. Although nasal discharge is initially serous, in the susceptible and young animal it becomes mucopurulent due to bacterial infection frequently caused by streptococcal species. Equine 1 causes a milder disease than equine 2, the latter having more pronounced pneumotropic properties. Within the respiratory tract, infection results in hyperemia, edema, desquamation, and focal erosions causing interruption of the mucous protective blanket and impairment of the clearance mechanism. This increases the likelihood of bacterial invasion and multiplication. In the susceptible animal with equine 2 infection, lower respiratory tract complications may lead to fatal pneumonia. In recent years, however, this has not been reported as horses are less susceptible either because of previous exposure or as a result of vaccination. Fatal pneumonia in foals results in necrosis of the brochiolar epithelium with considerable exudation of protein-rich fluid into the alveolar spaces. There is little cellular infiltration in the absence of bacterial infection. Respiratory sequelae that have been hypothesized to follow influenza infection include chronic obstructive pulmonary disease (COPD) and bronchopneumonia. More generalized problems include interstitial myocarditis and, very rarely, encephalitides.

Diagnosis

Virus can be isolated from nasopharyngeal swabs during the first 48 to 72 hours of illness. The virus is grown by inoculation of material into the amniotic cavity of 10- to 12-day-old chick embryos. The inoculated eggs are incubated for two to four days at 33° to 35° before the amniotic fluid is harvested and checked for the presence of virus by hemagglutination. Equine 2 viruses are recovered after one or two passages in eggs while equine 1 viruses are more difficult to isolate. Virus may also grow in Madin Darby canine kidney cell culture. Recent infection may be confirmed serologically by hemagglutination inhibition (HI), complement-fixation (CF), and radial hemolysis tests using acute and convalescent sera taken 14 to 21 days apart.

Epizootiology

Both equine 1 and 2 are common in horses throughout the world, although the disease has not been reported in South Africa, Australia, and New Zealand. The disease spreads very rapidly, with the short incubation period (one to three days) and the frequent coughing during the acute phase contributing to rapid dissemination of virus. Infected horses have been reported to shed virus for up to eight days. Previously unexposed horses are the most effective disseminators of virus and the ones from which influenza is most likely to be isolated.

The pathogenesis of influenza infection in the individual animal is influenced by the extent of prior exposure contributing to the level of immunity as well as the virulence of the virus, the level of exposure, and environmental conditions. Under experimental conditions it is difficult to reproduce the clinical disease as observed naturally. Because of the increased transport of horses, influenza has become widespread and outbreaks of the disease can occur at any time of the year. Most reported outbreaks occur in young horses when they are moved into large horse populations at training grounds, racetracks, and show grounds. Foci for the persistence of virus within the population have not been elucidated. Disease of epidemic proportions may develop when a few infected animals are introduced into a large group of susceptible horses.

Horses that have developed some immunity to influenza, either following natural exposure or as a result of vaccination, may become infected. These animals may show no signs of disease but are still capable of shedding virus. Clinical observation suggests that following natural infection immunity to both subtypes persists for at least one year.

Both locally produced secretory antibody in the respiratory tract and humoral antibody are important in protecting the horse against influenza infection. Cell-mediated responses are recognized; however, their significance is not understood. IgA antibody is the principal immunoglobulin in the secretions from the upper respiratory tract and the IgA concentration is correlated with resistance to infection. The presence of IgA antibody is transient, lasting only a few months, and IgA concentrations are independent of serum IgG neutralizing antibody levels. Serum neutralizing or HI serum antibody levels above 1/32 appear to give protection against the onset of clinical disease. However, great care must be taken with the interpretation of serologic data because the techniques for carrying out the tests may vary from one laboratory to another. Treatment of the hemagglutinin antigen with ether can improve the sensitivity of the HI test.

Treatment

Rest and confinement are essential for the rapid recovery of horses suffering from influenza. Training should not be resumed until at least a week after clinical signs have ceased and only if there is no coughing after initial exercise. Antimicrobial therapy should be reserved for those horses that develop secondary bacterial infections. Sulfonamide and penicillin are the most effective antibacterial agents. The importance of good stable hygiene with sufficient ventilation and freedom from dust needs to be strongly emphasized. The use of antiviral drugs has yet to find practical application in the treatment of equine influenza.

Prevention

Killed vaccines containing both equine 1 and 2 subtypes are commercially available. Most of the vaccines are complete disrupted virus vaccines combined with an adjuvant and administered by parenteral injection. Adequately vaccinated horses are protected from developing clinical disease attributable to equine influenza. Booster vaccination of already primed horses in the face of an outbreak is of benefit. Although little antigenic drift has occurred with equine 1, there is evidence of drift with equine 2 strains isolated from North America and Europe. As a consequence, most vaccines contain, in addition to the prototype Prague and Miami strains, either the equine 2 Kentucky/81 or Fontainbleau/79 strains. Subunit vaccines containing only the hemagglutinin and neuraminidase antigens have been developed but not extensively tested. These subunit vaccines should produce fewer side effects.

All inactivated vaccines require two primary injections given at intervals of 2 to 12 weeks. The vaccines may be administered to horses of any age although the response in foals under six months of age is poor due to the interference caused by maternal antibody. When the second primary vaccination is given after a 12-week interval, a heightened antibody response is obtained. In the young horse up to three years of age, it is preferable that booster vaccination is given at intervals of six months, thereafter annual boosters appear satisfactory. Following vaccination, horses should be put on the "easy list" for several days to minimize the possible adverse side effects. These may be manifested as a localized swelling at the site of injection or very infrequently as a generalized depression. Because the currently available killed vaccines provide immunity of a short duration and require regular boosters, there is an interest in the development of attenuated live vaccines. Studies have been undertaken with temperature-sensitive (ts) mutants of influenza virus that multiply only in the upper respiratory tract. They stimulate a local and humoral antibody response that may reduce the need for frequent revaccination.

EQUINE RHINOVIRUS

Equine rhinoviruses are members of the virus family picornaviridae, a number of which have been isolated from respiratory tract of the horse. They include equine rhinovirus type 1 (ERV-1), equine rhinovirus type 2 (ERV-2), equine rhinovirus type 3 (ERV-3), and an acid-stable picornavirus.

Rhinoviruses replicate in the upper respiratory tract and cause pyrexia, catarrh, and enlargement of the associated lymph glands, although signs may not always be observed. The incubation period is short, a matter of days, and viremia of five days' duration has been reported. ERV-1 has also been isolated from the alimentary tract. Clinical signs of ERV-1 infection range from severe pharyngitis with associated serous or mucopurulent discharge and pyrexia to transient fever with no other signs. A similar pathogenesis seems to exist for the other viruses in this group. Both ERV-2 and the acid-stable picornavirus have been isolated from apparently healthy horses.

Serum-neutralizing antibody to the equine rhinoviruses is readily detected as early as six days after infection, rising to a peak at 14 days and persisting for several years. Virus may be isolated in rabbit kidney and equine cell lines. However, attempts to isolate virus and to demonstrate a rise in antibody between acute and convalescent sera rarely are successful, as the antibody response may occur in advance of the onset of clinical signs.

Rhinoviruses may persist in the respiratory tract of individual horses indefinitely, suggesting that some horses are carriers of the virus and act as a source of infection to other susceptible horses. Young horses are especially susceptible when they congregate at sales and racetracks. Serologic studies have indicated that rhinoviruses are widely distributed among the equine population throughout the world. At present there are no vaccines available to control infection caused by equine rhinoviruses.

Supplemental Readings

Adenovirus

McGuire, T. C.; Poppie, M. J., and Banks, K. L.: Combined (B and T lymphocyte) immunodeficiency: A fatal genetic disease in Arab foals. J. Am. Vet. Med. Assoc., *164*:70, 1974.

African Horse Sickness

Erasmus, B. J.: The pathogenesis of African Horse Sickness. Proc. 3rd Int. Conf. Eq. Inf. Dis., 1972, pp. 1–11.

Equine Viral Arteritis

Mumford, J. A.: Preparing for equine arteritis. Equine Vet. J., *17*:6, 1985.

Equine Herpesvirus

Allen, G. P., and Bryans, J. T.: Molecular epizootiology, pathogenesis, and prophylaxis of Equine Herpesvirus-1 Infection. *In* Pandey, R. (ed.): Progress in Veterinary Microbiology and Immunology. Basel, S. Karger, 1985.

Campbell, T. M., and Studdert, M. G.: Equine Herpesvirus Type 1 (EHV-1). Vet. Bull., *53*:135, 1983.

Influenza

Gerber, H.: Clinical features, sequelae and epidemiology of equine influenza. Proc. 2nd Int. Conf. Eq. Inf. Dis., 1969, pp. 63–80.

Hinshaw, V. S., Naeve, C. W., Webster, R. G., Douglas, A., Skehel, J. J., and Bryans, J.: Analysis of antigenic variation in equine 2 influenza A virus. Bull. Wld. Hlth. Org., *61*:153, 1983.

Rhinovirus

Holmes, D. J., Kemem, M. J., and Coggins, L.: Equine rhinovirus infection—Serologic evidence of infection in selected United States horse populations. Proc. 4th Int. Conf. Eq. Inf. Dis., 1978, pp. 315–319.

Strangles

Ioana M. Sonea, EAST LANSING, MICHIGAN

Strangles is caused by *Streptococcus equi*, a gram-positive beta-hemolytic streptococcus that is an obligate parasite of Equidae. *S. equi* cell wall contains a species-specific M protein that is the antigen against which protective antibodies are formed. The M protein is antiphagocytic and may cause adhesions of the organism to epithelial cells, enhancing colonization and multiplication. *S. equi* frequently possesses a capsule that also is antiphagocytic: strains without a capsule are less virulent. Like other streptococci, *S. equi* is nearly always penicillin-sensitive.

PATHOGENESIS

S. equi initially invades the nasopharyngeal and oral mucosa, causing an acute pharyngitis and rhinitis. The organism then spreads to the regional lymph nodes. The retropharyngeal and submandibular lymph nodes are most commonly affected. These lymph nodes usually develop abscesses that rupture and drain, either to the exterior or into the pharynx or guttural pouches. In most cases, the infection remains localized and healing is uneventful once drainage of the abscesses has occurred.

After rupture and drainage of abscesses, *S. equi* is shed in the discharge for up to four weeks, contaminating pasture, equipment, and housing. It can remain viable in the environment for a month or more. Some apparently recovered horses may continue to shed *S. equi* intermittently for eight months or longer. In burros the disease does not follow the same course: *S. equi* produces a chronic caseous lymphadenitis with few clinical signs other than debility and weight loss.

In some cases the infection spreads to other lymph nodes ("bastard strangles"). Abscessation and rupture may occur with graver consequences, depending on the location of the affected lymph nodes. Furthermore, certain horses become sensitized to the streptococcal antigens and can develop purpura hemorrhagica, an immune-mediated vasculitis precipitated by persistence of streptococcal antigen in the face of high levels of circulating antibodies.

CLINICAL SIGNS

Anorexia, pyrexia (103 to 105° F, 39.5 to 40.5° C), and a serous nasal discharge that rapidly becomes mucopurulent appear after an incubation period of three to six days. In a previously unexposed population, morbidity may reach 100 per cent. Affected horses often hold the neck and head outstretched and have difficulty swallowing, presumably due to the severe pharyngitis. Dysphagia may be severe enough to mimic esophageal choke. A soft cough is often present and the larynx is painful on palpation.

The fever may subside but often returns when the submandibular lymph nodes begin to swell about two to three days after the initial fever. The lymph nodes are hot and painful and will usually rupture, draining thick creamy pus about 10 to 14 days after the onset of clinical signs. The nasal discharge at this time is abundant and purulent. The horse may be dyspneic or dysphagic, and is usually depressed and anorectic. Once the lymph nodes have started draining, recovery is generally uneventful.

Complications associated with strangles include guttural pouch empyema, aspiration pneumonia due to intratracheal drainage of abscessed lymph nodes, respiratory distress due to tracheal compression by abscesses, and pleuritis. Intra-abdominal abscessation can cause intermittent colic or chronic weight loss as a result of peritonitis and functional gastrointestinal disturbances. Myocarditis occurs with some frequency. Rarely, abscessation in other areas of the body causes meningitis, hepatic abscesses, or septic tendinitis. Mortality due to complications varies between 2 and 10 per cent.

Purpura hemorrhagica is uncommon (see p. 312), generally occurring two to three weeks after the appearance of respiratory signs. Affected horses are depressed, reluctant to move, and anorectic. Head and limb edema is common, as are urticarial plaques over the body. Edema may be severe enough to cause oozing of serum through the skin. Petechial hemorrhages may be seen on mucosal surfaces. Rectal temperature may be normal or elevated. Recovery generally occurs in four to seven days; fatalities are usually due to renal or hepatic failure or severe myositis.

Burros do not present with acute respiratory disease: chronic weight loss and debilitation are typical of *S. equi* infection in this species.

DIAGNOSIS

Clinical signs of fever, purulent nasal discharge, and enlarged or abscessed lymph nodes in the pharyngeal region are generally sufficient for a presumptive diagnosis of strangles. Bacteriologic culture of purulent material yielding *S. equi* confirms the diagnosis. Sometimes more than one culture is necessary. Endoscopic examination is useful in the detection of pharyngitis and guttural pouch empyema. Rectal examination, abdominocentesis, thoracocentesis, and thoracic radiography may be needed to diagnose bastard strangles.

In the early stages of the disease, strangles may be mistaken for any of the viral respiratory diseases. However, once enlargement and abscessation of lymph nodes nodes occur, these conditions are easily differentiated. *S. zooepidemicus* and *S. equisimilis* may also cause a respiratory disease with a purulent nasal discharge and occasionally abscessation of lymph nodes. Without bacteriologic culture, disease caused by other streptococcal organisms may be indistinguishable from strangles.

TREATMENT

Most cases of strangles are benign, and older horses with few systemic signs may not need any treatment other than nursing care. Although antibiotic therapy is somewhat controversial, current clinical evidence suggests that adequate antibiotic therapy before maturation of abscesses does not lead to a higher incidence of bastard strangles as was previously believed. Antibiotic therapy is indicated in severe cases. Penicillin remains the antibiotic of choice. If strangles is detected early and the case appears uncomplicated, procaine penicillin G at 22,000 IU per kg should be given twice daily intramuscularly until at least 5 to 10 days after the disappearance of signs or rupture of abscesses or both. If bastard strangles is suspected, more aggressive and prolonged treatment is recommended. Sodium penicillin (30,000 to 50,000 IU per kg four times a day intramuscularly or intravenously) may be given initially, followed by procaine penicillin G (22,000 to 45,000 IU per kg twice a day intramuscularly for two to six months). There is no advantage in using isoniazid. Although the drug penetrates abscesses effectively, it has no activity against *S. equi* or *S. zooepidemicus*.

Intravenous fluids and feeding through a nasogastric tube may be needed if dysphagia or anorexia is severe. Anti-inflammatory drugs (phenylbutazone, flunixin meglumine) can be given to reduce swelling and pain associated with pharyngitis and abscesses, or in cases with colic. A tracheostomy may be necessary if massive retropharyngeal or cervical abscessation produce severe respiratory distress.

Lancing and draining of mature abscesses is recommended. Guttural pouch empyema is best treated by frequent flushing of the pouch with large volumes of saline (see p. 614).

Purpura hemorrhagica should be treated with high doses of antibiotics to eliminate the persistent streptococcal antigens. Systemic corticosteroids (20 to 50 mg dexamethasone per 450 kg or 1 to 2 mg per kg prednisone or prednisolone daily) may be indicated. Furosemide, hand walking, and bandaging may be necessary to control edema.

PREVENTION

Strangles is difficult to prevent because of the presence of asymptomatic carriers and the prolonged persistence of the organism in the environment. On a farm, one month's quarantine of new arrivals will permit detection of most affected horses. However, this may be impractical in sale barns, racetracks, and brood mare farms where outbreaks are common.

Vaccination is of questionable value. S. equi is not strongly antigenic and protection following either natural infection or vaccination lasts only 6 to 12 months. Vaccination will reduce the incidence of strangles by about 50 per cent on farms where strangles is a constant problem and therefore may be recommended in some circumstances. Common vaccination-related complications include localized swelling, abscessation, and scarring at injection sites. Severe systemic reactions or purpura hemorrhagica may occur in previously vaccinated horses or those with previous exposure to the disease. Two types of vaccines exist: a bacterin* and an M protein fraction extract.† Both confer comparable immunity and have similar complications. The manufacturer's recommendation should be followed.

*Equibac II, Fort Dodge Laboratories Inc., Fort Dodge, IA
†Strepvax, Coopers Animal Health Inc., Kansas City, MO

Supplemental Readings

Hietala, S., and Knight, H. D.: Ineffectiveness of isoniazid against three equine pathogens. J. Am. Vet. Med. Assoc., 179:806, 1981.
Piche, C. A.: Clinical observations on an outbreak of strangles. Can. Vet. J., 25:7, 1984.
Reif, J. S., George, J. L., and Shideler, R. K.: Recent developments in strangles research: Observation on the carrier state and evaluation of a new vaccine. Proc. 27th Annu. Conv. Am. Assoc. Eq. Pract., 1981, pp. 33–40.
Rumbaugh, G. E., Smith, B. P. and Carlson, G. P.: Internal abdominal abscesses in the horse: A study of 25 cases. J. Am. Vet. Med. Assoc., 172:304, 1978.
Srivastava, S. K., and Barnum, D. A.: The serological response of foals to vaccination against strangles. Can. J. Comp. Med., 45:20, 1981.

Pleuropneumonia

Corinne Raphel Sweeney, KENNETT SQUARE, PENNSYLVANIA

Pleuritis and pleural effusion occur in association with a number of disease conditions, but most commonly with pneumonia or lung abscessation. In these instances the proper term for the condition is pleuropneumonia.

Pleuropneumonia often follows a stressful event such as transportation over an extended distance (travel time longer than two hours), recumbency under general anesthesia, recent illness from acute viral disease, or a combination of these. Although any age and type of horse may be affected with pleuropneumonia, it most commonly occurs in Thoroughbred and Standardbred racehorses. Aspiration of pharyngeal contents may play a significant role in the etiology of pleuropneumonia as suggested by the identification of anaerobes in the lungs of many of these horses. Racehorses may inhale dirt and sand from the racetrack. Transportation usually requires cross-tying of the head, preventing the horse from lowering its head in a more favorable position for mucus clearance. Inhalation of blood and bacteria from the upper respiratory tract during surgery and endotracheal intubation could also establish infection. This premise seems valid especially when one considers that general anesthesia by inhalants is known to depress normal respiratory tract clearance mechanisms. In addition, the use of anti-inflammatory agents such as phenylbutazone may suppress the clinical signs and allow the disease to progress before treatment is begun.

CLINICAL SIGNS

Clinical signs of pleuropneumonia include fever, anorexia, depression, cough, respiratory distress, tying up, lameness, weight loss, exercise intolerance, sternal or limb edema, and colic. In the acute stage of pleuritis, pain in the thorax may be elicited by applying pressure over the ribs or in the intercostal space. Pain is demonstrated by grunts, intercostal muscle spasms, or even escape maneuvers by the patient. Horses may abduct their elbows and a "catch" to inspiration may be visible. As more fluid accumulates in the pleural space, pain is less evident.

When horses with pleuropneumonia are forced to breathe deeply by either nostril occlusion or use of a rebreathing bag such as a large plastic garbage bag, no sounds or only bronchial or tracheal sounds are heard ventrally, while normal to harsh airway sounds are heard dorsally. Although pleural friction rubs heard during auscultation confirm the presence of pleuritis, they are too inconsistent to be a diagnostic criterion. Friction rubs are heard predominantly at the end of inspiration and the early part of expiration usually in the subacute stage of the disease when there is considerable inflammation of the pleura. Pleural friction rubs disappear as inflammation decreases or as pleural fluid accumulates. The cardiac sounds are often heard over a wider area of the chest than normal, probably as a result of enhanced conduction of sound through the fluid in the pleural space.

Thoracic percussion frequently confirms the impression gained from auscultation. The techniques for percussion and the landmarks for the caudal border of the lung field are described on p. 580. Pleural effusion causes a dullness of the ventral aspects of the lung field and is often delineated by a horizontal line. In chronic cases of pleuritis, percussion may reveal patchy areas of dullness caused by localized inflammation and adhesions between parietal and visceral pleura.

DIAGNOSTIC PROCEDURES

THORACOCENTESIS

If pleural effusion is suspected, thoracocentesis should be considered. In the acute stages of pleuropneumonia with small volumes of pleural effusion, thoracocentesis is not necessary if the horse is improving or is not showing signs of respiratory distress. Moderate amounts of pleural effusion may be resorbed quite readily. Although some clinicians believe that thoracocentesis is imperative to provide a specimen for bacterial culture, I think that culture of a tracheobronchial aspirate may be adequate. However, if fluid accumulates rapidly, if the horse is in respiratory distress, or if its condition deteriorates, thoracocentesis should be performed. Although the procedure is quick, easy, inexpensive, and considered safe, rare complications such as death due to cardiac puncture may occur. The preferred site is the sixth or seventh intercostal space just dorsal to the palpable costochondral junction. Choosing a site farther caudal may provide a sample but does not allow adequate drainage of the chest. When attempting to aspirate pleural fluid from a horse with a minimal amount of effusion, one should choose a space no farther back than the sixth or seventh intercostal space. The technique for thoracocentesis is described on p. 580. If the procedure has caused some trauma, the first fluid obtained may be blood-tinged, but this clears as more fluid is withdrawn. If the pleural fluid is blood-tinged because of the underlying disease process, the red coloration persists throughout the entire procedure. An aliquot of pleural fluid is transferred from the syringe into tubes containing anticoagulant solution (EDTA) so that appropriate laboratory evaluation may be performed. Part of the fluid should be saved in sterile containers with transport media for subsequent Gram stain and culture. Fluid should be removed as long as it flows freely. Both sides of the thorax should be tapped.

EXAMINATION OF PLEURAL FLUID

The color, turbidity, viscosity, and odor should be noted. Normal pleural fluid is clear and yellow; cloudiness reflects an increased number of white blood cells. Putrid-smelling pleural fluid is a hallmark of anaerobic infection; however, the absence of odor does not exclude anaerobic infection. In addition to the odor of the pleural fluid, the odor of the horse's breath should be noted, particularly after coughing. The majority of horses with anaerobic infections have a putrid odor associated with the pleural fluid or breath. These horses have a low survival rate.

The quantity of aspirated pleural fluid should be recorded to compare with subsequent thoracic drainage. While volumes may vary from 1 ml to 60 liters, the volume of fluid removed is not a prognostic indicator.

The white blood cell count of normal pleural fluid is generally less than 10,000 per μl. White blood cell count of pleural fluid in pleuropneumonia can range from 1,600 to 300,000 cells per μl, varying in the same pleural fluid sample between the beginning and the end of the thoracocentesis. There is no association between the white blood cell count in pleural fluid and survival. Pleural fluid protein is greater than 3 gm per dl in horses with pleuropneumonia, but this is also not a prognostic indicator.

Pleural fluid should be Gram-stained and cultured for bacteria. The Gram stain may provide tentative identification of the organism until the culture results are obtained. Both aerobic and anaerobic cultures should be performed. Anaerobes occur in 46 per cent of horses with pleuropneumonia. The pleural fluid used for anaerobic cultures should be transferred to the laboratory immediately after collection in a manner that prevents or minimizes exposure to air. Anaerobic transport medium* is commercially available and should be routinely used. Specimens submitted for isolation of anaerobes should not be refrigerated as many anaerobes are cold-intolerant. The most common aerobic isolates in equine pleuropneumonia are beta-hemolytic Streptococcus spp., Pasteurella spp., and *E. coli*. The most common anaerobes isolated are Bacteroides spp. (including *B. oralis*, *B. melaninogenicus*, and *B. fragilis*) and Clostridium spp. (including *C. beijerinchium* and *C. butyriciam*). Isolation of anaerobic bacteria from either the pleural fluid or tracheobronchial aspirate provides a poor prognosis. In one study 33 per cent of horses from which anaerobes were isolated survived, compared with a 67 per cent survival rate among those from which no anaerobes were isolated.

HEMATOLOGY

Hematologic findings in horses with pleuropneumonia are usually nonspecific and do not predict the outcome of the case. A low hematocrit (less than 30 per cent) usually reflects an anemia of chronic disease, while elevated total plasma proteins (greater than 8.0 per cent) is probably due to hypergammaglobulinemia. Both these findings suggest that the pleuropneumonia is chronic. White blood cell counts can be misleading, as not all affected horses have leukocytosis. Plasma fibrinogen appears to be a sensitive indicator of inflammation because it is elevated in almost all cases of pleuropneumonia.

TRACHEOBRONCHIAL ASPIRATE

A tracheobronchial aspirate (TBA) provides an excellent specimen for Gram stain and bacterial culture. The technique is described on p. 580.

OTHER DIAGNOSTIC TECHNIQUES

Thoracic radiography is often limited by the availability of facilities. However, lateral thoracic radiographs can often show small amounts of pleural effusion not detectable by either auscultation or percussion. Diagnostic ultrasonography can demonstrate small amounts of pleural fluid not easily detected by auscultation, percussion, or radiographs. However, volumes this small usually do not

need to be drained. Ultrasound can also detect pulmonary abscesses that are contiguous with the lung surface and pulmonary consolidation and atelectasis. Pleuroscopy, a procedure in which a flexible or rigid endoscope is introduced into the pleural space, is rarely indicated in bacterial pleuropneumonia. This technique is better reserved for equine patients with pleural effusion of undiagnosed etiology.

THERAPY

ANTIMICROBIAL THERAPY

The most important treatment of bacterial pleuropneumonia is the use of systemic antimicrobial agents. Ideally an etiologic agent is identified from either the tracheobronchial aspirate or the pleural fluid and antimicrobial sensitivity determined. Without bacterial culture results, broad-spectrum antibiotics should be used because many horses have mixed infections of both gram-positive and gram-negative organisms. Commonly used therapy is penicillin (procaine penicillin G,* 22,000 IU per kg intramuscularly, twice a day, or sodium penicillin G,† 20,000 to 40,000 IU per kg four times a day) combined with an aminoglycoside such as gentamicin,‡ (2.2 mg per kg intravenously or intramuscularly four times a day), trimethoprim and sulfamethoxazole§ (30 mg per kg orally, twice a day), or chloramphenicol‖ (20 to 50 mg per kg orally, four times a day). Because of the need for long-term therapy, initial intravenous or intramuscular therapy may need to be followed by oral antimicrobials. Preferably the oral antimicrobials are not administered until the horse's condition is stable and improving, because blood levels obtained by this route are not as high as those achieved following intramuscular or intravenous administration.

Treatment of anaerobic pleuropneumonia is usually empirical since antimicrobial susceptibility testing of anaerobes is difficult because of their fastidious nutritive and atmospheric requirements. Thus, familiarity with antimicrobial susceptibility patterns is helpful in formulating the treatment regimen in cases in which an anaerobe is suspected. The majority of anaerobic isolates are sensitive to relatively low concentrations of penicillin. *Bacteroides fragilis* is the only frequently encountered anaerobe that is routinely resistant to penicillin, although other members of the Bacteroides family are known to produce beta-lactamases and are potentially peni-

---

*Port-A-Cul, BBL Microbiology Systems, Becton-Dickinson, Rutherford, NJ

*Pfizer Inc., New York, NY
†Squibb, Princeton, NJ
‡Gentocin, Schering Corp., Kenilworth, NJ
§Tribrissen, Burroughs Wellcome Co., Research Triangle Park, NC
‖Anacetin, Bio-Ceutic Laboratories, St. Joseph, MO

cillin-resistant. Chloramphenicol is effective against most aerobes and anaerobes causing equine pleuropneumonia. However, because of human health concerns, the availability of chloramphenicol may decrease.

Metronidazole* has in vitro activity against a variety of obligate anaerobes including *Bacteroides fragilis*. Pharmacokinetic studies indicate a dose of 15.0 mg/kg intravenously or orally four times a day is necessary to maintain adequate serum levels Oral administration rapidly results in adequate serum levels and thus is an acceptable route of administration for horses with pleuropneumonia. However, there have been no reports of complications associated with either its oral or intravenous use in more than 30 horses. Metronidazole is not effective against aerobes and therefore should always be used in combination therapy.

Recent studies at the University of California have shown that trimethoprim-sulfa combinations are effective against most anaerobes isolated from horses with pleuropneumonia.

The aminoglycosides are ineffective in the treatment of anaerobic pleuropneumonia because the amount of the aminoglycosides needed to inhibit the growth of the anaerobic bacteria far exceeds the levels that are safely achieved in blood and tissue. Thus, aminoglycosides should not be considered for the treatment of pleuropneumonia caused by an anaerobe unless it is used in combination therapy—that is, with penicillin.

The use of intratracheal or intrapleural antimicrobials has not been critically evaluated in the horse. If they are used, they should *always* be combined with systemic administration of the same agent.

PLEURAL DRAINAGE

Following selection of an appropriate antimicrobial agent, the next decision to be made is whether to drain the pleural space. Ideally the decision is based on an examination of the pleural fluid. If the pleural fluid is thick pus, drainage using a chest tube should be initiated without delay. If the pleural fluid is not thick pus but the Gram stain is positive and white blood cell counts are elevated, pleural drainage is recommended. Another indication for therapeutic thoracocentesis is relief of respiratory distress secondary to a pleural effusion.

Drainage of a pleural effusion can be accomplished by thoracocentesis, by using a cannula, by indwelling chest tubes, or by thoracostomy. The latter is reserved for severe abscessation of the pleural space. Thoracocentesis (see p. 580) is easily accomplished in the field and may not need to be repeated unless considerable pleural effusion reac-

cumulates. I have not encountered any problem from thoracocentesis performed every 48 hours. Indwelling chest tubes are indicated when continued pleural fluid accumulation makes intermittent thoracocentesis impractical. If properly placed and managed they provide a method for frequent fluid removal and do not exacerbate the underlying pleuropneumonia or increase the production of pleural effusion. Human chest tubes are commercially available but often are not suitable for extensive subcutaneous tunneling in the horse. Brunswick or Levin feeding tubes and intravenous extension tubing (with end connectors removed) can be passed through an appropriately sized trocar into the pleural space as described for thoracocentesis. The cannula is then removed leaving the tube in the pleural space. If the tubing has its own stylet, a trocar is not necessary. Subcutaneous tunneling of the tubing provides a valve to minimize leakage of air into the chest and also secures the tube. A one-way flutter valve* may be attached to allow continuous drainage without leakage of air into the thorax. The chest entry site and end of the drainage tube must be maintained aseptic. If a chest tube is placed aseptically and managed correctly it can be maintained for several weeks. It should be removed as soon as it is no longer functional. Heparinization of tubing after drainage helps maintain patency. Local cellulitis may occur at the site of entry into the chest but is a minor complication. Bilateral pleural fluid accumulation requires bilateral drainage in most horses.

Open drainage or thoracostomy may be considered when tube drainage is inadequate. It is important not to begin open drainage too early in the disease. An incision is made in the intercostal space exposing the pleural cavity and causing a pneumothorax unless the visceral and parietal pleura adjacent to the drainage site have been fused by the inflammatory process. The wound is kept open for several weeks while the pleural space is flushed and treated as an open draining abscess.

OTHER THERAPY

Anti-inflammatory agents help reduce pain and may decrease the production of pleural fluid. This in turn may encourage the horse to eat and maintain body weight. Phenylbutazone (1 to 2 gm twice a day) or flunixin meglumine† (500 mg once daily) are commonly used for this purpose. I believe that corticosteroids are *contraindicated* in bacterial pleuropneumonia. Intrapleural instillation of 250,000 IU streptokinase diluted in 100 ml of normal saline is sometimes used to treat humans with pleuritis, but the value of intrapleural enzymes in

---

*Metronidazole Redi-infusion, Elkins-Sinn, Inc., Cherry Hill, NJ, or Metronidazole, Par Pharm, Inc., Upper Saddle River, NJ

*Heimlick, Bard-Parker, Rutherford, NJ
†Banamine, Schering Corp., Kenilworth, NJ

the treatment of equine pleuropneumonia has not been documented. Rest and the provision of an adequate diet are important components of the treatment of pleuropneumonia. Because the disease course and period of treatment are usually prolonged, attempts should be made to encourage eating.

PROGNOSIS

A guarded prognosis must always be given in cases of equine pleuropneumonia. Earlier studies reported that approximately 40 to 45 per cent of horses recover from pleuropneumonia and 50 per cent of the recovered group return to normal function. Others are well enough to use as breeding or pleasure horses. With the improved ability to treat the disease, survival rates are increasing to approximately 75 per cent.

Supplemental Reading

Arthur, R. M.: Subacute and acute pleuritis. Proc. 29th Annu. Conv. Am. Assoc. Equine Pract., 1983, pp. 65–69.
Mansmann, R. A.: The stages of equine pleuropneumonia. Chronic pneumonia. Proc. 29th Annu. Conv. Am. Assoc. Eq. Pract., 1983, pp. 61–63, 71–73.
Raphel, C. F., and Beech, J.: Pleuritis secondary to pneumonia and/or lung abscessation in 90 horses. J. Am. Vet. Med. Assoc., 181:808, 1982.
Raphel, C. F., and Beech, J.: Pleuritis and pleural effusions in the horse. Proc. 27th Annu. Conv. Am. Assoc. Eq. Pract., 1981, pp. 17–25.
Smith, B. P.: Disease of the pleura, Vet. Clin. North Am., (Large Anim. Pract.), 1:197, 1979.

Chronic Obstructive Pulmonary Disease

Frederik J. Derksen, EAST LANSING, MICHIGAN

The practitioner commonly encounters horses with a history of exercise intolerance and clinical signs of mild pulmonary disease, including abnormal secretions in the trachea and to the astute clinician, increased lung sounds. The condition of these animals is different from that in horses with complete exercise intolerance, chronic mucopurulent nasal discharge, hypoxemia, cyanosis, chronic cough, and inspiratory and expiratory dyspnea. The latter horses are often referred to as "heavy," or suffering from heaves. Between these two extremes a wide spectrum of clinical signs are recognized. This chapter will discuss the disease syndrome exemplified by these two conditions.

Attempts to categorize the variety of clinical manifestations of this disease syndrome into pathophysiologic entities have met with failure and have resulted in a confused nomenclature. Names such as chronic bronchitis, chronic bronchiolitis, chronic asthmoid bronchitis, allergic bronchitis, alveolar emphysema, and emphysema are pathologic diagnoses that the clinician, at the present state of the art, cannot establish with certainty. In any event, it may be that these pathologic changes are closely related and represent different stages of the same disease process. This does not imply that chronic obstructive pulmonary disease (COPD) has only one pathogenesis. It is more likely that a variety of causes lead to common pathologic and functional alterations. Presently it appears that subdivision of COPD on clinical grounds is unwarranted.

Chronic obstructive pulmonary disease is in large part a disease of domestication. The condition is uncommon in warm countries, where horses are kept on grass and spend most of their time in the fresh air. In temperate climates where most horses are kept in barns and fed hay for long periods, the disease is common. Mild forms of the disease are most evident in performance horses and occur in mature animals of all ages. The more severe forms with respiratory distress at rest are uncommon in horses under five years of age. Horses of all breeds and both sexes are affected.

HISTORY AND CLINICAL SIGNS

Mildly affected horses may show no signs at rest or during light exercise, but are unable to perform to capacity. Some horses cough when exposed to dust or cold air. They may work well in warm weather but perform poorly in winter months. Animals may have suffered from viral respiratory tract infection and never completely recovered. The more severely affected animal usually presents with a history of progressive deterioration from mild exercise intolerance to respiratory distress and coughing. Persistent bouts of coughing may be elicited when horses are exposed to dust or cold air. Often owners indicate that animals improve on pasture but exacerbations occur after indoor housing or work. In a few instances horses are presented with severe respiratory distress of acute onset. Careful questioning as to changes in management often reveals recent exposure to "new" antigenic material such as dust from chickens or molds. Animals may show an increased abdominal effort at end expiration or during the entire expiratory phase, a line of hypertrophy of the abdominal muscles often developing along the ventrocaudal edge of the rib cage (heave line). Nasal discharge may be slight and serous in nature or copious and mucopurulent. In the later stages, inspiratory respiratory distress with flaring of the nostrils may also be observed. The disease may result in anorexia, weight loss, depression, and inability to perform even the smallest task.

PATHOLOGY AND PATHOGENESIS

The primary pathologic lesion present in horses with clinical signs of COPD is bronchiolitis. In addition, mucous plugging of bronchioles, peribronchiolar fibrosis, bronchitis with diffuse epithelial hyperplasia and metaplasia, acinar overinflation (also called alveolar emphysema), emphysema with destruction of the alveolar walls, and right ventricular hypertrophy may also be present.

Although several hypotheses concerning the pathogenesis of COPD in the horse have been advanced, insufficient scientific data exist to confirm or refute their validity. It is likely that the syndrome describes several disease entities and therefore more than one mechanism may be involved in the generation of COPD. Possible etiologic factors include specific and nonspecific airway hypersensitivities, viral and bacterial infections, and diet.

Common management practices expose the respiratory system of the horse to large loads of organic and inorganic pollutants ranging from straw, hay, and racetrack dust to molds, ammonia, and ozone and sulfur dioxide from air pollution. Because a close correlation exists between exposure to organic dust and incidence of COPD, it has been postulated that animals have an inappropriate immune response to one or more antigens in the environment resulting in a specific hypersensitivity. Little is known about the immunopathology of this phenomenon, but studies in which horses with COPD were challenged with organic dust and antigens of *Micropolyspora faeni* and *Aspergillus fumigatus* support this hypothesis.

In experimental animals and humans, viral infections or chronic exposure to air pollutants may render airways hypersensitive to otherwise innocuous stimuli, such as cold or mechanical stimulation by rapid air flows. The hypersensitivity is nonspecific in that many different stimulants are effective in triggering bronchoconstriction. Clinical observations of exacerbation of signs of respiratory distress after exposure of some horses to dust, cold air, or exercise suggest that this mechanism may also be important in the pathogenesis of COPD in horses.

Many authors report that COPD commonly follows viral and bacterial respiratory tract infections. A similar correlation exists between infectious respiratory diseases and asthma in man. The significance of this correlation and the mechanisms whereby airway infections lead to COPD are presently unknown.

Dietary factors have been incriminated in the pathogenesis of COPD for centuries. Oral administration of 3-methylindole causes chronic bronchitis and obstructive pulmonary disease in the horse. 3-Methylindole is a metabolite of the amino acid L-tryptophan, and is present in the feces of domestic mammals. However, oral administration of the amino acid L-tryptophan results in hemolytic anemia, without pulmonary disease. Therefore, the role of 3-methylindole in the pathogenesis of COPD in horses is unknown as of this writing.

DIAGNOSIS

Auscultation and Percussion. Auscultation findings vary with the extent of lung disease. Horses with mild disease may be normal on auscultation. However, when the animal is forced to breathe deeply by occlusion of the nostrils for about 30 seconds, by use of a rebreathing bag, or after exercise, breath sounds are more evident than normal. Occasionally a wheeze is heard at the end of exhalation, suggesting airway obstruction. Percussion findings are normal. In more severely affected animals, auscultation may reveal a spectrum of abnormal lung sounds. Sounds associated with large bronchi are best heard at the beginning of exhalation when air flow rates are greatest, and sounds associated with small airways are most evident at the end of expiration, because in that part of the respiratory cycle small airways are narrowed. Percussion may be normal or suggest a caudal extension of the lung field beyond normal limits.

Endoscopy. Endoscopy is a valuable tool in assessment of chronic lung disease, especially in mildly affected horses when diagnosis is a challenge. The upper respiratory system is assessed on the way to the trachea and main stem bronchi. With the 180-cm endoscope now available, the entire trachea up to the carina can be observed in most 500-kg horses. Because of their poor cough reflex, most horses will allow passage of the fiberoptic endoscope without tranquilization. An occasional cough is normal, but when passage of the endoscope into the trachea results in paroxysmal bouts of coughing, a hyperirritable airway should be suspected. In horses suffering from COPD, variable amounts of yellow viscous exudate are present in the trachea, either in the form of tags along the wall or pooled on the floor of the trachea, most commonly near the thoracic inlet. Most if not all horses with COPD have accumulations of yellow viscous material in the trachea; however, the amount does not seem to correlate well with severity of clinical signs.

Transtracheal Wash. Transtracheal washing (p. 580) may be helpful to distinguish horses with COPD from animals with chronic pneumonia or other chronic lung diseases. Cultures of transtracheal washings of horses with COPD usually fail to grow pathogenic bacteria. Cytologic examination characterizes the fluid as a nonseptic neutrophilic exudate. Although a normal cytology excludes bronchitis and bronchiolitis, airway obstruction may still be present owing to functional bronchoconstriction. Transtracheal washings are not helpful in assessing the extent of lung damage in horses with COPD.

Transtracheal wash cytology needs to be interpreted with caution. It correlates poorly with the pulmonary cell population as assessed by either bronchoalveolar lavage or lung biopsy.

Bronchoalveolar Lavage. Bronchoalveolar lavage (p. 580) is a diagnostic tool that in human medicine has allowed classification of some chronic lung diseases into specific etiologic categories. Preliminary evidence suggests that the bronchoalveolar lavage fluid in a subgroup of horses with acute COPD contains large numbers of neutrophils, while in another subgroup the bronchoalveolar lavage fluid is characterized by large numbers of eosinophils. In the future, this information may allow subclassification of COPD and may allow recommendation of more reliable therapeutic regimens.

Radiography. Most practitioners do not have the radiographic equipment necessary to take diagnostic chest radiographs of mature horses. Even with the best equipment presently available, radiographic detail is poor. Variables such as the point in the respiratory cycle at which the film is taken are difficult to control. Generally radiography reveals increased density of the lung field with accentuation of the bronchial pattern. Thoracic radiographs are helpful in detecting focal or miliary lesions in the lung and distinguishing these cases from animals with COPD. Thoracic radiographs have not been helpful in assessing the severity of COPD for therapeutic and prognostic purposes.

Diagnostic Use of Bronchodilators. The clinician may wish to determine the role of airway narrowing caused by bronchospasm in the production of dyspnea. Isoproterenol,* a beta-adrenergic agonist, may be used to achieve airway smooth muscle relaxation. The drug (0.2 mg) is diluted in 50 ml of saline and administered intravenously until the heart rate doubles. Alternatively, atropine,† a parasympatholytic agent, at a dose of 4.0 μg per kg may be administered intravenously. Relief of respiratory distress and reversion of lung sounds toward normal constitute a positive response. This test does not distinguish between reversible and nonreversible lung disease, as has been supposed in the past. For example, in cases with bronchiolitis and mucous plugging of airways, atropine or isoproterenol may have no clinical effect, while the disease may be reversible if treated properly.

Lung Function Tests. Presently lung function tests are utilized in equine medicine on an experimental basis. With one exception, equipment necessary is generally not available to the practicing veterinarian. The simplest and so far perhaps the most sensitive test of lung function is measurement of the arterial blood oxygen tension. Arterial blood is most easily collected from the common carotid artery. Determinations of Pa_{O_2} can be made up to five hours after collection if blood is kept in a sealed glass syringe on ice. At sea level, Pa_{O_2} less than 83 mm Hg is considered abnormal. In normal animals arterial oxygen tension decreases with altitude; therefore, at higher altitudes, a lower Pa_{O_2} may be normal.

THERAPY

ALTERATION OF THE ENVIRONMENT

The most important factor in the development of COPD in the majority of cases appears to be exposure of the respiratory system to organic dust. Established management practices are so ingrained that despite this fact the main thrust of therapy is often directed toward drug administration with inevitably poor results. No therapeutic effort can succeed unless the horse's environment is altered and the exposure to dust or allergens is drastically reduced. This fact needs to be emphasized to owners, who otherwise may not be willing to follow recommendations. Damp, dusty barns with poor ventilation tend to exacerbate clinical signs of COPD, while the environment least likely to stress the respiratory system is a pasture with a modest shelter against inclement weather. If pasture is not available, horses with COPD should be housed in

---

*Isuprel, Winthrop-Breon Laboratories, New York, NY
†Fort Dodge Laboratories, Inc., Fort Dodge, IA

well-ventilated areas, with as little dust as possible. Animals may be bedded on moist wood shavings or clay. Pelleted feed should be substituted for hay and all feed should be moistened.

In mild cases of COPD, when bronchitis and bronchiolitis predominate, rest is an important part of the therapeutic regimen. Exercise to keep the animal in racing shape is not recommended. Although there is no scientific evidence to support this notion in the horse, it is my clinical impression that exercise resulting in high velocity of air flow through diseased airways is responsible for perpetuating airway irritation.

BRONCHODILATOR THERAPY

Since narrowing of airways by excess secretion of mucus, inflammation, or bronchospasm is characteristic of COPD in the horse, bronchodilators are potentially useful therapeutic agents. Bronchodilator drugs act by inducing airway smooth muscle relaxation through a variety of mechanisms (Fig. 1).

Anticholinergic Drugs. Some of the earliest remedies used in the treatment of heaves in horses contained anticholinergic drugs, related to atropine. Atropine is an important parasympatholytic drug that is particularly effective as a muscarinic blocker of neurotransmission by acetylcholine to smooth muscle. Thus, bronchodilation is one of the main effects of systemic administration. In addition, parasympathetic blockade results in decreased secretion by submucosal glands and drying of the respiratory mucosa. The effect of atropine as a pulmonary parasympatholytic drug illustrates two important

and discrete functions of the vagal supply to the lung, namely maintenance of bronchial tone and stimulation of airway secretions.

Atropine at a dose of 4.0 µg per kg body weight will decrease work of breathing and airway secretions in normal horses as well as in horses with COPD. The decreased work of breathing is not clinically evident in normal horses but can be demonstrated with pulmonary function tests. In horses with COPD, especially those in which vagally mediated bronchoconstriction plays a prominent role in the pathogenesis of dyspnea, clinical improvement is evident 20 minutes after treatment and persists for up to 12 hours. Drying of airway secretions may be advantageous in cases in which excessive secretion is observed but undesirable when expectoration is a goal of therapy. Side effects of atropine treatment include mydriasis, tachycardia, central nervous system excitation (especially in ponies), and bowel stasis. Short duration of action and its potentially serious side effects preclude its use as a therapeutic agent in the horse. Potentially, this class of drugs has great value in the treatment of COPD. New anticholinergic agents with more potent bronchodilator effect and fewer side effects are presently being evaluated in bronchodilator therapy in persons.

Sympathomimetic Agents. Sympathomimetic agents, including norepinephrine, isoproterenol, ephedrine,* and clenbuterol,† cause bronchodila-

---

*Ephedrine, Bristol Laboratories, Syracuse, NY
†Ventipulmin, Boehringer Ingelheim, Ridgefield, CT

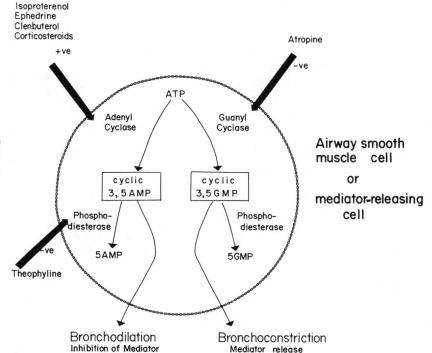

Figure 1. Schematic of the effect of therapeutic agents on airway smooth muscle tone and the release of mediators.

tion by stimulation of beta₂-adrenergic receptors in large and small airways. Airway smooth muscle relaxation is brought about by increased cyclic AMP production in the smooth muscle cell and mast cell. Bronchodilation occurs naturally by this mechanism when animals are stressed and sympathetic nervous system activity increases, but other receptors (alpha, beta₁) are then also stimulated in a variety of organ systems. Sympathomimetic bronchodilators were developed for their specific effect on beta₂-adrenergic receptors present in the bronchi, vascular beds, and uterus, thereby minimizing undesirable side effects on other organs such as the heart and gastrointestinal organs. In addition, a prolonged action is desirable. In some instances prolonged action is achieved by the preparation of slow-release formulations.

Ephedrine is a moderately active beta₂ stimulator; however, its main mechanism of action is through the release of stored norepinephrine. Consequently, it has both alpha and beta adrenergic properties. Therapeutic doses tend to cause depletion of the stored norepinephrine resulting in tolerance, so that progressively more drug is needed to achieve the same degree of bronchodilation. Although few controlled studies as to its efficacy are available, clinically the drug appears effective in some cases. Recommended dosage is 0.14 mg per kg twice a day orally for seven days.

Isoproterenol is a catecholamine with potent beta₂ activity. It has virtually no alpha-adrenergic properties but it has marked beta₁ effects. The drug is one of the most powerful bronchodilators and has a rapid onset of action. However, its bronchodilator effects may last only for an hour. When given intravenously, 0.2 mg of the drug should be diluted in 50 ml of saline, and the heart rate should be monitored continuously. Although the recommended dose is 0.4 μg per kg, infusion should be discontinued when the heart rate doubles. In humans, aerosol is more effective and achieves more selective bronchodilation; however, in horses this route of administration is not practical for long-term therapy because of the need for frequent treatments. Isoproterenol should not be administered orally, as absorption is erratic. Undesirable side effects are mainly due to its beta₁ adrenergic properties and include tachycardia, nervousness, tremors, and sweating. Isoproterenol may be useful in the treatment of acute exacerbations of bronchospasm; however, because of its short duration of action and side effects, it is undesirable for long-term therapy in the horse.

Clenbuterol is a specific beta₂ agonist as well as an expectorant. Its relaxant effects on the airway smooth musculature have been demonstrated in a series of studies in various animal species, including the horse. In the therapeutic dose range the drug has little effect on the smooth muscle of gastroin-testinal system and heart, and therefore side effects are minimal. Clenbuterol is well absorbed after oral administration and has a long duration of action. The drug can be administered orally or intravenously at a dose of 0.8 μg per kg twice a day. In Europe and Canada the drug has been on the market for several years, but in the United States it is not available. Several authors report that clenbuterol is efficacious in treatment of COPD.

Phosphodiesterase Inhibitors. Antiphosphodiesterases, of which the commonest member is theophylline,* act by inhibiting the breakdown of cyclic AMP, thereby promoting smooth muscle relaxation and interfering with the liberation of mediators that cause bronchospasm (Fig. 1). Presently theophylline is not available for use in the horse, but experience in this clinic indicates its effectiveness in most cases of COPD with a history of acute exacerbations when exposed to dust inside a barn. Empirically, the drug is given orally four times a day at a dose of 1.0 mg per kg body weight. Expense and the frequency of administration are the major deterrents. Scientific study as to proper dose levels, absorption, excretion, and efficacy of the drug is needed before usage can be recommended.

EXPECTORANT THERAPY

Expectorant therapy is controversial in the treatment of pulmonary disorders in humans and animals. Although it is commonly used to facilitate movement of respiratory tract secretions, few scientific reports confirm its efficacy. Since mucus plugging of airways is a common finding in horses with COPD, improved mucokinesis is a reasonable objective of therapy. Expectoration can be promoted by systemic administration of expectorants or by nebulization.

NEBULIZATION

The process of nebulization produces a particulate liquid suspension that, depending on particle size, electrical charge, and other characteristics, is deposited at various sites in the respiratory tract. Larger particles are trapped in the upper airway and trachea, while particles smaller than 5 μ may reach the lower respiratory system. Water and saline are the most commonly used solutions and serve to hydrate airway secretions, thereby promoting their removal. Water is more irritating than saline and may evoke coughing. Propylene glycol,† a hygroscopic agent, may be added to the solution in order to promote particle stability and penetration. A 2 per cent solution of propylene glycol is isotonic and nonirritating.

---

*Theo-dur, Key Pharmaceuticals, Miami, FL
†Propylene glycol, Burroughs Wellcome Co., Research Triangle Park, NC

Volatile oils are common ingredients in nebulization solutions. Although the scented fumes may have an esthetic appeal, no evidence for their effectiveness is forthcoming.

Acetylcysteine* is a true mucolytic agent that may be administered via nebulization. The drug ruptures the disulfide bridges of mucoprotein, thereby breaking the complex protein network into less viscous strands. The drug is not available for use in horses and I have had no experience with it.

Mucokinetic Agents. Iodides† are popular mucokinetic agents administered either orally or intravenously. Iodides are thought to act by direct stimulation of bronchial glands to increase secretion, thus liquefying the existing sputum. They may also stimulate secretion via a gastropulmonary reflex mediated through the vagus nerve, and also increase cilioexcitation. Adverse side effects include edema of the face and neck with laryngeal edema severe enough to cause difficult breathing. Iodides appear clinically useful in some cases of COPD and are in common use, although no controlled studies as to their efficacy are available.

Bromhexine‡ is a mucokinetic agent with a mechanism of action similar to the iodides. In Europe the drug has been marketed for several years and clinical studies have shown its efficacy.

Glyceryl guaiacolate,§ in combination with various salts such as ammonium chloride, ammonium carbonate, and potassium citrate, is a commonly used expectorant. The mechanism of action of this combination is mainly through the gastropulmonary mucokinetic reflex, mediated via the vagus nerve, although glyceryl guaiacolate is also thought to increase mucociliary clearance directly. Scientific evidence for its effectiveness in any species is scant. Clinical experience suggests that the compounds are not helpful in the treatment of COPD.

CORTICOSTEROIDS

Corticosteroids have a beneficial effect on most cases of COPD. It is presently thought that steroids stabilize the membranes of lysosomes, thereby preventing the release of their content of hydrolytic enzymes that would destroy the cell and cause an inflammatory response in the tissues. Although good evidence exists that this occurs in laboratory experiments, it is much less certain that this mechanism is of importance in vivo. Steroids may also inhibit cellular migration, potentiate the actions of beta$_2$ receptor stimulants, inhibit the enzyme catechol-O-methyl transferase (which breaks down catecholamines), and increase the availability of the enzyme cyclic AMP. The latter enzyme promotes airway smooth muscle relaxation and inhibits mediator release from lysosomes.

The undesirable side effects of steroid therapy are potentially serious and may develop weeks after initiation of treatment. Therefore, these drugs should be used with caution. Prolonged use of high dosages may lead to Cushing-like signs such as depression, muscle wasting, a long, dry hair coat, hyperglycemia, polydipsia, and polyuria. More commonly the immunologic status is impaired, resulting in the flare-up or establishment of respiratory or other infections. Exogenous steroids depress the release of ACTH from the posterior pituitary, resulting in adrenal cortical atrophy. Clinical signs of adrenal insufficiency may be evident after withdrawal of only two weeks of steroid therapy. Despite possible serious complications, steroid therapy has proven useful in the treatment of horses with COPD. In order to prevent steroid dependence, prednisolone* is administered orally every other day in the morning at a dose of 1 to 2 mg per kg. Endogenous blood steroid levels peak in the morning and decline to reach the lowest level in the early evening. When the drug is given every 48 hours in the morning, sufficient stimulation of the adrenal cortex occurs to prevent steroid dependence. After two weeks of steroid therapy, the response to treatment is evaluated and the dose level gradually reduced until a minimal effective dose is reached. Use of longer-acting steroids such as dexamethasone is not recommended because of the increased risk of adrenal cortical depression. Steroid therapy should not be initiated if concurrent infections are suspected.

ANTIBIOTICS

In animals affected with COPD, clearance of potential pathogens from the lung is likely to be impaired. Therefore, animals may be more susceptible to challenges by environmental pathogens resulting in the common concurrence of COPD and infectious bronchitis, bronchiolitis, and pneumonia.

Culture of transtracheal washings (p. 580) is an important tool in the detection of these cases. In vitro antibiotic sensitivity testing should be performed on isolates to determine the most effective and least expensive antibiotic. Cultures from tracheal washes often produce gram-positive cocci that are sensitive to procaine penicillin G† at a dose of 20,000 IU per kg body weight administered intramuscularly twice a day for at least two weeks. In all cases, adequate dosage and duration of the treatment regimen are important in maximizing therapeutic response and minimizing development of resistance.

---

*Mucomyst, Mead Johnson & Co., Evansville, IN
†Sodium Iodide, Haver-Lockhart, Shawnee, KS
‡Bisolvon, Boehringer Ingelheim, Ridgefield, CT
§Glycom, Bio-Ceutic Laboratories, St. Joseph, MO

---

*The Butler Co., Columbus, OH
†Pfizer, New York, NY

Isoniazid* is an antimicrobial agent, commonly used in the treatment of COPD in horses. Its reported efficacy is surprising because in vitro the agent has only antimycobacterial properties, without any effect on pathogens commonly encountered in the horse. Presently, no in vivo studies supporting the efficacy of isoniazid in the treatment of COPD are available. A commonly used oral dose is 2 mg per kg body weight for 30 to 90 days. However, undesirable side effects including anorexia, ataxia, incoordination, and apparent blindness have been observed at doses as low as 4 mg per kg. In view of its doubtful efficacy and its small safety margin, the use of isoniazid in the treatment of COPD cannot be recommended.

MISCELLANEOUS THERAPY

Antihistamines. Antihistamines† alone or in combination with other drugs have been used extensively in the treatment of COPD. Few scientific studies exist to evaluate the efficacy of antihistamine in the treatment of COPD in the horse, and in my experience these drugs are ineffective. Histamine may be only one of many mediators released in the lung and therefore antihistamines cannot be expected to produce significant improvement. Most antihistamines are used in combination with ephedrine in oral preparations,‡ and the efficacy of this combination may be attributed to the beta$_2$ agonist.

Anthelmintics. Two anthelmintic drugs, levamisol and diethyl carbamazine, have been commonly used in the treatment of COPD in horses. Levamisol§ is a known stimulator of cell-mediated immunity; its effectiveness in treatment of COPD in the horse is attributed to this mechanism. Therefore, when using the drug, the clinician should consider the relevance of immunomodulation in the disease process. It is not at all clear that cell-mediated immunity is important in the pathogenesis of COPD. Although successful treatment of advanced cases of COPD has been reported in the literature, levamisol's ineffectiveness in most cases may be related to the irrelevance of immunomodulation. The treatment regimen most commonly used is 5.5 mg per kg intramuscularly. The treatment may be repeated.

*Eli Lilly and Co., Indianapolis, IN
†A-H Solution, Jensen-Salsbery Laboratories, Kansas City, MO
‡Equi-Hist, Equine Products of Maryland, Pikesville, MD
§Levasole, Pitman-Moore, Inc., Washington Crossing, NJ

Diethylcarbamazine* inhibits production of a group of potent mediators of inflammation collectively called *leukotrienes*. The efficacy of diethylcarbamazine in the treatment of some horses with COPD may be attributed to this mechanism. However, it should be kept in mind that horses suffering from lungworm infection can exhibit clinical signs indistinguishable from those characteristic of COPD. In these cases, treatment with diethylcarbamazine is expected to result in remission of clinical signs. Clinical experience with diethylcarbamazine suggests limited efficacy in a few cases when used at a dose of 6.5 mg per kg orally for 14 days.

Cromolyn Sodium. Cromolyn sodium† is an antiasthmatic drug with no structural relationship to any other group of respiratory drugs. Its efficacy in the prevention of asthma is related to its ability to prevent mast cell degranulation. The drug has no direct effect on airway smooth muscle and has no direct antagonistic activity against mediators of inflammation such as histamine or prostaglandins. Therefore, in the treatment of asthma, cromolyn sodium is only effective prophylactically and is not effective as a therapeutic agent in cases of established disease. Anecdotal reports in horses suggest similar efficacy when 200 to 300 mg of cromolyn sodium are insufflated into the pharynx before exercise or exposure to allergens. The drug's effects last three to four hours and side effects have not been reported.

*Caricide, American Cyanamid Co., Princeton, NJ
†Intal, Fisons Co., Bedford, MA

Supplemental Readings

Beech, J.: Principles of Therapy. Vet. Clin. North Am. (Large Anim. Pract, 1:73, 1979.
Breeze, R. G.: Heaves. Vet. Clin. North Am. (Large Anim. Pract.), 1:219, 1979.
Calverley, A. H.: Levamisole phosphate as a treatment for heaves. Proc. 23rd Annu. Conv. Am. Assoc. Eq. Pract., 1977, pp. 363–365.
McPherson, E. A., Lawson, G. H. K., Murphy, J. R., Nicholson, J. M., Breeze, R. G., and Pirie, H. M.: Chronic obstructive pulmonary disease (COPD) in horses. Aetiological studies: Responses to intradermal and inhalation antigenic challenge. Equine Vet. J., 11:159, 1979.
Ziment, I.: Pharmacology of sympathomimetic agents. *In* Respiratory Pharmacology and Therapeutics, Philadelphia, W. B. Saunders Company, 1978, pp. 147–180.

Exercise-Induced Pulmonary Hemorrhage

Corinne Raphel Sweeney, KENNETT SQUARE, PENNSYLVANIA

Exercised-induced pulmonary hemorrhage (EIPH) is characterized by the presence of blood in the tracheobronchial tree following periods of competitive exercise. The most common terms used to describe this condition are bleeding and epistaxis, and horses with this condition are called bleeders. The prevalence of hemorrhage was reported to be low on the basis of observation of blood at the nares (between 0.5 and 2.5 per cent). However, use of the flexible fiberoptic endoscope has shown the prevalence of EIPH to be between 44 and 75 per cent in the racing Thoroughbred, 26 per cent in the racing Standardbred, 62 per cent in the racing Quarterhorse, 68 per cent in Steeplechasers, 67 per cent in timber racing horses, 40 per cent in three-day event horses, 10 per cent in pony club event horses, and 11 per cent in polo ponies.

EIPH is not a random event and EIPH-positive horses are more likely to have blood visible on subsequent examination than are EIPH-negative horses. Diagnosis of EIPH on the basis of clinical signs is difficult as horses with the condition show no pathognomonic signs and most affected horses show no clinical signs of respiratory disease. Horses returning from exercising or racing with blood at the nares most likely have EIPH. However, other sources of the hemorrhage, such as ethmoid hematoma, must be ruled out. Endoscopic examination demonstrating blood within the tracheobronchial tree allows for a definitive diagnosis of EIPH. The optimal time for this test is 30 to 120 minutes following exercise. I prefer examination at 60 minutes. If no blood is seen at the time of this examination, it should be repeated in approximately one hour. Cytologic examination of a tracheobronchial aspirate is a less specific way of diagnosing EIPH. The presence of macrophages containing hemosiderin indicates pulmonary hemorrhage but gives no indication of the time of its occurrence.

Although it has been the impression of many horsemen that EIPH is associated with diminished racing performance, its effect on performance is variable. No association has been demonstrated between finishing position in a race and the prevalence of EIPH in Thoroughbreds or Standardbreds. However, furosemide selectively improves the racing times of Thoroughbred racehorses diagnosed to have EIPH by endoscopic examination (see Furosemide in this chapter). This supports the contention that EIPH may impair performance. I believe that EIPH affects certain horses markedly, pre-venting them from obtaining racing speeds of which they were capable before its onset. However, other medical causes for the change in performance must be ruled out. Many horses continue to perform adequately despite repeated episodes of EIPH. Because of this variability each horse must be evaluated individually. In our hospital, several hundred horses with a history of EIPH are evaluated yearly to determine if any cardiopulmonary disease predisposes them to pulmonary hemorrhage. Medical evaluation (including physical examination, cardiac auscultation, auscultation and percussion of the thorax, cytologic and microbiologic examination of tracheobronchial aspirates, endoscopic examination of the respiratory tract, thoracic radiographs, and ultrasonograms) has rarely revealed a predisposing cause for EIPH. If an underlying cause is determined, such as atrial fibrillation, efforts should be directed toward its correction rather than only toward EIPH treatment. If clinical signs such as anorexia, fever, and depression accompany the EIPH one must consider that a respiratory disease such as pneumonia, pulmonary abscess, or pleuropneumonia may be either the result or the cause of EIPH.

THERAPY

Although many therapeutic regimens have been advocated to prevent EIPH in performance horses, most remedies have no proven efficacy. Until the cause or pathophysiology of EIPH is understood it is difficult to rationalize the use of most medications. This section will discuss current thoughts on selected therapeutic regimens including management changes, furosemide, bronchodilators, hesperidin and citrus bioflavinoids, estrogens, and coagulants.

MANAGEMENT

There is no consensus regarding the appropriate management of horses with EIPH. Little effort has been made to improve the stabling environment and to reduce air-borne irritants. Preliminary studies suggest that many racing Thoroughbreds have chronic bronchitis and bronchiolitis and thus any changes to improve ventilation or decrease exposure to hay, straw, and barn dust may be beneficial. Whether the association of chronic bronchitis and bronchiolitis with EIPH is significant remains a question, but environmental changes to decrease

603

the inhalation of irritants and allergens may improve respiratory function in general. Inhalation of water vapor–saturated air at above body temperature as delivered with the Equine Transpirator* may be effective in horses with EIPH through improved clearance of mucoid airway obstructions or a reduction in airway reactivity. Training methods for horses with EIPH also vary. Prolonged rest periods may be beneficial, but my experience suggests that after a return to the previous level of training or racing, EIPH will recur.

Supportive therapy to control the systemic effects of EIPH is usually not required. In most horses hemorrhage ceases within hours after racing. Although massive episodes of pulmonary hemorrhage may result in fatalities, the frequency of this occurrence is low. Fatal EIPH has occurred more commonly in horses with histories of mild to severe previous episodes. If massive nonfatal pulmonary hemorrhage occurs, prophylactic treatment with broad-spectrum antimicrobials is indicated to prevent secondary bacterial pneumonia. These horses should be rested for several weeks to months.

Furosemide. Furosemide† is the most popular drug used in the treatment of horses with EIPH. Clinical impressions and widespread use of the drug suggest that it is effective in preventing EIPH. The efficacy of furosemide in the *prevention* of EIPH has never been documented. However, recent studies indicate that furosemide may both decrease the apparent amount of pulmonary hemorrhage and improve the racing times of some bleeders. When furosemide's use is unrestricted by law the drug is usually administered at a dosage of approximately 150 to 300 mg intravenously 90 to 120 minutes before racing. However, most states that regulate the use of furosemide allow its administration only from 180 to 240 minutes before racing. In some states the dosage of furosemide is restricted to less than 250 mg intravenously while many states have no dosage restriction. In refractory cases of EIPH, some practitioners administer 350 to 500 mg of furosemide, divided into two doses, one at five or six hours and the other at three hours before racing. Furosemide does not improve racing times in normal horses but may cause an improvement in bleeders. It has no effect on hemostatic function.

The hemodynamic effects of furosemide last less than 120 minutes and are only apparent following larger doses than commonly used to treat EIPH. Thus the current time and dose restrictions placed on use of furosemide in some states may limit the effective use of the drug. Furosemide will dilute the urinary levels of water-soluble drugs and drug metabolites. Dilution is avoided by administering furosemide no less than 180 minutes before racing.

Bronchodilators. Limited studies on the pre-exercise use of parasympatholytic bronchodilators in three Thoroughbred race horses showed a decrease in the prevalence of EIPH. Atropine (15 mg intravenously), or ipratropium bromide* (10 ml of 1 per cent solution nebulized into a nasotracheal tube passed into the pharynx) was administered 60 minutes before exercise. Because of its undesirable cardiovascular effect, atropine is not recommended for therapeutic use in bleeders. The anticholinergic drug ipratropium has been developed as an aerosol bronchodilator drug in humans; at this time it is not approved for use in the United States. Other bronchodilators could also be considered in the therapy of EIPH on the basis of the preliminary results seen with atropine and ipratropium.

Hesperidin and Citrus Bioflavinoids. Because of the racing medication rules, some horse trainers have sought feed supplements that might have therapeutic value in the treatment of EIPH. A group of flavinoids that strengthens capillaries has been demonstrated in citrus and paprika. These flavinoids are thought to be essential for normal capillary integrity and to act synergistically with ascorbic acid. Citrus bioflavinoids, used in conjunction with ascorbic acid, reportedly enhance the efficacy of other therapeutic aids in controlling infection, stress, and nutritional deficiencies in humans even in cases in which there is no evidence of capillary weakness. Preoperative citrus bioflavinoids reduce capillary and venous bleeding in humans. Anecdotal reports have suggested that the bioflavinoids are helpful in preventing EIPH but controlled studies using an oral dose of 28 grams per day for over 90 days did not alter its prevalence.

Conjugated Estrogens. Another popular treatment for EIPH with unproven efficacy is conjugated estrogens. These substances reduce capillary bleeding and accelerate blood clotting in laboratory animals. As previously mentioned no coagulation defects have been noted with EIPH in horses; therefore no rationale exists for therapy with conjugated estrogens. Commonly used preparations are potassium estrone sulfate† or a mixture of sodium estrone sulfate and equilin sulfate.‡ These preparations are usually administered within one hour of racing at dosage rates of 0.05 to 0.1 mg per kg intravenously and 0.05 to 0.25 mg per kg intravenously, respectively. Estrogens are seldom used alone but rather in combination with furosemide.

Coagulants and Anticoagulants. A mixture of oxalic and malonic acids and a vitamin K preparation have both been used to treat EIPH. Because no

---

*Equine transpirator, Transpirator Technologies Inc., Somerset, NJ
†Lasix, American Hoechst Co., Somerville, NJ

*Boehringer Ingelheim, Ridgefield, CT
†Estro IV, Western Serum, Tempe, AZ
‡Premarin, Ayerst Laboratories, New York, NY

coagulation defect has been demonstrated, these treatments are unwarranted.

Supplemental Readings

Pascoe, J. R., and Raphel, C. F.: Pulmonary hemorrhage in exercising horses. Comp. Cont. Ed., 4:S411, 1982.

Pascoe, J. R., Ferraro, G. L., Cannon, J. H., Arthur, R. M., and Wheat, J. D.: Exercise-induced pulmonary hemorrhage in racing Thoroughbreds: A preliminary study. Am. J. Vet. Res., 42:703, 1981.

Raphel, C. F., and Soma, L. R.: Exercise-induced pulmonary hemorrhage in Thoroughbreds after racing and breezing. Am. J. Vet. Res., 43:1123, 1982.

Sweeney, C. R., and Soma, L. R.: Exercise-induced pulmonary hemorrhage in Thoroughbred horses: Response to furosemide and hesperidin-citrus bioflavinoids. J. Am. Vet. Med. Assoc., 185:195, 1984.

Sweeney, C. R., Soma, L. R., Bucan, C. A., and Ray, S. G.: Exercise-induced pulmonary hemorrhage in exercising Thoroughbreds: Preliminary results with pre-exercise medication. Cornell Vet., 74:263, 1984.

Tobin, T., Roberts, B. L., Swerczek, T. W., and Crisman, M.: The pharmacology of furosemide in the horse. III. Dose and time response relationships, effects of repeated dosing and performance effects. J. Equine Med. Surg., 2:216, 1978.

Sinusitis

Edward A. Scott, EAST LANSING, MICHIGAN

Sinus conditions in the horse are uncommon but are often diagnostic and therapeutic challenges. Sinusitis may result from primary infections or be secondary to dental problems, neoplasia, hematomas, cystlike lesions, traumatic injuries to the skull, and inflammatory brain disorders.

ANATOMY

Six pairs of paranasal sinuses communicate directly or indirectly with the nasal cavity: the maxillary, frontal, sphenopalatine, dorsal conchal, midconchal, and ventral conchal sinuses. Conchal sinuses are compartments or extensions of the turbinates. The dorsal conchal sinus communicates with the frontal sinus while the middle and ventral conchal sinuses communicate with the maxillary sinus. Clinically, the frontal and maxillary sinuses are of primary importance. External landmarks for the maxillary sinus are the facial crest, the medial canthus of the eye, and the infraorbital foramen. The maxillary sinus is the largest paranasal sinus and usually is divided into rostral and caudal compartments by an oblique septum, which is usually incomplete and variable in location. The septum is positioned perpendicular to the facial bones (maxilla, lacrimal, and zygomatic bones) roughly halfway between the orbit and cranial limit of the facial crest. The roots of all three molars and occasionally the last premolar are embedded in the floor of the maxillary sinus. In young horses, these roots extend dorsally and the maxillary sinuses are filled with these tooth roots covered only by a thin plate of bone. As the horse ages, the roots recede and the maxillary sinus increases in size. Rostral and caudal maxillary compartments communicate with the middle nasal meatus via openings located medially in both compartments. These openings are the routes of drainage for the sinus. The frontal sinus drains into the maxillary sinus via a large opening located between the roof of the caudal maxillary sinus and frontal sinus.

DIAGNOSIS

Clinical signs of sinusitis include copious foul-smelling purulent nasal discharge, facial malformation, difficulty breathing, epistaxis, exophthalmos, weight loss, and neurologic disturbances. One of the most consistent clinical signs associated with sinusitis is nasal discharge. Unilateral sinusitis results in an ipsilateral nasal discharge while bilateral nasal discharge occurs when right and left sinuses are involved or when separation of nasal passages is incomplete. The character of sinus drainage varies with the cause, chronicity, and complications. Sinusitis secondary to dental disease and tumor masses that invade sinus walls is characterized by a purulent foul-smelling and persistent nasal discharge. Serosanguinous exudate is typical of sinus cysts, slow-growing neoplasms, and certain stages of mycotic granulomas as well as hematomas. Copious quantities of exudate with considerable cellular debris can obstruct natural drainage and cause increased pressure within the affected sinus, resulting in facial distortion. Facial deformities may also result from inflammatory reaction of skin, subcutaneous tissues, teeth, and facial bone, and previous sinus surgery (Fig. 1). When facial distortion is seen, conchal distortion and narrowing of nasal passages should be expected. Exophthalmos when seen with clinical signs of sinusitis is suggestive of extension of sinusitis to the periorbital region.

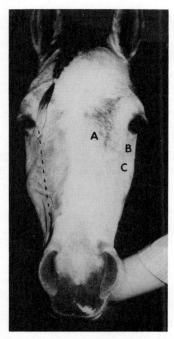

Figure 1. Frontal view of a horse with facial deformation due to sinusitis. Trephine sites are indicated (*A, B,* and *C*). Dotted line represents the nasolacrimal duct. *A,* Turbinate extension of the frontal sinus. *B,* Superior (posterior) compartment of the maxillary sinus. *C,* Inferior (anterior) compartment of the maxillary sinus.

Percussion of Sinuses. Normal percussion findings are established by experience with percussion of normal horses. I like to use the first two fingers of my right hand and start at the dorsal-caudal limit of the frontal sinus. This area is rarely fluid-filled and it serves as a reference point. Percussion is accomplished by striking the area sharply. Restraint of the head and operator safety should be kept in mind. A stethoscope may be used to listen for resonance or dullness. The frontal sinus should be evaluated first; then the maxillary sinus should be percussed from caudal to rostral compartments. Percussion in normal horses less than four years of age will be less resonant than in older horses because the tooth roots project into the maxillary sinus. Fluid or soft tissue densities filling sinus compartments result in duller percussion sounds. If facial bones are thickened from previous surgery, percussion is less reliable.

Endoscopy. Use of the endoscope in viewing nasal passages, turbinates, and ethmoid and pharyngeal regions is paramount in accurately defining pathologic changes in the areas. Guttural pouch empyema may look very much like an early case of primary sinusitis. These two conditions can be differentiated by both endoscopy and radiography. The endoscopic observation of exudate originating from the eustachian tube opening of a guttural pouch is evidence of guttural pouch empyema. Endoscopic findings of rhinitis and exudate from the turbinate area along the nasal passage in front of the ethmoids indicate the presence of drainage from a sinus compartment. Although the actual drainage site from maxillary sinus compartments is not visible endoscopically, exudate seen in the middle meatus below the dorsal conchal sinus indicates sinus disease. Turbinate distortion is accompanied by narrowing of nasal passages and deviation of the midseptum, which can be seen endoscopically. When doubt exists, comparison may be made with the opposite nasal passage or a normal horse.

Examination of the Oral Cavity. Dental disease of the upper arcade is the most probable cause of sinusitis. In order for dental disease to cause sinusitis, foreign material and/or septic material from the tooth or its alveolus must gain entrance into the sinus cavity. Dental conditions associated with sinusitis are fractured teeth, developmental anomalies (for example, patent infundibulum or agenesis), and displaced teeth. Anatomically the disease process must project into or lie adjacent to sinus cavities. Therefore, the teeth involved are most usually molars 1, 2, and 3. Extra or displaced diseased premolars may also affect a sinus. Visual inspection of the mouth can identify fractured and displaced teeth and patent infundibula. However, a patent infundibulum does not guarantee that this is the cause of sinusitis. To provide access of food material into the sinus, an infundibulum must be patent over its length. Food material will pack firmly into an infundibulum and it is difficult to determine its depth. An instrument with a right-angled sharp point is needed to check the depth of an infundibulum. A receding gum line, exudate around the affected tooth, and loosening of teeth in sockets indicate dental disease. The oral examination is extremely important. If necessary, the horse should be anesthetized for a thorough oral examination.

Radiography. Radiography of sinuses and the upper respiratory system is routinely used as a diagnostic aid. However, interpretation of radiographic findings may be challenging. Fluid levels, soft tissue and osseous densities, lytic changes, abnormalities of teeth and foreign bodies are definable radiographically. If sinusitis is primary, the radiographic appearance of the affected sinus may be a fluid-air interface in the involved compartments. If sinusitis is secondary to dental disease, abnormalities of teeth should be radiographically definable. Even with multiple radiographic views, the limits and distribution of a pathologic lesion may not be fully appreciated. This is an important consideration since surgical intervention in sinus cases is often full of surprises. If the surgeon is not prepared to handle the unexpected, both surgical and medical management will be less than optimal.

Culture, Cytology, and Biopsy. Differentiation of a soft tissue growth in a sinus compartment depends on histologic or cytologic examination. Cytologic examination can be performed on exudates from the nostril or material collected from the sinus compartment via a trephine hole. Since sinus lesions may not be homogenous, biopsy samples may be misleading.

THERAPY

In order to formulate an effective therapeutic plan, sinusitis must be categorized as primary or secondary. Primary sinusitis is inflammation of the sinus compartments without a predisposing cause, while secondary sinusitis has a defined predisposing cause such as diseased teeth or a space-occupying lesion. To resolve secondary sinusitis the underlying cause must be addressed. Techniques for surgical removal of teeth and dental and other tumors are covered in various references. When a predisposing cause of sinusitis is suspected but cannot be identified, a complete exploration of the sinus cavity and its content should performed using a "flap" technique.

Trephination of sinus compartments for both drainage and therapy is an important technique used in the treatment of sinusitis (Fig. 1). By location of appropriate sites for drainage and lavage, resolution of uncomplicated cases is expected. Use of large volumes of flush with antimicrobial action is important to dilute debris and to reduce bacterial populations. Continuous lavage of involved sinus cavities over a period of two to three days may be used. Continuous irrigation of sinuses is particularly effective postsurgically and is accomplished by a gravity flow system. I routinely lavage postoperative cases with 20 L of a 2 per cent povidone-iodine solution. This lavage is instituted after complete recovery from anesthesia when the horse is returned to the stall. Flow rates should be high initially to fill sinus compartments and lavage as much of the surface area as possible. Sinus lavage is discontinued while the horse eats and drinks. After the affected sinus has been lavaged for 48 to 72 hours, drainage tubes are removed. Flushing with small amounts (100 ml) of solution twice daily is continued until the trephine holes close. The maxillary-nasal opening must be patent for sinus lavage to be effective. If not, alternative routes of sinus drainage must be established. This is accomplished by a variety of surgical methods described in standard surgical texts.

Systemic medication may be used concurrently with local therapy. However, long-term systemic antimicrobial therapy as a sole therapeutic regimen for sinusitis in the horse is contraindicated. It can be costly and potentially harmful due to development of bacterial resistance. Trephine sites should be kept clean using head bandages or an orthopedic stockinette. Exercise and grazing may enhance drainage, and horses are routinely turned out to pasture as soon as possible after sinus lavage or surgery. Sinusitis in the horse may be expensive to treat and commonly is a long-term problem. Therefore, before starting treatment of sinusitis the owner should be aware of the time and cost required to treat the condition. An accurate diagnosis with full consideration of underlying causes is paramount if treatment is to be effective.

Supplemental Readings

Getty, R. (with Skull by D.J. Hillman): Sisson and Grossman's The Anatomy of the Domestic Animals, 5th ed. Philadelphia, W. B. Saunders Company, 1975, pp. 337–348.

Scott, E. A.: Surgery of the Oral Cavity. Vet. Clin. North Am. (Large Anim. Pract.), 4:3, 1982.

Diseases of the Pharynx and the Larynx

Gordon J. Baker, URBANA, ILLINOIS

The upper respiratory tract of the horse has evolved to function as an efficient conducting passage for air. In the change from quiet breathing at rest to air flow during maximal exercise, flow rates rise tenfold, providing minute volumes in excess of 1,000 L in a 400-kg horse. Since the horse is an obligatory nasal breather, effective expansion and streamlining of the nasal chambers, pharynx, and larynx are essential to accommodate the high flow rates of exercise. Therefore, lesions within this region often produce dramatic clinical effects by obstructing air flow and inducing dynamic airway collapse.

CLINICAL SIGNS

Lesions that obstruct or interfere with air flow result in turbulent air flow and produce noise during the breathing cycle. The degree of obstruction is reflected by the onset and nature of noise during exercise. An example is laryngeal hemiplegia, in which resting respiration is quiet but exercise results in a characteristic whistling or roaring noise on inhalation. Under other circumstances, airway obstruction may be dynamic and transient as is seen in dorsal displacement of the soft palate. In addition to making respiratory noise, such horses will stop as they attempt to swallow and reposition the free border of the palate. Riders and drivers refer to this phenomenon as "choking down" (see Dorsal Displacement of the Soft Palate).

In addition to causing noise and poor performance, an irritant focus such as a pharyngeal ulcer, cyst, or inflamed larynx may result in dysphagia. In extreme disease, for example, with a pharyngeal tumor or pharyngeal paralysis, the dysphagia may result in aspiration pneumonia.

In the past 15 years, major advances have been made in our ability to examine the upper respiratory tract of horses. Flexible fiberoptic endoscopes, radiographic techniques, and radiostethoscopes have given a better understanding of the etiology and pathogenesis of pharyngeal and laryngeal disease in the horse. At the same time the spectrum of recognized diseases is expanding. Inflammatory diseases of both the epiglottic and arytenoid cartilages of racehorses are emerging clinical problems even though their etiology and pathogenesis are unknown.

DIAGNOSIS AND CASE MANAGEMENT

Although it is not suggested that each horse with clinical signs of upper airway disease be subjected to all the diagnostic tests to be discussed, a complete history and physical examination are essential before a detailed upper respiratory examination is performed. It is important that a history be obtained from a knowledgeable source, and in many cases the exercise person or driver is the key to anamnestic clues.

Clients and trainers may request specific therapy such as pharyngeal curettage for pharyngeal lymphoid hyperplasia or laryngeal surgery for poor performance only to find that the horse also has sore shins, fractured carpal bones, pulmonary hemorrhage, or atrial fibrillation as the real disease. The practitioner should consider the diagnostic tests listed in Table 1 and make an accurate record of the clinical findings.

Medical and surgical treatment should then be discussed with the owner. Treatment of the competitive equine athlete should be discussed in relation to past performance and future hopes. Care should be taken to avoid suggesting that any medical or surgical cure will, by definition, mean success on the racetrack.

DISEASES OF THE PHARYNX

Congenital and Developmental Anomalies. Of these problems, cleft palate is perhaps the easiest diagnosed. The nasal return of milk during nursing in early life may be pathognomonic for this lesion. However, in some cases, minor palatine irregularities may not be diagnosed at an early age and may be confused with diseases such as acute upper

TABLE 1. DIAGNOSTIC TESTS USED IN EVALUATION OF HORSES
WITH UPPER RESPIRATORY TRACT DISEASE

Procedure	Comments
Accurate and complete history	Vaccination history, performance guides (times, etc.), and previous treatment
Compete physical examination at rest	
Palpation and auscultation of upper respiratory tract	
Endoscopic examination	This should be carried out without chemical restraint when possible—tranquilizers such as xylazine affect tone of pharyngeal walls
Radiographic examination	Only if indicated by the initial endoscopic examination: barium paste contrast radiography may be helpful in evaluating palatine, epiglottic, and laryngopharyngeal anomalies
Exercise tests	It may be necessary that the veterinarian either ride the horse or sit on the exercise bike with the driver to appreciate the full dynamics of noise at exercise or extent of poor performance
Repeat endoscopic examination after exercise	
Virology, microbiology, and serology	These should be used as indicated by history and physical findings; random nasal chamber bacteriology cultures in young race horses should be interpreted cautiously
Electrocardiogram	
Pre- and postexercise blood gases	Of limited value to the practitioner
Biopsy and histopathology	As indicated by diagnosed disease
Examination of stable mates	This examination may yield valuable information on the level of respiratory inflammatory disease in racetrack stables

airway infections. Palatine disease may remain asymptomatic until the horse comes into training. I believe that the surgical treatment of cleft palates in horses is an unrewarding exercise when the object is to produce an equine athlete (see p. 1).

Rostral displacement of the palatopharyngeal arch is an anomaly that has been reported in conjunction with dorsal displacement of the soft palate. It appears that rostral displacement of the palatopharyngeal arch is caused by an abnormal development of the laryngeal cartilages so that the arytenoid cartilages are caudal to the palatopharyngeal arch. Again the dynamics of air flow during exercise result in laryngopalatine dislocation and noise production.

In the young horse, subepiglottic and pharyngeal developmental cysts may arise either from remnants of the thyroglossal duct or as inclusion cysts within the aryepiglottic fold. Cysts are usually located on the oral surface of the epiglottis. The diagnosis is easy with endoscopic examination, and excision via a ventral midline pharyngotomy or laryngotomy affords good results.

Pharyngeal Lymphoid Hyperplasia. Pharyngeal lymphoid hyperplasia has been a topic of considerable interest in the past 10 years. Its "discovery" and "diagnosis" directly parallels the use of endoscopic equipment at the racetrack. A number of reports have been published dealing with the etiology and therapy of pharyngeal lymphoid hyperplasia in young horses. However, reports on the results of therapy are few.

Pharyngeal lymphoid hyperplasia is a normal phenomenon of all young horses. The condition is thought to be an immune response to a wide variety of environmental pollutions and infectious viral respiratory diseases, particularly rhinopneumonitis and equine influenza. One widely held opinion is that such disease problems can be dramatically altered by multiple vaccination programs and the development of a "hyperimmune state." Pharyngeal disease and pharyngeal inflammation in the young horse have been suggested to cause airway obstruction,

airway irritation, and induced lower airway spasm, or the production of pharyngeal secretions and induced functional pharyngeal obstruction. Such hypotheses are unproven. Recent evidence suggests that blood gases in some exercising horses affected by pharyngeal lymphoid hyperplasia are not altered.

Pharyngeal lymphoid hyperplasia has traditionally been diagnosed by endoscopic observation of the pharyngeal recess (pharyngeal tonsil) and the roof of the nasopharynx. Hypertrophy of the margins of the pharyngeal tonsil result in lymphoid tissue edema and the formation, in severe cases, of pedunculated tonsillar polyps. Tonsillar hypertrophy is accompanied by lymphoid follicle formation in the roof of the nasopharynx. Such follicles commonly coalesce and appear to "flow" out of the pharyngeal tonsil. Pharyngeal lymphoid hyperplasia can be graded by noting the extent of the nasopharyngeal follicles and the degree of exudate because the primary focus of pharyngeal lymphoid hyperplasia is the pharyngeal tonsil, that is, the lymphoid tissue localized within the pharyngeal recess. I would recommend a 1 to 4 grading system based on the endoscopic appearance of the pharyngeal recess (Fig. 1).

Stage 1. Hypertrophy limited to less than 180° of tonsillar margin.

Stage 2. Hypertrophy extends full circumference of tonsillar margin.

Stage 3. Hypertrophy makes midline contact.

Stage 4. Hypertrophic tonsillar tissue prolapses from pharyngeal recess.

Histopathology of hypertrophic tissue does not readily distinguish grades 1 to 4. There is epithelial edema, ulceration, and development of extensive lymphoid germinal follicles within the tonsillar tissue.

THERAPY. Because pharyngitis is a nonspecific inflammation, and because definitive information concerning its etiology and pathogenesis is unavailable, it is hardly surprising that therapeutic regimens for the treatment of this syndrome are diverse.

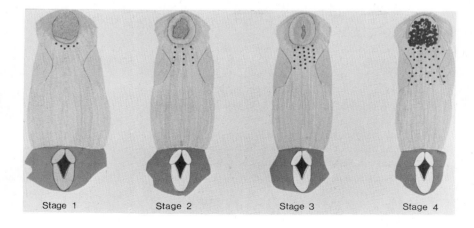

Figure 1. Pharyngeal lymphoid hyperplasia grading system. The pharyngeal tonsil is indicated by the circle at the top of the diagram and the dots represent follicles on the nasopharyngeal wall.

Stage 1   Stage 2   Stage 3   Stage 4

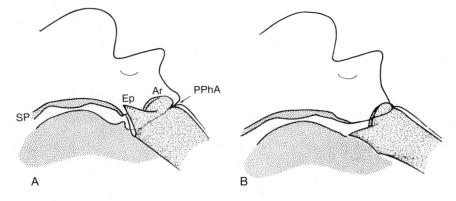

Figure 2. Dorsal displacement of soft palate. Relationship of normal (A) and displaced palate (B). Ar, arytenoid; EP, epiglottis; P Ph A, palato-pharyngeal arch; SP, soft palate.

They range from systemic antimicrobials to topical therapy. In recent years the use of procaine penicillin G (20,000 U per kg twice a day) and the potentiated sulfonamides have received wide support. The isolation of *Bordetella bronchiseptica* from some poorly performing young horses has encouraged such an approach. Topical therapy using a wide range of nasal sprays remains an unproven therapy. Lavage of the nasopharynx with 10 ml of a mixture of nitrofurazone and dimethylsulfoxide (DMSO) (3:1) solution with 0.2 per cent prednisolone acetate may be done three times daily. Local therapy using gentamicin in addition to prednisolone acetate has also been used.

In severe cases of pharyngeal lymphoid hyperplasia there is gross protrusion of hypertrophic material from the pharyngeal tonsil. Surgical curettage, suction, and Freon spray cause a dramatic, acute inflammatory response in the pharynx and may break the cycle of chronic recurrent inflammation.

A regular vaccination program has merit. Outbreaks of acute viral respiratory disease are usually associated with enhancement of pharyngeal lymphoid hyperplasia. Sixty-day interval vaccination against equine influenza and equine herpes virus I has been advocated for the high-risk horse. Such a program should be maintained until the animal is at least four years of age.

Dorsal Displacement of the Soft Palate. Numerous disease processes within the pharynx and larynx alter the stability of the relationship between the palatopharyngeal arch and the larynx. During exercise there may be a caudal retraction of the larynx and dislocation of the larynx from the palatopharyngeal arch. The soft palate then rises dorsally above the epiglottis and obstructs the additus laryngis (Fig. 2). Diseases such as epiglottic hypoplasia, rostral displacement of the palatopharyngeal arch, pharyngeal lymphoid hyperplasia, laryngeal chondroma, epiglottic cysts, and epiglottic entrapment may all lead to instability of the palatopharyngeal arch–larynx junction (Fig. 3). In a study using cineendoscopy and videofluoroscopy of pharyngeal and laryngeal function, the mechanics of dorsal displacement of the soft palate were demonstrated in 10 horses. Three main features were observed prior to dorsal displacement:

1. The lowering of the pharyngeal roof accompanied by contraction of the palatopharyngeal arch cranial to the arytenoid cartilages.

2. An elevation of the rostral portion of the soft palate.

3. Caudal retraction of the larynx.

These observations suggest that trainers who treat "choking" horses by using a tongue strap are, in effect, preventing caudal retraction of the larynx. Partial sternothyrohyoid and omohyoid myectomy used in the treatment of dorsal displacement of the soft palate also prevents caudal retraction of the larynx. In those horses that have displacement of the palate during the extremes of athletic effort and in which no predisposing disease can be found, partial sternothyroid and omohyoid myectomy has proven effective.

The procedure is carried out under general anesthesia with the animal on its back. A ventral midline skin incision extending some 10 cm caudal to a standard ventriculectomy is made. By blunt dissection, aided by coagulation, the hyoid insertions of the ventral throat muscles are divided and retracted caudally. Care is taken to preserve the jugular veins. A 10- to 12-cm section of each muscle is removed. If the procedure accompanies an exploratory laryngotomy or soft palate resection, the incision is only partially closed leaving ventral drainage. When surgery is limited to the myectomy, the muscle bellies

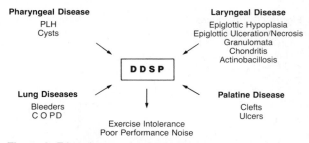

Figure 3. Etiopathogenesis of dorsal displacement of the soft palate (DDSP).

are sutured and the skin closed over a 2-cm Penrose drain.

DISEASES OF THE LARYNX

Laryngeal Hemiplegia. For more than two centuries veterinarians have recognized laryngeal hemiplegia in the horse. Inspiratory stridor during exercise, poor performance, and the characteristic roaring or whistling noises are the key clinical signs. The diagnosis is confirmed by endoscopic examination at rest, by the exercise test, and by postexercise endoscopy. As will be mentioned in a subsequent section, care should be taken in evaluating laryngeal malfunction in the horse in light of the increasing incidence of inflammatory disease of the arytenoid cartilage. If there is deformity of the arytenoid cartilage in addition to malfunction, the diagnostician should be suspicious of a complicated laryngeal paralysis. In general, laryngeal hemiplegia in the horse is a left-sided lesion and there is increasing evidence for an inherited etiology.

TREATMENT. The techniques of ventriculectomy, laryngoplasty, and partial arytenoidectomy have evolved over 150 years. Unfortunately, few critical studies have evaluated the effectiveness of these procedures and often the results have been expressed in terms of owner and trainer satisfaction rather than critical analysis of respiratory noise, air flow, blood gas analyses, and performance. Recent reports attempt to change this area of neglect. In one study, the earning capacity of 105 Thoroughbreds treated by left laryngoplasty was compared with age and racing class–matched controls. The results of surgery were reported as excellent. Of 326 horses treated surgically for laryngeal hemiplegia by ventriculectomy and laryngoplasty, 181 horses were available for re-evaluation at least six months after surgery. When ventriculectomy results were compared with those for combined laryngoplasty and ventriculectomy, it was found that ventriculectomy alone was less than 30 per cent effective in terms of noise reduction and endoscopic examination. Combined laryngoplasty and ventriculectomy gave good results in 60 per cent of the cases. A recent study reported changes in arterial blood gas oxygen tension in a horse with laryngeal hemiplegia and confirmed the efficacy of laryngoplasty in that case. A controlled study of the upper airway airflow mechanics in exercising horses before and after laryngeal neurectomy and laryngoplasty also confirmed efficacy of the surgery.

Laryngeal Chondritis. Irritation of the hyaline substance of the laryngeal cartilages in the horse results in dystrophic calcification, abscessation with subsequent formation of chondroma with discharging sinuses and airway obstruction. Such lesions were formerly only recognized following laryngeal surgery during which inadvertent damage was done to either the arytenoid cartilage (vocal process) or the cricoid cartilage.

In recent years, a spontaneous inflammatory disease of the arytenoid cartilage has been recognized. Affected horses are presented as poorly performing and noisy, with laryngeal obstruction due to abscessation and dystrophic calcification of the hyaline cartilage of the arytenoid. The enlargement of the arytenoid may make contact with the opposite cartilage and an induced "kissing" lesion may occur. The diagnosis of laryngeal chondritis is based upon thorough endoscopic examination and the recognition that in addition to malfunction or paralysis of the affected side there is distortion of the arytenoid cartilage. The disease in some very early stages can be treated by local laryngotomy and curettage. In general, however, the endoscopic examination should be regarded as the tip of the iceberg. Whatever disease is seen on the surface of the vocal process by the endoscopic examination represents only one fifth of the diseased cartilage. With this in mind, the technique of partial arytenoidectomy has been modified from the 19th century description and satisfactory results have been described in some 20 cases. The prognosis is less satisfactory in the presence of bilateral disease and in my experience also less satisfactory in the presence of atrophied laryngeal muscles.

EPIGLOTTIC DISEASE

Hypoepiglottis may be diagnosed on endoscopic examination and confirmed by radiographic evaluation of the larynx and pharynx. Specific treatment of this condition is not available.

Epiglottic Entrapment. Enlargement of the aryepiglottic fold may occur either spontaneously or in association with a small epiglottis or with inflammatory disease of the palatopharyngeal arch and epiglottis. The free margin of the aryepiglottic fold may become ulcerated and granulomatous and may result in subsequent erosion of the fold such that an entrapped epiglottis may, in time, become eroded. Obstruction to air flow, noise on exercise, and choking and coughing on exercise are clinical signs that accompany entrapment of the epiglottis by the aryepiglottic fold. Entrapment may be an incidental finding in some cases and may be truly asymptomatic. Therefore, surgical intervention should be considered only in cases in which the clinical signs support the diagnosis. The aryepiglottic fold may be trimmed by sharp dissection via a midline laryngotomy or pharyngostomy or by the oral approach using an ecraseur. Using fiberoptic endoscopy, the aryepiglottic fold can be excised with a wire knife in the standing, sedated horse.

Supplemental Readings

Baker, G. J.: Laryngeal hemiplegia in the horse. Comp. Cont. Ed., 5:S61, 1983.

Goulden, B. E., Anderson, L. J., Davies, A. S., and Barnes, G. R. G.: Rostral displacement of the palatopharyngeal arch: A case report. Equine Vet. J., 8:95, 1976.

Greet, T. R. C., Baker, G. J., and Lee, R.: The effect of laryngoplasty and pharyngeal function in the horse. Equine Vet. J., 11:153, 1979.

Haynes, P. F.: Dorsal dispalcement of the soft palate and epiglottic entrapment: Diagnosis, management, and interrelationship. Comp. Cont. Ed., 5:S379, 1983.

Heffron, C. J., and Baker, G. J.: Observations on the mechanism of functional obstruction of the nasopharyngeal airway in the horse. Equine Vet. J., 11:142, 1979.

Kester, W. O.: Equine pharyngitis report. Am. Assoc. Equine Pract. Newsletter, 3:19, 1976.

Raker, C. W., and Boles, C. L.: Pharyngeal lymphoid hyperplasia in the horse. J. Eq. Med. Surg., 2:202, 1978.

Speirs, V. C.: A retrospective survey of racing performance in Australian horses after surgery for carpal injuries and laryngeal hemiplegia. Proc. 26th Annu. Conv. Am. Assoc. Eq. Pract., 1980, pp. 335–344.

Stick, J. A., and Boles, C.: Subepiglottic cyst in three foals. J. Am. Vet. Med. Assoc., 177:62, 1980.

White, N. A., and Blackwell, R. B.: Partial arytenoidectomy in the horse. Vet. Surg., 9:5, 1980.

Diseases of the Auditive Tube Diverticulum (Guttural Pouch)

W. Robert Cook, NORTH GRAFTON, MASSACHUSETTS

The causes of guttural pouch tympany, empyema, and mycosis are unclear; therefore, treatment is less than perfect. Fortunately, diseases of the guttural pouch are uncommon. In order of frequency, mycosis occurs more often than tympany and the most uncommon is empyema. When these diseases do occur, however, all are serious and at least one is life-threatening.

ANATOMY AND PHYSIOLOGY

Although the anatomy of the auditive tube diverticulum or guttural pouch has been well described, the auditive tube itself has received little attention. A better understanding of the normal and abnormal anatomy of the auditive tube may be critical to managing guttural pouch disease.

The function of the diverticulum is unknown but the function of the auditive tube is the same in the horse as in other mammals, that is, equalization of air pressure on both sides of the membrana tympani. The pharyngeal opening of the auditive tube in humans is thought to be closed during respiration and to open mainly during swallowing. In the horse, although there is less information available, endoscopy confirms that the tube opens during swallowing. The mechanism whereby the pharyngeal orifice opens and closes has not been explained; it may be muscular, mechanical, or both. Some investigators suggested long ago that air enters the normal guttural pouch on expiration, but this has not been substantiated.

TYMPANY OF THE GUTTURAL POUCH

In this condition, which is also known as meteorism of the guttural pouch and bullfrog disease, the guttural pouch inflates with gas at greater than atmospheric pressure and becomes tympanitic. It also dilates, becoming emphysematous. Although tympany is always accompanied by emphysema, emphysema is occasionally seen without tympany. Secondary infection of the tympanitic pouch is common. However, for the disease to be classified as tympany rather than empyema, the predominating content of the pouch must be gas rather than pus. Tympany is generally a disease of foals and weanlings, whereas empyema is a disease of older horses.

Tympany of the guttural pouch is a disease of foals, especially fillies. In a series of about 20 cases that I have seen over 25 years, the disease has occurred in an unexpectedly high number of Arabian foals.

ETIOLOGY AND PATHOGENESIS

The disease can be either congenital or developmental (not noticed until after birth). Neither the mechanisms nor the cause is fully understood. A 4:1 female-to-male ratio suggests that a genetic factor may be involved. Tympany appears to be caused by too much air entering the guttural pouch during forced expiration. Once air is admitted, the excess pressure in the pouch presumably results in failure of the pharyngeal orifice of the auditive tube to open properly during deglutition, thus preventing air from escaping. Endoscopic observation of the pharyngeal opening in affected foals indicates that some movement of the medial lamina takes place during deglutition but, presumably, this fails to open the auditive tube gutter ventrally to allow communication with the diverticulum. I have observed defective pouches expanding during expiration while foals recovered from general anesthesia and inflating instantly when foals cough. This suggests that raising the air pressure in the nasopharynx on expiration, when the pharyngeal openings of the auditive tube are not airtight, leads to guttural pouch tympany.

In the early stages of the disease, the mucosa of the guttural pouch is probably normal. Once secondary infection becomes established, the mucosa becomes thickened and the tympanitic pouch tends to accumulate pus. This fluid does not stagnate and produce a true empyema. The purulent material seems to drain from the auditive tube in spite of the supposedly faulty pharyngeal opening. Rarely, some of the retained pus becomes inspissated.

The tympanitic pouch can obstruct the nasopharyngeal airway, especially during inspiration. In severe cases, the tympany may result in dysphagia and the cervical trachea may also be compressed. Although I have never known an affected foal to die from suffocation, temporary asphyxia does occur, especially during sleep or physical excitement. In hot weather, an affected foal may resort to mouth breathing.

CLINICAL SIGNS

Clinical signs include unilateral or bilateral parotid swelling, respiratory distress, dysphagia, nasal discharge, and cough. The disease has been recognized in a foal within two days of birth but, more commonly, clinical signs are not noticed until the foal is several weeks or months of age. A unilaterally affected foal first develops a swelling in the parotid region of the affected side and, as tympany increases, a swelling also appears on the healthy side. The latter is generally not so marked and may not extend lateral to the larynx. The foal often snores during inspiration when asleep, when excited in the stall, at exercise, and when the head is flexed. Some foals make a noise during feeding. The degree of tympany often increases after exercise in a paddock. Suckling can be tiring and difficult. The foal may cough and return some milk down its nostrils; dysphagia can lead to aspiration pneumonia. There may be a mucopurulent discharge at one or both nostrils, originating from a secondarily infected guttural pouch or from aspiration pneumonia.

In view of the abnormally high pressure in the auditive tube diverticulum, it is rather surprising that signs of middle ear disturbance are not observed.

DIAGNOSIS

The clinical history of respiratory distress in a foal, usually a filly, with a readily detectable parotid swelling on one or both sides, is often pathognomonic. If the skin over the swelling is flicked with finger and thumb, the percussion note is drumlike. Manual compression sometimes collapses the swelling and air escaping into the pharynx makes a sound. Lateral radiographs provide confirmation and a measure of the emphysema. A fluid level in the pouch may be noted on the radiographs, indicating secondary sepsis. Lateral and dorsoventral views may help to differentiate between unilateral and bilateral tympany. Contrast medium injected into both pouches can aid in identifying the most caudal extent of the medial compartment on both sides. An easier method of deciding this issue is to sedate the foal and introduce a metal catheter into the guttural pouch via the nostril. If catheterization of one guttural pouch results in instant deflation of the swelling on both sides, this confirms a unilateral condition. Subsequently, the pouch may be seen to reinflate during the expiratory phase of respiration.

TREATMENT

The objective of treatment is to re-establish normal communication between the diverticulum and the nasopharynx via the auditive tube. Dilation of the pouch persists, but emphysema does not constitute a problem if there is no tympany or secondary sepsis.

Reduction of pressure within the guttural pouch can be achieved, at least temporarily, by placing a self-retaining catheter in the diverticulum via the nostril. A mushroom-tipped catheter* provides better drainage than a Foley catheter, the cuff of which may leak and allow the catheter to fall out prematurely. If a catheter can be kept in for six or more weeks, some erosion of the medial cartilage or ventrolateral membrane of the auditive tube opening may take place, facilitating air exchange between guttural pouch and pharynx and providing a satisfactory long-term remedy for the disease. Even if this technique is not used as the permanent treatment it temporarily eliminates the clinical signs, prevents respiratory distress and further emphysema, and reduces the risk of aspiration pneumonia. To insert the catheter, the foal should be moderately sedated and the catheter introduced by stiffening its lumen with a metal stylet that has been bent distally. The catheter can be introduced blindly or under endoscopic vision. Deep sedation should be avoided as this can exacerbate the respiratory distress.

Fenestration of the medial septum, a surgical treatment that I introduced, permits the tympanitic guttural pouch to communicate with the healthy pouch by creating a fistula in the medial septum. An indwelling mushroom catheter should be inserted for a few days after surgery, to drain off the serous effusion that develops following this procedure.

---

*Malecot reinforced tip catheter, Bardex self-retaining drain, C. R. Bard, Inc., Murray Hill, NJ

In the case of bilateral tympany, long-term catheterization can be tried. Alternatively, a nasopharyngeal fistula into both guttural pouches can be created at the pharyngeal recess. Transendoscopic electrosurgery can be used to make the initial cuts or the fistula can be made by forcing a large uterine catheter through the pharyngeal recess. A mushroom catheter should be inserted through the new opening until the fistula is formed. The foal does not appear to suffer any discomfort as a result of having the auditive tube in free communication with the nasopharynx.

If aspiration pneumonia is present, it should be treated. Although continued dysphagia will be eliminated by prevention of further tympany, postural drainage and antibiotic therapy are indicated. Fluid in the lungs of the newborn foal can be drained by physically lowering the head and raising the hindquarters. Older foals should be encouraged to graze or eat at ground level.

Another surgical approach involves the "flap technique." In this technique, a membranous fold that lies on the floor of the pharyngeal opening of the auditive tube is trimmed away. It is likely that the fold resected is part of the normal anatomy—that it is the ventrolateral membranous lamina. The result of this operation is uncertain; anything less than a fairly complete removal of the membrane may fail to relieve the tympany. The operative site is difficult to approach, and for a unilateral tympany I prefer the simpler fenestration procedure.

PROGNOSIS AND PREVENTION

Without treatment tympany is permanent and emphysema is progressive. Remissions may occur but these are not permanent. With treatment the tympany can be eliminated, although the emphysema persists. In the absence of tympany the emphysema may be of no significance and so the prognosis is fair to good. Nevertheless, few long-term follow-up reports on how treated foals perform as adults have been published. It is questionable whether a Thoroughbred foal treated for guttural pouch tympany will ever develop into a top racehorse. If the disease is complicated by aspiration pneumonia, the outlook is guarded.

Until the cause is known, guttural pouch tympany cannot be prevented. There is some evidence that this is a familial disease.

GUTTURAL POUCH EMPYEMA

This condition is also known as pus in the guttural pouch, guttural pouch chondroids, and septic diverticulitis of the auditive tube. The word empyema implies that the normal air sac has been converted into an abscess cavity. Pus forms, fails to drain, stagnates, and eventually becomes inspissated. In most cases both the lateral and the medial compartments of the guttural pouch are filled with liquid or inspissated pus. I believe this condition is the true empyema, as opposed to a condition of the guttural pouch in which some mucus or fluid pus is present but the air space predominates. These latter cases are mostly infections secondary to a general infection of the whole of the respiratory tract, or complications of a tympanitic guttural pouch.

Guttural pouch empyema is uncommon and no sex incidence has been noted. The disease, which may be unilateral or bilateral, is more common in ponies than horses and in the older age groups rather than the younger.

ETIOLOGY AND PATHOGENESIS

Guttural pouch empyema is an end-stage disease. It may be secondary to abscess formation in the retropharyngeal lymph nodes; the inflammatory response causes a temporary closure of the pharyngeal opening of the auditive tube and establishes a self-perpetuating situation. Other cases may be caused by a congenital stenosis of the pharyngeal opening or an acquired stenosis from some inflammatory reaction. Empyema is also a complication of gunshot wounds or other foreign bodies, and an apparent sequel to fractures of the stylohyoid bone. Empyema of the lateral compartment may be secondary to abscess formation in the parotid lymph nodes, which lie within the substance of the parotid salivary gland.

If liquid pus is trapped in the guttural pouch for a period of time, it dries and becomes inspissated. The consistency of inspissated pus resembles dry cottage cheese. Over the passage of months or years the constant movement of the head molds this dry material into ovoid calculi, known as chondroids. An affected pouch may contain 30 or more chondroids, some quite large and others the size of small beans.

CLINICAL SIGNS AND DIAGNOSIS

Accumulated pus in the guttural pouch produces a parotid swelling. The swelling is not as large as with guttural pouch tympany, does not fluctuate, and is not resonant on percussion. Animals with guttural pouch empyema may show signs of airway obstruction on inspiration at exercise or at rest. If the swelling is large enough there may be some dysphagia, with coughing during attempts to eat and the return of food via mouth and nostrils. The dysphagia might also be caused by an accompanying pharyngitis. However, the presence of such a clinical sign needs to be interpreted with caution because, occasionally, guttural pouch empyema of long standing can also damage the pharyngeal plexus of nerves and result in pharyngeal paralysis.

Ponies or horses with guttural pouch empyema have a chronic, often malodorous nasal discharge that may be unilateral or bilateral, depending on the distribution of the condition. Nasal discharge from this disease is not noticeably exaggerated when the head is lowered, although this opinion has been frequently expressed in the past. Such a sign is much more characteristic of chronic bronchitis or some other pulmonary disease. The parotid swelling is doughlike in consistency and the head may be held stretched out, as though the horse is in discomfort. The linguofacial vein may be engorged and the area of Viborg's triangle tense and convex. Affected animals may retain good bodily condition or they may lose weight. Although it might be expected that the disease would be frequently accompanied by signs of middle ear disease, these are uncommon.

The signs and history are often highly suggestive of guttural pouch empyema. On physical examination, the dorsal landmarks of the larynx (the muscular process of the arytenoids and the caudal edges of the cricoid cartilage) are often obscured by chronic inflammatory swelling around the retropharyngeal lymph nodes. Endoscopy reveals a septic discharge from the affected auditive tube, and the roof of the nasopharynx is convex on the diseased side. The swelling in the roof and lateral wall of the nasopharynx may obscure a view of the ipsilateral arytenoid cartilage. Introduction of the endoscope into the affected guttural pouch may be difficult because of submucosal swelling or stenosis of the pharyngeal opening of the auditive tube. Even if one is successful in entering the guttural pouch, the chances are that nothing will be seen, as the air space is obliterated and pus covers the optics and light source of the endoscope. Lateral radiographs may reveal the complete absence of an air shadow in the guttural pouch. If chondroids are present, it is sometimes possible to recognize their shadows on the radiograph. When the retained pus is still liquid and it does not entirely fill the cavity, a fluid level will be seen. Ideally an otoscopic examination of the external ear, including the eardrum, should be part of the diagnostic work-up of these cases.

TREATMENT

The basis of treatment is removal of pus from the diverticulum and reestablishment of normal patency of the auditive tube. Drainage of a chronic abscess cavity is the prime need. An indwelling catheter coupled with daily irrigation of the abscess cavity is likely to be unsatisfactory if the pus is inspissated. Pus does not seem to liquefy again with irrigation. Inspissated pus acts like a foreign body and has to be removed under general anesthesia via a surgical opening in the cavity. I prefer a lateral approach to the pouch, ventral to the linguofacial vein. Compared with a ventral approach this is less likely to result in an iatrogenic postoperative pharyngeal paralysis. The pouch should be opened just wide enough to admit a long-handled spoon. Once the solid material has been removed, the pharyngeal opening of the auditive tube should be explored for patency and an indwelling mushroom catheter inserted via the nostril. Drainage into the nostril is encouraged rather than perpetuating drainage via the surgical wound, as the latter procedure may promote nerve damage. Postoperatively, irrigation should be carried out using not more than 30 ml of saline at a time, to avoid the danger of inhalation pneumonia. If a mushroom catheter is left in place for several weeks, this will generally ensure continued patency of the auditive tube once it is removed. Any concurrent sepsis of the middle and external ear should be treated.

There is generally no need to treat animals that have secondary catarrhal inflammation or secondary sepsis of the guttural pouch. These conditions will usually regress spontaneously when the primary condition has cleared up, especially if postural drainage can be encouraged. Fluid is not retained in the pouch, and on a lateral view radiograph, no fluid level is seen. Under these conditions irrigation of the guttural pouch is not necessary.

PROGNOSIS AND PREVENTION

The prognosis should be guarded but, if there is no pharyngeal paralysis, the outcome of surgery for guttural pouch empyema can be satisfactory. For the safety of other horses, the pus should be cultured to determine whether or not the infection is *Streptococcus equi*.

A reduction in the incidence of strangles by improved hygiene may have led to a similar reduction for guttural pouch empyema. When sepsis of the retropharyngeal lymph nodes is diagnosed, it may be better to let the abscesses mature naturally and rupture rather than risk aborting this process by giving antibiotics. Certainly, use of antibiotics at subtherapeutic doses for short periods seems to encourage chronic sepsis and tumefaction of the lymph nodes. In the face of a known retropharyngeal abscess, a better preventive measure would be to insert a mushroom catheter via the nostrils into each guttural pouch.

GUTTURAL POUCH MYCOSIS

This disease, also called guttural pouch diphtheria and gutturomycosis, is characterized by the presence of a mycelium. The mycelium grows on the mucosa of the pouch and subsequently invades submucosal tissues. Guttural pouch mycosis is the most common disease of the guttural pouch among horses admitted to teaching hospitals. However, a full-time equine practitioner may expect to see only one affected horse every two or three years.

There appears to be no particular breed or sex incidence, with occurrence in ponies as well as horses. It is encountered occasionally in foals, but more commonly it is seen in mature horses of any age. The disease is predominantly unilateral and sporadic and occurs over a wide geographic area. It has been observed only in stabled horses, less commonly in North America than in Europe, and has been infrequently reported from Australia. By the time clinical signs appear, the horse may have had the disease for several months.

ETIOLOGY AND PATHOGENESIS

The most commonly identified fungus is *Aspergillus nidulans*. The mycelium commonly originates in the roof of the medial compartment of the guttural pouch. It occurs on the mucosa overlying the bulla tympanica, at the point of articulation of the stylohyoid bone with the petrous temporal bone, on the dorsal third of the stylohyoid bone, and in the condyloid fossa. Because the guttural pouch mucosa lies directly over bone in these areas, it is colored yellow in a healthy guttural pouch. Once growth starts, the mycelium spreads in all directions. Rarely, a mycelium grows in the lateral compartment of the mucosa overlying the distal section of the external carotid artery, but it seldom originates at this site. The mycelium invades the submucosal nerves and blood vessels and causes a variety of neuropathies and vascular abnormalities. An intensive submucosal fibrous proliferation stimulated by the mycelium seems to result in deposition of new bone so that fusion of the stylohyoid and petrous temporal bones is not uncommon. Finally, as a sequel to this fusion, pathologic fractures of the petrous temporal bone can occur, leading to a new series of clinical signs associated with vestibular disturbance, facial paralysis, and dysphagia.

The majority of horses develop the mycelium in relation to the distal section of the internal carotid artery. Stenosis, followed by poststenotic aneurysm formation, is common. A few horses develop similar aneurysms on the external carotid artery. Even smaller numbers of horses have an aneurysm on the posterior auricular artery, which also courses around the lateral wall of the guttural pouch. The presence of numerous nerve trunks in the dorsal and caudal wall of the medial compartment of the guttural pouch explains why the disease so often causes cranial nerve damage. A horse with this disease may die of hemorrhage, of dysphagia followed by complete inability to swallow and inanition, or of aspiration pneumonia.

Guttural pouch mycosis probably is an opportunistic infection and some pre-existing circumstance provides the right environment for fungal growth. The guttural pouch is dark, warm, and humid, with minimal ventilation—factors favoring fungal growth. Generous exposure to spores occurs by housing horses in badly ventilated barns and feeding them spore-ridden hay in the warm damp climates of Europe and North America. However, some factor or factors in addition to these must be required for mycelium formation, otherwise this disease would occur in the majority of domesticated horses. It is necessary to understand why the mycelium is, anatomically, so specific in its point of origin.

The narrow equine auditive tube narrows even more at its tympanic opening. At this point it is a complete tube rather than a gutter and no more than 2 mm in diameter. Even when healthy, this is essentially a capillary space. Inflammation of the tubal mucosa, as part of an upper respiratory infection, may block the tympanic opening leading to absorption of air from the tympanic cavity of the middle ear and development of a negative pressure, followed by secretory otitis media. This sequence of events, beginning as a temporary obstruction of the tympanic opening, could produce a serous transudate from the middle ear into the guttural pouch. The serum would tend to lie on the mucosa in the roof of the medial compartment and would provide an ideal culture medium for the fungal spores constantly present in the horse's guttural pouch. The mycelium would form in the guttural pouch on and around the tympanic opening of the auditive tube, i.e., in exactly the area recognized as the predilection site for guttural pouch mycosis. This pathogenesis would explain, for example, why guttural pouch mycosis occurs as an apparent sequel to strangles in both the foal and the adult horse.

CLINICAL SIGNS

The disease can be asymptomatic. The presenting sign varies but it is often spontaneous epistaxis in a resting horse. Once this has occurred, however, many owners will report that the horse has had a unilateral catarrhal nasal discharge for several weeks. The episodes of nosebleeding are not generally precipitated by exercise and therefore differ from the common pulmonary hemorrhage of the racehorse. The amount of blood lost varies from just a trickle to several liters. A horse may survive two or three hemorrhages before suffering one that is fatal. For a few days after each hemorrhage, there is a mucosanguinous discharge at one nostril. Occasionally the parotid region is swollen because of blood accumulating in the pouch or in the extravascular spaces alongside the pouch, but this is the exception rather than the rule. However, extravasation of blood around the nerve trunks undoubtedly adds to the danger of nerve damage, and during the hemorrhages neurologic signs may be exaggerated. These signs include dysphagia, with regurgitation of food at one or both nostrils and reflux of water during drinking, Horner's syndrome, laryngeal hemiplegia, occasional and transient episodes of abdominal pain, facial nerve paresis, unilateral muscle atrophy of the tongue, head tilt, head shaking, ataxia, and nystagmus. Table 1 shows the neurologic signs correlated with the cranial nerves responsible.

It would be unusual for all the clinical signs to be present in any one case. Each affected horse usually shows three or four clinical signs. Potentially misleading cases are those involving ocular problems similar to periodic ophthalmia, and those in which epistaxis is not seen. The most common clinical signs are unilateral nasal catarrh, epistaxis, and pharyngeal paralysis.

DIAGNOSIS

The clinical history and signs are often characteristic of the disease. Physical examination supports the diagnosis if there is a pain reflex to digital palpation below the conchal cartilage on the diseased side, or evidence of an otitis externa. At pharyngoscopy there may be a catarrhal or mucosanguinous discharge into the nasopharynx from the auditive tube. If the problem is long-standing, the medial lamina of the pharyngeal opening may be eroded. Ipsilateral hemiplegia or pharyngeal paralysis may be evident—for example, dorsal displacement of the soft palate and food material in the nasopharynx or glottis.

The diagnosis is confirmed endoscopically, by showing the typical rough-surfaced diphtheritic lesion in one of the guttural pouches. Healthy mucosa is smooth and shiny. The presence of a mycelium can be shown histologically on a biopsy sample of the diphtheritic membrane collected transendoscopically. However, this is not strictly necessary. In some recovered horses, a cicatrized mucosa may

be present in the predilection site for the disease or there may be a thickening of the dorsal end of the stylohyoid bone. Survey radiographs are not normally necessary for diagnostic purposes but can provide useful information about secondary deposition of bone. Angiography of the carotid tree, however, is advisable in order to discover whether an aneurysm is present, as this affects prognosis and treatment. Angiography is done under general anesthesia and, if an aneurysm is present, ligation of the affected artery is carried out concurrently.

It follows from the hypothesis on etiology that the health of the tympanic cavity should be investigated in horses with guttural pouch mycosis. While the horse is anesthetized for angiography, an otoscopic examination of the eardrum should be carried out. Unfortunately, specialized endoscopic equipment necessary for the examination is not generally available. The external diameter of the endoscope should be not more than 4 mm and preferably less.

TREATMENT

In the absence of an aneurysm, the prime objective of treatment is to ventilate the affected pouch. This eliminates the predisposing factors and treats the mycelium, fresh air being a safe and effective fungicide. To promote maximum air exchange, a self-retaining mushroom-tipped catheter should be inserted in the diverticulum, using the largest bore available. In an adult Thoroughbred the proximal end of a 25 cm catheter lies just inside the nostril and, at each inspiration, air will be drawn into the auditory tube diverticulum. To ensure that the air is fresh the horse should be turned out, day and night, in a paddock. If housing is unavoidable, the horse should be maintained on dust-free stable management. The same precautions are necessary as recommended for the management of allergic bronchitis ("heaves"). Preferably the stall should be isolated and not one of several in a barn where other horses are kept under more traditional conditions. If fresh air ventilation of the diseased pouch

TABLE 1. NEUROLOGIC SIGNS OF GUTTURAL POUCH MYCOSIS

Clinical Signs	Affected Cranial Nerves
Dysphagia; dorsal displacement of soft palate; pain in region of atlanto-occipital joint and ventral to ear conchal cartilage	IX, X, XI
Horner's syndrome—i.e., ptosis, vasodilation of turbinate region causing nasal obstruction; patchy unilateral sweating especially around base of ear and more rarely, meiosis	Cervical sympathetic
Laryngeal paresis; abdominal pain	X
Paralysis of ear, eyelid, muzzle, lower lip	VII
Corneal opacity	V
Unilateral atrophy of tongue	XII
Head tilt, ataxia, abnormal head position, head shaking, nystagmus	VIII

is ensured, no topical or systemic fungicidal therapy is necessary.

Systemic fungicidal therapy is not justified. If topical treatment is employed, the irrigating fluid should be mild, nonirritant, and small in quantity. The medication must not irritate the already-damaged submucosal tissues and exposed nerves. Pharyngeal paralysis has been initiated by use of strong iodine solutions, hydrogen peroxide and disinfectants, even in guttural pouches with intact mucosa. Copious irrigation also involves the risk of causing an aspiration pneumonia. An acceptable protocol is infusion of a dilute povidone-iodine solution twice a day. The irrigating fluid should be made by taking a stock solution containing 0.5 per cent titratable iodine and diluting this with saline to produce a 1 per cent solution of the stock. During the infusion the horse's chin should be held high. Immediately after, with the head still in the raised position, the larynx should be gently balloted dorsally to splash the iodine solution onto the mycelium in the roof of the cavity. An alternative is to deliver the fungicidal solution into the guttural pouch by a nebulizer.

Management of secondary complications such as anemia and various effects of nerve paresis should be symptomatic. There is no cure for any cranial nerve damage if the paralysis is complete; however, some horses will either accommodate to or recover from a partial pharyngeal paralysis. Horner's syndrome may also regress in time. Horses that show dysphagia should graze and be encouraged to keep their heads down while eating or drinking. Aspiration pneumonia is a real danger. If given hay at ground level, the horse will simply drop its head momentarily to grasp a wisp and will then chew with its head raised. As there is a considerable time lag between onset of aspiration pneumonia and evidence of clinical signs, bronchoscopy is advisable for early detection of inhalation problems in horses with dysphagia.

If the arteriograms indicate that the horse already has an aneurysm, then the affected branch, generally the internal carotid artery, should be ligated on the cardiac side of the lesion. The surgery is an aseptic procedure and does not involve opening the guttural pouch. This technique is preferred to the insertion of a balloon catheter into the artery. Although it was originally thought that an internal carotid artery, when ligated on the cardiac side of the lesion only, represented a continuing hazard because of retrograde hemorrhage from the circle of Willis, this has not been the case. Proximal ligation probably reduces the arterial blood pressure and, if the horse lives for a few days postoperatively,

a thrombus fills the aneurysm and eliminates the likelihood of further arterial hemorrhages. There is possibly some risk of venous hemorrhage while an active mycelium is still present but this is not life-threatening.

PROGNOSIS

The future for a horse with no history of epistaxis, no signs of nerve damage, and no vascular changes is obviously far better than for a horse with these changes. The time to diagnose the disease is when the only clinical sign is a unilateral but persistent nasal catarrh. A horse showing one or more signs of Horner's syndrome has the next best prognosis. Dysphagia justifies a poor prognosis. If a horse is incapable of swallowing, even for a short period, this alone poses an immense management problem. However, if a horse with dysphagia has no pneumonia and can feed itself and maintain bodily condition, then it may be worth waiting six months for recovery. An aneurysm represents the danger of fatal hemorrhage until the offending vessel is ligated, after which the outlook is much improved. No horses I have seen have regained normal laryngeal movement once the recurrent laryngeal nerve has been damaged. Hypoglossal paralysis is also permanent. Many horses have recovered from what proved to be transient attacks of facial paralysis, vertigo, ataxia, torticollis, and headshaking.

Supplemental Readings

Colles, C., and Cook, W. R.: Carotid and cerebral angiography in the horse. Vet. Rec., *113*:483, 1983.

Cook, W. R.: Observations on the aetiology of epistaxis and cranial nerve paralysis in the horse. Vet. Rec., *78*:396, 1966.

Cook, W. R.: Clinical observations on the anatomy and physiology of the equine upper respiratory tract. Vet. Rec., *79*:440, 1966.

Cook, W. R.: The clinical features of guttural pouch mycosis in the horse. Vet. Rec., *83*:336, 1968.

Cook, W. R., Campbell, R. S. F., and Dawson, C.: The pathology and aetiology of guttural pouch mycosis in the horse. Vet. Rec., *83*:422, 1968.

Cook, W. R.: Diseases of the ear, nose and throat in the horse: Part I: The ear. *In* Grunsell, C. S. G. (ed.): Veterinary Annual, Vol 12. Bristol, John Wright, 1971, pp. 12–43.

Cook, W. R.: The auditory tube diverticulum (guttural pouch) in the horse: Its radiographic examination. J. Am. Vet. Rad. Soc., *14*:51, 1973.

Freeman, D. E., and Donawick, W. J.: Occlusion of internal carotid artery in the horse by means of a balloon-tipped catheter. Clinical use of a method to prevent epistaxis caused by guttural pouch mycosis. J. Am. Vet. Med. Assoc., *176*:236, 1980.

Heffron, C. J., and Baker, G. J.: Endoscopic observations on the deglutition reflex in the horse. Equine Vet. J., *11*:137, 1979.

Recurrent Urticaria
Due to Inhaled Allergens

Anne G. Evans, MENLO PARK, CALIFORNIA

Recurrent urticaria in the horse can be a frustrating diagnostic and therapeutic challenge. Inhaled allergens, in addition to drugs, ingested materials, and insect bites, must be included in the differential diagnosis of an urticarial eruption in the horse.

PATHOGENESIS AND CLINICAL SIGNS

It is theorized that a type I hypersensitivity reaction occurs when a sensitized horse is re-exposed to an inhaled allergen. The allergen bridges specific IgE antibodies fixed to the surface of tissue mast cells. The mast cells degranulate, releasing histamine and other pharmacologic mediators that in turn cause an acute urticarial reaction. The allergen(s) responsible for inhalant-induced urticaria may be found indoors (e.g., molds, feathers from roosting birds), outdoors (e.g., pollens), or in aerosolized feedstuffs.

Recurrent urticaria can be a cutaneous manifestation of inhalant allergies. An urticarial eruption involves the formation of multiple wheals that pit with pressure and range from 1 to 10 cm in diameter. The lesions tend to involve the cervical and craniolateral thorax, although they may become generalized. The horse may or may not be pruritic. Hair loss is not usually a feature of urticaria unless there has been serum leakage to the surface. An urticarial eruption that is due to inhaled allergens typically occurs within 12 to 24 hours after exposure to the inhalant(s) and resolves within 12 to 24 hours after exposure to the offending inhalant(s) ceases. Although the case numbers are too small to determine statistical significance, Arabians and Thoroughbreds appear to be predisposed to recurrent urticaria from inhaled allergens, with the onset occurring between 18 months and four years of age. There is no apparent gender predilection.

DIAGNOSIS

In the horse, the more commonly recognized causes of urticaria, other than inhaled allergens, include drugs and ingestants. Although insect bites are commonly incriminated, they are rarely a cause of urticaria in the horse.

HISTORY

The importance of obtaining accurate historical information cannot be overemphasized, since urticaria may result from several different allergic reactions. Important questions to be answered include:

1. Is this a steroid-responsive dermatosis? That is, do the lesions rapidly resolve with an anti-inflammatory dose of corticosteroids? A positive answer suggests an allergic etiology. If the lesions either slowly resolve or do not resolve, then other nodular diseases should be considered.

619

2. Does the occurrence of clinical signs correlate with administration of systemic or topical medications? A positive answer suggests a diagnosis of drug allergy.

3. Does the frequent application of fly repellents (twice or three times daily) result in resolution of the clinical signs? A positive answer suggests a diagnosis of insect bite hypersensitivity.

4. Does the occurrence of signs correlate with changes in feed? Feed exclusion trials may be necessary to answer this question. A positive answer suggests a diagnosis of ingestant allergy or inhalant allergy to feedstuffs. A negative answer rules out a diagnosis of ingestant allergy but does not rule out recurrent urticaria due to inhaled feed materials, because feeds present in other areas of a barn or paddock may be aerosolized and thus be inhaled by the affected horse. Since ingestants may persist within the horse for extended periods of time, a feed trial should be carried out for a minimum of four weeks. Ideally a feed trial restricted to oat hay should be performed and if no improvement is seen it should be followed by a feed trial restricted to alfalfa hay.

5. Is there clinical resolution within 12 to 24 hours after moving the horse from a stable to a paddock? A positive answer suggests recurrent urticaria due to inhaled molds or feather down of roosting birds.

6. Does clinical resolution occur with changes in season or within 12 to 24 hours after transportation to a region with different vegetation? A positive answer suggests a diagnosis of recurrent urticaria from inhaled pollens.

BIOPSY

Characteristic wheals that pit on pressure usually indicate a clinical diagnosis of urticaria. A biopsy of a lesion preserved in 10 per cent buffered formalin and submitted to a veterinary dermatohistopathologist may lend support to a clinical diagnosis. Typical histologic changes include an eosinophilic perivascular inflammatory infiltrate in the deep as well as the superficial dermis. Dermal edema may or may not be recognized histologically. There are few if any epidermal changes. Although these histologic findings are not helpful in determining the cause of the urticaria, they serve an important role in helping to rule out other nodular disease.

INTRADERMAL SKIN TESTING

Intradermal skin testing is the most definitive method for identifying an allergic inhalant basis for recurrent urticaria and defining the offending allergen(s). To perform the test an area approximately 20 cm by 30 cm on the lateral cervical region is clipped with a No. 40 blade. I test with 57 different *aqueous* (i.e., nonglycerinated) allergen extracts in addition to a positive (1:100,000 histamine) and a negative (saline) control (Table 1). Each allergen is

diluted to a concentration of 1000 protein nitrogen units (PNU) per ml. Mixed grain dust, which produces an irritant rather than an allergic reaction at 1000 PNU per ml, is diluted to 125 PNU per ml. The patient is sedated with 200 mg xylazine intravenously immediately before the test. Approximately 0.1 ml of each allergen is injected intradermally, in addition to the saline and histamine controls, and the subsequent local reactions are evaluated at 30 minutes, four hours, and 24 hours after injection. Saline is graded $0+$ and histamine is graded $4+$. All remaining reactions are graded relative to these controls. The size of the wheal and the steepness of its margins are taken into account when grading the reactions. A reaction greater than or equal to $2+$ is considered to be positive. In my

TABLE 1. ALLERGENS* USED FOR INTRADERMAL SKIN TESTING IN CALIFORNIA

Controls	Cultivated Farm Plants
Saline	Corn
Histamine (1:100,000)	Oat
Inhalants	Wheat
Cottonseed	Mustard
Mixed feathers (chicken,	Dusts
duck, goose)	Mixed grain
Pigeon feathers†	Smut Mixes
Tobacco	Grain smut mix
Pollens	Special Molds—Rusts
Red alder	Oat stem rust
White birch	Wheat stem rust
American elm	Molds
Fremont cottonwood	Penicillium mix
California live oak	Aspergillus mix
3 maple mix	Fusarium mix
Western sycamore	Mucor mix
Black willow	Rhizopus mix
Chinese elm	Monilia mix
Red cedar	*Alternaria tenuis*
Olive	*Curvularia spicifera*
California black walnut	*Pullaria pullans*
Arizona ash	*Cladosporium herborum*
Eucalyptus	
Red mulberry	
Box elder	
Acacia	
Almond†	
English walnut	
California black oak	
Arizona cypress†	
Monterey pine†	
Grass	
8 grass mix	
Bermuda	
Johnson grass	
Weeds	
Dandelion	
Western ragweed	
English plantain	
Russian thistle	
Sage mix	
Yellow dock	
Lambs quarter	
Red sheep sorrel	
Rough ragweed	

*Greer Laboratories, Inc., Lenoir, CA
†Hollister-Stier, West Haven, CT

experience, most reactions occur at 30 minutes after injection, are fading by 4 hours and have resolved by 24 hours.

A positive reaction does not necessarily mean that the patient has a clinical allergy to the injected allergen. Instead, a positive reaction indicates that the patient has skin-sensitizing IgE antibody to the allergen. Horses without clinical signs relating to allergy may have positive skin tests. This re-emphasizes the importance of accurate historical information to confirm the diagnosis of recurrent urticaria caused by inhaled allergens. False-negative intradermal skin tests may be caused by many factors. The most important is use of corticosteroids, antihistamines, or phenothiazine tranquilizers before testing. A horse that is to be skin tested should not have received phenothiazine tranquilizers for 72 hours before testing, antihistamines for three weeks before testing, and corticosteroids for a five-week period before testing.

THERAPY

ENVIRONMENTAL

Avoiding exposure to the allergen(s), if possible, results in rapid resolution of clinical signs. The horse should be kept in an open-air paddock if molds or feathers commonly found in barn are the allergens. If pollens are incriminated, the horse should be stabled in an area free from the offending vegetation and protected from winds that carry pollens, although often these environmental changes alone are insufficient. Since pollens can be airborne for hundreds of miles, successful avoidance may require transportation some distance to an entirely new habitat. If the allergens are aerosolized feeds, changing feeds, providing pelleted feeds, and thoroughly soaking hay in water before feeding are beneficial.

MEDICAL

A variety of medical therapies have been tried. Corticosteroids are most commonly employed. For a 450-kg horse, 400 to 600 mg of prednisone or prednisolone is given orally every morning until remission of clinical signs. The dose is then gradually decreased over a period of weeks to the lowest possible daily dose that will keep the clinical signs from recurring. The regimen is then altered so that twice the daily maintenance dose is given on alternate mornings. An attempt may be made to further decrease this alternate morning dose. Ideally, the urticaria should be controlled with 200 to 300 mg every other morning. Short-acting oral corticosteroids such as prednisone and prednisolone are preferable to dexamethasone or triamcinolone as they are less immunosuppressive and less likely to produce laminitis. Other agents that have been tried with minimal benefits include diethylcarbamazine, levamisole, and antihistamines.

TABLE 2. HYPOSENSITIZATION SCHEDULE

Day	Amount	Dosage
Vial 1–200 PNU/ml		
0	0.1 cc	20 PNU
2	0.2 cc	40
4	0.4 cc	80
6	0.8 cc	160
8	1.0 cc	200
Vial 2–2000 PNU/ml		
10	0.1 cc	200 PNU
12	0.2 cc	400
14	0.4 cc	800
16	0.8 cc	1,600
18	1.0 cc	2,000
Vial 3–20,000 PNU/ml		
20	0.1 cc	2,000 PNU
22	0.2 cc	4,000
24	0.4 cc	8,000
26	0.8 cc	16,000
28	1.0 cc	20,000
48	1.0 cc	"
68	1.0 cc	"
—*	1.0 cc	"
—*	1.0 cc	"
—*	1.0 cc	"
—*	1.0 cc	"

*Interval determined by clinical response of patient.

HYPOSENSITIZATION

Hyposensitization shows promise for the management of recurrent urticaria due to inhaled allergens. Selection of allergens to be used for hyposensitization is based on the grade of their skin test reaction in addition to historical information suggesting exposure of the horse to the allergen. A maximum of 10 aqueous allergen extracts are selected. The extracts are combined in a sterile vial to yield a concentration of 20,000 PNU per ml. Two serial dilutions are made to produce solutions of 2,000 PNU per ml and 200 PNU per ml. The initial dose is 20 PNU (0.1 ml of the 200 PNU per ml solution) administered subcutaneously. Subsequent doses are gradually increased as indicated in Table 2 over a 48-day period to a maintenance level of 20,000 PNU administered subcutaneously every 10 to 20 days. The dosage and frequency of the maintenance injections are varied on the basis of each patient's clinical response. Hyposensitization is continued throughout the horse's life.

Supplemental Readings

Halliwell, R. E., Fleischman, J. B., Mackay-Smith, M., Beech, J., and Gunson, D. E.: The role of allergy in chronic pulmonary disease of horses. J. Am. Vet. Med. Assoc., *174*:277, 1979.

Moschella, S. L.: Dermatology. Philadelphia, W. B. Saunders Company, 1975, pp. 228–233.

Nesbitt, G. H., Kedan, G. S., and Caciolo, P.: Canine atopy. Part II, Management. Comp. Cont. Ed., *6*:264, 1984.

Tizard, I. A.: Type I hypersensitivity: Allergies and anaphylaxis. *In* An Introduction to Veterinary Immunology, 2nd ed. Philadelphia, W. B. Saunders Company, 1982, pp. 258–275.

Ectoparasites

Valerie A. Fadok, GAINESVILLE, FLORIDA

Ectoparasites are an important and common cause of dermatitis in the horse. Two of the most common parasitic diseases, *Culicoides* hypersensitivity (p. 624) and onchocerciasis (p. 627), have been covered in other chapters. This chapter will cover biting flies, lice, ticks, chiggers, straw itch mites, and mange. The topic was also covered extensively on page 529 of the first edition of this book.

BITING FLIES

Horses are attacked by a variety of flies that cause annoyance and discomfort and whose bites may result in allergic reactions. Stable flies (*Stomoxys calcitrans*) in large numbers can attack horses. The bites are painful and bleed easily. The stable fly has vicious mouth parts that tear the skin, allowing them to feed on blood and tissue fluids. Horses can develop multiple papules and wheals. These may evolve into crusts on the back, chests, legs, and neck. These lesions may be caused by the irritating and toxic components of the saliva or may represent arthropod hypersensitivity. The stable fly is the intermediate host for *Habronema microstoma,* the larvae of which cause cutaneous habronemiasis, or "summer sores." Diagnosis of stable fly attack is made by physical examination; the diagnosis is indicated by improvement with stabling during the day, as stable flies are daytime feeders. Treatment involves the frequent application of fly repellents to the horse and good stable management. Insecticides containing synergized pyrethrins with repellents can be applied daily. One such product* is marketed with claimed residual activity of 14 days. Stable flies breed in decaying vegetation and manure; frequent cleaning of stalls and removal of soiled bedding and manure from the barn and surrounding areas are helpful.

Black flies (*Simulium*) are daytime feeders attacking sparsely haired areas on horses. Lesions are crusted papules that are pruritic. Alopecia, excoriations, and lichenification can result from self-mutilation. Lesions are seen in the intermandibular area, the pectoral area, the axillae, the ventral midline, and the inguinal area. These flies will also attack the ears, causing alopecia and crusting from self-trauma. Diagnosis can be made by physical examination and is indicated by response to stabling during the day. Intradermal skin testing with black fly extracts has shown positive reactions in some

but not all horses with this distribution of lesions. In the southeastern United States, *Culicoides* hypersensitivity may have a similar distribution; horses may be hypersensitive to both flies. Treatment involves stabling during the day, frequent application of insecticides and repellants, and corticosteroids if necessary to decrease pruritus (see *Culicoides* hypersensitivity, p. 624).

Horn flies (*Haematobia irritans*) cause a syndrome of focal ventral midline dermatitis in horses. This is a seasonal pruritic dermatitis characterized by one to many foci of alopecia, erythema, depigmentation, scaling, crusting, and excoriation centered on the umbilical area. The mouth parts of the horn fly tear the skin, so considerable physical damage results. The role of hypersensitivity is not known. Diagnosis is made by physical examination. This disease must be differentiated from the more diffuse ventral midline diseases caused by *Culicoides,* black flies, and onchocerciasis. Treatment involves clipping and cleansing the affected areas with a mild antiseptic and applying an antibiotic-corticosteroid cream to reduce inflammation. Fly repellents in a gel or ointment base provide a chemical and physical barrier against further bites.

Horse flies (*Tabanus, Hybomitra*) and deer flies (*Chrysops*) inflict painful bites on horses, which can result in large wheals. Control is difficult owing to the feeding habits and robust nature of these flies. Heavy and frequent applications of synergized pyrethrins with repellents may give some relief. These flies require water for breeding and egg deposition; therefore, drainage of breeding grounds or moving horses away from breeding areas may be helpful.

LICE

Horses can become infested with both biting (*Damalinia equi*) and sucking (*Haematopinus asini*) lice. In northern climates, clinical signs become apparent during the winter months when animals congregate for warmth, have longer coats, and are stressed by cold. In southern climates, lice can be seen year round. The primary sign is pruritus, as evidenced by alopecia, erythema, and excoriations. Infested horses may be restless and have a poor appetite. The coat is dull and scaly. Lice are host-specific and spend their entire life cycle on the host. They are transmitted by direct contact and through fomites such as brushes and tack. Diagnosis is made by physical examination and demonstration of adults and eggs (nits) cemented to the hairs. A

---

*McCullough-Cartwright, Inc., Barrington, IL

flashlight will facilitate examination in dark barns; the coat and skin require meticulous examination. Treatment involves at least two applications of insecticide sprays, dips, or powders at two-week intervals. Alternatively, ivermectin can be given orally at 200 μg per kg twice at two-week intervals. Studies in the bovine have shown that ivermectin is apparently effective against biting as well as sucking lice.

TICKS

A variety of ticks can parasitize horses. The spinose ear tick, *Otobius megnini*, affects the ear canal of horses. This is a soft-shell argasid tick, and only the larvae and nymphs are parasitic. The hard shell ixodid ticks that can affect the ear canal of the horse include the tropical horse tick, *Dermacentor nitens*, the Gulf coast tick, *Amblyomma maculatum*, and the lone star tick, *Amblyomma americanum*. Clinical signs include head shaking, ear rubbing, and the development of secondary bacterial otitis. Diagnosis is made by otoscopic examination, which usually requires sedation. Therapy involves insecticides applied to the ear canal; antibiotic-corticosteroid medications are indicated if bacterial infection is present.

A variety of ixodid ticks can infest the bodies of horses, resulting in reactions ranging from erythematous macules and papules that develop crusts to large nodules or "pseudolymphomas." Some species, such as *Ixodes*, have extremely long and tenacious mouth parts, making the tick difficult to remove. Diagnosis of tick infestation is by examination. Treatment involves use of dips and sprays. No effective repellent for ticks is available.

CHIGGERS

Horses may become infested with chiggers (harvest mites) during the summer and fall. Infestations are seen in pastured horses or those ridden through infested fields and woods. Lesions consist of papules that become crusted; they are distributed on the face, neck, chest, and extremities. Pruritus is variable. Diagnosis is based on clinical findings and supportive history. Early in the course of the disease the larvae may be present as small orange dots in the center of papules. Skin scrapings at this stage will enable identification of the larvae by microscopy. Treatment of chiggers is not usually necessary as the disease is self-limiting. The adults and nymphs are free-living and the larvae normally parasitize small rodents.

STRAW ITCH MITES

Straw itch mites (*Pyemotes tritici*) have been reported to infest horses. These mites normally parasitize the larvae of grain insects; however, when their natural food supply is reduced, they will infest man and animals. Lesions are nonpruritic papules that develop crusts. The source of infestation is contaminated hay or feed. Humans infested with these mites develop intensely pruritic papules and vesicles, and severe infestation can lead to systemic signs resembling anaphylaxis. Diagnosis is based on history, clinical signs, and finding the source of the mite. Treatment is not necessary, as the infestation is self-limiting. Straw itch mite infestation may be clinically similar to chigger infestation; history should help differentiate the two.

MANGE

Sarcoptic, psoroptic, chorioptic, and demodectic (p. 626) mange are infrequently seen in horses.

Clinical signs associated with sarcoptic mange, caused by *Sarcoptes scabiei* var. *equi*, are papules and vesicles. Alopecia, excoriations, crusts, scales, and lichenification can develop because of extreme pruritus. Lesions initially begin around the head and neck, then progress to cover the entire body. The horse may develop secondary bacterial infections and become systemically ill. Diagnosis is made by multiple skin scrapings; however, negative scrapes do not rule it out. Sarcoptic mange is contagious and readily transmissible to humans; it is a reportable disease.

Psoroptic mange, caused by *Psoroptes equi*, first presents with alopecia and papules at the base of the mane and tail and under the fetlock. Self-mutilation results in erosions, crusts, scales, and lichenification. Psoroptic mites in horses can cause pruritic otitis externa as the only clinical sign. Diagnosis is made by skin scrapings and ear swabs. These mites tend to be host specific and therefore do not affect man. Psoroptic mange is a reportable disease; it has been reported recently in cattle from the Midwest but has not been identified in horses as a generalized disease for several years.

Chorioptic mange, caused by *Chorioptes equi*, is also known as foot or leg mange. Alopecia, erythema, excoriations, and crusts occur on the pasterns and fetlocks. This disease is extremely pruritic; continued inflammation and self-mutilation cause lichenification and fissures. The disease can progress up the legs to involve the abdomen. Diagnosis is made by multiple skin scrapings. Chorioptic mange is one of the differential diagnoses for the syndrome "grease heel." The key feature for chorioptic mange is extreme pruritus. The disease has been seen sporadically in recent years in draft horses.

Treatment of sarcoptic, psoroptic, and chorioptic mange traditionally has involved the use of parasiticidal dips and sprays based on recommendations from state and federal authorities. Ivermectin has been shown to be effective against these mites in cattle; presumably, ivermectin could be used in horses at 200 µg per kg. The dosage may have to be repeated in two weeks, particularly if the paste is used, as blood levels persist for eight to ten days only. These mites generally have a life cycle of two to three weeks.

Supplemental Readings

Fadok, V. A.: Dermatologic diseases of horses. Part I. Parasitic dermatoses of the horse. Comp. Cont. Ed. Pract. Vet., 5:S615, 1983.
Fadok, V. A.: Parasitic skin diseases of large animals. Vet. Clin. North Am., 6:3, 1984.
Kunkle, G. A., and Greiner, E. C.: Dermatitis in horses and man caused by the straw itch mite. J. Am. Vet. Med. Assoc., 181:467, 1982.
McMullan, W. C.: The skin. In Mansmann, R. A., McAllister, E. S., and Pratt, P. W. (eds.): Equine Medicine and Surgery, 3rd ed., Vol. II. Santa Barbara, CA, American Veterinary Publications, 1982, pp. 789–843.

Culicoides Hypersensitivity

Valerie A. Fadok, GAINESVILLE, FLORIDA

A syndrome characterized by mane and tail rubbing has been recognized in horses throughout the world; common names include summer itch, muck itch, sweet itch, summer eczema, dhobie itch, kasen, and summer fungus, a misnomer because fungal organisms are not involved in the pathogenesis. Affected horses have allergic reactions to the bites of Culicoides insects, also known as "punkies," "no-see-ums," sand flies, and biting midges. By correlating the species of Culicoides feeding on horses with the development of pruritus on specific body regions and at particular times of the year, the individual species causing the dermatitis in specific geographic areas has been identified. The Culicoides species associated with equine dermatitis varies among different geographic areas; therefore, data cannot be extrapolated from country to country. Unfortunately, these studies have not been performed and published to date for pruritic horses in the United States.

There are over one hundred species of Culicoides in the United States. Each species has a characteristic habitat and preferred host for obtaining blood meals. In general, Culicoides breed in standing water—suitable habitats can include lakes, marshes, swamps, and irrigation canals, as well as water collecting in forks of trees, on the ground, and in watering troughs that are not cleaned regularly.

The pathogenesis of insect hypersensitivity is complex. The saliva of the biting flies contains many proteins that could be antigenic. Immediate hypersensitivity (type I hypersensitivity) mediated by reagin (IgE) very likely plays a role in Culicoides hypersensitivity, as intradermal skin testing with Culicoides extracts results in wheal formation within 20 minutes. This sensitivity can be passively transferred to normal horses by intradermal injection of serum from allergic horses (passive cutaneous anaphylaxis). The reactivity of the serum is destroyed by heat, suggesting an antibody very similar to IgE. The role of delayed hypersensitivity, as well as intermediate reactions such as cutaneous basophil hypersensitivity, needs further exploration.

HISTORY AND CLINICAL SIGNS

Clinical signs of Culicoides hypersensitivity are pruritus, alopecia, excoriations, crusts, and scaling. Bacteria can invade the traumatized skin, increasing the degree of exudation and crust formation. The classic body regions involved are the face, ears, mane, withers, rump, and tail. The severity of the disease is variable, ranging from slightly broken mane and tail hairs with scaling to severely eroded skin with lichenification, crusting, and scar formation. Affected horses may spend most of the day rubbing against trees, fences, and stalls. The entire dorsal midline may be involved in some horses. Some pruritic horses may also have lesions in the pectoral, ventral midline, inguinal, and lower limb regions. This distribution of lesions has been attributed to hypersensitivity to black flies. These horses may demonstrate variations of Culicoides hypersensitivity caused by species feeding in these areas, or they may have multiple insect hypersensitivities. Results of intradermal skin testing with extracts of Culicoides, mosquito, black fly, and horse fly suggest that both situations may occur.

Although seasonal at first, the dermatitis may

increase in severity and duration as the horse ages. Pruritus is usually noted during the fly season, which will vary in length depending on geographic location. Certainly affected horses in the southeastern United States suffer from almost year-round pruritus due to the lack of cold weather. Affected horses are usually three years or older; however, I have seen the disease in some yearlings and two-year-olds. Although in Britain and Denmark ponies are most commonly affected, many breeds of horses have been affected in the United States, including the Shetland pony, the Arabian horse, the Quarterhorse, the Thoroughbred, the Morgan, the Saddlebred, and many crossbreeds.

Factors influencing host response to arthropods are complex and can include host production of repellent pheromones as well as individual immunologic responses. There is some suggestion that the tendency to develop Culicoides hypersensitivity may be inherited, as the offspring of affected mares and stallions will often show clinical signs. I have seen this tendency particularly in Arabians and Quarterhorses; however, these breeds may be most frequently presented in Florida for problems that affect their appearance. The interaction of hereditary predisposition with degree of exposure to the insects needs to be explored. It is possible that high insect density and long insect seasons could be related to an increased prevalence of hypersensitivity.

Culicoides hypersensitivity, while not life-threatening, can be debilitating economically to the owner. Often, the discomfort and disfiguration associated with the disease prevents the animal from being used for show or riding. Affected horses are often sold for less than their worth. The possible hereditary implications can cause financial losses by removing valuable animals from a breeding program. These factors, coupled with the cost of topical and systemic therapy, are discouraging to owners.

DIAGNOSIS

The diagnosis of Culicoides hypersensitivity is made by correlating the historical findings of seasonal pruritus with the physical evidence of self-mutilation, particularly in the mane and tail. Histopathology of skin biopsies can lend support. The findings associated with arthropod hypersensitivity include superficial and deep eosinophilic and lymphocytic perivascular dermatitis. Epidermal changes can include acanthosis, hyperkeratosis, and crust formation. This pattern can be modified by aging of the lesion and erosions secondary to self-trauma. This pattern is *not* diagnostic for Culicoides hypersensitivity, as many arthropods can cause the same reaction.

Development of intradermal skin testing to explore and clarify pruritic dermatoses of the horse is recent. Preliminary results would suggest that some horses with mane and tail rubbing have positive reactions to multiple insects. The importance of these reactions to the etiology of equine pruritus has yet to be determined. Culicoides antigen is not commercially available as of this writing, but extracts of mosquito, horse fly, and black fly can be purchased.

Differential Diagnosis

Culicoides hypersensitivity is the most commonly recognized cause of mane and tail rubbing. Other insects may also play a role. Infestation with lice can cause generalized pruritus, as can infestation with stick-tight fleas. Pinworms (*Oxyuris equi*) cause pruritus restricted to the tail only. Psoroptic mange, although very rare, can cause pruritus of the dorsal midline. Food allergies have been diagnosed in horses and may involve generalized pruritus, with or without the development of urticaria. Pruritic ventral midline dermatitis can be caused by ventrally feeding Culicoides, horn flies, black flies, or onchocerciasis (p. 627). The latter is easily ruled out by treatment with ivermectin, which cures the disease.

TREATMENT

Treatment of Culicoides hypersensitivity involves reduction of insect exposure and concomitant use of anti-inflammatory medication, if necessary. Depending on geographic and climatic area, reduction of exposure to Culicoides may be difficult. Culicoides cannot fly long distances; estimates have included one quarter to one half mile. If possible, horses can be moved from close proximity to ponds, lakes, or irrigation canals to decrease exposure. In the northeastern United States where Culicoides can breed in small pockets of standing water in forests, moving horses to an open area at least one half mile from the trees may help. Water troughs or barrels should be inspected for algae or other signs that water stands for long periods. Frequent cleansing of water troughs will reduce the likelihood of their being used as breeding sites.

Since Culicoides feed primarily at dusk, night, and dawn, stabling horses during this time will reduce exposure. Stabling will be effective only if the barn can be closed. Barns with open stalls and alleys will not prevent the flies from attacking. Stalls can be screened with fine mesh, as ordinary screening will allow these tiny insects to pass through. Combinations of screening and frequent insecticide application to the screens has been helpful. Some owners have found that the installation of ceiling fans reduces exposure because Culicoides cannot fly well in brisk breezes.

Insecticide and repellents applied to the horse are a necessary part of disease control. Unfortunately, many of the insecticides and repellents sold for use on horses do not effectively repel Culicoides. The most useful products are those containing pyrethrins with synergists and repellents, which can be used on a daily basis. Examples include Equine Repellent Lotion* and Equi-shield Fly Repellent spray and gel.† These products are aesthetic and can be used daily. The Equi-shield gel is particularly effective in focal areas such as ears, base of the mane, and tail base. These products should be applied daily in the afternoon, before insect feeding begins. Many horse owners have reported success using a commercial bath oil‡ diluted 50:50 with water and applied as a wipe. This product also repels mosquitoes and Culicoides in humans; the effective ingredient is not known. A newly synergized pyrethrin and repellent spray has been formulated with 14-day residual activity.§ Personal experiences with the product suggest that duration of efficacy varies, but it is worth trying in those horses that cannot be sprayed daily.

Additional topical therapy can include once to twice weekly shampoos with tar or tar and sulfur shampoos. Many owners report that frequent bathing not only decreases scale and crust but also seems to decrease pruritus. Corticosteroid therapy may be required in horses that are exquisitely sensitive or when exposure to insects cannot be reduced effectively. Prednisone or prednisolone can be given at 1 mg per kg daily for seven to ten days then slowly decreased to the lowest dosage given on alternate days that will keep the animal comfortable. It is not unusual for some horses to require 400 to 500 mg every other day to keep pruritus controlled. This medication is acceptable to the horse; the tablets can be mixed with sweet feed. Possible side effects of steroids in the horse can include laminitis and altered mentation (hyperexcitability or placidity), but these seem rare.

---

*Adams Veterinary Research Laboratories, Inc., Miami, FL
†Carson Chemicals Inc., Newcastle, IN
‡"Skin-So-Soft" Bath Oil, Avon Products, Inc., New York, NY
§McCullough-Cartwright Corporation, Barrington, IL

Supplemental Readings

Baker, K.P., and Quinn, P.J.: A report on clinical aspects and histopathology of sweet itch. Equine Vet. J., *10*:243, 1978.
McMullan, W.C.: Allergic dermatitis in the equine. Southwest Vet., *24*:121, 1971.
Nelson, W.A., Bell, J.F., Clifford, C.M., and Keirans, J.E.: Interaction of ectoparasites and their hosts. J. Med. Ent., *13*: 389, 1977.
Quinn, P.J., Baker, K.P., and Morrow, A.N.: Sweet itch: Responses of clinically normal and affected horses to intradermal challenge with extracts of biting insects. Equine Vet. J., *15*:266, 1983.
Riek, R.F.: Studies on allergic dermatitis (Queensland itch) of the horse: The aetiology of the disease. Aust. J. Agric. Res., *5*:109, 1954.

Demodicosis

Danny W. Scott, ITHACA, NEW YORK

ETIOLOGY AND PATHOGENESIS

Demodicosis (demodectic mange, follicular mange) is a rare follicular dermatosis of horses. Demodectic mites are commonly found in small numbers as commensals of normal horse skin. The mites live in hair follicles and sebaceous glands, are host-specific, and complete their entire life cycle on the host. The life cycle of most demodicids has not been carefully studied but is assumed to be completed in 20 to 35 days. Horses possess two species of demodectic mites: *Demodex caballi* and *D. equi*. The former is long, has a thin body, and is found in the meibomian glands of the eyelids and in the pilosebaceous apparatus of the skin of the muzzle. *D. equi* is a short, plump parasite found in the pilosebaceous apparatus of the rest of the skin.

Under most environmental conditions, demodicids can survive only several minutes to a couple of days off the host. Studies in cattle and dogs have shown that: (1) demodectic mites are acquired during the first two to three days of life by direct contact with the dam, (2) animals delivered by cesarean section and raised away from other animals do not harbor demodectic mites, and (3) confining normal adult animals with severely infested and diseased animals for several months did not produce disease in the normal animals. In addition, attempts to transmit clinical demodicosis to horses by direct contact and by applying mites to the skin were unsuccessful. Thus, demodicosis is *not* thought to be a contagious disease in most instances.

Because demodectic mites are normal residents of the skin, it is likely that animals manifesting clinical disease from this parasite are in some manner immunocompromised. Demodicosis in dogs is known to occur as a result of immunosuppression by drugs and diseases and as a result of genetic predilection for selective immunodeficiency. In horses, many authors have theorized that clinical demodicosis probably occurs only in animals that are immunocompromised by concurrent disease, poor nutrition, or stress. Demodicosis has been reported in horses in association with chronic systemic glucocorticoid therapy.

CLINICAL SIGNS AND DIAGNOSIS

Equine demodicosis is worldwide but rare in occurrence and has no apparent age, breed, or sex predilections. Clinical signs consist of patchy alopecia and scaling, especially over the face, neck, shoulders, and forelimbs. A papulopustular eruption associated with variable pruritus may be seen.

The differential diagnosis includes other follicular dermatoses: staphylococcal folliculitis, dermatophytosis, and dermatophilosis. Definitive diagnosis is based on skin scrapings or skin biopsy or both. Skin lesions should be squeezed firmly and scraped deeply until blood is drawn. As an occasional demodectic mite may be seen in the skin scrapings from normal horses, large numbers of mites must be removed from lesions before diagnosis of demodicosis is made. Skin biopsy reveals hair follicles distended to varying degrees with demodectic mites and keratin. In addition, varying degrees of perifolliculitis, folliculitis, furunculosis, and foreign body granuloma formation may be seen.

Once the diagnosis of demodicosis is made, the clinician must carefully consider the possible roles of genetic predilection and endogenous and exogenous immunosuppression in the disease process.

MANAGEMENT

Because demodicosis is usually asymptomatic, may spontaneously regress, and has been refractory to most therapeutic agents and regimens, treatment is not usually attempted. Amitraz, currently used to treat demodicosis in dogs, appears to be an unacceptable acaricide for use in horses. Horses sprayed with 0.025 per cent amitraz developed somnolence, depression, ataxia, muscular weakness, and progressive large intestinal impaction beginning within 24 to 48 hours of treatment.

Considering the difficulties associated with treatment and the probable importance of genetic predilection in disease susceptibility, it may be best to cull severely affected animals and not use affected animals for breeding stock.

Supplemental Readings

Auer, D. E., Seawright, A. A., Pollitt, C. C., and Williams, S. G.: Illness in horses following spraying with amitraz. Aust. Vet. J., 61:247, 1984.
Bennison, J. C.: Demodicosis of horses with particular reference to equine members of the genus Demodex. J. Roy. Army Vet. Corps, 14:34, 1943.
Hopes, R.: Skin diseases in horses. Vet. Dermatol. News, 1:4, 1976.
Scott, D. W., and White, K. K.: Demodicosis associated with systemic glucocorticoid therapy in two horses. Equine Pract., 5:31, 1983.
Thomsett, L. R.: Skin diseases of the horse. In Practice, 1:15, 1979.

Cutaneous Onchocerciasis

Carol S. Foil, BATON ROUGE, LOUISIANA

Equine cutaneous onchocerciasis has been a difficult disease to define, the prevalence of *Onchocerca cervicalis* infection being much higher than the prevalence of cutaneous manifestations. This is one of the features of the disease that has led to the assumption that dermatologic signs develop in association with a hypersensitivity response, perhaps to dying microfilariae. The overlap of the clinical signs of onchocerciasis with hypersensitivity to various species of biting midges (Culicoides spp.), possibly including the vector of *O. cervicalis,* has led to confusion. The multifactorial etiology of seasonal ventral midline dermatitis has likewise contributed to confusion about the role of *O. cervicalis*

infection in that syndrome. Fortunately, the recent introduction of a drug (ivermectin) that is highly effective in the destruction of microfilariae and the demonstration that the skin disease resolves with administration of the drug will allow clinicians and researchers to better define the contribution of Onchocerca infection to equine skin diseases.

LIFE CYCLE

Onchocerca cervicalis is a long-lived filarid parasite of equids having a world-wide distribution and a high prevalence (Table 1). The adult worms reside

TABLE 1. REPORTED PREVALENCE OF *ONCHOCERCA CERVICALIS* INFECTIONS IN EQUIDS IN VARIOUS GEOGRAPHIC AREAS

Locale	Prevalence (%)
Eastern US	67
Midwestern US	77
Kentucky	52
US Gulf coast*	76
Louisiana	82
Texas	76
Western US	48
Northwestern US	26
Western Canada	12
Quebec	74
England	13
Japan	76
Australia	80

*Ponies.

in the ligamentum nuchae, while microfilariae reside in the skin and are responsible for cutaneous pathology. The vectors, *Culicoides variipennis, C. nubeculosus,* and perhaps other species of Culicoides, are obligate intermediate hosts. Microfilariae are produced in large numbers by mature females. The route of microfilarial migration to the dermis is thought to be through the subcutaneous tissue rather than by vessels. The microfilaria are ingested by the vector and undergo development and growth into the third-stage larvae (L_3) in approximately two weeks. The L_3 are introduced into the final hosts by breaking out of the vector mouth parts and entering the lesion caused by the feeding fly.

Microfilariae are not evenly distributed in the skin of infected horses. The highest numbers accumulate on the ventral midline around the umbilicus. High numbers are also found in the pectoral region, the withers, the skin of the medial upper thigh, and in the eyelids. Microfilaria are also unevenly distributed within the microscopic structures of the dermis. They have been reported to occur in nests or pockets and to have a seasonal variation in their distribution in the depth of the dermis. There may also be a seasonal variation in total numbers found in the skin.

PATHOGENESIS AND PATHOLOGY

The skin lesions in equine onchocerciasis are thought to represent hypersensitivity to microfilaria. Many horses harbor the parasites while manifesting no cutaneous disease, and neither the presence nor the severity of dermatitis is correlated to numbers of organisms present. The clinical signs are ameliorated by anti-inflammatory drugs as well as elimination of the organisms, but killing by

parasiticidal agents causes a temporary severe exacerbation of cutaneous disease in some patients.

Onchocerciasis can cause acute and chronic inflammation. The acute inflammation is mild to severe perivascular and periadnexal mononuclear and eosinophilic dermatitis. Proliferation of fibroblasts is characteristic. Fibrosis, including cicatricial alopecia, and depigmentation are characteristic of the chronic disease.

CLINICAL SIGNS

Cutaneous onchocerciasis is rare in horses less than two years old and is most common in horses older than five years. The disease is seasonal in some locales and nonseasonal in others. Skin lesions include alopecia, multifocal and coalescing crusting and shallow ulceration, scaling, macular depigmentation, and scarring. Pruritus varies from mild to severe, in which case excoriation of accessible affected skin may be seen.

The dermatitis involves characteristic parts of the body with the ventral midline being most commonly affected. The forehead (as opposed to the sides of the face) is characteristically involved, and the withers, pectoral area, and proximal limbs may be affected in severe cases. In distinction to Culicoides hypersensitivity dermatitis, the ears and the tailhead are not affected.

Horn flies (*Haematobia irritans*) are particularly prone to accumulate and feed on affected denuded skin. This may exacerbate and prolong the skin disease caused by onchocerciasis when flies are present in high numbers.

DIAGNOSIS

Demonstration of cutaneous microfilariae suggests, but does not prove, that they are the cause of skin disease. Several methods have been described for extraction of organisms from biopsy specimens obtained from the umbilical region. A simple extraction technique involves placing a coarsely minced punch biopsy in a small amount (1 to 3 ml) of normal saline in a covered Petri dish. The saline is examined microscopically after incubation at 37° C for 6 to 24 hours. Since some affected horses have low numbers of microfilariae, the 24-hour examination should be performed when earlier examinations have been negative.

Microfilariae can be demonstrated in histopathologic sections, although care must be taken to examine specimens closely when their numbers are low. Unfortunately, histopathologic changes in onchocerciasis are not specific. Presently, the most reliable diagnostic method for equine onchocerciasis is assessment of response to therapy. Ivermectin has been shown to be 100 per cent effective for temporary resolution of inflammatory disease within three weeks of treatment. Exacerbation of cutaneous disease for 24 to 72 hours after treatment is another supportive finding. Of course, scaling, scarring alopecia, and depigmentation do not resolve as quickly as inflammation.

Care should be taken to rule out dermatophytosis and infestation with sarcoptiform mites, as they may coexist with onchocerciasis and the latter will also respond to ivermectin treatment. Also, the presence of large numbers of horn flies may depress and delay the clinical response to therapy, so horses should be protected from horn flies for assessment of response.

THERAPY

There is no agent effective against adult *Onchocerca cervicalis,* and the long life span of these parasites (five years) dictates that microfilaricidal therapy must be administered repeatedly. Three drugs have been recommended for microfilarial treatment: diethylcarbamazine (DEC),* levamisole HCl,† and ivermectin.‡

Ivermectin oral paste is the treatment of choice. When administered at 0.2 mg per kg, it is 100 per cent effective within two to three weeks. Relapse of dermatitis after treatment is associated with the return of microfilariae to the skin and may occur two to nine months after therapy. Minor adverse reactions may occur in up to 25 per cent of horses after the use of ivermectin. The most common problem is ventral midline edema or pruritus or both within a few hours of administration. The reaction caused by death of microfilariae may be severe and be associated with limb edema, eyelid edema, or fever. Severe cases may be treated with short-acting corticosteroids (prednisone 0.5 mg per kg) or nonsteroidal anti-inflammatory drugs, but there is no good evidence that this hastens the resolution of the reaction, which subsides in 48 to 72 hours. It is probably not indicated to routinely pretreat with corticosteroids. Most horses do not experience adverse reactions on subsequent treatments with ivermectin when the drug is adminis-

tered regularly. Some evidence indicates that the ventral midline reaction is seen more often in horses (with or without dermatitis) with high microfilaria counts and in horses more than 10 years old. The presence or absence of dermatitis in horses with Onchocerca infection probably does not have any predictive value for this adverse reaction.

The more serious and occasionally fatal problem of clostridial abscess at the site of injection of ivermectin has been obviated by the introduction of the paste formulation. Neurologic reactions (mydriasis, ataxia, depression) are rare in horses and are generally associated with overdose. Signs of colic are occasionally reported.

Prior to the introduction of ivermectin, the drug of choice for cutaneous onchocerciasis was DEC. Ground tablets or liquid, mixed in sweet feed, is given daily at a dose of 1 mg per kg administered in 21-day cycles or continuously throughout the spring and summer. Ventral midline edema and pruritus are seen at the outset of therapy in many patients. Three to seven days of prednisone (0.5 mg per kg) or nonsteroidal anti-inflammatory drugs (NSAIDs) have been recommended to treat this problem. Diethylcarbamazine is not 100 per cent effective and relapses occur much more rapidly than after ivermectin therapy. It is a very safe drug, however.

Levamisole has been used in cutaneous onchocerciasis, especially in cases nonresponsive to DEC. It is administered mixed with syrup or peanut butter in sweet feed at 10 mg per kg daily for seven days along with prednisone or NSAID. Accurate dosing is important because the therapeutic index for this drug is not good. Side effects include the previously described ventral midline edema, sweating, colic, sound sensitivity, and head pressing.

Supplemental Readings

Anderson, R. R.: The use of ivermectin in horses: Research and clinical observations. Comp. Cont. Ed., 5:S516, 1984.

Fadok, V. A. and Mullowney, P. C.: Dermatologic diseases of horses. Part I. Parasitic dermatoses of the horse. Comp. Cont. Ed. 5:S615, 1983.

Herd, R. P., and Donham, J. C.: Efficacy of ivermectin against *Onchocerca cervicalis* microfilarial dermatitis in horses. Am. J. Vet. Res., 44:1102, 1983.

Karns, P. A., and Luther, D. G.: A survey of adverse effects associated with ivermectin use in Louisiana horses. J. Am. Vet. Med. Assoc., 185:782, 1984.

McMullan, W. C.: Onchocercal filariasis. Southwest Vet., 25:179, 1972.

Pascoe, R. R.: Equine dermatoses. Vet. Rev., No. 22. The University of Sydney Post-graduate Foundation in Veterinary Science, Sydney, 1981.

---

*Dirocide, Squibb, Princeton, NJ
†Levasole, Pitman-Moore, Washington Crossing, NJ
‡Eqvalan Paste 1.87%, MSD/AGVET, Rahway, NJ

Dermatophilosis

Vicki J. Scheidt, RALEIGH, NORTH CAROLINA

David H. Lloyd, LONDON, ENGLAND

Dermatophilosis is a moist, exudative dermatitis of horses and many other species caused by the actinomycetes *Dermatophilus congolensis.* Commonly referred to as "rain scald," lesions appear as tufts of matted hair and crusts over the dorsal aspects of the shoulders and back.

EPIDEMIOLOGY

Dermatophilosis occurs worldwide. It affects a wide variety of animal species and is particularly severe in regions of Africa and Australia. In humid tropical regions of Africa, serious losses in cattle have been reported.

Dermatophilosis is most prevalent during periods of heavy prolonged rainfall, primarily in the fall and winter. The zoospores of *D. congolensis* are released into the environment once activated by moisture. Under normal conditions, the stratum corneum is an effective barrier against invasion by the organism. With prolonged wetting, the outer layers of the skin are more susceptible to external trauma by such environmental factors as grooming tools and ectoparasites. Such abrasions or draining wounds provide an ideal environment for *D. congolensis,* especially when excessive weeping and moisture are present. Changes in atmospheric temperature and humidity are not directly associated with an increased susceptibility to infection. However, localized infections in profusely sweating horses may spread and become generalized. In most cases, dermatophilosis is self-limiting provided all inciting factors such as wetness, trauma, and insects have been eliminated.

The exact origin of the disease remains unknown. Transmission of the organism following contact with "reservoir" or contaminated fomites has been reported. Although isolation of the organism from the soil has not been documented, *D. congolensis* can persist in crusts or scabs from infected animals for 42 months. As a result, a contaminated farm may remain infected for years and have repeated outbreaks within a herd. Likewise, mechanical transmissions by the stable fly (*Stomoxys calcitrans*) and the housefly (*Musca domestica*) may contribute to enzootic infections on certain farms.

PATHOGENESIS

A degree of natural immunity to dermatophilosis exists in all domesticated animals and is felt to have a hereditary basis. Natural protection against dermatophilosis is dependent on the structure of the skin, nature of the hair coat, and inherent ability of the host to mount a rapid immune response to the organisms.

The underlying factors responsible for the severity of dermatophilosis in certain regions of the world remains obscure. Investigators have been unable to reproduce the severe generalized form that occurs naturally. Factors such as biting insects, environmental conditions, and concurrent disease play a significant role in lowering skin resistance and potentiating the infectious nature of the organism. Recent studies in cattle have shown that both the intact stratum corneum and the composition of the lipid film are important barriers to infection. The hair coat provides some additional protection to the epidermal and lipid barrier. Protection is directly related to the hair type, density, and length.

Penetration of the stratum corneum and invasion into the living epidermis by *D. congolensis* induces an acute inflammatory response primarily composed of neutrophils. As the disease progresses, the organism is unable to penetrate the neutrophilic barrier and is subsequently removed during re-epithelization and scab formation. Healing depends on prior exposure and the presence of both a high serum antibody titer and delayed type hypersensitivity. Although the antibody does not directly kill zoospores, it does enhance neutrophilic phagocytosis.

CLINICAL SIGNS

The appearance of *D. congolensis* infection varies, depending on the length of hair, age, and environment of the horse. Long-haired horses develop large plaques of matted hair and crusts, which tend to become more exudative in the later stages of the disease. Removal of scabs reveals a moist gray to pink indurated surface, similar in appearance to ringworm. Lesions may be painful but are rarely pruritic. Secondary infection with staphylococci, streptococci, or corynebacterium may develop in chronic cases.

In short-haired horses, lesions are smaller and occur as multifocal bumps covered with crusts or scale. These lesions are more readily palpated than visualized and vary in size from 1 to 2.5 mm. Examination of tufts of hair plucked from a nodular lesion reveals the typical scab of dermatophilosis adherent to the roots of the hair. Lesions commonly occur on the muzzle, distal extremities, around the eyes, and along the back. A similar distribution is observed in foals confined to wet stalls and yards. White-skinned areas are more sensitive to infection than dark areas.

Another form of the disease occurs in racing horses and horses grazing on flooded creeks or streams. Horses in training frequently develop abrasions as a result of track cinders striking the cranial surface of the hindlegs. These abrasions are ideal sites of infection by the organism. Numerous small scabs adherent to the base of hair follicles develop from the hocks to the coronet band. With excessive exudation, fissures and cracks may occur along the pastern and fetlocks, resulting in acute lameness.

DIAGNOSIS

In the acute stage of the disease, the organism is easily isolated and identified on impression smears made from the surface of an exudative lesion or the underside of a scab or crust. *D. congolensis* appears as branching mycelia or rows of coccoid bodies having a "railroad track–like" appearance when stained with new methylene blue, Giemsa, or Gram stain. In the late or chronic stages, dermatophilus may appear as fragmented filaments or chains of coccoid bodies. Impression smears from such lesions are commonly contaminated with secondary bacterial organisms, such as staphylococci.

D. congolensis can be isolated from acute lesions by culturing on blood agar. The organism does not grow on Sabouraud's medium or phenyl red indicator media. In chronic or secondarily contaminated cases, the following culture technique is recommended. Scabs from such lesions are placed in a 5 ml bijou screwtop bottle and moistened with approximately 1 ml of distilled water. Initially, bottles are incubated uncapped at room temperature for three and one half hours, and later for an additional 15 minutes in 20 per cent carbon dioxide. Using a bacteriologic loop, a final sample is collected and plated on 5 per cent ox blood agar and grown at 37° C in 20 per cent carbon dioxide for 24 to 48 hours. Small hemolytic brown colonies, which have a rough texture, are observed. Impression smears made from the colony growth confirm a diagnosis of *D. congolensis*.

TREATMENT

Successful treatment of *D. congolensis* infection in horses depends on elimination of the predisposing factors. Therefore, all affected animals should be confined in dry areas and kept out of the rain and wet pastures. Provided that the rainy season is

not prolonged, the disease is usually self-limiting within three to four weeks.

Loose crusts and scabs should be removed and the hair in the affected areas clipped. When scab removal is difficult or painful, lesions should be softened initially with either povidone-iodine soaks or a chlorhexidine solution. All scab material, hair, and crust should be adequately removed from the premises and the environment disinfected to prevent further reinfection.

Dermatophilosis is highly sensitive to most antibacterial agents and in mild cases only topical antiseptic therapy is needed. A 2 to 5 per cent lime sulfur solution, 3 per cent captan, or povidone-iodine can be applied as a spray or dip to the entire body and are very effective. Daily application is recommended for the first five to seven days and continued weekly until clinical remission is achieved. Other reportedly effective topical treatments include a 1 per cent potash alum, 1 per cent gentian violet in alcohol, 5 per cent salicylic acid and alcohol or copper sulfate (30 gm in 1 gallon of water).

Localized, superficial lesions respond well to a daily application of a 0.25 per cent aqueous chloramphenicol solution for five to seven days. Infections of nonpigmented areas such as the muzzle or lower extremities commonly crack or fissure, resulting in severe pain or lameness. Such dry, hard lesions respond best to a combined antibiotic-steroid cream such as a neomycin sulfate and hydrocortisone preparation. To reduce the secondary swelling and inflammation associated with an eczematous infection of the lower extremity, an astringent such as white lotion (20 gm zinc sulfate and 30 gm lead acetate in 50 ml water) can be applied daily for five days.

Horses with infections of the pastern and fetlock should be confined in stables with dry bedding. Bandages over these areas should be monitored closely, as wet bandages exacerbate the infection and cause further spread.

In severe or generalized cases, systemic antibiotics are recommended. A combination of penicillin (10,000 iu per kg) and streptomycin (10 mg per kg) given intramuscularly for three to five days is a common and highly effective treatment. Other antibiotics such as oxytetracycline used at normal therapeutic levels daily for three to five days have also been reported as an effective treatment.

Supplemental Readings

Kaplan, W., and Johnston, W. J.: Equine dermatophilosis (cutaneous streptotrichosis) in Georgia. J. Am. Vet. Med. Assoc., *149*:1162, 1966.
Lloyd, D. H.: Immunology of dermatophilosis: Recent developments and prospects for control. Prev. Vet. Med. 2:93, 1984.
McMullan, W. C.: The Skin. In Mansmann, R. A., McAllister,

E. S., and Pratt, P. W. (eds.): Equine Medicine and Surgery. Santa Barbara, CA, American Veterinary Publications, 1982.

Mullowney, P. C., and Fadok, V. A.: Dermatologic diseases of horses: Part II. Bacterial and viral skin diseases. Comp. Cont. Ed., 6:16, 1984.

Pascoe, R. R.: Further observations on dermatophilus infections in horses. Aust. Vet. J., 48:32, 1972.

Pascoe, R. R.: Dermatophilosis. In Robinson, N. E. (ed.):

Current Therapy in Equine Medicine. Philadelphia, W. B. Saunders Company, 1983.

Richards, J. L., and Pier, A. C.: Transmission of *Dermatophilus congolensis* by *Stomoxys calcitrans* and *Musca domestica*. Am. J. Vet. Res., 27:419, 1966.

Scanlan, C. M., Garrett, P. D., and Geiger, D.B.: *Dermatophilus congolensis* infection of cattle and sheep. Comp. Cont. Ed., 6:4, 1984.

Photosensitivity

Stephen D. White, NORTH GRAFTON, MASSACHUSETTS

Photosensitivity is an abnormal reaction of the skin when exposed to light. Photosensitivity in the horse is usually caused by a photodynamic agent in or on the skin that absorbs energy from light and transfers it to body cells. The activating light is usually in the ultraviolet A range (320 to 400 nm). Melanin in the skin screens ultraviolet light, thereby limiting photosensitivity reactions to the white and lightly pigmented areas of the body.

Photodynamic agents are either exogenous or endogenous. Exogenous agents may be ingested feedstuffs, contact photosensitizers found in certain plants, and drugs. A partial list of plants containing photodynamic agents is given in Table 1. The major endogenous agent in the horse is phylloerythrin, a porphyrin produced by bacterial degradation of chlorophyll in the intestine. Some phylloerythrin is normally absorbed into the portal circulation, removed by the liver, and excreted in the bile. In liver disease, the hepatic excretion of phylloerythrin is decreased. The subsequent excessive levels in the peripheral circulation eventually reach the skin, causing photosensitivity in approximately 25 per cent of horses with hepatic dysfunction. One of the most common causes of liver disease leading to elevated levels of phylloerythrin is the ingestion of plants containing pyrrolizidine alkaloids (Table 2). Other less common etiologies of liver disease to be considered are hepatotoxic drugs and biliary obstruction due to cholangiohepatitis or biliary calculi (see p. 112).

There are also plant species associated with photosensitization whose mechanisms of action are not understood (Table 3). Contact as well as ingested photodynamic agents may be involved.

Sunburn is a normal reaction of skin to excessive exposure to sunlight, especially in the ultraviolet B range (290 to 320 nm). Excessive exposure depends on both duration and pigmentation, and in the horse is usually seen in the white or lightly-pigmented animal.

Diagnosis of the etiology of photosensitivity is crucial for proper therapy and prognosis.

HISTORY AND CLINICAL SIGNS

Feedstuffs, environment, and drug exposure are the three important facets of the clinical history in cases of suspected photosensitivity. Ingested plants and feed should be noted and collected for future analysis. Environmental considerations include the type of pasture (or other material) with which the animal is in contact, the amount of time the animal is exposed to sunlight, any seasonality of the condition, and any other horses involved. A seasonal incidence would tend to negate liver disease; multiple horse involvement should arouse suspicion of an ingested or contact photosensitizer. A thorough history of recent drug therapy should be obtained. Oral, parenteral, and topical drugs may all cause photosensitivity. Although phenothiazine is often given as an example of drug-induced photosensitivity, the actual incidence is uncommon in the horse.

Physical examination usually reveals lesions limited to the hairless, white, or lightly pigmented

TABLE 1. PLANTS CONTAINING PHOTODYNAMIC AGENTS

Common Name	Scientific Name	Agent
St. Johnswort	*Hypericum perforatum*	hypericin
buckwheat	*Polygonum fagopyrum*	fagopyrin
perennial rye grass	*Lolium perenne*	perloline
whiteheads	*Spheociadium capitellatum*	unknown

TABLE 2. PLANTS CONTAINING PYRROLIZIDINE ALKALOIDS

Common Name	Scientific Name
common groundsel	*Senecio vulgaris*
ragwort, stinking Willie	*Senecio jacobaea*
tarweed	*Amsinckia intermedia*
rattleweed	*Crotalaria* spp
Salvation Jane	*Echium lycopsis*

TABLE 3. PLANTS CAUSING PHOTOSENSITIZATION THROUGH UNKNOWN MECHANISMS

Common Name	Scientific Name
rape	*Brassica rapa*
burr trefoil	*Medicago denticulata*
alfalfa	*Medicago sativa*
Alsike clover	*Trifolium hybridium*
lamb's tongue	*Erodium moschatum*

area of the skin. Initially the involved skin is erythematous, swollen, and often pruritic. The lesions may progress to serum exudation, thickening, fissuring, and in severe cases necrosis and sloughing. All of the nonpigmented areas will usually be involved in cases caused by ingested photodynamic agents, hepatic disease, or systemic drug administration. Involvement limited to the nonpigmented areas of the distal extremities and muzzle is suggestive of a contact photosensitizer, especially in the pasture, although occasionally hepatic disease may have this pattern. Sunburn will usually affect the dorsal and facial white areas. Unilateral or bizarre patterns of photosensitization are indicative of drug-induced photosensitization, especially topical therapy.

DIAGNOSIS AND THERAPY

Analysis of the feed, evaluation of liver function, and investigation of the environment are the most important diagnostic tools. Feed analysis should involve testing for the presence of plants known to contain pyrrolizidine alkaloids or photodynamic agents. Evaluation of liver function is discussed on page 111. Investigation of the environment should center on the type of pasture or other substances to which the animal has access. All drug therapy should be discontinued, if possible.

Histopathology of the affected skin will show variable changes, such as hyperkeratosis, parakeratosis, follicular keratosis, and a perivascular and/or perifollicular mixed inflammatory dermal infiltrate. These findings are not specific to any etiology of photosensitivity.

Therapy is obviously related to etiology. Treatment for hepatic disease is discussed on page 111; chronic liver disease carries a guarded prognosis. Removal of feedstuffs containing photodynamic agents, or removal of the horse from a pasture with plants containing these agents, will usually result in full recovery if the horse is also kept out of the sun for one to two weeks. Corticosteroids are helpful in controlling inflammation and pruritus. Oral prednisone or prednisolone given at a dosage of 1 mg per kg daily for a week, then halving the daily dosage for a second week, is an effective regimen. As prednisone must be metabolized by the liver into the active drug prednisolone, the latter is the preferred therapy in photosensitization due to liver disease.

Drug-induced photosensitivity may be long-lived, even after the drug has been discontinued. Avoidance of sunlight is important. Corticosteroids should be used to control clinical signs. Sites of application of suspected topical photosensitizers should be thoroughly cleaned with water, with care being taken to avoid spreading of the drug when the animal is washed. Sunburn cases often involve large areas of the body, rendering topical sunscreen application impractical. Avoiding excessive exposure to sunlight is the best therapy.

OTHER CONSIDERATIONS

The autoimmune skin diseases pemphigus foliaceus and bullous pemphigoid have been reported in the horse. While no exacerbation of these diseases by sunlight has thus far been noted, such adverse reactions have been seen in the dog and in humans. Neither systemic nor discoid lupus erythematosis have yet been reported in the horse, but photosensitivity could play an important part in the clinical presentation and therapy of these diseases. Finally, the porphyrias seen in cattle have not been documented in horses; however, the presence of photosensitivity in a neonatal or young horse should prompt inclusion of a congenital metabolic abnormality in the differential diagnoses.

Supplemental Readings

Blood, D. C., Radostits, O. M., and Henderson, J. A.: Veterinary Medicine. London, Bailliere Tindall, 1983, pp. 437–439.

Montes, L. F., and Vaughan, J. T.: Atlas of Skin Diseases of the Horse. Philadelphia, W. B. Saunders Company, 1983, pp. 152–155.

Stannard, A. A.: Some important dermatoses in the horse. Mod. Vet. Pract., 53:31, 1972.

Tennant, B., Evans, C. D., Schwartz, L. W., Gribble, D. H., and Kaneko, J. J.: Equine hepatic insufficiency. Vet. Clin. North Am. (Large Anim. Pract.), 3:279, 1973.

Nodular Skin Disease

Danny W. Scott, ITHACA, NEW YORK

A nodule is a circumscribed, solid, usually rounded mass greater than 1 cm in diameter. Nodules are usually elevated above the surface of the skin but may be intradermal or subcutaneous. Nodules may be produced by dermal or epidermal hyperplasia, by inflammatory or neoplastic infiltrates, or by lipid and amyloid products.

Single or multiple nodules are the most common equine skin lesions seen in my practice. When the frequency of equine nodular skin disease is viewed in light of the plethora of potential causes (Table 1), the clinician's plight is readily appreciated. A complete discussion of the differential diagnosis of equine nodular skin disease is beyond the scope of this article. Rather, I will focus on (1) the diagnostic approach to nodular skin disease, and (2) the clinicopathologic and therapeutic aspects of selected nodular dermatoses. The dermatoses selected for discussion were chosen on the basis of frequent occurrence, paucity of available literature, recent recognition, or frequent asymptomatic presentation.

DIAGNOSTIC APPROACH TO CUTANEOUS NODULES

HISTORY

The medical history in a patient with skin disease should obviously be obtained with the same care as exercised in a patient with any general medical or surgical illness. However, frequently it is not. Skin lesions are often too quickly assessed as trivial and unimportant. An adequate dermatologic history should include the following considerations: age, breed, gender, familial occurrence, geographic location, seasonal influences, environmental considerations, evidence of contagion, previous skin disease, previous medical or surgical problems, present noncutaneous symptomatology, previous and current therapy, inception and progression of the skin lesions, and the degree of pruritus.

PHYSICAL EXAMINATION

Inasmuch as a visual appreciation of skin lesions is the essential factor in dermatologic diagnosis, the examiner's eye is undoubtedly the most important instrument. The crucial determinations to be made during the examination of the skin are the type of lesions present and their configuration and distribution.

DIAGNOSTIC AIDS

Skin scrapings and Wood's lamp examination are rarely of diagnostic benefit in equine nodular dermatoses. Microscopic examination of plucked hairs suspended in mineral oil or 10 to 20 per cent potassium hydroxide may provide early evidence for the presence of dermatophytosis. Bacterial and fungal cultures of nodular dermatoses are best made by aseptically preparing a nodule and swabbing the cut surface with a culturette, or submitting part of the tissue in sterile transport medium for culture.

Exfoliative cytology is useful in equine nodular dermatoses. Nodules may be aspirated with 20- to 23-gauge needles attached to a 6- or 12-ml plastic syringe. Nodules with ulcerated surfaces or draining tracts may be sampled by impression smears. In either case, retrieved material is gently smeared on a glass microscope slide and stained with new methylene blue for microscopic examination.

Skin biopsy is the only way to achieve a definitive diagnosis in most equine nodular dermatoses. With small nodules, punch biopsies may be satisfactory. However, in most instances, excision biopsy is required. In general, selected nodules are gently clipped, cleansed, and anesthetized by infiltrating 2 per cent lidocaine under the lesion or in the form of a ring block. Excised nodules are placed in 10 per cent neutral buffered formalin and sent, ideally, to a veterinary dermatologist or veterinary pathologist with expertise in dermatohistopathology. The ability of either the dermatologist or pathologist to provide an accurate assessment of the biopsy specimen can be severely hampered by submission of inadequate information with the specimen.

TYPES OF NODULAR DERMATOSES

NODULAR COLLAGENOLYTIC GRANULOMA

Nodular collagenolytic granuloma, also called nodular necrobiosis and eosinophilic granuloma, is the most common equine nodular dermatosis in my practice. Its cause is unknown; a hypersensitivity reaction to insect bites has been suggested. There are no apparent age, breed, or gender predilections. The disease usually begins in warmer months. Lesions up to 5 cm in diameter may occur singly or multiply, and most commonly affect the neck, withers, and back. The nodules are usually rounded, well-circumscribed, firm, nonulcerative, nonpainful, and nonpruritic, and lacking alopecia. Occasionally, "cystic" or plaque-like lesions are seen. Affected horses are otherwise healthy.

Diagnosis is based on history, physical examination, exfoliative cytology, and biopsy, Direct smears may reveal numerous eosinophils, lymphocytes, and histiocytes. Skin biopsy reveals multifocal areas of

TABLE 1. DIFFERENTIAL DIAGNOSIS OF EQUINE NODULAR SKIN DISEASE

Disease	Common Site	Page No.
Bacterial		
Furunculosis (especially coagulase-positive staphylococci)	Saddle/tack areas	542, 1st edition
Ulcerative lymphangitis (especially *Corynebacterium pseudotuberculosis*)	Legs	31, 1st edition
Actinomycosis	Mandible, maxilla	
Nocardiosis	—	
Abscess (especially *C. pseudotuberculosis*)	Chest, abdomen	39, 1st edition
Botryomycosis (especially coagulase-positive staphylococci)	Legs, scrotum	
Tuberculosis	Ventral thorax and abdomen, medial thighs	29, 1st edition
Glanders	Medial hocks	
Fungal		
Dermatophytosis	Saddle/tack areas	—
Mycetoma (*Curvularia geniculata* = "black-grain", *Pseudoallescheria boydii* = "white-grain")	—	
Phaeohyphomycosis (*Dreschlera specifera, Hormodendrum* sp.)	—	
Sporotrichosis	Legs	555, 1st edition
Zygomycosis		
Basidiobolus haptosporus	Chest, trunk, neck, head	
Conidiobolus coronatus	Nostrils	
Alternariosis (*Alternaria tenuis*)	—	
Blastomycosis	—	34, 1st edition
Coccidioidomycosis	—	33, 1st edition
Cryptococcosis	—	33, 1st edition
Histoplasmosis farciminosi (*Histoplasma farciminosum*)	Face, neck, legs	33, 1st edition
Oomycosis (*Pythium* sp.)	Legs, ventral chest, abdomen	
Parasitic		
Hypodermiasis (*Hypoderma bovis, H. lineatum*)	Withers	
Habronemiasis (*Habronema muscae, H. majus, Draschia megastoma*)	Legs, ventrum, prepuce, medial canthus	560; also 551, 1st edition
Parafilariasis (*Parafilaria multipapillosa*)	Neck, shoulder, trunk	
Viral		
Viral papular dermatitis (variolalike poxvirus)	Trunk	
Immunologic		
Urticaria	Neck, trunk	619; also 535, 1st edition
Erythema multiforme	—	
Amyloidosis	Head, neck, chest, shoulder	636
Neoplastic		
Papilloma	Nose, lips	536, 1st edition
Aural plaques	Pinna	
Squamous cell carcinoma	Head, mucocutaneous junctions	
Sarcoid	Head, ventrum, legs	637; also 537 and 539, 1st edition
Apocrine gland adenoma	Pinna, vulva	
Fibroma	Head, neck, saddle area, legs	
Hemangioma	Legs	
Schwannoma	Eyelids, periorbital	
Mastocytoma	Head, legs	637
Melanoma	Perineum, perianal, ventral tail, base of ear	
Lymphosarcoma	—	314
Temporal teratoma	Base of ear	

collagen degeneration followed by granulomatous inflammation containing eosinophils, lymphocytes, and histiocytes. Older and larger lesions exhibit marked dystrophic mineralization and may be misdiagnosed as "calcinosis circumscripta" or "tumoral calcinosis." Cultures for bacteria and fungi are negative.

Horses with solitary lesions, or a few lesions, may be treated by surgical excision or glucocorticoid injections under the lesions. Triamcinolone acetonide (3 to 5 mg per lesion) or methylprednisolone acetate (5 to 10 mg per lesion) are effective. It has been recommended that no more than 20 mg triamcinolone acetonide be administered at once to any horse, as it may cause laminitis. Horses with multiple lesions may be treated with oral prednisone or prednisolone, 1 mg per kg once a day for two to three weeks.

Occasionally horses may suffer relapses and retreatment is successful. Some lesions undergo spontaneous regression. Older or larger lesions may be severely mineralized. Such lesions do not respond to glucocorticoid therapy, and surgical excision is required.

AXILLARY NODULAR NECROSIS

Axillary nodular necrosis or "girth galls," is a rare equine nodular dermatosis. The cause and pathogenesis are unknown. There are no apparent age, breed, or gender predilections. One or two well-circumscribed, firm, nonpainful nodules are present near the girth and axilla. Affected horses are otherwise healthy.

Diagnosis is based on history, physical examination, exfoliative cytology, and biopsy. Direct smears reveal suppurative to pyogranulomatous inflammation. Skin biopsy reveals focal dermal necrosis without collagen degeneration. Cultures for bacteria and fungi are negative. Surgical excision or sublesional glucocorticoid injections are effective treatment.

UNILATERAL PAPULAR DERMATOSIS

Unilateral papular dermatosis is an uncommon equine dermatosis of unknown cause. There are no apparent age or gender predilections. Initial descriptions of this condition suggested a genetic predisposition in Quarter horses, but I have also seen this condition in several other breeds.

Most horses develop lesions in spring and summer, the outstanding clinical feature being multiple (30 to 300) papules and nodules limited to one side of the trunk. The lesions are usually rounded, well-circumscribed, firm, and nonpainful. These horses are otherwise healthy.

Diagnosis is based on history, physical examination, exfoliative cytology, and biopsy. Direct smears reveal numerous eosinophils and skin biopsy reveals eosinophilic folliculitis and furunculosis. Cultures for bacteria and fungi are negative. Unilateral papular dermatosis usually undergoes spontaneous remission within several weeks to months. Because of this and the asymptomatic nature of the disease, treatment is not usually attempted. Oral prednisone or prednisolone, 1 mg per kg once a day for two to three weeks, is an effective treatment. Occasional horses suffer relapses.

AMYLOIDOSIS

Cutaneous amyloidosis is an uncommon dermatosis of unknown etiology. The condition appears to be a *primary* form of amyloidosis, in that concurrent inflammatory processes are not present, and amyloid deposition is restricted to the skin and occa-

sionally the regional lymphatics, regional lymph nodes, and upper respiratory mucosa.

There are no apparent age, breed, or gender predilections. Multiple cutaneous nodules, 2 to 10 cm in diameter, are found on the head, neck, chest, and shoulder. They are rounded, firm, well-circumscribed, and nonpainful. Occasionally the lesions are urticarial, with a rapid onset and spontaneous regression. However, remission is then followed by the reappearance of slowly developing lesions that do not regress. Horses with cutaneous amyloidosis may also have concurrent diffuse or nodular deposition of amyloid in the upper respiratory tract, especially the nasal mucosa. If severe, upper respiratory amyloidosis may result in respiratory distress. Horses with cutaneous or upper respiratory amyloidosis or both are usually otherwise healthy.

Diagnosis is based on history, physical examination, and skin biopsy, which reveals the diffuse deposition of a homogeneous, eosinophilic substance with an associated foreign body granuloma tissue response. Special stains such as Congo red, crystal violet, and thioflavin-T show the homogeneous, eosinophilic substance to be amyloid.

The course of cutaneous amyloidosis is progressive and prolonged, there being no effective treatment. Because certain forms of primary amyloidosis in humans have a genetic basis, it may not be advisable to use affected horses for breeding until more is learned about the genetics of the equine disorder.

STERILE NODULAR PANNICULITIS

Panniculitis is an uncommon, multifactorial inflammatory condition of subcutaneous fat. The lipocyte is vulnerable to trauma, ischemia, and neighboring inflammatory disease and when damaged liberates lipid, which undergoes hydrolysis into glycerol and fatty acids. Fatty acids are potent inflammatory agents and incite further inflammatory reactions.

The cause of the rare condition sterile nodular panniculitis is unknown. There are no apparent age, breed, or gender predilections. Lesions consist of deep-seated cutaneous nodules, which may occur singly or in crops, and be localized or generalized. The nodules may be firm and well-circumscribed or soft and ill-defined. They may or may not be painful, and may become cystic, ulcerative, and drain an oily yellow-brown to bloody substance. The chest, axillae, and shoulders are affected. Affected horses may have signs of systemic illness, including poor appetite, depression, lethargy, and pyrexia.

Diagnosis is based on history, physical examination, exfoliative cytology, culture, and biopsy. Direct smears reveal suppurative to pyogranulomatous inflammation with intra- and extracellular lipid droplets. Cultures are negative. Skin biopsy reveals pyogranulomatous to granulomatous panniculitis.

Treatment with oral dexamethasone, 20 mg once daily for two to three weeks, has been effective. Relapses may occur.

MASTOCYTOMA

Mastocytoma is an uncommon equine dermatosis. Although the cause and pathogenesis of this disorder are not known, it appears to be a reactive and hyperplastic process as opposed to a neoplastic one. Attempts to transmit the disease to other horses have been unsuccessful.

Although there are no apparent age or breed predilections, males appear to be affected about five times as frequently as females. Lesions are usually solitary and occur most commonly on the head and legs. Lesions on the head tend to be soft and well-circumscribed, while those on the legs tend to be hard and ill-defined. The nodules vary from 2 to 20 cm in diameter and may or may not be alopecic, ulcerative, painful, or pruritic.

Diagnosis is based on history, physical examination, exfoliative cytology, and biopsy. Direct smears reveal numerous mast cells and eosinophils. Skin biopsy reveals multinodular accumulations of normal mast cells, many eosinophils, multifocal areas of collagen degeneration, and coagulation necrosis. Older lesions show increasing dystrophic mineralization and fibrosis with fewer mast cells. Such lesions may be misdiagnosed as "calcinosis circumscripta" or "tumoral calcinosis."

Equine mastocytoma is self-limiting, with no metastases being recorded. Spontaneous regression has occasionally been reported. Surgical excision is the treatment of choice, and even with incomplete surgical excision, there have been no recurrences. Sublesional injections of glucocorticoid may also be effective.

Supplemental Readings

McMullen, W. C.: The skin. *In* Mansmann, R. A., McAllister, E. S., and Pratt, P. W. (eds.): Equine Medicine and Surgery. 3rd ed. Santa Barbara, CA, American Veterinary Publications, 1982, p. 789.

Mullowney, P. D.: Dermatologic diseases of horses part IV. Environmental, congenital, and neoplastic diseases. Compend. Cont. Ed., 7:S22, 1985.

Murray, D. R., Ladds, P. W. and Campbell, R. S. F.: Granulomatous and neoplastic diseases of the skin of horses. Aust. Vet. J., 54:338, 1978.

Scott, D. W., and Hackett, R. P.: Cutaneous hemangioma in a mule. Equine Pract., 5:8, 1983.

Scott, D. W., Walton, D. K., and Blue, M. G.: Erythema multiforme in a horse. Equine Pract., 6:26, 1984.

Scott, D. W.: Sterile nodular panniculitis in a horse. Equine Pract., 7:30, 1985.

Stannard, A. A.: The skin. *In* Catcott, E. J., and Smithcors, J. F. (eds.): Equine Medicine and Surgery. 2nd ed. Wheaton, IL, American Veterinary Publications, 1972, p. 381.

Stannard, A. A.: Equine dermatology, Proc. 22nd Ann. Conv. Am. Assoc. Eq. Pract., 273,1976.

Thomsett, L. R.: Skin diseases of the horse. In Practice, 1:15, 1979.

Walton, D. K., and Scott, D. W.: Unilateral papular dermatosis in the horse. Equine Pract., 4:15, 1982.

Immunotherapy for Sarcoids

William C. Rebhun, ITHACA, NEW YORK

Because equine sarcoids are notoriously likely to recur following sharp surgical removal, alternative forms of therapy have been sought for decades. Early forms of immunotherapy included foreign protein injections such as sterilized whole milk. Later efforts included autogenous vaccines produced by removal of sarcoid tissue and subsequent manufacture of crude vaccines from this tissue. These vaccines were then injected back into the affected animal. Currently, bacille Calmette-Guérin (BCG) immunotherapy is a popular and effective means of treatment for equine sarcoids. Immunotherapy with BCG or cryosurgery are the two most successful treatments for equine sarcoids at this time. This paper will address only immunotherapy with BCG; surgical therapy was described on page 537 of the first edition of this book.

Bacille Calmette-Guérin vaccines have been crudely manufactured from the cell wall of this specific mycobacterium for decades. Modern products have attempted to purify the protein derivatives of the cell walls to minimize potential foreign protein reactions and maximize mobilization of T cells to reject tumors such as the equine sarcoid by cellular immune mechanisms. When BCG is introduced into tumor cells, local immune mechanisms attempt to remove this foreign protein. In removing the foreign protein, the tumor cells containing the foreign protein are also recognized as foreign and destroyed. This is obviously an oversimplification but suffices as a clinical description of the mechanism of action.

Although live BCG vaccine is available, killed purified protein derivative vaccines are currently recommended and two commercial products are available.* Since these products are available to most practitioners, the recommendations for BCG usage to be described are based on my experience with these products.

PATIENT SELECTION

Immunotherapy with BCG should be considered only after a positive diagnosis of equine sarcoid has been established by biopsy. It must be emphasized that equine sarcoids have diverse clinical appearances, including wartlike or verrucous, nodular dermal, nodular ulcerative, and so-called "flat" sarcoids, which mimic epidermal crusts or ringworm lesions. A horse may have single or multiple sarcoids. When multiple sarcoids are present, they may vary in appearance. Sarcoids that have ulcerated through the skin may have a red granulation tissue surface that bleeds easily and may lead to an erroneous diagnosis of granulation tissue if too superficial a biopsy is obtained.

The anatomic area of involvement and size are important factors when considering immunotherapy with BCG. Large tumors in critical anatomic areas that might suffer from cicatricial damage due to cryosurgery are likely candidates for BCG. Tumors in areas such as the inguinal area or medial thigh that are difficult to inject without anesthesia might not be good candidates for BCG due to restraint problems. Very large tumors or multiple tumors that require a large volume of BCG are of concern since reactions to vaccination are more likely when large volumes (greater than 10 cc) are used. The best candidates for BCG therapy are horses with single or multiple nodular sarcoids less than 5.0 cm in diameter. Since the two most viable treatment alternatives for equine sarcoid are BCG and cryosurgery, the veterinarian should choose one of these alternatives on the basis of the specific location, size, and numbers of tumors in each patient. If one treatment is unsuccessful in obtaining tumor-free status, the alternative treatment is still available.

THERAPEUTIC TECHNIQUE

The injection of BCG products into an equine sarcoid may be more of an art than true science.

*Regressin, Ragland Research, Inc., Athens, GA, or Ribigen, RIBI Immunochem Research, Inc., Hamilton, MT

The reasons for this statement involve the viscous nature of the BCG solutions, the dense fibrous nature of this connective tissue tumor, variable recommendations as to how much BCG to inject, and restraint problems in some horses.

Although the currently available BCG products are not supposed to cause anaphylactic reactions, the veterinarian should remember that a foreign protein is being injected and therefore, theoretically, immune mediated reactions are possible. I recommend premedication of all horses with flunixin meglumine (1.1 mg per kg intravenously) and an antihistamine solution intramuscularly at the manufacturer's recommended dosage for the horse. In addition, tetanus prophylaxis should be current. Corticosteroids are contraindicated lest they interfere with the desired immunologic response.

The tumor site is clipped and prepared for surgery. If a large tumor is present or the surface is ulcerated and covered with granulation tissue, the tumor is debulked by sharp dissection down to the skin level. This is not necessary for solitary nodular sarcoids or flat sarcoids. The BCG is then reconstituted as recommended and injected with syringe and 18-gauge needle. Generally, smaller diameter needles are not useful because the solution is quite viscous and excessive plunger pressure becomes necessary. The solution should be injected into the tumor and intradermally immediately adjacent to the tumor. Approximately 1.0 cc of BCG solution should be injected per 1.0 to 2.0 cubic centimeter of tumor. I try not to inject more than 5.0 to 6.0 cc of BCG in any tumor.

Following the injection, localized edema, inflammation, and swelling occur within 24 to 48 hours. This is usually minimal following the first injection. Local reaction can be managed by warm compresses and, in some instances, 2.2 to 4.4 mg per kg phenylbutazone orally twice a day. Systemic reactions are rare. When observed, they consist of sweating, apprehension, mild fever and, in one instance, mild colic, diarrhea, and laminitis. If the tumor begins to regress or to slough over the next 14 days, only one treatment may be necessary. However, typically, at least one more injection of BCG 14 days after the initial injection is necessary to induce tumor regression or sloughing. In most cases, two to five injections at two-week intervals are necessary for resolution of the sarcoids. Each injection should be preceded by the local and systemic preparations as described. It is impossible to predict which sarcoids will respond to BCG immunotherapy or which sarcoids will simply regress as opposed to sloughing. When sloughing occurs, the lesions resemble tissue sloughing from cryosurgical destruction and the wound should be cleansed daily.

Depending upon the size, location, and numbers

of sarcoids present in each patient, tumor-free status may be obtained in 50 to 75 per cent of equine patients with available BCG products. If the patient become tumor free but has occurrence of sarcoids at the same or different anatomic areas months to years later, BCG can once again be utilized to treat the tumors.

Supplemental Readings

Murphy, J. M., Severin, G. A., Lavach, J. D., Hepler, D. I., and Lueker, D. C.: Immunotherapy in ocular equine sarcoid. J. Am. Vet. Med. Assoc., 174:269, 1979.
Wyman, M., Rings, M. D., Tarr, M. J., and Alden, C. L.: Immunotherapy in equine sarcoid: A report of two cases. J. Am. Vet. Med. Assoc., 171:449, 1977.

Burns

Susan L. Fubini, ITHACA, NEW YORK

Thermal injuries are relatively uncommon in domestic animals, especially large animals. For this reason, the veterinary literature is lacking in recent advancements made in the treatment of these cases. Most of the available information is extrapolated from human literature.

CLASSIFICATION

There are a variety of classifications of burns. In humans, burns are generally placed into three categories: first-degree burns are manifested by erythema, pain, and edema of the skin. Second-degree burns have similar signs, but the injury is more intense resulting in vesicle formation and, in some cases, necrosis of the epidermis. With third-degree burns there is destruction of cells and blood vessels in all layers of skin and loss of hair follicles and glandular structures. Cutaneous sensation is lost.

Application of this classification scheme to domestic animals is often difficult because there are less superficial vascular plexuses in animals and their skin does not blister as easily as that of humans. A simplified classification system may be used: partial-thickness (or minor) burns are those that have caused incomplete destruction of the skin and full-thickness (major) burns are characterized by complete destruction of all elements of skin, including adnexa and nerves.

Accurate evaluation of the amount of tissue damage sustained is difficult, especially immediately after the injury. The extent of the burn depends on the size of the area exposed. Its severity depends on the maximum temperature the tissue attains and the duration of overheating. A large amount of heat is required to raise the temperature of tissues; however, the heat is slow to dissipate. For this reason the duration of overheating extends beyond the contact time with the burning agent.

The most common cause of thermal injuries in horses are fires and lightning burns. Unfortunately, the latter are usually fatal. Thermal injury can also result from direct heat, friction, caustic chemicals, and electrical injuries.

PATHOPHYSIOLOGY

Following severe burns there are dramatic cardiovascular effects that have been called "burn shock." Before any change in blood or plasma volume a dramatic drop in cardiac output often occurs, probably caused by a circulating myocardial depressant factor. Very soon after a burn the vasculature in the area dilates, with a subsequent increase in capillary permeability resulting from the release of vasoactive amines. Tremendous loss of fluid and protein occurs. The inflammatory fluid accumulates within the interstitium, causing pressure on thin-walled vessels and lymphatics. Venous and lymphatic thrombosis may result. The protein loss causes a drop in oncotic pressure, which aggravates edema formation. The loss of albumin can lead to decreased transport capacity. This loss of plasma and extracellular fluid is most dramatic in the first 12 hours after the burn. The loss continues at a much slower rate over the next 6 to 12 hours.

An early anemia resulting from red cell hemolysis and splenic sequestration may be present but is often masked by hemoconcentration. Thrombocytopenia may result from platelet aggregation on damaged capillary endothelium. If damage is extensive a hemorrhagic diathesis may result from exhaustion of clotting factors. Immunoglobulin levels in the serum drop, with the lowest values at two days after a burn. Serious defects in neutrophil function such as a decrease in chemotaxis, random migration, impaired phagocytic rate, and impaired bactericidal capacity have also been observed in severely burned patients. The alveolar macrophage is initially hyperactive, and then for unknown reasons fails to undergo an increase in production resulting in severe pneumonitis.

Burns also destroy the lipid in the skin, allowing water transmission up to four times normal. The extent of water loss parallels the severity of the burn. This fluid loss results in an increase in heat loss from evaporation. The heat loss is, in part, responsible for an increase in oxygen consumption and metabolic rate, as the animal tries to generate heat. Depletion of fat stores and some endogenous protein supplies are two means by which metabolic compensation is achieved. In turn, this hypermetabolic rate leads to weight loss, a negative nitrogen balance, and retarded wound healing. Therefore, the nutritional condition of the patient at the time of burn injury is a prime prognostic consideration.

Renal function can be compromised by constriction of renal vessels, hypovolemia, and decreased cardiac output. Pneumonitis can be a complicating factor of severe burns due to the inefficiency of the alveolar macrophage. Invasion by bacteria (usually Pseudomonas) is common.

Burn wound sepsis is unfortunately very common. Burn tissue is a rich medium for growth of bacteria, especially Pseudomonas, Staphylococcus, Streptococcus, and Micrococcus. If dissemination occurs septicemia may result. Local and systemic sepsis from Candida and fungi has been reported.

THERAPY

Four primary objectives in treating thermal injury are (1) to save life, (2) to relieve pain, (3) to close the wound, and (4) to minimize or correct deformities. Superficial and partial-thickness (minor) burns are not life threatening and are not difficult to manage. With full-thickness burns attempts should be made to cool the affected skin using an ice or cold water bath. A water-based antibiotic ointment should be applied liberally to the affected areas. A bandage may be indicated to serve as a protective covering.

Partial-thickness burns are associated with vesicles and blisters, which should be left intact for the first 24 to 36 hours following formation. The fluid in a blister provides protection from infection and the presence of the blister is less painful than exposed surface. After this period of time the blister is partially excised and the area protected with either a dry plasma scab, an antibacterial protective dressing, or a xenograft. The most crucial area of the wound is the interface between the new migrating epithelium and the dermal edge beneath it. The bandage should be applied in a manner that permits drainage from the wound and does not allow for adherence. The dressing may need to be changed daily or more often depending on the nature of the wound and the amount of exudate.

Analgesics should be given because superficial wounds may be very painful.

Deep burns can be difficult to manage. A complete physical examination is performed and the patient's condition stabilized as rapidly as possible. Life-threatening problems encountered in managing these patients include shock, malnutrition, infection, reduced immunocompetency, and multiorgan system dysfunction.

The patient must have an adequate airway. Oxygen may be administered. A baseline hemogram, serum electrolytes, and BUN should be obtained. Intravenous fluid therapy should be instituted. Expansion of plasma volume in the immediate postburn period is dependent only on the rate of fluid administration regardless of the type of fluid being administered. For the first 24 hours a balanced isotonic sodium solution is given. An established rate is 2 to 4 ml per kg for each percentage of surface area burned. On the second day, when capillary integrity has been restored, the continued administration of the electrolyte solutions results in edema far in excess of any improvement in circulatory dynamics. For this reason treatment with colloid is recommended. The administration of these solutions not only produces a substantial elevation in cardiac output and plasma volume but also maintains them at these elevated levels.

As with minor burns, pain relief can be accomplished with nonsteroidal anti-inflammatory drugs or narcotics. Topical therapy in the form of cool compresses, cold water baths, and wound coverings may also provide some relief.

In order to control wound repair, early wound closure, topical antibiotics, and a clean environment are essential. If there has been little contamination, irrigation with large amounts of saline usually suffices to cleanse the wound surface. All the hair should be clipped from the burned area to make it easier to evaluate the extent of the damage and to help keep the area clean. All devitalized tissue should be debrided, initially as often as twice or three times a day. Whirlpool baths are effective in removing necrotic tissue and surface exudates. Systemic antibiotics are to be avoided in burn victims if at all possible. Systemic antimicrobials do not favorably influence mortality, fever, or rate of healing and can encourage emergence of resistant organisms. Furthermore, circulation to the burned areas is often compromised, making it highly unlikely that parenteral antibiotics can achieve adequate levels at the wound. If septicemia or pneumonia result antibiotics are indicated following a culture and sensitivity test.

The destruction of the dermis leaves a primarily collagenous structure called *eschar*. There are two different schools of thought on management of eschar. Dry exposure is a time-honored method of wound management that operates under the principle that bacteria do not thrive on a dry surface. The goals of therapy are to keep the wound dry and protected from mechanical trauma. The disadvantages of this method of therapy are the continued heat and water loss from the uncovered wound. Of those who favor the application of topical antimicrobials, some use an open technique (no protective covering), and others apply an overlying bandage. The latter method is the most practical for domestic animals.

Numerous topical products have been used on animals, thus suggesting that no one product is ideal. Nitrofurazone has a fairly narrow range of antibacterial activity, resistance can be developed to it, and it does not penetrate the eschar well. Mafenide is bacteriostatic, and Staphylococci and Pseudomonas may become resistant. It is irritating and painful when applied, does not penetrate deeply, and is not fungicidal. Suprainfection with Candida can be a problem. Mafenide is also a carbonic anhydrase inhibitor that can result in a metabolic acidosis. Chlorhexidine can be used as a solution or a cream but has questionable efficacy against gram-negative organisms. Povidone-iodine causes some patient discomfort but is effective against bacteria, yeasts, and fungi. It should not be used on extensive burns because of the possibility of systemic absorption and a resultant high level of serum iodine and severe metabolic acidosis. Gentamicin ointment is excellent for serious gram-negative infections but should be used only in selected cases because resistance can develop. It should not be used in patients with renal problems. Silver sulfadiazine is active against nearly all pathogenic bacteria and fungi and exerts a prominent antibacterial action against Pseudomonas. It may cause granulocyte depression, and is relatively expensive. Aloe vera cream from the aloe plant has been reported to relieve pain immediately, decrease inflammation, penetrate deeply, stimulate cell growth, kill bacteria and fungi, and have an anti-prostaglandin effect in burned tissue. It has been used in burned animals with success. Aloe vera and silver sulfadiazine would probably be a good first choice in antibiotic therapy for burns, and are used extensively in human medicine.

Closure of the burn wound allows for more rapid healing, pain relief, and prevention of loss of heat, water, and protein-rich exudate from the wound surface. A wound covering serves as a barrier to external invasive infections. Grafts can be extremely useful to provide wound closure and should be used early in the clinical course of a severely burned patient. Unfortunately, grafts are expensive and difficult to maintain. Autografts provide the most effective physiologic wound closure, although it may be necessary to use a different wound covering until a healthy granulation bed is formed and the patient's immunocompetence has improved.

Sterile starch graft copolymer dry flakes or sheets are available and when mixed with water form a moldable gel. This material absorbs about 30 times its weight in wound exudate, is soothing, molds to the contour of the wound, prevents eschar formation by keeping tissues moist, and will not interfere with topical antibiotics. These can be applied to the wound before gel application or mixed with the gel. Porcine heterografts have been shown to be effective biologic dressings and are available commercially.

Management of burns is expensive and time-consuming. Large animals require special consideration. Often there is involvement of large surface areas, increasing the loss of fluid, electrolytes, and protein. Many animals are pruritic and need to be restrained with crossties to prevent self-mutilation. Long-term hospitalization and daily patient monitoring are often necessary, requiring a sincere commitment on the part of the clinician and the client.

Supplemental Readings

Anderson, B. C.: Aloe vera juice: a veterinary medicant? Comp. Cont. Ed., 5:S364, 1983.

Cera, L. M., Heggers, J. P., Hagstrom, W. J., and Robson, M. C.: Therapeutic protocol for thermally injured animals and its successful use in an extensively burned rhesus monkey. J. Am. An. Hosp. Assoc., 18:633, 1982.

Geiser, D. R., and Walker, R. D.: Management of large animal thermal injuries. Comp. Cont. Ed., 7:S69, 1985.

Halbach, N., and DeYoung, D.: Treatment and management of major burns. Iowa State Vet., 3:120, 1979.

McKeever, P. J.: Thermal injury. In Kirk, R. W. (ed.): Current Veterinary Therapy VIII. Philadelphia, W. B. Saunders Company, 1983, pp. 180–183.

Valdez, H.: A hydrogel preparation for cleansing and protecting equine wounds. Equine Pract., 2:33, 1980.

Wound Care and Excessive Granulation Tissue

Llewellyn C. Peyton, GAINESVILLE, FLORIDA

Nolton Pattio, GAINESVILLE, FLORIDA

Wound care in the horse is almost synonymous with the control of excessive granulation tissue ("proud flesh"). The basic aspects of wound healing are similar in that all soft tissue wounds heal by the synthesis of connective tissue and the formation of a fibrous scar. There are three phases of repair.

Phase 1 is a vascular response. The immediate response to wounding is bleeding, which cleans the wound and provides cells that remove bacteria and tissue debris. Almost immediately there is a brief period of vasoconstriction in the wound edges; this aids hemostasis. Vasodilation and slowing of the blood flow follow vasoconstriction. This allows the polymorphonuclear neutrophil leukocytes to adhere to the walls of the capillaries. The ensuing increase in permeability of the capillaries allows plasma, white blood cells, and, to a limited extent, red blood cells to migrate through the capillary walls into the fibrin coagulum that has resulted from the initial bleeding and serves to unite the wound edges.

The cellular population of a wound consists primarily of neutrophils, monocytes, and fibroblasts. The number of neutrophils entering the wound increases during the first 48 hours. Very few are actively engaged in phagocytosis; rather, they release their cytoplasmic granules, which break down tissue debris and kill bacteria. The monocytes increase during the next few days until they are the dominant cells in the wound around the fifth day. These mononuclear macrophages are actively engaged in phagocytosis.

Fibroblasts also appear in the first phase of wound repair. These fibroblasts utilize the fibrin that was deposited earlier in the repair process as scaffolds to provide directional migration.

If the first phase of wound healing is prolonged because the wound is not adequately cleaned, the entire wound healing process is delayed. Healing problems developing in the first phase are identified by (1) an increased amount or prolonged appearance of purulent discharge and (2) a lack of granulation tissue formation.

The second phase of wound repair is the early proliferative phase, which begins around the fourth or fifth day after injury and lasts 7 to 14 days. Macrophages predominate early in this phase; however, fibroblasts continue to increase as wound healing progresses. Advancement of capillaries into the wound area also characterizes the proliferative phase. These capillaries are derived from endothelial buds that closely follow the fibroblast advancement into the wound. When the second phase of repair is fully established, the wound is filled with vascular granulation tissue. Clinically, this phase is characterized by the presence of a pink, soft-appearing, and very vascular tissue. The tissue has a somewhat granular-appearing surface owing to the new capillary growth. Upon reinjury of this tissue, the area bleeds diffusely as if the entire surface were oozing blood.

The end of the second phase and the beginning of the third phase (called the fibroplastic phase) are not as distinct as the transition between phases 1 and 2. Clinically, the transition is marked by a decrease in vascularity and an increase in wound collagen density. The final result is a relatively avascular scar composed of collagen fibers. Grossly a firm, light pink tissue can be observed that, when reinjured, bleeds sparsely. Often this tissue is raised above the wound epithelial margin, producing excessive granulation tissue.

Epithelial repair entails loosening of basal cells from their dermal attachment, multiplication of the cells at the wound edge, and migration and maturation of cell layers. The epithelial cells migrate only over viable tissues because they need the nutrition and blood supply acquired from the granulation tissue. Thus, the cells move onto the underlying tissue below the wound debris, blood clot, or eschar.

Epithelial repair can be recognized as a whitish-appearing tissue line around the wound margin extending out from the uninjured epithelium onto the granulation tissue. Contact inhibition may cause epithelialization to cease when granulation tissue extends above the wound edges. The presence of dirt and other debris also terminates migration. Therefore, therapeutic efforts should be made to maintain the granulation tissue below the level of the epithelium and also to keep the wound clean.

Wound contraction, or "wound shrinkage," moves all skin layers toward the center of the wound. The cells responsible for this active process are myofibroblasts. Any event that interferes with the viability of cells in the wound edge inhibits wound contraction.

FACTORS AFFECTING WOUND HEALING

Wound healing can be adversely affected by local (Table 1) or systemic (Table 2) factors. Malnutrition, hypoxia, uremia, and liver disease, which can all delay wound healing, will be detected on physical examination or by evaluation of diet and clinical laboratory data. Local factors, especially infection, are the most important and most easily identified factors that affect wound repair.

WOUND CARE

There are four management protocols available for wound care. *Primary closure* is the suturing of a wound within a few hours of injury. *Delayed closure* can be achieved before the appearance of granulation tissue (*delayed primary closure*) or following the appearance of granulation tissue at five to six days (*secondary closure*). *Second intention* healing allows the wound to heal by contraction and epithelialization. *Skin grafting* is necessitated by the lack of available skin for closure. A decision on the management protocol is based on clinical experience, the size, shape, and location of the wound, and the presence of pathologic modifications. For any of these processes to be successful, the wound must first be debrided. There are three procedures for debridement: sharp debridement, irrigation, and chemical debridement. These procedures can be combined and used simultaneously on the same patient.

Sharp debridement involves excision of the skin and subcutaneous tissue lining the edges of the wound and the removal of dead or devitalized

TABLE 1. LOCAL FACTORS AFFECTING WOUND HEALING

Local Factors	Effects
Surgical technique	All phases of healing
Blood supply	All phases of healing
Mechanical stress	Retards contraction of wound, increased fibrous phase
Suture materials	Increased inflammatory reaction, decreased wound resistance to infection
Suture technique	Can retard all aspects of healing
Radiation	Decreases inflammatory reaction, inhibits wound contraction; unstable epithelium; stops fibroblast proliferation; disturbance of collagen metabolism
Infection	Increases inflammatory reaction; retards all phases of healing

TABLE 2. SYSTEMIC FACTORS AFFECTING WOUND HEALING

Systemic Factors	Effects
Malnutrition	Decreased immunological response, decreased collagen synthesis
Vitamin C deficiency	Decreased collagen synthesis
Vitamin K deficiency	Impaired clotting mechanism
Other vitamin deficiencies	Little effect on wound healing
Zinc deficiency	Increased or decreased cell proliferation, fibroplasia, collagen synthesis, epithelialization
Trauma, hypovolemia, hypoxia, anemia	Decreased collagen synthesis, decreased immunologic response
Uremia	Decreased collagen synthesis, decreased growth of fibroblasts, decreased amount of granulation tissue
Malignant disease	No effects
Jaundice	Decreased fibroblast formation, decreased vascularization
Corticosteroid drugs	Decreased collagen synthesis, inhibits capillary proliferation, inhibits granulation tissue
Cytotoxic and antimetabolite drugs	Decreased cell proliferation

tissues. When the removal of tissue is not indicated or when a tissue of doubtful viability exists, the wound should be packed with gauze and a topical antibacterial solution. Periodic inspections are made of the wound for tissue viability and the presence of infection. When the wound is considered "clean," primary closure, skin graft, or other therapeutic regimen can be initiated. Criteria used to assess the status of the wound are (1) lack of purulent exudate or pyogenic membrane or both, (2) pink or red appearance of the granulation tissue and not the dark red or purple that denotes congestion, and (3) a quantitative bacterial count value of below 10^5 bacteria per gram of tissue (to be discussed later).

Wound irrigation requires delivery of fluids under pressure. A 60 cc disposable syringe and needle provide fluids at around 7 psi. A pressure of 10 to 15 psi removes approximately 80 per cent of the factors that lead to infection. Other factors important in wound irrigation include amount of fluid, type of fluid, and antibacterial additives. Sufficient fluid must be used to eliminate visible contamination of the wound bed. When the tissue begins to radiate a "gray hue" and the "cells" appear to be filled with fluid, we stop lavage. We refer to this as a water-logged tissue and we believe that at this point lavage has become detrimental to the healing process. We lavage with physiologic saline solution, often with 3 per cent povidone-iodine or 0.25 per cent neomycin solution for antimicrobial activity.

Our protocol is generally to lavage with a 3 per cent povidone-iodine solution in the acute stages of wounding and use a 0.25 per cent neomycin solution in the later stage. The 0.25 per cent neomycin is used primarily before closure or skin grafting is attempted. Povidone-iodine solution results in more tissue reaction than the neomycin; however, it provides a broader spectrum of antimicrobial activity and possibly aids more in the removal of infection-potentiating factors.

Chemical debridement should provide a simple rapid, safe debridement of irreparably damaged tissue without requiring anesthesia or surgery and with minimal blood loss. The debriding agent must be nontoxic and must have the capacity to differentiate between viable and nonviable tissue in its debriding action. Two debriding agents appear to offer some benefit, Sutitains ointment,* a *Bacillus subtilis* protease, and Oticlens,† a mixture of propylene glycol in an aqueous solution with a pH of 2.1 to 2.5. It is formulated to cause a larger variation in the degree of swelling between living and dead tissue. Consequently, a plane of cleavage develops, causing the dead tissue to slough.

Debriding agents do not require the repeated anesthesia frequently necessary to debride large wounds using sharp excision. Such agents can also better differentiate viable and nonviable tissue. These agents appear to be a safe topical means of removing devitalized tissue. They produce no clinically significant side effects when used before delayed closure or in skin grafting procedures.

MANAGEMENT OF EXCESSIVE GRANULATION TISSUE

The formation of excessive granulation tissue (also known as proud flesh or exuberant granulation tissue) often complicates the healing of equine skin wounds. Although excessive granulation tissue shows no age, sex, breed, or coat color predilection, it occurs most commonly on wounds of the distal extremities.

The etiology of excessive granulation tissue is unknown. It is often observed in wounds that lack underlying soft tissue, wounds that are subject to motion or tension, wounds that are treated with chemical irritants such as powdered medication or nonwater soluble–based medications, and wounds that are infected or contaminated with debris such as hair, dirt, and gravel. Many of the causes of proud flesh can be eliminated or minimized with good wound care.

Granulation tissue is pink to red colored, firm,

*Travase, Flint Laboratories, Morton Grove, IL
†Beecham Laboratories, Bristol, TN

and granular appearing. It becomes a problem when it is raised above and extends over the adjacent epithelium, delaying wound healing, particularly epithelialization and contraction. Other fibrovascular proliferative disorders such as cutaneous habronemias, phycomycosis, equine sarcoids (fibroblastic type), and squamous cell carcinomas may mimic excessive granulation tissue in their clinical appearance. Therefore, history, physical findings, lesion location, and gross appearance of the lesions should be carefully evaluated. Histopathologic studies may be needed for a definitive diagnosis.

TREATMENT

Many forms of therapy are used to remove or inhibit the formation of excessive granulation tissue. These include surgical excision, chemical cauterization, limb immobilization with a cast, corticosteroids, and radiation therapy. These modes of therapy have been used singularly or in combination depending on lesion location, size, and shape of the wound and involvement of underlying structures.

Surgical management is the treatment of choice for excessive granulation tissue. It produces less scarring and minimizes the inhibitory effects on the other phases of wound healing. Surgical excision of granulation tissue may be performed with the animal standing. Anesthesia of the wound is unnecessary since the fibrovascular proliferation has no sensory innervation. Physical and/or chemical restraint may facilitate work on the extremity of some horses. A scalpel is used to resect the excessive tissue in a distal to proximal direction. Because profuse hemorrhage occurs, resecting the lesion in a distal to proximal direction keeps the surgical field free of blood. Epithelialization occurs most efficiently when the granulation bed is excised just below the surface of the adjacent epithelium and care is taken to undermine the leading epithelial edges. This provides not only slight elevation of the epithelium above the granulation tissue, but it also reactivates epithelialization. Following surgical excision a pressure bandage or Robert Jones bandage is applied to control hemorrhage, immobilize the wound and to decrease or slow down the regrowth of the granulation tissue.

Chemical caustic agents, e.g., copper sulfate, zinc sulfate, antimony trichloride, and formalin, or corticosteroids are often applied topically to a wound under a bandage in an attempt to retard the growth of granulation tissue. These types of therapy not only suppress the growth of granulation tissue but also delay wound healing by suppressing epithelialization and wound contraction. This therapy is acceptable only when the clinical sequelae have been carefully considered beforehand. We believe that it offers no advantage over sharp excision.

Radiation therapy has been used to suppress

excessive granulation tissue. Like corticosteroids, radiation inhibits cell division and fibroblast proliferation. High cost and the retardation of wound healing make radiation therapy unacceptable.

The treatment of excessive granulation tissue by bandaging or casting appears to inhibit the growth of granulation tissue by minimizing movement. As casting results in more limb restriction, it has become a widely used method of treatment. Bandaging of leg wounds has had a routine place in wound therapy for many years. The inhibition of excessive granulation by bandages is thought to be associated with pressure on the wound and also restricted motion. Recent research has demonstrated that casting and bandaging may not be the treatment of choice to minimize excessive granulation tissue. However, the benefits that are derived from these methods, such as immobilization, minimizing of contamination, and reduction of tension, will result in bandaging and casting remaining an important part of wound care.

In the treatment of excessive granulation tissue, attention should be paid to the gross appearance of the tissue. Granulation tissue containing draining tracts, areas of tissue necrosis, or exposed bone may have an infected focus, foreign body, or bone sequestrum. In these cases medical therapy will be inadequate and surgical debridement or exploration is necessary.

Supplemental Readings

Hunt, T. K., and Van Winkle, W., Jr.: Normal repair. *In* Hunt, T. K., and Dunphy J. E. (eds.): Fundamentals of Wound Management. New York, Appleton-Century-Crofts, 1979.

Peacock, E. E., and Van Winkle, W.: Wound Repair, 2nd ed. Philadelphia, W. B. Saunders Company, 1976.

Pavletic J., and Peyton, L. C.: Plastic and reconstructive surgery in the dog and cat. *In* Bojrab, M. J., and Crane, S. W. (eds.): Philadelphia, Lea & Febiger, 1983.

Peyton, L. C.: Wound healing: The management of wounds and blemishes in the horse. Part 1. Comp. Cont. Ed. 6:S111, 1975.

Swaim, S. F., and Wilhalf, D.: The physics, physiology and chemistry of bandaging open wounds. Comp. Cont. Ed. Pract. Vet., 7:146, 1985.

Generalized Granulomatous Disease

Anthony A. Stannard, DAVIS, CALIFORNIA

Generalized granulomatous disease (GGD) is a recently recognized disease of horses characterized by skin lesions and widespread systemic involvement. The disease is infrequently encountered and there is no known sex or breed predilection.

ETIOLOGY AND PATHOGENESIS

The etiology of GGD is unknown. Cultures for aerobic, anaerobic, and acid-fast bacteria as well as for fungi have been negative. Special stains on tissue sections and laboratory animal inoculation with tissue suspensions from affected horses have failed to reveal an etiologic agent. Polarization of tissue sections and transmission electron microscopic examination have also failed to reveal an agent or any crystalline structures such as silicon that could account for the induction of a granulomatous response.

The pathogenesis of GGD is presumed to be an abnormal host response to the persistent presence of an unidentifiable antigen or antigens similar to that proposed for human sarcoidosis. The ingestion of the plant "hairy vetch" has been reported to produce a similar generalized granulomatous disease in horses and cattle, but none of the horses with GGD had any known exposure to it.

CLINICAL SIGNS

To date, all recognized cases of GGD have been presented with a primary complaint of skin disease. The skin lesions take two forms, the more common being generalized scaling and crusting associated with varying degrees of alopecia. Occasionally, the disease is focal or multifocal in distribution. Less frequently, the skin lesions consist of nodules or large tumorlike masses. The types of skin lesions may coexist.

In addition to skin lesions, the most frequent presenting complaints are weight loss, decreased appetite, and a persistent low-grade fever. There is a disparity between the extensive involvement of internal organs and the mildness or even absence of clinical signs. Lung lesions have been demonstrated in all cases by thoracic radiographs, percutaneous lung biopsies, or at necropsy. The lung involvement is manifested by exercise intolerance, increased resting respiratory rate, and mild dyspnea.

Although lymph node involvement has been demonstrated histologically in almost all cases, peripheral lymphadenopathy is only occasionally detected. Liver and gastrointestinal lesions are relatively common and may cause diarrhea or icterus. Kidney and spleen lesions are less common and generally not associated with clinical signs. Bone involvement in one horse was associated with lameness. Although ocular, cardiac, and central nervous system involvement occurs in human sarcoidosis, they have not been seen in the equine disease.

This discussion of GGD is based on cases presented to a dermatology service. Hence, all cases involved skin lesions. Only 30 per cent of humans with sarcoidosis have skin lesions; it is not known how many horses with "sterile granulomatous diseases" of internal organs represent examples of this syndrome.

HISTOPATHOLOGY

Regardless of the organ involved, the major histologic change is the presence of noncaseating granulomas consisting of aggregates of epithelioid cells and multinucleated giant cells. Neutrophils, lymphocytes, and plasma cells are present in small numbers. In the skin, the granulomas tend to be located in the superficial portion of the dermis.

DIAGNOSIS

Laboratory Findings. A complete blood count may reveal leukocytosis, increased fibrinogen, and hyperglobulinemia. In severe cases a modest degree of anemia may be seen. Depending on the degree of involvement, liver and kidney function tests may be abnormal.

A diagnosis of GGD is confirmed by demonstrating the typical granulomatous changes histologically and eliminating other causes of a granulomatous response. Generalized granulomatous disease is truly a "diagnosis of exclusion." Skin and peripheral lymph node biopsies are of greatest value. Percutaneous needle biopsies of lung or liver or both may also be helpful. In horses with lung involvement, thoracic radiographs reveal a widespread interstitial infiltrate.

The major dermatologic differential diagnoses include dermatophytosis, dermatophilosis, and pemphigus foliaceus. Potassium hydroxide preparations, bacterial and fungal cultures, and skin biopsies for conventional histopathology and direct immunofluorescence should rule out all these.

CLINICAL MANAGEMENT

Because of the small number of horses studied and the variability of clinical signs, response to therapy has not been well documented. Although a few horses with GGD have exhibited evidence of spontaneous regression, GGD appears to be a more severe disease than human sarcoidosis, justifying a guarded to poor prognosis.

The treatment of choice is the parenteral administration of corticosteroids, which hastens granuloma resolution. Initially, horses should receive 600 to 700 mg prednisone or prednisolone orally per day until symptomatic relief is noted. The daily dose is then gradually reduced and an alternate-day regimen instituted. Therapy should be maintained for six months or longer.

Photoactivated Vasculitis

Anthony A. Stannard, DAVIS, CALIFORNIA

Photoactivated vasculitis appears to be an unusual form of photosensitization in the horse. The disease is uncommon, affecting mature horses. There is no breed or sex predilection. The disease primarily occurs during the summer months in regions with abundant sunlight.

ETIOLOGY AND PATHOGENESIS

There appears to be little doubt that this disease is "photoactivated" and that the superficial blood vessels are involved. The nature of the photodynamic agent, however, remains unknown. Affected horses have had no known exposure to recognized photosensitizing compounds and their liver function is normal. In a few horses, direct immunofluorescence studies have shown the deposition of IgG or the C-3 portion of complement or both in the walls of affected vessels. Whether this represents evidence of an immune-complex disease or is simply nonspecific deposition as seen in the various forms of porphyria remains to be elucidated.

CLINICAL SIGNS

The disease is limited to the nonpigmented portions of the lower extremities. Photoactivated vasculitis occurs sporadically, only affecting an individual animal. Other susceptible horses on the premises, i.e., those with nonpigmented extremities, remain unaffected. The lesions consist of edema, erythema, oozing and crusting. Erosions and ulcerations may develop. The lesions are painful rather than pruritic. The most important feature of the disease is the edema, which is more extensive than would normally be expected with the degree of skin involvement.

DIAGNOSIS

Photoactivated vasculitis must be considered in the differential diagnosis of all inflammatory skin diseases limited to a nonpigmented extremity(ies). The major differential diagnoses are the more conventional forms of photosensitization, especially if other nonpigmented skin in addition to the lower leg(s) is involved. Liver function tests will rule out hepatogenous photosensitization. Contact photosensitization due to various plants (phytophotodermatitis) is an important differential diagnosis. A careful history should be taken for possible exposure to incriminated vegetation, either in the form of pasture plants or incidental exposure during trail rides.

Histopathology. The walls of many blood vessels in the superficial papillary dermis exhibit degenerative changes. Thrombosis is relatively common. The epidermis exhibits a variety of hyperplastic and degenerative changes depending on the stage of the disease. The dermis contains a mixed perivascular infiltrate.

CLINICAL MANAGEMENT

Management consists of preventing further exposure of the affected area(s) to ultraviolet radiation and reducing the inflammation. The patient should be stalled during the daylight hours. In addition, leg wraps may be used to further eliminate ultraviolet radiation of the affected skin. Parenteral administration of corticosteroids is required to reduce the inflammation. Topical corticosteroid or corticosteroid and antibiotic preparations are of limited value. Large doses of corticosteroids are required for at least two weeks. The dosage is then gradually reduced over the following two to four weeks. Symptomatic therapy may include clipping any excess hair in the region and the use of wet soaks to facilitate removal of crusts and debris. Irritating topical preparations should be strictly avoided.

The majority of cases of photoactivated vasculitis, if vigorously treated as outlined, will respond favorably and require no further therapy. In an occasional animal the disease will recur requiring additional therapy.

Hyperesthetic Leukotrichia
Anthony A. Stannard, DAVIS, CALIFORNIA

Hyperesthetic leukotrichia is a rare but highly characteristic skin disease of horses that to date has been described only in California. The disease affects mature horses and there is no known sex or breed predilection.

CLINICAL SIGNS

The lesions, which can be single or multiple, are limited to the dorsal midline from the withers to the base of the tail and consist of focal crusts ranging from 1 to 4 mm in diameter. The crusts are probably preceded by a papular or vesicular stage, although none has been noted. The most striking clinical feature is extreme pain. Affected animals react violently if the lesions are touched or even approached. In an occasional animal the pain appears to precede the development of clinically recognizable skin lesions. Within a few weeks white hairs appear in the area(s) of crusting. The disease runs a natural course of one to three months at which time the pain subsides and the crusts disappear. The leukotrichia, however, persists. In two horses the disease was recurrent.

ETIOLOGY AND PATHOGENESIS

The etiology and pathogenesis of hyperesthetic leukotrichia are not known. Severe subepidermal edema and intraepidermal vesiculation appear to be the primary changes. Although the pain resembles that in herpes zoster of humans, the clinical features are not similar.

DIFFERENTIAL DIAGNOSIS

Owing to the characteristic location of the lesions, the extreme pain, and the subsequent development of leukotrichia, the disease is not likely to be confused with many other dermatoses. The major differential diagnosis is reticulated leukotrichia, which occurs in young horses, is more extensive and not limited to the midline, and is not associated with any significant pain. Dermoid cysts involve the skin of the dorsal midline. They are nodular, have a normal skin surface, and are not painful. Culicoides hypersensitivity primarily involves the long hairs of the mane and tail and only to a lesser extent the short-haired regions. That disease is pruritic rather than painful. Dermatophilosis is usually much more widespread and any associated pain is minimal compared with that in hyperesthetic leucotrichia.

CLINICAL MANAGEMENT

There is no known therapy. Parenteral corticosteroids even at high doses appear to be of no value.

TOXICOLOGY

Edited by F. W. Oehme

Toxicoses Commonly Observed in Horses

Frederick W. Oehme, MANHATTAN, KANSAS

A knowledge of the common poisons in the practice area, the frequency of various toxicities, and the incidence of these poisonings during certain seasons of the year or during various activities helps the practitioner to narrow the potential range of poisonings from which a diagnosis may be made. In suspected poisoning, it is better to concentrate on common toxicities than to devote diagnostic and therapeutic efforts on a wide variety of potential toxins.

While each practitioner must learn the type and frequency of the chemical exposures possible in the practice area, certain groups of chemicals or toxin-containing materials frequently cause poisoning in horses. Tables 1 through 5 summarize the signs and therapy of the common toxicoses causing gastrointestinal, nervous system, and hematologic signs and those causing skin problems.

EMERGENCY TREATMENT

Urgency is of utmost importance in treating toxicoses. Three rules to follow are begin treatment promptly; retain samples of blood, urine, and feces for analysis; and keep the animal warm during therapy.

The practitioner must act to prevent further absorption of toxin. This can be simply accomplished by moving the horse to a different pasture or stall and supplying fresh food and water, i.e., preventing access to the toxin. In cases of skin exposure, a thorough washing with a mild detergent and plenty of water is necessary. In cases of ingested poisons a gastric lavage in the unconscious or anesthetized horse or a laxative of mineral oil (3 liters orally) should be used to empty the digestive tract.

Treatment should be followed by oral administration of an activated charcoal slurry (250 to 500 gm in 2 to 4 liters warm water). Administer a specific antidote, if known; otherwise treat the horse symptomatically. Assist the patient's respiration if necessary, keep the patient warm, and observe the initial signs carefully.

POISONOUS PLANTS

In horses other than those continually stabled and fed hay and commercial feed, the risk from injury due to poisonous or harmful weeds is a serious one. Pastures contain a variety of plants, often unrecognized, and plants growing along fences are often protected from mowing while still being accessible to the horse. Weather conditions may reduce the available pasture while weeds thrive. The clinical signs may be acute or subacute, but the effects are usually the result of animals consuming the plant material for several days and eventually showing the effects in one or more body systems.

Gastrointestinal problems, characterized by colic and diarrhea, may develop from plants such as castor bean (p. 673), oleander (p. 674), and bracken

TABLE 1. PRIMARY CLINICAL SIGNS ARE GASTROINTESTINAL

Toxin	Signs	Treatment
Acids	Corrosion of mucous membrane of upper GI tract; colic and purgation followed by acute shock	Milk of magnesia, 20–30 ml PO Flush externally with water; apply paste of sodium bicarbonate
Alkalis	As for acids	4–6 egg whites to 1 L tepid water followed by a cathartic Flush externally with water
Arsenic	Acute: abdominal pain, staggering gait, extreme weakness, trembling, salivation, diarrhea, fast, feeble pulse Subchronic: depression, anorexia, watery diarrhea, increased urination followed by anuria, dehydration, ataxia, trembling, stupor, cold extremities	Tannic acid, strong tea, or protein (egg white) to absorb; d-penicillamine, 11 mg/kg q.i.d. for 7–10 days PO; or sodium thiosulfate, 8–10 gm of 20% solution IV, and 20–30 gm plus 300 ml water PO; or dimercaprol (BAL), 3 mg/kg IM Repeat every 4 hours for 2 days, then q.i.d. on day 3, then b.i.d. until day 10 Supportive fluid and electrolyte therapy
Carbon tetrachloride	Loss of appetite, dullness, staggering gait, gastroenteritis, bloody feces, constipation followed by diarrhea, collapse, and death	Empty stomach, give high protein and carbohydrate diet; maintain fluid and electrolyte balance Do not give epinephrine
Petroleum distillates	Immediate bloat, shivering, and incoordination Anorexia	Mineral oil, 3 L PO; after ½ hr, 20% sodium sulfate, 250–1000 gm PO
Phenols and cresols	Gastroenteritis, painful abdomen, weakness and depression, sternal recumbency	Wash skin, apply sodium bicarbonate (0.5%) dressing Mineral oil, 3 L PO Activated charcoal, 250–500 gm PO
Plants: Crotolaria (alkaloid)	Acute: anorexia, gastric irritation, tenesmus, bloody feces	Supportive therapy
Oak (tannins)	Constipation, abdominal pain, hematuria, weakness	Symptomatic treatment, stimulants, blood transfusions, and fluid therapy
Ragwort (alkaloid)	Acute: dullness, weakness, abdominal pain, nervous excitement Chronic: prolonged poor condition, icterus, yawning, drowsiness, staggering gait	Symptomatic treatment

fern (p. 676). Damage to the liver, usually the result of continued plant ingestion for many weeks, produces an altered temperament, a dummy-like attitude, loss of weight, and hepatic cirrhosis. Fiddleneck (Amsinckia) (p. 672), groundsel (Senecio) (p. 672), and crotolaria (p. 672) are common plants that induce liver damage. Many horses with liver damage will exhibit central nervous system effects, assumed to result from the buildup of ammonia. This excitability and altered personality may be confused with direct central nervous system effects induced by another series of poisonous plants. Clinical signs of hyperexcitability, incoordination, paresis or paralysis, abnormal body movements or posturing, convulsions, and coma may result from yellow star thistle (p. 675), locoweed (p. 674), lupine, nicotine (p. 657), and the selenium-containing plants (p. 674). By the time central nervous system effects are observed, most horses are no longer treatable.

Sudden death may be due to cyanide-containing plants such as sorghums (p. 678) fed by owners unaware of the danger. A number of pasture plants contain awns and thistles that induce mechanical injury to the lips, gums, and tongues, of consuming horses. Others, such as vines and coarse plants, may provide a digestive tract obstruction.

INSECTICIDES AND RODENTICIDES

The organophosphate insecticides (p. 658) and chlorinated hydrocarbon insecticides (p. 657) are common poisons of horses. Chlordane, heptachlor, aldrin, dieldrin, isodrin, endrin, toxaphene, lindane, methoxychlor, and the variety of organophosphate compounds that are continually growing in number and in ingenuity of naming are highly toxic compounds that horses are exposed to topically or via ingestion.

The rodenticides that may produce poisoning in horses include strychnine (p. 661), ANTU (p. 661), compound 1080 (p. 661), warfarin (p. 660), arsenic (p. 662), barium (p. 663), thallium (p. 663), phosphorus (p. 663), and zinc phosphide (p. 662).

MEDICATIONS

Because of the variety of "health products" provided to horses by their proud and enthusiastic owners, toxicoses due to drugs and chemical products intended for maintaining and improving equine health are not uncommon. Vitamins, stimulants, analgesics, anthelmintics, and tranquilizers may all cause problems due to misuse through overappli-

TABLE 2. PRIMARY CLINICAL SIGNS ARE CENTRAL NERVOUS SYSTEM STIMULATION

Toxin	Signs	Treatment
Alkaloids	Nervousness, difficult breathing, loss of muscular control, excess salivation, convulsions	Potassium permanganate, 2–4 ml/kg (1:10,000 solution) gastric lavage or PO Physostigmine salicylate, 30–120 mg SC or IM
Insecticides:		
Carbamates	Profuse salivation, diarrhea, muscle fasciculation, hyperactivity, followed by posterior paresis	Atropine sulfate, 0.5–1.0 mg/kg IV or to effect (dry mucous membranes), repeat dose as needed
Chlorinated hydrocarbons	CNS stimulation, violent excitation, muscle fasciculations, cranial to caudal convulsions	External: wash thoroughly with soap and water Barbiturates or chloral hydrate to control seizures Activated charcoal 250–500 gm PO with 20% sodium sulfate, 250–1000 gm PO
Organophosphates	As for carbamates	Atropine sulfate, 0.5–1.0 mg/kg IV or to effect (dry mucous membranes) followed by pralidoxime chloride (2-PAM, protopam chloride), 2% solution, 25–50 mg/kg by slow IV, repeat as needed, usually every 8–12 hrs
Lead	Blindness, muscle twitching, ataxia, head pressing, convulsions; often appears as GI involvement (diarrhea, salivation, anorexia)	Activated charcoal, 250–500 gm PO with 20% sodium sulfate, 250–1000 gm PO Calcium disodium EDTA, 28.5 mg/kg q.i.d. for 5 days Initial dose IV, then SC as 10 mg/ml in 5% dextrose
Plants:		
Larkspur (alkaloid)	Hypersensitivity, muscular trembling, collapse, prostration, convulsions Constipation, bloat, excessive salivation sometimes noted	Physostigmine (2.2 grains) plus pilocarpine (4.4 grains) plus strychnine (1.1 grains) in 20 ml water given SC per 500 kg, use with caution
Locoweed (selenium plus others)	Very excitable and irritable, abnormal gait, separate from herd, head held peculiarly, disturbed vision, chronic loss of weight, weakness, prostration, convulsions	Laxative, sedatives, quiet
Lupine (alkaloid)	Nervousness, loss of muscular control, frothing at the mouth, convulsions	Sedatives, laxatives, see alkaloids
Oleander (glycoside)	Overstimulation of the vagus, abdominal pain, diarrhea, tremors, progressive paralysis, coma	Atropine sulfate, gastric lavage Symptomatic treatment
Water hemlock (resinoid)	Violent spasms resulting in rapid respiration and heart rate, coma	Symptomatic treatment Artificial respiration
White snakeroot (tremetol)	Marked trembling, incoordination, weakness, inability to stand Partial throat paralysis	Laxatives, stimulants
Yellow star thistle (unknown)	Lip twitching, involuntary chewing, mouth open, inability to swallow or hold food in mouth, mechanical damage to lips	Symptomatic treatment

TABLE 3. PRIMARY CLINICAL SIGNS ARE CENTRAL NERVOUS SYSTEM DEPRESSION

Toxin	Signs	Treatment
Mercury	Muscle incoordination, ataxia, hyperesthesia, tremor, convulsions, and coma Can appear as GI involvement (diarrhea, anorexia, emaciation)	Activated charcoal, 250–500 gm PO Dimercaprol (BAL), 3 mg/kg IM; repeat every 4 hrs for 2 days, then q.i.d. on 3rd day, then b.i.d. for 10 days until recovery Supportive fluid and electrolyte therapy
Plants: Black locust (glycoside)	Anorexia, depression, weakness, posterior paresis, irregular pulse, labored breathing	Digitalis Symptomatic treatment
Bracken fern (thiaminase)	Emaciation, incoordination, rapid progress to paralysis and inability to rise Chronic: emaciation and depression	Thiamine hydrochloride 100–200 mg SC daily for several days
Death camas (steroid alkaloid)	Stiff-leggedness, hypersensitivity, anxious expressions, dyspnea, weakness, posterior paresis, convulsions	Atropine sulfate (4.4 mg) plus picrotoxin (17.6 mg) in 5 ml water given IV per 100 kg; repeat every 2 hrs for 2–3 injections
Horsetail (thiaminase plus unknown)	Weakness, diarrhea, rapid weight loss, incoordination, coma	Thiamine hydrochloride 100–200 mg SC daily for several days
Milkweed (resinoid)	Incoordination, depression, shallow respiration, inability to stand, coma	Symptomatic treatment
Poison hemlock (alkaloid)	Incoordination, salivation, abdominal pain, weakness, shallow, irregular respiration, coma	Laxatives, tannic acid, stimulants Supportive treatment

TABLE 4. PRIMARY CLINICAL SIGNS ARE BLOOD ALTERATIONS

Toxin	Signs	Treatment
Chlorates, nitrites	Staggering, purging, abdominal pain, hematuria, hemoglobinuria, dyspnea, cyanosis Blood is dark brown	4% methylene blue 10 mg/kg IV; repeat at intervals of several hours
Cyanide Arrowgrass, corn, elderberry, prunus sp, sorghum sp	Initial excitement and muscle tremors followed by pronounced polypnea and dyspnea, salivation, lacrimation, and voiding of feces and urine Gasping for breath and clonic convulsions Blood is bright cherry red	20% sodium nitrite (10 ml) plus 20% sodium thiosulfate (30 ml), 0.09 ml/kg IV
Phenothiazine	Hemolysis, anemia, hemoglobinuria, weakness, anorexia, fever, icterus, colic, constipation, and diarrhea	Methylamphetamine 0.1–0.2 mg/kg IV for phenothiazine tranquilizers Symptomatic treatment

TABLE 5. PRIMARY CLINICAL SIGNS ARE EPITHELIAL DAMAGE

Toxin	Signs	Treatment
Plants: Horsebrush	Photosensitization	Topical ointments; symptomatic treatment Keep out of sun; graze at night
St. Johnswort	Photosensitization	See horsebrush
Foxtail	Mechanical injury	Symptomatic treatment
Cheatgrass	Mechanical injury	Symptomatic treatment
Needlegrass	Mechanical injury	Symptomatic treatment
Poverty grass	Mechanical injury	Symptomatic treatment
Crimson clover	Mechanical injury	Symptomatic treatment

cation or erroneous routes of administration. When several of these drugs are used concurrently, chemical interactions may occur, resulting in adverse drug reactions. The inherent sensitivity of the horse to foreign chemicals contributes further to the relatively high incidence of drug reactions in equine medicine.

SNAKE AND INSECT BITES

The sensitivity of horse skin and tissue, coupled with the environments in which many horses are housed or pastured, leads to a high incidence of insect (p. 622) or snake bites (p. 663). Localized and occasionally generalized reactions are common; fatalities occur if individual sensitivity is great or if bites evoke swelling that interferes with vital functions. Fortunately the incidence of snake and insect bite is seasonal and usually is restricted to specific regions.

MISCELLANEOUS TOXICOSES

Fungi are everywhere, and under appropriate conditions of moisture, temperature, and carbohydrate availability, they may grow in horse feeds. The presence of spoiled feed should remind the clinician of the possibility of fungal growth and the presence of mycotoxins. Aflatoxins produce pronounced liver damage, while other mycotoxins may induce colic, hemorrhagic gastroenteritis, kidney dysfunction, blood coagulation defects, and interference with immune status.

Gases may be generated under a variety of housing or environmental conditions. Carbon monoxide, hydrogen sulfide, nitrogen dioxide, ammonia, sulfur dioxide, carbon disulfide, and hydrogen cyanide are all toxic to horses in confined and poorly ventilated situations.

Supplemental Reading

Galitzer, S., and Oehme, F. W.: Emergency procedures for equine toxicoses. Equine Prac., *1*:49, 1979.

General Principles in Treatment of Poisoning

Frederick W. Oehme, MANHATTAN, KANSAS

The treatment of any poisoning is based upon a sound diagnosis. Except in emergency treatments, in which case general antidotal therapy is employed, every attempt should be made to utilize the available diagnostic information to formulate the most specific treatment for the poisoning.

DIAGNOSIS

The diagnosis of poisoning is based upon an adequate history, clinical evaluation of the patient, and a necropsy if death occurs and other animals are still involved. Since few poisonings have pathognomonic clinical syndromes or necropsy lesions, the history is often a key to diagnosis. Observation, an adept questioning procedure, and utilization of the practitioner's knowledge of management practices and personality quirks of the client assist greatly in generating diagnostic clues. The clinical signs in poisoned horses may involve a variety of body systems, with the central nervous system, digestive tract, liver, and blood frequently being affected. General signs of poisoning are lack of appetite, depression, weight loss, dehydration, colic, and frequent and difficult respiration. Hyperexcitability, incoordination, muscular twitching, abnormal posturing and body movements, and convulsions leading to prostration and coma may be suggestive of primary central nervous system effects or can be secondary to liver or digestive tract disturbance.

Diagnosis is especially difficult in chronic, low-grade poisonings that may involve biochemical or metabolic "interference syndromes" or may reflect the gradual accumulation of chemicals in various body systems and the eventual expression of their toxicity. The history and general physical appearance of the patient will often suggest a long-term process that may be at variance with the client's insistence that the horse "just got sick."

Whenever possible, a complete postmortem examination should be performed on animals dying from poisons. Although very few poisonings provide pathognomonic necropsy findings, there are many horses thought to have been poisoned that upon necropsy have a strangulation or torsion of the digestive tract, a discovery that warrants the effort involved in performing field necropsies. Although laboratory studies are frequently expensive, they are often the only definitive procedures to identify the cause of an intoxication. Unfortunately, the laboratory is not able to perform an all-encompassing screening test, and the clinician must suggest the most likely or suspected poison for laboratory assay. Suggestions for sample collection are given in the article on the etiologic diagnosis of sudden death (p. 685). In the living patient, blood and urine, as well as samples of suspected contaminated material, may be submitted for analysis.

The clinician should not rely upon the laboratory assay and should not wait for histopathologic or laboratory results before initiating therapy and suggesting management changes. "Tincture of time" is applicable only if the patient can spontaneously deal with the disease process. In cases of overwhelming intoxications or in instances of continuing ingestion and accumulation of a toxic compound, not waiting even a matter of hours before initiating treatment may mean the difference between recovery and death. There will be numerous instances in which an absolute diagnosis is not confirmed, but circumstantial, clinical, and perhaps gross pathologic evidence suggests a general group of poisons or a specific intoxication. Treatment should then be initiated promptly to prevent further absorption. Apply specific antidotes when possible, hasten elimination of the circulating toxin, and provide supportive therapy to the animal.

TREATMENT PRINCIPLES

It is useful to follow a general set of objectives in dealing with poisonings in horses. These general steps are stabilization of the patient (if necessary), prevention of further exposure to or absorption of the toxin, application of specific antidotes or therapy, increasing elimination of the absorbed poison, and supportive therapy to counteract the specific organ effects of the poisoning. To respond to these objectives requires not only prompt action but also the availability of appropriate and necessary equipment and medications. Table 1 is a listing of the suggested components of an emergency kit for poisonings. These items are fundamental to the treatment of equine poisonings and should always be available and fully stocked for immediate use by the clinician.

STABILIZATION OF THE PATIENT

Since a patient dying of respiratory failure is frequently not helped even by prompt administration of a specific antidote, it is most important to ensure that the horse does not die while the clinician is deciding upon the appropriate course of action. An adequate and patent airway should be ensured, and cardiac and respiratory function must be stabilized and maintained. Endotracheal intubation and artificial respiration may be coupled with cardiac stimulation to maintain these vital functions. Blood pressure should be adequate to ensure kidney perfusion and glomerular filtration. If in doubt, catheterization of the bladder should be performed and urinary flow monitored. Mechanical means may be used to stimulate vital signs and to maintain them, with drugs employed as necessary. When vital signs are stable, management of the poisoning may continue.

PREVENTION OF FURTHER EXPOSURE AND/OR ABSORPTION

In a situation in which horses are being exposed to the toxic material, they should either be removed from that environment or the toxic substance should be taken away. This may involve removal of the animals from a pasture or shed or may necessitate the cleaning of hay, grain, or water sources so that further consumption is halted. If the toxin has been applied to the skin, the animal should be washed with water and a mild detergent to remove the unabsorbed chemical. Abundant water should be used to wash the skin and to dilute any remaining toxin. Protective clothing should be worn by the veterinarian or animal handler during this process.

Absorption of toxins in the digestive tract may be limited by the use of adsorbents, such as activated charcoal, preferably of vegetable origin, used at a minimum of ½ lb (250 gm) for a foal, with up to 1½ lb (750 gm) used for an adult horse. Up to 1 gal (4 L) of warm water (depending upon the animal's size) should be used to make a slurry of the activated charcoal, which is then administered by stomach tube. The activated charcoal adsorbs many organic toxins but is relatively ineffective against inorganic and heavy metal poisons. The slurry should be left in the stomach for 20 to 30 minutes and then should be followed with a laxative to hasten removal of the charcoal and adsorbed chemical from the patient. Unless evacuated from the digestive tract, the poison may dissociate from the adsorbent and eventually may be absorbed by the patient. Although activated charcoal is probably the most effective adsorbent, other compounds such as bentonite, fuller's earth, and tannic acid may also be utilized to adsorb various toxic agents.

If no adsorbent is available, laxatives should be utilized to remove the toxic material from the digestive tract as soon as possible. Mineral oil (1 to 1½ gal, 4 to 6 l), 500 gm of magnesium sulfate or 1 mg of lentin (carbachol) may be administered to a mature horse. The sulfate laxatives (sodium or magnesium) are probably the most effective agents for evacuation of the digestive tract. If mineral oil

TABLE 1. EMERGENCY KIT FOR TREATMENT OF POISONING

Parenteral Solutions	Oral Medications	Equipment	Miscellaneous Items
Atropine sulfate	5% Acetic acid (vinegar)	Aspirator bulb	Mild detergent
Barbiturates (phenobarbital, pentobarbital)	Activated charcoal	Blankets	Oxygen
	Albumin (diluted egg white)	Endotracheal tubes, several sizes	Sodium bicarbonate paste
Calcium disodium EDTA	0.15% Calcium hydroxide	Enema kit	
23% Calcium gluconate	20% Magnesium sulfate solution	Gauze rolls and tape	
Digitalis		Intravenous catheters and stylets	
Dimercaprol (BAL)	Milk of magnesia	Mechanical respirator or compression bag	
Lactated Ringer's	Mineral oil		
4% Methylene blue	d-Penicillamine	Needles (hypodermic)	
Normal saline	1:10,000 Potassium permanganate solution	Stethoscope	
Physostigmine		Stomach tubes, several sizes	
Picrotoxin	20% Sodium sulfate	Syringes	
Pilocarpine	Tannic acid	Thermometers	
Pralidoxine chloride (2-PAM, Protopam chloride)	Vegetable oils, lard	Urinary catheters, various sizes	
Sedatives		Venotomy kit	
Thiamine hydrochloride			
1% Sodium nitrite			
20% Sodium nitrite			
20% Sodium thiosulfate			
Stimulants			
Strychnine			
Vitamin K_1			

is used initially, the use of a saline cathartic 30 to 45 minutes after oil administration will be an effective purgative. If the patient already has diarrhea due to the toxic syndrome, further administration of a purgative may add to the risk of dehydration.

SPECIFIC ANTIDOTES

If the poisoning is identified early and an antidote available, it should be used early in the treatment regimen, immediately following stabilization of the patient and prevention of further exposure and absorption. There are, however, very few poisons with specific antidotes, and it is frequently not possible to identify the toxic syndrome until later in the management of the patient. The specific antidotes given in Table 1 may be applied for such poisonings as insecticides, arsenic, cyanide, nitrite, and others. In some cases, doses are critical, but in most the animal is being titrated with the antidote against the body burden of the toxin. For example, in insecticide poisonings, atropine is given to effect by intravenous administration. As the clinical signs abate, the rate of atropine administration is diminished. In the absence of specific antidotes, application of sound therapeutic principles and common sense in further managing the poisoned patient is critical.

INCREASING ELIMINATION OF THE ABSORBED POISON

General nonspecific detoxicants may be used in the absence of specific antidotes. Intravenous administration of 100 to 500 ml of 20 per cent calcium gluconate, 500 to 1000 ml of 10 to 50 per cent dextrose, or 150 to 500 ml of 25 per cent sodium thiosulfate solution is useful.

Since absorbed toxins are usually excreted by the kidneys, renal excretion may be enhanced by the use of large volumes of intravenous fluids (electrolytes, 5 per cent dextrose, or saline) or by the use of diuretics, which should be carefully managed to avoid dehydration. Adequate renal function and hydration of the patient are vital concerns. If a urinary flow of 0.1 ml per kg per minute is not maintained by the patient, hydration of the affected horse should be improved.

SUPPORTIVE THERAPY

The final objective is to maintain the various body functions in a state compatible with detoxification of the poison and patient recovery. Central nervous system excitement may be managed by the use of sedatives, barbiturates, or combinations of tranquilizers, chloral hydrate, and magnesium sulfate. Convulsions are most effectively handled by pentobarbital administration, but care must be taken to ensure that respiration is not depressed. Although inhalation anesthetics are excellent for long-term management of central nervous system hyperactivity, prolonged anesthesia in horses is not without risk of gas exchange problems and muscle damage. Central nervous system depression is often complicated by respiratory depression, and both conditions must be managed. Artificial ventilation may support respiration while stimulants such as doxapram (5 to 10 mg per kg) pentylenetetrazol (6 to 10 mg per kg), or bemegride (10 to 20 mg per kg) may be administered intravenously to stimulate central nervous system activity. The action of the stimulants is of relatively short duration; hence, the clinician may wish to place more emphasis on artificial ventilation (see p. 475 of first edition of this book), since adequate respiratory support frequently stimulates recovery from central nervous system depression.

Effective respiratory support requires an adequate patent airway, which may be obtained by an endotracheal tube or by performing a tracheostomy. A mechanical respirator is of great value, but manual compression of the bag of an anesthetic machine may also be utilized with equal efficiency. In the event of cyanosis, oxygen may be necessary, but under most conditions, environmental air is adequate. A mixture of 50 per cent oxygen and 50 per cent environmental air may also be employed.

Support of cardiovascular function requires adequate heart function, appropriate circulating blood volume, and appropriate acid-base balance. Fluid volume and cardiac activity are of most immediate concern. Heart rate may be aided by the use of closed-chest cardiac massage and by the administration of therapeutic agents intravenously or directly into the heart. The slow administration of calcium gluconate has been useful in some instances. Digoxin, 0.2 to 0.6 mg per kg intravenously, may also be effective. Clinical judgment is important to determine the type and extent of cardiac stimulation to be pursued.

For decreased circulating volume, whole blood administration is a valuable procedure. Hypovolemia due to water loss alone may be treated by administering lactated Ringer's solution, saline, or 5 per cent dextrose solutions. Administration of 2 to 10 mg dexamethasone per kg intravenously is useful to prevent shock.

Acidosis is corrected by the administration of sodium bicarbonate, sodium lactate, or lactated Ringer's solution. Alkalosis is less commonly seen but may be reversed by the intravenous administration of physiologic saline (10 ml per kg) followed by 200 mg ammonium chloride per kg per day orally. Such therapy requires careful monitoring to ensure the administration of appropriate concentrations and volumes.

Animals with severe diarrhea may require very careful monitoring of water and electrolyte balance. Fluid requirements may be given via stomach tube or intravenously. Symptomatic care of gastrointestinal disturbances includes protectants such as Kaopectate* or bentonite.

Body temperature should be maintained within normal limits by protection from environmental cold or heat, by providing heat lamps to prevent hypothermia, or cold water enemas, cold water baths, or ice bags to reduce hyperthermia. Constant monitoring of the animal's body temperature is necessary to ensure that vital biochemical and physiologic detoxification processes are able to proceed at optimal physiologic temperatures. Since horses are extremely sensitive to pain, control of pain is important.

Although it is optimal to have all the suggested procedures operational in each poisoned individual, practicality dictates that the clinician select those measures most appropriate to the case being managed. Careful attention to the application of these objectives in the poisoned horse will ensure maximal therapeutic effectiveness.

---

*Kaopectate, Upjohn Co., Kalamazoo, MI

Supplemental Readings

Bailey, E. M.: Management and treatment of toxicosis. *In* Howard, J. L. (ed.): Current Veterinary Therapy, Food Animal Practice. Philadelphia, W. B. Saunders Company, 1981, pp. 378–388.

Osweiler, G. D., Carson, T. L., Buck, W. B., and Van Gelder, G. A.: Clinical and Diagnostic Veterinary Toxicology, 3rd ed. Dubuque, IA, Kendall/Hunt, 1985.

Insecticides

Frederick W. Oehme, MANHATTAN, KANSAS

Of all the chemicals to which horses might be exposed, insecticides constitute the largest and most potentially toxic group of compounds. They are chemicals that may either be intentionally applied for insect or parasite control in the animal, or they may be accidentally consumed via contamination of feed, forage, water, or the stable environment. These potentially hazardous situations make it imperative that the equine veterinarian be well informed of the dangers and safety of the various types of insecticides, and be prepared to diagnose and manage any instances of clinical intoxication.

There are three general groups of insecticide material to which horses may be routinely exposed:

The plant-origin insecticides, the chlorinated hydrocarbon insecticides, and the organophosphorus and carbamate materials.

PLANT-ORIGIN INSECTICIDES

This group includes insect control agents derived from plant materials and some that are now synthesized rather than extracted from plants. Rotenone and pyrethrins are materials applied topically directly to the horse and are essentially nontoxic. Clinical cases of rotenone or pyrethrin poisoning are extremely rare and are always due to massive ingestion of these insecticides rather than topical application. The materials are not absorbed from the skin and may be clinically considered of no hazard.

NICOTINE

Nicotine is an extremely toxic chemical, but fortunately, it is used only for mite control in buildings. Nicotine sulfate is never directly applied to horses. Toxicity is, therefore, limited to accidental contamination of feeding materials or water or of horses being housed in recently sprayed stables.

Clinical Signs

If toxicity does result from nicotine sulfate contact, the signs of poisoning occur within a few minutes. They are characteristically those of central nervous system stimulation, producing marked excitement, rapid respiration and salivation. If the animal consumed the nicotine, irritation of the oral mucosa is seen, with increased peristalsis and diarrhea occurring with the ingestion of low to moderate doses. The initial stimulation period is followed by depression, with the horse becoming incoordinated and ataxic and having a rapid pulse with shallow and slow respiration. This leads rapidly to a flaccid paralysis, with coma and death occurring within a few hours. Death usually occurs during a terminal convulsive seizure from paralysis of the respiratory muscles. Recovery from sublethal doses is usually complete within four to six hours after exposure. No characteristic postmortem lesions are found with nicotine sulfate other than cyanosis and congestion of internal organs. With oral ingestion, congestion of the digestive tract mucous membranes, particularly the upper portion of the small intestine, may be seen.

Therapy

Treatment of nicotine sulfate poisoning is usually not feasible because death occurs rapidly. However, spontaneous recovery may occur if only small amounts are ingested. Topical nicotine should be washed from the skin. The administration of laxatives, tannic acid, or potassium permanganate may help to eliminate ingested nicotine. General supportive care is aimed at prolonging life to allow biological detoxification.

CHLORINATED HYDROCARBON INSECTICIDES

Chlorinated hydrocarbon insecticides are slowly being removed from routine use as agricultural chemicals, but their application is still permitted on some non–food-producing animals, including horses. Although their environmental use has been reduced because of their biologic persistence, as a group these insecticides are effective agents. However, their slow metabolism and persistence in animal tissues causes biologic accumulation following repeated exposures. Horses may thus develop toxicity either from application of excessive concentrations or because of frequent, repeated applications of single recommended amounts. Because of their lipid solubility, all members of this class of insecticides are easily absorbed through the intact skin after topical application or close confinement of animals in recently sprayed housing areas.

Clinical Signs

The clinical signs of chlorinated hydrocarbon insecticide poisoning are intermittent, with colic and severe neurologic effects predominating. Hyperexcitability, hyperesthesia, and tonic-clonic convulsive seizures may alternate with periods of depression. The toxicity usually begins within an hour of application or exposure, with the animal initially being apprehensive. A period of hyperexcitability follows, characterized by exaggerated responses to stimuli and spontaneous muscle twitches and spasms. The muscle tremors usually originate in the head area and progress posteriorly to involve the neck, shoulder, back, and rear leg muscles. Early in the syndrome, the horse may develop these spasms while standing, but as they become more severe, the animal will collapse into lateral recumbency. The horse may have chewing movements, may twist or elevate its head, and may undergo abnormal posturing prior to the development of convulsions. Body temperature may be elevated during seizures. Intermittent respiratory paralysis occurs during the convulsions. The convulsions may last several hours, and the patient either dies during a severe seizure or recovers gradually, with the severity of each subsequent convulsion decreasing until body control and posture are once more regained. Recovered horses may have minor neurologic problems for a few days following recovery, with depression and partial loss of appetite remaining for three to five days. Most fatally affected horses will die within 12 hours after the onset of seizures. No characteristic postmortem lesions are observed in fatal cases other than those resulting from terminal convulsions and trauma due to the seizures.

Therapy

Although there is no specific treatment for chlorinated hydrocarbon poisoning, conscientious attempts should be made to remove all unabsorbed insecticide from the patient's body. Washing of the skin with soap and warm water is very important. In instances of oral ingestion of chlorinated hydrocarbon insecticide, large amounts of activated charcoal may given by stomach tube to bind the unabsorbed material. Oily laxatives should be avoided, but magnesium sulfate and similar cathartics can be given following the activated charcoal to empty the digestive tract of the contained insecticide. The neurologic effects may be diminished by the use of sedatives or anesthetics. Barbiturates seem to provide most effective control of the centrally originating seizures, but chloral hydrate and tranquilizers may also be used. Repeated dosing is required to control the seizures, and animals that recover need smaller doses as the severity of the convulsions diminishes. Intravenous fluids may be given in severe or prolonged cases to maintain hydration. Generally supportive care will hasten recovery.

Since a variety of chlorinated hydrocarbon insecticides are available, it may be important to determine the specific chemical involved in any poisoning and to establish its source so that future cases can be prevented. The most common chlorinated hydrocarbons used on horses are toxaphene and lindane. Benzene hexachloride, aldrin, endrin, dieldrin, methoxychlor, heptachlor, and chlordane are other chlorinated hydrocarbon insecticides that may be applied on and around horses. While each has its specific toxicity, individual horses may show hypersensitivity to the dose considered safe for the "average" horse. Young colts, weak and debilitated animals, and old horses with potential liver or kidney disease are especially at risk from exposure to the chlorinated hydrocarbon group of insecticides.

ORGANOPHOSPHORUS AND CARBAMATE INSECTICIDES

Unlike chlorinated hydrocarbons, the organophosphorus and carbamate insecticides have little environmental and biologic persistence and are, therefore, increasing in use. Their insecticidal properties depend upon an acute and overwhelming toxicity. Unfortunately, this same event often occurs in horses exposed to this group of chemicals.

As with the chlorinated hydrocarbon compounds, horses may be exposed by overzealous skin application, by spraying of the insecticide in confined areas containing horses, or by accidental contamination of forage, feed, or water. In addition, organophosphate compounds are also used for control of digestive tract parasites in horses, and toxicities occasionally result from this method of application. Horses with digestive tract lesions, animals with intestinal conditions that increase absorption (such as constipation or mucosal inflammation or irritation), or certain hypersensitive individuals are particularly likely to show clinical effects from the oral application of these compounds. The organophosphorus compounds include trichlorfon, dermeton, malathion, dichlorvos (DDVP), ronnel, Rulene, parathion, and diazinon. The carbamate group of insecticides is represented by carbaryl.

Clinical Signs

Both the organophosphorus and carbamate insecticides have their effect and cause their clinical signs by binding acetylcholinesterase, thereby permitting continuous cholinergic stimulation and excessive autonomic and muscular activity. Effects manifested within the first hour after exposure include frequent urination, increased peristalsis reflected as colic, and "patchy" sweating, particularly of the skin of the neck, shoulders, and rib cage of the affected horse. Salivation may be moderate to profuse, and the parasympathetic stimulation produces defecation, urination, and a general sense of anxiety or uneasiness in the patient. The heart rate is slow, respiratory efforts become exaggerated, and the animal may develop severe abdominal pains. A stiff-legged gait and muscle tremors of the face, neck, and other body muscles occur as the syndrome progresses. The muscular hyperactivity from organophosphorus and carbamate insecticides never develops into convulsions, as is so typical of the chlorinated hydrocarbon insecticides. Rather, the hyperactivity of the skeletal muscles is generally followed by muscle weakness, incoordination and ataxia, and prostration.

Respiratory failure is a sign of severe toxicity. Bronchoconstriction and pulmonary edema complicate respiratory efforts, and weakness of the respiratory muscles leads to difficult, frequent, and shallow respiratory efforts. Death is due to anoxia. Death may occur within minutes to several hours after the initial signs develop. Except in cases of oral absorption, when continuing absorption prolongs clinical signs, horses that do not die within 12 hours after exposure have a good chance of spontaneous recovery.

Some of the newer organophosphorus and carbamate insecticides are capable of producing variations in this clinical syndrome. All the described clinical signs may not be seen in any one horse, but several of the signs are usually present. In all instances, however, terminal muscle weakness and respiratory dysfunction are severe, and death is due to interference with and paralysis of respiratory efforts. If the diagnosis is in doubt, low blood cholinesterase activity will confirm the toxicity.

Interactions of organophosphorus and carbamate insecticides with other chemicals affecting the same enzyme systems are possible. Drugs working by this mechanism will have additive and sometimes synergistic clinical effects. Phenothiazine derivatives, such as the promazine tranquilizers, potentiate the effects of these cholinesterase-inhibiting insecticides. The administration of succinylcholine, carbachol, physostigmine, or neostigmine is contraindicated if horses have recently been exposed to organophosphorus or carbamate insecticides. The acetylcholinesterase inhibition persists for at least 14 days following organophosphorus insecticide exposure, and at least 30 days or more are required before normal circulating levels of acetylcholinesterase return in organophosphorus-exposed horses. The effects of carbamate insecticides are much shorter, but interaction with other anticholinesterase compounds is still possible if exposures occur within three to five days of each other.

Postmortem lesions associated with organophosphorus or carbamate poisoning are nonspecific. Excessive pulmonary fluids and evidence of excessive fluids in the mouth and digestive tract are supportive but not confirmatory for organophosphorus or carbamate poisoning. In some horses, the excessive peristaltic activity will result in pooling of the blood in "bands" in the small intestinal tract mucosa, and 1 to 7 cm wide areas of the mucosa of the small intestine will appear hyperemic. The bladder may be empty owing to excessive urination, and liquid feces may be found in the rectum. Final confirmation of death due to organophosphorus or carbamate insecticides depends upon the detection of significant plasma, brain, liver, or kidney concentrations of the suspected chemical. Excessively depressed plasma and red blood cell cholinesterase activity may also support a diagnosis.

Therapy

Fortunately for horses affected with organophosphorus or carbamate toxicity, an effective and specific treatment regimen is available. It involves providing respiratory assistance if death due to respiratory dysfunction is imminent, chemically antagonizing the signs produced by the excessive acetylcholine present at synapses, and aiding the dissociation of inhibited (complexed) acetylcholinesterase throughout the body.

All horses should be immediately treated intravenously with atropine sulfate. The approximate dosage of 1.0 mg per kg must be given to effect,

with mydriasis and an absence of salivation used as end points. Since the atropine administered is being titrated against the absorbed organophosphorus or carbamate, the actual amount of atropine required in any case will be variable. After the initial atropine administration, repeated doses may be given every 1½ to 2 hours as required. Additional doses of atropine may be administered subcutaneously. Intravenous atropine administration is also a useful diagnostic tool. Horses not showing decreased clinical effects (decreased anxiety and less evidence of dyspnea and colic) when atropine is administered are probably not suffering from organophosphorus or carbamate insecticide poisoning.

Although atropine dramatically counteracts the parasympathetic signs within a few minutes after administration, it will only minimally reduce the skeletal muscle and nervous system effects. It also will not counteract the insecticide-acetylcholinesterase binding, which is relatively resistant to spontaneous hydrolysis.

Oximes are utilized to increase release of the inhibited enzyme. These compounds (2-PAM, pralidoxime chloride, TMB-4, and the commercially available Protopam chloride) are effective in binding the organophosphorus compound and freeing it from the enzyme-phosphorus complex. This releases the previously inhibited acetylcholinesterase to return to its normal physiologic functions. At least 20 mg Protopam chloride per kg are required, but occasionally as much as 30 to 35 mg per kg may be necessary to secure lasting results. The compound is given intravenously and is repeated every four to six hours. It is important that early treatment with the oximes be instituted. After 18 to 20 hours of organophosphorus exposure, a stabilized enzyme insecticide complex has occurred. This complex is refractory to oxime therapy, which may need to be maintained for several days to be effective. The most effective results are observed with a combination of atropine and oxime treatment. In this way, the immediate clinical signs are treated, and the enzyme-organophosphorus complex is broken and directly antagonized.

Since oximes may have some deleterious effects in certain cases of carbamate poisoning, the routine use of oximes in cases not specifically known to be organophosphorus-produced is not recommended. In those instances, immediate treatment with atropine will provide life-saving effects. Since carbamate poisoning is short-lived owing to spontaneous dissociation of the complex and rapid biotransformation of the carbamate insecticide, repeated treatments with atropine are usually not necessary. Carbamate toxicity usually produces death within two hours, or spontaneous recovery occurs shortly thereafter. Provided that additional absorption of the carbamate insecticide does not occur through skin or the digestive tract, one or two treatments with atropine should be sufficient to manage carbamate toxicity. Rapid recovery should then follow.

To prevent additional absorption of the organophosphorus or carbamate insecticide, soap and water should be used to wash dermally exposed animals, and 1 to 2 lbs (0.5 to 1 kg) of activated charcoal should be administered orally in a water slurry to decontaminate the digestive tract of orally exposed horses. Osmotic laxatives should also be employed to empty the digestive tract.

The described specific therapy is usually quite adequate for routine cases of organophosphorus or carbamate toxicity. However, in severe instances or in episodes that are prolonged owing to delay in treatment or continuing exposure, clinical judgment must be used in the application of supportive therapy. Animals in life-threatening situations with severe respiratory embarrassment should be supported with artifical respiration where appropriate. Electrolyte and fluid therapy may be indicated in severely poisoned animals affected for several days. Whole blood and amino acid infusions may also be useful in ensuring the most effective management of these cases of insecticide toxicity.

Supplemental Readings

Carson, T. L., and Furr, A. S.: Insecticides. *In* Howard, J. L. (ed.): Current Veterinary Therapy, Food Animal Practice, Philadelphia, W. B. Saunders Company, 1981, pp. 475–477.

Clarke, M. L., Harvey, D. G., and Humphreys, D. J.: Veterinary Toxicology, 2nd ed. London, Bailliere Tindall, 1981, p. 97.

Van Gelder, G. A.: Insecticide poisoning. *In* Mansmann, R. A., McAllister, E. S., and Pratt, P. W. (eds.): Equine Medicine and Surgery, 3rd ed. Santa Barbara, CA, American Veterinary Publications, 1982, pp. 194–196.

Rodenticides

Frederick W. Oehme, MANHATTAN, KANSAS

Rodenticide toxicity in horses is relatively uncommon because most owners ensure that rodenticides are not placed in their horse's proximity. Should horses be exposed to rodenticides, the method of packaging and placement of bait usually result in the animal receiving less than a toxic dose. Since many of the commonly used anticoagulant rodenticides require several days of exposure, the potential for toxicity is further reduced.

In instances of feed contamination with highly toxic rodenticides, not only may a sufficient dosage be received, but also continual daily ingestion may result in accumulation of the toxic chemical. If the feed is being given to several horses, more than one animal may become ill, and a classic "outbreak" of poisoning may be seen. Environmental or feed contamination has produced poisoning from such rodenticides as warfarin and other anticoagulants, strychnine, ANTU, arsenic, fluoroacetate, zinc phosphide, and Vacor. In addition, potential toxic effects from phosphorus, thallium, barium chloride, and Castrix must also be considered whenever rodenticide toxicity in horses is discussed.

WARFARIN, PIVAL, AND OTHER ANTICOAGULANTS

Single doses of 75 to 100 mg per kg are toxic, but a dose of 2 mg or less per kg on a repeated daily basis is more likely and effective in producing poisoning. The anticoagulants antagonize vitamin K and produce coagulation system defects. Vascular shock may be seen with single large doses, but more commonly, mild to massive hemorrhages occur throughout the body. Nose bleeds, diarrhea with free blood in the stool, and subcutaneous hematomas (particularly over bony prominences and points of contact with hard surfaces) are typical signs. Lameness may occur due to hemorrhage into joint capsules, and soreness may be seen due to muscle hematomas. Occasionally, affected animals are first recognized by continual bleeding following owner or veterinary parenteral medication, and anemia may be observed upon examination of the mucous membranes or the performance of blood counts. The diagnosis is usually obvious upon the finding of elevated prothrombin times and clinical evidence of anemia and diffuse hemorrhagic foci. Occasionally in horses, acute death is seen due to massive hemorrhage into the thorax, abdominal cavity, or around the brain; these are obvious upon postmortem examination.

THERAPY

Treatment involves removal from the source of the anticoagulant, replacement of the inhibited coagulation factors, and supplying vitamin K to competitively antagonize the presence of the anticoagulant rodenticide. The horse should be removed from its immediate environment to prevent further exposure, or the source of the bait should be detected and removed. If ingestion of the anticoagulant has occurred within 24 hours, saline cathartics and activated charcoal may be administered. Whole blood (p. 317) will reverse anemia, will immediately replace missing coagulation factors, and will stabilize the horse against immediate life-threatening situations. Vitamin K_1 should be administered (1 mg per kg twice daily for five days). Synthetic vitamin K (menadione) is considerably less effective and should be reserved for less severe cases or for follow-up therapy by the owner (10 to 20 mg per kg for seven days orally or parenterally) following alleviation of the acute stage of the crisis. During the early stages of recovery, the horse should be kept quiet and should be handled as little as possible. Undue excitement and the potential for trauma carry the risk of producing internal or external hemorrhage that may be severe.

STRYCHNINE

At a dose of 0.5 to 1 mg per kg, horses may be poisoned with a single oral dose of strychnine. The rodenticide antagonizes inhibitory spinal cord neurons and allows excess activity of the central nervous system to cause convulsions and seizures in the patient. Acute onset of tetanus-like seizures is characteristic. The animal is hyperexcitable and hyperreflexic, so that wind, noise, and skin contact produce an aggravated reaction, often leading to muscle seizures, prostration, and tetanic convulsions. The syndrome is violent, with seizures progressing from moderate to fatal with 15 to 45 minutes. The seizure pattern is characteristic, and no significant postmortem lesions are found. A rapid onset of rigor mortis suggests strychnine poisoning.

THERAPY

No specific antidote is available, but seizures can be controlled with central nervous system depressants such as pentobarbital, chloral hydrate–magnesium sulfate combinations, or glyceryl guaiacolate (5 per cent solution intravenously, 212 mg per kg). The seizures are controlled by administering these compounds to effect and as often as necessary to control muscle activity. Care must be taken to avoid depressing the respiratory center with the central nervous system depressant, and the availability of respiratory support may be vital to recovery. Activated charcoal (0.5 to 1 kg per animal) should be administered orally to bind unabsorbed strychnine in the digestive tract and to prevent continual absorption and recurrence of signs. A laxative should be administered upon clinical recovery to hasten digestive tract elimination of the charcoal-bound strychnine. Healthy horses usually recover within 24 hours if treatment is conscientiously applied.

ANTU (Alpha-naphthylthiourea)

Although toxicity is not seen frequently in horses owing to the limited availability of this agent, this rodenticide produces dramatic lethal effects if consumed. The toxic dose varies from 25 to 75 mg per kg and produces its toxicity by increased permeability of the lung capillaries. Pulmonary edema is the outstanding clinical sign. The affected horse develops moist rales, increased respiratory efforts, muscle weakness, and severe dyspnea as pulmonary edema and hydrothorax cause anoxia and rapidly developing cyanosis. As the condition progresses, foamy froth bubbles from the nose and mouth of the laboring animal. Death occurs within hours after the beginning of signs, with the animal prostrate and large volumes of white frothy foam emanating from the nose and mouth. Postmortem observations reveal hydrothorax, pulmonary edema, and frothy edematous fluid filling the air spaces of the lung, trachea, nose and mouth.

THERAPY

No antidote is available to treat this rapidly fulminating condition. The animal should be kept as quiet as possible to reduce tissue oxygen demands, and sedation may be used if necessary. Oxygen should be administered. Osmotic diuretics (such as 50 per cent glucose or mannitol) and atropine administration (0.05 mg per kg) have been suggested to reduce pulmonary edema, but their effectiveness in field cases is not proven. Fluid balance should be ensured by monitoring skin tone and hemoconcentration. Secondary infections may be avoided by supplying broad-spectrum antibiotics during the stressful period of digestive tract irritation and inflammation.

FLUOROACETATE (Compound 1080)

This rodenticide is one of the most lethal based on a milligram dosage. The toxic dose ranges from approximately 0.25 to 1.5 mg per kg. The compound is converted to a metabolite that blocks the energy production cycle of the cell, producing cellular death due to lack of energy. When this affects the neurons of the central nervous system, dramatic major organ and central nervous system effects result. The chemical initially induces cardiac arrhythmias, a rapid, weak pulse, anxiousness, and hyperexcitability, with ventricular fibrillation, sudden excitement, and convulsions and death following quickly with sudden collapse. Because of the small quantity of toxin required to produce death, horses may consume sufficient amounts through feed or environmental contamination to become ill. The use of this chemical in range country for coyote and predator animal control may cause exposure to horses grazing native pastures. No significant post-mortem lesions are found, and the rapidity of this compound's action may lead the owner to report "sudden death" as the only observation.

THERAPY

No specific antidote is available, but seizures and excessive nervous activity should be controlled with short-acting barbiturates given to effect. Activated charcoal may be given orally to reduce further absorption of fluoroacetate. Glycerol monoacetate (0.1 to 0.5 mg per kg intramuscularly) may be given every hour for several doses, but its effectiveness has only been shown if given before or at the same time that clinical signs develop. The clinician must use common sense and knowledge of respiratory physiology to manage horses affected with fluoroacetate poisoning. Recovery from this toxicity is not common once clinical signs have developed.

ARSENIC

This compound is used as a rodent and insect control agent, as well as being employed as a herbicide in agricultural weed control programs. The toxic dose ranges from 2 to 7 mg per kg. Arsenic is a very irritating heavy metal and produces digestive tract irritation within hours after the ingestion of a toxic dose. Horses have signs of colic and excessive peristaltic activity and exhibit typical signs of digestive tract obstruction or irritation. After several hours, diarrhea develops, which is at first fluid and mucoid. After 12 hours, the diarrhea becomes blood-tinged owing to bleeding into the digestive tract. Affected horses may become rapidly dehydrated from arsenic toxicity and may often be misdiagnosed as having colitis or a digestive tract obstruction. A careful physical examination will reveal congestion of most mucous membranes and obvious pain upon external and rectal palpation. The continuing excessive peristaltic activity followed by the appearance of bloody feces may help in the diagnosis.

THERAPY

Dimercaprol (BAL) is the specific antidote for arsenic. It is given intramuscularly four times daily at the rate of 3 to 4 mg per kg. Sodium thiosulfate (20 per cent solution, 30 to 40 mg per kg intravenously) may be given two or three times daily in lieu of BAL. Since BAL is inherently nephrotoxic, it should only be given for three to four days. Sodium thiosulfate may then be administered until recovery. In severe acute cases, the combination of BAL and sodium thiosulfate may be valuable in providing additional sulfur for binding and detoxification of the arsenic. Since dehydration is a frequent complication of arsenic poisoning, the administration of electrolytes and glucose should be considered. Fluid balance should be ensured by monitoring skin tone and hemoconcentration. Secondary infections may be avoided by supplying broad-spectrum antibiotics during the stressful period of digestive tract irritation and inflammation.

ZINC PHOSPHIDE

With toxic doses of 20 to 40 mg per kg, zinc phosphide produces toxicity by being broken down in the acid of the stomach to phosphine. The toxicity of this compound is greater when the stomach is full owing to the additional acidity present during the digestive process. The phosphine generated produces irritation of the mucous membranes of the digestive tract, pulmonary edema, and cardiovascular collapse. The animal affected with toxicity becomes depressed, colicky, and dyspneic. Occasionally horses will develop convulsive seizures. The digestive tract hyperemia is seen on postmortem examination together with excessive pulmonary fluid.

THERAPY

The acidity of the intestinal tract may be neutralized by administering 2 to 4 L of 5 per cent sodium bicarbonate. This should be repeated as needed together with laxatives to purge the digestive tract of the unabsorbed zinc phosphide. Supportive treatment may be utilized, but no specific antidote is available.

VACOR

This rodenticide was very popular during the past several years but has recently been removed from the market owing to unexpected chronic adverse effects in dogs, cats, and humans. The toxic dose is in the range of 300 mg per kg. The compound is a general metabolic toxin and produces effects in the gastrointestinal tract and nervous system by apparently affecting biologic oxidation-reduction reactions. Affected horses may show colic, mental confusion and uneasiness, increased peristalsis, and some difficulty in vision.

THERAPY

Because of the high dose required for lethal toxicity, most affected horses recover spontaneously, but affected animals should be treated with cathartics and supportive care to replace fluid loss and to control any nervous activity that might inflict damage to the horse or property. Nicotinamide is a specific antidote used in dogs and humans. It may be employed in horses by giving 1 gm per kg every four hours for two days, followed by 1 gm of nicotinamide per day orally for seven more days.

PHOSPHORUS

Phosphorus is a systemic poison that has a toxic dose of 1 to 4 mg per kg. White and yellow phosphorus are the toxic forms capable of producing digestive tract, liver, and kidney damage. The early signs of toxicity are abdominal pain and a fluid, hemorrhagic diarrhea. After several days, generalized depression, icterus, and hepatorenal failure develop, followed shortly thereafter by death. A saline cathartic may be administered early in the syndrome to evacuate the digestive tract. Liver damage is obvious. Treatment is supportive and symptomatic, since no direct antidote is available. Glucose and lipotrophic agents (such as methionine) may be beneficial in hepatotoxic conditions (pp. 111 and 113).

THALLIUM

Although no longer used extensively as a rodenticide, thallium is notoriously toxic to all body systems. It has a toxic dose of 10 to 15 mg per kg, with about 50 mg per kg required to kill. Almost all body systems are affected, but the digestive tract, skin, and respiratory and nervous systems are the most severely involved. The clinical onset of signs is usually delayed 24 to 48 hours after ingestion, but once signs occur, the digestive tract becomes severely damaged. A hemorrhagic gastroenteritis is present, together with difficult respiration, fever, and inflammation of the gums and eyelids. Chronic skin lesions, hair loss, tremors, or muscular seizures develop later.

THERAPY

Evacuation of the digestive tract with laxatives and purgatives is indicated. Glucose, parenteral vitamins, antibiotics, and general supportive therapy are employed as needed. The use of dithizone, as recommended in small animals, has not been evaluated in horses, nor has the use of Prussian blue as an adsorbing agent in the digestive tract.

BARIUM CHLORIDE

This infrequently used rodenticide is a generalized poison that produces digestive tract irritation, generalized depression, and prostration following consumption of doses in excess of 150 mg per kg. The toxicity is sufficiently nonspecific to make diagnosis difficult. Symptomatic and supportive therapy may be utilized to counter the digestive tract irritation and the general toxicity of this compound.

CASTRIX

Castrix is a convulsive rodenticide that requires only 25 mg or less per kg to produce effects. Affected animals become anxious and then nervous, with muscular tremors leading to convulsions and prostration in extreme cases. The horse should be sedated and orally administered activated charcoal and purgatives provided to bind the unabsorbed rodenticide and flush the digestive tract.

Supplemental Readings

Fowler, M. E.: Toxicity of rodenticides. *In* Catcott, E. J., and Smithcors, J. F. (eds.): Equine Medicine and Surgery, 2nd ed. Wheaton, IL, American Veterinary Publications, 1972, p. 200.
Osweiler, G. E., and Hook, B. S.: Rodenticides. *In* Howard, J. L. (ed.): Current Veterinary Therapy, Food Animal Practice. Philadelphia, W. B. Saunders Company, 1981, pp. 478–480.

Snake Bite

Frederick W. Oehme, MANHATTAN, KANSAS

Probably several hundred horses are bitten by poisonous snakes in the United States each year with a mortality ranging from 10 to 30 per cent. The most dangerous snake for horses is the large rattlesnake of the genus Crotalus. Other pit vipers that may bite horses are copperheads and water moccasins. The venom from these three types of snakes is mainly hemotoxic and proteolytic and produces extreme local swelling with marked tissue and red blood cell destruction and a direct effect on the heart. The fourth most common poisonous snake seen in the United States is the coral snake, found primarily in the southeast. This snake is not a major source of equine snake bite because of its shy nature and its distribution in areas where horses are not used. The coral snake venom is a rapidly acting neurotoxin.

CLINICAL SIGNS

Most snake bites in horses occur during the warm days of the spring and throughout the summer when snakes are out and active. Horses are bitten most frequently on the nose, head, and neck. They are less frequently bitten on the legs and chest, although exposure of the legs is common, especially if horses are moving through tall grass. Because of the lack of abundant muscle or connective tissue on the lower limbs, snake bites in those areas are occasionally not detected owing to minimal injection of venom and limited tissue swelling. Bites of the nose and head are extremely serious because of the rapid swelling that follows a bite. The bitten area becomes edematous, and the tissue reaction spreads throughout the head and neck. If the horse is bitten on the nose, the nose and nasal mucosa swells, and blood-stained exudate may drain from each nostril. The eyelids and ears may also swell, producing a deformed appearance. Swelling of the throat may produce stridor and life-threatening respiratory distress, which may require emergency tracheotomy. The effects of the bite may be sufficiently severe to cause depression and muscular weakness.

The severity of the snake bite is usually related to the size of the snake involved, the size of the bitten horse, the amount of venom injected, the site of the bite, and prior physical condition of the horse. Most bitten horses will not die, but sometimes, swelling of the throat or a massive injection of venom by a large rattlesnake in a tissue site producing rapid absorption may produce a fatal outcome. However, even with limited mortality, the tissue necrosis and prolonged recovery period required for healing are of considerable concern.

THERAPY

A variety of treatments may be employed for bitten horses, depending upon the site and severity of the bite, the time elapsed since the horse was bitten, and the value of the individual animal. If the horse is in respiratory distress, tracheotomy or other respiratory assistance is required. Anti-inflammatory compounds, such as corticosteroids, are of considerable value in reducing tissue swelling and necrosis. Although no work has been reported using antihistamines in horses, studies in mice and dogs have indicated that antihistamines are contraindicated in snake bite. Antivenom specific for the snake thought to be involved may be used systemically or via injections at the site of the bite. The risk of anaphylactic reactions must be considered, since antivenom is made from horse serum. Antivenom is most useful when given early in the clinical course. Antibiotics, particularly broad-spectrum ones, are indicated because bacteria are injected during the bite. Tetanus antitoxin is always indicated in snake bites in horses.

Additional treatments that may be considered by the clinician, depending upon the circumstances, are fluids to combat shock or dehydration, epinephrine to reduce the risk of circulatory collapse, calcium gluconate to limit hemolysis of red blood cells, and the injection of proteolytic enzymes to reduce tissue swelling.

If the time between bite and initiation of treatment warrants, an incision may be made over the fang marks and suction applied. If the bite is on an extremity, a tourniquet may be placed above the bite area for 15- to 20-minute intervals. Cold water packs applied to the bite area may prevent swelling, but the direct application of ice or other frozen materials is contraindicated, as it causes additional tissue damage.

It is important that the animal be treated as soon as possible and that the veterinarian see the patient either by going to the location of the bitten horse or meeting the animal and owner at some mutually determined location. The time that elapses between the bite and initiation of treatment appears to be the most important factor in reducing tissue damage and the risk of mortality.

Supplemental Reading

Burger, C. H., and Van Gelder, G. A.: Snakebite. *In* Mansmann, R. A., McAllister, E. S., and Pratt, P. W. (eds.): Equine Medicine and Surgery, 3rd ed. Santa Barbara, CA, American Veterinary Publications, 1982, pp. 215–216.

Carbon Tetrachloride

Frederick W. Oehme, MANHATTAN, KANSAS

Occasionally carbon tetrachloride enters the equine diet by accident or through its misuse as an anthelmintic. The compound is volatile and has a peculiar odor, which may result in horses rejecting feed containing this compound. Atmospheric concentrations of less than one part per million are detectable by the healthy horse's nose.

The toxicity of this drug may be expressed in several ways. Inhalation or absorption of large quantities of carbon tetrachloride can cause central nervous system depression and narcosis. Ingestion of carbon tetrachloride results in rapid absorption from the digestive tract and a toxic effect upon the liver cells, producing fatty degeneration in small quantities and centrilobular necrosis if larger amounts are absorbed. Because repeated administration of small quantities of carbon tetrachloride produces no toxic signs and since fatal cases of poisoning usually reveal kidney damage to a greater extent than liver pathology, the hepatic effects of carbon tetrachloride most likely must be accompanied by severe renal failure to produce clinical signs of toxicity and death. Local application of carbon tetrachloride, such as the parenteral injection of carbon tetrachloride in oil, produces localized tissue necrosis and may lead to lameness.

The toxic dose of carbon tetrachloride for horses is variable, with as little as 0.25 ml per kg producing serious liver damage in some animals, while 3 ml per kg may produce no signs in other individuals. Poisoning in horses, however, is usually acute, with signs manifesting themselves within the first 24 to 36 hours. Occasionally, severe signs may be delayed for another 48 hours, but eventually depression, muscle weakness, and ataxia follow the initial loss of appetite. Constipation is followed by diarrhea with the passage of blood-stained feces. Total collapse occurs terminally, with death usually occurring within 24 hours of the onset of severe signs. Gastroenteritis of the upper digestive tract is a consistent postmortem finding. The liver and kidneys are congested with gross evidence of degeneration and necrosis, hemorrhages, and focal areas of fatty degneration. Microscopically, the liver has centrilobular necrosis, and the kidneys have cloudy swelling and necrosis of the tubular epithelium. Repeated administration of moderate doses of carbon tetrachloride may produce liver fibrosis and cirrhosis. This circumstance would be unusual in horses owing to the finicky appetite of this species.

A specific antidote for carbon tetrachloride is not available. The general principles of treating poisoning (p. 653) should be followed, with special attention to eliminating further exposure and reducing additional absorption by the use of activated charcoal adsorbent and the use of laxatives and saline purges to rapidly empty the digestive tract. General supportive and symptomatic care is useful in allowing the patient time to detoxify and excrete the absorbed carbon tetrachloride. Horses showing clinical signs of carbon tetrachloride toxicity are best given a guarded prognosis, since the extent of liver and/or kidney damage in individual cases is unpredictable based upon the known carbon tetrachloride exposure or the degree of clinical signs seen.

Supplemental Reading

Clarke, E. G. C., and Clarke, M. L.: Veterinary Toxicology. Baltimore, Williams & Wilkins, 1975.

Phenothiazine

Frederick W. Oehme, MANHATTAN, KANSAS

The use of phenothiazine as an anthelmintic is complicated by its toxicity, the mechanism of which is not understood. The toxicity of phenothiazine varies greatly between individuals, young and debilitated animals being most susceptible. Toxicity depends on absorption from the gastrointestinal tract, and therefore small particle size, digestive tract stasis, and other factors increasing absorption favor toxicity. Multiple small doses are less likely to be toxic than a single large dose. Horses receiving more than 30 gm are likely to exhibit toxic signs. In general, single doses should not exceed 67 mg per kg.

The urine of horses receiving phenothiazine is red. This is because some phenothiazine is absorbed from the digestive tract as phenothiazine sulfoxide, which is metabolized in the liver, and the metabolites are excreted in urine, where they turn red on exposure to air.

CLINICAL SIGNS

Toxic signs are usually seen within hours of drug administration but occasionally develop in one to two days. The most common signs are anorexia and depression of rapid onset followed by hindleg weakness and a staggering gait. Digestive tract pain and colic are also common. The absorbed phenothiazine and/or its metabolites may also induce hemolysis of red blood cells, leading to anemia, icterus, and hemoglobinuria. Extreme cases may progress to dyspnea, a weak, rapid pulse, and prostration. There may be no postmortem lesions, but if present, they usually are an enlarged liver, swollen kidneys and spleen, generalized icterus of subcutaneous tissues, and dark red urine in the bladder.

Phenothiazine-induced photosensitivity, due to the metabolite phenothiazine sulfoxide, is uncommon in horses.

THERAPY

Oral administration of mineral oil and general symptomatic care of colic are important. When red blood cell hemolysis is evident, whole blood transfusion should be employed. Corticosteroids may be employed, but other treatments, such as stimulants and intravenous glucose, have not been of value for treating the phenothiazine-induced hemolysis of red blood cells.

The photosensitization is best avoided by keeping affected horses in the shade and out of direct sunlight for three to five days after dosing. Eye or skin lesions may be treated with topical ointment or salves.

The general problem of phenothiazine toxicity in horses can best be avoided by not using phenothiazine in those situations producing a high risk of poisoning. Doses should be carefully calculated. Dosing of horses with digestive tract problems should be postponed, and use of phenothiazine in horses with conditions favoring increased digestive tract absorption of the drug should be avoided.

Supplemental Reading

Clarke, M. L., Harvey, D. G., and Humphreys, D. J.: Veterinary Toxicology, 2nd ed. London, Bailliere Tindall, 1981, pp. 98–99.

Petroleum Products

Frederick W. Oehme, MANHATTAN, KANSAS

Horses generally avoid feed, forage, or water containing petroleum products. However, horses with a depraved appetite or those confined to areas containing petroleum products may ingest these materials. Various petroleum products may be applied by owners to control insects or to treat skin conditions with "home remedies."

Petroleum products include kerosene, gasoline, and other fuel oils, waste crankcase oil, and crude oil or partially refined petroleum materials. Petroleum distillates may also be used as vehicles for the application of insecticides or other environmental sprays. Waste oily materials are used to reduce dust in arenas. The used petroleum materials may contain contaminants, such as lead, pentachlorophenol (PCP), or tetrachlorodibenzodioxine (TCDD). Inhalation of spray may occur when stables are sprayed with petroleum products.

CLINICAL SIGNS

The clinical signs of petroleum product toxicity depend upon the type of product being applied, its contaminants, and the route of exposure. Ingestion of the petroleum products may produce blistering of the muzzle and mouth, salivation, colic, mild to moderate diarrhea, and one to three days of reduced appetite.

When petroleum products are applied to the skin, local irritation with some hair loss results. The horse may rub the involved area, producing additional inflammation and possibly bleeding. Inhalation of droplets of petroleum products will result in mild respiratory tract irritation. Coughing, sneezing, increased respiratory rate, and pulmonary congestion may develop following heavy exposure.

The application to the skin of petroleum products containing lead results in significant lead absorption. If repeatedly applied, lead accumulation in tissues may result in signs of lead poisoning. PCP- or TCDD-containing petroleum products will induce chronic weight loss and a rough hair coat. The usual exposure to such products is moderate, and only in extreme cases will permanent or lethal damage result.

THERAPY

The treatment for petroleum product toxicity varies with the type and extent of exposure. In many instances, conservative and supportive therapy is sufficient, while in other situations, such as aspiration pneumonia from petroleum product droplet inhalation, even the most vigorous antibiotic and supportive therapy is ineffectual. In general, the petroleum material should be removed from contact with the animal as soon as possible. Laxatives (particularly the osmotic variety) may be used to empty the digestive tract, and soap and water should be used on the skin to remove topically applied petroleum materials. Provision of soft feed will reduce irritation to the mouth and digestive tract. With severe gastrointestinal irritation, parenteral fluid therapy or nasogastric tube feeding may be necessary. Soothing ointments may be used topically to protect irritated skin, and antibiotics may be employed to reduce the potential for systemic infections. Although cases of petroleum product toxicity in horses are rare and most are minimally toxic, the clinician must always recognize the potential for more severe reactions and, therefore, should support the animal to hasten recovery.

Supplemental Reading

Rowe, L. D.: Crude oils, fuel oils, and kerosene. *In* Howard, J. L. (ed.): Current Veterinary Therapy, Food Animal Practice. Philadelphia, W. B. Saunders Company, 1981, pp. 517–520.

Lead

Frederick W. Oehme, MANHATTAN, KANSAS

Lead poisoning in horses is uncommon. However, when horses are placed in environments where lead is available, toxicity can result. The equine clinician should therefore monitor the environment of patients to ensure that lead is not a factor in any neurologic disease.

Lead almost always enters the body via the digestive tract, although smaller amounts may be inhaled into the lung and by phagocytosis will enter the circulation. Reported cases of lead poisoning in horses have usually resulted from environmental contamination from industrial smelting operations. Effluents from such mining and ore-producing activities contain large amounts of lead that are distributed by prevailing wind patterns to contaminate surrounding pastures and animal holding areas. In addition, leadbase paints may be improperly used around horse facilities, and batteries, used motor oil, putty and caulking compounds, grease, or linoleum, may provide additional sources for ingestion. Horse pastures near heavily traveled highways may develop high lead concentrations from automobile engine exhaust systems. In areas of hard water tending toward an acidic pH, lead water pipes or lead connections in water lines provide a source for lead in the water. In areas of marginal management, poor-quality pastures may allow animals access to dump sites, which could contain a variety of sources of lead. Except in instances of massive exposure to lead-containing materials (such as partially used containers of lead-base paint), chronic and continuing exposure to the lead is required for many days or weeks before toxicity is evident. Depending upon the method of exposure, as much as 500 gm may be required to produce fatalities, while daily exposure to 2.4 mg of lead per kg of body weight has been suggested as a chronic cumulative fatal dose.

CLINICAL SIGNS

Lead toxicity in horses is manifested by a variety of signs, mostly related to a peripheral neuritis. This is demonstrated by general weakness, a knuckling of the fetlocks and pharyngeal paralysis with laryngeal hemiplegia. Incoordination may be seen in advanced cases. In some horses, anemia with basophilic stippling of red blood cells is seen. Joint enlargement and stiff joints may also be observed, particularly in young horses, especially if there are complicating intoxications with other heavy metals.

The most characteristic and life-threatening effect of lead is laryngeal hemiplegia resulting from damage to the recurrent laryngeal nerve. Inspiratory dyspnea and respiratory sounds are easily detected upon moderate exercise. Affected horses may collapse and die of respiratory insufficiency after only minimal exertion. The presence of severe unexplained respiratory difficulties following mild exercise should suggest laryngeal damage and the possibility of lead intoxication. In extreme instances, food and water may be regurgitated from the nostrils following feeding.

DIAGNOSIS

Diagnosis is based upon blood lead analysis in the living animal. While clinical cases have been reported with blood lead concentrations as low as 0.3 parts per million (ppm), many horses with blood lead levels of 0.4 to 0.6 ppm or greater may exhibit no clinical signs. After death, liver or kidney lead concentrations of at least 15 ppm will support a lead poisoning diagnosis. Necropsy observations are usually nonspecific and are not helpful in the diagnosis.

THERAPY

Since almost all cases of lead poisoning in horses are chronic, removal of the animals from the source of the lead is an important first step in the treatment of poisoning. Removal of the source early enough in the syndrome may allow spontaneous improvement and eventual recovery. For severely affected animals, the intravenous administration of calcium di-sodium edetate (calcium EDTA or calcium versenate) is essential. Treatment is administered slowly in saline or 5 per cent dextrose at the rate of 75 mg calcium EDTA per kg daily for four to five days. The dosage may be divided into two or three administrations over a day's time. Treatment is then stopped for two days, and the sequence is then repeated for another four to five days.

Adequate nutritional intake should be ensured, and any anorectic horses should be fed by stomach tube until appetite returns. While treatment may be beneficial in early or mild cases of lead poisoning, the damage to the recurrent laryngeal and other peripheral nerves can be permanent in severe cases, and complete recovery may not always occur.

Supplemental Readings

Burrows, G. E.: Lead toxicosis in domestic animals: A review of the role of lead mining and primary lead smelters in the United States. Vet. Human Toxicol., 23:337, 1981.

Burrows, G. E., Sharp, J. W., and Root, R. G.: A survey of blood lead concentrations in horses in the North Idaho lead/silver belt area. Vet. Human Toxicol., 23:328, 1981.

Sexton, J. W., and Buck, W. B.: Lead. In Howard, J. L. (ed.): Current Veterinary Therapy. Food Animal Practice. Philadelphia, W. B. Saunders Company, 1981, pp. 498–500.

Van Gelder, G. A.: Lead Poisoning. In Mansmann, R. A., McAllister, E. S., and Pratt, P. W. (eds.): Equine Medicine and Surgery, 3rd ed. Santa Barbara, CA, American Veterinary Publications, 1982. pp. 191–192.

Arsenic

Frederick W. Oehme, MANHATTAN, KANSAS

Horses may be exposed to arsenic on farms through the use of pesticides, defoliants, and drugs. Horses may consume forage previously contaminated with arsenical pesticides or weed killers, or may graze in areas where arsenic-containing baits or rubbish have been burned. Arsenic is not flammable and will remain in the ash. Arsenic-containing insecticides and rodenticides may contaminate feed or be placed in areas to which horses have access, or horses may accidently gain access to containers of arsenicals. Air-borne arsenicals from industrial operations or smelters can contaminate feed or water supplies. Also, horses may chew wooden fences or stalls that have previously been treated with preservatives containing arsenic.

The various formulations and chemical combinations in which arsenic may be presented to the horse makes estimation of a specific lethal dose difficult; however, a range from 1 to 25 mg per kg body weight is a reasonable estimate. Most arsenic exposures occur through the digestive tract, although some insecticide formulations containing arsenic may be absorbed in significant quantities through the skin. Arsenic in the digestive tract is usually absorbed to a significant degree and has the potential to produce toxicosis. It damages epithelial cells, producing skin irritation and necrosis, as well as necrosis of the mucosal cells of the digestive tract. Damage to the capillary endothelium results in loss of blood or plasma. Following absorption, the arsenic primarily affects tissues with high oxidative activity, such as the liver, kidney, and lung, and leads to vital organ damage. Excretion is largely by the kidneys and to a lesser degree through bile. When further arsenic exposure is limited, horses excrete arsenic rapidly if fluid balance and kidney function are maintained for two to four days following toxic exposure. Failure to excrete arsenic in urine may be life-threatening in weak, debilitated, or dehydrated animals with reduced renal function.

CLINICAL SIGNS

The clinical effects of arsenic toxicity in horses are dramatic, with a sudden onset of severe signs. Damage to the epithelial structures, particularly the digestive tract mucosa and capillary endothelium, produces edema of the digestive tract, increased fluid content of the bowel, and increased gastrointestinal motility. The fluid loss also causes dehydration, hypotension, and shock. Severely affected horses may die of circulatory failure without showing signs of digestive tract irritation or diarrhea. Initially feces are fluid but become bloody after the first 12 to 18 hours. Shreds of intestinal tract mucosa may be mixed with the bloody diarrhea. The affected horse rapidly progresses through the initial stages of weakness and shock to incoordination, muscular trembling, severe colic and abdominal pain, cardiovascular collapse, and death within hours to one day of the initial onset of signs. If the horse survives the acute effects of arsenic, it remains depressed, weakened, and dehydrated, with the circulating arsenic now producing liver and kidney damage, which may eventually be terminal. The kidney damage often compromises urine flow and decreases the excretion of arsenic, increasing the toxic effects on other organs. The intestinal tract damage, coupled with the horse's weakened condition, may lead to septicemia. During the last stages of arsenic toxicity, two or more days following the initial clinical signs, the body temperature becomes subnormal as body functions are compromised.

Postmortem findings are representative of the caustic action of the arsenical. Horses dying rapidly will have excessive fluid in the digestive tract accompanied by edema of the intestinal mucosa. Horses surviving several hours to a few days show more characteristic effects of the cauterizing arsenical properties. The digestive tract mucosa is invariably hyperemic with areas of hemorrhage and necrosis (often with mucosal shreds sloughing into the lumen) and with excessive fluid content. If the disease process has progressed further, the intestinal contents are dark, bloody, and foul-smelling. Hemorrhage and necrosis into the intestinal tract mucosa are easily verified by microscopic examination, as are fatty change and necrosis of the liver cells and toxic degeneration of the renal tubules. With continuing survival time, the liver and kidney changes are more dramatic.

In addition to the characteristic postmortem findings, laboratory analysis of liver and kidney tissues will confirm the diagnosis of arsenic poisoning. Arsenic concentrations greater than 10 parts per million (ppm) (on a wet weight basis) are diagnostic, although some horses, particularly those that survive for three or more days, may have liver or kidney levels at 5 or less ppm. The final diagnosis is based upon an evaluation of the history, clinical observations, postmortem findings, and the chemical analysis results. Differentiation must be made between arsenic toxicity and other causes of acute abdominal pain. These include blister beetle toxicity (p. 120), the ingestion of various caustic plants including castor bean (p. 673), acute salmonellosis (p. 88), colitis (p. 94), intestinal torsion (p. 47), and anterior mesenteric artery thrombosis (p. 70).

THERAPY

The treatment of arsenic toxicity is complicated by the often peracute nature of the syndrome, the necrotizing effects of arsenic on the epithelial cells and resulting fluid loss and shock, and the toxic nephrosis and hepatosis in surviving animals. Although so-called "specific antidotes" are available for treating arsenic poisoning, the results of therapy in horses are often disappointing. Once arsenic toxicity is diagnosed, treatment should be started immediately to afford the patient the best opportunity for recovery. Severe damage will likely have already occurred to the epithelial cells of the skin or digestive tract mucosa, but intensive efforts should be made to remove or inactivate any remaining unabsorbed material. Topically applied arsenicals should be washed from the skin using mild detergents or soap. Emptying of the digestive tract should be encouraged by use of laxatives, but since the intestinal mucosa is already irritated and undergoing necrosis, severe purgatives or other forms of aggravating irritants should be avoided. Liberal use of mineral oil is laxative, soothes and protects the intestinal mucosa, and may offer a barrier to further arsenic absorption. Oral use of sodium thiosulfate (50 to 75 gm every 6 to 8 hours) will bind to unabsorbed arsenic still in the digestive tract and allow it to be excreted in the feces. Continuing fluid and electrolyte therapy is necessary to prevent dehydration.

The intravenous administration of 25 to 30 gm of sodium thiosulfate given as a 20 per cent solution in distilled water may counteract absorbed arsenic. Sodium thiosulfate may be repeated every 8 to 12 hours as needed. Dimercaprol (BAL) is the classical arsenic antidote. However, its effectiveness for horses is greatly reduced by the acute nature of the disease, the usual delay of several hours before treatment is initiated, and the necessity for administration of BAL intramuscularly. Most veterinary practitioners do not have access to sufficient quantities of this antidote for its practical use. If available, however, 5 mg per kg should be administered intramuscularly initially and 3 mg per kg repeated every six hours the remainder of the first day. A dosage of 1 mg per kg is then administered intramuscularly every six hours for two or more additional days, as needed. Because the BAL is in an oil solution, the intramuscular injections are especially painful. Experimental work suggests that thioctic acid given intramuscularly alone or together with BAL may be of therapeutic value in arsenical toxicities. However, the product is not available in a formulation ready for administration, nor has its benefit been proved in field cases. Successful clinical experiences and the commercial availability of this product may stimulate its practical use in the future.

At the present time, early initiation of therapy together with liberal use of protective digestive tract laxatives, oral and intravenous application of sodium thiosulfate, possible employment of BAL, and enthusiastic fluid and supportive therapy are the most useful procedures in treating arsenic toxicity in horses. Despite these measures, successful treatment and resolution of equine arsenic toxicity cases is uncommon. Of greater value to the horseman is the careful search for, identification, and removal of the source of the arsenic to prevent future poisoning.

Supplemental Readings

Buck, W. B.: Arsenic poisoning. *In* Mansmann, R. A., McAllister, E. S., and Pratt, P. W., (eds.): Equine Medicine and Surgery, 3rd ed. Santa Barbara, CA, American Veterinary Publications, 1982, pp. 189-191.
Osweiler, G. D., Carson, T. L., Buck, W. B., and Van Gelder, G. A.: Clinical and Diagnostic Veterinary Toxicology, 3rd ed. Dubuque, IA, Kendall/Hunt, 1985, pp. 72-79.

Selenium

Frederick W. Oehme, MANHATTAN, KANSAS

Selenium poisoning in horses occurs primarily in the midwest plains states. It is associated with the presence of naturally occurring selenium in soils. Because rainfall leaches much of the selenium from the native soils, selenium toxicity is largely seen in the region west of the Mississippi River to the western slope of the Rocky Mountains.

Selenium toxicity may be due to water supplies that contain 0.5 parts per million (ppm) or more of selenium, but more commonly it is due to the consumption of plants that are grown on soils containing selenium. The majority of cases of selenium toxicity are due to the consumption of secondary accumulator plants, which extract soil selenium normally unavailable to most range plants. These accumulator plants are found on seleniferous soils that contain greater than 5 ppm selenium and are less commonly found on soils with lower selenium content.

Plants that require high-selenium-content soils for survival are called "indicator plants" or "obligate accumulators" and generally build up 100 times or more of the selenium levels of other plants in the same area. Facultative or "secondary selenium accumulators" do not require high-selenium-content soils for survival, but when growing on seleniferous soils, they accumulate concentrations found in accumulator plants in the same area.

While these accumulator plants may build up high concentrations of selenium that will induce relatively acute toxic syndromes in horses consuming them, plants such as cereal crops grown in seleniferous soils will passively build up soluble selenium in their plant matrices. These crop plants may contain more than 5 ppm selenium, the tolerance limit for selenium in the diet of livestock.

Plants of the species of Astragalus (vetch) are most commonly associated with selenium toxicity in horses. However, other plants of species of Xylorrhiza (woody aster), Oonopsis (goldenweed) and Stanleya (prince's plume) also contain members that can produce selenium poisoning. These seleniferous plants are toxic when consumed fresh as well as when they are foraged in the dormant or dry state. They are, therefore, toxic during all seasons. Some plants have a higher selenium concentration when large than when small, but others seem to have smaller selenium concentrations as they mature in the growing season. Although horses generally avoid poisonous species of selenium-containing plants when good forage is available, moderate starvation may result in these plants being consumed. Once seleniferous plants are eaten, horses may subsequently seek them out even when adequate forage is made available.

CLINICAL SIGNS

Selenium poisoning may be acute or chronic. Ingestion of plants containing large concentrations of selenium results in death in several hours to a day. Signs indicate nervous, digestive, cardiovascular, and respiratory system involvement. Depression, diarrhea, labored breathing, rapid prostration, and death due to respiratory failure make this condition difficult to diagnose owing to its complexity of signs and rapidity of action.

The subacute form of toxicity results from the ingestion of moderate amounts of selenium-containing material and is characterized by signs of liver and brain involvement over several days to several weeks. A depressive mania that causes blindness, straying from a group of animals, muscle weakness,

SELENIUM—continued / 671

and finally paralysis is usually unresponsive to therapy and results in death. The blindness and central nervous system disturbance have led to this syndrome being called "blind staggers."

Chronic selenium poisoning, or the lay term "alkali disease," occurs if low doses somewhat in excess of 5 to 10 ppm selenium are consumed and accumulated in the body over a period of several weeks to several months. This chronic disease manifests the basic mechanism by which selenium interacts with biologic tissues, that is, binding of the selenium with sulfur-containing tissue compounds. The affected horses gradually lose weight and are only moderately depressed. Appetite may vary, but anorexia is not usual. There is loss of hair from the mane and tail, and the hoof wall on one or more feet develops a break at the coronary band. As this break grows out, the hooves become cracked and roughened, and the breaking off of portions of this weakened wall may give the hoof a ragged appearance. Affected animals are lame and tender in the feet. The loss of hair and breaks in the hoof wall are due to the altered chemical content of these sulfur-containing structures. Fatalities are rare with chronic selenium poisoning, but affected animals are often destroyed or sold because owners often become impatient and discouraged by the chronic and apparently unresponsive syndrome. Horses on selenium-containing water supplies (with as little as 0.1 to 2.0 ppm selenium) are especially sensitive to chronic selenium poisoning owing to the continued ingestion of low concentrations of the element.

Acute selenium poisoning produces minor internal hemorrhages following the terminal convulsions. Subacute selenium toxicity, because of its longer duration, induces internal congestion, moderate hyperemia of the digestive tract, and some fatty degeneration and focal necrosis of the liver. Lesions of chronic selenium poisoning are observed when one or more affected animals are sacrificed as an aid for diagnosis. Anemia, fatty atrophy of the heart, paleness and firmness of the liver with cirrhosis seen on microscopic examination, moderate and diffuse gastroenteritis, and joint erosions due to the disturbed gait are all characteristic of this long-term syndrome.

Selenium concentrations of 8 to 20 ppm in the hooves, 1 to 4 ppm in blood, and 11 to 45 ppm in hair are associated with chronic selenium poisoning. In more acute syndromes, the hoof and hair selenium concentrations are less than in the chronic syndrome, whereas concentrations in blood and liver are significantly greater.

THERAPY

There is no effective treatment for selenium poisoning, although animals seen before death should be managed symptomatically. In subacute cases, the administration of 4 to 6 mg strychnine sulfate per 600 to 800 lbs (275 to 375 kg) subcutaneously every two to three hours has been suggested as beneficial. However, the overall value of therapy must be carefully weighed against the low rate of eventual recovery, and the equine clinician is urged to balance any additional therapeutic expenditure against the low probability of recovery in this situation.

Chronic cases have a 50 per cent chance of recovery. The liver damage, as reflected in the weight loss and poor condition, and the damage to joints and hooves require long-term therapy. Arsenic in the form of sodium arsenite may be added to water or salt to biochemically protect the sulfur-containing structures in the body. Approximately 5 ppm of inorganic arsenic are recommended in drinking water, with salt containing 35 to 40 ppm arsenic recommended as a useful supplement. Naphthalene (4 to 5 gm orally per day) for five days has also been utilized for treating horses affected with chronic selenium poisoning. The dose is repeated for five additional days after a rest period of five days between dosing sequences.

The altered hoof conformation associated with chronic selenium poisoning requires corrective hoof trimming at frequent intervals. Acrylic may be used to support the weakened hoof wall or to replace damaged and nonfunctional portions of the wall. Careful attention to the animal's hoof structure is necessary to avoid chronic damage to the sensitive laminae and to joint surfaces. Horses being treated for chronic selenium toxicity should be confined away from exposure to the responsible selenium-containing plant. A high-quality balanced ration must be made available to the recovering patient.

Supplemental Readings

Hulbert, L. C., and Oehme, F. W.: Plants poisonous to livestock, 3rd revised ed. Manhattan, KS, Kansas State University, 1984, pp. 56–57.
Hultine, J. D., Mount, M. E., Easley, K. J., and Oehme, F. W.: Selenium toxicosis in the horse. Equine Pract., 1:57, 1979.

Plant Toxicities*

Frederick W. Oehme, MANHATTAN, KANSAS

This chapter reviews the toxic plants affecting horses, describing the clinical syndromes and suggesting the conditions under which the horse may encounter the plant.

The etiology of many toxic syndromes in horses is never determined. Plant poisoning should be considered in any sudden onset of illness, especially if it is accompanied by gastrointestinal disorders, nervous signs, sudden collapse, or death. There may be a history of exposure to a toxic plant. Many chronic toxicities may also have sudden onset of signs, sometimes well after the animal stops eating the toxic plant. Determining the etiologic agent is often difficult. A good history is imperative in the diagnosis of plant poisoning. Where an animal has been, changes in feed in the past six months, and alterations in environment must all be carefully considered.

Many animals coexist with poisonous plants without harm, grazing the surrounding herbage with impunity. A stress such as introduction of a newcomer to the herd may precipitate the ingestion of unfamiliar plants, including toxic species. When forage is scarce or under conditions of overcrowding, animals may seek out any green plant, including those that are poisonous. A common link in the history of some acute poisonings is the introduction of plant clippings into the horse's pen by an unsuspecting gardener.

The age of the animal and the amount of plant consumed affect an animal's susceptibility. The time of year, soil type, and climatic conditions alter production of the plant toxin. Methods and times of harvesting of contaminated pasture will also affect the ultimate toxicity of the plant.

PLANTS PRODUCING GASTROINTESTINAL EFFECTS

RAGWORTS (Senecio sp): STINKING WILLIE (S. jacobaea); COMMON GROUNDSEL (S. vulgaris); FIDDLENECK (Amsinckia sp); TARWEED (A. intermedia); RATTLEWEED (Crotalaria sp); SALIVATION JANE (Echium lycopsis)

Toxic Principle. A variety of pyrrolizidine alkaloids are toxic principles.

Location of the Plant. Senecio is found throughout much of the southern United States, the Pacific Northwest, and parts of New England. Crotalaria is used extensively as a cover crop in the South as far

west as Texas. Amsinckia is a common hay and pasture contaminant and is native to the Pacific Coast states.

Conditions of Toxicity. The majority of the pyrrolizidine alkaloid–containing plants are unpalatable and are only eaten when other forage is scarce or when baled in hay or pelleted. The weeds grow in winter and early spring and are therefore found in first cutting hay. Owing to the management practices of hay making in California, it has been estimated that no more than 4 per cent of the state's total acreage is contaminated at any time.

The effects of the alkaloids are cumulative, and ingestion occurs over a period of weeks before the liver is damaged enough to cause clinical signs of disease. Clinical cases are usually recognized in the late summer to early winter months. If ingestion has been sporadic, animals may develop signs months after the first exposure, and the offending hay may no longer be available to aid in diagnosis. Hay with 15 per cent Amsinckia or Senecio content will kill a horse over a period of time, but perhaps 50 to 150 lbs of weed must be ingested before signs appear.

Although most farm animals are susceptible to the pyrrolizidine alkaloids, there is some species variation . The horse is certainly the most sensitive to the effects of the toxin. The different plant genera cause a wide variety of signs in the different animal species. For the most part, the four plant genera that contain pyrrolizidine alkaloids cause a similar set of signs in the horse. Although clinical toxicities from *Echium lycopsis* have only been reported in Australia, the plant's recent advent in a limited area of California makes exposure a possibility.

Clinical Signs. In rare cases, ingestion of at least 20 lbs of pyrrolizidine alkaloid–containing plant at one time has caused acute toxicity characterized by extreme excitement and violence, gastrointestinal signs, pupillary dilation, and increased heart rate.

Toxicity from chronic ingestion of pyrrolizidine alkaloid—containing plants is much more common. Overt signs of chronic ingestion also appear abruptly, although weight loss and anorexia may have developed slowly over at least a month prior to clinical recognition of the disease. The alkaloids damage the liver, and elevations in the icteric index, alkaline phosphatase, sorbitol dehydrogenase, and prothrombin time may all occur. Bromsulphalein retention half time is consistently elevated, and liver biopsy is usually diagnostic. Neutrophilia with a toxic left shift has been seen. Signs of hepatoencephalopathy due to increased blood ammonia levels resulting from a malfunctioning liver are typical.

*This article has been compiled with the assistance of several authorities.

672

A horse may be depressed or drowsy, may yawn, and may keep its head down or may press it against stationary objects. The uncoordinated, staggering gait sometimes gives the disease the name "sleepy staggers." Circling or aimless walking is seen in 80 per cent of clinical cases. Lack of obstacle avoidance and apparent blindness have also been noted.

Chronic liver damage may lead to the accumulation in the skin of phototoxic substances and signs of photosensitization in the lightly pigmented areas of the face or legs. Other signs related to liver disease are ascites or subcutaneous edema secondary to hypoalbuminemia and portal hypertension. The mouth may be ulcerated and may have an offensive odor; abdominal pain and diarrhea may be present.

In the last two weeks of life, the animal often goes through a rapid progression of signs. A hemolytic crisis may be clinically demonstrated by the presence of hemoglobinuria. Terminally, the mucous membranes may be congested, and icterus may no longer be recognizable as severe anemia develops. The horse commonly dies quietly but may undergo delirium, collapse, and convulsions before death.

Pathology. Pyrrolizidine alkaloid–intoxicated horses are often emaciated, have decreased muscle mass, and show jaundice. The liver is usually enlarged, weighing more then 7 kg, and has a mottled appearance with an accentuated lobular pattern. It is so firm that it cannot be crushed with the fingers. Occasional reports suggest a pale, small liver, but firmness is a consistent finding. The kidneys may be enlarged and congested, as are the adrenals. Widespread petechial and ecchymotic hemorrhages may be seen with subendocardial, gastrointestinal tract, mesenteric, and urinary bladder hemorrhages. Edema occurs in the lungs or brain. Cytotoxic edema in the central nervous system is the basis for the neurologic signs seen with advanced liver disease; however, the central nervous system lesions in the horse are not as extensive as those in other animals with hepatoencephalopathy.

Liver histopathology is diagnostic. Megalocytosis with increased nuclear size, bile duct hyperplasia, and perilobular fibrosis are the classic findings. The kidneys may show megalocytosis and mild nephrosis. Veno-occlusion has been reported in horses eating Crotalaria sp but is thought to be just another manifestation of the general effects of pyrrolizidine alkaloids on the liver. Proliferation of collagen and subendothelial swelling of central or hepatic veins lead to narrowing of the vessel walls. The veno-occlusion may lead to an increase in portal pressure and the congestion seen in the liver and gastrointestinal tract.

Treatment. Once clinical signs appear in a horse, the prognosis for survival is poor. The use of a methionine and dextrose saline drip was reported to be effective in two horses poisoned by ingesting Senecio but was ineffective in cases of *Crotalaria retusa* poisoning. Recent reports suggest that intravenous infusion of glucose and branched-chain amino acids may help considerably. Recovery rates of 30 to 40 per cent have been reported. Herbicides are useful when the plants are in the rapidly growing stages, and the cinnabar moth, *Tyria jacobalae*, has been reported as an effective control for ragwort.

Castor Bean (*Ricinus communis*)

Toxic Principle. The seeds contain a phytotoxin, ricin.

Location of the Plant. The plant is grown in the southwestern and the southeastern United States.

Conditions of Toxicity. Although unpalatable, the seeds or castor bean byproducts may be consumed when mixed with other feedstuffs. The horse is very susceptible to ricin, and 25 gm of castor bean is a lethal dose.

Clinical Signs. Phytotoxins are antigenic plant proteins that may act as potent proteolytic enzymes, causing signs of gastrointestinal irritation. If enough of the toxin is absorbed, signs of anaphylaxis and shock predominate. Usually a latent period of several hours to two days occurs before the onset of signs, which are rapidly progressive. Initially there are dullness, slight incoordination, and profuse sweating, possibly with muscular spasms in the neck and shoulders. The respiratory and heart rates are increased. The heart contractions may be so strong that the entire body shakes, and the pounding of the heart against the thorax may be seen from 10 feet away. Usually a nonhemorrhagic watery diarrhea occurs and is accompanied by colic. Early signs are accompanied by a fever spike and a left shift in the hemogram. As the episode progresses, leukopenia and a progressive rise in hematocrit due to dehydration are observed. Death occurs within 36 hours, and terminal convulsions are seen.

Pathology. Congestion of internal organs occurs. Inflammation and hemorrhage in the gastrointestinal tract, epicardium, and endocardium are common along with pooling of fluid in the intestine and engorgement of the right heart.

Treatment. The horse should be treated for shock and sedatives given.

Oak (Quercus sp)

Acorn poisoning has not been recorded in horses in the United States, but there have been several reports from England. Signs of colic and hematuria were noted in two horses about one week after they had access to clippings of oak leaves (*Quercus rubra*).

PLANTS PRODUCING CENTRAL NERVOUS SYSTEM STIMULATION

LOCOWEED (Astragalus sp and Oxytropis sp)

Toxic Principle. These plants contain locoine, an incompletely characterized extract with alkaloidal properties.

Location of the Plant. Astragalus sp that accumulate selenium are found throughout the western United States, and those that produce locoism are found in most of the same states. Oxytropis sp are more restricted to the central United States.

Conditions of Toxicity. The "loco" syndrome is produced by many of the Astragalus and Oxytropis sp and affects all species of livestock. The entire plant is poisonous at any time of the year. Many of the more than 300 Astragalus are toxic, but the toxicity of the plants varies among years and locations. Certain members of Astragalus grow only on seleniferous soils and accumulate selenium, causing a syndrome characteristic of selenium toxicity. A few Astragalus sp, known commonly as milkvetch, cause an acute syndrome in sheep evident when the animals are stressed or driven. The clinical signs are primarily related to damage to the respiratory system. Poisoning of this type in horses has not been reported in the United States but has been described in British Columbia. Signs develop less than one week after ingestion of the plant and include roaring, staggering, salivation, and sudden death.

Horses are the species most susceptible to the "loco" syndrome. The ingestion of 30 per cent of their body weight in plants is required over six weeks. The most severe signs may not be noted until after the animal has ceased to ingest the plant. Although animals are not usually attracted to the plant when better forage is available, once it is eaten, horses will seek out the plant, even when dry, to the exclusion of other plants.

Clinical Signs. In the early stages, "loco" syndrome may cause the animal to be unpredictable and dangerous to ride. Affected horses may separate themselves from other animals and may carry the head in abnormal ways, in part owing to the apparent visual disturbances and altered perception of spatial relationships, thereby running into objects or over cliffs. Locomotor ataxia has been reported with staggering or circling, incoordination, and abnormal or exaggerated movements of the limbs. Unsuccessful attempts to rear may result in the horse falling back on its haunches. Although generally the horse is listless and depressed, excitation aggravates these locomotor signs and may precipitate nervousness, trembling, and the classical description of wild behavior. The course of the disease is chronic, progressing to locomotor paralysis and

difficulty in prehension, causing weakness and starvation. Convulsive death may follow an episode of excitement. Recovery in some cases is incomplete owing to irreversible brain damage, and the animal is at best suitable only for reproduction.

A second syndrome associated with Astragalus ingestion is known as "blind staggers" but is seen more often in cattle. Straying, muscular weakness or partial paralysis, and visual impairment have been noted. The selenium-accumulating species of Astragalus have been referred to as poison vetches. These plants, as well as the woody aster (*Xylorrhiza purryi*) and others, are called "indicator" plants because they grow only on selenium-containing soils. When these plants contain enough selenium to make toxicity a possibility, they are generally unpalatable. However, chronic selenium toxicity can occur from eating forages grown on selenium-rich land. Chronic selenium toxicity, "alkali disease," is characterized in horses by loss of mane and tail hair and lameness caused by damage to the coronary band (p. 670).

Pathology. Generalized emaciation and hypertrophy of the thyroid gland, kidney, liver, and adrenal gland have been described. Transitory edematous vacuolization of brain cells and other organ systems occurs. In the central nervous system, these lesions are replaced in time by small eosinophilic argyrophillic bodies called spheroids and may account for the residual neurologic effects. The parenchymal organs can repair themselves if the animals are removed from exposure to the offending plant before the onset of clinical signs. Most signs of the disease can be explained by the brain lesions, but damage to the other organs can account for many of the problems with assimilation and metabolism of ingesta. Vacuoles in the retina and lacrimal gland explain visual impairment and the decreased lacrimation that gives the eye a dull appearance.

Acute selenium toxicity is characterized pathologically by hemorrhages and congestion in many organs. The liver and kidneys undergo degenerative changes.

Treatment. There is no antidote for locoism. A clinical response to reserpine has been reported but has not been confirmed.

OLEANDER (*Nerium oleander*)

Toxic Principle. Oleandrin and nerioside glycosides akin to digitoxin are the toxic principles.

Location of the Plant. Oleander is found primarily in the southern United States from coast to coast.

Conditions of Toxicity. The entire plant is toxic. Toxicity may occur at any time of the year but is most likely when animals are given plant trimmings to eat. Horses will rarely eat the fresh plant, but the wilted or dried leaves are less bitter and more palatable. Thirty or 40 green or dry leaves, about

¼ lb, are fatal. Death occurs less than 12 hours after ingestion.

Clinical Signs. Depression and a profuse catarrhal, watery, or bloody diarrhea and colic occur within a few hours of ingestion. Alternating bradycardia and tachycardia are accompanied by a variety of arrhythmias and murmurs that cannot be localized to any heart area. Peripheral vessel constriction may cause pallor of the mucous membranes and coldness of the extremities. Sweating may be profuse. Muscle anoxia may give rise to tics. Ultimately, horses become comatose and die.

Pathology. There are no characteristic lesions. A mild gastroenteritis with hemorrhage into the gut lumen, onto various body organs, and on visceral pleura, the epicardium, and endocardium has been observed. Ascites has been seen.

Treatment. Horses may die without showing signs of sickness, making treatment impossible. Laxatives and enemas should be helpful in sublethal poisonings. Atropine in conjunction with propranolol has also been advocated.

WATER HEMLOCK, COWBANE (Cicuta sp)

Toxic Principle. Cowbane contains cicutoxin, a resin.

Location of the Plants. Found in wet areas and ditches, Cicuta sp are common from the upper Midwest westward to the Pacific.

Conditions of Toxicity. Poisonings are most frequently seen in cattle, often when ground is reclaimed. The majority of livestock deaths occur in spring when leaves are most palatable and when the root can be easily pulled up and digested. As the leafy plant matures in summer and fall and when found in hay, it has a lower toxicity. The roots are the most toxic part of the plant and remain so even when dried. Eight ounces of the root are lethal to mature horses.

Clinical Signs. Signs occur between 10 and 60 minutes after ingestion and are due to the toxin's irritant action in nerve cells, which results in central nervous system stimulation. The horse shows signs of apprehension with pupillary dilation and slight muscle tics of the neck, which progress to contractions of major muscle groups. The animal thereafter has difficulty maintaining its balance and may back up. Breathing rapidly becomes labored, and the animal falls down and convulses. Death due to respiratory paralysis occurs less than 30 minutes after ingestion of a lethal dose of water hemlock.

Pathology. There are no characteristic lesions at necropsy.

Treatment. If a lethal dose is ingested, death is an inevitable consequence, but gastric lavage and anticonvulsive therapy may otherwise be helpful. Livestock that survive for five to six hours seem to recover without ill effects. The plant can be controlled with 2,4-D.

WHITE SNAKEROOT (Eupatorium rugosum)

Toxic Principle. The primary toxic component is the higher alcohol tremetol, which is incapable of producing the clinical disease when completely dried. Since it is excreted slowly, tremetol exerts a cumulative effect.

Location of the Plant. Snakeroot is found throughout the Midwest and parts of the South.

Conditions of Toxicity. Poisonings occur in the late summer and fall. Although toxicity decreases with drying, the plant in hay retains enough toxicity to cause problems. The lethal plant dose in the horse is 2 to 10 lbs. Tremetol is accumulated in the milk, and this can be an indirect route for toxicity in suckling animals. The rayless goldenrod (*Isocoma wrightii*), another North American plant, also contains tremetol and can produce a similar syndrome.

Clinical Signs. The onset of signs varies from less than two days to three weeks after ingestion and may be precipitated by any type of stress. If a toxic dose has been consumed, enzymatic damage to the heart muscle occurs, precipitating a bout of rapid shaking, especially in the flanks and rear legs, hence the name "trembles." If the animal is not stressed, the only signs are reluctance to move, sluggishness, stiffness of gait, or ataxia. Horses are the least likely of the domestic animals to tremble and may die without doing so. Partial throat paralysis and severe sweating have been reported in horses. The disease in horses tends to run a shorter clinical course than in other animals, with death occurring in about two days.

Pathology. Hemorrhages in the heart, gastrointestinal tract, and other organs occur as a result of heart failure. The most consistent lesion is congestion of the liver, kidneys, or central nervous system. There is also fatty degeneration of the liver.

Treatment. Since the disease is usually recognized late in its clinical course, treatment is usually frustrating and ineffective. Mineral oil laxatives offer the best approach. Plants may be controlled with 2,4-D.

YELLOW STAR THISTLE (Centaurea solstitialis); RUSSIAN KNAPWEED (C. repens) (C. picris)

Toxic Principle. The toxic principle is an unidentified alkaloid.

Location of the Plant. C. *solstitialis* grows primarily in California and the other Centaurea sp are a source of poisoning in the other Pacific Coast states and as far east as Colorado. C. *repens* is more toxic than C. *solstitialis*, and a horse must consume 59 to 71 per cent and 86 to 200 per cent of its body weight, respectively, in fresh plant before signs of the disease occur. Continuous ingestion over an average of 54 days for C. *solstitialis* and 30 days for C. *repens* is required to exceed the toxic threshold. Although ingestion of either the dried or fresh plant causes clinical signs, the majority of cases occur between October and November or in June and July. At these times in California, yellow star thistle may be the only available forage on dry pasture. Younger animals are said to be most commonly affected and seem to acquire a taste for the weed despite its spines.

Only horses are affected by the plant's toxin. Donkeys with access to the weed do not seem to be affected. Ruminants can eat the thistle without suffering any ill effect. Experimental attempts to reproduce the disease in other animal species have been unsuccessful.

Clinical Signs. Signs develop acutely and are usually fully evident at the time of clinical presentation. Horses are at that time in good flesh. The primary clinical sign is an inabiliity to hold or chew food with a concomitant inabilty to eat or drink and a characteristic facial dystonia. The upper lip is hypertonic, the cheeks are drawn tightly against the mandible, and the corners of the mouth may be held halfway open with the tongue moving awkwardly in an attempt to retain food in the mouth. Horses may immerse their heads up to their eyes and get water in this manner, as they can swallow if food or water is placed far enough back in the throat. Chewing, yawning, or head tossing may be seen. Most frequently, horses stand with their heads down in their frustrated attempts to get food. The development of severe facial edema is common. At other times, they may appear depressed or inattentive but can easily be aroused. Gait is not generally affected, although some horses may walk aimlessly or may show slight hypermetria or stiffness in the walk. Occasionally, central nervous sytem disorders such as head pushing, walking through obstacles, or excitement to the extent of self-induced trauma may be seen.

Signs are the most severe for the first day or two but thereafter subside to a static level. In a few cases, unilateral signs predominate, such as unidirectional circling or reluctance to be turned in one direction. Signs are irreversible, and if the animal is not destroyed, it will eventually die of dehydration, starvation, or aspiration pneumonia.

Pathology. Liquefactive necrosis of the substantia nigra and globus pallidus sections of the brain is the pathognomonic lesion of the disease; hence, the name equine nigropallidal encephalomalacia. Prior to seven days of the clinical course, only discoloration of these brain areas may be seen. The specific lesions are most often bilateral, although any or all of the four sites may be affected. Other more subtle brain lesions have been demonstrated in experimental horses. Traumatic lesions or signs of secondary complications may also be present.

Treatment. No treatment is available, although slight symptomatic relief has been obtained with massive doses of atropine. Although horses have been kept alive for months by tube feeding, euthanasia is recommended.

YEW (Taxus sp)

Toxic Principle. The alkaloid taxine is found in most Taxus sp.

Location of the Plant. The plant is found as an ornamental throughout most of the United States.

Conditions of Toxicity. The plant is poisonous year-round, but toxicity occurs when animals are given access to the trimmings, usually in the spring or summer. The horse is the species most susceptible to the alkaloid's toxicity, and one mouthful can be lethal. Drying or storage does not lessen toxicity. One veterinary diagnostic laboratory attributed 50 per cent of horse deaths from toxic agents to the ingestion of Japanese yew (*Taxus caspictata*).

Clinical Signs. Taxine depresses cardiac conduction. Death in donkeys and horses can be so sudden that few abnormalities are noted before collapse and extensor rigidity or muscle spasms. Animals are most often found lying next to the Taxus source, as death can occur within five minutes after ingestion.

Pathology. There are no characteristic lesions. Postmortem diagnosis is best confirmed by finding plant fragments within the stomach. This may be difficult in horses and requires the use of a dissection microscope owing to the complete mastication of plants by the horse.

Treatment. Death comes so rapidly that there is no time to treat the animal symptomatically, and there is no known antidote.

PLANTS PRODUCING CENTRAL NERVOUS SYSTEM DEPRESSION

BRACKEN FERN (Pteridium aquilinum)

Toxic Principle. The toxic principle is thiaminase.

Location of the Plant. Bracken fern is especially abundant in forested areas, burns, or abandoned sandy fields throughout the northwestern and northern United States to the upper Midwest.

Conditions of Toxicity. Toxicity can occur at any time of the year, depending on climatic conditions. Horses usually consume bracken fern in the late summer when other forage is scarce, although horses can acquire a taste for the plant in pasture or when it is used as bedding. Toxicity due to ingestion of hay containing 20 per cent or more bracken is most common in the winter months. Levels of thiaminase in the plant peak in the late summer. Thiaminase is destroyed by heat but not by drying. The entire plant is toxic.

Clinical Signs. Horses generally must consume bracken fern for 30 to 60 days before signs of toxicity are observed. Signs can appear even if horses have not ingested bracken fern for two to three weeks. On presentation, blood thiamine levels are low. Clinical signs are due to myelin degeneration in peripheral nerves; generalized weakness and muscle problems are related to a buildup of pyruvates. Animals lose weight progressively starting several days after exposure to the plant.

The first gait abnormality seen is an unsteady walk about 30 days after the first ingestion of bracken. This incoordination progresses over the next week or so to overt staggering, hence, the name "bracken staggers." The animal stands peculiarly with the back arched and the feet based widely in the back. There may be crossing of the front legs when the animal is in motion and wide action in the rear. Severe muscle tremors and weakness appear, especially when animals are forced to work. Bradycardia with cardiac arrhythmias is not uncommon early in the course of the disease, but tachycardia occurs terminally, accompanied by a rise in temperature. At this time, the animal usually becomes recumbent and may exhibit clonic spasms and the typical opisthotonus of thiamine deficiency. Without treatment, death occurs within 2 to 10 days after the onset of clinical signs. There has been a clinical report of a hemolytic crisis associated with bracken fern ingestion.

Pathology. Although postmortem lesions are not diagnostic, enteritis with some pericardial and epicardial hemorrhages is observed.

Treatment. The prognosis for full recovery is good if the disease is recognized before the animal becomes recumbent. Thiamine hydrochloride (0.25 to 0.5 mg per kg) should be administered daily either intravenously or intramuscularly.

HORSETAIL, MARESTAIL, SCOURING RUSH (*Equisetum arvense*)

This plant is found in wetter and colder areas than bracken fern and over a wider geographic range. The toxic principle is the same, and signs are virtually identical to those of bracken fern poisoning. Cases are usually associated with ingestion of the plant in hay.

DEATH CAMAS (Zigadenus sp)

Toxic Principle. A steroidal glycosidal alkaloid, zygadenine, is the toxic principle.

Location of the Plant. Zigadenus sp are found west of the Mississippi on sandy plains and in the foothills of the Rocky Mountains.

Conditions of Toxicity. Although many Zigadenus sp are toxic, only *Z. nuttallii*, which is more geographically restricted, has been reported as a cause of toxicity in horses. Colic and salivation in a group of pack mules in the California Sierras was, however, attributed to another Zigadenus sp. Poisonings are most likely to occur in the spring on ranges where other forages are scarce, since the plant is unpalatable to horses. Less than 10 lbs of the plant need to be ingested to produce signs of a frequently fatal toxicity.

Clinical Signs. Signs begin within several hours of ingestion, although death may not occur for up to several days. Depression, staggering, profuse salivation, pupillary constriction, and decreased heart and respiratory rate have all been observed.

Pathology. There are no distinctive lesions.

Treatment. An effective treatment described for sheep is 4 mg atropine sulfate and 8 mg picrotoxin in 10 ml of water per 100 kg of body weight subcutaneously as needed to ameliorate signs. Atropine sulfate (33 mg) and carbachol (0.25 to 0.5 mg) have been recommended for horses. Clinical success has been less effective than with sheep.

POISON HEMLOCK (*Conium maculatum*)

Toxic Principle. A number of alkaloids, the most toxic being N-methyl conine, are toxic principles.

Location of the Plant. Poison hemlock is a ubiquitous weed found throughout the United States.

Conditions of Toxicity. The plant appears in early spring, and most toxicities occur at this time when the plant is palatable. The level of N-methyl conine increases as the plant matures, and the root becomes toxic only later in the year. Drying seems to neutralize the toxic principle, and the plant is not a problem in hay. Four to five pounds of fresh leaves have been lethal to horses.

Clinical Signs. Conine acts similarly to nicotine, causing first stimulation, then depression of the autonomic ganglia. Signs occur within about two hours of eating the plant. Horses may fall without signs of approaching paralysis and retain normal corneal reflexes but lack awareness. Variable signs of apprehension with mydriasis and posterior muscle incoordination to the point of extensive trembling have preceded falling episodes. The clinical course may continue over several hours to a day or two, and the animal may be comatose for part of this time, but this in itself may not be fatal. Death in severe cases occurs within 5 to 10 hours of the onset of signs.

Pathology. There are no diagnostic postmortem findings, although the toxin is eliminated via the kidneys and lungs, giving the urine and exhaled air a characteristic mousey odor.

Treatment. Adequate nursing of recumbent animals and administration of laxatives may aid in successful recovery. Tannic acid can be used to neutralize the active principle, and stimulants such as strychnine, atropine, or metrazol have been reported to be effective.

BLACK NIGHTSHADE (*Solanum nigrum*)

Toxic Principle. The glycoalkaloid solanine is the toxic principle.

Location of the Plant. The plant is found east of the Rocky Mountains.

Conditions of Toxicity. Toxicity usually occurs in late summer and early fall when other forages are lacking. All parts of the plant are toxic, especially the berries. The concentration of toxic alkaloid varies with soil, climate, season, and region. One to 10 lbs may be lethal.

Clinical Signs. Although several poisoning syndromes are recognized, horses usually exhibit central nervous system signs of depression, dullness, weakness, and prostration. In addition, the toxin has a direct irritant effect on the gastrointestinal mucosa, causing signs of colic and pain. Copious diarrhea is said to be a good prognostic sign.

Pathology. The primary pathologic sign is a slight gastroenteritis.

Treatment. There is no antidote for solanine. Good nursing care is required. Plants should be controlled with herbicides.

BLACK LOCUST (*Robinia pseudoacacia*)

The black locust (*Robinia pseudoacacia*) which is found in the eastern United States, contains a phytotoxin that is extremely toxic. Horses may become poisoned when tied to the tree and allowed to strip the bark. Horses usually show weakness, posterior paralysis, anorexia, and depression. Mydriasis, mild colic, diarrhea, a rapid, irregular heartbeat, or diaphragmatic flutter may be noted. Animals may die in a few days or may survive, depending on the amount ingested.

SCOTTISH BROOM (*Cytisus scoparius*)

Mild signs of central nervous system depression and increased urination are seen when horses ingest large amounts of Scottish broom (*Cytisus scoparius*).

PLANTS AFFECTING BLOOD

CHOKECHERRY (*Prunus virginiana*)

Toxic Principle. Chokecherry contains the cyanogenic glycosides amygdalin in the fruit and prunasin in the leaves.

Location of the Plant. Chokecherry is found in most of the United States in a variety of climates.

Conditions of Toxicity. Because the cyanogenic compounds are located in one part of the plant's cells and the enzymes needed for degradation are located in another part, the cherry and other cyanogenic plants do not easily release free cyanide. Unusual field conditions such as drought, frost, wilting, or stunting of the plants combined with maceration by the animal are necessary to release lethal levels of cyanide. Great potential for toxicity occurs in immature or rapidly growing varieties. If much of the plant is ingested, the cyanide blocks

cytochrome oxidase, preventing oxygen uptake by tissues. Clinical signs are due to tissue anoxia despite adequate blood oxygen content, which gives the cherry red color of the blood.

Clinical Signs. Death occurs within minutes to an hour of ingestion of the offending plant. The progression of signs following the eating of large amounts of wild cherry leaves is as follows: Dyspnea with flaring of the nostrils occurs almost immediately. Lifting of the tailhead is seen, and involuntary micturition or defecation has been described. Central nervous system signs of agitation, including trembling, ataxia, and muscular contractions, are pronounced. Finally the horse becomes prostrate and kicks and flails its legs. Respiratory arrest occurs minutes before cardiac arrest.

Pathology. Mucous membranes often appear red and well oxygenated, but this is not a consistent clinical finding. Hemorrhages in the heart and other organs are a result of violent death.

Treatment. Although the veterinarian usually arrives too late to institute treatment, intravenous administration of 4 ml per 45 kg of body weight of a mixture of 1 ml of 20 per cent sodium nitrite and 3 ml of 20 per cent sodium thiosulfate can be effective. An additional 20 gm of sodium thiosulfate given orally will fix free cyanide in the stomach. Sodium nitrite forms methemoglobin, which reacts with free cyanide to form nontoxic cyanmethemoglobin. Thiosulfate reacts with cyanide and with enzymatic catalysis forms thiocyanate, which is eliminated in the urine.

Determination of cyanide-associated deaths in the field can be performed by testing suspect plants or abdominal contents. The material should be crushed and placed in a jar with some water and a few drops of chloroform and sulfuric acid. Strips of filter paper wetted with a preformed mixture of 4 gm sodium bicarbonate and 0.5 gm picric acid in 100 ml water are suspended in the jar without contacting the plant material. This is heated for 5 to 10 minutes. If cyanide is present, the paper will turn a brick red color in a few minutes.

SORGHUM SP

Toxic Principle. A cyanogenic glycoside, which can be hydrolyzed to free cyanide, is the toxic principle.

Location of the Plant. Sorghum is found in the Southwest and in much of the eastern United States.

Conditions of Toxicity. Milo and Sudan grass are both members of the Sorghum sp and are excellent forage plants. *S. halpense* or Johnson grass, though not unique in containing the glycoside, is the most toxic of the sorghums alone or in hybrid pastures and is often considered a weed. It is, however, used in some of the Southern states as a forage crop. As with other cyanogenic-containing plant species, the sorghums may have increased toxic potential under certain environmental conditions (see Choke-cherry).

Pastures rather than hays are most commonly associated with clinical toxicity, as mature plants have far less toxic potential. Many of the Sorghum sp have been bred for low cyanogenic potential. Two syndromes seen in horses grazed on sorghum pastures bear similarities to the lathyrism syndrome in humans and may be related to chronic exposure to low levels of cyanide or the accumulation of lathyrogenic principles or both.

Lathyrism occurs in the underdeveloped countries, in people consuming poor-quality legumes, including Lathyrus sp, some peas, Vicia sp, and vetches. These plants are cyanogenic. With long-term ingestion, some cyanide is metabolized to neurolathyrogenic compounds, which cause focal axonal degeneration and demyelination of the lumbar and sacral parts of the spinal cord with a concomitant paresis or paralysis. Additionally, osteolathyrogenic compounds may be produced.

Clinical Signs. Several syndromes have been described in horses on sorghum pasture. The commonest syndrome is acute cyanide toxicity, which causes loss of livestock, especially on sorghum hybrid pastures, which are more toxic than the pure varieties of the plant. Signs of acute cyanide toxicity are described under chokecherry poisoning.

A condition unique to horses grazing sorghum pastures has been recognized in the southwestern United States. Equine sorghum cystitis ataxia is characterized by posterior ataxia with curious incoordination of the hindlegs, especially when the animal is backed, turned, or trotted. Urinary incontinence and cystitis with bladder atony are observed in 50 per cent of horses. Urine scalds may cause loss of hair, and the urine may be thick and may puddle owing to the large amount of sediment. Death in adult horses is usually due to pyelonephritis. Pregnant mares grazing these pastures may abort or may give birth to deformed foals. Articular ankylosis or arthrogryposis in these foals may cause dystocia.

A condition very similar to the sorghum cystitis ataxia syndrome has been reported following ingestion of baled hay containing caley pea (*Lathyrus hirsutis*) in California. Initially the animals seem to be in pain and carry all their body weight on the forelegs with the hindlegs "camped under." The animals are uncoordinated but are not paretic and remain alert, retaining normal vital signs. Residual signs may be seen for years after the initial plant insult, and the horse may develop a "stringhalt-like gait" in which the hindlimbs are primarily affected. The leg is, however, held in prolonged flexion, and the gait abnormalities are most marked when the animal is moved out or backed. No pain is associated with this stage of the disease, and cystitis has not been observed.

Pathology. The lesions characteristic of the cystitis ataxia syndrome are acute fibrinopurulent cystitis, chronic ulcerative sclerosing cystitis with accumulation of bladder sediment, and degeneration of the spinal cord as described earlier for neurolathyrism.

Treatment. Treatment of acute cyanide poisoning is described under chokecherry poisoning. There is no specific treatment for the chronic syndromes.

RED MAPLE (*Acer rubrum*)

Toxic Principle. The toxic principle(s) in red maple has not been identified, but on the basis of its biologic properties it is believed to be an oxidant.

Location of the Plants. The red maple tree is native to the eastern United States and to Canada. It may be found as far north as Nova Scotia and as far west as Texas and the Rocky Mountains. The full grown maple is a large tree that may exceed 100 feet in height and have a similar limb spread.

Conditions of Toxicity. Poisonings are reported in horses most commonly from the ingestion of wilted red maple leaves, either from the normal shedding process in autumn or from consuming leaves from fallen branches or trimmings thrown into pastures. Toxicity has been reproduced experimentally with twigs and bark from red maple; however, it is unlikely that field circumstances will result in cases developing from this source. The incidence of red maple leaf toxicity is highly seasonal, with cases occurring in summer and fall (June through October). Fresh red maple leaves have not been shown to be toxic.

Clinical Signs. Clinical signs develop one or more days after horses consume significant amounts of the red maple leaves. Experimentally, 1.5 gram of dried red maple leaves per kilogram of body weight delivered by stomach tube has reproduced the syndrome. Anorexia, depression, obvious methemoglobinemia, and weakness are observed early, followed in approximately 24 hours by intravascular and extravascular red blood cell hemolysis, anemia, Heinz body formation, and prominent hemoglobinuria. Icterus, cyanosis, and respiratory distress are common results of the underlying physiologic changes. Severely affected horses become comatose about the fourth or fifth day, and may die spontaneously or be euthanatized at the owner's request. Death loss is significant, and it is common to have 50 to 75 per cent of clinically affected horses die. Animals with mild signs or undergoing spontaneous recovery may appear clinically normal 7 to 14 days following the onset of signs.

Pathology. The postmortem lesions are characteristic of widespread red blood cell hemolysis, and include diffuse marked icterus, splenomegaly, moderate swelling and brownish discoloration of the liver, and swollen dark kidneys, often with a metallic sheen. Coffee-colored urine may be found in the bladder. Splenic hemosiderosis, moderate centrilobular necrosis of the liver, and nephrosis characterized by hemoglobin in renal tubular epithelial cells and in the tubular lumen are microscopic findings compatible with the severe hemolytic anemia.

Treatment. Effective therapy for red maple leaf toxicity in horses is not available. The response of equine methemoglobinemia to methylene blue is not as effective as in other livestock, but intravenous methylene blue administration may be attempted and could be useful in early stages of the disease before significant methemoglobinemia has occurred. The administration of isotonic fluids and perhaps blood transfusions may offer replacement therapy during the hemolytic crisis. Hypoxia can be assisted by providing oxygen. Other symptomatic therapy can be applied as needed. Horses with severe signs of red blood cell destruction, methemoglobinemia, and hemoglobinuria must be given a grave prognosis.

WILD ONIONS (*Allium canadense*)

Ingestion of wild onions has also caused acute hemolytic anemia with hemoglobinuria and icterus.

PLANTS PRODUCING EPITHELIAL OR SKELETAL DAMAGE

ST. JOHNSWORT (*Hypericum perforatum*)

Toxic Principle. The primary photosensitizing agent hypericin is the toxic principle.

Location of the Plant. St. Johnswort is found as a pasture weed in parts of the Pacific Coast and the Atlantic Coast toward the Southeast.

Conditions of Toxicity. Primary photosensitization is a rare occurrence in horses but is much more commonly reported in sheep and cattle. St. Johnswort and others contain photodynamic agents that reach the skin after absorption from the digestive tract. When the animal is subsequently exposed to sunlight, the compounds cause cellular damage at the skin level. Species of clover (Trifolium), vetches (Vicia), and buckwheat (Fagopyrum) have all been incriminated in primary or contact photosensitivity. *Trifolium hybridum* may also cause liver disease in horses. Photosensitizing plants seem to cause the problem when they are in the lush green stage and are growing rapidly. In the case of St. Johnswort, large amounts need to be eaten, and the plant is not very palatable, so cases of toxicity are rare.

Clinical Signs. The first signs of photosensitivity may be seen within four to five days of ingestion. Erythema and edema of the white or lightly pig-mented areas occur first. The eyelids may be swollen, and keratitis and conjunctivitis may be present. Within a few days, the affected areas blister and the skin sloughs, opening an avenue for secondary bacterial infection. The horse will seek out shade and may resent having the affected areas touched.

Pathology. There are no pathognomonic lesions.

Treatment. Horses will make a full recovery in one to two weeks if kept out of the sun and removed from the source of the plant. Corticosteroids may be helpful to decrease some of the inflammatory response. Antibiotics are useful to control bacterial infection. Open wounds should be given routine care.

BLACK WALNUT (*Juglans nigra*)

Toxic Principle. Black walnut contains juglone (5-hydroxy-1,4-naphthoquinone). This compound is also available from commercial sources through synthetic preparation.

Location of the Plants. The black or American walnut is native to the United States and is well distributed along the eastern seacoast, west to Michigan and throughout most of the midwestern states. It is a large tree that gains a height of 30 to 65 feet at maturity. The wood is aromatic and it and the nut kernel contain an oil that is fast drying, yellow in color, and, particularly when taken from the nut kernel, is used for artist's paints.

Conditions of Toxicity. Poisonings occur in horses when shavings containing 20 to 25 per cent or more from black walnut wood are used for stall bedding. The dark walnut shavings are easily seen in contrast to the other lighter-colored sources of wood shaving bedding, such as pine.

Clinical Signs. Clinical signs may occur as soon as 12 to 18 hours after initial exposure to the black walnut–containing shavings. Commonly, 24 hours elapse before toxicity is seen. Effects may be noted when the animals consume portions of the wood shavings or merely when they are bedded in the shavings and move through or stand in the material continuously. Affected horses become reluctant to move, are slightly depressed, and show early signs of laminitis with slight to severe edema in all limbs. A few horses may have edema but may not be depressed or have severe lameness. When present, the edema is marked distally. The laminitis may be demonstrated by a reluctance to move and by strong resistance to efforts made to lift the affected animal's feet. Increased respiratory rate and labored breathing may also be seen.

Pathology. Other than edema of the lower portions of the limbs, no lesions are seen. This disorder is not fatal.

Treatment. Affected horses should be removed promptly from further contact with black walnut shavings. Cooling of the hooves and edematous portions of the limbs may limit the severity of effects, but this treatment is not necessary for recovery. Horses seen to be eating the shavings may be given mineral oil as a laxative to evacuate the shavings from the digestive tract. Most affected horses will be markedly improved within 24 hours after removal from the black walnut shavings, and almost all clinical signs will have disappeared from the affected animals within 48 hours. No sequelae to this condition have been reported.

WILD JASMINE (*Cestrum diurnum*)

Toxic Principle. A steroidal glycoside that acts like vitamin D is the toxic principle.

Location of the Plant. Cestrum is found in waste ground in Texas and Florida.

Conditions of Toxicity. *Cestrum diurnum* produces a vitamin D–like factor that bypasses the usual feedback regulation of normal vitamin D metabolism in the horse. When a horse ingests the plant and is also on a ration containing adequate calcium and phosphorus, more calcium is absorbed than can be physiologically accommodated. Although hypercalcemia is moderate to severe, phosphorus levels are usually normal. The elevated calcium levels cause sustained secretion of calcitonin, which contributes to osteopetrosis. Hypercalcemia also decreases parathyroid activity, which can be seen histologically. The exact amount of the plant required to cause toxicity is unknown, but Cestrum is toxic at all times of the year.

The South American *solanum malacoxylon* is associated with the disease enteque seca, which causes signs very similar to those of jasmine poisoning. Hyperphosphatemia occurs with hypercalcemia, and there is calcification of soft tissue, for example, in the lungs, diaphragm, and kidney. *Solanum sodomauim* in Hawaii has been implicated in a similar syndrome in cattle. *Trisetum flavescens* in Germany has also been reported to cause vitamin D–like toxicity.

Clinical Signs. Horses that have ingested *C. diurnum* retain normal appetites but invariably demonstrate weight loss over two to six months. As the disease progresses, lameness increases in severity, and the animals develop a humped-up appearance and a short choppy gait. Animals lie down frequently. Pain around the flexors and suspensory ligaments with overextension of the fetlock joint has been observed.

Pathology. Dystrophic calcinosis of the elastic tissues of the heart, major arteries, tendons, and ligaments is seen.

Treatment. Regression of the disease can occur when animals are moved to clean pastures and are carefully nursed.

SLEEPY GRASS (Stipa sp)

Sleepy grass (Stipa sp) can cause mechanical damage to the mouth owing to the plant's physical characteristics. Ingestion of the New Mexico variety can produce a transient drowsiness that may last as long as two days, making movement of the animals difficult.

Supplemental Readings

Adams, L. G., Dollahite, J. W., Romane, W. M., Bullard, T. L., and Bridges, C. H.: Cystitis and ataxia associated with sorghum ingestion by horses. J. Am. Vet. Med. Assoc., 155:518, 1967.

Alden, C. L., Fasnaugh, C. J., Smith, J. B., and Mohan, R.: Japanese yew poisoning of large domestic animals in the midwest. J. Am. Vet. Med. Assoc., 170:314, 1977.

Clarke, E. G. C., and Clarke, M. L.: Veterinary Toxicology. Baltimore, Williams & Wilkins, 1975.

Cordy, D. R.: Nigropallidal encephalomalacia in horses associated with ingestion of yellow star thistle. J. Neuropathol. Exp. Neurol., 13:330, 1954.

Cordy, D. R.: Nigropallidal encephalomalacia (chewing disease) in horses on rations high in yellow star thistle. Proc. 91st Annu. Meet. Vet. Med. Assoc., 1954, pp. 149–154.

Divers, T. J., George, L. W., and George, J. W.: Hemolytic anemia in horses after the ingestion of red maple leaves. J. Am. Vet. Med. Assoc., 180:300, 1982.

Duncan, C. S.: Oak leaf poisoning in two horses. Cornell Vet., 51:159, 1961.

Evers, R. A., and Link, R. P.: Poisonous plants of the midwest. Special Publication 24, Urbana, IL, College of Agriculture, University of Illinois, 1972.

Fowler, M. E.: Nigropallidal encephalomalacia in the horse. J. Am. Vet. Med. Assoc., 147:607, 1965.

Fowler, M. E.: Plant poisoning. In Mansmann, R. A., McAllister, E. S., and Pratt, P. W. (eds.): Equine Medicine and Surgery, 3rd ed. Santa Barbara, CA, American Veterinary Publications, 1982, pp. 204–215.

Harries, W. N., Baker, F. P., and Johnston, A.: An outbreak of locoweed poisoning in horses in southwestern Alberta. Can. Vet. J., 13:141, 1972.

Hulbert, L. C., and Oehme, F. W.: Plants Poisonous to Livestock, 3rd revised ed. Manhattan, KS, Kansas State University, 1984.

Keeler, R. F., Van Kampen, K. R., and James, L. F.: Effects of Poisonous Plants on Livestock. New York, Academic Press, 1978.

Kelleway, R. A., and Geovjian, L.: Acute bracken fern poisoning in a 14-month old horse. VM SAC, 73:295, 1978.

Kingsbury, J. M.: Poisonous Plants of the United States and Canada. Englewood Cliffs, NJ, Prentice-Hall, 1964.

Krook, L., Wasserman, R. H., Shively, J. N. Tashjian, A. H., Brokken, T. D., and Morton, J. F.: Hypercalcemia and calcinosis in Florida horses: Implication of the shrub "Cestrum diurnum" as the causative agent. Cornell Vet., 65:26, 1975.

Larson, K. A., and Young, S.: Nigropallidal encephalomalacia in horses in Colorado. J. Am. Vet. Med. Assoc., 156:626, 1970.

Long, P. H., and Payne, J. W.: Red maple-associated pulmonary thombosis in a horse. J. Am. Vet. Med. Assoc., 184:977, 1984.

McCunn, J.: Castor bean poisoning in horses. Vet. J., 101:136, 1945.

Mettler, F. A., and Stern, G. M.: Observations on the toxic effects of yellow star thistle. J. Neuropathol., 22:164, 1963.

Osweiler, G. D., Carson, T. L., Buck, W. B., and Van Gelder, G. A.: Clinical and Diagnostic Veterinary Toxicology, 3rd ed. Dubuque, IA, Kendall/Hunt Pub. Co., 1985.

Pierce, K. R., Joyce, J. R., England, R. B., and Jones, L. P.: Acute hemolytic anemia caused by wild onion poisoning in horses. J. Am. Vet. Med. Assoc., *160*:323, 1972.

Pritchard, J. T., and Voss, J. L.: Fetal ankylosis in horses associated with hybrid Sudan pastures. J. Am. Vet. Med. Assoc., *150*:871, 1967.

Ralston, S. L., and Rich, V. A.: Black walnut toxicosis in horses. J. Am. Vet. Med. Assoc., *183*:1095, 1983.

Tennant, B., Dill, S. G., Glickman, L. T., Mirro, E. J., King, J. M., Polak, D. M., Smith, M. C., and Kradel, D. C.: Acute hemolytic anemia, methemoglobinemia, and Heinz body formation associated with ingestion of red maple leaves by horses. J. Am. Vet. Med. Assoc., *179*:143, 1981.

Tru, R. G., and Lowe, J. E.: Induced juglone toxicosis in ponies and horses. Am. J. Vet. Med. Res., *41*:944, 1980.

Wasserman, R. H.: Active vitamin D–like substances in *Solanum malacoxylon* and other calcinigenic plants. Nut. Rev., *33*:1, 1975.

Wharmby, M. J.: Acorn poisoning. Vet. Rec., *99*:343, 1976.

Young, S., Brown, W. W., and Klinger, B.: Nigropallidal encephalomalacia in horses caused by the ingestion of weeds of the genus Centaurea. J. Am. Vet. Med. Assoc., *157*:1602, 1970.

Water Quality

Frederick W. Oehme, MANHATTAN, KANSAS

Good-quality water is an essential part of horse management, but because of the variable conditions under which horses are kept and the variety of sources from which horses receive their water, there are possibilities for deterioration in water quality and potential harm to the horses consuming it.

Water sources for horses may come from public water supplies originating from reservoirs or community or public deep wells, from open ponds, springs, or streams, from dug or drilled wells on the farm or premises where the horses are kept, or from local collections of rain or spring water in ponds, dirt-lined pools, or metal containers. In some cases, the water being collected and offered to horses is from heated springs originating deep in various layers of mineral-rich rocks or from water that has percolated through disrupted soils and mine tailings rich in minerals and metals. Superheated water from springs (geothermal water) is usually contaminated with underground elements in concentrations from a few hundred mg per liter to many thousands of mg per liter. The most common chemicals are sodium, potassium, lithium, calcium, magnesium, ammonium, silica, chloride, fluoride, borate, sulfate, carbonate, bicarbonate, hydrogen sulfide, carbon dioxide, and some particularly toxic elements, such as arsenic, molybdenum, selenium, and a variety of other heavy metals. These substances may occur as suspended solids, in solution, or as combinations of the two forms.

In certain areas of the Rocky Mountain plateau and the Mississippi Valley, mining and ore recovery operations are common. Disrupted soils and processed rock are readily available to be leeched by rains, carrying dissolved chemicals to water collection basins or streams that might be used to water horses. Tailings are finely ground rock and minerals that have been processed to remove the commercially desirable ores. Excessive concentrations of soluble salts are present in many tailings and may also be leeched out of piles of tailings into horses' drinking water supplies. Most mine tailing materials contain various sulfides, which may oxidize to form acid and thus lower the water pH and increase solubility of heavy metals. The hazard of pollution of water supplies with heavy metals, therefore, increases as tailing waters age and oxidize.

The numerous sources of water for use by horses and the variable conditions under which it may be collected and stored result in numerous physical, chemical, and microbiologic contaminants potentially present in the final product offered to horses. Agricultural practices, particularly those used in intensive land use, increase the frequency with which agricultural chemicals appear in such waters. The most potentially hazardous contaminants in horses' water supplies are microorganisms, dissolved solids and salts, nitrates and nitrites, fluoride, heavy metals (such as arsenic, cadmium, copper, iron, lead, mercury, selenium, and zinc), and the variety of pesticides used in daily farming operations.

BACTERIAL MICROORGANISMS

The presence of potentially pathogenic microorganisms is usually tested by evaluating the degree of bacterial contamination from animal or human wastes. Laboratory tests examine for indicator organisms rather than for actual pathogens; the coliforms are the principal indicators of the suitability of a particular water supply. However, specific bacterial examinations for other disease-producing organisms may also be performed by appropriately equipped laboratories. The usual limitations placed on animal waters are that the coliform count should not exceed 5000 per 100 ml of water. Contamination of horses' water supplies is more likely to occur if fecal wastes are draining into the water supply or if wells receive water from nearby feedlots or animal holding areas. Surface waters open to sunlight and oxygen may present less of a hazard owing to the sterilizing effects of ultraviolet light.

DISSOLVED SOLIDS AND SALTS

Salinity is the concentration of solids in water and is an expression of the amount of dissolved salts in a particular water supply. The ions most commonly involved in high saline waters are calcium, magnesium, sodium, bicarbonate, chloride, and sulfate. Water hardness is the tendency of water to precipitate soap or form scale on heated surfaces. It is generally expressed as the sum of calcium and magnesium, but other cations, such as iron, strontium, aluminum, zinc, and manganese, also contribute to hardness. Although water with cation concentrations above 120 mg per L is classified as hard, the hardness of water in itself is not a problem in horses' drinking water. Rather, the concentration of dissolved salts (sodium, magnesium, calcium, bicarbonate, sulfate, and chloride) is of much greater concern. Soluble salt concentrations of less than 7000 mg per L in horses' drinking water are considered safe. Between 7000 and 10,000 mg soluble salts per L in drinking water present mild risks for pregnant or lactating horses and thus should be avoided if possible in those stress situations. Waters with soluble salt concentrations greater than 10,000 mg per L present greater risks and are not recommended for consumption by horses, although field experience suggests that in most cases the major effect is transient diarrhea. Soluble salt concentrations considerably greater than 10,000 mg per L (for example, greater than 12,000 mg per L) present considerably greater risks and should not be made available for consumption by horses.

NITRATES AND NITRITES

Nitrates and nitrites are extremely water-soluble and move easily with ground water. The most common source of contamination for horses' water supplies is surface water runoff from high organic matter–containing soils or grounds heavily fertilized with nitrogen. Nitrates are not significantly toxic to horses, since horses lack the ability to rapidly reduce nitrates to the more toxic nitrite. However, if water supplies have high levels of nitrite, this ion oxidizes the iron in hemoglobin to the trivalent state, forming methemoglobin. The result is acute methemoglobinemia and potentially rapid death. Levels of nitrite in water for horses should not exceed 10 mg per L. Some evidence suggests that low levels of nitrate in waters may produce chronic effects on mares stressed with late pregnancy or on foals beginning to supplement nursing with available water supplies. Among the suggested effects from low-level nitrate are infertility and late-term abortions, poor growth rate in young animals, vitamin A deficiency, interference with iodine metabolism, and increased susceptibility to infections. Although good experimental evidence substantiating these field observations is lacking, clinicians may wish to consider recommending alternate water sources in instances in which patients have one or more of these observed effects and nitrate levels in available waters exceed 90 mg per L. If other obvious etiologic factors have been ruled out, instances of rapid improvement have occurred in such circumstances two to three weeks after implementing a water change.

FLUORIDE

Fluoride in water at concentrations of 3 mg per L or more will cause mild fluorosis and mottling of developing teeth. In some areas of the country, horses' water supplies may considerably exceed this level, resulting in badly worn and discolored teeth and bone changes. Soreness of the teeth and sensitivity to heat and cold, quidding of feed, and intermittent lameness are effects of chronic exposure to fluoride. There is little fluoride accumulation in soft tissues. Following removal of the fluoride-containing water, the lameness problems will improve, but the bone and teeth changes are permanent.

HEAVY METALS

Heavy metals in water seldom present problems to horses because they usually do not occur at high levels. However, under unusual instances of chemical spills, drainage through dump sites, or leeching from mining operations, hazardous levels of certain heavy metals may appear in water offered to horses. Aluminum, beryllium, boron, chromium, cobalt, copper, iodide, iron, manganese, molybdenum, and zinc are examples of such potential metal contaminants. Suggested acceptable limits for these metals and other potential contaminants in livestock waters are listed in Table 1.

Some heavy metal elements may be of special hazard to horses because of their inherent toxicity or tissue accumulation. Arsenic may induce digestive tract irritation. Cadmium is potentially a neph-

TABLE 1. RECOMMENDED LIMITS OF CONCENTRATION OF SOME POTENTIALLY TOXIC
SUBSTANCES IN DRINKING WATER FOR LIVESTOCK*

Substance	Safe Upper Limit of Concentration (mg/L)		
	For Humans U.S. EPA	For Animals U.S. EPA	NAS
Aluminum	—	5.0	—
Arsenic	0.05	0.2	0.2
Barium	1.0	—	NE
Beryllium	—	No Limit†	—
Boron	—	5.0	—
Cadmium	0.01	0.05	0.05
Chromium	0.05	1.0	1.0
Cobalt	—	1.0	1.0
Copper	—	0.5	0.5
Fluoride	—	2.0	2.0
Iron	—	No Limit	NE
Lead	0.05	0.1	0.1
Manganese	—	No Limit	NE
Mercury	0.002	0.001	0.01
Molybdenum	—	No Limit	NE
Nickel	—	—	1.0
Nitrate	45	100	440
Nitrite	—	33	33
Selenium	0.01	0.05	—
Vanadium	—	0.1	0.1
Zinc	—	25.0	25.0

*Modified from Carson, TL: Water quality for livestock. *In* Howard, J. L. (ed.): Current Veterinary Therapy, Food Animal Practice. Philadelphia, W. B. Saunders Company, 1981, pp. 420–424.

†No limit/not established (NE). Experimental data available are not sufficient to establish definite limits or recommendations.

EPA = Environmental Protection Agency

NAS = National Academy of Sciences

rotoxic compound if high concentrations are consumed. Copper may induce liver damage owing to its biologic accumulation in that organ, with red blood cell destruction occurring during a "hemolytic crisis." Lead accumulates in all tissues, particularly the liver and kidneys. The peripheral nervous system of horses is particularly sensitive to this metal. Respiratory distress on moderate exercise is an early indication of lead toxicity in horses. Mercury is more readily absorbed in the organic form than in the metallic state. Digestive tract irritation and later kidney and central nervous system effects may be seen, depending upon its form and concentration in consumed water supplies. Selenium is an essential element, but in some areas of the United States, it is present in water at concentrations sufficient to produce chronic selenium toxicity. Levels in excess of 0.5 parts per million (ppm) may induce weight loss, loss of long hair of the mane and tail, and changes in the hoof wall. Zinc is also an essential element but may induce digestive tract disturbances or arthritic problems in horses consuming abnormal amounts in water.

PESTICIDES

Agricultural chemicals, such as pesticides, enter water from soil runoff, spray drift, rainfall, direct application to ponds or lakes, accidental spills, or faulty waste disposal techniques. High levels present in water owing to accidental spills may produce acute toxicity, either nervous signs from the chlorinated hydrocarbon insecticides or excessive salivation and digestive tract activity with moderate peripheral nervous signs from organophosphate or carbamate insecticides. Levels in waters sufficient to produce intoxication in consuming horses will always produce fish kills, since fish are considerably more sensitive to insecticide concentrations than are horses. Chronic toxicity is infrequent, except in the instance of chlorinated hydrocarbon exposures, when persistent residues may accumulate in equine tissues. Biodegradation of the organophosphate and carbamate insecticides is rapid, and chronic exposures are unlikely. In general, water concentrations of pesticides less than 0.1 mg per L are acceptable for equine use.

CLINICAL SIGNS

The clinical effects likely to be seen in horses consuming poor-quality water vary considerably with the type and concentration of the contaminant. In some instances, one chemical entity may be responsible for a clinical syndrome. Acute toxicities may result from the release of large amounts of soluble pollutants as a result of pond failure or the washing of chemicals through rainfall from highly contaminated soils. In other instances, chemical spills will produce massive contamination and effects similar to those observed with direct application or consumption of specific compounds. Chronic intoxication may occur by small amounts of drainage from contaminated soils or through constant environmental pollution. The equine clinician must evaluate each situation critically and must relate the disease syndrome to water exposure and concentrations of hazardous materials in the equine water source.

TREATMENT AND PREVENTION

Until a definitive diagnosis is available, treatment of affected horses can only be symptomatic and supportive. Once an accurate diagnosis has been made, the most appropriate therapy and management should be employed. Such management should always include removal of horses from the contaminated water supply and determination that the replacement water supply does not present other hazards. Balanced and adequate mineral sup-plementation is imperative, since the intake of chemical elements via water often results in mineral imbalances. Salt hunger or depraved appetite due to mineral inadequacies may induce horses to seek out hazardous water supplies to satisfy cravings. In most instances, water quality hazards are a chronic management problem that develops over a period of many months. Their resolution may also require considerable effort and adequate time for patient recovery.

Preventing horses from having to utilize poor-quality water is important. In quality equine practices, the periodic chemical analysis of water supplies may be a useful safeguard against future health problems.

Supplemental Readings

Carson, T. L.: Water quality for livestock. *In* Howard, J. L. (ed.): Current Veterinary Therapy, Food Animal Practice. Philadelphia, W. B. Saunders Company, 1981, pp. 420–424.

Oehme, F. W.: Water quality as related to animal health. Quality Water for Home and Farm. St. Joseph, MO, American Society of Agricultural Engineers, Pub. 1–79, 1979, pp. 21–29.

Shupe, J. L., Peterson, H. B., and Olson, A. E.: Toxicants in geothermal waters and in mine tailings. *In* Howard, J. L. (ed.): Current Veterinary Therapy, Food Animal Practice. Philadelphia, W. B. Saunders Company, 1981, pp. 424–428.

The Etiologic Diagnosis of Sudden Death

Frederick W. Oehme, MANHATTAN, KANSAS

The horse that dies quickly or is found dead with no premonitory signs is both an emotional and diagnostic problem: Reactions of disbelief, shock, or amazement may turn to guilt, defensiveness, anger, or an emotional demand for action and answers. The equine clinician may be confronted by an excited and anxious client.

A human tendency is for the clinician to grasp at the first opportunity to pacify the client. The "catch-all" diagnosis of "poisoning" may provide an easy way out until the client asks, "Poisoned how?" Since there are many possible reasons for horses dying suddenly, it is the ethical responsibility of every veterinarian to conscientiously inform clients of the potential causes of the situation. If the client is willing to stand the expense and effort, a thorough diagnostic program should be initiated to resolve the many questions raised by the sudden death. Much harm, both morally and professionally, has been done by hasty diagnoses being suggested and accepted by emotionally distraught clients.

The causes of sudden death must be explored in the same way that any other equine disease is investigated. Not only toxic but also nutritional, metabolic, infectious, and even accidental causes of death should be considered in a differential diagnosis. Circulatory collapse due to cardiovascular failure, lightning stroke or electrocution, anaphylaxis, trauma producing brain and spinal cord damage, acute digestive tract torsion or displacement, and even fatal gunshot wounds are just as viable initial possibilities for producing sudden death as are infectious or chemical etiologies. The history surrounding the circumstance and the events leading up to the finding of the dead horse are critical. Because the owner is often upset, a history obtained by the owner's observations should be carefully reviewed. The "facts" may be inaccurate and should be considered suspect if the physical findings and observations of the clinician do not support the history provided by the client.

Following a detailed history and examination of

the environment and circumstances of the incident, a thorough postmortem examination should be performed. Despite the awkwardness and frequent inconvenience of such examinations, all body systems and organs should be observed. Minor lesions in the digestive tract, central nervous system, or circulatory system may suggest conditions that further scrutiny will prove contributory to death. All abnormalities should be carefully recorded, and specimens of selected body tissues should be collected and preserved for microbiologic, histopathologic, or chemical examination. Environmental samples of water, feed, pasture content, or other suspected etiologic sources should be collected for possible later laboratory study.

At the conclusion of the clinical investigation, the veterinarian should present initial impressions to the client. If evidence is strong supporting one cause, the client may be satisfied and the issue may be resolved. In many instances, more than one potential cause of death is apparent, and the clinician should then provide the client with options for additional action. Costs involved (for toxicology examinations, these are significant) and the time interval before reasonable responses may be expected should be realistically presented and discussed. The client should also recognize that despite the expenditure of considerable time, money, and effort, the results of the laboratory examinations may not be conclusive and that an absolute final diagnosis may not be possible despite the best of intentions. At whatever point the client and veterinarian decide to cease further evaluations, all parties should feel confident that all practical options and alternatives have been considered. The veterinarian should also make sure that the client has had the best available opinion as to what caused the sudden death of the horse and that the client has also been offered recommendations to prevent this disaster in the future.

CHEMICAL CAUSES OF SUDDEN DEATH

Chemically caused sudden death in previously apparently healthy horses may follow exposure to lethal amounts of highly toxic chemicals, exposure to single large doses of poisons, the misapplication of drugs and chemicals producing unusual exposure situations, or individual animal hypersensitivity or idiosyncrasies resulting in unique toxic reactions. The latter circumstances are especially popular diagnoses when routine examinations of individual sudden deaths produce negative results. In some cases, there is indeed foundation for suggesting such a cause-and-effect relationship, but an absolute diagnosis of such may be very difficult to confirm.

FAILURE OF OXYGEN TRANSPORT IN BLOOD

Toxins that produce an inability of the blood to properly oxygenate vital tissues produce dramatic and sudden death. Cyanide toxicity, produced by ingestion of plants such as sorghum (p. 678), wild cherry (p. 678), and arrowgrass, and nitrite and chlorate ingestion may cause death within 5 to 10 minutes. Cyanide poisoning produces bright cherry-red blood and tissues, while nitrite and chlorate poisoning produces chocolate-brown methemoglobinemia.

TOXIC GASES

Environments that favor the presence of toxic gases can induce fatalities within minutes after exposure. Some housing environments may result in fatalities overnight from faulty air circulation or the accumulation of waste gases. Carbon monoxide induces pink-red blood and results from exposure to heater or automobile exhaust fumes. Chloroform and hydrogen sulfide are central nervous system and cardiovascular depressants, producing sudden death by respiratory failure.

INSECTICIDES

The insecticides are all toxic in small quantities and are capable of inducing fatalities within minutes to hours after exposure. The organophosphate and carbamate insecticides are the most lethal (p. 658). Chlorinated hydrocarbon insecticides produce convulsions and violent death, which may not be observed (p. 657). Nicotine, applied as nicotine sulfate for insects in housing structures, is rapidly absorbed with fatality due to peripheral and central nervous system dysfunction (p. 657).

PLANT TOXINS

Of the numerous plant toxins, several are extremely lethal and are capable of producing almost immediate fatalities. Blue-green algae may induce sudden death in horses consuming water with algae in it. Japanese yew induces muscle weakness, tremors, and death minutes after consumption (p. 676). Cicuta (water hemlock) induces violent seizures and almost immediate fatality (p. 675). Oleander (Nerium) is a rapid cardiovascular toxin (p. 674). Castor bean (Ricinus) contains a plant protein that induces a shock reaction in horses that consume it (p. 673). The plants containing high levels of oxalates (Halogeton, Sarcobatus) dramatically lower circulating calcium levels, with sudden death due to hypocalcemia.

BACTERIAL TOXINS

Bacterial toxins, such as those formed by *E. coli*, may induce autointoxication and sudden death due to digestive tract absorption of ingested or digestive tract–formed bacterial poisons (p. 81). Dietary changes or excesses are important circumstances leading to such fatalities.

VENOMS

The venom of insects contains complex neurotoxins, and some contain irritating substances such as formic acid. Stings from bees, wasps, and ants induce not only local reactions but also a rapid and generalized effect producing collapse. Death may occur if repeated stings are received. Blister beetles (p. 120) may induce sufficient digestive tract irritation to cause shock and early death. Bites from snakes, such as the rattlesnake, produce massive tissue reaction. If this reaction interferes with respiration, death due to suffocation is possible (p. 663).

DRUGS

A variety of drugs are potentially fatal. Curare may induce immediate respiratory failure. Overdosage of intravenous antimicrobial agents can produce shock and death. Improper administration of parenteral medication (with drugs intended for intramuscular injection being given intravenously) is an unfortunate cause of prompt fatality. Individual horse hypersensitivity or allergy to therapeutic agents can produce sudden death. Fortunately, immediate administration of epinephrine is an effective emergency treatment for these situations.

FEED CONTAMINATION

Accidental or intentional contamination of feed with acutely toxic chemicals is a human factor that is occasionally responsible for sudden horse deaths. Arsenic and strychnine may be accidentally included in horse feeds or may be added maliciously. Rumensin is acutely toxic in small doses to horses and may be in cattle feeds that are later offered to horses.

SAMPLE COLLECTION AND SUBMISSION

Tissue selection and collection for chemical analysis and its proper submission to testing laboratories are important scientific and legal procedures to secure meaningful analytical results. Samples collected from horses dying suddenly from suspected poisoning should include liver, kidney, stomach or intestinal contents, urine, and whole blood. At least 10 ml of whole blood should be submitted together with 50 ml or more of urine and at least 100 gm each of liver and kidney. At least 200 gm of digestive tract contents should be collected if available. In specific suspected intoxications, the collection of other selected organs may also be indicated. The entire brain, 100 gm or more of body fat and spleen, and generous samples of hair or hoof and bone may be of special value in certain circumstances.

Often overlooked is the submission of samples from suspected sources of the poison. Feed, water, weeds in the area, and suspected sources or baits are excellent samples for determining the possible origin of a toxicity. Generous portions (in excess of 200 gm and preferably 2 kg) of each sample should be provided. Table 1 lists the suggested specimens and amounts desired for the toxicologic tests likely to be considered in evaluating causes of sudden death in horses.

Specimens should be taken free of chemical contamination and debris and should not be washed because of the possibility of contaminating the specimen or removing residues of the toxic material. Clean glass or plastic containers that can be tightly sealed are excellent for collecting specimens. Each sample should be preserved separately in an individual container labeled with the owner's and animal's identification and the type of tissue or specimen in the container. Preservatives, such as formalin, should never be added unless there is a specific reason for doing so. In those cases, such information should be included on the specimen label. Samples of the preservative, if used, should also be submitted separately for possible analytical reference. Serum or blood samples should be kept refrigerated, while tissue specimens are best frozen. They should be packaged so that they arrive at the laboratory while still frozen.

The importance of supplying a complete account of history, signs, and lesions observed cannot be overemphasized. This should all be a part of the fundamental information supplied to the laboratory with the samples. The clinician's name and address, the owner's name and address, and the horse's breed, sex, age, and weight should be basic information. Additional facts should include the number of other horses in the field or on the farm, whether other animals were affected or died, the type of management, feeding program, history of past illness or problems, and immunization records. Other facts that would be helpful to the laboratory include the period of time that the horse had been eating the last batch of prepared feed, the type of pasture, the presence of trash, dumps, old motors, or farm machinery and their accessibility to the animal, descriptions of the clinical signs and postmortem findings, including negative observations, length of time since the horse was last observed, its condition at the last observation, medications that were given before death, and any treatments for parasites. All such information is equally important when analyses originally requested are negative and the need for

TABLE 1. SPECIMENS REQUIRED FOR SELECTED TOXICOLOGIC TESTS

Analysis Requested	Specimen Required	Amount of Specimen Desired	Special Precautions
Aflatoxin	Food	200 gm	Keep dry and cool
Ammonia	Whole blood, urine	5 ml	Maintain air-tight
	Stomach contents	100 gm	Freeze until tested
ANTU	Stomach and intestinal contents, liver	200 gm	Must be tested 12-24 hours after ingestion
Arsenic	Liver, kidney	50 gm	
	Food, stomach contents	100 gm	
	Urine	50 ml	
Carbon monoxide	Whole blood	15 ml	
Chlorinated hydrocarbon insecticide	Whole blood	10 ml	Keep tissues separate and free of contamination; use only chemically clean glass jars to package
	Body fat, stomach contents	100 gm	
	Liver, kidney	50 gm	
Cholinesterase	Whole blood	10 ml	Keep refrigerated
Copper	Whole blood	10 ml	
	Liver, kidney	50 gm	
	Feces	100 gm	
Ethylene glycol	Serum, urine	10 ml	Fix in formalin for histopathologic examination
	Kidney	Both kidneys	
Fluoroacetate (1080)	Stomach contents	All available	Freeze until tested
	Kidney	One whole	
	Urine	50 ml	
	Liver	50 gm	
	Bait, source	100 gm	
Lead	Whole blood	10 ml	Use only heparin or citrate as anticoagulant
	Liver, kidney	50 gm	
Methemoglobin	Whole blood	10 ml	
Nitrate, nitrite	Water	50 ml	
	Source	100 gm	
Organophosphorus insecticide, carbamate insecticide	Body fat, stomach contents	50 gm	
	Whole blood	10 ml	Use only heparin as anticoagulant
	Urine	50 ml	
	Food	100 gm	
Oxalate	Kidney	Both kidneys	Fix in formalin for histopathologic examination
Phenothiazine or derivative	Food or other source	50 gm	
Strychnine	Stomach contents, urine	All available	
	Liver	50 gm	
Thallium	Urine	10 ml	
	Liver, kidney	50 gm	
Warfarin	Liver, food, source	100 gm	
Zinc	Liver, kidney	50 gm	
	Source	100 gm	

Modified from Oehme, F. W.: Laboratory diagnosis of chemical intoxications. Vet. Clin. North Am., 6:723, 1976.

intelligently suggesting and selecting other analytical procedures becomes obvious. If adequate specimen material and a detailed history of circumstances, signs, necropsy lesions, and other appropriate history are available, the laboratory toxicologist is in an excellent position to provide alternatives for assay and to offer optimal assistance and service. The recording of this information also documents specific facts and responsibilities in the event that legal action is later taken.

If a concurrent histopathologic examination is requested, samples for histopathology should be preserved in 10 per cent buffered formalin and shipped in containers separate from those being used for the chemical analysis. Since the tissues for chemical assay are usually frozen, separate specimens and separate packages for the histopathologic studies should be provided so that the formalinized tissues do not also undergo freezing.

Plastic bags, cardboard, newspaper, and various forms of ice are good for packing specimens. Liquids should be shipped in leakproof containers and individually wrapped in packing material to prevent leakage and contamination of other specimens or accompanying mail. Ideally, the best method for submitting samples to a laboratory is by personal messenger. Often the owner of the deceased animal is sufficiently concerned to make the delivery. Bus and truck services may also be used, as well as the postal service. In all instances, delivery time should be anticipated so that holidays and weekends are avoided.

Proper interpretation of the laboratory test results is important for accurate assessment of the etiologic cause of sudden death. Frequently too much emphasis is placed on individual laboratory values when many factors in the patient's biology and the exposure circumstances are capable of producing variations. In addition, laboratory variations inherent in any procedure add to the variability of results. A competent laboratory should provide a normal range of values and comments indicating those results considered abnormal.

THE FINAL EVALUATION. . . . POISONING?

All the available data and information must now be taken into consideration to evaluate whether a poisoning was the cause of the horse's sudden death. The mere presence of a suspected toxicant is not always sufficient to confirm poisoning, nor is a negative finding conclusive evidence that a toxicosis did not occur. The persistence of certain compounds, such as heavy metals and chlorinated hydrocarbon insecticides, and their common environmental occurrence ensure that these chemicals are usually detected in most horse tissues regardless of the cause of death. Other rapidly metabolized toxins, such as the organophosphate and carbamate insecticides, may not be detected on postmortem chemical analysis owing to postmortem decomposition or rapid biodegradation to metabolites. The clinician's previous experience with poisoning should help in evaluating the analytical results, but tissue levels of poisons must be related to concentrations normally found in healthy animals. Thus, it is important to establish that the chemical concentrations detected are meaningful and indeed dose-related to the specific sudden death. An experienced toxicologist is of potential value in helping to relate the field and laboratory data to the clinical circumstances. The clinician should not hesitate to contact such individuals for assistance at this crucial time.

Given a complete clinical and environmental history, the physical and pathologic observations from the horse, the results of clinical chemistry, histopathology, and chemical analysis, and perhaps the benefit of consultation, the clinician should be able not only to properly interpret the results of chemical analysis but also to put into focus the history, clinical signs, and other examination results. The responsibility for the definitive or most likely diagnosis (or alternative diagnoses) should be assumed by the equine clinician after all the circumstantial, clinical, postmortem, pathologic, and laboratory findings have been carefully and competently evaluated.

Supplemental Readings

Barkan, B. A., and Oehme, F. W.: A classification of common Midwestern animal toxicoses. Vet. Toxicol., *17*:34, 1975.
Buck, W. B.: Use of diagnostic laboratories. *In* Howard, J. L. (ed.): Current Veterinary Therapy, Food Animal Practice. Philadelphia, W. B. Saunders Company, 1981, pp. 369–376.
Fowler, M. E.: Poisoning syndromes associated with sudden collapse and death. *In* Catcott, E. J., and Smithcors, J. F. (eds.): Equine Medicine and Surgery, 2nd ed. Wheaton, IL, American Veterinary Pub., 1972, p. 197.
Harvey, D. G.: Has it been poisoned? Br. Vet. J., *137*:317, 1981.
Oehme, F. W.: Laboratory diagnosis of chemical intoxication. Vet. Clin. North Am., *6*:723, 1976.

Sample Collection for Diagnosis of Drug Abuse in Horses

Frederick W. Oehme, MANHATTAN, KANSAS

Veterinarians may become involved with equine drug abuse by their professional work at race tracks or trail rides, or through owners requesting that veterinarians administer, prescribe, or sell various drugs for their horses. On occasion, veterinarians may be asked to give drugs to cover up physical defects before a horse sale. These are usually intended as deceptive activities and in most instances may be illegal and at best unethical for the veterinarian to participate in.

Drugs such as short-acting stimulants (amphetamine) or narcotics may be given to horses to influence their winning ability in competitive events. Depressants such as sedatives or tranquilizers may be given to reduce the chances of the animal being successful. Vitamins or anabolic steroids may be given for weeks or months between competitive events to improve general body condition. Occasionally, a highly excitable horse may receive a small dose of a tranquilizer or depressant to ease its handling and better channel its competitive characteristics. In the case of acute or chronic injury, various medications may be used to restore or maintain normal locomotion and performance. Antiinflammatory drugs such as phenylbutazone and corticosteroids injected intra-articularly to diminish joint pain are common choices. Local anesthetics for nerve or joint blocks may be misused for this purpose. A variety of drugs may be administered to interfere with the detection of other illegal drugs, and diuretics such as furosemide may be given to produce diuresis and thwart the analysis of urine for illegal medication by dilution. Bicarbonate administration and the autoadministration of red blood cells are other techniques to gain competitive advantage for the racing horse. Unintentional exposure to drugs that may produce test results interpreted as doping can result from the administration of procaine penicillin (and the detection of procaine in urine) and from animals consuming feed containing cocoa residues and caffeine appearing in tested urine. Some equine testing programs permit the controlled use of selected medications. In these instances, phenylbutazone and its derivatives, furosemide, and intra-articularly injected corticosteroids may be permitted.

SAMPLES AVAILABLE FOR COLLECTION

Several biologic fluids are collected from competitive horses for drug testing. The most common sample collected is urine, but it is difficult and time consuming to secure. The veterinarian must wait until the horse spontaneously voids, and although many horses urinate within minutes after the stimulation of competition, others may take one or more hours to produce a sample. Continuous attention must be given to the animal to ensure collection of the 200 to 600 ml sample in a clean container suitable for laboratory submission. The difficulty in obtaining such a collection has resulted in only a selected number of horses from any given event being tested. But because of the sensitivity with which urine can be assayed for various drugs, and the duration for which illegal drugs may be detected in urine, urine collection remains a most important part of the equine drug abuse testing program.

Blood samples are also available for collection and have the advantage that procedures other than drug detection may be performed on the single sample obtained. Collection of 10 to 20 ml does the horse no harm when proper technique is used. Although drug concentrations in blood are usually lower than those in urine, the parent form of the drug is usually detected and the specific significance of particular drug blood levels is more easily interpreted. Blood samples may be collected both before and after the competitive event.

Saliva has historically been used as a drug testing

medium from horses. Because of the few types of drugs that may be detected in saliva, it is much less commonly used for drug testing in horses than is urine and blood. Sweat may also be sampled but is not usually available until after the race or event. Sweat analysis suffers from the inability to rule out skin contaminants in the sweat. Sweat is therefore also rarely used in routine equine drug testing programs.

COLLECTION PROCEDURES

Veterinarians may be asked to collect samples either before a race or competitive event or immediately after it. Prerace testing involves a blood sample being withdrawn from all competing horses within two hours of the event. The analysis is usually performed in a laboratory on the premises or immediately adjacent. Any positive samples found result in the animal being withdrawn from the event. Blood testing before an event is almost always followed by urine testing after completion of the competition.

The more common collection of samples from horses occurs after the race or performance. Blood or urine samples are collected immediately after the event from winners and commonly also from second-place horses, favorites that did not place, and any other horses that might be selected by the officials. An area is designated for holding the animals after the event until the blood and urine are collected. As with the blood sample, collected before the event, these are sealed and clearly identified by the veterinarian or other responsible official. The postevent samples are usually refrigerated and then sent to more elaborately equipped laboratories for analysis. Since time is not a factor for testing after the event, the limited nearby facilities used for the pre-event testing program to ensure rapid results are bypassed in favor of more sophisticated facilities capable of more sensitive and specific analytic procedures.

EQUINE DRUG TESTING AND THE VETERINARIAN'S RESPONSIBILITIES

The veterinarian associated with an equine drug testing program has great professional and ethical responsibilities. The required samples must be collected properly and with no harm to the horses and minimal inconvenience to the attending personnel. Proper amounts of the desired samples must be collected in appropriate containers, sealed promptly, and adequately and correctly identified. The samples must then be carefully stored until they are directly transferred to the next responsible individual. This latter step is extremely important to document that a legal "chain of evidence" is in place in the event of a judicial challenge to the finding of illegal drugs in one or more samples.

The samples will eventually be placed in the hands of an analytic chemist who will utilize modern detection techniques to check for minute quantities of several hundred possible illegally used chemicals. The blood sample collected before the event will be subjected to rapidly performed and moderately sensitive procedures to provide an early result for evaluation. The samples collected following the event (usually blood and urine) are subjected to considerably greater scrutiny using modern elaborate instrumentation that will not only detect minute quantities of medications but will also identify metabolites of these drugs and quantify these compounds to nanogram sensitivities. A variety of chromatography procedures (thin-layer, gas, and high-performance liquid chromatography) are commonly employed, and are usually coupled with mass spectrometry, often as a single gas chromatography–mass spectrometry instrumentation unit. In addition, ultraviolet spectrometry, radioimmunoassay, and even testing of microcrystals of the suspected drug may be employed. To ensure validity and accuracy, usually two or more separate tests detecting any one drug in a sample must be shown "positive" before the horse is considered illegally medicated.

All veterinarians, whether officially involved with drug testing programs and sample collection or not, have the ethical responsibility to control the availability of drugs that might potentially be used to affect horses' performances in races and other competitive events. Although it is often difficult to refuse to sell such medication to a favorite client, or to decline to administer a drug to a horse in preparation for competition, the veterinarian has the responsibility to provide each horse with an equal opportunity for success. The veterinarian also must guard the horse's health and protect the injured animal from the use of drugs that mask injuries and place both the animal and the rider at risk during competition.

IS IT ALL WORTH IT?

The continuing conflict between the veterinarian's ethical and professional desires and the horse owner's wish to "get the edge" on the competition presents many challenges. Does it really matter and affect performance if drugs are administered? In spite of the widely held impression that a significant difference in performance results from equine drug abuse, the scientific evidence in support of this is controversial. Stimulants have not been clearly shown to improve the racing performance of horses. Although some may stimulate running response, at higher doses incoordination results. The use of anti-inflammatory drugs to restore normal performance does not generally result in improved performance. Toxicity from the extended use of all these medications is a realistic danger. The use of furosemide is common to reduce bleeding from the lungs of racing horses, but research studies show that use of the drug does not improve performance.

Perhaps of more practical import is the potential damage that could result to the veterinarian and the sport of horse racing and other horse competition if illegal use of drugs in horses is not continually challenged. The idea of veterinarians affecting horse performance and arbitrarily influencing the outcome of events is one that produces nightmares. Attempts to affect the outcome of equine competitive events by the use of drugs is filled with danger. Veterinarians should know their professional role and must approach clinical practice with an ethical and patient-oriented set of values.

Supplemental Reading

Tobin, T.: Medication of performance horses. *In* Mansmann, R.A., McAllister, E.S., and Pratt, P.W. (eds.): Equine Medicine and Surgery, 3rd ed. Santa Barbara, CA, American Veterinary Publications, 1982, pp.158–172.

URINARY TRACT DISEASES

Edited by W. M. Bayly

Acute Renal Failure

Ragan Adams, GAINESVILLE, FLORIDA

A diverse group of clinical states including intensive support therapy, prolonged anesthesia, long-term therapy with potential nephrotoxins, and strenuous exercise have all been associated with acute compromise of renal function. Regrettably, information concerning the pathophysiology of equine renal disease has not been generated at the same rate at which the clinical condition has been diagnosed. Much of this chapter will emphasize the etiology and diagnosis of acute renal failure to assist the clinician in recognizing and managing these often difficult cases.

Acute renal failure is the sudden, theoretically reversible inability of the kidney to perform the major functions of clearing nitrogeneous waste products from the blood and maintaining fluid and electrolyte homeostasis. Azotemia, or the accumulation of nitrogeneous waste products in the blood, is the hallmark of this disease, but may also result from other nonrenal conditions. Azotemia is diagnosed when serum creatinine normally less than or equal to 1.7 mg per dl serum or urea nitrogen normally equal to 10 to 20 mg per dl serum become elevated. This occurs when approximately two thirds to three fourths of the nephrons are not functioning properly. Obviously, some degree of renal dysfunction may be present prior to an elevation of serum creatinine and urea nitrogen. Three categories of azotemia have been defined.

Prerenal azotemia is caused by any event that diminishes perfusion of the kidneys and impairs glomerular filtration. Renal function should resume immediately upon restoration of perfusion, because the kidney itself is not damaged. However, severe or prolonged hypoperfusion may lead to ischemic injury to the kidney, which is a common cause of acute renal disease. *Renal azotemia* occurs if the kidney is damaged. *Postrenal azotemia* results when the patency of the urinary collecting system is sufficiently impaired to modify urine excretion. Because the kidney is not affected, once urine flow resumes, azotemia resolves. However, if back pressure from a lower urinary tract obstruction depresses glomerular filtration and renal blood flow sufficiently, kidney damage may occur.

ETIOLOGY

Prerenal causes of azotemia include hypovolemia, reduced cardiac output secondary to cardiac failure or low blood pressure, and vascular thromboses. Renal injury is commonly caused by hemodynamic, toxic, or inflammatory insults. Inadequate blood flow to the kidney can decrease glomerular filtration and cause ischemic injury, tubular dysfunction, and even necrosis. When blood flow is shunted from medullary to cortical nephrons during times of low perfusion, alterations in tubular function may occur because of the inherent specialization of the individual nephrons.

The effects of circulating endotoxins on renal blood flow have not been documented in the horse; however, endotoxins are associated with systemic coagulopathies, vascular damage, and thromboses that can involve renal tissue. The administration of prostaglandin synthetase inhibitors such as phenylbutazone and flunixin meglumine may compromise the kidney's ability to autoregulate blood flow.

Many compounds are considered potentially nephrotoxic (see p. 704); however, the mechanism of their toxicity in the horse is not well documented. Nephrotoxins can be classified according to their primary site of nephron damage. If more sensitive clinical tests were available to diagnose glomerular, proximal tubular, or distal tubular dysfunction, renal failure might be averted by early recognition of dysfunction and removal of the offending toxin.

Bacterial infections within the kidney are usually difficult to diagnose until fulminant. Bacteria may ascend from the lower urinary tract or enter the kidney hematogenously. In patients with chronic inflammatory conditions such as *Corynebacterium equi* pneumonia, streptococcal abscesses, equine infectious anemia, or Leptospira infections, deposits of circulating antibody-antigen complexes can cause glomerular damage and lead to acute renal failure. However, this condition as well as the formation of antibodies against glomerular basement membrane is usually associated with chronic renal insufficiency.

Postrenal azotemia is caused by abnormalities in the lower urinary tract. Rupture of the bladder most commonly occurs in neonates but has been documented in postparturient mares. These patients as well as those patients with urethral or ureteral tears may be anuric, azotemic, dehydrated, hyponatremic, hyperkalemic, and hypochloremic. These clinical signs usually resolve after surgical repair of the lesion and resumption of urine flow.

If an obstruction occurs in only one ureter and affects only one kidney, clinical signs may not develop because of compensation by the other kidney. More frequently, calculi in the horse form in the bladder and become lodged in the urethra. Dysuria, stranguria, hematuria, and an enlarged urinary bladder are the clinical signs that enable the diagnosis to be made before the condition causes severe renal dysfunction.

In summary, renal dysfunction may be caused by any number of factors, but it is frequently an accumulation of renal insults that triggers failure. A thorough examination of the patient as well as a complete medical history including environment, diet, water source, medical problems, and treatments including dosage, time interval, and duration must be assessed to understand the reasons a particular individual has developed acute renal failure. Its pathogenesis in the horse is controversial; thus, information on which to base clinical judgments is limited. Finally, the antemortem diagnosis of renal dysfunction or failure may not be obviously supported by significant gross or histologically observed pathology.

CLINICAL SIGNS

The clinical signs of acute renal failure are nonspecific. Commonly, horses are anorectic, depressed, and weak. They may show signs of decreased performance, mild colic, or intermittent fevers. Physical examination can reveal dehydration, abnormal frequency or volume of urination, increased water intake, edema, thrombosis, and hypertension. Diarrhea and laminitis may predispose the patient to renal failure or develop following its onset. Evaluation of kidney size on rectal palpation is highly subjective. Although the kidneys are often enlarged and may be painful, normal size or lack of pain does not rule out renal dysfunction.

It is often difficult to accurately estimate urine production, normally 1 to 2 ml per kg per hr in an adult, without access to a specialized collecting apparatus. In adult horses, anuria, dysuria, and stranguria usually suggest an obstructive urinary tract problem. Oliguria often occurs in the early stages of renal disease from hemodynamic causes, but polyuria is most common with aminoglycoside-induced acute renal failure or during the reparative stage of tubular disease.

LABORATORY FINDINGS

The important clinical laboratory findings can be obtained from three sources: a whole blood sample for hemogram and simultaneously obtained serum and urine samples that are taken before or just after the start of fluid therapy. Unfortunately, no one laboratory test is pathognomonic, and all data must be scrutinized in light of the patient's physical examination and medical history. Table 1 reviews reference values for tests used in the diagnosis of acute renal failure. However, reference values should be established for each laboratory.

Serum levels of sodium, potassium, and chloride are often within a normal range in the early stages, but hyponatremia and hypochloremia may develop with diarrhea or polyuria. Marked intracellular ionic potassium deficits can develop in anorectic patients

TABLE 1. REFERENCE VALUES FOR NORMAL ADULT HORSES

Serum chemistries*	Calcium (mg/dl) 12.3–13.9
	Chloride (mEq/L) 98–100
	Creatinine (mg/dl) 1.1–1.7
	Phosphorus, inorganic (mg/dl) 2.6–3.6
	Potassium (mEq/L) 3.9–4.5
	Sodium (mEq/L) 133–139
	Serum urea nitrogen (mg/dl) 10–20
Fractional excretion ratios[2]	Na 0.02–1%
	K 15–65%
	PO$_4$ 0–0.5%
Urine GGT/Urine Creatinine Ratio†	25

*From reference values used at the University of Florida Veterinary Medical Teaching Hospital, Gainesville, Florida.

†Adams, R., McClure, J. J., Gossett, K. A., Koonce, K. L., and Ezigbo, C.: Evaluation of a technique for measurement of gamma-glutamyltranspeptidase in equine urine. Am. J. Vet. Res., 46:147, 1985.

GGT = gamma glutamyl transpeptidase.

with diarrhea. More often, serum phosphorus and calcium levels are deranged. Various patterns of derangement can be seen in the adult horse with renal disease, although hypercalcemia and hypophosphatemia have been observed in bilaterally nephrectomized ponies.

The urine sample can be obtained by free catch or catheterization. Furosemide-induced samples and those taken while the patient has been on prolonged fluid therapy should not be used. Catheterization of the bladder in the male or female is not difficult, but aseptic technique is mandatory. In certain cases when the bladder is full and can be visualized sonographically, cystocentesis might be considered. The urine sample should be split into three aliquots and submitted for urinalysis, bacterial culture, and biochemistry tests.

Urinalysis includes measurement of specific gravity, quick test strips for pH, glucose, protein, blood, urobilinogen, bilirubin, and nitrates, as well as sediment analysis. Specific gravity of the urine should be measured before initiation of fluid therapy if possible. Low specific gravity (less than 1.020) in a dehydrated, azotemic adult horse is good evidence of intrarenal disease. However, specific gravity may be misleading, for it can be driven down by extrarenal causes such as excessive water intake, fluid diuresis, and hyperglycemia, as well as by intrarenal causes. The water deprivation test can be used in the horse to differentiate obligatory from compensatory polyuria but is not recommended for azotemic animals.

Changes in urine color are not specific for acute renal failure because horse urine varies widely in color from light yellow to dark brown. Reddish-brown urine is indicative of myoglobinuria following muscle damage. Hematuria or hemoglobinuria is suspected when urine is red, although the administration of phenothiazine may cause urine to turn red when exposed to the light. Equine urine is normally alkaline (7.5 to 8.5). Trace or low levels of protein in alkaline urine are often measured by dipstick analysis, but this is usually a false positive because of the analytic method. Bilirubinuria occurs in cases involving obstructive hepatic disease; however, the inherent orange color of many equine urine samples may lead to the interpretation of false positives when the dipstick analysis method is used.

Sediment analysis must be performed soon after collection because alkaline urine can dissolve casts. Because equine urine contains a large amount of mucus and crystals, casts, bacteria, and cellular material can be missed. A sample collected with sterile technique should be submitted for culture even if bacteria or large numbers of leukocytes are not seen in the sediment. White blood cells may appear in normal free catch samples; in high numbers they are indicative of an infectious process in the urinary tract. Red blood cells often appear in catheterized samples, and a low number of transitional epithelial cells is considered normal. Casts form in the distal tubules of the nephron and their presence in the urine usually indicates renal disease. Calcium carbonate crystals in alkaline (pH 7.5 to 8.5) and triple phosphate crystals in more neutral or acidic urine (pH <7) are normally found abundantly. Although the presence of many calcium oxalate crystals is an abnormal finding, they are not pathognomonic for an oxalate-induced nephropathy. The characteristic slimy texture of equine urine is due to mucus produced in glands of the renal pelvis.

Urine supernatant from a centrifuged sample can be analyzed for creatinine, phosphorus, sodium, and potassium to calculate creatinine clearance and the fractional excretion of electrolytes (Table 2). Although these single-sample calculations are not as precise as 24-hour clearance calculations and are potentially affected by diet, fluid therapy, and hormonal influences, they provide additional information on the patient's electrolyte status. As with any laboratory data, interpretation of abnormal values must be made in view of the particular clinical case. In my experience, an elevation of fractional excretion of phosphorus occurs in most adult equine patients with suspected tubular dysfunction. The kidney is the primary organ responsible for phosphorus homeostasis, and early alterations in renal perfusion resulting in tubular dysfunction may be reflected by inefficient phosphorus handling. On the other hand, some authors suggest that an elevation in fractional excretion of sodium should be used as the criterion to differentiate renal from prerenal azotemia. However, in human patients

TABLE 2. FORMULAS USED FOR CALCULATION OF INDICES OF URINARY TRACT FUNCTION

Index	Formula
Fractional excretion of substance "x" Fx"X"	$FxX = \dfrac{(UrX)}{(SX)} \times \dfrac{(SCr)}{(UrCr)} \times 100$
Creatine clearance	$CrC = \dfrac{(urine\ creatinine)}{(serum\ creatinine)}$
Urine GGT/urine creatine	$UrGGT/UrCr = \dfrac{UrGGT\ (IU/L)}{UrCr\ (mg/dl) \times 0.01}$

Cr = creatine, GGT = gamma glutamyl transpeptidase, S = serum, Ur = urine.

urine sodium output varies depending on the cause of acute renal failure and, in my experience, several horses with renal failure have had normal sodium excretion.

The measurement of enzyme activities in the urine can be used to monitor renal damage. In contrast to electrolytes, which are concentrated in the urine after being filtered from the plasma, the enzymes measured in urine are not filtered but released from the damaged renal tissue into the urine. In the horse only gammaglutamyltranspeptidase (GGT) has been studied. This enzyme is relatively stable in refrigerated urine supernatant for up to 48 hours and can be assayed by any laboratory using the technique for serum GGT.* A ratio of urinary GGT activity to urine creatinine levels is calculated from a single sample to account for changes in urine flow. Ratios of less than 25 are considered within normal limits. Elevations of the ratio are presumed to indicate some degree of proximal tubular cell damage. An elevated urine GGT/creatinine ratio does not provide prognostic information but merely reveals that active tubular cell damage is occurring.

OTHER STUDIES

Ultrasonic Evaluation. Sonographic evaluation of equine kidneys is a promising field and offers the most accurate noninvasive method to estimate renal size or identify causes of acute renal failure when renal structure is grossly distorted.

Renal Biopsy. With the advent of ultrasound-guided biopsy techniques, the accuracy of percutaneous renal biopsy has improved. Still, the procedure may result in renal hemorrhage; hematuria and red blood cell casts appear for 24 to 48 hours following the biopsy. The biopsy is most helpful prognostically to differentiate the subclinically diseased kidney that has acutely failed from one with minimal pathologic changes in which the disease process is truly acute and more likely to respond to

*Spin Chem, Glutamyltranspeptidase, Smith Kline Instruments, Inc., Philadelphia, PA

treatment. In acute renal failure renal tissue may appear relatively normal as evaluated by light microscopy despite laboratory data indicating severe dysfunction.

THERAPY

Once acute renal failure is recognized, four principles of therapy should be followed regardless of cause: (1) correction of fluid, electrolyte, and acid-base abnormalities; (2) identification and treatment of any underlying disease process such as septicemia, endotoxemia, rhabdomyolysis, hemolysis, heat stress, and dehydration; (3) discontinuation or modification of nephrotoxic drugs and administration of antidotes for identified toxins; and (4) support of the patient while the renal tissue is regenerating.

FLUIDS

Administration of fluids and electrolytes is the cornerstone of therapy for acute renal failure (Table 3). In principle, the type of replacement fluid administered is based on the needs of the individual patient as determined by the physical examination, medical history, state of hydration, and serum electrolyte levels. The amount of fluid is dictated by estimating the state of hydration using packed cell volume, total plasma protein, heart rate, capillary refill, and skin turgor, as well as the rate and route of fluid loss. In contrast to the dog or cat, the adult horse usually tolerates the administration of fluids when the hydration status is questionable.

The administration of oral fluids via nasogastric tube is the easiest and most convenient method for the practitioner to deliver large volumes of fluid. A nasogastric tube is passed and if no gastric reflux is obtained, 6 to 8 liters of warm water or isotonic electrolyte solution may be given to the 400-kg adult horse. This volume can be repeated every 30 to 60 minutes if the stomach is checked for distention before administration. Recipes for electrolyte mixtures may be tailored to the requirements of the patient.

If the patient requires more rigorous therapy or if gastric distention is present, sterile fluids must be given through an intravenous catheter. Delivery systems based on gravity flow, hand mechanical pumps, or catheterization of two veins simultaneously can be used to increase the rate of fluid administration. A 450-kg horse that is 10 per cent dehydrated will need 45 liters of fluid simply for rehydration. This volume can be given rapidly at 10 L per hr. Once the patient appears to be rehydrated but is still anuric or oliguric, fluid administration should be restricted to the individual's daily fluid requirements and losses (10 to 15 liters in an adult). These requirements can be provided at up to 5 L per hr. Daily body weight measurements, auscultation of the lungs for sounds consistent with pulmonary edema, and observation for the development of dependent edema are practical methods to check the patient for overhydration. If possible, central venous pressure is monitored and maintained at 5 to 10 cm water. Patients with tubular damage may be oliguric at presentation, but are frequently polyuric during the reparative stage. The patient generally loses sodium, chloride, phosphorus, potassium, and glucose in the tubular filtrate.

Serum electrolytes and acid-base status should be closely monitored to guide the selection of appropriate replacement fluids. However, the limitation of these values should be appreciated. Serum sodium levels are influenced by total body water as well as potassium. Serum potassium levels must be interpreted in conjunction with the acid-base status. Experimental data are greatly needed to clarify the proper rate and type of replacement fluid appropriate for equine patients with various types of dehydration and electrolyte imbalance. At this time, the most sensible approach is to tailor the basic principles of fluid therapy to the individual's response.

NUTRITION

If the horse with acute renal failure is anorectic, feeding via nasogastric tube may be necessary to minimize breakdown of endogenous protein (see p. 421). Supplementation with oral potassium chloride and sodium chloride may be made in the feed mix or in an oral solution and is especially important in the polyuric animal with diarrhea. One to two mEq potassium chloride per kg per day may be safely given orally. Ample clean fresh drinking water as well as an appropriate electrolyte mixture should be offered to the patient. Often after initial fluid deficits are corrected by intravenous fluid administration, the horse will resume drinking and maintain hydration on oral fluids.

MEDICATIONS

Therapy for the septicemic, endotoxic, diarrheic, and laminitic horse includes potentially nephrotoxic antibiotics and cyclooxygenase inhibitors as antiinflammatories. Practically, the use of these agents often cannot be avoided. Although means of adjusting dosages for drugs excreted by the kidney in the patient with renal dysfunction are controversial, one can either decrease the daily dosage or increase the time interval between treatments. Bacteriostatic antibiotics with long half-lives should be adjusted by increasing the dosing interval, whereas bactericidal antibiotics with short half-lives should be given in lower dosages. Potentially detrimental effects of phenylbutazone therapy may be minimized if the patient is properly hydrated. Flunixin meglumine is effective against endotoxemia at 0.25 mg per kg three to four times a day, a lower dose than the manufacturer recommends.

The horse that remains anuric after fluid deficits have been restored and circulatory volume re-established presents a major problem for the veterinarian. Some investigators believe tubules are blocked and therapy should be aimed at flushing out the debris. Furosemide, 20 per cent mannitol, and hyperosmolar solutions (10 per cent dextrose) are administered until the patient begins to produce urine. There are no scientifically based dosage reg-

TABLE 3. COMPOSITION OF COMMON INTRAVENOUS FLUIDS AND ORAL ELECTROLYTE SUPPLEMENTS

Fluid	Sodium (mEq/L)	Potassium (mEq/L)	Chloride (mEq/L)	Bicarbonate (mEq/L)	Calories (KCal/L)
Saline	154	—	154	—	—
Lactated ringer's	130	4	109	28	9
5% dextrose	—	—	—	—	170
5% sodium bicarbonate	600	—	—	600	—
Oral Supplements	**(mEq)**	**(mEq)**	**(mEq)**	**—**	**Kcal**
Sodium chloride 1 tbs (16.6 gm)	284	—	284	—	—
Potassium chloride 1 tbs (16.2 gm)	—	217	217	—	—
Lite Salt 1 tbs (16.9 gm)	144	113	256	—	—
Eltrad* 8 oz packet	570	39	415	—	724

*Haver-Lockhart, Elwood, KS

imens for this therapy. Others believe that intrarenal vascular dynamics control the glomerular filtration rate and they give dopamine to open renal vessels, increase blood flow, and thus glomerular filtration. Again, no dosage has been established for the horse in acute renal failure. A third group proposes that glomerular filtration ceases when the tubule of that nephron is unable to reabsorb the filtered sodium load. If this is true, it emphasizes the importance of diagnosing renal failure early in its course and minimizing the manipulation of the self-healing process. I believe that the first line of treatment should be provision of sufficient if not liberal volumes of balanced electrolyte solutions and minimal manipulation of renal blood flow.

The response to treatment varies depending on the duration of the condition before the beginning of treatment, the severity of the initial insult, the development of secondary complications such as diarrhea, laminitis, thrombophlebitis, and the patient's renal functional reserve capacity. Serum creatinine should stabilize or decline after initial rehydration, yet several days to weeks may be needed for serum creatinine values to fall to within normal range. Although serum electrolyte values may normalize rapidly, fractional excretion values for sodium and especially phosphorus take longer to revert to normal, suggesting a lag in tubular repair. Urinary GGT activity is only elevated in the acute phase of injury, and reduction of this value does not necessarily indicate resolution. Renal biopsies may provide helpful prognostic information. If marked histologic damage is apparent, the patient's renal reserve is probably diminished. Thus, even with repair and resolution of existing signs, future renal insults may be more likely to trigger exacerbation of dysfunction.

RENAL DYSFUNCTION IN THE NEONATE

The physiology of the neonatal equine kidney is even more poorly understood than that of the adult horse. Congenital abnormalities including renal cysts and ectopic ureters should be included in the list of potential disease etiologies. Hypoxic incidents in utero or during parturition have been linked to pathology in the nervous system of newborn foals, and may affect kidney function as well. Upon necropsy examination of septicemic foals that have signs of antemortem renal dysfunction, renal abscesses as well as acute tubular necrosis have been identified. Postrenal lesions such as ruptured bladders or urethral tears are more frequent in newborn foals than older animals.

Reference values for urine enzymes, urine volume, and urine electrolytes have not been established for neonatal foals less than seven days of age. Thus, diagnosis is more difficult than in the adult. Apparently healthy foals have very dilute, hyposthenuric urine with urine specific gravity as low as 1.006. Serum creatinine levels are often surprisingly high shortly after birth but should decrease to normal adult levels by day 2. The significance of this type of azotemia is not known. Foals with postrenal lesions involving tears in the ureter, bladder, or urethra vary in their presentation according to the severity and duration of the lesion (see p. 717). Commonly, these foals are azotemic, hyperkalemic, hyponatremic, and hypochloremic. Elevation of peritoneal fluid creatinine aids in the diagnosis. Sonography of the abdomen, contrast radiography, and injection of dye into the bladder followed by peritoneal taps can help localize the urinary tract lesion.

Therapy is based on the same four principles covered in the section on the adult horse. Volume and rate of fluid administration should be closely monitored, for it is easier to overhydrate the smaller newborn animal than an adult horse.

Supplemental Readings

Carlson, G. P.: Response of the horse to oral or intravenous fluids. In Proc. from 5th Annu. Meeting of Eq. Sports. Med., 1985, p. 102.

Coffman, J. R.: Equine Clinical Chemistry and Pathophysiology. Bonner Springs, KS, Veterinary Medical Publishing Co., 1981.

Rose, R. J.: A physiological approach to fluid and electrolyte therapy in the horse. Equine Vet. J., *13*:7, 1981.

Solez, K., and Whelton, A.: Acute Renal Failure: Correlations between Morphology and Function. New York, Marcel Dekker, 1984.

Stern, A.: Drug metabolism in renal failure. Comp. Cont. Ed., 5:913, 1983.

Chronic Renal Failure

Thomas J. Divers, KENNETT SQUARE, PENNSYLVANIA

Chronic, progressive renal disease causes continued loss of nephron function or population. Renal disease does not equal renal failure. Clinical signs of renal failure are not usually observed until two thirds or more of the nephron function is lost; polysystemic signs may not occur until there is 75 per cent loss. Only a few diseases of the kidney such as renal neoplasia and focal septic nephritis noticeably affect body condition without causing renal failure.

Chronic renal failure in the horse may be divided by clinical and pathologic findings into two broad classifications: primary glomerular disease and primary tubulointerstitial disease. Since the nephron is a single functioning unit, a disease process in one portion of an individual nephron will usually affect function of the entire nephron. Clinical and laboratory findings, diagnosis, and treatment of chronic renal failure resulting from primary tubulointerstitial disease are the focuses of this chapter.

PATHOPHYSIOLOGY

Renal disease may cause total destruction and absence of function in some nephrons while causing partial damage and decreased function in others. As the nephron number or function or both decrease there is a decline in glomerular filtration rate (GFR), and those solutes eliminated mostly by glomerular filtration or tubular secretion are retained in the body. The most significant of these solutes are byproducts of protein and amino acid metabolism such as urea, creatinine, and guanidine. Loss of nephron function also results in a failure to properly catabolize certain hormones and polypeptides such as parathyroid hormone, insulin, and glucagon. Abnormally high plasma concentrations of these protein byproducts and hormones are thought to exert toxic effects on virtually all organ systems. The clinical condition caused by this multisystemic toxic effect is called uremia.

Retention of potassium, hydrogen, calcium, and magnesium may be gradual because of compensatory increases in tubular secretion or decreased reabsorption in remaining functional nephrons. Plasma electrolytes such as sodium, chloride, and phosphorus, which are normally reabsorbed across the tubules, may decrease below normal in horses with polyuric chronic renal failure. Increased solute filtration and diuresis in surviving nephrons, along with concurrent tubular disease and dysfunction, impede normal resorption of water. This inability to concentrate urine causes polyuria, and the animal compensates by increasing water intake—polydipsia. The syndrome of polyuria and polydipsia is abbreviated PU/PD. Severely uremic horses may not maintain adequate fluid intake, allowing dehydration and hypovolemia to complicate the already life-threatening decline in GFR. Oliguria, when present in normovolemic horses with chronic renal failure, is usually terminal.

Horses with chronic renal failure and increased urine production may have increased concentrations of sodium, chloride, and phosphorus in the urine. If electrolyte-deficient water or feed is provided to these patients, a relative imbalance between body water and electrolytes results.

Systemic acid-base values are variable in horses with uremia. There may be a decreased reabsorption of bicarbonate and decreased hydrogen excretion causing metabolic acidosis and acidemia. Organic anions may also accumulate as a result of the decreased GFR and nephron function. However, a severely hypochloremic horse may have metabolic alkalosis.

The uremic effects on body systems may be observed either clinically or by laboratory evaluation or by both. Anemia that is usually of moderate severity is thought to be caused by toxic effects on the red blood cells and by decreased erythropoietin production. Within the grastrointestinal tract, increased amounts of urea may be excreted in the salivary secretions, causing a uriniferous odor of the breath, abnormal oral flora, and excessive dental tartar. Uremic toxins may also cause focal ulceration of the oral and intestinal mucosa. Normal intracellular shifting of sodium, potassium, and free water may be disrupted by the effect of uremic toxins on cell membranes, resulting in the ultimate demise of the animal.

Hyperlipemia occurs frequently in horses with chronic renal failure. Azotemia may inhibit peripheral removal of triglyceride from the blood and this, plus the lipolysis occurring with anorexia, results in hyperlipemia.

CAUSES

In most instances, the etiology of renal disease is unknown. Tubulointerstitial disease may occur as a chronic sequela to acute tubular necrosis, caused for example by aminoglycosides, vitamin K_3, heavy metals, pigments, hypovolemia, or ischemia. Pyelonephritis, hydronephrosis, and primary interstitial nephritis can also cause tubulointerstitial disease as can papillary necrosis, but the latter rarely causes renal failure. If the cause is no longer present when the horse is examined, a pathologic diagnosis of chronic interstitial nephritis or fibrosis may be all that can be provided.

History of previous sepsis, drug administration, acute or chronic diarrhea, myositis, fevers, and pyuria may provide clues to the etiology. Ultrasonography, urinalysis, and microscopic examination of urine may help in formulating a more specific diagnosis such as nephrocalcinosis, nephrolithiasis, hydronephrosis, and pyelonephritis.

Nephroliths are not uncommon in horses with chronic renal failure, their passage into a ureter causing an acute exacerbation of uremia. Nephroliths are usually calcium salts resulting from previous pyelonephritis or mineralizing interstitial fibrosis. Abnormally high mineral excretion by functional nephrons and change in solubility of the calcium complexes could also play a role in nephrolith formation. However, it is uncertain whether the nephroliths are a cause or a result of the condition.

CLINICAL SIGNS

The most pronounced and frequent clinical sign of chronic renal failure caused by tubulointerstitial disease is weight loss. Inappetence is the second most common finding. Unfortunately, the veterinarian may not be called to examine some horses with chronic renal failure until both of these clinical signs are present. Polyuria and polydipsia are likely present in most horses with renal failure that are not anorectic, but this usually goes unnoticed by the owner. Dysuria, urinary scalding, and fever may be observed in horses with urinary tract infections. The color of the urine is usually unremarkable. Oral ulceration and excessive dental tartar are infrequently observed.

Rectal examination of the left kidney and both ureters should be carefully performed. With chronic, nonseptic, and nonobstructive tubulointerstitial disease, the kidney is usually smaller than normal. In contrast, ureteral obstruction, active pyelonephritis, and renal carcinoma may produce enlargement of the kidney and/or ureter. Obstructing ureteral stones are often felt near the bladder, necessitating careful palpation of this area when ureteral obstruction is suspected. Enlarged kidneys may cause signs of colic. Horses with renal carcinomas often have hematuria resulting in severe anemia. Nephroliths may also cause gross hematuria, especially after exercise, but this is not common.

LABORATORY FINDINGS

The laboratory findings in horses with chronic renal failure are highly variable. Although azotemia, an abnormally high concentration of blood urea nitrogen or creatinine or both, is almost always present, it may be modest in horses that continue to eat well. Sudden exacerbation of the azotemia in these animals should suggest a prerenal abnormality such as dehydration or a postrenal problem such as ureteral obstruction. If prerenal factors are present in addition to the intrinsic renal dysfunction or if the patient is severely cachectic, the ratio of blood urea nitrogen to serum creatinine may increase to more than 15:1.

Electrolyte abnormalities most frequently include hyponatremia and hypochloremia. Serum potassium and magnesium are often normal but may be increased. Hypercalcemia and hypophosphatemia are somewhat unique to the equine patient with chronic renal failure. Hypercalcemia, which is probably present in less than one half of horses with chronic renal failure, is most commonly observed when horses ingest moderate- or high-concentration calcium diets. The hypercalcemia is possibly caused by a decreased urinary calcium excretion. Occasionally, however, a horse with chronic renal failure that has not eaten for several days and therefore has minimal calcium intake may be found to be hypercalcemic. Failure of the kidneys to adequately excrete parathyroid hormone has not been proved as a mechanism of the hypercalcemia, which may be of sufficient magnitude to cause blood to clot when collected in EDTA.

The urine of horses with chronic renal failure resulting from tubulointerstitial pathology is usually within or close to the isosthenuric range. Tubulointerstitial disease and pyelonephritis cause minimal proteinuria unless hematuria is present. Casts may not be observed in urine sediment. More than five white blood cells per high power field and bacteria are usually observed in pyelonephritis. Urine culture of a midstream voided or catheterized sample should have 10^4 or more organisms per ml of urine to confirm a diagnosis of pyelonephritis. Microscopic hematuria may be frequently observed with renal calculi.

A moderate anemia (hematocrit = 20 to 30 per cent) is usual and may be more pronounced in horses with renal carcinomas. The plasma protein concentration is usually normal but may be increased with chronic pyelonephritis. Leukocytosis is frequent in horses with chronic renal failure regardless of the cause.

DIAGNOSIS

The diagnosis is based on appropriate clinical findings and laboratory results supportive of renal dysfunction. Horses with chronic renal failure due to tubulointerstitial disease usually are azotemic and have urine specific gravity close to the isosthenuric range. Knowledge of the patient's serum and urine osmolality allows accurate assessment of tubular concentrating ability in azotemic patients. Urine to serum osmolality ratio is less than 3:1 in patients with tubulointerstitial disease and greater than 3:1 when azotemia is from prerenal causes. Rarely a horse may be examined with some clinical signs such as weight loss and PU/PD that are consistent with renal failure, but the animal is not azotemic. Repeated measurements should reveal that, although still within accepted range for the horse (less than 2 mg per dl), the serum creatinine is significantly higher than in other comparable stablemates on similar diets and in similar training programs. The urine specific gravity and/or ratio of urine to serum osmolality in this patient should reflect an inability to properly concentrate urine. If further diagnostic tests are required to more accurately determine urinary concentrating abilities, 60 IU antidiuretic hormone per 450-kg horse may be administered intramuscularly every six hours for three injections. Urine should be collected at different intervals during this time to determine maximum urine concentration.

Glomerular filtration rate in nonazotemic horses may be estimated by serial changes in serum creatinine, by the creatinine clearance test (normal = 1.39 to 1.87 ml per min per kg), or by the sodium sulfanilate clearance test.

Once a diagnosis of renal failure has been confirmed, an attempt should be made to identify an etiologic or pathologic diagnosis. Diagnosis can be based on clinical findings, history, and microscopic examination of a sample of the kidney acquired by renal biopsy. Fever, leukocytosis, hyperfibrinogenemia, pyuria, and white blood cell casts in urine sediment support a diagnosis of pyelonephritis. Gross hematuria along with a palpable or ultrasonically identified renal mass would arouse suspicion of a renal carcinoma. Ultrasonic examination with two-dimensional ultrasound is also helpful in estimating kidney size, presence of nephroliths, renal parenchymal mineralization, or distended ureter and calyces. Ultrasonic examination may also improve the safety and success of acquiring an adequate sample during renal biopsy.

A renal biopsy should be performed only if it is likely to be important in making an etiologic or pathologic diagnosis and if the results may dictate a change in therapy or prognosis. Serious hemorrhage is a real possibility after renal biopsy. Although a pathologic description may be acquired, an etiologic diagnosis is seldom derived.

THERAPY

The chronic progressive loss of nephron function makes successful long-term therapy unlikely in most equine patients with chronic renal failure. Treatment is most likely to succeed if there is an acute reversible component exacerbating the condition. Therefore, it is imperative in managing such horses to first determine if there is an acute component to the disease. An acute exacerbation is most likely to be a result of a concurrent disease such as diarrhea, sepsis causing volume depletion, upper urinary tract infection, obstruction of the urinary tract, or the ingestion or administration of a nephrotoxic product. These complications should be corrected rapidly in the hope of preventing irreversible chronic renal failure and uremia. If an acute component is present, this should be treated as suggested for acute renal failure in the horse.

In all cases of chronic renal failure it is important to determine if the patient has the polyuric or the oliguric form. Those with oliguric chronic renal failure without an acute exacerbating component can only be managed for an extended period of time by hemodialysis or peritoneal dialysis. Peritoneal dialysis is the more practical of the two procedures but is difficult in the horse because of frequent omental plugging of the catheters. Although hemodialysis can be performed in the horse the procedure is not readily available. In most cases, both methods of dialysis are impractical because even if performed successfully they would only prolong the life of the patient by a short time.

Supportive therapy in polyuric stabilized patients passing more than 18 ml of urine per kg per day may substantially prolong life. The most important general principle is to provide sufficient fluids, electrolytes, and nutritional support. Water should be available at all times in the hope of maintaining normovolemia and acceptable renal blood flow. Salt blocks should be provided as long as edema or hypertension is absent. If edema develops, salt should be restricted even in the face of hyponatremic plasma. Blood samples should be taken routinely to monitor plasma sodium, potassium, calcium, and bicarbonate concentrations. If the plasma bicarbonate is less than 18 mEq per L, up to 225 grams (8 ounces) per day of sodium bicarbonate powder may be added to the feed or water. If the plasma bicarbonate is more than 24 mEq per L and the chloride concentration decreased, additional sodium chloride should be added to the diet. If plasma calcium is increased, removal of calcium-rich feeds such as alfalfa hay may result in a return of calcium to normal values. Although there is no published evidence that the hypercalcemia is harmful, a persistent hypercalcemia can predispose to nephroliths. The associated decrease in plasma phosphorus in horses with hypercalcemia and chronic renal failure may prevent excessive mineralization of soft tissues. Nevertheless, there appears to be no cause for vitamin D supplementation in horses with chronic renal failure. Anabolic steroids and B vitamins may be administered routinely. If the horse maintains a good appetite, anabolic steroids may decrease muscle wasting and increase the hematocrit. If hyperlipemia is marked, heparin (40 to 100 IU per kg subcutaneously twice daily) may decrease plasma lipids. This treatment should be used cautiously, as it may cause a further decline in hematocrit and potentiate bleeding tendencies.

Nonsteroidal anti-inflammatory drugs are best avoided. If these are essential in treating a complicating disease such as laminitis, they should not be used until any systemic volume deficits are corrected (see p. 118).

Horses with CRF and obvious weight loss are

best fed with gradually increasing amounts of fats and carbohydrates. Proteins should be limited so that the ratio of serum urea nitrogen to serum creatinine does not greatly exeed 15:1. If the horse is anorectic, several types of feed, especially grass, should be offered several times daily. If the horse refuses to eat, force feeding via nasogastric tube should be attempted (see p. 421).

Sudden stressful changes in diet, housing, and exercise should be avoided. Surgery may be indicated when uroliths disrupt urine flow.

Supplemental Readings

Brenner, B. M., and Lazarus, J. M.: Chronic renal failure: Pathophysiology and clinical considerations. *In* Petersdorf, R. G.,Adams, R. D., Braunwald, E., Isselbacher, K. J., Martin, J. B., and Wilson, J. D. (eds.): Harrison's Principles of Internal Medicine. New York, McGraw-Hill, 1983.

Brobst, D. F., and Bayly, W.M.: Response of horses to a water deprivation test. J. Equine Vet. Sci., *2*:51, 1982.

Brobst, D. F., Bramwell, K., and Kramer, J. W.: Sodium sulfanilate clearance as a method of determining renal function in the horse. J. Equine Med. Surg., *2*:500, 1978.

Brobst, D. F., Bayly, W. M., Reed, S. M., et al.: Parathyroid hormone evaluation in normal horses and horses with renal failure. J. Equine Vet. Sci., *2*:150, 1982.

Divers, T. J.: Chronic renal failure in horses. Comp. Cont. Ed., *5*:S310, 1983.

Morris, D. D., Divers, T. J., and Whitlock, R. H.: Renal clearance and fractional excretion of electrolytes over a 24-hour period in horses. Am J. Vet. Res., *45*:2431, 1984.

Naylor, J. M., Kronfeld, D. S., and Acland, H.: Hyperlipemia in horses: Effects of undernutrition and disease. Am. J. Vet. Res., *41*:899, 1980.

Tennant, B., Bettleheim, P., and Kaneko, J. J.: Paradoxic hypercalcemia and hypophosphatemia associated with chronic renal failure in horses. J. Am. Vet. Med. Assoc., *180*:630, 1982.

Glomerulonephritis

Debra Deem Morris, KENNETT SQUARE, PENNSYLVANIA

Glomerulonephritis is a common cause of chronic renal insufficiency in horses. Clinical signs usually occur in horses over five years of age. Necropsy findings suggest that the prevalence of renal glomerular lesions in horses is higher than the prevalence of resulting clinical renal disease.

Glomerulonephritis is believed to be immunologically mediated by one of two mechanisms. In the most common form, circulating immune complexes are deposited along the epithelial side of the glomerular basement membrane (GBM). Viral, bacterial, and parasitic infections have been incriminated as sources of antigen; however, only the equine infectious anemia virus has been definitively associated with immune complex glomerulonephritis in horses. More rarely, glomerulonephritis may be an autoimmune disease, in which antibodies are formed against antigens in the GBM. Both mechanisms result in complement activation, increased vascular permeability, leukotaxis, release of lysosomal enzymes from neutrophils, activation of the coagulation system, and subsequent glomerular capillary destruction. Capillary wall damage leads to fibrin leakage into Bowman's spaces and crescent formation. Proliferation of endothelial and mesangial cells follows in an attempt to repair the damage. If the process continues, glomerular sclerosis and interstitial fibrosis result in end-stage renal disease.

CLINICAL SIGNS

Clinical signs of glomerulonephritis depend on the stage and severity of the pathologic process. Pitting ventral edema often develops subsequent to hypoproteinemia from massive urinary protein loss via damaged glomerular capillaries. Edema precedes other signs of renal failure, when hypoproteinemia occurs before there has been sufficient destruction of the nephron population to cause azotemia. Once renal insufficiency has developed, chronic weight loss ensues, often accompanied by depression, anorexia, polyuria, and polydipsia.

LABORATORY FINDINGS

The most consistent laboratory abnormality of glomerulonephritis is persistent proteinuria. Because the alkaline pH of horse urine interferes with the protein indicator on commercial urine dipsticks, the sodium sulfosalicylic acid test must be performed to accurately assess the presence of urinary protein. Hypoproteinemia or hypoalbuminemia or both generally result if urinary protein loss has been massive or prolonged. Microscopic hematuria may accompany acute glomerulitis but is generally absent in the chronic stages of the disease. The urine may be isosthenuric (specific gravity 1.008 to 1.012) if there are insufficient nephrons for adequate urine concentration; however, conclusion of the latter must be based on a water deprivation test or clinical evidence of dehydration or both. Once renal insufficiency develops, plasma concentrations of creatinine and urea nitrogen are elevated. Mild hypokalemia, hypochloremia, hyponatremia, and hypercholesterolemia are frequently observed. Hypercalcemia and hypophosphatemia develop in some horses with chronic renal failure, depending on the diet, plasma albumin concentration, and/or stage of disease. Moderate nonresponsive anemia generally develops late in the disease process.

PATHOLOGY

Significant necropsy findings in horses with glomerulonephritis are generally confined to the kidneys, which grossly are reduced in size, pale, and may be firm with a thickened capsule and an irregular surface. Histologic lesions depend on the type and stage of the disease process. By the time most horses are examined, their lesions reflect end-stage renal disease and cannot be accurately classified. Thickening of the GBM, as well as glomerular hypercellularity and increased mesangial matrix, are common in horses with chronic glomerulonephritis. Other evidence of chronic renal disease includes sclerosis, glomerular adhesions, and interstitial fibrosis. Immunofluorescent microscopy using stains for antiequine gamma globulin or complement or both is usually positive. A granular staining pattern is characteristic of the immune complex deposition, whereas a linear pattern identifies the more rare anti-GBM disease.

DIAGNOSIS

A tentative diagnosis of glomerulonephritis is based on the presence of persistent proteinuria, without hematuria, and is further supported by accompanying ventral pitting edema or chronic weight loss or both. Isosthenuria and elevated plasma concentration of creatinine confirm the presence of renal insufficiency. Although rare in horses, renal amyloidosis also causes proteinuria without urinary sediment abnormalities and usually progresses to renal failure. Although glomerulonephrotic kidneys are often small, with an irregular surface, these changes are not easily detected by rectal palpation of the left kidney. Ultrasonography may be useful in estimating renal size.

Definitive antemortem diagnosis of glomerulonephritis is made by renal biopsy. Tissues should be fixed in formalin for histopathologic examination and frozen for immunofluorescence testing. Since renal biopsy is attended by the risk of severe hemorrhage and results rarely change the mode of therapy or prognosis, it generally is not warranted.

THERAPY

No mode of treatment will effectively correct the underlying disorder in glomerulonephritis. Immunosuppressive therapy with corticosteroid or cytotoxic drugs or both has produced mixed results in humans and dogs with glomerulonephritis. Recently, encouraging results have been seen with methylprednisolone pulse therapy or plasma exchange in humans. In pulse therapy, methylprednisolone sodium succinate* is given intravenously, once daily, at a dosage of 30 mg per kg for three days, followed by oral prednisone,† at 2 mg per kg, tapered over several months. Although a similar approach has not been verified in horses it could be tried. Since the antigen source is rarely recognized and cannot be eliminated, immunosuppression would have to be long-term, which is complicated by the threat of severe sepsis. Plasma exchange may be an alternate mode of therapy for valuable horses, although there is no experience in using this technique to treat immune-complex glomerulonephritis in this species. Plasmapharesis is expensive and very few veterinary hospitals are equipped to provide this treatment.

Glomerulonephritis is generally not diagnosed in horses until renal insufficiency and attendant chronic weight loss have developed; therefore, treatment must include supportive care to correct fluid and electrolyte imbalances and encourage the intake of a high-quality carbohydrate diet. Roughage and grain should contain less than 10 per cent protein. A good-quality timothy or grass hay with grain mix, including corn and oats with molasses, are optimal feeds. Plasma transfusions are helpful in the short-term control of edema. Although the clinical course of glomerulonephritis can be unpredictable, the prognosis is usually grave, especially once chronic renal insufficiency has developed.

---

*Solu-Medrol, Upjohn Co., Kalamazoo, MI
†Deltasone, Upjohn Co., Kalamazoo, MI

Supplemental Readings

Banks, K. L., and Henson, J. B.: Immunologically mediated glomerulitis of horses. II. Antiglomerular basement membrane antibody and other mechanisms in spontaneous disease. Lab. Invest., 26:708, 1972.

Divers, T. J.: Chronic renal failure in horses. Compend. Cont. Ed. Vet., 5:S310,1983.

Sabnis, S. G.,Gunson, D. E., and Antonovych, T. T.: Some unusual features of mesangioproliferative glomerulonephritis in horses. Vet. Pathol., 21:574, 1984.

Toxic Nephropathies

David G. Schmitz, COLLEGE STATION, TEXAS

Endogenous substances, drugs, industrial by-products, environmental pollutants, certain plants, and other natural compounds such as aflatoxins can all cause renal damage (Table 1). Most nephrotoxins cause acute tubular necrosis, although the tubular basement membrane generally remains intact. Clinically this is often manifested by signs of acute renal failure (see p. 693). Nephrotoxins seldom damage only the kidney and often cause lesions in other organ systems. Systemic disorders can also produce substances toxic to renal tissue. Although nephrotoxins are reported to be a major cause of acute renal failure, chronic exposure to certain toxic substances may lead to chronic renal failure and end-stage kidney disease.

CAUSES

MEDICATIONS

Aminoglycosides. The aminoglycoside antibiotics are most often incriminated as causes of nephropathy. Streptomycin is least toxic, neomycin is most

TABLE 1. SOME IMPORTANT EQUINE NEPHROTOXINS

Medications
  Antibiotics
    Aminoglycosides
    Amphotericin B
    Cephaloridine
    Sulfonamides
    Polymyxin B
    Vancomycin
  Phenylbutazone, other nonsteroidal anti-inflammatories (?)
  Vitamin D_2, D_3
  Menadione sodium bisulfite (synthetic vitamin K_3)
Endogenous substances
  Hemoglobin
  Myoglobin
Toxic plants
  See Table 2
Mycotoxins
  Aflatoxin B_1
  probably others
Heavy metals
  Mercury
  Arsenic
  Selenium
  Cadmium
  Gold
  Uranium
Miscellaneous
  Cantharidin (blister beetle)
  Tetrachlorodibenzodioxin (dioxin)
  Endotoxin
  Oxalates

nephrotoxic, and gentamicin and kanamycin are of intermediate nephrotoxicity. Gentamicin is probably used most frequently and therefore is more commonly associated with acute nephrotoxicity in horses.

Because aminoglycosides are eliminated primarily by the kidney, reduced renal function increases the serum concentration of the drug and thus the potential for nephrotoxicity. Toxicity of gentamicin is also enhanced by acidosis, dehydration, hypovolemia, endotoxemia, increased dosage or frequency of drug administration, and simultaneous use of other nephrotoxic agents such as nonsteroidal anti-inflammatory agents. Concurrent use of furosemide may enhance nephrotoxic potential by producing volume depletion. Foals are somewhat more susceptible to toxicity than adults.

Gentamicin nephrotoxicity is initially manifested by a reduced ability to concentrate urine, polyuria, proteinuria, hematuria, and cylindruria. This is followed by an increase in serum urea nitrogen and creatinine. Monitoring urine for protein, blood, and casts is the most sensitive means of detecting early drug toxicosis. Proteinuria may be detected as early as three days after treatment is initiated. Casts are reported up to nine days before elevation of serum creatinine.

Treatment of aminoglycoside nephrotoxicosis is aimed at maintenance of normal blood volume and glomerular filtration rate by volume diuresis and drug withdrawal. Urinary alkalinization may exert a protective effect against nephrotoxicosis. Toxic effects can be minimized by giving a recommended dosage of aminoglycoside, and periodic evaluation of urine for protein and casts, especially in pediatric and geriatric patients. If aminoglycosides are essential in patients with renal dysfunction, toxic potential can be reduced by increasing the time interval between doses or by giving a reduced total dosage divided three or four times daily.

Cephalosporins. Of the cephalosporin antibiotics, cephaloridine is most nephrotoxic. Cephaloridine accumulates within the proximal tubular cells and results in tubular necrosis. Because tubular damage is dose-dependent, recommended dosages should be used.

Polyene Antibiotics. The polyene antibiotic amphotericin B exerts a lytic effect on distal tubular cells and lysosomal membranes of kidney cells. Amphotericin B combines with sterols within these membranes and results in leakage of cytosol and cell death. Renal vasoconstriction may also play a role in the nephrotoxicity of this compound. The direct injury to the distal tubular epithelium is dose-related and leads to excessive loss of potassium, bicarbonate, and water into the urine. Hypokalemia and metabolic acidosis may develop in these patients. Treatment of amphotericin B nephrotoxicity involves adequate hydration and reduced dosage or drug withdrawal. In dogs, the concomitant use of mannitol appears to reduce its toxicity.

Sulfonamides. Sulfonamides have historically been incriminated as a cause of renal dysfunction. These agents may precipitate in the tubular lumen, causing obstruction and anuria or tubular epithelial necrosis. The modern sulfonamides, including trimethoprim-sulfa combinations, have much greater urine solubility, so nephropathy is relatively uncommon. The potential for sulfa nephropathy may still exist in the patient that is dehydrated or hypovolemic or has other renal dysfunction.

Vitamin D. Vitamin D is a nephrotoxin that is likely to cause chronic renal failure. Both vitamin D_2 (ergocalciferol) and D_3 (cholecalciferol) are potentially toxic. However, vitamin D_3 is much more active in the horse and results in more severe lesions with wider tissue distribution than does an equivalent dose of Vitamin D_2. The toxicity of vitamin D is related to the dosage and the duration of treatment. High dietary concentration of calcium may exacerbate the effects of large amounts of vitamin D.

Although the horse's requirement for vitamin D has not been established, the minimum daily allowance of 6.6 IU per kg body weight is currently recommended by the National Academy of Science–National Research Council subcommittee on horse nutrition. Toxicosis is usually iatrogenic, resulting from the overzealous use of vitamin supplements. Ingestion of *Cestrum diurnum* found in the southeastern United States can also result in vitamin D toxicity. This plant contains a metabolically active glycoside of 1,25-dihydroxycholecalciferol and causes lesions and signs similar to those of vitamin D toxicosis.

Serum phosphorus concentration appears highly sensitive to increased amounts of vitamin D. In experimental studies, hyperphosphatemia was a consistent finding in horses given toxic amounts of vitamin D. Hypercalcemia was invariably present in this same study. Measurement of serum phosphorus and calcium may be of value in the diagnosis of vitamin D toxicity. The lesion of vitamin D toxicosis is disseminated soft tissue mineralization. In the kidney, mineralization of the basal lamina and epithelial cells of the tubules occurs.

Treatment of vitamin D toxicosis should include removal of all exogenous sources of vitamin D. Diuresis may be necessary and adequate water intake should be encouraged. Cation chelators such as sodium phytate* may be beneficial in reducing intestinal absorption of calcium, but its efficacy has not been determined. Recovery may take several months.

Vitamin K. Menadione sodium bisulfite, synthetic vitamin K_3, has produced signs of toxicity in experimental animals when given at the recommended dosage of 2.2 to 11 mg per kg intravenously or intramuscularly. Clinical signs of depression, colic, strangury, and sometimes hematuria have occurred within six hours of injection. Pathologic lesions are those of acute tubular necrosis, although the mechanism by which this occurs is unknown. Interstitial fibrosis with renal failure may occur in severe cases. Treatment of affected horses is largely symptomatic.

Phenylbutazone. Phenylbutazone is potentially toxic to various organ systems including the kidneys (see p. 118). Doses of 8 to 10 mg per kg may produce toxicity if given on several consecutive days. Lesions consist of necrosis of the tubular epithelium and medullary crest. Phenylbutazone should be used with caution in horses exhibiting hypovolemia, dehydration, or pre-existing renal dysfunction. Concurrent use of other nephrotoxic medications should be avoided.

PIGMENTS

Hemoglobin and myoglobin are two endogenous substances that can produce acute renal failure. Myoglobin nephrosis may be seen following severe muscle damage. Possible etiologies include extensive crushing or bruising injuries, extensive burns (see p. 639), heat stroke (see p. 482), and exertional rhabdomyolysis (see p. 487) or "tying-up." Hemoglobin nephropathy is the usual result of extensive intravascular hemolysis. Possible causes of intravascular hemolysis include incompatible blood transfusions and acute hemolytic anemia due to *Babesia caballi* or *B. equi* (see p. 299), equine infectious anemia (see p. 297), neonatal isoerythrolysis (see p. 244), phenothiazine toxicosis, onion toxicosis (*Allium* spp.), and ingestion of withered red maple (*Acer rubrum*) leaves (see p. 679).

Pigment nephropathy should be suspected when the affected animal exhibits clinical signs of acute renal failure, and blood, hemoglobin, or myoglobin appears in the urine. Affected horses typically void red to brown-tinged urine. The discoloration of the urine can be of variable intensity.

Toxicosis due to phenothiazine or ingestion of onions or red maple leaves results in formation of Heinz bodies within the erythrocytes. Affected erythrocytes then undergo extravascular hemolysis within the reticuloendothelial system. This pro-

---

*Sodium Phytate, City Chemical Corporation, New York, NY

duces more hemoglobin, which may add to the toxic burden of hemoglobin already presented to the kidney.

The pathogenesis of tubular nephrosis seen in pigment nephropathy is not known, although hemoglobin by itself is probably nontoxic. Experimental studies in rats indicate that nephrosis is due to erythrocyte stromal elements rather than hemoglobin. Hemoglobin casts are present within tubules in affected horses and may result in ischemic injury to renal tubules. It has also been proposed that hemoglobin and myoglobin may cause renal ischemia so that nephropathy develops in hypovolemic but not in normovolemic horses. Additional factors that seem to be required for the development of pigment nephropathies include dehydration, circulatory failure, endotoxemia, acidosis, and hypoxia.

No specific therapy is indicated in pigment nephropathies other than maintaining renal perfusion. In cases of severe hemolytic anemia, compatible blood transfusions may be required. Horses should be denied exposure to onions and red maple leaves when possible. Methylene blue is relatively ineffective in reducing the methemoglobin formed in red maple leaf intoxication. Methylene blue also enhances Heinz body formation and therefore its use may be contraindicated in such patients.

PLANTS

A variety of plants are toxic to animals. Table 2 includes a list of plants that result in some degree of nephrosis. Most of these plants will affect other body organs in addition to the kidney. In general, toxic plants are unpalatable to animals. Toxicity usually arises when pastures are overgrazed or an adequate food supply is not available. Since some toxic plants become more palatable following herbicide application, caution should be exercised to prevent access of horses to such plants.

Treatment of suspected plant toxicity involves removal of the offending plant from the diet and symptomatic care. Affected horses should be placed on an adequate diet. Many horses affected with acute toxicity will recover. In a few instances chronic renal failure may be the end result and treatment is unrewarding.

MYCOTOXINS

Mycotoxins have worldwide distribution and are known to affect many animal species. They often cause dysfunction of more than one body organ. Documented cases of equine renal disease due to mycotoxins are rare, but many of these compounds may be nephrotoxic to the horse. Aflatoxins are a group of metabolites produced by two species of fungi—*Aspergillus flavus* and *A. parasiticus*. Cereal grains are highly susceptible to aflatoxin contamination and most animal toxicoses result from ingestion of contaminated grain. In the horse, aflatoxin B_1 produces a fatty degeneration of the proximal tubular epithelium. Reported cases involved horses eating moldy corn.

Diagnosis may be difficult but involves recovering aflatoxin from suspect feed or body organ specimens. Serum sorbitol dehydrogenase activity is not specific for renal dysfunction but has been used as an indicator of aflatoxicosis in experimentally affected horses. Therapy should be supportive, as there is no known specific therapy for aflatoxin nephropathy. However, a good-quality ration may be protective against small-dose aflatoxin exposure.

TABLE 2. PLANTS CAUSING RENAL DYSFUNCTION

Plant	Common Name	Toxic Principle	Renal Lesion
Quercus spp.	oak	tannins (?) polyphenols (?)	tubular necrosis
Halogeton glomeratus	halogeton	Na^+, K^+ oxalates	tubular necrosis, obstruction, anuria (oxalate nephropathy)
Sarcobatus vermiculatus	black greasewood	Na^+, K^+ oxalates	tubular necrosis, obstruction, anuria (oxalate nephropathy)
Astragalus spp.	loco, poisonvetch	selenium (chronic exposure)	nephritis
Eupatorium rugosum	white snakeroot	tremetol	tubular necrosis
Isocoma wrightii	rayless goldenrod	tremetol	tubular necrosis
Cestrum diurnum	day-blooming jessamine, day cestrum, wild jasmin	glycoside of 1,25-dihydroxycholecalciferol	tubular mineralization, soft tissue calcinosis
Acer rubrum	red maple tree	unidentified oxidant	tubular nephrosis (pigment nephropathy)
Allium canadense	wild onion	n-propyl disulfide	tubular nephrosis (pigment nephropathy)
A. validum	wild onion	n-propyl disulfide	tubular nephrosis (pigment nephropathy)
A. cepa	cultivated onion	n-propyl disulfide	tubular nephrosis (pigment nephropathy)

HEAVY METALS

Equine heavy metal intoxication is infrequently diagnosed. Although tubular degeneration and necrosis result, the mechanism of action of individual metals differs.

Mercury. Mercury intoxication is probably the most common of the heavy metal nephropathies. Both organic and inorganic mercury are toxic to the horse, with organic mercury degraded in the body to the inorganic form. All forms of mercury may be converted to methylmercury, which results in toxicity.

Both acute and chronic toxicity can occur in the horse. The toxic dose of inorganic mercury in the adult horse is 8 to 10 gm. However, chronic toxicity can be produced by ingestion of 0.4 mg per kg per day over a period of several weeks. Mercury nephropathy appears to be a function of the amount of protein-bound mercury concentrated in the kidney. Bound mercury can persist in the kidney for several weeks after the last exposure.

Poisoning is usually associated with ingestion of feed or seed grain contaminated with an organic mercurial seed preservative. Certain cutaneous "counterirritants" manufactured for use in the horse contain inorganic mercuric iodide and may serve as a source of exposure.

Diagnosis is confirmed by measuring the amount of residue in renal specimens. Inorganic mercury is concentrated to high levels within the proximal tubules. The metal binding protein metallothionein binds mercuric ions within the endoplasmic reticulum of the tubular epithelial cells and slowly releases mercury, causing continual damage to the tubule. Mercury complexes with sulfhydryl groups within cells. As a result, sulfhydryl enzyme systems essential to cellular metabolism and respiration are inhibited, and cell death may occur. Acute toxicity results in massive tubular necrosis and clinical signs of acute renal failure. Chronic exposure to mercury causes renal interstitial fibrosis and may result in chronic renal failure.

Treatment of acute and chronic toxicity involves removing the source. In acute toxicity, evacuation of the bowel with a mild laxative may be helpful. Activated charcoal* (500 gm) given orally might help block absorption of mercury, but the efficacy of this product in the horse has not been documented. Circulating mercury may be inactivated by the injection of dimercaprol.† Dimercaprol should be given intramuscularly at a dosage of 3 mg per kg every four hours for the first two days, four times on the third day, and twice daily for the next ten days until recovery is complete. Treatment of

---

*Humco Laboratories, Texarkana, TX
†BAL in Oil, Hynson, Westcott & Dunning, Div. of Becton-Dickinson and Co., Baltimore, MD

chronic mercury intoxication is usually unrewarding.

Arsenic. Arsenic poisoning usually results from ingestion of rodenticides or industrial herbicides. Arsenic is rapidly excreted through the urine and toxicosis typically produces signs of acute nephropathy. Diagnosis of arsenic nephropathy depends on finding the chemical in liver, stomach, and intestinal contents, and/or urine. The mechanism of action of arsenic nephrotoxicity is similar to that of mercury.

Specific therapy for arsenic toxicosis should include large doses of saline purgative to remove the unabsorbed material from the gastrointestinal tract. Sodium thiosulfate* should be given orally and intravenously. Adult horses are given 20 to 30 gm orally in a small amount of water and 8 to 10 gm intravenously as a 10 to 20 per cent solution. Dimercaprol may be effective and can be dosed as described for mercury toxicity. The prognosis is poor, even if an early diagnosis is made.

Selenium. Chronic selenium intoxication usually is the result of ingestion of selenium-concentrating plants. Signs of toxicity are usually referable to other body systems, but nephritis is an ancillary finding. Renal dysfunction is probably not an important aspect of selenium toxicosis.

Selenium apparently exerts its toxic effect by enzymatically inhibiting oxidation-reduction systems in the body. A high-protein diet may protect an animal from the adverse effects of selenium.

Cadmium. Cadmium toxicity has been reported in the horse as a result of ingestion of contaminated forage near a smelting operation. Renal lesions include nephrocalcinosis, interstitial fibrosis, and deposition of calcium and phosphate crystals within the renal tubules.

MISCELLANEOUS

Other substances that may cause nephropathy include cantharidin and tetrachlorodibenzodioxin (dioxin). Both substances cause tubular necrosis of mild to moderate severity. Nephrotoxicity is only one aspect of these agents, and death is usually attributable to other organ dysfunction in affected horses. Endotoxin is harmful to the kidney by producing renal ischemia. Acute renal failure is often a secondary condition following endotoxemia.

Oxalate nephropathy is a relatively rare occurrence in the horse. Potential sources of oxalate include the plants *Halogeton* and *Sarcobatus*, and ethylene glycol. Oxalates are derived from the degradation of ethylene glycol. Oxalate crystals precipitate within the tubular lumen and result in obstruction and focal necrosis of the epithelial cells. Tubular obstruction, if severe, results in anuria and acute renal failure.

---

*MCB Manufacturing Chemists, Inc., Cincinnati, OH

TREATMENT

Most cases of nephrotoxicity result in clinical signs of acute renal failure. Treatment is aimed at maintaining fluid balance, correction of any acid-base or electrolyte disorders, and general symptomatic care. The reader is referred to page 693 for a more detailed discussion of treatment of acute renal failure.

Identification and removal of the toxin source are of primary importance in treating any toxic condition. In some instances this may necessitate moving the horse from a contaminated environment to clean premises. In any event, adequate forage and ample fresh water should always be available to the affected horse.

Specific therapy for certain nephropathies has already been discussed. More specific therapeutic regimens can be found in the section dealing exclusively with toxicologic problems (p. 649).

PROGNOSIS

The prognosis of nephrotoxic acute tubular necrosis depends upon the clinical setting surrounding its development. In general the prognosis is much better when toxin has not caused serious damage to other organs. If the toxic source is removed and further renal damage is inhibited, the intact basement membrane will often regenerate tubular epithelial cells. This may result in at least partial return of renal function.

Supplemental Readings

Aller, W. W., Edds, G. T., and Asquith, R. L.: Effects of aflatoxins in young ponies. Am. J. Vet. Res., *42*:2162, 1981.
Anderson, G. A., Mount, M. E., Vrins, A. A., and Ziemer, E. L.: Fatal acorn poisoning in a horse: Pathologic findings and diagnostic considerations. J. Am. Vet. Med. Assoc., *182*:1105, 1983.
Buck, W. B., Osweiler, G. D., and Van Gelder, G. A.: Clinical and Diagnostic Veterinary Toxicology. Dubuque, IA, Kendall/Hunt, 1973.
Divers, T. J., George, L. W., and George, J. W.: Hemolytic anemia in horses after the ingestion of red maple leaves. J. Am. Vet. Med. Assoc., *180*:300, 1982.
Gunson, D. E., Kowalczyk, D. F., Shoop, C. R., and Ramberg, C. F.: Environmental zinc and cadmium pollution associated with generalized osteochondrosis, osteoporosis, and nephrocalcinosis in horses. J. Am. Vet. Med. Assoc., *180*:295, 1982.
Harrington, D. D., and Page, E. H.: Acute vitamin D$_3$ toxicosis in horses: Case reports and experimental studies of the comparative toxicity of vitamins D$_2$ and D$_3$. J. Am. Vet. Med. Assoc., *182*:1358, 1983.
Kimbrough, R. D., Carter, C. D., Liddle, J. A., Cline, R. E., and Phillips, P. E.: Epidemiology and pathology of a tetrachlorodibenzodioxin poisoning episode. Arch. Environ. Health, *32*:77, 1977.
Kingsbury, J. M.: Poisonous Plants of the United States and Canada. Englewood Cliffs, NJ, Prentice-Hall, Inc., 1964.
Mackay, R. J., French, T. W., Nguyen, H. T., and Mayhew, I. G.: Effects of large doses of phenylbutazone administration to horses. Am. J. Vet. Res., *44*:774, 1983.
Olson, C. T., Keller, W. C., Gerken, D. F., and Reed, S. M.: Suspected tremetol poisoning in horses. J. Am. Vet. Med. Assoc., *185*:1001, 1984.
Pierce, K. R., Joyce, J. R., England, R. B., and Jones, L. P.: Acute hemolytic anemia caused by wild onion poisoning in horses. J. Am. Vet. Med. Assoc., *160*:323, 1972.
Read, W. K.: Renal medullary crest necrosis associated with phenylbutazone therapy in horses. Vet. Pathol., *20*:662, 1983.
Rebhun, W. C., Tennant, B. C., Dill, S. G., and King, J. M.: Vitamin K$_3$-induced renal toxicosis in the horse. J. Am. Vet. Med. Assoc., *184*:1237, 1984.
Riviere, J. E., and Coppoc, G. L.: Selected aspects of aminoglycoside antibiotic nephrotoxicosis. J. Am. Vet. Med. Assoc., *178*:508, 1981.
Warner, A. E.: Methemoglobinemia and hemolytic anemia in a horse with acute renal failure. Comp. Contin. Ed., *6*:S465, 1984.
Webb, R. F., and Knight, P. R.: Oxalate nephropathy in a horse. Aust. Vet. J., *53*:554, 1977.

Cystitis and Pyelonephritis

David R. Hodgson, PULLMAN, WASHINGTON

CYSTITIS

Inflammation of the bladder, which is rare in the horse, is usually caused by bacterial infection. Affected animals may manifest evidence of strangury, dysuria, or pollakiuria. Inflammatory cells, bacteria, and possibly blood are commonly demonstrated in urine samples. Many cases are chronic and refractory to therapy.

ETIOLOGY AND PATHOPHYSIOLOGY

Under normal circumstances the bladder is relatively resistant to infection and bacteria are quickly eliminated by the normal flow of urine. As a result, cystitis is rarely a primary disease in horses. However, any condition causing stagnation of urine such as urolithiasis, late pregnancy, dystocia, or bladder paresis or paralysis will usually predispose the bladder to infection and result in cystitis. Cystic calculi invariably produce a secondary cystitis. Horses fed Sudan grass or those grazing hybrid sorghum pastures have an increased incidence of bladder paralysis or paresis with associated urine retention and subsequent cystitis. Improper technique used to perform urinary catheterization, chronic or repeated placement of the catheter, and various other conditions such as chronic vaginitis and anatomic abnormalities may also predispose horses to bladder infections.

Most cases of cystitis are the result of ascending infections, although descending infection in horses suffering from embolic suppurative nephritis (renal abscess) has been reported. Females are more commonly affected than males, probably because females have a relatively short urethra. Cystitis is usually the result of bacterial infection, and the most commonly implicated species include *Escherichia coli*, Proteus, Klebsiella, Pseudomonas, streptococci, staphylococci, and very rarely *Corynebacterium renale*.

Cystitis associated with the grazing of Sudan grass or Sudan-sorghum hybrids has been reported in the southwest United States and in northern Australia. The condition occurs most commonly during the growing season when horses consume young, rapidly growing hybrid crosses of Sudan grass. Horses eating well-cured Sudan hay are apparently not affected. Hindlimb ataxia and incoordination, the result of myelomalacia, are among the earliest and most frequently observed signs of this disease. Approximately half those patients showing neurologic abnormalities may subsequently develop signs consistent with cystitis. This cystitis is probably the result of urine stasis, sediment accumulation, and bacterial growth.

CLINICAL SIGNS

Most cases of cystitis are chronic and many of the clinical signs associated with the disease reflect the degree of chronicity. Affected animals may dribble urine (pollakiuria) and make frequent attempts to urinate, usually the result of urethritis that often accompanies cystitis. Pain and grunting may occur in association with micturition and only small volumes of urine may be voided. In mares, pollakiuria may cause perineal scalding and alopecia, skin scaling, and the accumulation of sediment on the hindlimbs. In addition, these animals may appear to be in estrus. Various degrees of penile relaxation often accompany cystitis in males, particularly those affected with "Sudan-sorghum cystitis." Those horses with relatively severe and acute cases may show some systemic signs of infection, including depression, fever, and anorexia. Urine is often more turbid than normal and hematuria may be observed. In chronic cases, rectal examination often reveals a thickened bladder wall. Cystoscopic examination

may reveal a thickened bladder wall with a rough and coarsely granular mucosal surface. Soft masses of calcium carbonate and large mucosal ulcers may be observed in the bladder of horses with Sudan-sorghum cystitis. Sudan-sorghum cystitis is usually associated with hindlimb ataxia and incoordination, and when forced to back, these animals may assume a dog-sitting posture.

LABORATORY FINDINGS

Although alterations in urine quality may be obvious macroscopically in some patients, microscopic examination for leukocytes, erythrocytes, and desquamated epithelial cells, carried out on centrifuged or sedimented deposits, and bacteriologic examination may be necessary to confirm the diagnosis. It is of the utmost importance that samples for bacteriologic examination be collected aseptically via a catheter, as the presence of contaminating organisms in the sample may produce misleading culture results. In addition, if at all possible the animal should not have been treated with antibiotics in the 48 to 72 hours preceding sample collection. These agents may dramatically alter the activity of many organisms in vitro, which in turn may reduce the efficacy of laboratory culture and sensitivity techniques. These alterations in the in vitro characteristics of certain bacteria will often occur following exposure to a particular antibiotic, even if the organisms are not sensitive to that agent in vivo. If facilities allow, quantitative culture techniques provide the best reflection of the bacterial population in the bladder, while the determination of minimum inhibitory concentrations of potential therapeutic agents against suspected pathogenic bacteria will aid in the selection of the most appropriate antibiotic.

TREATMENT

As most cases of cystitis occur as a sequel to some primary disease process, a major goal for successful treatment often involves identification and elimination of the predisposing cause. For example, in animals suffering from urolithiasis and an associated mild cystitis, removal of the calculi is often sufficient for the bladder to return to normal function and for the cystitis to clear spontaneously. However, in many other horses in which the condition is more chronic or severe, or in which a primary predisposing factor cannot be identified and/or eliminated, specific therapy directed at controlling the cystitis is required.

Successful medical therapy often involves prolonged treatment with the appropriate antimicrobial agent(s). However, several factors will directly influence the selection of an antimicrobial agent. Some of these include sensitivity of the organisms to the agent, percentage of the drug excreted by the kidneys and its activity in the urine, pH of the urine, whether the agent is inactivated within the gastrointestinal tract, expense, and ease and frequency of administration. If possible, urine samples should be submitted for bacteriologic examination and culture and sensitivity testing (as described previously) before antibiotic therapy is begun. Such practices maximize the chances of identifying the causative organism(s) and selecting the most appropriate antibiotic, leading to therapeutic success. In acute cases when the animal is showing signs of systemic disease, a Gram stain of the deposit from a centrifuged urine sample will often provide useful information for the selection of initial therapy while culture and sensitivity tests are processed. Indiscriminate use of broad-spectrum antibiotics or the initiation of so-called "shotgun" antibiotic therapy in the absence of appropriate bacteriologic examinations is in most cases contraindicated. It is nearly impossible to predict the bacterial species involved in the disease without such tests, and contrary to some suggestions, many of the pathogens known to be involved in equine cystitis may not be sensitive to these agents. Information regarding some commonly employed antibiotics for the treatment of equine urinary tract infections may be found in Table 1.

Antimicrobial therapy should be continued for a minimum of seven to 10 days in mild and relatively uncomplicated cystitis, and for at least one month in horses with chronic forms of the disease. Urine samples should be checked for bacterial counts at least once during the treatment, after 10 to 14 days,

and if possible again two to four weeks following cessation of therapy.

Additional therapeutic aids in treatment of cystitis include irrigating the bladder with large volumes of isotonic fluid to flush out urinary sediment and remove cellular debris. Although the repeated use of this precedure has been largely discarded as a routine method of treatment, it may provide some benefits when performed at the initiation of therapy, particularly in cases of Sudan-sorghum cystitis in which accumulations of calcium carbonate are found in the bladder. Urinary acidifiers such as mendelic acid, methenamine, hexamine, and possibly ammonium chloride are believed to have bacteriostatic effects within the urine. Although not necessarily useful as therapeutic agents when administered alone, these drugs may potentiate the effects of some antimicrobial agents within the urine such as penicillin, nitrofurantoin, and oxytetracycline. Horses demonstrating systemic signs of disease resulting in reduced water intake may require fluid administration to ensure that adequate urine flow is maintained. Oral fluids administered by stomach tube will, in the majority of cases, provide the most simple, inexpensive, and physiologic means of supplementation.

The underlying cause of Sudan-sorghum cystitis is bladder paralysis resulting from myelomalacia. Treatment of bladder paralysis is described on p. 712.

The prognosis in cases of chronic cystitis is often poor, as there may be great difficulty in completely eradicating the infection from small foci in the

TABLE 1. ANTIMICROBIAL AGENTS SUITABLE FOR USE IN URINARY TRACT INFECTIONS OF THE HORSE

Drug	Dosage Rate	Route of Administration	Specific Comments

Penicillin
  Crystalline (Na$^+$ or K$^+$)
  Procaine G
	20,000–50,000 U/kg q.i.d.
	20,000–40,000 U/kg b.i.d.
		IV or IM
		
		IM
			Rapidly excreted; Na$^+$ salt may give superior tissue levels when administered IM; well concentrated in urine; procaine salt prolongs absorption of injected dose

Ampicillin Na$^+$	10–20 mg/kg t.i.d.	IV or IM	May have synergistic effects with gentamicin in some situations
Cloxacillin Na$^+$	30 mg/kg t.i.d.	IV or IM	Increased activity against β-lactamase–producing organisms; should only be used when specifically indicated
Ticarcillin	20–30 mg/kg q.i.d.	IV	Possibly has increased activity against Pseudomonas infections; should only be used when specifically indicated
Gentamicin	2 mg/kg b.i.d.–q.i.d.	IM	Excretion in urine often prolonged; should only be used when culture and sensitivity show no other drugs to be effective
Amikacin	6 mg/kg b.i.d.–t.i.d.	IM	Excretion in urine often prolonged; should only be used when culture and sensitivity show no other drug to be effective
Chloramphenicol	40–50 mg/kg q.i.d.	PO	Bacteriostatic; definitive public health risk; reserve for use when no alternatives exist
Nitrofurantoin	2.5 mg/kg	PO	Urinary antiseptic; concentrated and more effective in acid urine; most active against gram-negative organisms
Oxytetracycline	5 mg/kg b.i.d.	IV	Bacteriostatic; diarrhea reported in horses in association with this drug; anaphylaxis reported following IV injection; effective in acid urine
Cephalothin	11 mg/kg q.i.d.	IV	Active against β-lactamase–producing organisms, specifically staphylococci; well concentrated in urine; may be nephrotoxic

bladder wall. Therefore, although horses with cystitis will often demonstrate a good initial response to therapy, recrudescence of the disease is not uncommon.

PYELONEPHRITIS

Pyelonephritis is an ascending infection that may develop as the result of any lower urinary tract infection or obstruction. Urinary stasis, allowing multiplication and migration of bacteria up the urinary tract, is reported as being an invariable and important influence on the development of this disease. Although relatively rare in the horse when compared to cattle and pigs, pyelonephritis does occur and is often refractory to therapy.

ETIOLOGY AND PATHOPHYSIOLOGY

Any condition involving infection of the lower urinary tract and urinary stasis has the potential to cause pyelonephritis. This allows multiplication and progression of infection up the tract, a process believed to be enhanced by reflux of urine up the ureters from the bladder. Urinary stasis and infection may occur as the result of any of the conditions described in the previous section dealing with cystitis, with most cases being reported in postparturient females. Infective organisms ascend the ureters and invade the renal pelvis. Bilateral involvement may occur, although lesions need not necessarily be symmetrical. Pathologic changes develop predominantly in the papillae and renal medulla, with cortical involvement being a more infrequent finding. All the bacterial species implicated in the etiology of cystitis have been identified in association with pyelonephritis.

CLINICAL SIGNS

Pyelonephritis often presents as a chronic disease process causing weight loss, anorexia, depression, elevated temperature, pulse rate, and respiratory rate, and at times evidence of abdominal pain. Dysuria, pollakiuria, and pain on micturition are frequently observed, the result of cystitis and urethritis that commonly occur in association with this disease. Rectal examination may reveal changes including enlarged ureters, an abnormal left kidney, and other changes consistent with cystitis. Alterations in the size and consistency of the kidneys may often be visualized using abdominal ultrasound techniques. In addition to rectal and ultrasound examinations, ureteral catheterization via cystoscopy is very useful in determination of unilateral or bilateral involvement. Intravenous pyelograms may be useful in determining the extent of upper urinary tract compromise in foals.

LABORATORY FINDINGS

Pyuria and hematuria are frequent findings in horses with pyelonephritis, and in some cases may be obvious macroscopically. The presence of erythrocytes, leukocytes, protein, and desquamated epithelial cells is usually confirmed with urinalysis. Bacteria are frequently present in urinary sediment and leukocytes. Identification of the species of organism and its sensitivity to various antimicrobial agents can often be determined using bacteriologic techniques. Although there is some risk of disseminating the infective organisms, renal aspirates or biopsies or both may aid in identification of the causative bacteria.

Hematologic and plasma biochemical examinations may reveal evidence of mild anemia, leukocytosis, and elevated fibrinogen levels. In horses with marked renal compromise there may be evidence of uremia, dehydration, electrolyte disturbances, and possibly other signs consistent with chronic renal disease.

TREATMENT

Any therapeutic plan for the treatment of pyelonephritis is likely to be similar to that adopted for cystitis. Of primary concern is identification and elimination of any predisposing cause for the disease. Unfortunately the disease is often well established by the time it is diagnosed, and severe impairment to renal function is not uncommon. On the basis of results of bacteriologic tests the most appropriate antimicrobial agent can be selected and therapy commenced. Although information is available on the concentrations achieved by many antibiotics within the urine, there is a relative dearth of information, particularly for the horse, on tissue levels of these drugs. As a result, it is difficult to determine whether bacteria sequestered within the renal parenchyma are in fact being exposed to adequate concentrations of the particular agents to ensure favorable results. Therapy should be continued for at least two to four weeks and possibly longer, with bacterial counts being checked during and again several weeks after cessation of therapy. Information about some antibiotics available for the treatment of urinary tract diseases in the horse may be found in Table 1. Antimicrobial therapy may halt the progression of the disease and reduce the number of bacteria in the lower urinary tract, which in turn may remove a possible source of reinfection. However, as most cases of pyelonephritis are chronic in nature, often associated with relatively severe renal change and localized pockets of infection, the results of medical therapy are often very poor. Surgical extirpation of the involved kidney in cases of chronic severe unilateral pyelonephritis has become a popular method of management in other species. Although not widely practiced in equine medicine this mode of therapy may be of potential value for this type of case.

Additional therapy for horses with pyelonephritis may involve supportive therapy for the uremia, toxemia, and impairment of renal function. More detailed descriptions of these therapeutic protocols may be found in the appropriate sections elsewhere in the text (see p. 693).

As this condition is usually chronic and insidious in nature, the prognosis for patients with well-established forms of the disease is usually poor.

Supplemental Readings

Divers, T. J.: Urinary tract—Horse, Cow. In Johnston, D. E., (ed.): The Bristol Veterinary Handbook of Antimicrobial Therapy. Syracuse, Bristol Laboratories, 1982, pp. 84–91.

Romane, W. M., Adams, L. G., Bullard, T. L., and Dollahite, J. W.: Cystitis syndrome of the equine. Southwest Vet., 19:95, 1966.

Van Kampen, K. R.: Sudan grass and sorghum poisoning of horses: A possible lathyrogenic disease. J. Am. Vet. Med. Assoc., 156:629, 1970.

Paralytic Bladder

Jill J. McClure, BATON ROUGE, LOUISIANA

CLINICAL SIGNS

The hallmark of paralytic bladder is urinary incontinence characterized by intermittent or continuous dribbling of small volumes of urine. Neurogenic damage that results in loss of reflex emptying of the bladder is followed by passive overflow of urine when the bladder distends to maximal capacity. Exercise and coughing, which increase intraabdominal pressure, often cause urine spurting. Rectal examination reveals an enlarged bladder that may be displaced ventrally and cranially in the abdomen by the weight of the urine. Large quantities of urine sediment tend to accumulate in the bladder, and secondary bacterial cystitis frequently complicates the condition. Scalding of the perineal area and rear limbs may be present in mares.

Paralytic bladder is seldom an isolated finding and is usually observed in conjunction with other neurologic deficits. These include analgesia or hyperalgesia of the perineum, paralysis of the tail, rectum, penis, vulva, urethral sphincter and anal sphincter, pelvic limb weakness, and atrophy of gluteal and other pelvic limb muscles. Colic is occasionally a presenting sign caused by impaction of the rectum with fecal material. The presence of other neurologic signs is an important feature in differentiating neurogenic from non-neurogenic causes of urinary incontinence.

ETIOLOGY

Causes of paralytic bladder include neuritis of the cauda equina (equine polyradiculoneuritis, polyneuritis equi), equine herpesvirus I myeloencephalitis, sorghum ataxia-cystitis (enzootic equine ataxia-cystitis), fractures, osteomyelitis or neoplasia involving the lower lumbar, sacral, or upper coccygeal vertebrae, and iatrogenic alcohol "tail blocks."

Neuritis of the cauda equina is usually insidious in onset and slowly progressive. The condition is characterized by an inflammatory reaction of unknown etiology involving nerve roots and peripheral nerves. Involvement is not limited to the sacrococcygeal area; cranial nerve deficits, often asymmetrical, are commonly present. No definitive antemortem test is available for confirmation of diagnosis. Gross necropsy lesions include discoloration and thickening of the epidural nerve roots on the cauda equina. There is no known effective form of treatment and the condition is ultimately fatal.

Sorghum or Sudan grass ataxia-cystitis is associated with ingestion of plants of the genus Sorghum, which are believed to contain hydrocyanic acid. Focal axonal degeneration and demyelination occur in the lumbar and sacral segments of the spinal cord, resulting in varying degrees of neurologic deficits including rear limb weakness, ataxia, and paralytic bladder. Abortions and birth of foals with arthrogryposis have been associated with the intoxication. Clinical improvement may follow removal of the offending forage from the diet; however, total recovery has not been observed.

Equine herpesvirus I myeloencephalitis is described on page 345.

Traumatic, inflammatory, or neoplastic lesions that impinge on the lumbosacral spinal cord or regional peripheral nerves may produce paralytic bladder. Rectal examination is sometimes useful to identify displaced fractures. Radiography and ultrasound are also useful diagnostic procedures.

Permanent neurologic deficits including paralytic bladder have been observed following administration of alcohol tail blocks to prevent "tail wringing" in show horses. Since the procedure is clearly unethical it is difficult to document whether the neurologic damage results from the actual deposition of the substance epidurally (intentionally or otherwise) or whether it occurs because of ascending diffusion of the substance from more distal sites.

THERAPY

In most cases, there is no specific treatment for the cause of the neurologic lesion, the possible exception being a focal abscess or osteomyelitis that might respond to antimicrobial therapy. In equine herpesvirus I myeloencephalitis, prednisone (0.5 to 1 mg per kg orally) may be administered every other day for eight to ten days. If the patient's condition improves, the dosage may be tapered off sooner. In acutely recumbent patients, initial administration of dexamethasone (0.1 mg per kg) may produce a more profound effect.

In general, treatment is designed to provide temporary support for the patient to allow time for lesions to resolve spontaneously. The bladder may be intermittently or continuously drained by catheterization to relieve distention; however, many chronically affected horses seem to do quite well without repeated drainage. Ascending bacterial cystitis and pyelonephritis are potential secondary complications, particularly with repeated catheterization; antimicrobial therapy is useful in their management. Application of petroleum jelly to the rear limbs will help prevent urine scalding. Frequent manual evacuation of feces from the terminal rectum is often necessary to prevent impaction colic. Diets that promote soft stools (e.g., bran supplements) and intermittent administration of mineral oil are also helpful in management.

Cystotomy or urethrostomy to evacuate the massive quantities of urine sediment that accumulate in the bladder have met with little success. The sediment is difficult to remove without contamination of the surgical field. Degenerative changes in the bladder wall and inflammatory changes caused by concurrent bacterial cystitis also contribute to failure.

Obstructive Urinary Tract Disease

Richard M. Debowes, MANHATTAN, KANSAS

The frequency of obstructive urinary disease in the horse is generally considered to be low. When present, urinary tract obstructions are usually attributed to a form of urolithiasis, the cystic or vesicular calculus being the most common. Reports have identified nephrolithiasis and ureterolithiasis as potentially obstructive diseases of the urinary tract. While it is conceivable that neoplastic, granulomatous, or inflammatory disease of the urinary tract could obstruct urine outflow, such conditions are extremely rare and are usually diagnosed as an incidental finding on necropsy examination.

CYSTIC CALCULI

While there are no definitive predisposing causes for their formation, these calculi are most frequently diagnosed in middle-aged or older male horses. The greater frequency of diagnoses in stallions and geldings has been attributed to anatomic differences between the male and female urethra.

Cystic calculi classically contain a variety of hydrated salts of calcium carbonate, calcite being the most common. Typically, these calculi may be found in one of two general forms: the first is a soft concretion of mucoproteins and salts organized loosely into a friable spiculated yellow urolith. The second form is a firm, smooth, white concretion that is very resistant to physical disruption. The physical presence of these calculi, particularly those of the spiculated form, abrades the mucosa of the bladder, resulting in traumatic cystitis. Occasionally, conditions of the bladder that result in atony permit the accumulation of a soft conglomerate of calcium carbonate crystals, mucoproteins, and urinary epithelial cells, which can contribute to or produce a urinary tract obstruction.

CLINICAL SIGNS

Clinical signs associated with the presence of cystic calculi include strangury, dysuria, pollakiuria, and hematuria. Strangury and dysuria are probably related to the posterior displacement of the calculus into the neck of the bladder during micturition. Clinically, affected horses adopt the posture for micturition and maintain it for variable periods of time before voiding urine. These animals may grunt or show mild signs of colic during this time. Hematuria, a frequent observation in affected animals, may be explained by the traumatic cystitis typically found in these cases. Fresh blood may be seen either in the last fraction of urine voided from a resting horse or in any part of the urinary stream voided shortly after exercise. While the disease may be asymptomatic initially, the signs of impaired micturition are eventually observed. With chronicity, weight loss, soiling of the medial hindlimbs, low-grade abdominal pain, or an altered hindlimb gait may be evident.

The presumptive diagnosis of cystic calculus is readily confirmed by rectal examination. Palpation of a vesicular calculus is enhanced by an empty bladder. Passage of a urinary catheter will permit decompression of the bladder while simultaneously establishing the patency of the distal urethra. In most instances, a firm, ovoid intravesicular mass can be palpated immediately caudad to the brim of the pelvis. Urinalysis may be performed in these cases; however, the results confirm only the presence of a traumatic cystitis without providing a definitive diagnosis of an intravesicular calculus.

Cystoscopic examination may provide additional information regarding the diagnosis and prognosis of a given case of urolithiasis. Direct inspection of the bladder and urethra utilizing a flexible fiberoptic endoscope* permits an assessment of the vesicular mucosa and the gross appearance of the calculus. Cystoscopy also affords the opportunity to observe the patency of both ureteral openings and to identify any additional pathology of the lower urinary tract. While the diagnosis of vesicular calculi is usually available from the history, physical, and rectal examination, cystoscopy is a valuable ancillary aid in the diagnosis and subsequent selection of cases for surgical management.

THERAPY

The treatment of cystic calculi is primarily surgical. The use of dietary modifications with urinary acidifiers or other forms of conservative therapy has received minimal attention in the literature. The use of ammonium chloride as a urinary acidifier (20 mg per kg) may be attempted; however, the response to such daily medical therapy has usually been unsatisfactory. Options for surgical management include the use of the midline or paramedian laparocystotomy, subischial urethrotomy, pararectal cystotomy, and urethral sphincterotomy. The selec-

tion of a particular surgical procedure may be influenced by the size, number, and characteristics of the calculi as well as the sex and physical condition of the patient. (The reader is referred to standard surgical texts for the specific details of individual surgical procedures.) Recent improvements in equine surgery and general anesthesia have made the laparocystotomy the most acceptable method of calculus removal in the healthy male equine patient. Essential to the success of this technique is the maintenance of continuous digital traction on the bladder for several minutes to facilitate delivery of this organ into the operative field. After the bladder has been exposed, minimal traction with stay sutures is necessary to maintain the exposure for cystotomy. The location of the trigone above the brim of the pelvis precludes direct efforts to visualize the ureteral openings during a laparocystotomy. This technique permits the surgeon to inspect much of the bladder and lavage the vesicular mucosa under direct visualization—operative advantages not available when utilizing other techniques.

The pararectal cystotomy and subischial urethrotomy are best reserved for use in male patients whose condition will either not permit a general anesthesia and laparocystotomy or in those situations when appropriate facilities for general abdominal surgery are unavailable. Both techniques may be performed under epidural anesthesia and tranquilization in the standing animal. In the female patient, the short distensible urethra may be enlarged by urethral sphincterotomy to facilitate removal of a cystic calculus. Tranquilization and regional anesthesia are usually the only forms of chemical restraint necessary. The urethral sphincterotomy is usually the procedure of choice in most female patients.

URETERAL AND RENAL CALCULI

Ureteral and renal calculi are infrequently described in the veterinary literature; this suggests that their incidence is probably quite low. Several reported cases of renal and ureteral calculi have been made primarily as incidental findings on postmortem. When present, these diseases appear to be either asymptomatic or possibly accompanied by mild signs of abdominal discomfort or lumbar pain. Rectal palpation of multiple uroliths and a grossly distended ureter is possible when such pathology is located in the distal ureter. Palpation of a hydronephrotic kidney may also be possible; however, diagnostic sonography provides an improved imaging modality for evaluation of the equine kidneys. Ultrasonic scanning of the kidneys, when available, may provide additional information on the dimensions of the kidney, fluid distention of the renal

---

*Flexible Endoscope, Mod SIF, Type B, Olympus Corp., Medical Instr. Div., Strongsville, OH

pelvis, or the presence of an acoustic shadow attributable to a sound-dense urolith. Cystoscopy also provides an opportunity to evaluate the patency of the proximal urinary tract. By positioning a flexible fiberoptic endoscope at the neck of the bladder, the ureters may be observed for the periodic discharge of urine. The ureters of clinically normal horses sedated with xylazine hydrochloride* have been noted to empty urine from the ureteral openings in a pulsatile fashion. This seems to occur at a frequency of one to two discharges per minute. When urine is emptied from the ureter, the ureteral orifice at the trigone dilates and is quite obvious on cystoscopic examination. Visual observation of this phenomenon would confirm the patency of the associated renal pelvis and ureter and is more feasible than attempts to visualize the trigone during the surgical procedure. Special diagnostic studies such as intravenous pyelography or excretory urography are unfortunately difficult to impossible in all but the pediatric equine patient.

The treatment of ureteral and renal calculi is usually a surgical exercise. The surgical approach for a nephrectomy involves the resection of the 18th rib to permit access to the kidney and proximal ureter. This procedure is quite difficult and carries the attendant risks of pneumothorax and continued

---

*Rompun, Haver-Lockhart, Shawnee Mission, KS

hemorrhage. Given the difficulty of this surgical procedure, an alternative approach involves the use of fiberoptic cystoscopy. With the appropriate cystoscopic instrumentation, it is possible with the guidance of digital manipulation through rectal palpation or a laparotomy incision to position a Dormia basket* within the distal ureter for removal of a ureteral calculus. Nephrectomy may still be required if significant hydronephrotic damage has occurred.

---

*Dormia Stone Dislodger, V. Mueller Co., Division of American Hospital Supply Co., Chicago, IL

Supplemental Readings

DeBowes, R.M., Nyrop, K.A., and Boulton, C.H.: Cystic calculi in the horse. Comp. Cont. Ed., 6:S268, 1984.

Hackett, R.P., Vaughan, J.T., and Tennant, B.C.: The urinary system. *In* Mansmann, R.A., McAllister, E.S., and Pratt, P.W. (eds.): Equine Medicine and Surgery, 3rd ed. Santa Barbara, CA, American Veterinary Publications, 1982.

Macharg, M.A., Foerner, J.J., Phillips, T.N., and Barclay, W.P.: Two methods for the treatment of ureterolithiasis in a mare. J. Vet. Surg., 13:95, 1984.

Trotter, G.W., Bennett, D.G., and Behm, R.J.: Urethral calculi in five horses. J. Vet. Surg., 10:159, 1981.

Walker, D.F., and Vaughan, J.T.: Surgery of the urinary tract. *In* Walker, D.F., and Vaughan, J.T. (eds.): Bovine and Equine Urogenital Surgery, 2nd ed. Philadelphia, Lea & Febiger, 1980.

Urinary Bladder Displacement

Conrad H. Boulton, PULLMAN, WASHINGTON

Displacement of the equine urinary bladder through the vulvar lips of the mare is a rare occurrence presenting in one of three forms: urinary bladder prolapse, bladder eversion, and bladder prolapse associated with vaginal prolapse. The most common of these is bladder eversion in which the bladder is everted through the urethral opening. Since the bladder is "turned inside out," the whitish mucosal surface is presented to the observer as well as two readily observable ureteral openings on the dorsal surface, from which urine is periodically expressed (Fig. 1). The everted bladder may be pear-shaped or round. In cases of urinary bladder prolapse the reddened, round serosal surface of the bladder can be seen. The bladder has most often passed through a tear in the vaginal floor located anterior to the urethral opening and is "flipped" posterior, thus sharply kinking the intact urethra and preventing discharge of urine from the bladder (Fig. 2). In the third form, the bladder is prolapsed

within a vaginal prolapse and the tissue protruding between the vulvar lips is the vaginal floor with the urinary bladder being contained within the prolapsed vagina (Fig. 3). Discussion of this displacement is more appropriate in a discussion of primary vaginal prolapse. In most cases the type of displacement can be identified by (1) examination of the surface presented, (2) identification to determine the presence or absence of ureteral openings, and (3) most importantly, careful digital palpation of the origin of the prolapsed tissue.

The exact causes of bladder displacement are speculative; however, a consistent factor is excessive abdominal straining. Such straining is generally associated with parturition but has also been noted in cases of colic and vaginitis, and subsequent to repair of third-degree perineal lacerations. Displacements have not been associated with urinary bladder paralysis, cystic calculi, and enlarged urethras. The occurrence and type of displacement are

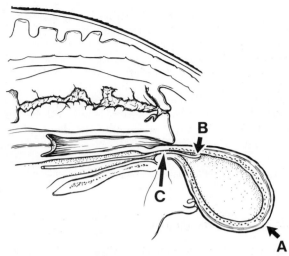

Figure 1. A drawing of a median plane section of a urinary bladder eversion. The bladder is "turned inside out." *A,* Exposed mucosal lining of bladder; *B,* intact ureter within everted bladder; *C,* everted urethral opening through which the bladder has passed.

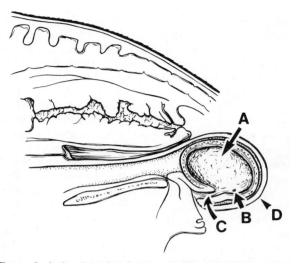

Figure 3. A drawing of a median plane section of a urinary bladder prolapse associated with prolapse of the vaginal floor. *A,* Mucosal lining of the bladder; *B,* ureteral opening; *C,* urethra; *D,* visible prolapsed vaginal floor surrounding associated bladder prolapse.

related to the ratio of abdominal pressure to urethral sphincter strength, and/or the relative strength of intra-abdominal vaginal and vesicular supporting structures.

Although the bladder is fixed at its neck, the distensible body is only loosely held to the lateral pelvic walls by remnants of the umbilical artery and to the pelvic floor by remnants of the umbilical veins. These structures are not strong and are damaged or avulsed when the bladder is displaced.

THERAPY

Following identification of the displacement type, repositioning is most often accomplished by manual

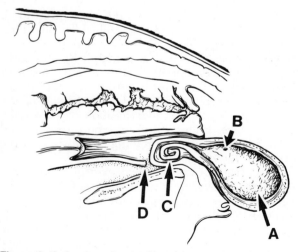

Figure 2. A drawing of a median plane section of a urinary bladder prolapse. *A,* Mucosal lining of bladder; *B,* ureteral opening within the prolapse not visible from the exposed surface; *C,* intact urethra; *D,* edge of tear through which the bladder has passed.

reduction. When associated with parturition, reduction should be done before delivery of the fetus. The use of epidural anesthesia to reduce straining during reduction is often necessary in even the simplest cases, while general anesthesia has been used in the difficult or complicated case. With general anesthesia the animal should be placed in dorsal or lateral recumbency with the hindquarters elevated. Raising of the hindquarters by standing the horse on a slope also aids reduction in the standing horse.

Initially the displaced tissue and associated perineal area are cleansed with a disinfectant and liberal lavage, and then assessed for viability. If a true prolapse is present the cleansed surface must be returned to its original intra-abdominal position with the associated risk of peritonitis. Although more common in the cow, eversion of a bladder with constriction as it passes through the urethra may result in strangulation and loss of viability. These factors, combined with self-inflicted trauma, may seriously complicate the otherwise simple case.

Reducing the size of the displaced bladder is recommended before its repositioning is attempted. This is best accomplished by centesis of the displaced tissue using a 20-gauge, 1½ inch needle. In cases of urinary prolapse this will result in the removal of urine. In cases of eversion a peritoneal transudate is often removed, thus greatly reducing the size of the structure and aiding repositioning. Remaining tissue may also be treated with massage and circumferential pressure or the topical application of 50 per cent dextrose to reduce edema, if needed. Following these procedures the bladder is generally shrunken enough to accomplish manual repositioning. The average adult mare urethra can be dilated to approximately 8 cm diameter. If insufficient dilation is obtained for repositioning an eversion, a dorsal urethral sphincterotomy may aid replacement. Repair of the sphincterotomy following replacement is accomplished with an interrupted suture pattern of absorbable suture. In cases of bladder prolapse the bladder must be replaced through a vaginal tear and then closure of the tear with an interrupted pattern of absorbable suture is recommended.

Cases of eversion may be seriously complicated by the prolapse of bowel within the everted bladder. This is most often the pelvic flexure and is subject to incarceration, edema, and infarction. Swelling may physically prevent reduction, thus requiring general anesthesia, dorsal recumbency, and a posterior midline celiotomy. One operator may then provide gentle traction while a second tries to replace the bladder and associated bowel. At times, cystotomy and intestinal resection have been indicated in order to accomplish reduction.

Following replacement, the bladder should be dilated with saline via the urethra to ensure that it is properly repositioned. In cases in which general anesthesia has been used or in which the cause of abdominal straining cannot be alleviated, a pursestring suture of nonabsorbable suture may be placed in the external urethral orifice, thus limiting it to approximately a 1½ cm diameter. This suture is left in place for five to ten days. If straining is severe and pharmacologic control unobtainable, a tracheotomy is indicated to reduce the intra-abdominal pressure associated with abdominal contraction. Another recognized complication is rupture of the devitalized bladder wall in severe cases before or during replacement. Such a case requires resection of devitalized tissue and closure of the bladder wall. Success is possible if the ureteral openings are not compromised.

Successful treatment may be related to an early diagnosis, correction within hours of occurrence, and alleviation of the cause of abdominal straining. Complications that should be anticipated include cystitis, ascending pyelonephritis, bladder paresis, and fatal peritonitis. Immediate recurrence has been noted in occasional cases but has not been documented in subsequent pregnancies in otherwise normal mares. Use of a systemic antibiotic that is eliminated via the urine is encouraged, and appropriate tetanus prophylaxis is mandatory.

Supplemental Readings

Frank, E.R.: Affections of the tail, anus, rectum, vagina and penis. *In* Veterinary Surgery, 7th ed. Minneapolis, Burgess Publishing Co., 1964.

Haynes, P.F., and McClure, J.R.: Eversion of the urinary bladder: A sequel to third-degree perineal laceration in the mare. Vet. Surg., 9:66, 1980.

Vaughan, J.T., and Walker, D.F.: Surgery of the urinary tract. *In* Bovine and Equine Urogenital Surgery. Philadelphia, Lea & Febiger, 1980.

Rupture of the Urinary Bladder

David R. Hodgson, PULLMAN, WASHINGTON

Cystorrhexis, or rupture of the urinary bladder, occurs most frequently in neonates. However, this condition has been reported in adult horses, usually as a sequel to urinary tract obstruction or following parturition. Diagnosis is usually based on the history, clinical signs, and laboratory profile of the patient. Treatment often involves metabolic support and surgical correction of the bladder defect.

ETIOLOGY AND PATHOPHYSIOLOGY

Cystorrhexis is reported to occur in approximately 0.05 to 1.0 per cent of foals and is believed by many to be the result of parturient trauma. It is observed predominantly in male foals, possibly due to the small diameter of the urethral exit. Theoretically, this allows excessive pressure to build up within the distended bladder during foaling, usually rupturing the body of the bladder (corpus vesicae) dorsal to the apex, which is its weakest point. Others have suggested that some cases of cystorrhexis may be the result of congenital defects in the bladder wall, often associated with a concomitant patent urachus. In such cases, little if any hemorrhage or inflammation of the defect is observed.

CLINICAL SIGNS

Affected foals are frequently reported to have uncomplicated births and usually appear to behave normally immediately after birth. Clinical signs are often present within 24 to 36 hours, although veterinary attention may not be sought for several days. Initially, foals become depressed, lose the desire to nurse, and make frequent attempts to urinate, with only small amounts of urine being voided. Tachycardia, tachypnea, and progressive abdominal distention are common findings. Tactile percussion and auscultation of the abdomen may reveal fluid accumulation. As the condition progresses, foals may exhibit signs of abdominal irritation and respiratory distress. After several days, affected foals may become severely depressed and dyspneic, develop cardiac arrythmias, and demonstrate signs consistent with central nervous system derangement, such as blindness and lack of awareness of their surroundings.

LABORATORY FINDINGS

Hematology often reveals evidence of stress, reflected by elevations in the packed cell volume and a neutrophilic leukocytosis. Severe hyponatremia, hypochloremia, and hyperkalemia are frequent findings and are valuable diagnostic indices in cases of cystorrhexis. For example, values in the range of 110 to 125 mEq per L, 4.5 to 7.0 mEq per L, and 70 to 95 mEq per L for plasma sodium, potassium, and chloride, respectively, are commonly encountered in foals with this disorder. Abdominocentesis usually yields a large volume of pale yellow fluid of low specific gravity. Serum urea nitrogen and creatinine concentrations are often normal or only moderately elevated in affected foals, and although the concentration of urea nitrogen and creatinine in the abdominal fluid may be elevated this is by no means a consistent finding in these animals. However, if values for abdominal fluid urea nitrogen and creatinine concentrations are found to be more than twice those found in the serum, this is regarded as being suggestive of cystorrhexis. Infusion of relatively nonirritant dyes such as methylene blue into the bladder via a urinary catheter and subsequent demonstration of the dye in abdominal fluid samples may aid in confirmation of the diagnosis. Similarly, contrast radiography may reveal defects in the integrity of the bladder wall. In adult horses, the demonstration of the urinary crystals, such as calcium carbonate in abdominal fluid samples, may also help in confirming the diagnosis.

TREATMENT

Correction of the defective bladder wall necessitates surgical intervention (p. 714). However, foals often require medical therapy before surgery in order to correct many of the metabolic derangements associated with this condition. This usually involves drainage of the extravasated urine to remove pressure from the diaphragm and aid in the relief of respiratory embarrassment. I have found

that use of a sterile teat cannula, inserted through the posteroventral abdominal wall lateral to the umbilicus, provides a safe and effective means of abdominal drainage. Commonly, many liters of fluid may be drained from the abdomen using this technique. As the rapid drainage of large volumes of fluid may result in circulatory compromise, it is advisable to remove the fluid over a period of one hour or longer. In addition, institution of intravenous fluid therapy before and during abdominal drainage will aid in avoiding such complications. Electrocardiographic monitoring of foals with severe metabolic derangements may also be indicated, allowing for early detection and appropriate action if cardiac arrhythmias develop.

Intravenous fluid therapy is usually indicated to aid in the correction of the electrolyte abnormalities associated with this condition. Normal saline administered intravenously is often the fluid of choice as this will aid in correction of the hyponatremia and hypochloremia. As a rule, fluids containing potassium should not be used in the initial course of therapy. Addition of dextrose, constituting 5 to 10 per cent of the final solution, may also be of value as a limited source of calories for the foal, and may also aid in reducing the hyperkalemia that often accompanies this condition. Initial infusion rates of between 10 to 25 ml per kg per hour are commonly employed. If facilities allow, frequent reassessment of the foal's fluid and electrolyte balance is advised, with the therapeutic plan being modified accordingly. In acidotic foals, judicious bicarbonate therapy may be indicated. A means of estimating the amount of bicarbonate required can be obtained from the following equation:

$$\frac{\text{bicarbonate required}}{\text{(mEq per L)}} = \frac{\text{foal's body weight (kg)} \times 0.4}{\times \text{ bicarbonate deficit (mEq per L)}}$$

Bicarbonate deficit is measured by the blood gas analysis or with the Harleco apparatus (see p. 36). Half this deficit is administered initially, over a period of several hours. This often provides additional reductions in the serum potassium concentration. Appropriate medical management of foals with cystorrhexis before surgical intervention will reduce the risks associated with anesthesia, thus improving the chances of a successful resolution of the problem.

Supplemental Readings

Behr, M. J., Hackett, R. P., Bentinck-Smith, J., Hillman, R. B., King, J. M., and Tennant, B. C.: Metabolic abnormalities associated with rupture of the urinary bladder in neonatal foals. J. Am. Vet. Med. Assoc., *178*:263, 1981.

Darbishire, H. B.: Operation to repair rupture of the bladder in a young foal. Vet. Rec., *73*:693, 1961.

Johnson, J. H.: Surgical considerations of the abdomen: newborn foals. *In* Turner, A. S. (ed.): Some Techniques and Procedures in Equine Surgery. Edwardsville, KS, Veterinary Medicine Publishing Co., 1983, pp. 125-127.

Conditions of the Urethra

James T. Robertson, COLUMBUS, OHIO

Examination of the urethra is part of a complete urinary tract examination, and in the male includes external inspection of the penis, urethral process, and the fossa glandis, rectal palpation of the pelvic urethra and accessory glands, catheterization of the urethra to obtain an uncontaminated urine sample and to check urethral patency, and an endoscopic examination. These examinations are best performed under sedation. In the mare, the external urethral orifice is visualized per vaginum through a speculum. A sterile lubricated hand can be introduced into the vestibule to allow digital palpation of the urethra, which is short and very distensible.

A 100-cm flexible endoscope is adequate to examine the length of the urethra in the male. The endoscope should be cleansed thoroughly before the examination and should be well lubricated. In the male, distention of the urethra with air allows excellent visualization of the mucosa. The short urethra of the mare cannot be distended in such a fashion. The horse may become uncomfortable when the bladder distends; air should be allowed to escape around the endoscope when the horse strains. In the pelvic urethra of the male, ducts of the bulbourethral glands and more anteriorly the colliculus seminalis are visible on the dorsal surface of the urethra.

Specific indications for examination include a history or clinical evidence of hematuria, cystitis, urethritis, cystic or urethral calculi, urethral obstruction, masses involving the penis and urethral process, urethral trauma, and hemospermia.

URINARY CALCULI

Urinary calculi occur infrequently in horses. Cystic calculi are the most common type, with urethral calculi being much less prevalent. Urethral calculi are found in colts, geldings, and stallions but are unheard of in females due to the short length and distensibility of the urethra. The point of obstruction is likely to be in the pelvic portion of the urethra, near the ischial arch, or in the distal urethra. Once the calculus lodges in the urethra and the bladder fills, the horse will strain, prolapse the penis, and make repeated attempts to urinate and perhaps dribble small amounts of urine. The diagnosis can be confirmed by rectal examination if the stone is in the pelvic urethra. If the stone is in the distal urethra, the distended bladder and pelvic urethra are palpable per rectum. Passage of a urinary catheter or flexible fiberoptic endoscope will allow localization and identification of the calculus. Prolonged obstruction may produce urethral necrosis or lead to rupture of the bladder.

Calculi in the pelvic urethra can be removed by ischial urethrotomy under epidural anesthesia in the standing horse. The urethral incision can be left to heal by secondary intention. Distal urethral calculi may be dislodged in the tranquilized horse with the aid of a catheter or an instrument such as a hemostat or sponge forceps. Surgical removal of distal urethral calculi is accomplished through a ventral approach to urethrotomy, which requires dorsal recumbency and general anesthesia.

GRANULOMAS AND TUMORS

Granulomas and tumors that involve the glans and the mucous membranes of the urethral process can produce inflammation, ulceration, bleeding, and obstruction. Diagnosis is confirmed by biopsy of the affected tissue. Cutaneous habronema granulomas are treated with ivermectin or topical and/or systemic application of organophosphates. Surgical resection of the urethral process is indicated in chronic refractory cases. Neoplasms, such as squamous cell carcinoma, may be treated with cryosurgery or surgical excision. Invasive neoplasms necessitate penile amputation.

URETHRITIS

Urethritis may be: (1) secondary to a cystitis or a cystic calculus, (2) the result of repeated catheterizations or endoscopic examinations, or (3) primarily bacterial in nature. Other reported causes of urethritis include necrosis of the urethra as a result of pressure from a stallion ring, vesicular urethritis, and stricture formation. An active urethritis in the breeding stallion will reduce semen quality, may produce hemospermia, and is associated with a reluctance to cover mares because of the associated pain that increases in intensity with ejaculation. The bleeding is probably from subepithelial vessels that have prolapsed into the urethral lumen at sites of ulceration. Urethral swabs should be obtained for culture and sensitivity before treatment. Double-contrast urethrography may be beneficial in identifying pseudomembranous urethritis, ulceration, fistulas, protrusion of subepithelial vessels into the lumen and strictures. Bacterial urethritis, particularly Pseudomonas infection, is very difficult to treat, even with high levels of antibiotics. In addition to systemic antibiotics, therapy for urethritis includes rest from mating activity and suppository inserts, which are placed through a perineal urethrotomy incision into the proximal urethra.

TRAUMA

Blunt trauma to the penis may produce urethral obstruction as a result of the surrounding inflammation and paraphimosis or a hematoma of the corpus spongiosum as seen with a contusion below the ischial arch. Anti-inflammatory medication and urinary drainage are indicated. Lacerations of the urethra, depending on their location and the condition of the wound, may be sutured or left to heal by secondary intention, around an indwelling urinary catheter if the laceration is fully circumferential. Suture material used to close urethral mucosa

should be absorbable; surrounding tissue must be adequately drained. A sequela to urethral wounding is stricture formation.

Supplemental Readings

Hacket, R. P., Vaughan, J. T., and Tennant, B. C.: The urinary system. *In* Mansmann, R. A., McAllister, E. S., and Pratt, P. W., (eds.): Equine Medicine and Surgery, 3rd ed., vol. II, Santa Barbara, CA, American Veterinary Publications, 1982, pp. 921-922.
Neely, D. P.: Physical examination and genital diseases in the stallion. *In* Morrow, D. (ed.): Current Therapy in Theriogenology. Philadelphia, W. B. Saunders Company, 1980. pp. 694-706.
Sullins, K. E., and Traub-Dargatz, J. L.: Endoscopic anatomy of the equine urinary tract. Comp. Cont. Ed., 6:S663, 1984.
Trotter, G. W., Bennett, D. G., and Behm, R. J.: Urethral calculi in five horses. Vet. Surg., 10:159, 1981.
Voss, J. L., and Wotowey, J. L.: Hemospermia. Proc. 18th Annu. Conv. Am. Assoc. Eq. Pract., 1972, pp. 103-112.
Walker, D. F., and Vaughan, J. T.: Bovine and Equine Urogenital Surgery. Philadelphia, Lea & Febiger, 1980, pp. 105-114; 170-177.

Neoplastic and Anomalous Conditions of the Urinary Tract

Polly Modransky, BLACKSBURG, VIRGINIA

NEOPLASIA

Renal adenocarcinoma and transitional cell carcinoma of the bladder have been reported in the horse. Early diagnosis, however, is difficult. Clinical signs often are not evident until the tumor mass has enlarged significantly or metastasis to other organs has occurred. These neoplasms may produce syndromes in which involvement of the urinary tract is not always recognized. Chronic weight loss, colic, ascites, anemia, hematuria, and lameness have been associated with neoplasia of the equine urinary tract.

Perirenal masses or tumor implants on the serosa of palpable abdominal organs or both can be detected on rectal examination. Evaluation of urine sediment for the presence of tumor cells should be performed. Neoplastic cells will not always be present within the sediment; therefore, a neoplastic process should not be ruled out on the basis of the absence of tumor cells.

Ultrasonography is a very useful diagnostic aid. The kidneys can be examined two-dimensionally and their sizes determined. Internal architecture can be evaluated and areas of abnormal echogenicity can be detected. Endoscopy has been shown to be

a feasible method of evaluating the urethra, bladder, and ureters in horses. A standing flank laparotomy provides a means of establishing or confirming a diagnosis of neoplasia.

Surgical removal of the tumor is usually not attempted. By the time an antemortem diagnosis can be reached, involvement of surrounding structures either because of adhesions or metastasis is quite extensive and total excision of the neoplastic process is impossible.

The most common neoplasm involving the penis, distal urethra, and prepuce is squamous cell carcinoma. Focal pedunculated lesions are usually surgically excised or removed with cryotherapy. The prognosis is considered good provided that metastases have not occurred. Diffuse, more invasive involvement of the penis or prepuce necessitates radical excision of all involved tissues and possibly penile amputation. Metastasis to regional lymph nodes is characteristic of this tumor. Metastatic involvement of the lungs has also been reported. Cases having extensive neoplastic involvement carry an extremely guarded prognosis. Other neoplasms occurring in this area include sarcoid, squamous papilloma, melanoma, and hemangioma.

ECTOPIC URETERS

Faulty differentiation of the mesonephric and metanephric ducts in the developing embryo results in one or both ureters terminating in sites other than the trigone of the bladder. Some degree of hydronephrosis and hydroureter will be present in animals with ectopic ureter(s). Other abnormalities of the urogenital system such as ureteral duplication, persistent hymen, renal hypoplasia, cryptorchidism, and hypoplasia of the bladder may also be evident.

The most common presenting complaint in fillies is urinary incontinence. Affected colts, however, are usually presented for persistent urinary tract infections and rarely incontinence. This may be due to a retrograde flow of urine from the ureteral openings back into the bladder.

A definitive diagnosis of ureteral ectopia can be made by retrograde cystography or excretory urography. These procedures are relatively safe and can be performed using standard contrast agents. Good-quality radiographs of the abdomen and pelvis are essential and can be achieved by using general anesthesia, high-speed screens, and high-ratio grids. Generally, these techniques are limited to use in foals because of the difficulties encountered in obtaining diagnostic abdominal radiographs in large animals.

Once a diagnosis is made, treatment for ureteral ectopia is surgical transpositioning of the ureter(s) into the bladder, or nephrectomy. A urinalysis and bacteriologic culture of the urine should be performed in affected animals to discover any existing infection before surgical intervention. On the basis of the results of the microbial culture, appropriate antibiotic therapy should be initiated preoperatively.

If the condition is unilateral, surgical removal of the affected kidney and ureter can be performed provided that the contralateral kidney is normal. General anesthesia is essential. The animal is positioned in lateral recumbency. Resection of the 18th rib and deep retraction allow adequate surgical exposure to remove the affected organ.

Postoperative complications of this technique include hemorrhage and pneumothorax. Careful ligation of renal vessels and hemostasis will help minimize the likelihood of severe hemorrhage and formation of retroperitoneal hematomas. Pneumothorax can occur if the incision into the retroperitoneal space inadvertently invades the caudal extension of the pleural cavity. Closure and restoration of negative intrathoracic pressure should be performed as soon as the problem is identified.

Bilateral ectopic ureters can be surgically reimplanted into the bladder. Either a side-to-side anastomosis of the ureter to the bladder or a submucosal tunneling technique is effective in re-establishing a functional urinary system. Postoperative complications include formation of peritoneal adhesions, peritonitis, and stenosis of the anastomotic sites. Gentle handling of tissues, maintenance of aseptic technique, and utilization of nonreactive suture materials will help in minimizing these potential problems. Systemic and/or intraperitoneal heparin may also be beneficial in preventing adhesion formation following abdominal surgery in these cases. Persistent hydroureter and hydronephrosis, as well as hypoplasia of the bladder, should be considered if there is incontinence following surgery.

PATENT URACHUS

During fetal development, the urachus serves as a connection between the bladder and the allantoic cavity. At birth or shortly thereafter, spontaneous closure of the structure normally occurs. Failure of this process is caused by excessive torsion placed on the umbilical cord in utero (congenital patency) or is the result of omphalophlebitis (acquired patency).

In most instances, diagnosis of this condition can be made on the basis of history, clinical signs, and physical examination. Affected foals present with urine dribbling from the umbilicus. Urine scald around the navel may also be present if the condition has persisted for several days. Septicemia can result from an ascending infection of the umbilicus since the patent urachus serves as an excellent portal of entry for opportunistic organisms. Organisms commonly incriminated in neonatal infections are beta-hemolytic streptococci, *Escherichia coli*, and *Actinobacillus equuli*.

Once the condition is diagnosed, treatment should be prompt. Therapy should be directed toward promoting rapid closure of the defect and preventing infection. Parenteral antibiotics should be administered. Choice of antibiotic should be based on culture and sensitivity results if possible. This is especially important in foals with an apparent infection such as "joint ill." If culture and sensitivity results are not available, a good broad-spectrum antibiotic regimen should be instituted. The foal's environment should be kept as clean as possible until closure of the urachus occurs.

Cauterization of the urachus with 90 per cent phenol, Lugol's solution, or silver nitrate sticks has reportedly been successful in many cases if treatment was begun early. The urachus should be treated for a distance of 3 to 4 cm once or twice daily for several days. If closure does not occur within three to five days, the urachus should be resected surgically to prevent abscessation, ascending infection, and septicemia.

General anesthesia is recommended. Systemic antibiotics should be administered preoperatively and continued for five to seven days postoperatively. The bladder is emptied via a urethral catheter and a ligature is placed around the urachal opening before the surgical preparation in an attempt to minimize contamination. An elliptical skin incision is made around the navel and extended into the abdominal cavity. The umbilical vessels should be identified and examined closely for signs of infection. The umbilical arteries, extending caudally toward the bladder, are transfixed at the level of the bladder and severed. The umbilical vein extends cranially toward the liver. The vessel should be ligated proximal to any signs of infection, if possible. Surgical exposure may limit access to the most proximal extent of the infected umbilical vein.

The urachus and a portion of the bladder apex are usually resected. The bladder wall is closed with absorbable suture material in two inverting layers. Following closure of the bladder, it should be evaluated for any areas of leakage before the abdominal incision is closed.

Postoperative complications include suture line leakage, peritonitis secondary to intraoperative contamination, incisional problems, and persistent septicemia-related problems. Prognosis depends on duration of the condition, effectiveness of the antibiotic therapy, and the immune competence of the animal.

UROPERITONEUM

Ruptured bladder (see p. 717) is the most common cause of uroperitoneum. Other causes include ureteral or urachal defects or both types. Clinical signs are the same as for a ruptured bladder. Colts are more commonly affected than fillies. Affected foals are usually normal at birth but within 48 hours, strangury, labored breathing, and abdominal distention develop. Ballottement of the abdomen may elicit a distinguishable fluid wave. Evaluation of the abdominal fluid reveals urinelike material with urea nitrogen and creatinine values generally two or more times higher than those in serum. Hyponatremia, hypochloremia, and hyperkalemia are consistent electrolyte abnormalities in these foals.

Injection of sterile dye solution such as fluorescein or methylene blue via a urethral catheter into the bladder followed by appearance of the dye in the peritoneal fluid confirms the presence of an intraperitoneal defect of the urinary tract. An alternative method for field diagnosis is injection of air through a urethral catheter with simultaneous auscultation of air as it escapes into the abdominal cavity.

Positive contrast cystography is considered an extremely reliable diagnostic technique in small animals with ruptured bladders. However, it has been of limited use in foals, especially under field conditions.

Surgical repair of the defect is indicated (see p. 718).

Supplemental Readings

Hackett, R. P.: Rupture of the urinary bladder in neonatal foals. Comp. Cont. Ed., 6:488, 1984.

Haschek, W., King, J. M., and Tennant, B. C.: Primary renal cell carcinoma in two horses. J. Am. Vet. Med. Assoc., 179:992, 1981.

Modransky, P. D., Wagner, P. C., Robinette, J. D., et al: Surgical correction of bilateral ectopic ureters in two foals. Vet. Surg., 12:141, 1983.

Sullins, K. E., and Traub-Dargatz, J. L.: Endoscopic anatomy of the equine urinary tract. Comp. Cont. Ed., 6:663, 1984.

Traub, J. L., Bayly, W., Reed, S. M., et al: Intra-abdominal neoplasia as a cause of chronic weight loss in the horse. Comp. Cont. Ed., 5:526, 1983.

Renal Tubular Acidosis

Ellen L. Ziemer, KENNETT SQUARE, PENNSYLVANIA

Renal tubular acidosis (RTA) is a newly recognized syndrome in horses. It is well documented in humans and has been reported in dogs and a cat.

PATHOPHYSIOLOGY

Renal tubular acidosis accompanies renal tubular dysfunction. Three classifications of RTA are described in humans: types 1, 2, and 4. Type 1 RTA involves distal renal tubular dysfunction, with a failure to obtain or maintain a hydrogen ion gradient between the extracellular fluid and the intratubular lumen. Type 2 involves the proximal renal tubule, with a reduction in renal tubular reabsorption of filtered bicarbonate so that urinary wastage of this anion occurs. Type 2 is often associated with a complex dysfunction of the proximal tubule, such as the Fanconi syndrome in humans. Type 4 involves the distal renal tubule, with the cation exchange segment of the distal nephron affected so that decreased secretion of hydrogen and potassium ions occurs. Two extensively studied equine RTA cases appeared to be type 1.

CLINICAL SIGNS AND PATHOLOGY

Horses with RTA are depressed and weak and may have chronic weight loss. Ataxia, lethargy, and collapse due to hypokalemia have also been described. Physical examination may be normal except for poor body condition. Bradycardia and mild epistaxis are also reported.

Hyperchloremic metabolic acidosis is typical of all types of RTA. Types 1 and 2 RTA are usually nonazotemic, and may be either normokalemic or hypokalemic. An alkaline urinary pH may be noted in the face of severe metabolic acidosis in both types 1 and 2. However, type 2 patients can acidify urine in response to an oral acid load such as ammonium chloride, while type 1 patients are unable to acidify urine to any significant extent with the same treatment.

Type 4 RTA patients may be azotemic; hyperkalemia is usually present, and urinary pH may be normal. It is wise to remember that alkaline urine is normal in herbivores. Estimation of acid-base status by blood gas analysis or estimation of total carbon dioxide* may reveal a severe metabolic acidosis with plasma bicarbonate concentrations below 10 mEq per L.

DIAGNOSIS

Diagnosis of RTA is primarily by exclusion of other causes of metabolic acidosis. Hyperchloremia has been a consistent feature. Acidosis may be transient, with recovery in approximately one week. However, in several instances withdrawal of bicarbonate therapy causes recurrence of hyperchloremic metabolic acidosis. Renal biopsy results do not appear to be diagnostic.

TREATMENT

Treatment is based on correction of the acid-base and electrolyte abnormalities. Therapy may be intravenous or oral, although a combination of these routes may be preferable in severe cases. Bicarbonate replacement must be coupled with potassium therapy in cases with a normokalemia or hypokalemia, or a life-threatening hypokalemia may result. Correction of the acidosis may be gradual. In human cases of RTA, the bicarbonate deficit is calculated using the formula:

$$\text{body weight (kg)} \times 0.5 \times \text{base deficit (mEq/L)}$$

Half of the calculated deficit is administered over 24 hours, and the remainder is given over 36 hours. This appears applicable to equine cases; however,

*S/Pecial Chem CO_2 Apparatus Set, American Scientific Products, McGraw Park, IL

more bicarbonate supplementation may be necessary to obtain correction of acid-base status than originally calculated.

To correct the calculated deficit, sodium bicarbonate may be given intravenously in the form of 5 per cent bicarbonate solution, or powdered sodium bicarbonate may be added to a normal or half-strength saline solution. Sodium bicarbonate may also be administered by stomach tube or by dose syringe in small, frequent amounts (50 to 100 gm or 600 to 1200 mEq) four to six times a day, if necessary.

Total body potassium deficiencies are difficult to determine, particularly in the face of metabolic acidosis. Intravenous supplementation with potassium chloride should not exceed 100 to 150 mEq per hour for an adult horse. A safe way to supplement large amounts of potassium, vital in equine RTA cases, is to administer potassium chloride orally. Forty grams (533 mEq K^+) diluted in several liters of water may be administered by stomach tube two to three times a day. Care must be taken, however, when administering potassium chloride and sodium bicarbonate orally that osmotic diarrhea is not induced.

Once acid-base and electrolyte stabilization occurs, appetite normally resumes. At this point, potassium supplementation is generally no longer necessary, since hay contains large amounts of potassium. If the horse relapses after bicarbonate therapy is withdrawn, oral sodium bicarbonate therapy, 2 to 4 mEq per kg divided into twice daily dosages, may be sufficient to maintain stabilization for long periods of time. Sodium bicarbonate has been successfully mixed with feed and water. Frequent monitoring of acid-base status is recommended until a precise bicarbonate dosage is established. Periodic monitoring is recommended after stabilization.

PROGNOSIS

All cases of RTA in horses have been of undetermined etiology. Most have been transient, with treatment required from three days to 28 months. Some patients are currently under long-term bicarbonate replacement.

Supplemental Readings

Carlson, G. P.: Fluid therapy in horses with acute diarrhea. Vet. Clin. North Am. (Large Anim. Pract.), 1:313, 1979.

Morris, R. C., and Sebastian, A.: Renal tubular acidosis and Fanconi syndrome. *In* Stanbury, J. B. et al (eds.): The Metabolic Basis of Inherited Disease, 5th ed. New York, McGraw Hill, 1983, pp. 1808-1843.

Thornhill, J. A.: Renal tubular acidosis. *In* Kirk, R. W. (ed.): Current Veterinary Therapy, VI. Philadelphia, W.B. Saunders Company, 1977, pp. 1087-1097.

Section 18

APPENDICES

Normal Clinical Pathology Data

Duane F. Brobst, PULLMAN, WASHINGTON

B. W. Parry, PULLMAN, WASHINGTON

The data presented are derived from the literature and our own laboratory. Some factors such as age, sex, breed, training and temperament can cause variation in normal values. Different methods of performing a particular laboratory procedure may also influence the result.

TABLE 1. HEMATOLOGY VALUES

	Hot-Blooded Horses	Cold-Blooded Horses
Total erythrocytes ($\times 10^6/\mu$l)	6–12	5.5–9.5
Packed cell volume (%)	32–52	24–44
Hemoglobin (gm/dl)	11–19	8–14
Mean corpuscular volume (fl)	34–58	40–48
Mean corpuscular hemoglobin concentration (gm/dl)	32–38	32–38
Total leukocytes ($\times 10^3/\mu$l)	5.5–12.5	6–12
Band neutrophils ($\times 10^3/\mu$l)	0–0.1	0–0.1
Segmented neutrophils ($\times 10^3/\mu$l)	2.7–5.8	2.5–6.2
Lymphocytes ($\times 10^3/\mu$l)	1.5–6.0	1.2–5.0
Monocytes ($\times 10^3/\mu$l)	0–0.6	0.1–0.8
Eosinophils ($\times 10^3/\mu$l)	0–0.9	0.1–1.0
Basophils ($\times 10^3/\mu$l)	0–0.2	0–0.2
Platelets ($\times 10^5/\mu$l)	1–3.5	1–3.5

For conversion to SI units:
  Conventional Units (above) $\times$ Correction Factor = SI Units
    Total erythrocytes $\times$ 10^6 = Erythrocytes $\times$ 10^{12}/L
    Packed cell volume $\times$ 10^{-2} = L/L
    Hemoglobin $\times$ 0.62 = mmol/L
    Mean corpuscular volume: fl = 10^{-15}L
    Mean corpuscular hemoglobin concentration $\times$ 0.62 = mmol/L
    Leukocytes $\times$ 10^6 = Leukocytes $\times$ 10^9/L
    Platelets $\times$ 10^6 = Platelets $\times$ 10^9/L

Modified from Krehbiel, J. D.: Normal Clinical Pathology Data. *In* Robinson, N. E. (ed.): Current Therapy in Equine Medicine, 1st ed. Philadelphia, W. B. Saunders Company, 1983.

TABLE 2. PLASMA PROTEINS AND HEMOSTATIC PARAMETERS

Test	Values	Significance/Interpretation
Fibrinogen* (Factor I)	0.20–0.40 gm/dl	May increase with dehydration and inflammation; may decrease in fulminant hepatic failure and DIC§
Total plasma protein (TPP)†	6.0–8.5 gm/dl	May increase with dehydration and inflammation; may decrease with renal loss, gut loss or failure of hepatic synthesis
TPP/fibrinogen ratio	≥15:1 ≤10:1	Normal or dehydration. Absolute hyperfibrinogenemia, i.e., inflammation
Activated coagulation time (ACT)‡	100–215 seconds (at 37°C)	Prolongation implies deficiency or inhibition of Factors XII, XI, X, IX, VIII, V, II, and/or I and/or severe thrombocytopenia
Prothrombin time (PT)‡	8.2–10.6 seconds	Prolongation implies deficiency or inhibition of Factors VII, X, V, II, and/or I
Activated partial thromboplastin time (APTT, PTT)‡	27.0–39.4 seconds	Prolongation implies deficiency or inhibition of Factors XII, XI, X, IX, VIII, V, II, and/or I
Fibrin/fibrinogen degradation products (FDP)	0–10 µg/ml (0 to +)	Increased in DIC§

*Microhematocrit, heat precipitation method.
†Refractometer.
‡Analyze patient and control (normal horse) samples in parallel.
§Disseminated intravascular coagulation.

RENAL FUNCTION EVALUATION

1. **Urinalysis**
   Urine specific gravity (USG).
   Following water deprivation sufficient to produce 12% decrease in body weight, 95% of normal horses have a USG ≥1.042.
   Significance: Useful in determining renal concentrating ability. Do not perform a water deprivation test on azotemic horses.

2. **Urine/Plasma (U/P) ratios**
   Technique: U/P ratios are determined from paired blood and urine samples.
   a. U/P osmolality ratio = 2–6.
      Significance: An important preliminary indicator in differentiating prerenal azotemia and acute tubular disease. Values in horses with renal azotemia range from 0.8 to 1.7 and in horses with prerenal azotemia range from 1.7 to 3.4.
   b. U/P urea nitrogen ratio = 20–124.
      Significance: An important preliminary indicator in differentiating prerenal azotemia and acute tubular disease. Values in horses with renal azotemia range from 2 to 14 while those in horses with prerenal azotemia range from 15 to 44.
   c. U/P creatinine ratio = 2–344.
      Significance: An important preliminary indicator in differentiating prerenal from renal azotemia. Values in horses with renal azo-temia range from 3 to 37 while those in horses with prerenal azotemia range from 51–242.

3. **Fractional excretion (FE) of electrolytes**
   Technique: Values for FE of each electrolyte are based on single samples of plasma and urine collected at the same time with electrolyte excretion related to creatinine (Cr) excretion. Computed by:

   $$FEx = \frac{(Cr)p}{(Cr)u} \times \frac{(X)u}{(X)p} \times 100$$

   Where
   $(Cr)p$ = concentration of plasma Cr (mg/dl)
   $(Cr)u$ = concentration of urine Cr (mg/dl)
   $(X)u$ = concentration of urinary electrolyte (mEq/L)
   $(X)p$ = concentration of plasma electrolyte (mEq/L)

   a. FE_{Na} = 0.032–0.52%.
      Significance: To differentiate prerenal and renal azotemia. Excessive Na excretion occurs in renal azotemia.
   b. FE_K = 23.3–48.1%.
      Significance: Excretion of K is dependent upon glomerular filtration rate (GFR). Low FE_K may imply the need for K replacement therapy.
   c. FE_{Cl} = 0.59–1.86%.
      Significance: Directly correlated with excretion of Na.

d. FE_{Ca} = 0.0–6.72%; >2.5% when horses are fed adequate Ca.
 Significance: Permits assessment of Ca nutrition in horses.

e. FE of inorganic phosphorus (FE_{Pi}) = 0 to >20% depending on amount of dietary phosphate.
 Significance: FE_{Pi} >4% suggests excessive phosphate intake.

4. **Urine γ-glutamyltranspeptidase (uGGT)/urine creatinine (uCr) ratio**
 Technique: Determined on a single urine specimen. May be stored at 4°C or 25°C (never frozen), assays performed within 72 hours of collection.

$$uGGT/uCr = \frac{GGT\ (IU/L)}{Cr(mg/dl) \times 0.01} = 1\text{-}20$$

 Significance: Horses with various types of renal insults have ratios >25.

5. **Renal clearance**
 Technique: Performed on pooled and timed urine collection. Clearance is computed by:

 C_X = (Ux/Px) × Vu/time/kg BW
 where Ux = concentration of x in urine
 Px = concentration of x in plasma
 Vu = volume of urine in number of minutes of urine collection
 Kg BW = body weight in kilograms

Significance: A measure of GFR and thus useful in differentiating prerenal and renal azotemia.

  a. Creatinine clearance (C_{cr}).
   Horses = 0.96–2.80 ml/min/kg (24-hour clearance).
   Ponies = 0.31–3.59 ml/min/kg (24-hour clearance).
  b. Sodium clearance (C_{Na}) = 0.003–0.009 ml/min/kg.
  c. Potassium clearance (C_K) = 0.538–1.05 ml/min/kg.
  d. Chloride clearance (C_{Cl}) = 0.013–0.031 ml/min/kg.

TABLE 3. ACID-BASE, BLOOD GAS ANALYSIS

	Arterial (carotid)	Venous (jugular)
pH	7.347–7.475	7.345–7.433
PO_2 torr	80–112	37–56
PCO_2 torr	36–46	38–48
HCO_3 mEq/L	22–29	22–29
Base excess mEq/L	−1.7–+3.9	−2.7–+4.1
Anion gap* mEq/L		7–15
Lactate mg/dl		3.6–14.5

*Anion gap = ([Na] + [K]) − ([Cl] + [HCO_3])

1 torr = 1 mm Hg

With appropriate compensation in acid-base disorders, the following changes will probably occur:

Acute respiratory acidosis	[HCO_3^-] increases 1 mEq/L for every 10 torr increase in PCO_2.
Chronic respiratory acidosis	[HCO_3^-] increases 3 to 4 mEq/L for every 10 torr increase in PCO_2.
Acute respiratory alkalosis	[HCO_3^-] decreases 1 to 3 mEq/L for every 10 torr decrease in PCO_2.
Chronic respiratory alkalosis	[HCO_3^-] decreases 5 mEq/L for every 10 torr decrease in PCO_2.
Metabolic acidosis	PCO_2 decreases 1.2 torr for every 1 mEq/L reduction in [HCO_3^-].
Metabolic alkalosis	PCO_2 increases 0.6 to 1.0 torr for every 1.0 mEq/L increase in [HCO_3^-].

Modified from Blackmore, D. J., and Brobst, D.: Biochemical Values in Equine Medicine. Newmarket, England, Animal Health Trust, 1981; and Brobst, D. F., Pathophysiologic and adaptive changes in acid-base disorders. J. Am. Vet. Med. Assoc., *183*:773, 1983.

CEREBROSPINAL FLUID (CSF)

1. *Appearance:* Clear, colorless.

2. *Cellularity:* <8 nucleated cells/μl, all mononuclear cells.

3. *Chemistry:*
  a. Total protein 32–48 mg/dl, mostly albumin.
  b. Glucose 48–57 mg/dl, varies directly with blood glucose concentration and is usually 60–80% of the latter (may be 35–75% of blood value if both are collected shortly after tranquilization/anesthesia). Paired blood and CSF glucose determinations are recommended.
  c. Creatine (phospho)kinase (CK, CPK) 0–8 IU/L.

TABLE 4. BLOOD CHEMISTRY VALUES (ADULT HORSES)

	"Conventional" Values	MF to get SI Unit Value	SI Values	MF to get "Conventional" Value
Alkaline phosphatase*	83–283 IU/L	ND		
Albumin	2.8–3.2 gm/dl	10	28–32 gm/L	0.1
Amylase	9–34 IU/L	ND		
Aspartate aminotransferase†	153–411 IU/L	ND		
Bilirubin: Total	0.1–2.5 mg/dl	17.1	1.7–42.8 μmol/L	0.0585
Indirect	0–2.2 mg/dl	17.1	0.0–37.6 μmol/L	0.0585
Direct	0.1–0.3 mg/dl	17.1	1.7–5.1 μmol/L	0.0585
Calcium	10.9–12.8 mg/dl	0.250	2.7–3.2 mmol/L	4.01
Chloride	99–109 mEq/l	1.0	99–109 mmol/L	1.0
Cholesterol	31–85 mg/dl	0.0259	0.80–2.20 mmol/L	38.7
Cortisol	0.4–6.6 μg/dl	27.6	10.8–182.2 nmol/L	0.362
Creatine (phospho)kinase	92–307 IU/L	ND		
Creatinine	0.7–1.8 mg/dl	88.4	62–159 μmol/L	0.0113
γ-Glutamyltranspeptidase	11–44 IU/L	ND		
Glucose	53–83 mg/dl	0.0555	2.9–4.6 mmol/L	18.0
Lipase	40–78 IU/L	ND		
Magnesium	1.3–2.5 mEq/L	0.411	0.53–1.02 mmol/L	2.43
Osmolality	270–300 mOsm/kg	Unnecessary		
Phosphate*	1.6–4.5 mg/dl	0.323	0.52–1.45 mmol/L	3.10
Potassium	2.4–4.7 mEq/L	1.0	2.4–4.7 mmol/L	1.0
Sodium	132–146 mEq/L	1.0	132–146 mmol/L	1.0
Sorbitol dehydrogenase	3–14 IU/L	ND		
Total protein‡	5.9–8.4 gm/dl	10	59–84 gm/L	0.1
Thyroxine (T₄)*	0.9–2.9 μg/dl	12.9	5.1–48.9 nmol/L	0.0777
Triiodothyronine (T₃)	24–187 ng/dl	0.0154	0.37–2.87 nmol/L	65.1
Urea nitrogen	10–24 mg/dl	0.357	3.6–8.6 mmol/L	2.80

MF Multiplication Factor; ND Not done; IU/L usually used.
All enzymes measured at 37°C.
*Age dependent; higher in foal
†Formerly glutamic oxaloacetic transaminase (GOT).
‡Age dependent; lower in foal.

TABLE 5. RECOMMENDED COLLECTION TUBES FOR VARIOUS TESTS*

Collection Tube	Specimen Used	Tests Performed
Anticoagulant		
Ethylenediamine tetraacetic acid	Whole blood	Hemogram, blood crossmatch, platelet count
(EDTA)	Whole fluid,	Cytology (including cell counts)
	Plasma	Blood urea nitrogen, cortisol, refractometric protein, fibrinogen
Heparin	Whole blood	Blood pH and gases
	Synovial fluid	Mucin clot test
	Plasma	Electrolytes, osmolality
Fluoride/Oxalate	Plasma	Glucose, lactate
Citrate	Plasma	Partial thromboplastin time, prothrombin time, specific factor analysis
None	Serum	Electrolytes, osmolality, virtually all chemistries,† electrophoresis, T₄, T₃
Procoagulant		
Siliceous earth	Whole blood	Activated coagulation time
Thrombin‡ (+ proteolytic inhibitor)	Serum	Fibrin/fibrinogen degradation products

*Specimen requirements for some tests may vary among laboratories.

†Several enzymes are heat-labile and activity may decrease if assay is not performed soon after collection. Glucose concentration can be measured in serum, but concentration may decrease up to 10% per hour if serum is not separated from cells. Fluoride inhibits such glucose metabolism.

‡Special tube provided with kit (Thrombo-Wellcotest, Burroughs Wellcome Co., Research Triangle, NC).

PERITONEAL FLUID

1. *Appearance:* Transparent, colorless to yellow fluid, which does not clot.
2. *Cellularity:* Usually approximately $2-4 \times 10^3$ nucleated cells/μl (always $<10 \times 10^3/\mu$l), with about 45–90% neutrophils, 7–47% mononuclear/mesothelial type cells, 4–26% lymphocytes and 0–2% eosinophils.
3. *Chemistry:*
   a. Fibrinogen <10 mg/dl (Heat precipitation technique).
   b. Total protein 0.7–2.0 gm/dl.
   c. Glucose 90–115 mg/dl in peritoneal fluid
       71–104 mg/dl in blood
       Blood value always less than peritoneal fluid value.
   d. Lactate 3–9 mg/dl in peritoneal fluid
       4–15 mg/dl in blood
       Blood value always greater than peritoneal fluid value.
   e. Urea nitrogen 11–23 mg/dl in peritoneal fluid
       8–25 mg/dl in blood.

PLEURAL FLUID

1. *Appearance:* Clear to slightly turbid yellowish fluid, which does not clot.
2. *Cellularity:* Approximately $1-10 \times 10^3$ nucleated cells/μl, with about 32–90% neutrophils, 5–66% mononuclear/mesothelial type cells, 0–16% lymphocytes, and 0–5% eosinophils.
3. *Chemistry:* Total protein 0.2–4.0 gm/dl

SYNOVIAL FLUID

1. *Appearance:* Highly viscous, clear to pale yellow fluid. Exhibits reversible thixotrophy if undisturbed.
2. *Cellularity:* <500 nucleated cells/μl, with $>90\%$ mononuclear cells (lymphocytes and nonreactive macrophages), $<10\%$ neutrophils and $<10\%$ vacuolated or phagocytic macrophages. "No" cartilage fragments present (possibly a few superficial fragments in $<10\%$ of clinically normal horses).

3. *Chemistry*
   a. Total protein 0.6–2 gm/dl
   b. Hyaluronic acid 0.3–0.4 gm/dl
4. *Other tests*
   a. Mucin clot test (subjective) always produces a tight ropey clot.
   b. Relative viscosity 23–66.

TRANSTRACHEAL WASH

1. *Appearance:* Virtual absence of mucoid or purulent material.
2. *Cellularity:* <1000 nucleated cells/μl, with most being ciliated columnar epithelial cells and alveolar macrophages. Some neutrophils, nonciliated columnar and cuboidal epithelial cells, and lymphocytes. Occasional to rare eosinophils and goblet cells. Possibly large numbers of hemosiderin-laden macrophages.

Supplemental Readings

Adams, R., McClure, J. J., Gossett, K. A., Koonce, K. L., and Ezigbo, C.: Evaluation of a technique for measurement of γ-glutamyltranspeptidase in equine urine. Am. J. Vet Res., 46:147, 1985.

Brobst, D. F., and Bayly, W. M.: Responses of horses to a water deprivation test. J. Equine Vet. Sci., 2:51, 1982.

Brownlow, M. A., Hutchins, D. R., and Johnston, K. G. Reference values for equine peritoneal fluid. Equine Vet. J., 13:127, 1981.

Caple, I. W., Doake, P. A., and Ellis, P. G.: Assessment of the calcium and phosphorus nutrition in horses by analysis of urine. Aust. Vet. J., 58:125, 1982.

Coles, E. H. Cerebrospinal fluid. *In* Kaneko, J. J. (ed.): Clinical Biochemistry of Domestic Animals, 3rd ed. New York, Academic Press, 1980, p. 719.

Duncan, J. R., and Prasse, K. W.: Veterinary laboratory medicine. Ames, IA, Iowa State University Press, 1977.

Grossman, B. S., Brobst, D. F., Kramer, J. W., Bayly, W. M., and Reed, S. M.: Urinary indices for differentiation of prerenal and renal azotemia in horses. J. Am. Vet. Med. Assoc., 180:284, 1982.

Morris, D. D., Divers, T. J., and Whitlock, R. H.: Renal clearance and fractional excretion of electrolytes over a 24-hour period in horses. Am. J. Vet. Res., 45:2431, 1984.

Tew, W. P., and Hotchkiss, R. N.: Synovial fluid analysis and equine joint disorders. J. Equine Vet. Sci., 1:163, 1981.

Whitwell, K. E., and Greet, T. R. C.: Collection and evaluation of tracheobronchial washes in horses. Equine Vet. J., 16:499, 1984.

Table of Common Drugs: Approximate Doses

N. Edward Robinson, EAST LANSING, MICHIGAN

Name of Drug	Dose	Route
Acepromazine	0.04–0.10 mg/kg	IV or IM
Acetylsalicylic acid	15–100 mg/kg s.i.d.	PO
Alfaprostol	3 mg/450 kg for luteolysis; 2 doses 14–18 days apart	IM
Altrenogest	0.044 mg/kg s.i.d. for 8–12 days; for estrus synchronization follow with luteolytic dose of prostaglandin $F_{2\alpha}$	PO
	0.044 mg/kg s.i.d. for aggression	PO
Amikacin sulfate	6.6 mg/kg b.i.d.	IV or IM
Aminophylline	4–7 mg/kg t.i.d.	PO
Aminopropazine fumarate	0.5 mg/kg b.i.d.	IM or IV
Aminopyrine	2.5–10 mg/450 kg	IV or IM
Amphotericin B	0.3 mg/kg in 5% dextrose	IV
Ampicillin sodium	10–50 mg/kg t.i.d.	IV or IM
Ampicillin trihydrate	5–20 mg/kg b.i.d.	IM
Atropine	0.02–0.1 mg/kg	IV, IM, or SC
Atropine	1–4% solution	Topical
Benzathine penicillin G	4000 U/kg every 2 days	IM
Bismuth subsalicylate suspension	0.5 ml/kg for foal diarrhea	PO
	1–2 liters/450 kg b.i.d.	PO
Boldenone undecylenate	1 mg/kg repeated at 3-wk intervals	IM
Bromhexine	30 mg/kg	PO
Butorphanol	0.02–0.05 mg/kg	IV
Calcium disodium edetate	1 mg 6.6% solution/kg daily in 3 divided doses	IV
Calcium gluconate	To effect	IV
	100–300 ml 20% solution for synchronous diaphragmatic flutter	IV
Cambendazole	20 mg/kg (not in 1st trimester of pregnancy)	PO
Captan	3% solution	Topical
Carazol	.015 mg/kg 10 min before mating; for ejaculation failure, combine with alpha-adrenergic agonist	IV
Carbenicillin	100 mg	Subconjunctival
Carbon disulfide	24 mg/450 kg	PO
Casein (iodinated)	5 gm s.i.d.	PO
Cefazolin	50 mg	Subconjunctival
Cefazolin sodium	11 mg/kg q.i.d.	IM or IV
Cephalexin	25 mg/kg q.i.d.	PO
Cephalothin sodium	11–18 mg/kg q.i.d.	IM or IV
Charcoal (activated)	2–8 oz/450 kg b.i.d.	PO
Chloral hydrate	7% solution to effect (usually 50–100 ml)	IV
	50–60 gm/450 kg	PO
Chloramphenicol	10–50 mg/kg q.i.d.	PO
Chloramphenicol palmitate	20–50 mg/kg q.i.d.	PO
Chloramphenicol sodium succinate	20–50 mg/kg q.i.d.	IM or IV
	40 mg	Subconjunctival
Cimetidine HCl	1000 mg divided b.i.d. or t.i.d. in foals	PO, IV, or IM
Clenbuterol	200 µg for uterine relaxation	IM or slow IV
	0.8 µg/kg b.i.d.	IV or PO
Cloxacillin sodium	30 mg/kg t.i.d.	IM or IV
Corticotropin	1 unit/kg	IM
Coumaphos	0.06% wash, 0.1% dust	Topical
Cromolyn sodium	200–300 mg	Insufflated into the pharynx
Danthron	15–30 ml/450 kg	PO
Dantrolene sodium	15–25 mg/kg q.i.d. for acute rhabdomyolysis	Slow IV
	2 mg/kg s.i.d. for prevention of rhabdomyolysis	PO
Detomidine HCl	8 mg/kg	IV
Dexamethasone	0.05–0.2 mg/kg s.i.d.	IV, IM, or PO
Dextran	8 gm/kg as 6% solution daily for up to 3 days	IV
Diazepam	0.05–0.4 mg/kg (repeat in 30 min if necessary)	IV
Dichlorvos	10–35 mg/kg	PO

Name of Drug	Dose	Route
Dichlorvos	0.93% solution	Topical
Diethylcarbamazine citrate	6.5 mg/kg s.i.d. for 14 days for chronic obstructive lung disease	PO
	1 mg/kg s.i.d. for 21 days for onchocerciasis	PO
Digitalis or digitoxin	0.03–0.06 mg/kg for digitalization, 0.01 mg/kg maintenance	PO
Digitalis tincture	0.03–0.6 ml/kg for digitalization; 0.05–0.1 ml/kg maintenance	PO
Digoxin	0.06–0.08 mg/kg for digitalization; 0.01–0.02 mg/kg maintenance	PO
Dihydrostreptomycin	5–15 mg/kg t.i.d.	IM
Dimercaprol	3 mg/kg q 4 hr for 2 days, q.i.d. on day 3, then t.i.d. for 10 days	IM
Dimethylsulfoxide	50% solution	Topical
	1 gm/kg as 20% solution in saline s.i.d. for 3 days, then alternate days for 6 days for spinal cord injury	IV
	0.9 gm/kg as 10% solution in polyionic fluids for cantharidin poisoning	IV
Dinoprost tromethamine	10 mg/450 kg	IM
Dioctyl sodium sulfosuccinate	7.5–30 gm/450 kg	PO
Dioxathion	0.15% wash	Topical
Diphenylhydantoin	1–10 mg/kg q 2–4 hr	IV, IM, or PO
Dipyrone	22 mg/kg	IV or IM
Dobutamine	2–10 µg/kg/min	IV
Dolophine HCl	0.2–0.4 mg/kg	IM
Dopamine	2–5 µg/kg/min	IV
Doxapram	0.5–1.0 mg/kg at 5 min intervals (do not exceed 2 mg/kg in foals)	IV
	0.02–0.05 mg/kg/min for neonatal foal resuscitation	IV
Ephedrine sulfate	0.7 mg/kg b.i.d.	PO
Epinephrine 1:1000	3–5 ml/450 kg	IM or SC
	0.1 ml/kg for foal resuscitation	IV
Erythromycin	10 mg/kg t.i.d.	IV or IM
Erythromycin estolate	25 mg/kg q.i.d.	PO
Estradiol cypionate	5–10 mg/450 kg	IM
Estrone sulfate	0.05–0.1 mg/kg for epistaxis prevention	IV
Ethylene diamine dihydriodide	0.5–1.5 gm/450 kg s.i.d.	PO
Febantel	6 mg/kg	PO
Fenbendazole	5 mg/kg	PO
	10 mg/kg s.i.d. for 5 days for *S. vulgaris* in foals	PO
Flumethasone	1.0–2.5 mg/450 kg	IV or IM
Flunixin meglumine	1 mg/kg s.i.d. or b.i.d.	IV, IM, or PO
9-Fluoroprednisolone acetate	5–20 mg/450 kg	IM
Fluprostenol	250 µg/450 kg	IM
Follicle-stimulating hormone	10–50 mg	IV, IM, or SC
Furazolidone	4 mg/kg t.i.d.	PO
Furosemide	1 mg/kg	IV
	0.3–0.6 mg/kg 60–90 min before racing for epistaxis prevention	
Gentamicin	1–3 mg/kg q.i.d.	IM
	20 mg	Subconjunctival
Glycerol	0.5–2.0 gm/kg for brain edema	IV
Glyceryl guaiacolate	3.0 mg/kg for expectoration	PO
	100 mg/kg for anesthesia combined with barbiturate in 5% dextrose (5% solution)	IV
Gonadotropin-releasing hormone (Buserelin)	0.04 mg 6 hr before mating to induce ovulation	IM
Griseofulvin	10 mg/kg s.i.d.	PO
Heparin	50 U/kg added to intraperitoneal lavage fluid	
	40–100 U/kg b.i.d.	SC or IV
Hesperidin–citrus bioflavinoids	28 gm/450 kg	PO
Human chorionic gonadotropin	2500 USP units	IV
	10,000 USP units	IM or SC
Hydrocortisone sodium succinate	1.0–4.0 mg/kg	IV drip
Imidocarb diproprionate	2 mg/kg s.i.d. for 2 days for *B. caballi*	IM
	4 mg/kg q 3 days for 4 treatments for *B. equi*	IM
Imipramine HCl	0.55 mg/kg	IM or IV
Insulin	0.4 U/kg	IM or SC
Insulin–protamine zinc	0.15 IU/kg b.i.d.	IM or SC
Iodochlorhydroxyquin	10 gm/450 kg (repeat for 3–4 days, then gradually reduce dose if response is obtained)	PO
Iron cacodylate	1 gm	IV
Isoniazid	5–20 mg/kg s.i.d.	PO
Isoproterenol HCl	0.4 µg/kg by slow infusion (discontinue when heart rate doubles)	IV
	0.05–1.0 µg/kg/min for foal resuscitation	IV
Isoxsuprine lactate	0.5 mg/kg b.i.d.	IM

Table continued on next page

Name of Drug	Dose	Route
Ivermectin	0.2 mg/kg	PO
	0.2 mg/kg twice at 4-day intervals for lice and mange	PO
Kanamycin sulfate	5–10 mg/kg t.i.d.	IM
Kaopectate	2–4 qt/450 kg b.i.d.	PO
Ketamine	2 mg/kg	IV
Levallorphan tartrate	0.02–0.04 mg/kg	IV
Levamisole	2–5 mg/kg	PO or IM
	10 mg/kg s.i.d. for 7 days for onchocerciasis	PO
Levothyroxine	10 mg in 70 ml Karo syrup s.i.d.	PO
Lidocaine	1–1.5 mg/kg bolus or slow drip	IV
Lindane	3% spray	Topical
Magnesium sulfate	100–400 gm/450 kg	PO
Malathion	0.5% wash, 5% dust	Topical
Mannitol	0.25–2.0 mg/kg as 20% solution by slow infusion	IV
Mebendazole	8.8 mg/kg	PO
	15–20 mg/kg s.i.d. for 5 days for lungworms	
Meclofenamic acid	2.2 mg/kg	PO
Megestrol acetate	65–85 mg/450 kg s.i.d.	PO
Meperidine HCl	2.2–4.0 mg/kg	IM
	0.2–0.4 mg/kg (may cause excitement)	IV
Metaclopramide HCl	10 mg/kg	IV
Metamucil	2 kg in 4–6 liters of water	PO
Methadone	0.05–0.1 mg/kg	IV
Methicillin	5 mg	Subconjunctival
Methionine, dl	22 mg/kg s.i.d. for 1st wk; 11 mg/kg s.i.d. for 2nd wk; 5.5 mg/kg s.i.d. for 3rd wk	PO
Methocarbamol	15–25 mg/kg slow infusion	IV
Methoxychlor	0.5% wash	Topical
Methylcellulose flakes	0.25–0.5 kg in 8–10 L water/450 kg	PO
Methylprednisolone	0.5 mg/kg	PO
Methylprednisolone acetate	20–40 mg	Subconjunctival
Methylprednisolone sodium succinate	0.5 mg/kg	IV or IM
	10–20 mg/kg for shock	IV
Metronidazole	7.5 mg/kg q.i.d.	IV or PO
Miconazole	1–2% solution	Topical
	10 mg	Subconjunctival
Mineral oil	3–4 L/450 kg	PO
Morphine sulfate	0.2–0.4 mg/kg	IM
	0.02–0.04 mg/kg	IV
Naloxone	0.01–0.02 mg/kg	IV
Naproxen	10 mg/kg	PO
Neomycin	5–15 mg/kg s.i.d.	PO
Neostigmine	0.4–2 mg/100 kg	SC
Niclosamide	100 mg/kg	PO
Nitrofurantoin	2.5–4.5 mg/kg t.i.d.	PO
Norepinephrine	0.01 mg/kg	IM
Ouabain	2.5–3.0 mg/450 kg q 1½ to 2 hr until heart rate slows or intoxication develops; do not exceed 10 gm total	IV
Oxacillin	25–50 mg/kg b.i.d.	IM or IV
Oxfendazole	10 mg/kg	PO
Oxibendazole	10 mg/kg	PO
Oxymorphone	0.02–0.03 mg/kg	IM
Oxytetracycline	5–10 mg/kg b.i.d.	IV
Oxytocin	5–40 U/450 kg as bolus	IV
	80–100 U in 500 ml saline by slow infusion	IV
	20–150 U/450 kg	IM
	1–3 U/450 kg for milk letdown	IV
Pencillin G, potassium	5000–50,000 IU/kg q.i.d.	IV
Penicillin G, procaine	5000–50,000 IU/kg b.i.d.	IM
Penicillin G, sodium	5000–50,000 IU/kg q.i.d.	IV
	250,000 U	Subconjunctival
Pentazocine	0.3 mg/kg slow injection	IV
	0.3 mg/kg	IM
Pentobarbital	3–15 mg/kg	IV
Phenobarbital	1–10 mg/kg	IV
Phenothiazine	55 mg/kg; 27.5 mg/kg with piperazine	PO
Phenoxybenzamine	0.66 mg/kg in 500 ml saline	IV

Name of Drug	Dose	Route
Phenylbutazone	2–4 gm/450 kg s.i.d.	PO
	1–2 gm/450 kg s.i.d.	IV
	To avoid toxicity in horses use 4.4 mg/kg b.i.d. on day 1, 2.2 mg/kg b.i.d. for 4 days, then 2.2 mg/kg s.i.d.	
	To avoid toxicity in ponies use 4.4 mg/kg s.i.d. for 4 days, then 4.4 mg/kg on alternate days	
Phenylephrine	10% solution	Topical
Phenytoin	1–10 mg/kg q 2–4 hrs	IV, IM, or PO
Piperazine salts	88 mg base/kg	PO
	44 mg base/kg with carbon disulphide	
	55 mg base/kg with thiabendazole	
Potassium iodide	0.5–5.0 mg/kg s.i.d.	IV
Potassium permanganate	1% solution for mouthwash	
Povidone-iodine	10% volume/volume solution	
Prednisolone acetate	0.25–1.0 mg/kg	IM
	10–25 mg	Subconjunctival
Prednisolone sodium succinate	0.25–1.0 mg/kg	IV
Prednisolone tabs	0.25–1.0 mg/kg	PO
Prednisone	0.25–1.0 mg/kg	IM
Primidone	1 gm/foal b.i.d.–q.i.d.	PO
Progesterone	100 mg/450 kg/day in oil for abortion prevention	IM
Progesterone	150–200 mg/450 kg/day in oil to inhibit follicular development	IM
	Can be combined with 10 mg/450 kg estradiol 17β	
Progesterone	100 mg/450 kg/day in oil with 1 mg/450 kg estradiol 17β for 5 days to cause uterine involution	IM
Progesterone (repositol)	1000 mg/450 kg once weekly for abortion prevention	IM
Promazine HCl	0.4–1.0 mg/kg	IV or IM
Propantheline bromide	0.014 mg/kg	IV
Propranolol	150–350 mg/450 kg b.i.d.	PO
	25–75 mg/450 kg b.i.d.	IV
Prostaglandin $F_{2\alpha}$	2.2 mg/100 kg	IM
	5 mg/450 kg, 2 doses 14–18 days apart for synchronizing estrus	
Prostalene	2 mg/450 kg, 2 doses 2 wks apart	SC
Pyrantel pamoate	6.6 mg (base)/kg	PO
	13.2 mg (base)/kg for cestodes	PO
Pyrilamine maleate	1 mg/kg	IV, IM, or SC
Quinidine gluconate	1% solution at 50 ml/min until fibrillation converts to sinus rhythm (monitor EKG, total dose 5–20 gm)	IV
Quinidine sulfate	5 gm test dose, then 10 gm b.i.d., increasing to 15 gm q.i.d. on day 10	PO
Ranitidine	0.5 mg/kg b.i.d.	PO
Rifampin	5 mg/kg b.i.d.	PO
Ronnel	2.5% spray	Topical
Selenium (sodium selenite)	5.5 mg/450 kg	IM
Sodium iodide	20% solution, 10–40 ml/day	IV
Sodium thiosulfate	20–30 g/450 kg q.i.d.	PO
	plus 8–10 gm (10–20% solution)	IV
Spectinomycin	20 mg/kg t.i.d.	IM
Stanozolol	0.5 mg/kg, up to 4 doses 1–2 wks apart	IM
Stilbestrol	30 mg/450 kg	IM
Stirofos	1% wash	Topical
Streptomycin	5–15 mg/kg t.i.d.	IM
Sucralfate	2 mg/kg t.i.d.	PO
Sulfonamides	100–200 mg/kg on day 1; 50–100 mg/kg subsequently; check individual products for specific dosage	IV, SC, or PO
Terbutaline sulfate	3.3 µg/kg	IV
Tetramethrin	0.4% solution, wipe on	Topical
Theophylline	1.0 mg/kg q.i.d.	PO
Thiabendazole	44 mg/kg; 440 mg/kg larvicidal	PO
Thiamine	0.5–5 mg/kg	IV, IM, or PO
Thiamylal sodium	2–4 mg/kg	IV
Thiopental	8–12 mg/kg	IV
Thyroxine (1)	0.01 mg/kg s.i.d.	PO
Ticarcillin	44 mg/kg q 5 hrs	IV
	44 mg/kg t.i.d.	IM
Toxaphene	0.5% wash	Topical

Table continued on next page

Name of Drug	Dose	Route
Triamcinolone acetonide	0.1–0.2 mg/kg	IM or SC
	3–6 mg	Subconjunctival
Trichlorfon	35 mg/kg	PO
Trichlorfon	90% powder	Topical
Trichlormethiazide	200 mg/450 kg	PO
Trimethoprim-sulfadiazine	15 mg/kg sulfadiazine divided into equal doses	IM
	25 mg/kg sulfadiazine s.i.d.	PO
Tripelennamine hydrochloride	1 mg/kg	IM
Tylosin	10 mg/kg b.i.d.	IM
Vitamin E	50 mg/450 kg	IM
Vitamin K_1	40–50 mg/450 kg	SC
Warfarin	30–75 mg/450 kg	PO
Xylazine	0.5–1.0 mg/kg	IV

This table was composed primarily from doses recommended by authors. It is recommended that the manufacturer's literature be checked before a drug is used. Not all drugs have been approved for use in horses.

IM = intramuscular, IV = intravenous, PO = by mouth, SC = subcutaneous.

INDEX

Page numbers in italics refer to illustrations; page numbers followed by a "t" refer to tables.